IASLC Thoracic Oncology

SECOND EDITION

IASLC Thoracic Oncology

SECOND EDITION

Executive Editor:

Harvey I. Pass, MD

Stephen E. Banner Professor of Thoracic Oncology
Vice Chairman of Research
Department of Cardiothoracic Surgery
New York University Langone Medical Center
New York, New York

Editors:

David Ball, MD, FRANZCR

Director
Lung Cancer Stream
Victorian Comprehensive Cancer Centre
Parkville Professional Fellow
The Sir Peter MacCallum Department of Oncology
The University of Melbourne
Melbourne, Australia

Giorgio V. Scagliotti, MD, PhD

Professor of Medical Oncology
Head of Department of Oncology at San Luigi Hospital
University of Turin
Orbassano, Turin, Italy

Deborah Whippen
Managing Editor
Editorial Rx, Inc.

ELSEVIER

ELSEVIER

1600 John F. Kennedy Blvd.
Ste 1800
Philadelphia, PA 19103-2899

IASLC THORACIC ONCOLOGY, SECOND EDITION   ISBN: 978-0-323-52357-8

Notices

Knowledge and best practice in this field are constantly changing. As new research and experience broaden our understanding, changes in research methods, professional practices, or medical treatment may become necessary.

Practitioners and researchers must always rely on their own experience and knowledge in evaluating and using any information, methods, compounds, or experiments described herein. In using such information or methods they should be mindful of their own safety and the safety of others, including parties for whom they have a professional responsibility.

With respect to any drug or pharmaceutical products identified, readers are advised to check the most current information provided (i) on procedures featured or (ii) by the manufacturer of each product to be administered, to verify the recommended dose or formula, the method and duration of administration, and contraindications. It is the responsibility of practitioners, relying on their own experience and knowledge of their patients, to make diagnoses, to determine dosages and the best treatment for each individual patient, and to take all appropriate safety precautions.

To the fullest extent of the law, neither the Publisher nor the authors, contributors, or editors, assume any liability for any injury and/or damage to persons or property as a matter of products liability, negligence or otherwise, or from any use or operation of any methods, products, instructions, or ideas contained in the material herein.

Previous edition copyrighted in 2014.
Library of Congress Cataloging-in-Publication Data

Names: Pass, Harvey I., editor. | Ball, David (David L.), editor. |
   Scagliotti, Giorgio V., editor. | International Association for the Study
   of Lung Cancer, issuing body.
Title: IASLC thoracic oncology / executive editor, Harvey I. Pass ; editors,
   David Ball, Giorgio V. Scagliotti.
Other titles: The IASLC multidisciplinary approach to thoracic oncology. |
   Thoracic oncology | International Association for the Study of Lung Cancer
   thoracic oncology
Description: Second edition. | Philadelphia, PA : Elsevier, [2018] | Preceded
   by: The IASLC multidisciplinary approach to thoracic oncology / executive
   editor, Harvey I. Pass ; editors, David Ball, Giorgio V. Scagliotti.
   [2014] | Includes bibliographical references and index.
Identifiers: LCCN 2017004620 | ISBN 9780323523578 (hardcover : alk. paper)
Subjects: | MESH: Thoracic Neoplasms
Classification: LCC RC280.C5 | NLM WF 970 | DDC 616.99/494--dc23 LC record available at
https://lccn.loc.gov/2017004620

Content Strategist: Kayla Wolfe
Director, Content Development: Taylor Ball
Publishing Services Manager: Patricia Tannian
Senior Project Manager: Sharon Corell
Book Designer: Brian Salisbury

Printed in China.

Last digit is the print number: 9 8 7 6 5 4 3 2 1

Contributors

Alex A. Adjei, MD, PhD
Professor
Head
Early Cancer Therapeutics Program
Director
Global Oncology Program
Mayo Clinic
Rochester, Minnesota, USA

Mjung-Ju Ahn, MD, PhD
Professor
Division of Hematology/Oncology
Department of Medicine
Samsung Medical Center
Sungkyunkwan University School of
    Medicine
Seoul, South Korea

Chris I. Amos, PhD
Associate Director for Population
    Sciences
Department of Biomedical Data Science
Geisel School of Medicine
Dartmouth College
Hanover, New Hampshire, USA

Alberto Antonicelli, MD
Section of Thoracic Surgery
Department of Surgery
Yale University
New Haven, Connecticut, USA

Hisao Asamura, MD
Professor of Surgery
Chief
Division of Thoracic Surgery
Keio University School of Medicine
Tokyo, Japan

Todd Atwood, PhD
Department of Radiation Medicine and
    Applied Sciences
University of California, San Diego
La Jolla, California, USA

Paul Baas, MD, PhD
Professor
Department of Thoracic Oncology
The Netherlands Cancer Institute
Amsterdam, The Netherlands

Joan E. Bailey-Wilson, PhD
Co-Chief and Senior Investigator
Computational and Statistical Genomics
    Branch
National Human Genome Research
    Institute
National Institutes of Health
Baltimore, Maryland, USA

David Ball, MD, FRANZCR
Director
Lung Cancer Stream
Victorian Comprehensive Cancer Centre
Parkville Professional Fellow
The Sir Peter MacCallum Department of
    Oncology
The University of Melbourne
Melbourne, Australia

Fabrice Barlesi, MD, PhD
Professor
Oncologie Multidisciplinaire et
    Innovations Thérapeutiques
Aix Marseille University
Assistance Publique Hôpitaux de Marseille
Marseille, France

Jose G. Bazan, MD, MS
Assistant Professor
Department of Radiation Oncology
The Ohio State University
Columbus, Ohio, USA

José Belderbos, MD, PhD
Department of Radiation Oncology
The Netherlands Cancer Institute—
    Antoni van Leeuwenhoek
Amsterdam, The Netherlands

**Andrea Bezjak, BMedSc, MDCM, MSc,
FRCPC**
Professor
Department of Radiation Oncology
University of Toronto
Princess Margaret Cancer Centre
Toronto, Ontario, Canada

**Lucinda J. Billingham, BSc, MSc, PhD,
CStat**
Professor of Biostatistics
Cancer Research UK Clinical Trials Unit
Institute of Cancer and Genomic
    Sciences
University of Birmingham
Birmingham, United Kingdom

Paolo Boffetta, MD, MPH
Professor
Tisch Cancer Institute
Icahn School of Medicine at Mount Sinai
New York, New York, USA

Martina Bonifazi, MD
Department of Byomedic Sciences and
    Public Health
Polytechnic University of Marche Region
Pulmonary Diseases Unit
Azienda Ospedali Riuniti
Ancona, Italy

Julie R. Brahmer, MD
Associate Professor of Oncology
Director of Thoracic Oncology
Sidney Kimmel Comprehensive Cancer
    Center
The Johns Hopkins University
Baltimore, Maryland, USA

Elisabeth Brambilla, MD, PhD
Professor of Pathology
Grenoble University Hospital
Grenoble, France

Fraser Brims
Institute of Respiratory Health
Department of Respiratory Medicine,
    Sir Charles Gairdner Hospital
Curtin Medical School
Faculty of Health Sciences
Curtin University
Perth, Australia

Alessandro Brunelli, MD
Consultant Thoracic Surgeon
Honorary Senior Lecturer
St. James's University Hospital
Leeds, United Kingdom

Ayesha Bryant, MSPH, MD
Assistant Professor
Section of Thoracic Surgery
University of Alabama School of
    Medicine
Birmingham, Alabama, USA

Nicholas Campbell, MD
Clinical Assistant Professor
NorthShore University HealthSystem
Kellog Cancer Center
Evanston, Illinois, USA

Brett W. Carter, MD
Assistant Professor
Department of Diagnostic Radiology
Division of Diagnostic Imaging
The University of Texas MD Anderson
    Cancer Center
Houston, Texas, USA

**Robert Cerfolio, MD, MBA, FCCP,
FACS**
Professor
Section of Thoracic Surgery
University of Alabama School of
    Medicine
Birmingham, Alabama, USA

Byoung Chul Cho, MD, PhD
Associate Professor
Yonsei Cancer Center
Yonsei University College of Medicine
Seoul, Republic of Korea

William C. S. Cho, PhD, Chartered Scientist, FIBMS
Department of Clinical Oncology
Queen Elizabeth Hospital
Hong Kong, China

Hak Choy, MD
Professor
Department of Radiation Oncology
University of Texas Southwestern
Dallas, Texas, USA

Chia-Yu Chu, MD, PhD
Associate Professor
Department of Dermatology
National Taiwan University Hospital and
    National Taiwan University College of
    Medicine
Taipei, Taiwan

Glenda Colburn, EMBA
National Director
Thoracic Cancers and Rare Lung
    Diseases
General Manager
Research
Lung Cancer National Program
Lung Foundation Australia
Queensland University of Technology
Milton, Australia

Henri Colt, MD
Professor Emeritus
School of Medicine
University of California, Irvine
Orange, California, USA

Rafael Rosell Costa, MD
Director
Cancer Biology and Precision Medicine
    Program
Catalan Institute of Oncology
Germans Trias i Pujol Health Sciences
    Institute and Hospital
Associate Professor of Medicine
Autonomous University of Barcelona
    (UAB) Campus Can Ruti
Barcelona, Spain

Gail E. Darling, MD, FRCSC, FACS
Professor
Division of Thoracic Surgery
Department of Surgery
University of Toronto
Toronto, Ontario, Canada

Mellar Davis, MD, FCCP, FAAHPM
Director of Palliative Care
Geisinger Medical System
Danville, Pennsylvania, USA
Professor of Medicine
Cleveland Clinic Lerner School of
    Medicine
Case Western Reserve University
Cleveland, Ohio, USA

Patricia M. de Groot, MD
Associate Professor
Department of Diagnostic Radiology
Division of Diagnostic Imaging
The University of Texas MD Anderson
    Cancer Center
Houston, Texas, USA

Harry J. de Koning, MD, PhD
Professor
Department of Public Health
Erasmus University Medical Center
Rotterdam, The Netherlands

Paul De Leyn, MD, PhD
Professor and Chief
Department of Thoracic Surgery
University Hospitals Leuven
Leuven, Belgium

Dirk De Ruysscher, MD, PhD
Maastricht University Medical Center
Department of Radiation Oncology
    (Maastro Clinic)
GROW School
Maastricht, The Netherlands
Katholieke Universiteit Leuven
Radiation Oncology
Leuven, Belgium

Ayşe Nur Demiral, MD
Professor
Department of Radiation Oncology
DokuzEylül University Medical School
Izmir, Turkey

Jules Derks, MD
Department of Pulmonology
Maastricht University Medical Center
Maastricht, The Netherlands

Frank C. Detterbeck, MD
Professor
Section of Thoracic Surgery
Department of Surgery
Yale University
New Haven, Connecticut, USA

Siddhartha Devarakonda
Fellow
Division of Medical Oncology/Hematology
Department of Medicine
Washington University School of
    Medicine
St. Louis, Missouri, USA

Anne-Marie C. Dingemans, MD, PhD
Pulmonologist
Department of Pulmonology
Maastricht University Medical Center
Maastricht, The Netherlands

Jessica S. Donington, MD, MSCr
Associate Professor
Department of Cardiothoracic Surgery
New York University School of Medicine
New York, New York, USA

Carolyn M. Dresler, MD, MPA
President
Human Rights and Tobacco Control
    Network
Rockville, Maryland, USA

Steven M. Dubinett, MD
Professor
Division of Pulmonary and Critical Care
    Medicine
David Geffen School of Medicine at UCLA
UCLA Clinical and Translational
    Science Institute
Los Angeles, California, USA

Grace K. Dy, MD
Associate Professor
Department of Medicine
Roswell Park Cancer Institute
Buffalo, New York, USA

Jeremy J. Erasmus, MD
Professor
Department of Diagnostic Radiology
Division of Diagnostic Imaging
The University of Texas MD Anderson
    Cancer Center
Houston, Texas, USA

Alysa Fairchild, BSc, MD, FRCPC
Associate Professor
Department of Radiation Oncology
University of Alberta
Cross Cancer Institute
Edmonton, Alberta, Canada

Dean A. Fennell, PhD, FRCP
Professor of Thoracic Medical Oncology
Cancer Research UK Centre
University of Leicester and University
    Hospitals of Leicester NHS Trust
Leicester, United Kingdom

Hiran C. Fernando, MBBS, FRCS, FRCSEd
Co-Director
Thoracic Oncology
ISCI Thoracic Section
Department of Surgery
Inova Fairfax Medical Campus
Falls Church, Virginia, USA

Pier Luigi Filosso, MD
Associate Professor of Thoracic Surgery
University of Turin
Turin, Italy

Raja Flores, MD
Professor
Department of Thoracic Surgery
Mount Sinai Medical Center
New York, New York, USA

Kwun Fong, MBBS (Lon), FRACP, PhD
Department of Thoracic Medicine
The Prince Charles Hospital
University of Queensland Thoracic
    Research Centre
Brisbane, Australia

Jesme Fox, MB, ChB, MBA
Medical Director
Roy Castle Lung Cancer Foundation
Liverpool, United Kingdom

David R. Gandara, MD
Professor
Thoracic Oncology Program
Division of Medical Oncology
University of California Davis
    Comprehensive Cancer Center
Sacramento, California, USA

Leena Gandhi, MD, PhD
Director of Thoracic Medical Oncology
Laura and Isaac Perlmutter Cancer Center
New York University Langone Medical
    Center
New York, New York, USA

Laurie Gaspar, MD, MBA, FACR, FASTRO
Professor
Department of Radiation Oncology
University of Colorado
Aurora, Colorado, USA

Stefano Gasparini, MD, FCCP
Head Respiratory Diseases Unit
Department of Byomedic Sciences and Public Health
Polytechnic University of Marche Region
Pulmonary Diseases Unit
Azienda Ospedali Riuniti
Ancona, Italy

Adi F. Gazdar, MD
Professor
Hamon Center for Therapeutic Oncology Research and Department of Pathology
The University of Texas Southwestern Medical Center
Houston, Texas, USA

Giuseppe Giaccone, MD, PhD
Professor of Medical Oncology and Pharmacology
Associate Director for Clinical Research
Georgetown University
Lombardi Comprehensive Cancer Center
Washington, DC, USA

Nicolas Girard, MD, PhD
Professor
Respiratory Medicine Service
Hospices Civils de Lyon
Claude Bernard Lyon 1 University
Lyon, France
Thorax Institute Curie Montsouris
Curie Institute
Paris, France

Peter Goldstraw, MD, FRCS
Emeritus Professor
Academic Department of Thoracic Surgery
Royal Brompton Hospital
Imperial College London
London, United Kingdom

Elizabeth M. Gore, MD
Professor of Radiation Oncology
Department of Radiation Oncology
Medical College of Wisconsin
The Zablocki VA Medical Center
Milwaukee, Wisconsin, USA

Glenwood Goss, MD, FCP(SA), FRCPC
Professor of Medicine, University of Ottawa
Director of Clinical Research
The Ottawa Hospital Cancer Centre
Chair
Thoracic Oncology Site Committee
Canadian Cancer Trials Group
Ottawa, Canada

Ramaswamy Govindan, MD
Professor
Department of Medicine
Division of Oncology
Washington University School of Medicine
St. Louis, Missouri, USA

Alissa K. Greenberg, MD
Pulmonary Group
Northeast Medical Group, Inc.
New York, New York, USA

Dominique Grunenwald, MD, PhD
Professor
University of Paris
Paris, France

Matthias Guckenberger, MD
Department of Radiation Oncology
University Hospital Zurich
Zurich, Switzerland

Swati Gulati, MD
Division of Pulmonary Allergy and Critical Care Medicine
University of Alabama at Birmingham
Birmingham, Alabama, USA

Raffit Hassan, MD
Senior Investigator
National Cancer Institute
National Institutes of Health
Bethesda, Maryland, USA

Christopher Hazzard, MD
Department of Thoracic Surgery
Icahn School of Medicine at Mount Sinai
New York, New York, USA

Fiona Hegi, MBBS, FRANZCR
Radiation Oncologist
Radiation Physics Laboratory
The University of Sydney
Sydney, Australia

Thomas Hensing, MD
Clinical Associate Professor
University of Chicago
NorthShore University HealthSystem
Kellogg Cancer Center
Evanston, Illinois, USA

Roy Herbst, MD, PhD
Ensign Professor of Medicine (Medical Oncology) and Professor of Pharmacology
Chief of Medical Oncology
Yale Cancer Center and Smilow Cancer Hospital
New Haven, Connecticut, USA

Fred R. Hirsch, MD, PhD
Professor
Professor of Medicine and Pathology
Department of Medicine
Department of Pathology
University of Colorado Cancer Center
Aurora, Colorado, USA

Nanda Horeweg, MD
Junior Researcher
Erasmus University Medical Center
Department of Public Health
Department of Pulmonary Diseases
Erasmus University Medical Center
Rotterdam, The Netherlands

David M. Jablons, MD
Professor and Chief Thoracic Surgery
UCSF Department of Surgery
Nan T. McEvoy Distinguished Professor of Thoracic Surgical Oncology
Ada Distinguished Professor of Thoracic Oncology
Program Leader Thoracic Oncology
UCSF Helen Diller Family Comprehensive Cancer Center
San Francisco, California, USA

James R. Jett, MD
Professor Emeritus
Department of Medicine
Division of Oncology
Cancer Center
National Jewish Medical Center
Denver, Colorado, USA

Andrew Kaufman, MD
Assistant Professor
Department of Thoracic Surgery
Mount Sinai Medical Center
New York, New York, USA

Paul Keall, PhD
Professor
Radiation Physics
The University of Sydney
Sydney, Australia

Karen Kelly, MD
Professor
Division of Hematology and Oncology
UC Davis Comprehensive Cancer Center
Sacramento, California, USA

Feng-Ming (Spring) Kong, MD, PhD
Professor of Radiation Oncology and Medical and Molecular Genetics
Director of Clinical Research/Clinical Trials
Radiation Oncology
Co-Leader of Thoracic Oncology Program
IU Simon Cancer Center
Indiana University School of Medicine
Indianapolis, Indiana, USA

Kaoru Kubota, MD
Department of Pulmonary Medicine and Oncology
Graduate School of Medicine
Nippon Medical School
Tokyo, Japan

Ite A. Laird-Offringa, PhD
Associate Professor
Department of Surgery
Department of Biochemistry and Molecular Biology
USC/Norris Cancer Center
Keck School of Medicine of USC
Los Angeles, California, USA

Primo N. Lara, Jr, MD
Professor of Medicine
University of California, Davis
School of Medicine
Acting Director
UC Davis Comprehensive Cancer Center
Sacramento, California, USA

Janessa Laskin, MD, FRCPC
Associate Professor
Department of Medicine
Division of Medical Oncology
British Columbia Cancer Agency
Vancouver, British Columbia, Canada

Quynh-Thu Le, MD, FACR, FASTRO
Professor and Chair
Department of Radiation Oncology
Stanford University
Stanford, California, USA

Cécile Le Péchoux, MD
Gustave Roussy, Hopital Universitaire
Radiation Oncology Department
Villejuif, France

Elvira L. Liclican, PhD
Scientific Officer
UCLA Clinical and Translational
    Science Institute
Los Angeles, California, USA

Yolande Lievens, MD, PhD
Associate Professor
Radiation Oncology Department
Ghent University Hospital
Ghent University
Ghent, Belgium

Chia-Chi (Josh) Lin, MD, PhD
Clinical Associate Professor
Department of Oncology
National Taiwan University Hospital
Taipei, Taiwan

Billy W. Loo, Jr., MD, PhD
Associate Professor
Radiation Oncology – Radiation Therapy
Stanford Cancer Institute
Stanford University
Stanford, California, USA

Michael Mac Manus, MB, BCh, BAO, MD, MRCP, FRANZCR
Professor
The Sir Peter MacCallum Department of
    Oncology
Peter MacCallum Cancer Centre
The University of Melbourne
Melbourne, Australia

Homer A. Macapinlac, MD
Professor
Department of Nuclear Medicine
Division of Diagnostic Imaging
The University of Texas MD Anderson
    Cancer Center
Houston, Texas, USA

Fergus Macbeth, MA, DM, FRCR, FRCP, MBA
Professor
Wales Cancer Trials Unit
School of Medicine
Cardiff University
Cardiff, United Kingdom

William J. Mackillop, MB, ChB, FRCR, FRCPC
Professor
Departments of Oncology and Public
    Health Sciences
Division of Cancer Care and
    Epidemiology
Queen's Cancer Research Institute
Queen's University
Kingston, Canada

Christopher Maher, PhD
Assistant Professor
Department of Medicine
Division of Oncology
Washington University School of
    Medicine
St. Louis, Missouri, USA

Isa Mambetsariev
Research Assistant
Department of Medical Oncology and
    Molecular Therapeutics
City of Hope Comprehensive Cancer
    Center and Beckman Research
    Institute
Duarte, California, USA

Sumithra J. Mandrekar, PhD
Professor of Biostatistics and Oncology
Division of Biomedical Statistics and
    Informatics
Mayo Clinic
Rochester, Minnesota, USA

Aaron S. Mansfield, MD
Assistant Professor
Medical Oncology
Mayo Clinic
Rochester, Minnesota, USA

Lawrence B. Marks, MD
Dr. Sidney K. Simon Distinguished
    Professor of Oncology Research
Chairman
Department of Radiation Oncology
University of North Carolina
Lineberger Comprehensive Cancer
    Center
Chapel Hill, North Carolina, USA

Céline Mascaux, MD, PhD
Associate Professor
Assistance Publique Hôpitaux de
    Marseille
Oncologie Multidisciplinaire et
    Innovations Thérapeutiques
Aix Marseille University
Marseille, France

Pierre P. Massion, MD
Professor
Thoracic Program at the Vanderbilt
    Ingram Cancer Center
Vanderbilt University School of Medicine
Nashville, Tennessee, USA

Julien Mazieres, MD, PhD
Professor
Toulouse University Hospital
Universite Paul Sabatier
Toulouse, France

Annette McWilliams, MBBS, FRACP, MD, FRCPC
Fiona Stanley Hospital
Department of Respiratory Medicine
University of Western Australia
Murdoch, Australia

Tetsuya Mitsudomi, MD, PhD
Professor
Division of Thoracic Surgery
Department of Surgery
Kinki University Faculty of Medicine
Osaka-Sayama, Japan

Tony Mok, MD
Professor
Department of Clinical Oncology
The Chinese University of Hong Kong
Hong Kong, China

Daniel Morgensztern, MD
Associate Professor
Department of Medicine
Division of Oncology
Washington University School of Medicine
St. Louis, Missouri, USA

Francoise Mornex, MD, PhD
Université Claude Bernard, Lyon1, EMR
    3738, Department de Radiotherapie
CHU Lyon, France

James L. Mulshine, MD
Dean
Graduate College (Acting)
Vice President
Rush University
Chicago, Illinois, USA

Reginald F. Munden, MD, DMD, MBA
Professor and Chair
Department of Radiology
Wake Forest School of Medicine
Winston-Salem, North Carolina, USA

Kristiaan Nackaerts, MD, PhD
Associate Professor
Department of Pulmonology/Respiratory
    Oncology
University Hospital Gasthuisberg
Leuven, Belgium

Shinji Nakamichi, MD
Department of Pulmonary Medicine and
    Oncology
Graduate School of Medicine
Nippon Medical School
Tokyo, Japan

Masayuki Noguchi, MD, PhD
Professor
Department of Pathology
University of Tsukuba
Tsukuba, Japan

Krista Noonan, MD, FRCPC
Medical Oncologist
Division of Medical Oncology
British Columbia Cancer Agency
Surrey, British Columbia, Canada
Clinical Assistant Professor
University of British Columbia
Vancouver, British Columbia, Canada

Silvia Novello, MD, PhD
Full Professor of Medical Oncology
Thoracic Oncology Unit
San Luigi Hospital
University of Turin
Orbassano, Turin, Italy

Anna K. Nowak, MBBS, FRACP, PhD
Professor
School of Medicine
University of Western Australia
Crawley, Australia

Kenneth J. O'Byrne, MD
Professor, Medical Oncology
Princess Alexandra Hospital
Queensland University of Technology
Queensland, Australia

Nisha Ohri, MD
Department of Radiation Oncology
Mount Sinai Hospital
New York, New York, USA

Morihito Okada, MD, PhD
Department of Surgical Oncology
Research Institute for Radiation Biology
    and Medicine
Hiroshima University
Hiroshima, Japan

Jamie S. Ostroff, PhD
Professor and Chief, Behavioral Sciences
    Service
Department of Psychiatry and Behavioral
    Sciences
Memorial Sloan Kettering Cancer Center
New York, New York, USA

Mamta Parikh, MD
University of California, Davis
School of Medicine
Sacramento, California, USA

Elyse R. Park, PhD
Associate Professor
Psychiatry and Mongan Institute for
    Health Policy
Harvard Medical School
Massachusetts General Hospital
Boston, Massachusetts, USA

Keunchil Park, MD, PhD
Professor
Division of Hematology/Oncology
Department of Medicine
Samsung Medical Center
Sungkyunkwan University School of
    Medicine
Seoul, Korea

Harvey I. Pass, MD
Stephen E. Banner Professor of Thoracic
    Oncology
Vice-Chairman of Research
Department of Cardiothoracic Surgery
New York University Langone Medical
    Center
New York, New York, USA

Nicholas Pastis, MD, FCCP
Associate Professor of Medicine
Fellowship Program Director
Division of Pulmonary and Critical Care
Medical University of South Carolina
Charleston, South Carolina, USA

Luis Paz-Ares, MD, PhD
Head of Medical Oncology Department
University Hospital Doce de Octubre
Professor
Complutense University, Medicine
    Campus
Madrid, Spain

Nathan Pennell, MD, PhD
Associate Professor
Department of Hematology and Medical
    Oncology
Cleveland Clinic Taussig Cancer
    Institute
Cleveland, Ohio, USA

Maurice Perol
Centre Leon Berard
Department of Medical Oncology
Lyon, France

Rathi N. Pillai, MD
Assistant Professor
Department of Hematology and
    Oncology
Winship Cancer Institute
Emory University
Atlanta, Georgia, USA

Pieter E. Postmus, MD
Professor of Thoracic Oncology
Clatterbridge Cancer Centre
Liverpool Heart and Chest Hospital
University of Liverpool, United Kingdom

Suresh S. Ramalingam, MD
Professor of Hematology and Medical
    Oncology
Roberto C. Goizueta Chair for Cancer
    Research
Deputy Director
Winship Cancer Institute
Emory University School of Medicine
Atlanta, Georgia, USA

Sara Ramella, MD
Associate Professor
Radiation Oncology Department
Campus Bio-Medico University
Rome, Italy

Ramón Rami-Porta, MD, PhD, FETCS
Attending Thoracic Surgeon
Department of Thoracic Surgery
Hospital Universitari Mutua Terrassa
University of Barcelona and CIBERES
    Lung Cancer Group
Terrassa, Barcelona, Spain

Martin Reck, MD, PhD
Professor
Department of Thoracic Oncology and
    Department of Clinical Trials
Lungen Clinic Grosshansdorf
Grosshansdorf, Germany

Mary W. Redman, PhD
Associate Member
Clinical Biostatistics
Clinical Research Division
Lead Statistician
SWOG Lung Committee
Fred Hutchinson Cancer Research Center
Seattle, Washington, USA

Niels Reinmuth, MD, PhD
Professor
Department of Thoracic Oncology
Lungen Clinic Grosshansdorf
Member of German Center for Lung
    Research (DZL)
Grosshansdorf, Germany

Umberto Ricardi, MD
Full Professor Radiation Oncology
Department of Oncology
University of Turin
Turin, Italy

David Rice, MD
Professor
Department of Thoracic and
    Cardiovascular Surgery
The University of Texas MD Anderson
    Cancer Center
Houston, Texas, USA

Carole A. Ridge, FFRRCSI
Consultant Radiologist
Department of Radiology
Mater Misericordiae University Hospital
Dublin, Ireland

William N. Rom, MD, MPH
Professor
Division of Pulmonary, Critical Care,
    and Sleep Medicine
Department of Medicine
Department of Environmental Medicine
New York University School of Medicine
New York University College of Global
    Public Health
New York, New York, USA

Kenneth E. Rosenzweig, MD, FASTRO, FACR
Professor and Chairman
Department of Radiation Oncology
Icahn School of Medicine at Mount Sinai
New York, New York, USA

Enrico Ruffini, MD
Associate Professor
Section of Thoracic Surgery
Department of Surgery
University of Turin
Turin, Italy

Valerie W. Rusch, MD, FACS
Attending Surgeon
Thoracic Service
Vice Chair
Clinical Research
Department of Surgery
Miner Family Chair in Intrathoracic
    Cancers
Memorial Sloan Kettering Cancer Center
New York, New York, USA

Ravi Salgia, MD, PhD
Professor and Chair
Associate Director for Clinical Sciences
Department of Medical Oncology and
   Therapeutics Research
City of Hope Comprehensive Cancer
   Center
Duarte, California, USA

Montse Sanchez-Cespedes, PhD
Head of the Genes and Cancer
   Laboratory
Cancer Epigenetics and Biology Program
Bellvitge Biomedical Research Institute-
   IDIBELL
Hospital Duran i Reynals
Barcelona, Spain

Anjali Saqi, MD, MBA
Professor
Department of Pathology and Cell
   Biology
Columbia University Medical Center
New York, New York, USA

Giorgio V. Scagliotti, MD, PhD
Professor of Medical Oncology
Head of Department of Oncology at
   San Luigi Hospital
University of Turin
Orbassano, Turin, Italy

Selma Schimmel†
Founder
Vital Options International, Inc
Studio City, California, USA

Ann G. Schwartz, PhD, MPH
Deputy Center Director and Professor
Department of Oncology
Karmanos Cancer Institute
Wayne State University
Detroit, Michigan, USA

Suresh Senan, MRCP, FRCR, PhD
Professor of Clinical Experimental
   Radiotherapy
Department of Radiation Oncology
VU University Medical Center
Amsterdam, The Netherlands

Francis A. Shepherd, MD, FRCPC
Professor of Medicine
University of Toronto
Scott Taylor Chair in Lung Cancer
   Research
Department of Medical Oncology and
   Hematology
University Health Network
Princess Margaret Cancer Centre
Toronto, Ontario, Canada

Jill M. Siegfried, PhD
Professor and Head
Department of Pharmacology
Frederick and Alice Stark Endowed Chair
Associate Director for Translation
Masonic Cancer Center
University of Minnesota
Minneapolis, Minnesota, USA

Gerard A. Silvestri, MD, MS, FCCP
Professor
Vice Chair of Medicine for Faculty
   Development
Division of Pulmonary and Critical Care
Medical University of South Carolina
Charleston, South Carolina, USA

George R. Simon, MD
Professor
Department of Thoracic/Head and Neck
   Medical Oncology
The University of Texas MD Anderson
   Cancer Center
Houston, Texas, USA

Egbert F. Smit, MD, PhD
Professor
Department of Pulmonary Diseases
Vrije Universiteit VU Medical Centre
   and Department of Thoracic Oncology
Netherlands Cancer Institute
Amsterdam, The Netherlands

Stephen B. Solomon, MD
Chief
Interventional Radiology Service
Department of Radiology
Memorial Sloan Kettering Cancer Center
New York, New York, USA

Laura P. Stabile, PhD
Research Associate Professor
Department of Pharmacology and
   Chemical Biology
University of Pittsburgh
Pittsburgh, Pennsylvania, USA

Matthew A. Steliga, MD
Associate Professor of Surgery
Division of Cardiothoracic Surgery
University of Arkansas for Medical
   Sciences
Little Rock, Arkansas, USA

Thomas E. Stinchcombe, MD
Duke Cancer Institute
Durham, North Carolina, USA

Nicholas S. Stollenwerk, MD
Associate Clinical Professor
UC Davis Comprehensive Cancer Center
VA Northern California Health Care
   System
Sacramento, California, USA

Jong-Mu Sun, MD, PhD
Clinical Assistant Professor
Division of Hematology/Oncology
Samsung Medical Center
Sungkyunkwan University School of
   Medicine
Seoul, Korea

Anish Thomas, MD
Developmental Therapeutics Branch
National Cancer Institute
National Institutes of Health
Bethesda, Maryland, USA

Ming-Sound Tsao, MD, FRCPC
Professor
Department of Laboratory Medicine and
   Pathobiology
Department of Medical Biophysics
University of Toronto
Consultant Pathologist
University Health Network
Princess Margaret Cancer Centre
Toronto, Ontario, Canada

Jun-Chieh J. Tsay, MD, MSc
Assistant Professor
Division of Pulmonary, Critical Care,
   and Sleep Medicine
Department of Medicine
New York University School of Medicine
New York, New York, USA

Paul Van Houtte, MD, PhD
Professor Emeritus
Department of Radiation Oncology
Institut Jules Bordet
Université Libre Bruxelles
Brussels, Belgium

Paul E. Van Schil, MD, PhD
Chair
Department of Thoracic and Vascular
   Surgery
Antwerp University Hospital
Edegem, Belgium

Nico van Zandwijk, MD, PhD, FRACP
Professor University of Sydney
Director Asbestos Diseases Research
   Institute
Rhodes, Australia

J. F. Vansteenkiste, MD, PhD
Professor Internal Medicine
Respiratory Oncology Unit (Department
   of Respiratory Medicine)
University Hospital KU Leuven
Leuven, Belgium

Marileila Varella-Garcia, PhD
Professor
Department of Medicine
Division of Medical Oncology
University of Colorado Anschutz Medical
   Campus
Aurora, Colorado, USA

Giulia Veronesi, MD
Division of Thoracic Surgery
Director of Robotic Thoracic Surgery
Humanitas Research Hospital
Rozzano, Italy

Shalini K. Vinod, MBBS, MD, FRANZCR
Associate Professor
Cancer Therapy Centre
Liverpool Hospital
Sydney, Australia

Everett E. Vokes, MD
John E. Ultmann Professor
Chairman
Department of Medicine
Physician-in-Chief
University of Chicago Medicine and
   Biologic Sciences
Chicago, Illinois, USA

---

†Deceased.

Heather Wakelee, MD
Associate Professor of Medicine
Division of Oncology
Stanford Cancer Institute
Stanford, California, USA

Tonya C. Walser, PhD
Assistant Professor
Division of Pulmonary and Critical Care
    Medicine
David Geffen School of Medicine at UCLA
Los Angeles, California, USA

Shun-ichi Watanabe, MD
Department of Thoracic Surgery
National Cancer Center Hospital
Tokyo, Japan

Walter Weder, MD
Professor
Department of Thoracic Surgery
University Hospital
Zurich, Switzerland

Benjamin Wei, MD
Assistant Professor
Section of Thoracic Surgery
Division of Cardiothoracic Surgery
Department of Surgery
University of Alabama-Birmingham
    Medical Center
Birmingham, Alabama, USA

Ignacio I. Wistuba, MD
Professor
Chair
Department of Translational Molecular
    Pathology
Anderson Clinical Faculty Chair for
    Cancer Treatment and Research
The University of Texas MD Anderson
    Cancer Center
Houston, Texas, USA

James Chih-Hsin Yang, MD, PhD
Professor and Director
Graduate Institute of Oncology
College of Medicine
National Taiwan University
Director
Department of Oncology
National Taiwan University Hospital
Taipei, Taiwan

David F. Yankelevitz, MD
Professor
Department of Radiology
Mount Sinai Medical Center
Mount Sinai Hospital
New York, New York, USA

Kazuhiro Yasufuku, MD, PhD
Director of Endoscopy
University Health Network
Director
Interventional Thoracic Surgery Program
Division of Thoracic Surgery
Toronto General Hospital
University Health Network
Toronto, Ontario, Canada

Ken Y. Yoneda, MD
Professor
Clinical Internal Medicine
UC Davis Comprehensive Cancer Center
VA Northern California Health Care
    System
Sacramento, California, USA

Gérard Zalcman, MD, PhD
CHU Caen
Interne des Hopitaux de Paris
Ile-de-France, France

Caicun Zhou, MD, PhD
Professor
Shanghai Pulmonary Hospital
Tongji University
Shanghai, China

Yang Zhou, PhD, MPH
Program Manager
Yale Comprehensive Cancer Center
Yale School of Medicine
New Haven, Connecticut, USA

Daniel Zips, MD
Chair
Professor Radiation Oncology
Director
CCC Tübingen-Stuttgart
University Hospital Tübingen
University Department of Radiation
    Oncology
Tübingen, Germany

Preface

Reference texts for the management of cancer are only as good as their information, and the information must be relevant to clinical practice and must be current. Moreover, lung cancer and other thoracic malignancies remain an international problem. Lung cancer is not only the greatest cause of cancer death but also a major cause of disability and suffering.

For the past 40 years the **International Association for the Study of Lung Cancer** has remained the only society totally dedicated to the study and treatment of lung cancer and other thoracic malignancies. These cancers are notoriously complicated, as was recently pointed out by their mutational burdens and histologic heterogeneity. New discoveries, novel trials, and changes in the standard of care are happening at an extraordinary rate, and medical, surgical, and radiation oncologists, as well as respiratory physicians, nurses, physician's assistants, and social workers, need reliable and up-to-date sources of information filtered by experts in the field. The IASLC represents international and multidisciplinary expertise at every level: basic science, epidemiology, respiratory medicine, medical and radiation oncology, surgery, and palliative care, as well as nursing and advocacy. The IASLC, however, has recognized that this expertise must be channeled toward a mission of education. At the foundational level of education is a reference text that is thorough, timely, and readily available to all practitioners who are confronted with patients with thoracic malignancy.

That is why the organization published the first edition of *The IASLC Multidisciplinary Approach to Thoracic Oncology* in 2014 with the hope that this would be the first step in consolidating this information in one comprehensive source. The plan was always to be able to update, amend, and incorporate new ideas in later editions so that the basics were retained but new discoveries were discussed by the "discoverers" themselves. That is the reason why we now have a new edition of the reference text, *IASLC Thoracic Oncology*. However, we never imagined the explosion of information that would happen over a 2-year period that would need to be presented to the reader. The genomic phenotyping of lung cancer has expanded remarkably, necessitating the discovery and validation with new trials of third-generation targeted agents. The staging system for the disease has been modified and externally validated. Histologic classification of the disease has helped to define high-risk patients in early-stage disease. Radiation techniques are being expanded with greater implementation in oligometastatic disease as well as for early-stage patients, and, most dramatically, immunotherapeutic strategies, not limited solely to check point inhibition, now dominate many of the novel trials for metastatic disease as well as for neoadjuvant and adjuvant therapy.

Can you cover everything and be "au courant" with a textbook? It's a formidable task; however, the editors, along with our previous dedicated group of chapter writers, have been extraordinarily fortunate to add new experts and the most recent data from meetings in the fourth-quarter of 2016. The textbook remains a "work in progress" with online capabilities, which the IASLC and its publishing partner, Elsevier, hope to use to get information to the "treaters" in the future as early as "real time." Future updates available for selected chapters online will give readers access to the latest news as well as innovations for many of the disciplines. Just as the IASLC has matured and is growing, it is hoped that these chapters will mature so that the reader will alter his or her practice quickly due to a more rapid delivery of timely evidence-based information.

But for now, this second edition, which represents updated material for more than 50 percent of the book, will help manage the wealth of new data so that the word gets out in a comprehensive multispecialty coordinated fashion. Novel findings are presented "hot off the press" in a way that academics and nonacademics alike can keep up with thoracic cancer diagnostics and therapeutics so that the ultimate beneficiary is the patient. This endeavor calls for one international society and one book or information source that is born and keeps on growing, just like the society

As with the first edition, there is absolutely no way that this project would have been completed essentially in less than 2 years without our managing editor, Deborah Whippen. Deb has always been the binding glue for this book, as well as every single IASLC publication, and without her, every page would have scattered to the wind. Physicians are notoriously unorganized, and physician editors fall right into that category. Therefore the momentum for getting this task accomplished, from keeping updates about the status of the chapters to copyediting to indexing to even organizing what the cover would look like, fell to Deb and her cadre of book-producing experts at Elsevier including Taylor Ball and Sharon Corell. We are the luckiest editors in the world to be able to work with and listen to these dedicated manuscript aficionados.

The editors are also indebted to the Board of the IASLC for allowing us to expand this portion of the IASLC educational portfolio. Although the IASLC has been extraordinarily successful with conferences, webinars, consensus meetings, and publications, including the *IASLC Staging Manual in Thoracic Oncology* and the *IASLC Atlas of ALK and ROS1 Testing in Lung Cancer*, the updating of this 62-chapter textbook has proceeded on schedule for many reasons. We felt that our authors are dedicated to the mission, and this devotion is very different from the usual heartaches that come with editing a book. The commitment of the authors to write the most informative chapters was obvious from the beginning to the end of the task.

IASLC Thoracic Oncology is meant to provide both the practitioner and the fellow with an updated reference source that will be useful in dealing with lung cancer. It is also meant to further unify the international community through recognition that wars are won by forming allies, and in the battle against lung and other thoracic cancers, the IASLC stands for such an alliance. The battle is not only fought in the clinics and the hospitals but also on the educational front in order to supply the troops with successful plans for therapy. The editors' most profound wish is that the knowledge available in the book and all of its associated future ventures will help to move the survival curves upward and toward the right.

Harvey I. Pass
Giorgio V. Scagliotti
David Ball

Contents

SECTION I
Lung Cancer Control and Epidemiology

1   Classic Epidemiology of Lung Cancer, 1
Paolo Boffetta

2   Tobacco Control and Primary Prevention, 9
Matthew A. Steliga and Carolyn M. Dresler

3   Assessing and Treating Tobacco Use in Lung Cancer Care, 18
Jamie S. Ostroff and Elyse R. Park

4   Lung Cancer in Never-Smokers: A Different Disease, 23
Adi F. Gazdar and Caicun Zhou

5   Gender-Related Differences in Lung Cancer, 30
Silvia Novello, Laura P. Stabile, and Jill M. Siegfried

6   Genetic Susceptibility to Lung Cancer, 46
Ann G. Schwartz, Joan E. Bailey-Wilson, and Chris I. Amos

7   Screening for Lung Cancer, 52
Annette McWilliams, Fraser Brims, Nanda Horeweg, Harry J. de Koning, and James R. Jett

8   Preclinical Biomarkers for the Early Detection of Lung Cancer, 59
Jun-Chieh J. Tsay, Alissa K. Greenberg, William N. Rom, and Pierre P. Massion

9   Chemoprevention of Lung Cancer and Management of Early Lung Cancer, 69
Swati Gulati, James L. Mulshine, and Nico van Zandwijk

SECTION II
Lung Cancer Molecular Carcinogenesis

10   Copy Number Abnormalities and Gene Fusions in Lung Cancer: Present and Developing Technologies, 82
Marileila Varella-Garcia and Byoung Chul Cho

11   Mutational Events in Lung Cancer: Present and Developing Technologies, 95
Daniel Morgensztern, Siddhartha Devarakonda, Tetsuya Mitsudomi, Christopher Maher, and Ramaswamy Govindan

12   Epigenetic Events in Lung Cancer: Chromatin Remodeling and DNA Methylation, 104
Ite A. Laird-Offringa and Montse Sanchez-Cespedes

13   Stem Cells and Lung Cancer: In Vitro and In Vivo Studies, 117
Dean A. Fennell and David M. Jablons

14   Microenvironment and Lung Cancer, 121
Tonya C. Walser, Elvira L. Liclican, Kenneth J. O'Byrne, William C.S. Cho, and Steven M. Dubinett

15   MicroRNAs as Biomarkers for Lung Cancer, 129
William C.S. Cho

SECTION III
Immunology

16   Humoral and Cellular Immune Dysregulation and Lung Cancer, 137
Anish Thomas, Julie R. Brahmer, and Giuseppe Giaccone

SECTION IV
Pathology

17   Classic Anatomic Pathology and Lung Cancer, 143
Ignacio I. Wistuba, Elisabeth Brambilla, and Masayuki Noguchi

18   Molecular Testing in Lung Cancer, 164
Celine Mascaux, Ming-Sound Tsao, and Fred R. Hirsch

19   Management of Small Histologic and Cytologic Specimens in the Molecular Era, 178
Anjali Saqi and David F. Yankelevitz

SECTION V
Clinical and Radiologic Presentation of Lung Cancer

20   Clinical Presentation and Prognostic Factors in Lung Cancer, 186
Kristiaan Nackaerts, Keunchil Park, Jong-Mu Sun, and Kwun Fong

21   Conventional Imaging of Lung Cancer, 199
Patricia M. de Groot, Brett W. Carter, and Reginald F. Munden

22   Positron Emission Tomography Imaging of Lung Cancer, 219
Jeremy J. Erasmus, Feng-Ming (Spring) Kong, and Homer A. Macapinlac

SECTION VI
Diagnosis and Staging of Lung Cancer

23   Diagnostic Workup for Suspected Lung Cancer Confined to the Chest, 233
Nicholas Pastis, Martina Bonifazi, Stefano Gasparini, and Gerard A. Silvestri

24   Preoperative and Intraoperative Invasive Staging of the Mediastinum, 241
Gail E. Darling, Ramón Rami-Porta, and Kazuhiro Yasufuku

25   The Eighth Edition of the Tumor, Node, and Metastasis Classification of Lung Cancer, 253
Ramón Rami-Porta, Peter Goldstraw, and Harvey I. Pass

SECTION VII
Surgical Management of Lung Cancer

26 Preoperative Functional Evaluation of the Surgical Candidate, 265
Alessandro Brunelli and Pieter E. Postmus

27 Results of Video-Assisted Techniques for Resection of Lung Cancer, 274
Frank C. Detterbeck, Alberto Antonicelli, and Morihito Okada

28 Robotic Surgery: Techniques and Results for Resection of Lung Cancer, 283
Ayesha Bryant, Benjamin Wei, Giulia Veronesi, and Robert Cerfolio

29 Extent of Surgical Resection for Stage I and II Lung Cancer, 289
Hisao Asamura and Dominique Grunenwald

30 Extended Resections for Lung Cancer: Chest Wall and Pancoast Tumors, 295
Valerie W. Rusch and Paul E. Van Schil

31 Extended Resections for Lung Cancer: Bronchovascular Sleeve Resections, 304
Shun-ichi Watanabe

32 Multiple Nodules: Management of Synchronous and Metachronous Lung Cancers, 308
Jessica S. Donington

33 Surgical Management of Patients Considered Marginally Resectable, 314
Hiran C. Fernando and Paul De Leyn

SECTION VIII
Radiotherapeutic Management of Lung Cancer

34 Technical Requirements for Lung Cancer Radiotherapy, 318
Fiona Hegi, Todd Atwood, Paul Keall, and Billy W. Loo, Jr.

35 Radiobiology of Lung Cancer, 330
Jose G. Bazan, Quynh-Thu Le, and Daniel Zips

36 Patient Selection for Radiotherapy, 337
Dirk De Ruysscher, Michael Mac Manus, and Feng-Ming (Spring) Kong

37 Stage I Nonsmall Cell Lung Cancer and Oligometastatic Disease, 342
Suresh Senan, Umberto Ricardi, Matthias Guckenberger, Kenneth E. Rosenzweig, and Nisha Ohri

38 Ablation Options for Localized Nonsmall Cell Lung Cancer, 355
Carole A. Ridge and Stephen B. Solomon

39 Radiotherapy for Locally Advanced Nonsmall Cell Lung Cancer Including Combined Modality, 363
Paul Van Houtte, Hak Choy, Shinji Nakamichi, Kaoru Kubota, and Francoise Mornex

40 Radiotherapy in the Management of Small Cell Lung Cancer: Thoracic Radiotherapy, Prophylactic Cranial Irradiation, 374
Sara Ramella and Cécile Le Péchoux

41 Palliative Radiotherapy for Lung Cancer, 382
Andrea Bezjak, Alysa Fairchild, and Fergus Macbeth

42 Acute and Late Toxicities of Thoracic Radiotherapy: Pulmonary, Esophagus, and Heart, 393
José Belderbos, Laurie Gaspar, Ayse Nur Demiral, and Lawrence B. Marks

43 Neurotoxicity Related to Radiotherapy and Chemotherapy for Nonsmall Cell and Small Cell Lung Cancer, 409
Thomas E. Stinchcombe and Elizabeth M. Gore

SECTION IX
Chemotherapy and Targeted Agents for Lung Cancer

44 Frontline Systemic Therapy Options in Nonsmall Cell Lung Cancer, 418
Suresh S. Ramalingam, Rathi N. Pillai, Niels Reinmuth, and Martin Reck

45 Systemic Options for Second-Line Therapy and Beyond, 434
Glenwood Goss and Tony Mok

46 Maintenance Chemotherapy for Nonsmall Cell Lung Cancer, 448
Maurice Perol, Heather Wakelee, and Luis Paz-Ares

47 Pharmacogenomics in Lung Cancer: Predictive Biomarkers for Chemotherapy, 466
George R. Simon, Rafael Rosell Costa, and David R. Gandara

48 New Targets for Therapy in Lung Cancer, 479
Aaron S. Mansfield, Grace K. Dy, Mjung-Ju Ahn, and Alex A. Adjei

49 Management of Toxicities of Targeted Therapies, 490
James Chih-Hsin Yang, Chia-Chi (Josh) Lin, and Chia-Yu Chu

50 Immunotherapy and Lung Cancer, 501
Leena Gandhi, Johan F. Vansteenkiste, and Frances A. Shepherd

51 Adjuvant and Neoadjuvant Chemotherapy for Early-Stage Nonsmall Cell Lung Cancer, 512
Giorgio V. Scagliotti and Everett E. Vokes

52 Treatment of Extensive-Stage Small Cell Lung Cancer, 525
Mamta Parikh, Karen Kelly, Primo N. Lara, Jr., and Egbert F. Smit

SECTION X
Other Thoracic Malignancies

53 Malignant Mesothelioma, 536
Paul Baas, Raffit Hassan, Anna K. Nowak, and David Rice

54 Mediastinal Tumors, 550
Christopher Hazzard, Andrew Kaufman, and Raja Flores

55 Neuroendocrine Tumors of the Lung Other Than Small Cell Lung Cancer, 555
Krista Noonan, Jules Derks, Janessa Laskin, and Anne-Marie C. Dingemans

56 Thymic Tumors, 569
Enrico Ruffini, Walter Weder, Pier Luigi Filosso, and Nicolas Girard

SECTION XI
Symptom Management and Complications

57   Lung Cancer Emergencies,   590
Ken Y. Yoneda, Henri Colt, and Nicholas S. Stollenwerk

58   The Role of Palliative Care in Lung Cancer,   608
Mellar Davis and Nathan Pennell

SECTION XII
Clinical Trials

59   Clinical Trial Methodology in Lung Cancer: Study
Design and End-Point Considerations,   620
Sumithra J. Mandrekar, Mary W. Redman, and Lucinda J. Billingham

60   How to Promote and Organize Clinical Research in
Lung Cancer,   628
*Fabrice Barlesi, Julien Mazieres, Yang Zhou, Roy Herbst, and
Gérard Zalcman*

SECTION XIII
Thoracic Oncology Advocacy

61   The Role of Advocacy Groups in Lung Cancer,   635
Glenda Colburn, Selma Schimmel[†], and Jesme Fox

62   The Role of Health Services Research in Improving
the Outcomes for Patients With Lung Cancer,   639
William J. Mackillop, Shalini K. Vinod, and Yolande Lievens

Appendix

Diagnostic Algorithms,   651
Thomas Hensing, Isa Mambetsariev, Nicholas Campbell, and Ravi Salgia

[†] Deceased.

1 Classic Epidemiology of Lung Cancer

Paolo Boffetta

SUMMARY OF KEY POINTS

- Lung cancer incidence and mortality has declined among men in many countries, following a decline in the prevalence and level of smoking. Among women, lung cancer incidence and mortality is still increasing in many countries and has become the main cause of cancer death.
- Despite important advances in lung cancer screening, primary prevention through tobacco control remains the main approach in the fight against lung cancer, especially in low-income countries.
- Occupational factors, passive smoking and other indoor pollutants, including radon, and air pollution are other important modifiable causes of lung cancer; nutritional factors and infectious agents are additional potential risk factors. Control of exposure to lung carcinogens other than tobacco, in both the general and the occupational environment, has had a substantial impact in several high-risk populations.
- Lung cancer in never-smokers is not an uncommon disease. While there is an interaction between tobacco smoking and other lung carcinogens, several agents have been shown to cause lung cancer also in never-smokers.
- Lung cancer was the most important epidemic of the 20th century, and it is likely to remain a major public health problem in the 21st century. It is also a paradigm of the importance of primary prevention and a reminder that scientific knowledge is not sufficient per se to ensure human health.

The history of lung cancer epidemiology parallels the history of modern chronic disease epidemiology. In the 19th century, an excess of lung cancer was observed among miners and some other occupational groups, but otherwise the disease was very rare. An epidemic increase in lung cancer began in the first half of the 20th century, with much speculation and controversy about its possible environmental causes.

Among both women and men, the incidence of lung cancer is low in persons under 40 years of age, it increases up to age 70 or 75 years (Fig. 1.1), and it declines thereafter. The decline in incidence in the older-age groups can be explained, at least in part, by incomplete diagnosis or by a generation (birth cohort) effect.

Methodologically, epidemiologic studies of lung cancer have been straightforward because the site of origin is well defined, progressive symptoms prompt diagnostic activity, and the predominant causes are comparatively easy to ascertain. Novel approaches to the classification of lung cancer based on molecular techniques will likely bring new insights into its etiology, especially among nonsmokers.

DESCRIPTIVE EPIDEMIOLOGY

Lung cancer, a rare disease until the beginning of the 20th century, has become the most frequent malignant neoplasm among men in most countries and the main neoplastic cause of death in both men and women. In 2012, lung cancer accounted for an estimated 1,242,000 new cancer cases among men, which is 17% of all cancers excluding nonmelanoma skin cancer, and 583,000, or 9%, of new cancers among women. After nonmelanocytic skin cancer, lung cancer is the most frequent malignant neoplasm in humans and the most important cause of neoplastic death. Approximately 58% of all cancers occur in developing countries.[1]

The geographic and temporal patterns of lung cancer incidence are determined chiefly by consumption of tobacco. An increase in tobacco consumption is paralleled a few decades later by an increase in the incidence of lung cancer, and a decrease in consumption is followed by a decrease in incidence. Other factors, such as genetic susceptibility, poor diet, and indoor air pollution, may act in concert with tobacco smoking in shaping the descriptive epidemiology of lung cancer.

The pattern found today in men (Fig. 1.2) is composed of populations at high risk, in which consumption of tobacco has been persistently high for decades, and populations at low risk, either because tobacco consumption has not been increasing for long (e.g., China, Africa) or because a decrease in consumption has been present for several decades (e.g., Sweden).

In countries with populations made up of different ethnic groups, differences in lung cancer rates are frequently observed. For example, in the United States, the rates are higher among black men than among other ethnic groups (Table 1.1).

Over the past 25 years, the distribution of histologic types of lung cancer has been changing. In the United States, squamous cell carcinoma, which was formerly the predominant type, is decreasing, whereas adenocarcinoma has increased in both genders.[2] In Europe, similar changes are occurring in men, whereas in women, both squamous cell carcinoma and adenocarcinoma are increasing.[3] Although the increase in the incidence of adenocarcinoma may be due, at least in part, to improved diagnostic techniques, changes in composition and patterns of tobacco consumption (deeper inhalation of low-nicotine and tar tobacco smoke) are additional explanations.[4]

RISK FACTORS

Tobacco Smoking

The evidence is very strong that tobacco smoking causes all major histologic types of lung cancer. A carcinogenic effect of tobacco smoke on the lung has been demonstrated in epidemiologic studies conducted since the early 1950s and has been recognized by public health and regulatory authorities since the mid-1960s. Tobacco smoking is the main cause of lung cancer in most populations, and the geographic and temporal patterns of the disease largely reflect tobacco consumption during the previous decades. Because of the high carcinogenic potency of tobacco smoke, a major reduction in tobacco consumption would result in the prevention of a large fraction of human cancers.[5,6]

The excess risk among continuous smokers relative to the risk among never-smokers is on the order of 10-fold to 20-fold. The overall relative risk reflects the contribution of the different aspects of tobacco smoking: average consumption, duration of smoking, time since quitting, age at start, type of tobacco product, and inhalation pattern, as well as the absolute risk in never-smokers.

Several large cohort and case–control studies have provided detailed information on the relative contributions of duration and amount of cigarette smoking to excess lung cancer risk. Doll and Peto[7] analyzed data from a large cohort of British doctors and concluded that the excess lung cancer risk rises in proportion to the square of the number of cigarettes smoked per day but to the fourth power of the duration of smoking. Therefore duration of smoking should be considered the strongest determinant of lung cancer risk in smokers. Analysis of the same cohort after 50 years of follow-up confirmed these results.[8]

An important aspect of tobacco-related lung carcinogenesis is the effect of cessation of smoking. The excess risk sharply decreases in ex-smokers, starting approximately 5 years after quitting, and an effect is apparent even for cessation late in life. However, an excess risk throughout life likely persists even in long-term quitters.[6]

The risk of lung cancer is lower among smokers of low-tar cigarettes than among smokers of high-tar cigarettes and lower among smokers of filtered cigarettes than among smokers of unfiltered cigarettes. Smokers of black (air-cured) tobacco cigarettes are at twofold to threefold higher risk of lung cancer than smokers of blond (flue-cured) tobacco cigarettes.[6] Tar content, the presence or absence of a filter, and the type of tobacco are not independent, however. High-tar cigarettes tend to be unfiltered, and in countries where both black and blond tobacco are used, cigarettes are more frequently made from black tobacco.

Although cigarettes are the main tobacco product smoked in Western countries, an exposure–response relationship with lung cancer risk has also been shown for cigars, cigarillos, and pipes, indicating a carcinogenic effect of these products as well.[6] An increased risk of lung cancer has also been shown after consumption of local tobacco products, such as bidi and hookah in India, khii yoo in Thailand, and water pipe in China.[6] Limited data suggest an increased lung cancer risk after consumption of other tobacco products, such as narghile in western Asia and northern Africa and toombak in Sudan.

Differences in the Effect of Tobacco Smoking According to Histology, Gender, and Race

Although the evidence is abundant that tobacco smoking causes all major histologic types of lung cancer, the associations appear to be stronger for squamous cell and small cell carcinoma and weaker for adenocarcinoma. The incidence of adenocarcinoma has greatly increased during the past decades. Some of the increase may be attributable to improved diagnostic techniques,

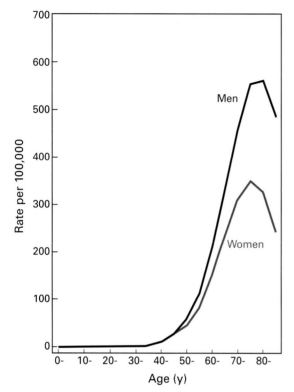

Fig. 1.1. Age-specific incidence rate of lung cancer per 100,000, by gender, according to the US Surveillance, Epidemiology End-Result (SEER) database for 2003–2007.[1]

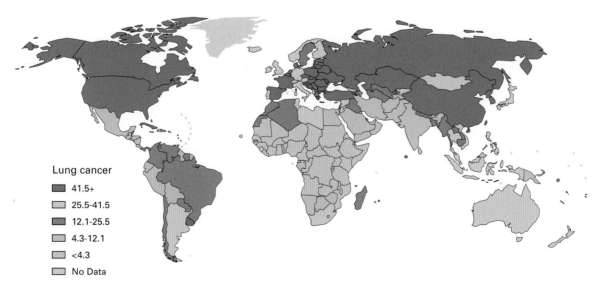

Fig. 1.2. Estimated age-standardized rate (ASR) of lung cancer in men per 100,000 men, by country, 2012
Ferlay J1, Steliarova-Foucher E., Lortet-Tieulent J., et al. Cancer incidence and mortality patterns in Europe: estimates for 40 countries in 2012. Eur J Cancer. 2013 Apr;49(6):1374–1403. http://dx.doi.org/10.1016/ j.ejca.2012.12.027. Epub 2013 Feb 26. (Reprinted from International Agency for Research on Cancer. GLOBOCAN 2012. Estimated Cancer Incidence, Mortality, and Prevalence Worldwide in 2012. http:// globocan.iarc.fr/Default.aspsx. 2012.)

but aspects of tobacco smoking may also have played a role; it is unclear, however, which aspects of smoking might explain these changes.

A few studies have suggested a difference in the risk of lung cancer between men and women who have smoked a comparable amount of tobacco,[9] but most of the available evidence does not support this gender difference.[6]

The higher rate of lung cancer among the black population compared with the rates in other ethnic groups in the United States is probably explained by the higher tobacco consumption in that population.[10] The lower risk of lung cancer among smokers in China and Japan compared with the risks among smokers in Europe and North America may be due to the relatively recent beginning of regular heavy smoking in Asia, although differences in the composition of traditional smoking products and in genetic susceptibility may also play a role.[11]

Secondhand Tobacco Smoke

The epidemiologic evidence and biologic plausibility support a causal association between secondhand exposure to cigarette smoke and lung cancer risk in nonsmokers.[12] The evidence of a high relative risk in the original studies[13,14] has been challenged on the basis of both possible confounding by active smoking, diet, or other factors and possible reporting bias. However, when these factors were taken into account, the association was confirmed, and the excess risk was on the order of 20% to 25%.[12,15]

The effect of involuntary smoking appears to be present for both household exposure, mainly from the spouse, and workplace exposure.[16,17] By contrast, little evidence has been found for an effect of childhood involuntary smoking exposure.[18]

Confounding Effects of Tobacco Smoking

The importance of tobacco smoking in the causation of lung cancer complicates the investigation of the other causes of this disease because tobacco smoking may act as a powerful confounder. For example, a population of industrial workers exposed to a suspected carcinogen may smoke more than the unexposed comparison population. An excessive lung cancer risk in the exposed group, especially if small, might be due to the difference in smoking rather than to the effect of the occupational agent. One solution is to restrict the investigation to lifetime nonsmokers. However, they may represent a selected group, with low prevalence of exposure to many agents of interest. An alternative is to collect detailed information on smoking habits and to compare the effect of the suspected carcinogens across different groups of smokers. This approach has shown that tobacco smoking as a confounder rarely completely explains excess risks larger than about 50%.[19]

Interaction Between Tobacco Smoke and Other Lung Carcinogens

Other carcinogens may interact with tobacco smoke in the determination of their carcinogenic action on the lung. In other words, the absolute or relative risk from exposure to another agent may be greater (or smaller) among heavy smokers compared with the corresponding risk among light smokers and nonsmokers. The interaction may take place at the stage of exposure; that is, the other agent has to be absorbed on the tobacco particles to penetrate the lung. Or it may take place at some stage of the carcinogenic process, for example, on induction of common metabolic enzymes or activation of common molecular targets. The empirical evidence for an interaction between tobacco smoking and other agents is scanty, mainly because of lack of data among light smokers and nonsmokers.[20] The interaction between asbestos exposure and tobacco smoking falls between the additive and the multiplicative model.[21] The interaction between radon exposure and tobacco smoking best fits a submultiplicative model; data for other agents are too sparse to allow conclusions.

Use of Smokeless Tobacco Products

Few studies have investigated the risk of lung cancer among users of smokeless tobacco products. In two large cohorts of US volunteers, the relative risk of lung cancer associated with spit tobacco use among nonsmokers was 1.08 (95% confidence interval [CI], 0.64–1.83) and 2.00 (95% CI, 1.23–3.24).[22] In a Swedish cohort, the relative risk of lung cancer for every use of snus was 0.80 (95% CI, 0.61–1.05).[23] In a large case–control study from India, the relative risk of lung cancer for every use of tobacco-containing chewing products was 0.74 (95% CI, 0.57–0.96).[24] Overall, the evidence of an increased risk of lung cancer from use of smokeless tobacco products is weak; the apparent protective effect detected in studies including smokers may be due to uncontrolled negative confounding.

Dietary Factors
Vegetables and Fruits

There is some evidence that a diet rich in vegetables and fruits probably exerts a protective effect against lung cancer.[25] Although a protective effect of high vegetable and fruit intake was found in most case–control studies, results of prospective studies with detailed information on dietary intake are less consistent in showing a similar effect. Possible reasons for the inconsistent results include bias from retrospective dietary assessment, misclassification and limited heterogeneity of exposure in cohort studies, residual confounding by smoking, and variability in food composition. Among specific types of fruits and vegetables, the evidence is stronger for cruciferous vegetables,[26] but even in this case it is unlikely that this group of foods represents a strong protective factor against lung cancer.

Meat and Other Foods

It has been suggested that high intake of meat, in particular fried or well-done red meat, increases the risk of lung cancer,[27] although the available evidence does not support this hypothesis.[25] If real, the association may be explained by the formation of nitrosamines during cooking of the meat,[28] as well as by the saturated fat content of meat (as discussed later). Although risk estimates for the intake of other foods, such as cereals, pulses, eggs, milk, and dairy products, have been specified in some studies, these results are inadequate for a judgment of the evidence of an effect.[25]

Coffee and Tea

In a few studies, high consumption of coffee has been associated with an increased risk of lung cancer.[29] However, residual confounding by tobacco smoking is a distinct possibility, and no conclusion can be drawn at present.[25] There is some evidence of a chemopreventive effect of tea, notably green tea, in smokers.[30] The overall evidence, however, is not consistent.

TABLE 1.1 Age-Standardized Incidence Rates of Lung Cancer per 100,000 by Gender and Ethnic Group[a]

Ethnic Group	Men	Women
Asian and Pacific Islander	31.6	17.5
Black	66.8	35.5
Hispanic white	25.0	16.5
Non-Hispanic white	51.2	38.1

[a]Data from the US Surveillance, Epidemiology End-Result database for 2003–2007.[1]

TABLE 1.2 Preventive Trials on Supplementation of Beta-Carotene and Lung Cancer Risk

Author	Setting, Population, Age (y)	Follow-up	Daily Dose (mg)	RR	95% CI
Kamangar et al. (2006)[30a]	Linxian (China), 29,584, 40–69	1986–2001	15[a]	0.98	0.71–1.35
ATBCCP Study Group (1994)[30b]	Finland, 29,133 male smokers, 50–69	1985–1993[b]	20	1.18	1.03–1.36
Hennekens et al. (1996)[30c]	United States, 22,071 male physicians, 40–84	1982–1995	25[c]	0.93	NA
Omenn et al. (1994)[30d]	United States, 18,314 smokers or asbestos workers, 45–74	1985–1995	30	1.28	1.04–1.57

[a]Combined with selenium (50 µg) and alpha-tocopherol (30 mg).
[b]Follow-up for cancer incidence.
[c]50 mg on alternate days.
CI, confidence interval; *NA*, not available; *RR*, relative risk.

Lipids

In several ecologic studies, a positive association was found between total lipid intake and lung cancer risk that appears to be independent of the risk of tobacco consumption.[31] The analytic studies that have addressed this association, however, have produced mixed results. Although no study has provided evidence of a protective effect of total lipid intake, an increased risk was shown only in case–control studies, whereas a pooled analysis of eight cohort studies provided no evidence of an increased risk of lung cancer for high intake of either total fat or saturated fat.[32]

Carotenoids

Many studies have addressed the risk of lung cancer in relation to estimated intake of either beta-carotene or total carotenoids (which in most cases correspond to the sum of alpha- and beta-carotene).[33] Five cohort and 18 case–control studies published up to 1994 provided 28 risk estimates in different populations; with one notable exception,[34,35] 25 of these estimates indicated a protective effect of high beta-carotene intake. The protective effect provided a 30% to 80% reduction in the risk of lung cancer between the highest and lowest intake categories.[31] The risk decreased for all major histologic types of lung cancer in many countries, in both genders, and in both smokers and nonsmokers. Similar results have been obtained in studies based on measurement of beta-carotene in prospectively collected sera.[36] The evidence of a protective effect from most observational studies has been refuted by the results of randomized intervention trials based on beta-carotene supplementation (Table 1.2). In two of these trials, which included smokers or workers exposed to asbestos, a significant increase in the incidence of lung cancer was observed in the treated groups; in the remaining studies, no effect was ascertained. The difference in results between observational studies and preventive trials can be explained by confounding by cancer-protective factors in fruits and vegetables other than beta-carotene or by the possibility that high, nonphysiologic doses of beta-carotene may cause oxidative damage, especially among smokers.[37]

Other Micronutrients

For none of the antioxidant vitamins or the other micronutrients is there conclusive evidence of a protective effect against lung cancer. The data for selenium, vitamin A, lutein, and lycopene, in particular, are inconclusive.[25,38] The results of studies of serum level of these micronutrients are insufficient for an evaluation. There is evidence from observational studies that low levels of vitamin D are associated with lung cancer risk;[39] results of randomized trials, however, do not provide supportive evidence, arguing for caution in drawing conclusions.

Isothiocyanates

Isothiocyanates are a group of chemicals with cancer-preventive activity in experimental systems and may be responsible for the

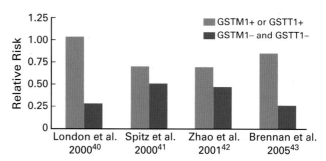

Fig. 1.3. Interaction between high intake of isothiocyanates and polymorphism in glutathione S-transferase mu 1 (GSTM1) and glutathione S-transferase theta 1 (GSTT1) in four case–control studies of lung cancer.

possibly reduced risk of lung cancer associated with high intake of cruciferous vegetables. The enzymes glutathione S-transferase M1 and T1 are involved in their metabolism. As indicated, these enzymes are polymorphic, with 5% to 10% of Europeans and 30% to 40% of Asians being carriers of a deletion in both. In four studies it has been shown that the protective effect of a high intake of isothiocyanates is stronger in carriers of both deletions than in other noncarriers (Fig. 1.3).[40–43] No final conclusions can be drawn, but this effect is an example of a possible gene–environment interaction in lung carcinogenesis.

Alcohol

Given the strong correlation between alcohol drinking and tobacco smoking in many populations, it is difficult to disentangle the contribution of alcohol to lung carcinogenesis while properly controlling for the potential confounding effect of tobacco. Meta-analyses have demonstrated that the increased risk of lung cancer observed among alcoholics is mainly attributable to such residual confounding, but some evidence of a smoking-adjusted association with high alcohol consumption was found.[44,45] This conclusion was confirmed by a pooled analysis of seven cohort studies.[46] Overall, it may be premature to conclude that an association between alcohol drinking and lung cancer has been confirmed by the available data. If the association is causal, alcohol may act as a solvent for carcinogens such as the ones in tobacco smoke. In addition, alcohol can induce metabolic enzymes or act through direct DNA damage via the active metabolite acetaldehyde.[47]

Hormones

Estrogen and progesterone receptors are expressed in the normal lung and in lung cancer cell lines, and estradiol has a proliferative effect on lung cancer cells. Although an effect of estrogens on lung carcinogenesis has not been demonstrated, estrogens may act via formation of DNA adducts and activation of growth factors.[48] Data on risk of lung cancer after the use of hormone replacement therapy have been reported from five case–control studies, two cohort studies, and one randomized trial.[49–56] A small increased risk of lung cancer has been found in the early studies, whereas a decreased risk was detected in the more recent studies. No effect was observed in the only randomized trial.[53] Although the different results may be explained by changes in the formulations used for replacement therapy, the lack of an effect in the only study with an experimental design argues against an effect of this type of exposure on lung cancer.

Three cohort studies and one case–control study were included in a meta-analysis of serum insulin-like growth factor 1 level and lung cancer. The overall relative risk was 1.01 (95% CI, 0.49–2.11).[57] The results for insulin-like growth factor–binding protein 3 level were also negative (summary relative risk, 0.83; 95% CI, 0.38–1.84), although exclusion of a deviant study resulted in a decreased risk of lung cancer for a high level of insulin-like growth factor–binding protein 3 (relative risk, 0.53; 95% CI, 0.34–0.83).

Anthropometric Measures

There is some evidence for association between a reduced body mass index and an increased risk of lung cancer.

However, this inverse association can be explained, at least in part, by negative confounding by smoking,[58] and no clear association has been demonstrated among never-smokers. Subsequent studies have supported this conclusion that the apparent association is due to confounding.[59]

Evidence suggests a direct association between height and lung cancer risk.[60] Subsequent studies have supported this finding,[61,62] although the evidence is not fully consistent.[63,64]

Infections

People with pulmonary tuberculosis have been found to be at increased risk of lung cancer.[65] A similar association was reported from community-based studies among smoking and nonsmoking women.[49,66–68] In the most informative study, involving a large cohort of people with tuberculosis from Shanghai, China,[69] the relative risk of lung cancer in the whole cohort was 1.5 and it was 2.0 20 years after the diagnosis of tuberculosis; a correlation was also seen with the location of the tuberculosis lesions. Whether the excess risk is caused by the chronic inflammatory status of the lung parenchyma or by the specific action of the *Mycobacterium* is not clear. A role of isoniazid, a widely used tuberculosis drug that causes lung tumors in experimental animals, was excluded in one large study.[70]

Chlamydia pneumoniae is a cause of acute respiratory infection. Six studies have been published on the risk of lung cancer among individuals with markers of *C. pneumoniae* infection. A positive association was detected in all six studies.[71] However, studies based on prediagnostic samples had lower risk estimates than studies based on postdiagnostic samples. An association between infection with human papilloma virus and lung cancer, in particular the adenocarcinoma type, has been suggested by the results of an analysis of series of cases and by the growing evidence of an increased risk among workers potentially exposed to this agent, such as butchers.[72] The results are insufficient to draw a conclusion about the presence or absence of a causal association. Other biologic agents that have been suggested as playing a role in lung carcinogenesis include simian virus 40 and the fungus *Microsporum canis*.[73,74]

Ionizing Radiation

There is conclusive evidence that high exposure to ionizing radiation increases the risk of lung cancer.[75] Atomic bomb survivors and patients treated with radiotherapy for ankylosing spondylitis

or breast cancer are at moderately increased risk of lung cancer (relative risk, 1.5–2.0 for cumulative exposure in excess of 100 rad).[76] The association with high doses of ionizing radiation was stronger for small cell carcinoma than for other histologic types of lung cancer. Studies of nuclear industry workers exposed to relatively low levels of ionizing radiation, however, provided no evidence of an increased risk of lung cancer.[75]

Underground miners exposed to radioactive radon and its decay products, which emit alpha particles, have been consistently found to be at increased risk of lung cancer.[77] The risk increased with estimated cumulative exposure and decreased with attained age and time since cessation of exposure.[78] In a pooled analysis of 11 cohorts, an apparently linear, approximately 6% risk increase per working-level year of exposure was estimated.[78] Evidence was also found that for comparable cumulative exposure, the risk is greater for lower rates over a longer period and that smoking modifies the carcinogenic effect of radon.[78,79] Today the main concern about lung cancer risk from radon and its decay products comes from residential rather than occupational exposure. In a pooled analysis of 13 European case–control studies, a relative risk of 1.084 (95% CI, 1.030–1.158) per 100 Bq/m³ increase in measured indoor radon was found.[80] After correction for the dilution caused by measurement error, the relative risk was 1.16 (95% CI, 1.05–1.31). The exposure–response relationship was linear with no evidence of a threshold. The same conclusion was reached from a similar analysis of North American studies.[81] These results suggest that indoor radon exposure may be an important cause of lung cancer, in particular among nonsmokers unexposed to occupational carcinogens.

Occupational Exposures

The important role of specific occupational exposures in lung cancer etiology has been well established in reports dating back to the 1950s. The risk of lung cancer is increased among workers employed in a number of industries and occupations (Table 1.3).[82,83] The responsible agents have been identified for several, but not all, of these high-risk workplaces. Evidence for the carcinogenicity of many occupational agents has been reviewed.[19] Estimates of the proportion of lung cancer cases attributable to occupational agents in France (12.5% in men and 6.5% in women) and the United Kingdom (14.5% overall) have been reported in two studies, published in 2010 and 2012, respectively.[84,85] Although asbestos remains the most important occupational lung carcinogen, the precise role of silica, radon, heavy metals, and polycyclic aromatic hydrocarbons (PAHs) in the burden of occupational cancer is uncertain. The remaining occupational lung carcinogens are likely to play a lesser role in terms of disease burden.

Asbestos

The first evidence of increased risk of lung cancer after inhalation of asbestos fibers dates back to the 1950s.[86] All forms of asbestos—chrysotile and amphiboles, including crocidolite, amosite, and tremolite—are carcinogenic to the human lung, although chrysotile's potency may be lower than that of other types.[87] Although asbestos has been banned in many countries, a substantial number of workers are still exposed, mainly in the construction industry. In many low-resource and medium-resource countries, occupational exposure is widespread. Asbestos is responsible for a large number of occupationally related lung cancers in many countries.

Metals

Exposure to inorganic arsenic, known as a lung carcinogen since the late 1960s, occurs mainly among workers employed in hot smelting; other groups at increased risk are fur handlers,

TABLE 1.3 Occupational Agents, Groups of Agents, Mixtures, and Occupations Classified as Human Carcinogens (Group 1) by the IARC Monographs Program, Volumes 1–100, Which Have the Lung as Target Organ (Cogliano et al.[82])[a]

Agents, Mixtures, Occupations	Main Industry, Use
AGENTS AND GROUPS OF AGENTS	
Arsenic and inorganic arsenic compounds	Glass, metals, pesticides
Asbestos	Insulation, filters, textiles
Beryllium and beryllium compounds	Aerospace
Bis(chloromethyl)ether and chloromethyl methyl ether	Chemical intermediate
Cadmium and cadmium compounds	Dye/pigment
Chromium-b compounds	Metal plating, dye/pigment
Involuntary tobacco smoking	Hospitality
Nickel compounds	Metallurgy, alloy, catalyst
Plutonium	Defense
X-ray radiation and gamma radiation	Medical
Radon-222 and its decay products	Mining
Silica, crystalline	Stone cutting, mining, glass, paper
MIXTURES	
Coal-tar pitch	Construction, electrodes
Soot	Pigments
OCCUPATIONS	
Aluminum production	NA
Coal gasification	NA
Coke production	NA
Hematite mining (underground)	NA
Iron and steel founding	NA
Painting	NA
Rubber production industry	NA

[a]Since the publication of this source, diesel engine exhausts (mainly used in mining and transportation) have been added to the list (Benbrahim-Tallaa et al.[83]).

IARC, International Agency for Research on Cancer; *NA,* not available.

manufacturers of sheep-dip compounds and pesticides, and vineyard workers.[88] Chromium VI compounds increase the risk of lung cancer among chromate-production workers, chromate-pigment manufacturers, chromium platers, and ferrochromium producers. No such risk has been detected among workers exposed only to chromium III compounds. An increased risk of lung cancer has been found in studies of nickel miners, smelters, electrolysis workers, and high nickel alloy manufacturers.[88] Agreement is lacking on whether all nickel compounds are carcinogenic for humans; the available evidence does not allow a clear separation of the effects of the different nickel salts to which workers are exposed. An increased risk of lung cancer has been demonstrated among workers in cadmium-based battery manufacturing industries, copper–cadmium alloy industries, and cadmium smelters. The increased risk does not seem to be attributable to concomitant exposure to nickel or arsenic. In US studies, an excess risk of lung cancer has been found among workers exposed to beryllium in the early technologic phase of the industry,[89] although the relevance of these results to the current exposure situation has been debated.[90]

Silica

An increased risk of lung cancer has been consistently reported in cohorts of people with silicosis.[91] Many authors have investigated workers exposed to crystalline silica in foundries, pottery making, ceramics, diatomaceous earth mining, brick making, and stone cutting, in some of whom silicosis may have developed. An increased risk of lung cancer was found in some, but not all, studies, and in the positive studies the increase was small, with evidence of an exposure–response relationship.[92]

Polycyclic Aromatic Hydrocarbons

PAHs are a complex and important group of chemicals formed during combustion of organic material. They are widespread in the human environment; for most people, diet and tobacco smoke are the main sources of exposure to PAHs. A number of occupational settings entail exposure to high levels of PAHs. These chemicals, however, occur inevitably as complex mixtures of variable composition; an assessment of the risk from individual PAHs is therefore difficult. An increased risk of lung cancer has been demonstrated in several industries and occupations entailing exposure to PAHs, such as aluminum production, coal gasification, coke production, iron and steel founding, tar distillation, roofing, and chimney sweeping.[93] An increase has also been suggested in a few other industries, including shale oil extraction, wood impregnation, road paving, carbon black production, and carbon electrode manufacture, with an exposure–response relationship found in the studies with detailed exposure information. Motor vehicle and other engine exhausts represent an important group of mixtures of PAHs because they contribute significantly to air pollution. The available epidemiologic evidence shows an excess risk among workers with high occupational exposure to diesel engine exhaust.[94]

Medical Conditions and Treatment

In addition to tuberculosis and lung fibrosis from chronic exposure to high levels of fibers and dusts (both discussed in earlier sections), chronic respiratory diseases have been associated with lung cancer risk. People with chronic bronchitis and emphysema are at moderately increased risk, and after adjustment for tobacco smoking, this risk is greater for squamous cell carcinoma than for other cancers.[66,94,95] The roles of shared exposures, namely, tobacco smoking and chronic inflammation, have not been fully elucidated. A meta-analysis of studies of lung cancer and asthma in never-smokers showed a summary relative risk of 1.8 (95% CI, 1.3–2.3);[96] the results were similar when the analysis was restricted to studies that controlled for smoking. However, because the evidence is based mainly on case–control studies, selection and recall bias cannot be fully excluded.[97]

The risk of lung cancer is increased in individuals surviving other tobacco-related and lifestyle-related cancers.[98] Commonality of risk factors, long-term effects of radiotherapy, and increased susceptibility probably interact in the causation of second primary cancers. The effect of chemotherapy and radiotherapy on the risk of a second primary lung cancer has been extensively investigated among long-term survivors of breast cancer; lung cancer develops in 2% to 9% of this group.[99] The increased risk is restricted to patients receiving radiotherapy. Among them, a clear exposure–response relationship has been shown, together with an interactive effect of tobacco smoking.

Several studies have assessed lung cancer risk among regular users of aspirin and other nonsteroidal anti-inflammatory drugs. A meta-analysis of 15 studies resulted in a pooled relative risk of 0.86 (95% CI, 0.76–0.98).[100] However, there was heterogeneity among the different studies, likely owing in part to differences in the definition of the exposure. The protective effect was stronger for case–control studies (relative risk, 0.74; 95% CI, 0.57–0.99) than for cohort studies (relative risk, 0.97; 95% CI, 0.87–1.08), suggesting a role for recall bias. In particular, in a large cohort study of 1 million US volunteers, a reduction in risk was not found.[101] However, in a meta-analysis of eight aspirin trials, the risk of lung cancer was reduced during the first 10 years after the end of the trial (relative risk, 0.68; 95% CI, 0.50–0.92).[102]

Indoor Air Pollution

Indoor air pollution is thought to be the main determinant of the elevated risk of lung cancer among nonsmoking women living in

TABLE 1.4 Results of Selected Cohort Studies on Fine Particle Exposure and Risk of Lung Cancer

Study; Population; Reference	No. and Sex	RR	95% CI	Exposure Contrast[a]	Basis for Exposure Assessment	Range or Mean (SD) or Both, µg/m³
Seventh-Day Adventists; USA, 1977–1992 (McDonnell et al., 2000)[102a]	6338, M	2.23	0.56–8.94	per 24.3 µg/m³ PM$_{2.5}$	Residential history 1966–1992 and local monthly pollutant estimates based on airport visibility data 1966–1992	Mean (SD) PM$_{2.5}$, 59.2 (16.8)
ASC/CPS-II; USA, 1982–1998 (Pope et al., 2002)[102b]	500,000, M + F	1.08	1.01–1.16	per 10 µg/m³ PM$_{2.5}$	City of residence in 1982. Pollutant average of 1979–1983	Mean (SD) PM$_{2.5}$, 21.1 (4.6); range, roughly 5–30 µg/m³
Six Cities; USA, 1975–1998 (Laden et al., 2006)[102c]	8111, M + F	1.27	0.96–1.69	per 10 µg/m³ PM$_{2.5}$	City of residence in 1975. Pollutant average 1979–1985	Range PM$_{2.5}$, 34.1–89.9 µg/m³
ESCAPE; Europe; 1990s–2000s[a] (Raaschou-Nielsen, 2013)[102d]	273,838, M + F	1.18	0.96–1.46	per 5 µg/m³ PM$_{2.5}$	Place of residence at enrollment. Pollutant average 2008–2011	Range of cohort-specific mean PM$_{2.5}$, 6.6–31.0 µg/m³

[a]Pooled analysis of 14 cohorts, enrollment mainly in the 1990s, follow-up until late 2000s.
CI, confidence interval; *F*, female; *M*, male; *NA*, not available; *PM*, particulate matter; *RR*, relative risk; *SD*, standard deviation.

several regions of China and other Asian countries. The evidence is stronger for coal burning in poorly ventilated houses, but evidence also exists for burning of wood and other solid fuels, as well as for the fumes from high-temperature cooking using unrefined vegetable oils, such as rapeseed oil.[103] A positive association between various indicators of indoor air pollution and lung cancer risk has also been reported in populations exposed to less extreme conditions than the ones encountered by some Chinese women, for example, populations in Central Europe and Eastern Europe and other regions.[104,105]

Outdoor Air Pollution

There is abundant evidence that lung cancer rates are higher in cities than in rural settings.[106] However, this pattern, may result from confounding by other factors, notably tobacco smoking and occupational exposures, rather than from air pollution. Cohort and case–control studies are limited by difficulties in assessing past exposure to the relevant air pollutants. The exposure to air pollution has been assessed either on the basis of proxy indicators—for example, the number of inhabitants in the community of residence, residence near a major pollution source—or on the basis of actual data on pollutant levels. These data refer to total suspended particulates, sulfur oxides, and nitrogen oxides, which are not likely to be the agents responsible for the carcinogenic effect, if any, of air pollution.[107] Furthermore, the sources of data may cover quite a wide area, masking small-scale differences in exposure levels.

The combined evidence suggests that urban air pollution may confer a small excess risk of lung cancer on the order of 50%, but residual confounding cannot be excluded. In four cohort studies, assessment of exposure to fine particles was based on environmental measurements (Table 1.4). The results of these studies suggest a small increase in risk among people classified as most highly exposed to air pollution. In 2013, the International Agency for Research on Cancer classified outdoor air pollution as an established cause of lung cancer in humans.[108]

Drinking Water Contamination

An increased risk of lung cancer has been consistently reported among people exposed to arsenic in drinking water. Investigations include ecologic studies from Argentina, Chile, and Taiwan and case–control and cohort studies from Taiwan—in particular, in areas endemic for blackfoot disease, caused by chronic arsenic poisoning—Japan, the United States, and Chile.[109] An exposure-response relationship was observed in most of these studies. In particular, in a cohort study from a contaminated area in Taiwan, the relative risk of lung cancer according to cumulative estimated exposure to arsenic from drinking water was 4.0 for 20 or more milligrams per liter of drinking water contamination compared with uncontaminated water.[110]

CONCLUSION

Given the poor prognosis of lung cancer and the lack of effective screening procedures, primary prevention remains the main weapon against this neoplasm and control of tobacco smoking is by far the most important preventive measure. Although the effects of tobacco control on the incidence of the disease can be demonstrated in several populations, much remains to be done, especially among women and in low-income countries. Control of exposure to other lung carcinogens, in both the general and the occupational environment, is another measure that has been taken and, at least in some instances, has had substantial effects. Priorities for the prevention of lung cancer, in addition to tobacco control, include understanding the carcinogenic and preventive effects of dietary and other lifestyle factors, control of occupational exposures, avoidance of high exposure to outdoor and indoor pollution, and elucidation of conditions that entail increased genetic predisposition to lung cancer.

Lung cancer in never-smokers is not a rare disease. Occupational factors, passive smoking, and indoor exposure to radon explain a portion of these cases, and nutritional, infectious, and genetic factors are receiving attention as additional risk factors.

Lung cancer was the most important epidemic of the 20th century, and it is likely to remain a major public health problem in the 21st century. It is ironic that this cancer causes more deaths than any other malignancy in the world, even though epidemiologic research has led to the identification of more than 10 causes of the disease, including the quantitatively dominant cause, tobacco smoking. Lung cancer is also a paradigm of the superiority of prevention over treatment and a reminder that scientific knowledge is not sufficient per se to ensure human health.

KEY REFERENCES

5. Peto R, Lopez AD, Boreham J, Thun M, Heath Jr C. Mortality from tobacco in developed countries: indirect estimation from national vital statistics. *Lancet.* 1992;339(8804):1268–1278.
7. Doll R, Peto R. Cigarette smoking and bronchial carcinoma: dose and time relationships among regular smokers and lifelong nonsmokers. *J Epidemiol Community Health.* 1978;32(4):303–313.
8. Doll R, Peto R, Boreham J, Sutherland I. Mortality in relation to smoking: 50 years' observations on male British doctors. *BMJ.* 2004;328(7455):1519.

15. Hackshaw AK, Law MR, Wald NJ. The accumulated evidence on lung cancer and environmental tobacco smoke. *BMJ*. 1997;315(7114):980–988.
37. Greenwald P. Beta-carotene and lung cancer: a lesson for future chemoprevention investigations? *J Natl Cancer Inst*. 2003; 95(1):E1.
80. Darby S, Hill D, Auvinen A, et al. Radon in homes and risk of lung cancer: collaborative analysis of individual data from 13 European case-control studies. *BMJ*. 2005;330(7485):223.
84. Rushton L, Hutchings SJ, Fortunato L, et al. Occupational cancer burden in Great Britain. *Br J Cancer*. 2012;107:S3–S7.
85. Boffetta P, Autier P, Boniol M, et al. An estimate of cancers attributable to occupational exposures in France. *J Occup Environ Med*. 2010;52(4):399–406.

102. Rothwell PM, Fowkes FG, Belch JF, Ogawa H, Warlow CP, Meade TW. Effect of daily aspirin on long-term risk of death due to cancer: analysis of individual patient data from randomised trials. *Lancet*. 2011;377(9759):31–41.
105. Hosgood 3rd HD, Boffetta P, Greenland S, et al. In-home coal and wood use and lung cancer risk: a pooled analysis of the International Lung Cancer Consortium. *Environ Health Perspect*. 2010;118(12):1743–1747.
107. Straif K, Cohen A, Samet J. *Air Pollution and Cancer. IARC Scientific Publication No. 161*. Lyon, France: International Agency for Research on Cancer; 2013:161.

See Expertconsult.com for full list of references.

2 Tobacco Control and Primary Prevention

Matthew A. Steliga and Carolyn M. Dresler

SUMMARY OF KEY POINTS

- Smoking is the predominant risk factor for development of lung cancer. As tobacco is introduced to societies, common patterns emerge. Typically, it is first used in men, then later in women. A 20- to 25-year lag between smoking rates and lung cancer rates reflects this.
- The World Health Organization (WHO) Framework Convention on Tobacco Control (FCTC) provides a comprehensive global tobacco-control strategy. Six key concepts are described with the mnemonic "MPOWER."
  - **M**onitor Tobacco Use and Prevention Policies: The WHO has standardized surveys and metrics to make comparisons possible between societies and over time.
  - **P**rotect People from Tobacco Smoke: Secondhand smoke is a risk factor for lung cancer. Implementation of public smoking bans has been linked to decreased disease from tobacco smoke (asthma exacerbations, acute coronary events, etc.).
  - **O**ffer to Help Quit Tobacco Use: Physician advice, pharmacotherapy, and tobacco quitlines improve cessation rates, but are underutilized.
  - **W**arn About the Dangers of Tobacco: Public service messages are effective. Written and graphic warning labels on tobacco packages reach each user and are effective at decreasing use.
  - **E**nforce Bans on Tobacco Advertising, Promotion, and Sponsorships: Often tobacco marketing targets youth and socioeconomically disadvantaged populations. Restricting marketing prevents initiation and decreases use.
  - **R**aise Taxes: Taxation suppresses use while raising money; unfortunately, most tobacco tax funds do not support other tobacco-control measures.

Many lives have been saved by tobacco control over the past 50 years. However, due to ongoing use of tobacco, millions of preventable deaths have occurred. Tobacco use has steadily grown and spread across the globe to such a degree that tobacco-induced death and disability have attained epidemic proportions. Many diseases and conditions attributable to smoking, such as cerebrovascular disease, heart disease, emphysema, and cancer—especially lung cancer—have led to death and disability. This chapter highlights the growth, spread, and current status of the tobacco epidemic worldwide; global efforts to curb the use of tobacco; and the potential impact of control measures on outcomes, specifically lung cancer–related mortality.

As tobacco use is encouraged, promoted, and perpetuated with a variety of mechanisms, there is a need to intervene and provide tobacco prevention and cessation in multiple dimensions. Various tobacco-control strategies have been used in the past, with varying degrees of success across different populations. The WHO FCTC provides a unified multidimensional approach to tobacco control for the 21st century, with a structure to discuss implementation of comprehensive tobacco control. Although societies around the globe differ widely in terms of language, cultural norms, economic resources, and smoking rates, nearly all societies are afflicted with the tobacco epidemic, and a concerted effort involving the use of evidence-based strategies has the potential to save millions of lives.

HISTORICAL CONTEXT OF THE TOBACCO EPIDEMIC

Tobacco is indigenous to the Americas, and, prior to its European discovery in 1492, tobacco was unknown in the rest of the world. After Europeans were introduced to tobacco—and nicotine addiction—consumption steadily grew in Europe. Despite its popularity, King James I of England issued "A Counterblaste to Tobacco" as one of the first documented efforts of tobacco control. In 1604, he not only stated the harm to the smoker as being "… hatefull to the Nose, harmefull to the braine, dangerous to the Lungs …" but also discussed the implications of second-hand smoke in the context of a woman whose husband smokes and "resolve[s] to live in a perpetuall stinking torment."[1] One of the first documented tobacco-control policies was his accompanying "Commissio pro Tabacco," which levied a tax on tobacco importation.[2] In these early years of the spread of tobacco, much of its use was in the form of chew tobacco, pipe tobacco, cigars, or snuff. Tobacco was even touted as medicinal. Despite the proclamation from King James I, government taxation, and various religious edicts, tobacco use continued to grow throughout Europe.

The Industrial Revolution included the development of cigarette-rolling machines in the late 1800s, which not only spawned mass production and increased the use of tobacco but also shifted the bulk of tobacco use to cigarette smoking. Cigarettes are smoked with deeper inhalation than pipe tobacco or cigars, leading to absorption in the pulmonary parenchyma rather than in buccal and pharyngeal parenchyma. As a result of pulmonary delivery, a much more rapid and intense peak in nicotine levels leads to a greater addiction potential. This more addictive product, combined with industrialization, global transportation, and aggressive marketing to men, women, and children across the globe, led to an explosion in tobacco use and a highly profitable industry.

The epidemiologic relationship between smoking rates in a population and death rates attributable to smoking has been extensively analyzed on a global scale, and fascinating patterns tend to recur predictably from one society to another. Lopez et al.[3] noted that the rise in the prevalence of cigarette smoking was reflected in the rise in the death rate caused by smoking-related illnesses, with an approximately 20-year to 25-year lag.[3] Overall, it has been demonstrated that death rates from tobacco-induced disease occur at a rate of roughly half of the smoking rate, given this time lag (e.g., for a population with a 60% smoking rate, 30% of the deaths 20 years later are secondary to smoking). Stage I of a smoking epidemic represents initiation, with low smoking rates and very low death rates due to smoking (Fig. 2.1). Stage II consists of a rapid rise in the smoking prevalence among men to its peak, with the beginning of a rise in deaths. During this time, smoking among women just starts to increase, but there are few deaths. Stage III consists of a decline in smoking among men, with a continued increase in smoking among women. During this time, the death rate among men continues to rise following the 20-year to 25-year lag from the peak in smoking, and the death

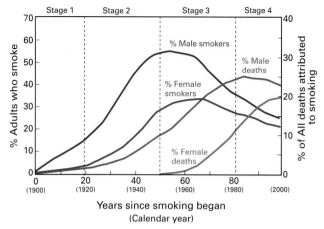

Fig. 2.1. Lopez curve from 1994 demonstrating the stages of the tobacco epidemic in countries with developed economies as indicated by the rates of smoking and smoking-attributable deaths (based on lung cancer data) for men and women. *(Reprinted with permission from Thun M, Peto R, Boreham J, Lopez AD. Stages of the cigarette epidemic on entering its second century. Tob Control. 2012;21(2):96–101.)*

rate among women also begins to increase. Stage IV consists of a decline in smoking rates among men and a plateau or fall in smoking rates among women, with an eventual decline in death rates. The Lopez model has been applied to many societies, and, in general, developing nations tend to be represented by stages I and II, whereas many industrialized nations have experienced their peak in smoking rates and deaths, particularly among men, and are in stages III or IV.

This rise and fall in the number of smoking-related deaths closely parallels the rise and fall in lung cancer incidence and mortality rates in the United States. Smoking was relatively uncommon before 1900, correlating with Lopez stage I. The smoking rate among men in the United States increased from the 1900s and peaked around 1965 (stage II). After the Surgeon General's report of the link between smoking and cancer,[4] smoking rates among men decreased, yet smoking-related deaths among men continued to increase (stage III). This increase in male smoking prevalence eventually led to a peak and decrease in lung cancer–related deaths among men approximately 20 years later. During this time, the smoking rate among women rose and plateaued. In the late 1990s and beyond, the death rate among women was just beginning to decrease (stage IV). According to the Lopez model, the incidence of lung cancer and lung cancer–related mortality should continue to fall for men and women in the United States as smoking rates have declined.

This descriptive model has also been applied to many other societies. Rates of smoking in China and Japan have risen for men, and the rates of smoking-attributable deaths continue to rise in these societies (stage II). However, countries such as Australia, New Zealand, the United Kingdom, and Sweden have progressed through all phases of the Lopez model and are in stage IV, with declining rates of smoking-related deaths among men and women. Despite the decrease in tobacco use in some of the aforementioned countries, tobacco use is growing in other countries, particularly India, Japan, and China, where societal and cultural shifts are leading to growing numbers of people who smoke, particularly women. The growth of the global population, the spread of tobacco use to more countries, and the rising rates of smoking among women are all contributing to a projected rapid global increase in tobacco use and tobacco-induced deaths. The toll of tobacco is considerable, with an estimated 100 million deaths globally in the 20th century; currently, 5 million deaths

TABLE 2.1 Measures to Assist With Implementation of Effective Tobacco Control
Monitor tobacco use and prevention policies
Protect people from tobacco smoke
Offer help to quit tobacco use
Warn about the dangers of tobacco
Enforce bans on tobacco advertising, promotion, and sponsorship
Raise taxes on tobacco

are reported annually, with 1 billion deaths projected globally in the 21st century if the trajectory is not changed.[5]

As smoking rates have declined in some countries, they have stabilized or increased in other countries as a result of aggressive marketing by the tobacco industry and lax or nonexistent tobacco-control policies. With the irrefutable evidence that this aggressively marketed, addictive product leads to premature death and disability among people who smoke (with one in two people who continue to smoke dying of tobacco-related disease) and illness in people exposed to secondhand smoke, tobacco control not only can be seen as a public health crisis but also can be viewed from ethical and human rights perspectives.[6,7] By the end of the 20th century, the tobacco epidemic had steadily grown into a massive global crisis in which, currently, 5 million people die annually as a result of its use. Attempts at tobacco control have varied among different countries, and often by state or province within a country. The production, marketing, and distribution of cigarettes are predominantly controlled by a few international corporations: Philip Morris, Altria, British American Tobacco, Japan Tobacco, R. J. Reynolds, and China National Tobacco. The production, marketing, and distribution of cigarettes had become a globally organized network, and although the battle was being fought on many fronts, there was no global consensus on measures of tobacco control, and unified countermeasures to combat this problem were lacking.

21ST CENTURY TOBACCO-CONTROL MEASURES

The need for a comprehensive, unified, and enforceable global strategy to combat this global epidemic was initially conceptualized by Roemer and Taylor in 1993.[8] These authors subsequently presented a strategy for a FCTC to the WHO in 1995. Persistent efforts led to adoption of the WHO FCTC at the World Health Assembly in 2003. The WHO FCTC came into force in 2005 as the first international treaty adopted under the WHO and was ratified by 177 parties in 2013. The United States notably remains a nonparty. This unprecedented agreement between party nations became the first international legal instrument for a unified approach to combat the global tobacco epidemic. The multidimensional treaty delineates universal standards declaring the dangers of tobacco and outlines strategies for limiting its use worldwide through provisions regarding education, production, advertisement, distribution, sale, and taxation.

The details of the entire WHO FCTC are beyond the scope of this chapter, but the WHO produced an internationally applicable summary of the essential elements of a tobacco-control strategy, publicized as the mnemonic "MPOWER," which includes six components (Table 2.1). Examples of successful tobacco-control strategies are discussed here using these categories as a construct.

Monitor Tobacco Use and Prevention Policies

If an epidemic is to be treated, it must first be measured. It is crucial to dramatically improve global surveillance of tobacco use among adults and youths. Until recently, the extent of the epidemic has not been well documented, particularly in developing countries. Differences among nations with regard to the tools that have been used to measure this epidemic have made comparisons difficult. The WHO Global Tobacco Surveillance System is a uniform comprehensive format for measuring the epidemic and gauging the impact of measures when implemented. The system comprises three school-based components (the Global Youth Tobacco Survey, the Global School Personnel Survey, and the Global Health Professions Student Survey) and one adult component (the Global Adult Tobacco Survey). These surveys contain the same basic data fields in all queries, and individual countries can add other specific points if they wish. Uniformity is necessary to compare one society and/or time point with another. The system involves three sequential phases: a survey workshop, data analysis, and a programmatic workshop that is designed to determine the needs and priorities to suit that area at that time. The surveys are intended to be conducted shortly after the implementation of control measures and then repeated every few years. Monitoring with reliable tools to obtain accurate data is the only way to truly determine where tobacco control is most needed, what type of tobacco control is most appropriate, who the target audience should be, and the outcomes of any implemented policies.

Protect People From Tobacco Smoke

The harm that smoking causes to people who smoke has been a driving force for tobacco control, but the effects of smoking on nonsmokers has led to another arm of tobacco control: protecting all people from tobacco smoke. Secondhand smoke, also known as environmental tobacco smoke or passive smoking, is a risk factor for asthma, bronchitis, and respiratory infections and also has been demonstrated to be a risk for the development of lung cancer and cardiovascular disease. Rates of lung cancer are higher for women who have never smoked but have husbands who smoke, with a relative risk ranging from 1.3 to 3.5.[9] Rates are higher for women with husbands who are "heavy" smokers (>20 cigarettes per day), suggesting a dose–response relationship.[9]

Mackay et al.[10] and Pell et al.[11] reported on the effect of a 2006 policy to prohibit smoking in all enclosed places in Scotland on health conditions related to secondhand smoke. In analyzing hospital data, the authors found that the rate of hospitalizations for childhood asthma was increasing 5.2% per year before the policy and fell by 18.2% per year after the policy took effect; this change was noted for both preschool and school-age children. In addition, after implementation of the policy, the rate of admissions for acute coronary syndrome decreased by 14% among active smokers, by 19% among former smokers, and by 21% among individuals who had never smoked. When the 12-month periods before and after implementation of the policy were compared, the rate of admissions for acute coronary syndrome fell by 17%. In comparison, during that time in England (where there were no smoke-free laws), the rate fell by only 4%, and during the preceding decade in Scotland, the rate decreased by an average of 3% per year. Serum cotinine was measured in patients during this time. The self-reported exposure to secondhand smoke decreased among nonsmokers, and this decrease was validated on the basis of lower cotinine levels in those individuals.[11] Many other examples demonstrate the impact of smoke-free laws on public health, and it is not surprising that improved outcomes are seen among nonsmokers, but it is encouraging that improved outcomes can be found among smokers as well, likely as a result of a reduction in tobacco use despite the fact that they are still smoking.

Offer Help to Quit Tobacco Use

Many people who use tobacco may not actively seek assistance with cessation because of either a lack of interest in quitting, the perceived futility of cessation efforts, the stigma associated with tobacco use, or a lack of willingness to invest the time and financial resources to support their desire to quit. The International Association for the Study of Lung Cancer conducted a survey regarding the smoking-cessation practices among its members (response rate, 40.5%).[12] According to the survey, 90% of respondents believe that current smoking affects clinical outcomes and that cessation should be a standard part of care; 90% ask their patients about smoking at the time of the initial visit; 81% advise their patients to quit (but only 40% discuss pharmacotherapy); and 39% provide cessation assistance. These survey results likely represent a best-case scenario for cancer providers, as the respondents were members of an international multidisciplinary lung cancer organization who were motivated to respond to the survey and because the survey responses were self-reported. By contrast, the rates of primary physician queries about smoking and advice on cessation have been disappointingly low, likely driven by the perceived of lack of efficacy of such efforts among practitioners.

However, although many people who smoke may not quit on the basis of their physician's advice, brief counseling from primary physicians at every visit could have a substantial impact. In one of the first landmark studies on this subject, published in 1979, researchers from London found that physician practices such as asking patients about tobacco use, advising patients to stop smoking, providing informational pamphlets, and telling patients they will be called for follow-up yielded a 5.1% quit rate at 1 year.[13] Although this quit rate was modest, it was significantly higher than the rate for the control group (0.3%; $p < 0.001$). This finding suggests that active cessation interventions by primary care physicians could substantially impact the number of people who would quit. Unfortunately, as yet, primary care providers often do not follow the most basic steps of asking patients about smoking, advising them to stop smoking, and referring them to a cessation service such as a telephone quitline or other resource.

In many countries, quitlines are able to offer assistance with cessation. In the United States, many, but not all, of the quitlines run by individual states provide pharmacotherapy such as nicotine-replacement therapy. However, most countries are not able to afford this type of intervention. For many people who smoke, the cost of the nicotine-replacement therapy can exceed the cost of cigarettes. The convenience of the quitline, the availability of nicotine-replacement therapy, and the free-of-charge service would lead one to think that quitlines are popular, but the penetrance of quitlines is low, even in developed countries. For example, Australia has extremely aggressive and successful tobacco-control programs, with the quitline number displayed in all retail outlets, on every package of cigarettes, and in advertisements as part of a mass media campaign, yet one study demonstrated that only 3.6% of people who smoke used the service in 1 year, suggesting that many people who smoke may not initiate the call for help in quitting and may not be interested in asking for help.[14]

Compared with face-to-face counseling with a physician or other health-care provider, quitlines are more convenient, less costly, and more easily approached by reluctant smokers. A cost analysis of a national quitline in Sweden demonstrated a 31% self-reported 1-year quit rate with an estimated cost of $1052 to $1360 per quitter and of $311 to $401 per life year saved, indicating that the quitline was less costly than other modalities that were analyzed, such as counseling by a general practitioner, a community mass media campaign, and bupropion treatment.[15]

Warn About the Dangers of Tobacco

Education regarding the addictive and harmful nature of smoking can be delivered in multiple ways, including (but not limited to) physician–patient interactions, education in schools, public announcements on television and radio, warning labels on cigarettes, and print and outdoor advertisements related to the effects of tobacco. One of the simplest and least expensive ways to distribute education about tobacco is through mandatory warning labels on tobacco packaging. A 2006 study conducted in four countries (the United States, the United Kingdom, Australia, and Canada) demonstrated that larger warnings and graphic warnings were more effective for communicating the risks of smoking compared with the very inconspicuous United States warnings.[16] Another report on warnings in these same countries was published in 2009, after the use of graphic warnings had been implemented in Australia. The impact of health warnings was evaluated by comparing graphic warnings from Australia and Canada with text-only warnings from the United Kingdom and the United States.[17] The new graphic warnings in Australia increased smokers' salience (reading and noticing), cognitive reactions (thinking about harm and quitting), and behavioral responses (forgoing cigarettes and avoiding the warnings).

Clearly, graphic warning labels are important means of communication in areas with lower literacy rates, but, even for populations with higher literacy rates, the graphic labels have greater impact and are associated with lower smoking rates. While public media campaigns and advertisements that warn about the dangers of tobacco have been shown to be effective, they do require financial resources for the creation and distribution of the messages and ongoing funding for maintenance. The implementation of policies regarding enlarging warning labels and including graphic warnings does not require ongoing cost to the government and literally puts an effective warning message in the hands of every tobacco user.

Enforce Bans on Tobacco Advertising, Promotion, and Sponsorship

The tobacco industry spends tens of billions of dollars annually to promote its product, which in turn kills up to half of its users. The industry depends on promotion to maintain its current customer base and to recruit "replacement smokers," that is, to replace the minority of smokers who successfully quit and the masses who die of tobacco-related diseases. An Article of the WHO FCTC states that all parties must implement comprehensive restrictions on tobacco advertising, promotion, and sponsorship within 5 years.[13] In many countries, particularly those with developing economies, tobacco use among women traditionally has not been high and women are viewed as a growth market by industry because of growing financial and social independence. It is unsurprising that women and minors have been the targets of many tobacco advertising, promotion, and sponsorship activities, with the rate of smoking among women expected to double between 2005 and 2025.[18] Because of this selective targeting, tobacco control also needs to be gender and age based in its approach. Exposure to tobacco advertising, promotion, and sponsorship is associated with a higher prevalence of smoking, and a comprehensive ban on such activities leads to lower exposure to these messages, a finding that has held true across different socioeconomic groups.[19] Bans on tobacco advertising, promotion, and sponsorship have been shown to decrease smoking rates in both developed and developing countries.[20,21]

Raise Taxes on Tobacco

"Of all the concerns, there is one—taxation—that alarms us the most. While marketing restrictions and [restrictions on] public and passive smoking do depress volume, in our experience taxation depresses it much more severely."[22]

These words from the tobacco industry, written more than 25 years ago, still hold true today. A 10% rise in retail price will result in a 4% decrease in cigarette sales through both increased cessation and reduced consumption by active smokers in developed nations and in an estimated 8% decrease in middle- to lower-income countries.[23] The fact that tobacco disproportionately affects lower socioeconomic groups that are linked with a greater elasticity (i.e., reduced sales with increased price) makes increasing the cost a logical tobacco-control strategy, particularly with respect to these lower socioeconomic groups. While some tobacco-control policies (e.g., media campaigns and cessation-support services) require ongoing financial resources and others (e.g., clean indoor air policies and policies banning advertisement) are fairly inexpensive to implement, taxation has the unique ability to effectively suppress tobacco use and generate revenue. Unfortunately, of the $133 billion globally generated by tobacco taxation, less than 1% of revenues collected in tobacco taxes are reinvested in prevention or cessation efforts.[24] A progressive approach to tobacco taxation was implemented in Costa Rica in 2012, with a rise in tobacco taxes of approximately $0.80 per pack. This change increased total taxes from approximately 56% to 71% of the cost of a pack of cigarettes, and all of the new tax revenue was earmarked for cancer treatment, tobacco-prevention and cessation services and research, support of the nation's Health Promotion Act, and other health-related measures. Although not all of these measures are directly related to tobacco control, some of the increased funds will directly benefit prevention, cessation, treatment, and patient-support efforts. A provision of this act is that taxes will automatically increase annually to keep pace with inflation.[25] Taxes passed as a flat tax amount per quantity of tobacco will be eroded by inflation over time unless levied as a percentage of the price or adjusted for inflation.

Combinations of Measures

Typically, successful tobacco control is implemented not as a single measure but rather as part of a more comprehensive multifaceted approach involving several of the aforementioned concepts; therefore it may be difficult to distill the impact of one measure on smoking rates when several are implemented in combination. For example, in California, clean indoor air legislation was accompanied by increased tax and antitobacco advertising. This combination resulted not only in a lower smoking prevalence but also lower per capita cigarette consumption. Reducing smoking is the aim of these programs, but the deeper overall goal is to improve public health, and therefore outcomes such as the lower mortality from heart disease and the decreased rates of bladder cancer and lung cancer that were found following the implementation of the California comprehensive tobacco program[26,27] further strengthen the need for multidimensional tobacco-control programs.

Some of the strongest tobacco-control measures that have an impact on several of the aforementioned categories have been developed in Australia. For example, the implementation of plain packaging regulations in Australia acts in several dimensions by providing health warnings and the quitline number while also eliminating brand image and advertising and promotion on the packaging itself. This approach not only has resulted in the distribution of warnings and the promotion of quitlines but has also been shown to decrease the appeal of smoking and to increase thoughts about quitting.[28]

Impact of Tobacco Control on Lung Cancer Mortality

As described in the previous section, effective tobacco-control efforts have been well defined and have a strong evidence base. The MPOWER strategy was developed by the WHO to assist countries in implementing the FCTC. The impact of tobacco-control efforts on the incidence of and mortality resulting from lung cancer is demonstrated by the Lopez curves describing the stages of the smoking epidemic and the consequent epidemic of lung cancer (Fig. 2.1).[29] Unfortunately, only a few of the more economically developed countries heeded the epidemiologic news from the 1950s that smoking causes lung cancer.[30,31]

Doll et al.[32] demonstrated significantly improved survival for British male physicians who were nonsmokers (Fig. 2.2) and also significant benefits for physicians who had smoked but quit. Predominantly because of this cessation, Britain was also the first country to have a drop in lung cancer rates among men (Fig. 2.3).[29] Australia and the United States were close behind, but, interestingly, the decline was slower. Unfortunately, the lung

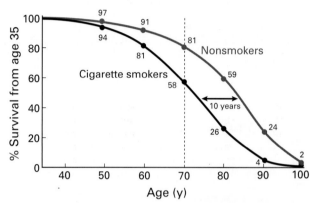

Fig. 2.2. Survival after 35 years of age for continuing smokers and nonsmokers among male physicians in the United Kingdom (born between 1900 and 1930). The values indicate the percentage of individuals in each group who were still alive at each decade of age. *(Reprinted with permission from Doll R, Peto R, Boreham J, Sutherland I. Mortality in relation to smoking: 50 years' observations on male British doctors. BMJ. 2004;328(7455):1519.)*

cancer rates among women do not replicate the rates among men in different countries because of the variety of cultural influences on smoking prevalence. These changes in the United States and the United Kingdom were primarily driven by smoking cessation as a result of epidemiologic evidence linking disease to smoking. In the United States, the peak prevalence of male smokers started to decline after the 1930 birth cohort as a result of smoking cessation (Fig. 2.4).[33] In the United Kingdom, the rates of smoking among both male and female individuals and the annual rates of lung cancer–related death (Fig. 2.5) declined.[34] These changes indicate that smoking cessation occurs as a result of public education about the risks of smoking in the years following these early epidemiologic studies on lung cancer.

In both the United Kingdom and the United States, large-cohort epidemiologic studies were established to quantify the risk of lung cancer with continued smoking and the markedly decreased risk with cessation. Data from the United Kingdom demonstrate that the decrease in lung cancer mortality depends on the age at the time of tobacco cessation (Fig. 2.6).[34] These data indicate that even middle-aged individuals who stop smoking before they have incurable lung cancer or another fatal disease avoid most of their risk of being killed by tobacco. Smoking cessation before middle age reduces the risk further.[33]

As already noted, education can lead to cessation, which results in fewer people smoking and a decrease in the incidence of lung cancer. Sharing of educational information with the public was the first demonstration of how tobacco-control efforts could affect the incidence of tobacco-related disease, such as lung cancer. Subsequently, other countries implemented policies that have an impact on the incidence of lung cancer.

Another mechanism to reduce smoking levels was introduced in Sweden, where the GOTHIATEK standard for the manufacturing of a smokeless tobacco product (Swedish snus) was instituted in the 1980s and 1990s.[35] The transition to the GOTHIATEK standard was an incremental process and was influenced by regulatory oversight by the Swedish Food

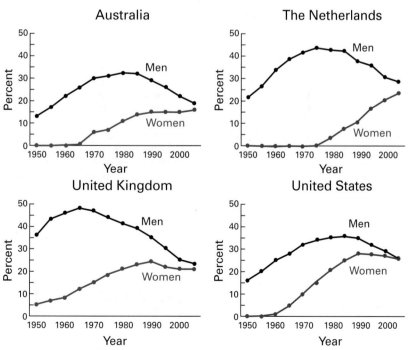

Fig. 2.3. Smoking-attributable deaths as estimated from lung cancer rates. The values are expressed as the percentage of all deaths. *(Reprinted with permission from Thun M, Peto R, Boreham J, Lopez AD. Stages of the cigarette epidemic on entering its second century. Tob Control. 2012;21(2):96–101.)*

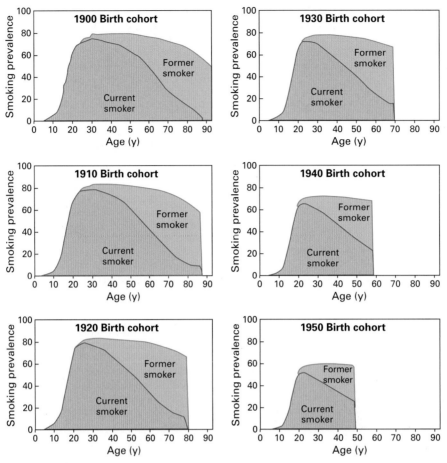

Fig. 2.4. Age-specific prevalence of current and former smoking according to birth cohort for white male individuals in the United States. *(Reprinted with permission from International Agency for Research on Cancer (IARC). IARC Handbooks of Cancer Prevention, Tobacco Control, Vol. 11, Reversal of Risk After Quitting Smoking. Lyon, France: IARC Press; 2007.)*

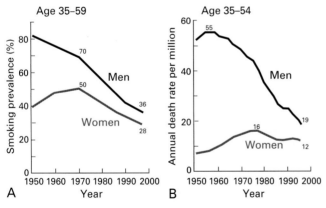

Fig. 2.5. (A) Trends in smoking prevalence and (B) change in the annual rate of lung cancer–related deaths.[34] *(Reprinted with permission from Peto R, Darby S, Deo H, Silcocks P, Whitley E, Doll R. Smoking, smoking cessation and lung cancer in the UK since 1950: combination of national statistics with two case-control studies. BMJ. 2000;321(7257):323–329.)*

Authority in the 1970s. Smokeless tobacco products were initially manufactured by the government-controlled Swedish tobacco industry, but, since the 1990s, the manufacturing was privatized into the company Swedish Match North Europe AB. As a result of marketing efforts, lower price, social pressure, or,

most likely, some combination of these influences, men in Sweden began to use more Swedish snus than combusted tobacco (as in cigarettes).

Snus is a smokeless product that has been manufactured in Sweden since the 1800s and has since spread to other, mostly Scandinavian, countries. Snus also has migrated to the United States and is now manufactured by several different tobacco companies, although Swedish Match notes that these products are not analogous to Swedish snus because they are not made with adherence to the GOTHIATEK standard. The GOTHIATEK standard was developed to be consistent with Swedish food standards and, through the adherence to several manufacturing standards, provides for low levels of microbiologic growth, heavy metals, and nitrosamines. As a result of Swedish men switching to snus in the 1970s, the rate of smoking among Swedish men decreased (Fig. 2.7).[35] Between 1980 and 2010, smoking rates in Sweden dropped from 36% to 12% among men and from 29% to 13% among women.[36,37] During those same years, the prevalence of snus use increased from 16% to 20% among men and from 1% to 4% among women,[36,37] which subsequently had an effect on the incidence of lung cancer and the trend in lung cancer–related mortality (Figs. 2.8 and 2.9).[38,39] Switching to a tobacco product that causes fewer deaths among men, particularly deaths from lung cancer, is a type of smoking cessation, but this change resulted from both educational awareness of tobacco-induced mortality and the marketing of a smokeless tobacco product manufactured according to GOTHIATEK standards, which allowed for a substantial change of the addictive habit from a combusted to a noncombusted nicotine-delivery product. Women in Sweden have been slower than men to switch to snus or to stop smoking.

The next movement in tobacco control was the push for smoke-free environments. The rationale for smoke-free environments was based on data demonstrating that exposure to secondhand smoke is also detrimental to health, with increased asthma attacks and more deaths from conditions related to

secondhand combusted tobacco or from lung cancer–related deaths among individuals exposed to secondhand smoke than individuals not exposed. The intention of these laws was built on the evidence that eliminating exposure to secondhand smoke would benefit the health of those who had been previously exposed. Although many localities established second-hand smoke laws, Ireland was the first country to implement a comprehensive ban on smoking in the workplace. Other regions restrict where smoking is allowed, specifying that smoking is not allowed in such locations as the workplace, public spaces, or outdoor venues (e.g., stadiums, parks, or beaches). These restrictions have had an impact on how much individuals smoke; as a result of smoke-free workplace policies, cigarette consumption has decreased in the United States, Germany, and Japan.[40–42] It is important to note, however, that the risk of lung cancer is more strongly related to the duration of smoking than to the number of cigarettes smoked per day.[43,44] Other tobacco-control policies as delineated by MPOWER also will decrease the number of people who smoke or use other tobacco products. Price controls (usually through increased taxes), restrictions prohibiting advertising and marketing, and measures designed to help people to quit are a few of the major policies that have been recommended. Different countries are in various stages of implementing these policies, and the strength and breadth of their implementation and enforcement will have an impact on the rates of smoking and, as a direct consequence, the rates of lung cancer.

Various grading systems have been developed to illustrate the relationship between the degree of tobacco-control implementation and lung cancer. A tobacco-control scorecard was proposed by Levy et al.[45] in 2004 to assess the success of implemented policies. Joossens and Raw,[46] in a report prepared for the Association of European Cancer Leagues, described the use of The Tobacco Control Scale to examine policies across countries in the European Union. Interestingly, the United Kingdom and Ireland were considered to have the best tobacco-control policies among the participating countries in the European Union, whereas Sweden was ranked ninth, despite having the lowest rates of male individuals who smoke and the lowest rates of lung cancer for men among developed countries. Thus the correlation between tobacco-control policies and smoking prevalence is not yet tight.

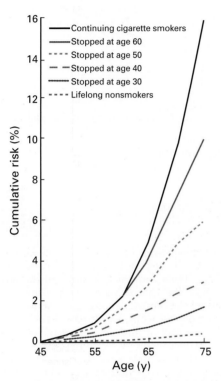

Fig. 2.6. Cumulative risk of smoking cessation at different ages in the United Kingdom. *(Reprinted with permission from Peto R, Darby S, Deo H, Silcocks P, Whitley E, Doll R. Smoking, smoking cessation and lung cancer in the UK since 1950: combination of national statistics with two case-control studies. BMJ. 2000;321(7257):323–329.)*

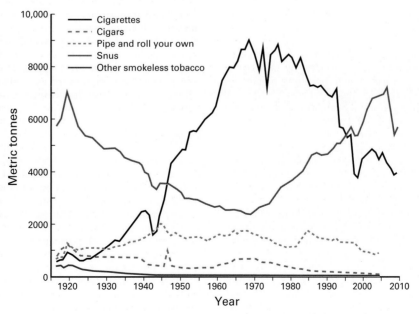

Fig. 2.7. Changes in Swedish smoking and snus use over time.

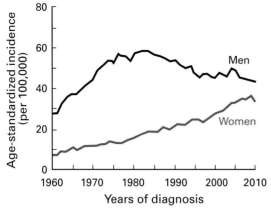

Fig. 2.8. Age-standardized incidence of lung cancer in Sweden. *(Reprinted with permission from Cancer Incidence in Sweden. http://www.socialstyrelsen.se/Lists/Artikelkatalog/Attachments/ 18530/2011-12-15.pdf. 2010.)*

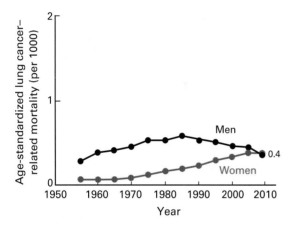

Fig. 2.9. Age-standardized rate of lung cancer–related deaths among individuals aged between 35 years and 69 years in Sweden. *(Reprinted with permission from Peto R, Lopez AD, Boreham J, et al. Mortality from smoking in developed countries 1950–2005. [The additional appendix to this article (and www.ctsu.ox.ac.uk) updates these 1990–2000 estimates to the years 2005–2009]. New York, NY: Oxford University Press; 1994.)*

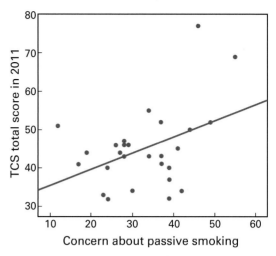

Fig. 2.10. Correlation between concern for health effects of secondhand smoke and stronger tobacco-control policies ($p = 0.006$). *TCS, Tobacco Control Scale. (Reprinted with permission from Willemsen MD, Kiselinova N. Concern about passive smoking and tobacco control policies in European countries: an ecological study. BMC Public Health. 2012;12:876.)*

More recently, denormalization of tobacco use has been considered as a potential powerful driver for decreasing tobacco use (smoking or using smokeless tobacco) and increasing support for tobacco-control policies. Willemsen and Kiselinova[47] compared the European Union Tobacco Control Scale with each country's smoking rates, and the only significant finding was the correlation between concern for the health effects of secondhand smoke and stronger tobacco-control policies (Fig. 2.10). In turn, there was an association between strong tobacco-control policies and lower smoking rates, although the association was not significant. The achievement of significance was based entirely on the data from the United Kingdom and Ireland. Both of those countries have strong tobacco-control polices and lower smoking rates. As noted earlier, the decline in smoking in the United Kingdom, particularly among male individuals, started as a result of the epidemiologic studies from the 1950s, and Ireland was the first country to institute a strong secondhand smoking law (in 2004) that had strong societal support. Willemsen and Kiselinova[47] suggested that denormalization of tobacco use in a society is a result of education and internalization of the harms of secondhand smoke and leads to stronger tobacco-control policies and, probably, to lower smoking rates.

To address the question of whether tobacco-control policies, which do decrease tobacco use, also will decrease the incidence of lung cancer, Thun and Jemal[48] estimated that decreases in smoking rates in the United States resulted in 146,000 fewer lung cancer–related deaths among men between 1991 and 2003. Building on that study, six universities developed models to address the impact of tobacco-control policies on smoking rates and lung cancer mortality.[49] In the development of these models, the authors considered what would have happened if there had been no tobacco-control efforts and the smoking rates of the 1950s had persisted. Next, they considered the impact of the changes resulting from tobacco-control efforts and the actual decreases in smoking rates in the United States. Lastly, they considered what the lung cancer mortality rates would have been if there had been so-called complete tobacco control; that is, all smoking stopped abruptly as of the 1965 Surgeon General Report. The findings are striking (Fig. 2.11). The results of this modeling suggested that 795,851 deaths were prevented between 1975 and 2000 (552,574 in men and 243,277 in women) as a result of actual tobacco-control efforts. Although the number of deaths prevented alone is remarkable, the total number of preventable deaths with optimal tobacco control is three-fold greater. If complete tobacco control had been achieved, 2,504,402 deaths from lung cancer could have been prevented between 1975 and 2000.

CONCLUSION

Various tobacco-control strategies have been used with various degrees of success across populations. The WHO FCTC outlines an international collaborative front to this globally spreading epidemic. Although societies around the globe differ widely in language, cultural norms, economic resources, and smoking rates, nearly all societies are afflicted with the tobacco epidemic, and a concerted effort using evidence-based strategies can alter the future course of this epidemic, with the potential to save millions of lives. One cannot truly consider the magnitude of the effect of good tobacco control (or even complete tobacco control) and its impact on global morbidity and mortality from lung cancer without questioning why we are not doing much, much more than we already are.

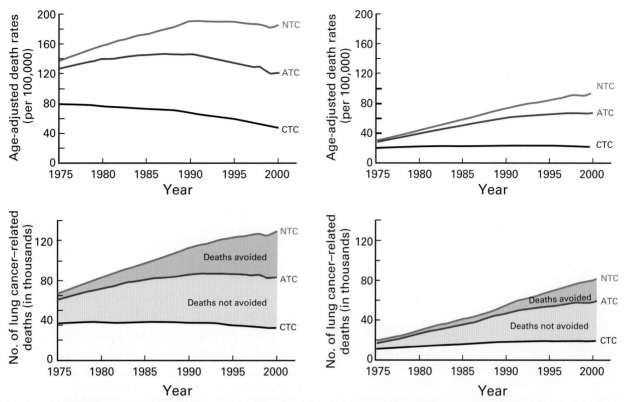

Fig. 2.11. Lung cancer–related deaths among men (left) and women (right) aged between 30 years and 84 years in the United States. *ATC,* actual tobacco control; *CTC,* complete tobacco control with no smoking after 1965; *NTC,* no tobacco control. *(Reprinted with permission from Moolgavkar SH, Holford TR, Levy DT, et al. Impact of reduced tobacco smoking on lung cancer mortality in the United States during 1975–2000.* J Natl Cancer Inst. *2012;104(7):541–548.)*

KEY REFERENCES

3. Lopez AD, Collishaw NE, Piha T. A descriptive model of the cigarette epidemic in developed countries. *Tob Control.* 1994;3(3): 242–247.
5. World Health Organization. Tobacco Free Initiative: tobacco facts. http://www.who.int/tobacco/mpower/tobacco_facts/en/index.html.
8. Roemer R, Taylor A, Lariviere J. Origins of the WHO Framework Convention on Tobacco Control. *Am J Public Health.* 2005;95(6): 936–938.
10. Mackay D, Haw S, Ayres JG, Fischbacher C, Pell JP. Smoke-free legislation and hospitalizations for childhood asthma. *N Engl J Med.* 2010;363(12):1139–1145.
12. Warren GW, Marshall JR, Cummings KM, et al. Practice patterns and perceptions of thoracic oncology providers on tobacco use and cessation in cancer patients. *J Thorac Oncol.* 2013;8(5):543–548.
16. Hammond D, Fong GT, McNeill A, Borland R, Cummings KM. Effectiveness of cigarette warning labels in informing smokers about the risks of smoking: findings from the International Tobacco Control (ITC) Four Country Survey. *Tob Control.* 2006;15(suppl 3):iii19–iii25.
17. Borland R, Wilson N, Fong GT, et al. Impact of graphic and text warnings on cigarette packs: findings from four countries over five years. *Tob Control.* 2009;18(5):358–364.
26. Barnoya J, Glantz S. Association of the California Tobacco Control Program with declines in lung cancer incidence. *Cancer Causes Control.* 2004;15(7):689–695.

28. Wakefield MA, Hayes L, Durkin S, Borland R. Introduction effects of the Australian plain packaging policy on adult smokers: a cross-sectional study. *BMJ Open.* 2013;(7):3.
29. Thun M, Peto R, Boreham J, Lopez AD. Stages of the cigarette epidemic on entering its second century. *Tob Control.* 2012;21(2): 96–101.
32. Doll R, Peto R, Boreham J, Sutherland I. Mortality in relation to smoking: 50 years' observations on male British doctors. *BMJ.* 2004;328(7455):1519.
34. Peto R, Darby S, Deo H, Silcocks P, Whitley E, Doll R. Smoking, smoking cessation and lung cancer in the UK since 1950: combination of national statistics with two case-control studies. *BMJ.* 2000;321(7257):323–329.
44. Peto R. Influence of dose and duration of smoking on lung cancer rates. *IARC Sci Publ.* 1986;74:23–33.
48. Thun MJ, Jemal A. How much of the decrease in cancer death rates in the United States is attributable to reductions in tobacco smoking? *Tob Control.* 2006;15(5):345–347.
49. Moolgavkar SH, Holford TR, Levy DT, et al. Impact of reduced tobacco smoking on lung cancer mortality in the United States during 1975–2000. *J Natl Cancer Inst.* 2012;104(7):541–548.

See Expertconsult.com for full list of references.

3

Assessing and Treating Tobacco Use in Lung Cancer Care

Jamie S. Ostroff and Elyse R. Park

SUMMARY OF KEY POINTS

- Addressing tobacco dependence in patients with cancer increases the quality of care by reducing their risk for treatment complications, improving their prognosis, and reducing the risk of disease recurrence and second primary cancers.
- Smoking cessation after a diagnosis of lung cancer has been shown to have a beneficial effect on performance status.
- Many patients with cancer who smoke want to quit but unfortunately do not receive support and evidence-based tobacco treatment.
- Further provider training and research are needed to determine strategies to implement best practices for treating tobacco dependence among patients with cancer.
- In the absence of tobacco cessation interventions, lung cancer specialists are encouraged to follow general clinical practice guidelines for treating tobacco use and dependence.
- Lung cancer screening provides an invaluable opportunity to promote tobacco cessation.
- There is much debate and little data as to whether e-cigarettes or other electronic nicotine delivery devices will facilitate or impede smoking cessation.

In 1964, the landmark US Surgeon General's report, Smoking and Health, first linked smoking to lung cancer. This irrefutable knowledge about the harms of tobacco spawned five decades of tobacco prevention and control research and policy, resulting in a rich compendium of comprehensive national and international evidence-based, population-based, and clinical practice guidelines aimed at reducing tobacco-related morbidity and mortality.[1–3] Smoking not only has a causal link with disease and death but also has adverse effects on outcomes for patients with a wide range of chronic diseases, including cancer.[4] Now more than ever, tobacco cessation is firmly within the purview of modern oncology. By highlighting the specific adverse effects of persistent tobacco use on cancer outcomes, this chapter provides justification for why lung cancer specialists should assess and treat tobacco use and direction for how lung cancer specialists can help their patients stop smoking.

WHY LUNG CANCER SPECIALISTS SHOULD HELP THEIR PATIENTS STOP TOBACCO USE

Cigarette smoking is the primary risk factor responsible for 87% and 70% of lung cancer deaths in men and women, respectively,[5] making tobacco prevention and cessation essential goals for lung cancer prevention and control. Despite five decades of national and international public health accomplishments in reducing the morbidity, mortality, and economic costs of tobacco-induced diseases, there are currently an estimated 42.1 million current smokers (18.1% of all adults) in the United States alone and at least one billion smokers worldwide.[6,7] Tobacco kills nearly six million people each year; more than five million of those deaths are the result of direct tobacco use, and more than 600,000 are the result of nonsmokers being exposed to secondhand smoke. Unless urgent action is taken, the annual death toll could rise to more than eight million by 2030.[8]

Risks of Persistent Smoking and Benefits of Cessation on Lung Cancer Outcomes

Health-care providers who treat patients with cancer may assume that it is too late after diagnosis to intervene about smoking. However, an emerging body of evidence demonstrates that smoking is associated with several adverse outcomes for patients with cancer, such as increased complications from surgery, increased treatment-related toxicity, decreased treatment effectiveness, poorer quality of life, increased risk of recurrence, increased risk of second primary tumors, increased noncancer-related comorbidity and mortality, and decreased survival.[9–11] Although the number of clinical studies on the effects of smoking cessation in patients with cancer is limited, the existing data suggest that many of the adverse effects of smoking can be reduced with cessation.[12]

Although these adverse outcomes are applicable to patients diagnosed with a wide range of cancers, much of this research has focused on identifying the adverse effects of smoking for patients diagnosed with lung cancer.[12,13] Continued smoking after the diagnosis of lung cancer has been associated with treatment delays and increased complications from surgery, radiotherapy, and chemotherapy.[14] Adverse effects from continued smoking at the time of surgery include complications from general anesthesia, increased risk of severe pulmonary complications, and detrimental effects on wound healing. Complications from smoking while receiving radiotherapy include reduced treatment efficacy and increased toxicity and side effects. Smoking while receiving chemotherapy alters the metabolism of many chemotherapy drugs, decreases the effectiveness of treatment, and increases drug toxicity.[15–20] Smoking cessation before lung cancer treatment reduces the risk of recurrence and the development of additional smoking-related cancers.[21,22] Although further research is needed to examine the beneficial effects of smoking cessation in patients with cancer, smoking cessation after a diagnosis of lung cancer has been shown to have a beneficial effect on quality of life and performance status.[23,24]

Prevalence of Persistent Smoking Among Patients With Lung Cancer

Despite these risks, at least 15.1% of all adult cancer survivors report current cigarette smoking.[25] Patients with lung cancer tend to be motivated to quit smoking at higher rates than patients diagnosed with other cancers.[26,27] Focusing exclusively on the prevalence of smoking in lung cancer, 90.2% of patients with lung cancer report ever-smoking. At the time of diagnosis, 38.7%

of patients with lung cancer report current smoking, whereas 5 months after diagnosis, at least 14.2% of patients with lung cancer report current smoking.[28] Despite heavy encouragement to quit smoking and strong intentions to quit, continued tobacco use after diagnosis and resumption of smoking after initial quit attempt remains a problem in this patient population, with an estimated 10% to 20% of all patients with lung cancer smoking at some point after diagnosis.[28–32]

FACTORS ASSOCIATED WITH PERSISTENT SMOKING AMONG PATIENTS WITH LUNG CANCER

Physicians who treat patients with cancer, especially lung cancer specialists, may not understand why some patients continue to smoke. A few studies have examined factors associated with persistent smoking and smoking relapse after quit attempts.[33–35] For patients with lung or head and neck cancer who were smoking within the week before surgery, smoking relapse in the following year was predicted by lower baseline quitting self-efficacy, higher tendency for depression, and greater fears about cancer recurrence; whereas among patients who had stopped smoking before surgery, higher perceived difficulty quitting and lower cancer-related risk perceptions predicted smoking relapse.[33] In another longitudinal study of patients with early-stage lung cancer, low household income, exposure to environmental tobacco smoke at home, and evidence of depression were positively associated with return to smoking.[34] In a particularly noteworthy study, Park et al.[28] also examined factors associated with continued smoking among patients with lung cancer enrolled in the national, population-based Cancer Care Outcomes Research and Surveillance (CanCORS) cohort; at 4 months after diagnosis, younger age, more advanced disease, history of cardiovascular disease, lower social support, poorer perceived health, higher fatalism, greater pain, and depression were all identified as significant factors associated with continued smoking ($p < 0.05$).

ASSESSING TOBACCO USE AND INTEGRATING EVIDENCE-BASED TOBACCO TREATMENT IS AN INDICATOR OF HIGH-QUALITY ONCOLOGY CARE

Addressing tobacco dependence in patients with cancer increases the quality of care by reducing their risk for treatment complications, improving their prognosis, and reducing the risk of disease recurrence and second primary cancers. Clinicians have a responsibility to their patients to provide them with the best quality of care possible, and this care should include cessation treatment for those patients who smoke.[36,37] Growing awareness of the cancer-specific health risks, the emerging lines of evidence that quitting smoking may improve the prognosis for patients with cancer, and the prevalence of persistent smoking provide a strong argument for providing evidence-based treatment of tobacco dependence as a standard of quality care in cancer settings.[35,38,39] In fact, there is a growing consensus among oncology leadership organizations that assessment of tobacco use and treatment should be a metric for quality of care.[40–43] As such, oncologists are encouraged to assess smoking status and advise cessation for patients who smoke.[10,44,45] In keeping with this quality-of-care perspective, the American Society of Clinical Oncology's Quality Oncology Practice Initiative (ASCO QOPI) includes documentation of current smoking status and counseling for all smokers, by the second office visit, as a core quality indicator.[42,46,47] In recognition of the few number of clinical trials that assess tobacco use, a National Cancer Institute-American Association for Cancer Research (NCI-AACR) Task Force on Tobacco Use and Assessment has recommended assessment of tobacco use in cancer clinical trials.[48]

DELIVERY OF EVIDENCE-BASED TOBACCO DEPENDENCE TREATMENT IN CANCER SETTINGS IS CURRENTLY SUBOPTIMAL

Many patients with cancer who smoke want to quit but do not receive support and evidence-based tobacco treatment. During cancer treatment, many smokers are not even advised to quit, and after cancer treatment is completed, tobacco use is often not addressed.[49,50] In a recent survey of ASCO members, the ASCO Tobacco Subcommittee found that oncologists provide quitting advice to 25% of their patients.[51] In addition, most cancer care settings have not yet established tobacco cessation treatment as standard care; a 2012 survey found that 97% of NCI-designated comprehensive cancer centers in the United States said that having a tobacco treatment program was "very important," but only half had any type of tobacco treatment program.[52]

Most germane to determining the current status of assessing and treating tobacco dependence among patients with lung cancer are the findings of an online survey of International Association for the Study of Lung Cancer (IASLC) members, which addressed the practices, perceptions, and barriers to tobacco assessment and cessation in patients with thoracic cancer.[53] More than 90% of the 1507 physician respondents (representing 40.5% of all IASLC members) said that current smoking affects outcome and that cessation should be a standard part of clinical care. At the initial patient visit, 90% said they ask patients about tobacco use, 79% said they ask patients whether they will quit, and 81% said they advise patients to stop tobacco use, but only 40% said they discuss medication options, and 39% said they actively provide cessation assistance; fewer respondents said they address tobacco use at follow-up. Respondents identified pessimism regarding their ability to help patients stop using tobacco (58%) and concerns about patient resistance to treatment (67%) as the leading barriers. Only 33% said they felt adequately trained to provide cessation interventions.

These survey findings highlight the need to examine barriers to tobacco treatment delivery in cancer care. Barriers to addressing tobacco use include patient-related factors (shame, helplessness, addiction), physician-related barriers (lack of training and referral options, beliefs about patients' lack of interest or ability to quit), and system-level factors (inadequate identification of smokers, costs) that impede the delivery of effective tobacco programs.[54] In recognition of this problem, the NCI convened a conference to review the state of tobacco treatment at NCI-designated comprehensive cancer centers and formulate recommendations for improvement.[55] The survey findings underscore the considerable need for further provider training and research aimed at determining strategies to implement best practices for treating tobacco dependence among patients with cancer.

TREATMENT OF TOBACCO DEPENDENCE IN LUNG CANCER CARE

As summarized in a recent review, randomized controlled trials of pharmacologic and counseling interventions for cessation conducted with tobacco-dependent patients with cancer have generally not shown significant treatment effects, with 6-month point abstinence rates ranging from 14% to 30% among patients assigned to the intervention conditions.[56] Few randomized controlled trials have been conducted to test the effectiveness of cessation pharmacotherapy for patients with cancer who smoke. Schnoll et al.[57] conducted a placebo-controlled trial to evaluate the efficacy of bupropion and found benefit (reduced withdrawal symptoms and increased abstinence rates) only for the subset of patients with cancer who had symptoms of depression. In a pilot study, Park et al.[58] found significantly higher quit rates among patients with thoracic cancer who received varenicline and intensive counseling than among patients who received usual (unspecified) care (smoking abstinence at 3 months: 34.4% vs. 14.3%; $p = 0.18$). Ostroff et al.[27] examined the utility of adding a presurgical tapering regimen to nicotine-replacement therapy and cessation counseling by telephone and found a 32% rate of smoking abstinence at 6-month follow-up for both interventions. In terms of optimal timing for the delivery of tobacco treatment, it appears that the closer to the time of diagnosis that smoking cessation treatment is delivered, the higher the likelihood for continued smoking abstinence.[59,60] These findings illustrate the need for continued development and evaluation of novel smoking cessation interventions that are acceptable and efficacious for patients with cancer and are feasible to deliver across a wide range of cancer care settings. In the absence of tobacco cessation interventions tailored and targeted to patients with cancer, lung cancer specialists are encouraged to follow general clinical practice guidelines for treating tobacco use and dependence.[61]

Guidelines for Treating Tobacco Use

Most recently updated in 2008, the US Public Health Service Treating Tobacco Use and Dependence Clinical Practice Guideline (PHS guideline) recommends that evidence-based tobacco treatment be delivered to all smokers in health-care settings.[3] Specifically, these guidelines recommend that a combination of medication and counseling be used, that counseling involve multiple sessions, and that clinicians use the five As: ask, assess, advise, assist, and arrange. Clinicians, especially thoracic cancer specialists, are encouraged to ask all their patients about their smoking status at every encounter. Once current smokers are identified, clinicians should assess their readiness to quit in order to determine what forms of assistance are needed. Smokers' quitting readiness is commonly classified as either precontemplation (no immediate plans to quit), contemplation (plan to quit within 6 months), preparation (planning to quit within a month), action (quitting for less than 6 months), or maintenance (staying quit for at least 6 months). Clinicians should strongly advise their patients against smoking, providing a personalized risk of persistent smoking and benefits of cessation in relation to the patient's disease and treatment. The next A, assist, speaks to the active role the clinician should play in his or her patients' cessation efforts by providing education, addressing barriers to quitting (such as concerns about coping), suggesting behavioral strategies that may help them overcome these barriers, developing a quit plan, and prescribing pharmacotherapy, as needed. For patients who are reluctant to quit, clinicians need to provide motivational counseling in an effort to encourage them to at least reduce their daily cigarette consumption. Considering the high rate of smoking relapse, patients who have recently quit (maintenance phase) should be reassessed for smoking lapses and given prolonged support and encouragement to remain abstinent from smoking. Lastly, clinicians are encouraged to arrange follow-up support, such as reevaluation of the smoking status during subsequent visits or referrals to other resources, such as quit-lines or onsite tobacco treatment specialists.

Pharmacotherapy

The PHS guideline strongly recommends that pharmacotherapy be used along with counseling in order to optimize cessation outcomes. Several medications are safe and effective for smoking cessation: nicotine-replacement therapies (in the form of a patch, gum, lozenge, nasal spray, or inhaler), bupropion, and varenicline (Table 3.1).

Because they are well-tolerated and acceptable to most patients, nicotine-replacement therapies should be recommended to all smokers except for patients in whom these treatments are contraindicated. Bupropion is an antidepressant that reduces withdrawal symptoms and, although it is not limited to patients

with cancer, it may be especially useful in such patients who have depression. Varenicline is a partial nicotinic agonist that reduces the urge to smoke by binding to the nicotine receptors in the brain. Neuropsychiatric adverse events (e.g., depression, agitation, suicidal ideation) are rare, but patients should be monitored closely for this and other adverse effects.

It has been shown that combination pharmacotherapy may be more effective than single-agent treatment for tobacco dependence. Nicotine-replacement therapies may be combined, with a long-acting treatment such as the patch, used to maintain a steady level of nicotine and thus decrease cravings and withdrawal symptoms throughout the day, and a short-acting treatment, such as a lozenge, gum, or inhaler, used as needed. In comparison to monotherapy, the use of combination nicotine-replacement therapies increases the likelihood of achieving long-term smoking abstinence.[3] Nicotine-replacement therapies may also be used in conjunction with sustained-release bupropion.

After completion of cancer treatment, resumption of smoking is common and therefore it is essential for clinicians to reassess smoking status during follow-up visits and provide motivational counseling to help patients remain abstinent. For patients who decline pharmacotherapy support or in whom cessation drugs are contraindicated, counseling should still be included as part of treatment.

SPECIAL CONSIDERATIONS IN TREATING TOBACCO DEPENDENCE IN PATIENTS WITH CANCER

Considering the negative effects of smoking for patients with cancer,[62] oncologists should include cessation as part of treatment planning and address barriers to quitting. Because most patients will have made prior quit attempts, clinicians must provide empathy and support for their patients' quitting efforts. Some unique barriers that may exist for patients are ambivalent motivation, self-blame and internalized stigma, nihilism ("why bother?"), psychologic distress, and living with other smokers. Encouraging patients to seek psychosocial support services acknowledges the need for assistance in developing alternative strategies for coping with the stress of cancer and its treatment. Little progress has been made to integrate these guidelines into cancer care settings and there is a paucity of data on how best to promote cessation among patients with cancer.

FUTURE DIRECTIONS

Two emerging hot topics relevant to tobacco treatment and lung cancer warrant further attention from lung cancer specialists: lung cancer screening and e-cigarettes.

Lung cancer screening provides an invaluable opportunity to promote tobacco cessation. The findings from the National Lung Cancer Screening Trial and the release of the US Preventive Services Task Force recommendations for annual low-dose computed tomography screening for lung cancer for adults aged 55 to 80 years old who are at high risk for lung cancer because of their age and smoking history provide a compelling opportunity for the delivery of smoking cessation treatment.[63,64] Because lung cancer screening programs are being developed for people with a longstanding history of heavy tobacco use, these programs provide an exciting vehicle for integrating smoking cessation efforts into lung cancer screening protocols. Several studies have reported cessation rates ranging from 6.6% to 42% following enrollment in lung cancer screening programs.[65–73] The authors of a 2012 review describe these studies as collectively providing much promise for lung cancer screening as a so-called teachable moment for reaching smokers and promoting cessation through the delivery of evidence-based tobacco cessation treatment.[74] Although smokers seeking lung cancer screening appear motivated to quit,[71] the use of evidence-based smoking cessation

TABLE 3.1 Pharmacotherapy for Smoking Cessation

Pharmacotherapy	Dosage	Duration (wks.)	Availability	Precautions/ Contraindications	Adverse Effects	Patient Education
Nicotine patch	If smoking ≥11 cigarettes/d: 21 mg/24 h 14 mg/24 h 7 mg/24 h If smoking ≤10 cigarettes/d: 14 mg/24 h 7 mg/24 h	6 2 2 6 2	Over the counter	Uncontrolled hypertension	Skin irritation (redness, swelling, itchiness) Sleep disruptions (nightmares, vivid dreams)	Rotate patch site daily Remove patch before bedtime if sleep is disrupted and bothersome
Nicotine polacrilex gum	If smoking ≤24 cigarettes/d: 2 mg If smoking ≥25 cigarettes/d: 4 mg	Up to 12	Over the counter	Poor dentition Xerostomia	Hiccups Upset stomach Jaw ache	Chew gum on a fixed schedule Chew each piece of gum and then place between the gums and cheek for 30 min (so-called chew and park) Avoid eating or drinking anything except water 15 min before chewing and during chewing Do not exceed 24 pieces of gum in 24 hours
Nicotine lozenge	If smoking first cigarette more than 30 min after waking up: 2 mg If smoking first cigarette within 30 min after waking up: 4 mg	Up to 12	Over the counter	Xerostomia	Local irritation to mouth and throat Upset stomach	Avoid eating or drinking anything except water 15 min before and during use of a lozenge The lozenge will take 20–30 min to dissolve Do not use more than 20 lozenges in 24 h
Nicotine inhalation system	6–16 cartridges/d	Up to 26	Prescription		Local irritation to mouth and throat Upset stomach	Each cartridge will take 80–100 inhalations over 20 min Puff on inhaler like a cigar
Nicotine nasal spray	0.5 mg/inhalation/ nostril 1–2 times/h (or as needed)	Up to 12	Prescription	Sinus infections	Irritation to nose, eye, or upper respiratory system	Nasal irritation may become less bothersome with continued use
Bupropion	Days 1–3: 150 mg daily Thereafter: 150 mg twice daily	12	Prescription	History of seizures History of eating disorders (bulimia, anorexia)	Insomnia Xerostomia Restlessness Dizziness	Overlap with smoking for 1–2 weeks Do not need to be tapered off drug
Varenicline	Days 1–3: 0.5 mg daily Days 4–7: 0.5 mg twice daily Day 8–end of treatment: 1 mg twice daily	12[a]	Prescription	Kidney problems or treatment with dialysis Pregnancy or plan to become pregnant Breastfeeding	Mild nausea Sleep problems Headaches	Take medication with a full glass of water after eating a meal Allow 8 h between each dose Take medication a few hours before bedtime to avoid restlessness

[a]If the patient has quit smoking, treatment for another 12 weeks may be given to prevent smoking relapse.

treatments among screening enrollees is low, and the rate of persistent smoking is high 1 year after enrollment. All smokers seeking lung cancer screening should be advised to quit and provided with access to evidence-based cessation treatments.[75] Further research examining the development and evaluation of tobacco treatment interventions for smokers seeking lung cancer screening is needed.

Identified as a so-called disruptive technology in the field of tobacco control,[76] e-cigarettes are battery-powered devices that mimic the hand-to-mouth sensory experience of smoking and typically deliver nicotine to the user. Cigarette smokers report using e-cigarettes to manage nicotine cravings and withdrawal symptoms, to reduce daily smoking consumption, and to quit smoking or avoid smoking relapse.[77] Given the increasing popularity and availability of e-cigarettes in the general population and the strong advice to quit smoking traditional cigarettes at the time of diagnosis, patients with cancer are likely to consider use of e-cigarettes.

There is much debate and little data as to whether e-cigarettes will facilitate or impede smoking cessation and reduction of known hazards of traditional cigarettes and other combustible tobacco products.[66] One recent observational study found no evidence that the use of e-cigarettes promoted smoking cessation among patients with cancer who were referred to a hospital-based smoking cessation program.[78] On the other hand, promising results were reported in two clinical trials conducted among smokers from the general population. Cessation outcomes were comparable with those observed in trials of nicotine replacement therapies.[79,80] Until more is known about the risks and benefits of e-cigarettes for patients with cancer, oncologists are likely to struggle with these complexities and face challenges in how to respond to patient inquiries. In 2014, the IASLC Tobacco Control and Smoking Cessation Committee published a commentary providing guidance to oncologists about what to recommend to their patients who may be struggling to stop smoking or wondering about e-cigarettes.[81] According to this guidance, oncologists should advise smokers to quit smoking traditional cigarettes, encourage the use of FDA-approved cessation medications, refer patients for tobacco-cessation counseling, and provide education about the potential risks and lack of known benefits of e-cigarette use with regard to long-term cessation. These recommendations are quite similar to those made by an AACR-ASCO Task Force on electronic cigarettes and other electronic nicotine delivery systems.[82]

CONCLUSION

There is a strong rationale for assessing tobacco use and promoting smoking cessation among patients with cancer. The risks of persistent smoking for patients diagnosed with lung cancer are well established and include adverse outcomes such as treatment toxicities, cancer recurrence, second primary malignant tumors, decreased survival, and poorer quality of life. Given the cancer-specific health risks and the availability of clinical practice guidelines for treating tobacco dependence, oncologists are encouraged to assess smoking status and advise cessation for patients who smoke. Further research examining patient-, provider-, and system-related strategies for engagement and retention of smokers into evidence-based tobacco treatment is needed.

KEY REFERENCES

4. U.S. Department of Health and Human Services. *The Health Consequences of Smoking—50 Years of Progress: a Report of the Surgeon General*. Atlanta, GA: U.S. Department of Health and Human Services, Centers for Disease Control and Prevention, National Center for Chronic Disease Prevention and Health Promotion. Office on Smoking and Health; 2014.
5. Centers for Disease Control and Prevention (CDC). Smoking-attributable mortality, years of potential life lost, and productivity losses—United States, 2000–2004. *MMWR Morb Mortal Wkly Rep*. 2008;57(45):1226–1228.
10. Toll BA, Brandon TH, Gritz ER, Warren GW, Herbst RS. Assessing tobacco use by cancer patients and facilitating cessation: an American Association for Cancer Research policy statement. *Clin Cancer Res*. 2013;19(8):1941–1948.
11. Ferketich AK, Niland JC, Mamet R, et al. Smoking status and survival in the national comprehensive cancer network non-small cell lung cancer cohort. *Cancer*. 2013;119(4):847–853.
16. McBride CM, Ostroff JS. Teachable moments for promoting smoking cessation: the context of cancer care and survivorship. *Cancer Control*. 2003;10(4):325–333.
23. Baser S, Shannon VR, Eapen GA, et al. Smoking cessation after diagnosis of lung cancer is associated with a beneficial effect on performance status. *Chest*. 2006;130(6):1784–1790.
27. Ostroff JS, Burkhalter JE, Cinciripini PM, et al. Randomized trial of a presurgical scheduled reduced smoking intervention for patients newly diagnosed with cancer. *Health Psychol*. 2014;33(7):737–747.
38. National Comprehensive Cancer Network. NCCN practice guidelines in oncology–v.1.2007: genetic/familial high-risk assessment: breast and ovarian. http://www.nccn.org/professionals/physician_gls/default.asp; 2007.
44. Hanna N, Mulshine J, Wollins DS, Tyne C, Dresler C. Tobacco cessation and control a decade later: American Society of Clinical Oncology policy statement update. *J Clin Oncol*. 2013;31(25):3147–3157.
59. Schnoll RA, Zhang B, Rue M, et al. Brief physician-initiated quit-smoking strategies for clinical oncology settings: a trial coordinated by the Eastern Cooperative Oncology Group. *J Clin Oncol*. 2003;21(2):355–365.
63. Aberle DR, Adams AM, Berg CD, et al. Reduced lung-cancer mortality with low-dose computed tomographic screening. *N Engl J Med*. 2011;365(5):395–409.
79. Bullen C, Howe C, Laugesen M, et al. Electronic cigarettes for smoking cessation: a randomised controlled trial. *Lancet*. 2013;382(9905):1629–1637.

See Expertconsult.com for full list of references.

4 Lung Cancer in Never-Smokers: A Different Disease

Adi F. Gazdar and Caicun Zhou

SUMMARY OF KEY POINTS

- The known or suspected etiologic factors for lung cancer arising in never-smokers are weak carcinogens or rare factors, which cannot explain the relatively high frequency of cancer in never-smokers. This also applies to environmental tobacco smoke.

- Genetic factors play an increasing role in the etiology of lung cancer in never-smokers. These include rare high penetrance mutations in crucial genes such as the T790M mutation in the *EGFR* gene. However, high-frequency, low-penetrance variations in susceptibility genes are playing an increasingly prominent role. These include loci that predispose to smoking as well as those that may contribute directly to cancers arising in smokers and never-smokers.

- The molecular alterations in lung cancers arising in smokers and never-smokers are very different. Smoke related tumors are associated with high numbers of mutations, especially C:G>A:T transversions, while never-smoker tumors are associated with low numbers of mutations targeting C:G>T:A transitions.

- The specific mutational targets are also different in smoker and never-smoker tumors. Thus *KRAS* mutations are more frequent in ever-smoker tumors, while *EGFR* mutations and *ALK* translocations are more frequent in never-smokers. Paradoxically, the number of therapeutic actionable mutations is more frequent in never-smoker tumors.

- Lung cancers arising in never-smokers show major differences based on ethnicity, gender, and histology. The ethnic differences point out the importance of genetic susceptibility loci in the development of lung cancers.

- The major clinical, ethnic, gender, and histology differences between lung cancers arising from smokers and never-smokers, coupled with their different etiologic factors and major molecular differences, indicate that they represent very different tumor types, confirming that lung cancers in never-smokers represent a different form of cancer.

Lung cancer is the leading cause of cancer-related mortality worldwide, with about 1.4 million deaths each year.[1] In 2008, lung cancer was the most commonly diagnosed cancer globally, the leading cause of cancer-related death in men, and the fourth most commonly diagnosed cancer and second leading cause of cancer-related death in women.[1] The lung cancer incidence rate for men in East Asia ranks as the fifth highest in the world, after Eastern and Southern Europe, North America, Micronesia, and Polynesia, with an age-standardized incidence rate by gender and area of the world of 45.0 per 100,000 cases.[1] For women, the third highest lung cancer incidence rate is found in East Asia, Australia, and New Zealand, with 19.9 per 100,000 cases.[1] Interestingly, the lung cancer incidence rate for women is higher in China (21.3 cases per 100,000 women) than in Germany (16.4) and Italy (11.4), although adult smoking prevalence is substantially lower in China (4% vs. 20%).[2]

The World Health Organization estimates that lung cancer is the cause of 1.37 million deaths globally per year, or 18% of all cancer deaths.[1] An estimated 71% of lung cancers are caused by smoking, indicating that about 400,000 deaths each year are caused by lung cancer in lifetime never-smokers.[1] It has been estimated that 15% of men and 53% of women with lung cancer worldwide are never-smokers.[3] Thus, lung cancer in never-smokers is among the seven or eight most common causes of cancer death. However, lung cancer in never-smokers is often grouped together with lung cancer in ever-smokers. In this chapter, we describe the clinical-pathologic and molecular differences between these two types of lung cancer. Although several review articles have addressed this topic,[4–6] this chapter focuses on lung cancer in never-smokers in East Asian countries, where the incidence rate is higher than in other geographic regions. In addition, we discuss molecular differences between lung cancer in never-smokers and ever-smokers. For these purposes, we use standard definitions as follows:

KEY TERMS

Ever-smoker. An individual who has smoked 100 or more cigarettes during his or her lifetime.

Never-smoker. An individual who has smoked fewer than 100 cigarettes during his or her lifetime.

Current smoker. An individual who is currently smoking or who has quit smoking during the past 12 months.

Former smoker. An ever-smoker who quit more than 12 months earlier.

EPIDEMIOLOGY OF NONSMOKING-RELATED LUNG CANCER

Although numerous articles on lung cancer in never-smokers in Asia have been published, some data are inconsistent and other data are suspect, as the definitions of never-smokers are not uniform, and the quality of some of the data is questionable. Also, smoking incidence rates differ among women even within a single country. For example, the smoking incidence rates among women in northeastern China are considerably higher than the rates among women in southern China.[7] For these reasons, we extensively cite reviews or meta-analyses that combine data from multiple published reports and from cancer registries. By doing so, we can avoid some of the biases from small, individual studies, and we can place ethnic, gender, and geographic differences in their proper context. Findings from a case–control study on epidemiologic risk factors for lung cancer in never-smokers are described in a 2010 article by Brenner et al.[8]

A review of published studies on the epidemiology of lung cancer (18 studies, comprising 82,037 people) showed a marked gender bias that lung cancer among never-smokers appears to affect women more frequently than men, irrespective of geography ($p < 0.0001$).[5] The proportion of women with lung cancer who reported never having smoked regularly is particularly high in East Asia (61%)[9–14] and South Asia (83%),[15,16] whereas only

15% of women with lung cancer in the United States are never-smokers.[17-21] In contrast, only 11% of men with lung cancer in East Asia are never-smokers.[5]

Thun et al.[7] published an analysis of 13 cohorts and 22 cancer registry studies with data from nearly 2.5 million never-smokers and from cancer registries in 10 countries covering several decades. Some of the key findings from this comprehensive analysis regarding lung cancer in never-smokers include the following:

- death rates from lung cancer were higher among men than women across all age and racial groups
- incidence rates among men and women were similar, with some variation by age
- death rates were higher among East Asian individuals (but not among those living in the United States) and black Americans than among white Americans
- no temporal trends were seen for American women
- lung cancer incidence rates were higher and more variable among East Asian women.

KNOWN OR SUSPECTED ETIOLOGIC FACTORS FOR LUNG CANCER IN NEVER-SMOKERS

Because tobacco use is a powerful carcinogen and the major cause of lung cancer, most attention has focused on environmental tobacco exposure as the major cause of lung cancer in lifetime never-smokers. Although environmental tobacco exposure has been identified as a contributing factor for lung cancer in never-smokers since 1986, the Surgeon General of the United States 2006 report confirmed that environmental tobacco exposure modestly increased the risk of lung cancer.[22] However, the odds ratios for the development of lung cancer in the United States indicated that such exposure is a very weak carcinogen compared with active smoking, as cited in the Surgeon General's report.[22,23] According to that report, the odds ratio is 1.0 for never-smokers who do not have environmental tobacco exposure and 1.2 for never-smokers who do have such exposure; in contrast, the odds ratio is 40.4 for ever-smokers.[23] Thus, if environmental tobacco exposure is a weak carcinogen and cannot be the major cause of lung cancer in never-smokers, other known or suspected factors should be considered, such as indoor air pollution, environmental and occupational toxins (e.g., arsenic, radon, asbestos), and human papillomavirus (HPV) infection (and possibly other infections). Genetic factors should also be considered, and these are discussed later.

Indoor Air Pollution

The relatively high burden of lung cancer among women in China who have no history of regular smoking is attributed to indoor air pollution from coal smoke generated by unventilated coal-fueled stoves, volatilization of oils from cooking at high temperatures in open woks, and secondhand smoke.[7,24-29] A meta-analysis of seven studies from China and Taiwan of never-smokers found that cooking oil vapors are the risk factor associated with lung cancer for women, and indoor coal and wood burning is a risk factor for both women and men.[30] Indeed, a retrospective study on the association of household stove improvement and risk of lung cancer in rural China indicated that changing from unvented fire pits to stoves with chimneys was associated with a subsequent reduction in the lung cancer incidence rate.[31] Other factors thought to contribute to higher lung cancer incidence among rural Chinese women who are never-smokers include a higher prevalence of nonsmoking women in Asian countries and viral factors of HPV infection.[32]

Environmental and Occupational Toxins

Exposure to some environmental and occupational toxins has been shown to increase the risk of lung cancer for smokers and, to a lesser extent, for never-smokers.[11,29,33] These toxins include arsenic, radon, asbestos, chromium, organic dust, and others.[34-36]

As summarized in a meta-analysis,[34] several studies indicate that high levels of arsenic in the major source of drinking water of highly defined geographic regions (southwestern Taiwan, the Niigata Prefecture, Japan, and northern Chile) were associated with increased incidence of lung cancer, both for smokers and never-smokers. The authors of the meta-analysis concluded: "Despite methodologic limitations, the consistent observation of strong, statistically significant associations from different study designs carried out in different regions provide[s] support for a causal association between ingesting drinking water with high concentrations of arsenic and lung cancer."[34]

Present in soil and groundwater, radon is a gaseous decay product of uranium-238 and radium-226, which is capable of damaging respiratory epithelium by emitting alpha particles.[40,41] The increased risk of lung cancer among uranium miners has been more clearly established and is thought to be caused by radiation from radon,[42] although most miners are ever-smokers.[40] The role of radon in the home is more difficult to assess.

An analysis of occupational asbestos exposure in the Netherlands found a relative risk of lung cancer of 3.5 after controlling for age, smoking, and other factors.[37] In a French study of 1493 cases, some occupational exposure was identified in 9.4% and 48.6% of female and male never-smokers, respectively, in whom lung cancer developed.[38] In a Canadian case–control study, the odds ratio for lung cancer risk from occupational exposures in never-smokers was 2.1 (95% confidence interval [CI], 1.3–3.3) but was higher for exposure to solvents, paints, or thinners (odds ratio, 2.8; 95% CI, 1.6–5.0).[8] A meta-analysis that focused on lung cancer risk for painters demonstrated a relative risk of lung cancer for all painters of 1.35 (95% CI, 1.29–1.41), but 2.0 (95% CI, 10.9–3.67) among never-smokers.[39]

Human Papillomavirus

Several studies have found that HPV infection is associated with lung cancer, particularly in China and Taiwan. Cheng et al.[44] reported a high incidence of HPV infection among never-smoking women in Taiwan. Results of a case–control study (141 cases and 60 controls) in Taiwan showed that the prevalence of HPV16 and HPV18 infection was significantly higher among never-smoking women with lung cancer who were older than 60 years; HPV 16 and HPV 18 infection was thought to be associated with the high lung cancer incidence and death rates among never-smoking women in Taiwan.[44] Results of a similar study in Wuhan, China, indicated that no association with clinical-pathologic features was noted.[45] However, the role of HPV infection in lung cancer pathogenesis in never-smokers might be restricted to certain geographic areas because the incidence rate of lung cancer associated with HPV infection varies widely based on geographic location and is reported to be low in Australia, Europe, and North America.[46-48]

CLINICAL-PATHOLOGIC FEATURES OF LUNG CANCER IN NEVER-SMOKERS

Adenocarcinoma is the most common form of nonsmall cell lung cancer (NSCLC) in most parts of the world and the predominant form of lung cancer in never-smokers worldwide,[5] followed by large cell carcinoma, which may represent an undifferentiated form of adenocarcinoma. Squamous cell carcinoma is rare among never-smokers with lung cancer, and small cell lung cancer almost never occurs. However, another neuroendocrine tumor, the bronchial carcinoid, may be slightly more common among never-smokers, although no relationship to smoking status has been shown.[49]

The age at which lung cancer is diagnosed varies according to geographic location and smoking status. Studies from East Asian countries, such as Singapore and Japan, as well as Hong Kong, demonstrate an earlier age at the time of diagnosis among never-smokers compared with smokers,[9,12,33] whereas the same or older age at the time of diagnosis among never-smokers has been found in studies from the United States and Europe.[1,18,21,50–52] The possible reasons for this geographic variation include the greater contribution of risk factors other than active smoking in East Asian countries, much later age of initiation of smoking among East Asians with a smoking history compared with individuals from Western countries, and different degrees of detection bias between countries.[53]

A retrospective study in Singapore comparing differences in the epidemiologic characteristics and survival outcomes between never-smokers and former and current smokers showed that never-smoker status was associated with a significantly better performance status, younger age at the time of diagnosis (10 years and 5 years earlier, respectively), higher proportion of women (68.5% vs.12% to 13%), and more advanced stage at the time of diagnosis.[9] The variation in disease stage at the time of diagnosis might be explained by late presentation of symptoms and delayed diagnosis by physicians. The survival outcome for never-smokers was significantly better than that for smokers, with a 5-year overall survival rate of 10.8% and 7.7%, respectively ($p = 0.0003$).[9] Differences in treatment response and survival outcome between never-smokers and smokers with lung cancer may be attributed to differences in pathogenesis and tumor biology.

THE GENETICS OF LUNG CANCER

Inherited cancer syndromes are associated with rare and highly penetrant single-gene mutations, but genetic factors also play a role in sporadic cancers, as reported in numerous family-based studies. About 100 genes with mendelian inheritance cause an even smaller number of cancer syndromes, but these syndromes provide an explanation for only a minor part of the familial clustering of common cancers.[54] Linkage analyses of high-risk families may identify other rare high-penetrance genes, and such studies have identified a lung cancer susceptibility locus on chromosome 6q.[55] Smoking appeared to increase the susceptibility. Further studies indicated that the regulator of G-protein signaling 17 (RGS17) gene at this location was a major candidate for lung cancer susceptibility.[56]

The major mechanism of acquired resistance to tyrosine kinase inhibitors in lung cancers with epidermal growth factor receptor (EGFR) gene mutations is the appearance of a second activating mutation, T790M (substitution of threonine 790 with methionine).[57] However, T790M may be inherited as a rare familial mutation.[58] Our recently published study of a large family with an inherited T790M mutation and lung cancer, combined with analysis of published cases, indicates that inherited T790M predisposed lifetime never-smokers (and women) to lung cancer.[59] These findings have, in part, been independently confirmed.[60] Of interest, although EGFR mutations occur more frequently among East Asians, no case of an inherited T790M mutation has been described among East Asians. However, V843I, an even rarer inherited EGFR gene mutation that predisposes to lung cancer, has been reported in both Asian and non-Asian families.[61,62] Another recent report described a Japanese family with an autosomal inherited germline mutation in human epidermal growth factor receptor 2 (HER2) associated with lung cancer risk, which may also target women and light or never-smokers.[63]

It is now believed that alleles with high frequency (typically greater than 10%) and low penetrance (typically less than a twofold increased lifetime risk) contribute substantially to susceptibility to many diseases, including lung cancer. Genome-wide association studies (GWAS) using population-based designs have identified many genetic loci associated with risk of a range of complex diseases, including lung cancer;[54] however, each locus exerts a very small effect, and combinations of genes are required to exert a significant effect on risk. GWAS are often based on large microchip analyses of single nucleotide polymorphisms (SNPs), and more than one million SNPs can be analyzed on a single microchip. These studies of weak associations often consist of many thousands of cases and controls, and meta-analyses may be required for confirmation. In lung cancer, more than 150 GWAS have been published. Although some findings are widely accepted, others are controversial or require confirmation. In 2008, three studies identified three potential susceptibility loci for lung cancer.[64,65] Two of these loci, on chromosomes 15q25 and 5p15.33—the site of the telomerase reverse transcriptase (TERT) gene, essential for telomerase activation—have been confirmed, but the cancer-associated role of the locus on 6p21-6p22 remained more controversial; however, it may be histology related.[64] Additional studies, including a meta-analysis, confirmed that the major susceptibility locus was on 15q25, encoding several genes, including the nicotinic acetylcholine receptor (nAChR) genes: cholinergic receptor, nicotinic, beta 4 (neuronal) (CHRNB4), alpha 5 (neuronal) (CHRNA5), and alpha 3 (neuronal) (CHRNA3).[66] Because the variants at 15q25 are also associated with nicotine dependence, they may influence lung cancer risk at least in part through an effect on smoking behavior rather than a direct effect on lung carcinogenesis. A large meta-analysis of lung cancer in female never-smokers in six Asian countries showed no evidence of association for lung cancer at 15q25 in that population, which the authors said provided "strong evidence that this locus is not associated with lung cancer independent of smoking."[67] Other studies, including meta-analyses, have identified additional variants associated with increased risk, such as smoking, ethnicity, gender, and histology.[64,66–71] Thus, although genetic variation of the TERT locus appears to be involved in susceptibility to all lung cancers, the 15q25 locus predisposes to smoking, the cyclin-dependent kinase inhibitor 2A (CDKN2) locus at 9p21 may influence susceptibility to squamous cell carcinomas, and the tumor protein p63 (TP63) locus may influence susceptibility to lung adenocarcinoma in East Asian populations.

As confirmed by the GWAS cited previously, nicotine and its derivatives, by binding to nAChR on bronchial epithelial cells, can regulate cellular proliferation and apoptosis by activating the protein kinase B (PKB/Akt) pathway. Lam et al.[72] found different nAChR subunit gene expression patterns between NSCLCs from smokers and nonsmokers, and a 65-gene expression signature was associated with nonsmoking nAChR alpha-6 beta-3 expression.

MOLECULAR CHARACTERISTICS OF NONSMOKING EAST ASIAN INDIVIDUALS WITH LUNG CANCER

With the development of molecular genetic therapies for lung cancer, the molecular profile of East Asian individuals with lung cancer was found to differ from that of white individuals with lung cancer. Mutations in Kirsten rat sarcoma viral oncogene homolog (KRAS) and EGFR genes are mutually exclusive and demonstrate striking frequency differences related to ethnicity. EGFR mutation is the first specific molecular alteration associated with lung cancers arising among never-smokers. A relatively high incidence of somatic mutations in EGFR has been found in a specific subpopulation: women, never-smokers, patients with adenocarcinoma, and Asians. In the First Line Iressa versus Carboplatin/Paclitaxel in Asia (Iressa Pan-Asia Study [IPASS]) study, with 1214 (99.8%) of 1217 patients of East Asian origin and 1140 (93.7%) of 1217 never-smokers, the incidence rate of EGFR mutation was 59.7% in the 437 patients evaluable for EGFR mutation.[73] A recent multinational study demonstrated variations in the EGFR gene mutation rates in Asian countries, with the lowest frequencies from India.[74,75]

Nevertheless, a review of nine published studies showed that the frequency of *EGFR* mutation among US never-smokers with NSCLC was substantially lower (20%).[76] In addition, even in an unselected population, the frequency of *EGFR* mutation among East Asian individuals with NSCLC was also considerably higher than that for white individuals. In the review, which included an analysis of data on 2347 patients for whom ethnicity was noted, the frequency of *EGFR* mutations among East Asian patients was significantly higher compared with non-Asian patients (33% vs. 6%; *p* < 0.001).[77] Unlike *EGFR* mutations, *KRAS* mutations occur less commonly in lung cancers among individuals from East Asia and more frequently in lung cancers among smokers.[76]

In pooled data summarizing three published studies comprising 1536 patients with NSCLC, *EGFR* and *KRAS* were shown to be mutually exclusive in the same tumors.[76,78,79] *KRAS* mutations were detected in 20% of patients with NSCLC, particularly patients who smoked or who had adenocarcinoma.[77] A study investigating the *EGFR* and *KRAS* status of 519 unselected patients with NSCLC showed that *KRAS* mutations were present more frequently in smokers than never-smokers (10% vs. 4%; *p* = 0.01), among non–East Asians than East Asians (12% vs. 5%; *p* = 0.001), and among patients with adenocarcinoma than patients with nonadenocarcinoma histologies (12% vs. 2%; *p* < 0.001).[76] Several studies found that *KRAS* mutations were present in 20% to 30% of white patients with lung adenocarcinoma but only 5% of patients with lung adenocarcinoma from East Asia.[80–82] In addition, in previous studies from Hong Kong and Taiwan, *KRAS* mutations were found in 13% to 19% of men with adenocarcinoma but in none of the women studied.[83,84] A potential explanation for the distinction between genders may be that the vast majority of Chinese female patients were never-smokers.

A Japanese case–control study assessing the impact of smoking and gender on the risk of NSCLC with or without *EGFR* mutation demonstrated that ever-smoking was a substantial risk factor for NSCLC without *EGFR* mutation but not for NSCLC with *EGFR* mutation.[85] Cumulative exposure to smoking was associated with a linear increased risk of NSCLC without *EGFR* mutation only. This finding was consistent for both men and women. Age at the start of smoking among ever-smokers and years since quitting smoking among former smokers also showed a strong correlation between NSCLC without *EGFR* mutation and smoking. *EGFR* mutation was present more frequently among patients who smoked no more than 20 pack-years. Similarly, in another Japanese study, *EGFR* mutation was found more frequently among patients who quit smoking at least 20 years before the date of lung cancer diagnosis.[86] These findings suggest an inverse correlation between *EGFR* mutation and exposure dose of cigarette smoking.

Smoking status is a risk factor affecting not only *EGFR* mutations but other somatic mutations as well. The authors of a Korean study screened genetic tests for *EGFR* mutations, *KRAS* mutations, and enchinoderm-microtubule-associated protein-like 4-anaplastic lymphoma kinase (*EML4-ALK*) fusions in 200 fresh surgical specimens of primary lung adenocarcinoma by polymerase chain reaction (PCR), Sanger sequencing, and fluorescence in situ hybridization. They then performed high-throughput RNA sequencing in 87 lung adenocarcinoma specimens that were negative for the three known driver mutations (three samples with insufficient RNA quality were excluded). The results showed that people who had a smoking history of at least 40 pack-years harbored significantly more somatic point mutations than did people who had a smoking history of fewer than 40 pack-years or of never-smoking. In addition, important differences in mutation patterns exist between lung cancer in never-smokers and ever-smokers.[87]

Given the difference in the incidence rate of *EGFR* mutations between East Asian and white populations, several studies have investigated ethnic differences in *ALK*, c-ros oncogene 1 receptor tyrosine kinase (*ROS1*), and ret proto-oncogene (*RET*) fusions after these three novel driver fusions were identified in NSCLC. Most studies showed that *ALK* fusions occurred in 2.4% to 5.6% of NSCLC cases,[88–91] and no differences in incidence rate between Asian and non-Asian populations have been identified to date. However, a Chinese study screening *ALK* fusions by rapid amplification of complementary DNA ends (RACE)-coupled PCR sequencing found that *ALK* fusions existed in 12 (11.6%) of 103 individuals with NSCLC, 10 (16.13%) of 62 individuals with adenocarcinomas, and 10 (19.23%) of 52 never-smokers.[92] This high incidence of *ALK* fusions in a selected East Asian population may be explained by the relatively small sample size and use of a different screening method. Unlike ethnicity, smoking status is regarded as an important factor affecting the incidence rate of fusion genes. Similar to *ALK* fusions, *ROS1* and *RET* fusions appear to occur more frequently among never-smokers.[93,94] Given a very low frequency of *ROS1* as well as *RET* fusions identified in NSCLC, a large sample study is warranted to prove the role of smoking status in the occurrence of fusion genes.

Several Chinese studies have demonstrated the previously described differences in the molecular profile of lung cancer between never-smokers and smokers. An et al.[95] screened for candidate driver genes in 524 Chinese patients with NSCLC with the use of several methods, including sequencing, high-resolution melt analysis, quantitative PCR, or multiplex PCR and RACE, and analyzed the differences in driver gene alterations among a subgroup based on histology and smoking status (Table 4.1).[95] The findings demonstrated that the driver gene alterations in nonsmokers differ completely from driver gene alterations in smokers, irrespective of histologic type. In adenocarcinoma, *EGFR*, phosphatase and tensin homolog (*PTEN*), and phosphatidylinositol-4,5-bisphosphate 3-kinase, catalytic subunit alpha (*PIK3CA*) mutations and *ALK* fusions were present more frequently among never-smokers, whereas *KRAS* and serine/threonine kinase 11 (*STK11*) mutations were present more frequently among smokers. The met proto-oncogene methylated CpG (mCpG) sequences (*MET*) and v-raf murine sarcoma viral oncogene homolog B (*BRAF*) mutations did not differ substantially by smoking status. As expected, fewer squamous cell carcinomas were present, and discoidin domain receptor tyrosine

TABLE 4.1 Driver Mutations in Lung Cancers Among Chinese Never-Smokers and Ever-Smokers Adjusted for Histologic Type and Smoking Status[95]

ADENOCARCINOMA (*n* = 347)		
Gene	**Never-Smokers (66%)**	**Ever-Smokers (34%)**
EGFR	49.8	22.0
PTEN	9.9	2.6
ALK	9.3	4.5
PIK3CA	5.2	2.1
STK11	2.7	11
KRAS	4.5	12
C-MET	4.8	4
BRAF	1.9	3.1
SQUAMOUS CELL CARCINOMA (*n* = 144)		
Gene	**Never-Smokers (35%)**	**Ever-Smokers (65%)**
DDR2	0	4.4
FGFR2	0	2.2

ALK, anaplastic lymphoma receptor tyrosine kinase; *BRAF*, v-raf murine sarcoma viral oncogene homolog B; *C-MET*, growth factor receptor c-Met; *DDR2*, discoidin domain receptor tyrosine kinase 2; *EGFR*, epidermal growth factor receptor; *FGFR2*, fibroblast growth factor receptor 2; *KRAS*, Kirsten rat sarcoma viral oncogene homolog; *PIK3CA*, phosphatidylinositol-4,5-bisphosphate 3-kinase, catalytic subunit alpha; *PTEN*, phosphatase and tensin homolog; *STK11*, serine/threonine kinase 11.

kinase 2 (*DDR2*) and fibroblast growth factor receptor 2 (*FGFR2*) mutations, although infrequent, were present only in tumors from smokers.

In another Chinese study limited to lung cancers from never-smokers, Li et al.[96] identified driver mutations in 89% of the tumors (Table 4.2). Of interest, these mutations were mutually exclusive, consistent with their driver status. Although the mutation figures may be lower among lung cancers in never-smokers in Western countries, most of these tumors contain potentially actionable driver mutations. In conclusion, driver gene alterations in NSCLC are shown to be associated with smoking status rather than gender.

GENOME-WIDE MOLECULAR CHANGES

Although we have discussed specific genes mutated in lung cancer in never-smokers or ever-smokers, some genome-wide changes also are characteristic of both forms of lung cancer. Point mutations may represent changes involving purine to pyrimidine or pyrimidine to purine (transversions) or purine to purine or pyrimidine to pyrimidine (transitions). At the turn of the 21st century, it was noted that the point mutations in the tumor protein p53 (*TP53*) gene present in lung cancer were of a different pattern than the point mutations seen in most other types of solid tumor. The most frequent mutation change in the *TP53* gene in lung and other tobacco-associated cancers (head and neck or bladder) represented a G to T transversion.[97–99] These mutations frequently occur at mCpG hotspots. 5-Methylcytosine in DNA is genetically unstable, and mCpG sequences frequently undergo mutation resulting in a general depletion of this dinucleotide sequence in mammalian genomes. In human genetic disease-relevant and cancer-relevant genes, mCpG sequences are mutational hotspots.[99] Although initial attention focused on the *TP53* gene, whole genome sequencing studies have confirmed that G to T transversions are the most frequent type of point mutation in tobacco-associated cancers, and G to A transitions are the most common type of point mutation in lung cancers among never-smokers.[87,100]

Seo et al.[87] extensively analyzed the transcriptomes of 87 lung adenocarcinoma specimens from Korean patients. The authors found that the expression signature, as well as the mutation pattern, was highly related to active smoking. In another study of nontumorous lung tissues, Bosse et al.[101] compared gene expression levels between never-smokers and current smokers, as well as time-dependent changes in gene expression in former smokers. A large number of genes (3223 transcripts) were differentially expressed between the groups. Moreover, some genes showed very slow or no reversibility in expression, including serpin peptidase inhibitor, clade D (heparin cofactor), member 1 (*SERPIND1*), which was found to be the gene that was most

consistently permanently altered by smoking. Thus, their findings indicate that smoking deregulates many genes, many of which reverse to normal after smoking cessation. However, a subset of genes remains altered even decades after smoking cessation and may account, at least in part, for the residual risk of lung cancer among former smokers. In another study, Lam et al.[102] evaluated the expression patterns of a small number of cell lines established from smokers and never-smokers in Hong Kong. These authors identified 71 genes that were differentially expressed or showed class predictive significance.

Whole genome sequencing has shown that the number of synonymous and nonsynonymous mutations in lung cancer in ever-smokers is remarkably high and that this lung cancer is among the cancers with the highest number of such mutations.[103]

However, major differences exist between lung cancer in never-smokers and ever-smokers with respect to the number of mutations and complexity of molecular changes, with this number being 10-fold or less in never-smokers.[87,100] These findings indicate that exposure to tobacco carcinogens induces DNA instability, resulting in the formation of numerous driver and passenger mutations. By contrast, although the number of driver mutations may be similar, the etiologic agents associated with lung cancer in never-smokers induce a more modest total number of changes.

PRENEOPLASTIC CHANGES

For more than a decade, we have known that the development of invasive lung carcinoma is preceded by numerous and widespread molecular alterations in the respiratory tree that commence in histologically normal epithelium.[104,105] However, similar studies on the development of *EGFR* mutant lung cancers indicate a far more modest field effect, largely limited to the field immediately surrounding the invasive carcinoma.[106] Although these observations may be partly due to differences in the field effects of centrally arising squamous cell carcinomas compared with peripherally arising adenocarcinomas, they also suggest that smoking induces much or all of the respiratory epithelium to undergo molecular changes very early in lung cancer pathogenesis, whereas lung cancers arising in never-smokers have much more restricted field effects.

DNA METHYLATION

Although most molecular studies have focused on genetic changes, epigenetic differences in lung cancer between ever-smokers and never-smokers demonstrate multiple differences in the overall methylation pattern and in methylation (and occasionally downregulation) of several genes. However, some studies describe contradictory findings and others are unconfirmed. One study of 59 matched lung adenocarcinoma/nontumor lung pairs, with genome-scale verification on an independent set of tissues, used the older Infinium HumanMethylation27 platform (Illumina, San Diego, CA, USA).[107] Although more than 700 genes were found to be differentially methylated between tumor and nonmalignant lung tissue, comparison of DNA methylation profiles between lung adenocarcinomas of current smokers and never-smokers showed modest differences, identifying only the lectin, galactoside-galactoside binding, soluble, 4 (*LGALS4*) gene as significantly hypermethylated and downregulated in smokers. *LGALS4*, encoding a galactoside-binding protein involved in cell-cell and cell-matrix interactions, is a known tumor suppressor. Other studies have examined individual or small numbers of genes, which have included Ras association (RalGDS/AF-6) domain family member 1 (*RASSF1A*), cyclin-dependent kinase inhibitor 2A (*CDKN2A*), and others (Table 4.3).[108–115] The association between *CDKN2A* methylation and active smoking was confirmed by meta-analysis.[116] The association between inactivation of *CDKN2A* and inactivation by any mechanism and its

TABLE 4.2 Driver Mutations in Lung Adenocarcinomas Among Chinese Never-Smokers[96]

Driver Mutation[a]	Percentage (%) of Patients (*n* = 202)
EGFR	75
HER2	6
ALK fusion	5
KRAS	2
ROS1 fusion	1
BRAF	0
No mutation	11
Any mutation	89

[a]Mutations were mutually exclusive.

ALK, anaplastic lymphoma receptor tyrosine kinase; *BRAF*, v-raf murine sarcoma viral oncogene homolog B; *EGFR*, epidermal growth factor receptor; *HER2*, human epidermal growth factor receptor-2; *KRAS*, Kirsten rat sarcoma viral oncogene homolog; *ROS1*, c-ros oncogene 1, receptor tyrosine kinase.

TABLE 4.3 Summary of Major Differences Between Lung Cancers Arising in Ever-Smokers and Never-Smokers

FACTOR	LC IN EVER-SMOKERS	LC IN NEVER-SMOKERS
Clinical and Pathologic Factors		
Major etiologic factor	Cigarette smoking	Unknown or diverse
Major histologic types	NSCLC and SCLC	Largely adenocarcinoma
Field effects	Widespread	More limited
Stage at time of diagnosis	More advanced in never-smokers	
Response to therapy and overall survival	Improved in never-smokers	
Age at time of diagnosis	Younger for never-smokers (especially in East Asia)	
Gender	Higher ratio of women among never-smokers (worldwide)	
Genetics		
RGS17 locus (chromosome 6q)	Lung cancer susceptibility locus for ever-smokers	
Polymorphisms	Patterns differ according to smoking status and ethnicity. *CHRNA5* predisposes to smoking	
Molecular Changes		
Total number of mutations	Much higher In ever-smokers	
Most frequent mutation	G to A transitions	G to T tranversions
Specific mutations	*KRAS, STK11, SMARCA4*	*EGFR, ALK, PTEN, PIK3CA*
Percentage of cancers with potential targets for treatment	Approximately 60% (East Asia)	More than 90% (East Asia)
Gene expression signatures	More deregulation of gene expression in lung tumors and adjacent tissue in ever-smokers	
DNA methylation	Multiple genes show differential methylation, predominantly affecting cancers in never-smokers	
Methylated genes (some are unconfirmed)	*RASSF1A, CDKN2A, MTHFR, HtrA3, LGALS4*	*NFKBIA, TNFRSF10C, BHLHB5, BOLL*

ALK, anaplastic lymphoma receptor tyrosine kinase; *BHLHB5,* basic helix-loop-helix domain containing, class B5; *BOLL,* boule-like RNA-binding protein; *CDKN2A,* cyclin dependent kinase inhibitor 2A; *CHRNA5,* cholinergic receptor, nicotinic, alpha 5 (neuronal); *EGFR,* epidermal growth factor receptor; *HtrA3,* HtrA serine peptidase 3; *KRAS,* Kirsten rat sarcoma viral oncogene homolog; *LC,* lung cancer; *LGALS4,* lectin, galactoside-binding, soluble, 4; *MTHFR,* methylenetetrahydrofolate reductase (NAD(P)H); *NFKBIA,* nuclear factor of kappa light polypeptide gene enhancer in B-cells inhibitor, alpha; *NSCLC,* nonsmall cell lung cancer; *PIK3CA,* phosphatidylinositol-4,5-bisphosphate 3-kinase, catalytic subunit alpha; *PTEN,* phosphatase and tensin homolog; *RASSF1A,* Ras association (RalGDS/AF-6) domain family member 1; *RGS17,* regulator of G-protein signaling 17; *SCLC,* small cell lung cancer; *SMARCA4,* SWI/SNF (switching/sucrose nonfermenting) related, matrix associated, actin dependent regulator of chromatin, subfamily a, member 4; *STK11,* serine/threonine kinase 11; *TNFRSF10C,* tumor necrosis factor receptor superfamily, member 10c, decoy without an intracellular domain.

relationship to smoking has been demonstrated, with one interesting study examining gene promoter methylation assayed in exhaled breath and finding differences between smokers and individuals with lung cancer.[117]

CONCLUSION

We focused on lung cancer in never-smokers in East Asia because this type of lung cancer occurs most frequently in this geographic region. However, East Asia is a vast region, containing 10 countries and the Asian Pacific islands. It encompasses more than one-fifth of the world's population. Thus, lung cancer differences among heterogeneous East Asian subpopulations may also occur. We believe that the observations and findings summarized in this chapter demonstrate conclusively that lung cancers arise as a result of complex interactions among several factors, including exposure to tobacco through either active smoking or secondhand smoke, gender, ethnicity, and genetic predisposition. For lung cancer in never-smokers, other largely unknown environmental carcinogens or lifestyle factors may be contributors; however, no single factor or combination of factors identified to date can be responsible for the majority of cancers.

As a result, major clinical, pathologic, demographic, gender, ethnic, molecular, and genetic predisposition factors differ between lung cancers in smokers and never-smokers. We summarize many of the important differences between these two groups of lung cancers (Table 4.3). Studies have conclusively demonstrated that lung cancers arising in ever-smokers and never-smokers are very different and should be regarded as separate tumors with different pathogeneses and their own clinical, genotypic, and phenotypic features.

However, many questions remain, in particular regarding the major etiologic cause or causes of lung cancer in never-smokers. There may be no simple or universal answers, with this type of cancer remaining a heterogeneous cancer with a pathogenesis influenced by genetics, ethnicity, environmental tobacco exposure, other environmental or occupational carcinogens, and geography.

KEY REFERENCES

5. Sun S, Schiller JH, Gazdar AF. Lung cancer in never smokers—a different disease. *Nature Rev Cancer.* 2007;7(10):778–790.
6. Subramanian J, Govindan R. Lung cancer in never smokers: a review. *J Clin Oncol.* 2007;25(5):561–570.
7. Thun MJ, Hannan LM, Adams-Campbell LL, et al. Lung cancer occurrence in never-smokers: an analysis of 13 cohorts and 22 cancer registry studies. *PLoS Med.* 2008;5(9):e185.
8. Brenner DR, Hung RJ, Tsao MS, et al. Lung cancer risk in never-smokers: a population-based case–control study of epidemiologic risk factors. *BMC Cancer.* 2010;10:285.
21. Wakelee HA, Chang ET, Gomez SL, et al. Lung cancer incidence in never smokers. *J Clin Oncol.* 2007;25(5):472–478.
22. US Department of Health and Human Services. Cancer among adults from exposure to secondhand smoke. In: *The Health Consequences of Involuntary Exposure to Secondhand Smoke: A Report of the Surgeon General.* Atlanta, GA: US Dept of Health and Human Services, Centers for Disease Control and Prevention, National Center for Chronic Disease Prevention and Health Promotion, Office on Smoking and Health; 2006. chap 7. http://www.surgeongeneral.gov/library/reports/secondhandsmoke/chapter7.pdf.
40. Samet JM. Radiation and cancer risk: a continuing challenge for epidemiologists. *Environ Health.* 2011;10(suppl 1):S4.

42. Wakelee H. Lung cancer in never smokers. UpToDate. http://www .uptodate.com/contents/lung-cancer-in-never-smokers. Updated January 13, 2014.

50. Dibble RLW, Bair S, Ward J, Akerley W. Natual history of non-small cell lung cancer in non-smokers. *J Clin Oncol*. 2005;23(16s):7252. [abstract].

54. Gazdar AF, Boffetta P. A risky business—identifying susceptibility loci for lung cancer. *J Natl Cancer Inst*. 2010;102(13):920–923.

55. Bailey-Wilson JE, Amos CI, Pinney SM, et al. A major lung cancer susceptibility locus maps to chromosome 6q23-25. *Am J Hum Genet*. 2004;75(3):460–474.

59. Gazdar A, Robinson L, Oliver D, et al. Hereditary lung cancer syndrome targets never smokers with germline EGFR gene T790M mutations. *J Thor Oncol*. 2014;9:456–463.

69. Dong J, Hu Z, Wu C, et al. Association analyses identify multiple new lung cancer susceptibility loci and their interactions with smoking in the Chinese population. *Nat Genet*. 2012;44(8):895–899.

75. Gazdar AF. EGFR mutations in lung cancer: different frequencies for different folks. *J Thorac Oncol*. 2014;9:139–140.

76. Shigematsu H, Lin L, Takahashi T, et al. Clinical and biological features associated with epidermal growth factor receptor gene mutations in lung cancers. *J Natl Cancer Inst*. 2005;97(5):339–346.

96. Li C, Fang R, Sun Y, et al. Spectrum of oncogenic driver mutations in lung adenocarcinomas from East Asian never smokers. *PLoS One*. 2011;6(11):e28204.

99. Pfeifer GP. Mutagenesis at methylated CpG sequences. *Curr Top Microbiol Immunol*. 2006;301:259–281.

100. Govindan R, Ding L, Griffith M, et al. Genomic landscape of non-small cell lung cancer in smokers and never-smokers. *Cell*. 2012;150(6):1121–1134.

106. Tang X, Shigematsu H, Bekele BN, et al. EGFR tyrosine kinase domain mutations are detected in histologically normal respiratory epithelium in lung cancer patients. *Cancer Res*. 2005;65(17):7568–7572.

See Expertconsult.com for full list of references.

5 Gender-Related Differences in Lung Cancer

Silvia Novello, Laura P. Stabile, and Jill M. Siegfried

SUMMARY OF KEY POINTS

- Epidemiology of lung cancer is still changing: in the last 10 years lung cancer became the first cause of cancer-related deaths in both men and women in many countries, while having previously been a rare disease in females.
- Smoking is the first cause of lung cancer also among women: no conclusive data are present in the literature about female smokers and their susceptibility to develop lung cancer, compared with their male counterparts.
- The risk of lung cancer is 2.5 times more common in female lifetime nonsmokers compared with male non-smokers with different geographic distribution: in Asia the proportion of female lung cancer patients who are never-smokers ranges from 61% to 83%.
- Several publications describe a more favorable prognosis of lung cancer in women than in men, and this is regardless of a longer life expectancy or the influence of other factors.
- Population studies and preclinical studies suggest that steroid hormone pathways, as well as progesterone receptors, are involved in the biology of lung cancer: these pathways are consequently promising targets for lung cancer therapy.
- From a molecular biology point of view, lung cancer in women should be considered a specific entity, and this fact must be taken into account in diagnosis and therapeutic approaches.

For several decades, lung cancer has been considered a neoplastic disease affecting mainly men; however, during the past 40 years, the incidence of the disease has increased exponentially among women. From 1990 through 1995, in many Western countries, the incidence of lung cancer among men has gradually declined as a result of antitobacco campaigns, which, in turn, led to a progressive reduction in incidence rates for men and women, with a projection of equal incidences by 2020.[1]

The mortality rate for lung cancer among women shows a clear inverse trend compared with most other cancers. Whereas deaths from gastric and uterine cancer have plummeted in the past four decades and deaths from breast cancer have steadily declined since a peak in 1990, deaths from lung cancer have continued an upward trajectory, reflecting the consequences of tobacco smoking among women. Overall, lung cancer causes death for more women than the combination of the three most common cancers among women (breast, colorectal, and ovarian cancer).[2]

Whether women are more or less susceptible than men to the carcinogenic effects of cigarette smoking is controversial. Compared with men, women are less likely to have a smoking history and are more likely to be younger at the time of diagnosis and to have a better survival at any stage (Fig. 5.1).[3] Adenocarcinoma of the lung is the most common histologic subtype among women.

EPIDEMIOLOGY

Worldwide, lung cancer accounts for the most cancer diagnoses (1,600,000 new cases; 12.4% of total new cancer cases) and is the leading cause of cancer-related deaths in both men and women (1,378,000 deaths; 17.6% of total cancer deaths).[2] The estimated number of lung cancer cases worldwide has increased by 51% since 1985 (a 44% increase in men and a 76% increase in women).[4]

The World Health Organization (WHO) estimates that worldwide lung cancer deaths will continue to increase, largely as a consequence of an increase in global tobacco use, primarily in Asia. Despite efforts to curb tobacco smoking, there are approximately 1.1 billion smokers around the world, and if the current trends continue, that number will increase to 1.9 billion by 2025.[5,6]

United States

In the United States, it is estimated that 118,080 men and 110,110 women were diagnosed with lung cancer in 2013, and 87,260 men and 72,220 women died of the disease. The age-adjusted death rate for the period from 2006 to 2010 was 63.5/100,000 and 39.2/100,000 for men and women per year, respectively.[3]

The most common cancers expected to occur in men in 2013 included prostate, lung and bronchus, and colorectal, which account for about 50% of all newly diagnosed cancers (prostate cancer alone accounted for 28%, or 238,590 of all new cases).[2] In women, the three most commonly diagnosed types of cancer in 2013 were breast, lung and bronchus, and colorectal, accounting for 52% of estimated cancer cases (breast cancer alone accounted for 29%, or 232,340 of all new cases). These cancers continue to be the most common causes of cancer death (Fig. 5.2).[2] In 2013, lung cancer was expected to account for 26% of all cancer-related deaths among women and 28% of all cancer-related deaths among men.[2] Of the 2,437,163 deaths recorded in the United States in 2009, 567,628 were caused by cancer. Lung cancer is the leading cause of death among men aged 40 years and older and is the leading cause of cancer-related deaths among women aged 60 years and older.[2]

The Hispanic/Latino population is the largest and fastest growing major demographic group in the United States, accounting for 16.3% (50.5 million/310 million) of the US population in 2010. In 2012, an estimated 112,800 new cases of cancer were diagnosed and 33,200 cancer-related deaths occurred among Hispanic individuals.[7] The incidence and mortality rates for all cancers combined and for the four most common cancers (breast, prostate, lung and bronchus, and colorectal) are lower for the Hispanic population than for the non-Hispanic white population, but the incidence and mortality rates are higher for cancers of the stomach, liver, uterine cervix, and gallbladder. These differences in rates reflect greater exposure to cancer-related infectious agents, lower rates of screening for cervical cancer, differences in lifestyle and dietary patterns, and possibly genetic factors.[7]

The considerable efforts in implementing tobacco-control strategies in the United States since the 1950s and the subsequent favorable changes in smoking behaviors in 1975 to 2000 have averted more than 240,000 lung cancer-related deaths in women.[8] However, it is estimated that 20.6% of all American

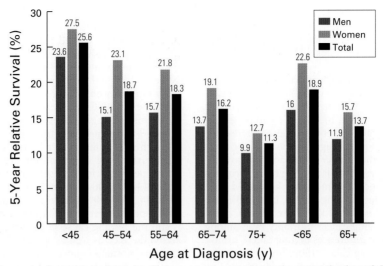

Fig. 5.1. Five-year relative survival of people with lung cancer according to the age at the time of diagnosis. Based on data from 2001 to 2008 in 17 areas covered by the US Surveillance, Epidemiology and End Results (SEER) database.[1]

Estimated New Cases*

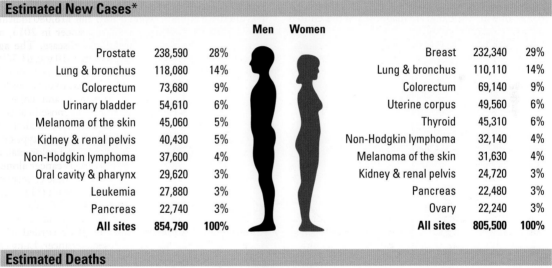

Men				Women		
Prostate	238,590	28%		Breast	232,340	29%
Lung & bronchus	118,080	14%		Lung & bronchus	110,110	14%
Colorectum	73,680	9%		Colorectum	69,140	9%
Urinary bladder	54,610	6%		Uterine corpus	49,560	6%
Melanoma of the skin	45,060	5%		Thyroid	45,310	6%
Kidney & renal pelvis	40,430	5%		Non-Hodgkin lymphoma	32,140	4%
Non-Hodgkin lymphoma	37,600	4%		Melanoma of the skin	31,630	4%
Oral cavity & pharynx	29,620	3%		Kidney & renal pelvis	24,720	3%
Leukemia	27,880	3%		Pancreas	22,480	3%
Pancreas	22,740	3%		Ovary	22,240	3%
All sites	**854,790**	**100%**		**All sites**	**805,500**	**100%**

Estimated Deaths

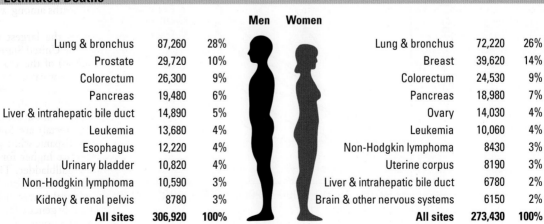

Men				Women		
Lung & bronchus	87,260	28%		Lung & bronchus	72,220	26%
Prostate	29,720	10%		Breast	39,620	14%
Colorectum	26,300	9%		Colorectum	24,530	9%
Pancreas	19,480	6%		Pancreas	18,980	7%
Liver & intrahepatic bile duct	14,890	5%		Ovary	14,030	4%
Leukemia	13,680	4%		Leukemia	10,060	4%
Esophagus	12,220	4%		Non-Hodgkin lymphoma	8430	3%
Urinary bladder	10,820	4%		Uterine corpus	8190	3%
Non-Hodgkin lymphoma	10,590	3%		Liver & intrahepatic bile duct	6780	2%
Kidney & renal pelvis	8780	3%		Brain & other nervous systems	6150	2%
All sites	**306,920**	**100%**		**All sites**	**273,430**	**100%**

Fig. 5.2. Estimated number of new cases and deaths for the 10 leading types of cancer in men and women in the United States for 2013. (*Estimates are rounded to the nearest 10 and exclude basal cell and squamous cell skin cancers and in situ carcinoma, except urinary bladder.) *(Modified with permission from Siegel R, Naishadham D, Jemal A. Cancer statistics, 2013. CA: Cancer J Clin. 2013;63:11–30.)*

adults 18 years and older continue to smoke, a percentage that has changed slightly since approximately 1997.[9] Smoking prevalence in the United States has decreased from a high of 53% for men and 32% for women in 1964 to rates of 21.6% for men and 16.5% for women in 2011.[10]

Large geographic differences in public policies against tobacco use and socioeconomic factors affect the distribution of lung cancer mortality rates across states. California has been a leader in introducing public policies designed to reduce cigarette smoking. It was the first state to establish a comprehensive state-wide tobacco-control program in 1988 through increased excise taxes on cigarettes, and as early as the mid-1970s it had local government ordinances for smoke-free work places. As a result, progress in reducing smoking prevalence and mortality associated with smoking-related diseases, including lung cancer, has been much greater in California than in the rest of the United States. Jemal et al.[1] evaluated state-specific lung cancer mortality rates among white women to assess regional differences in lung cancer trends. The decrease in age-specific lung cancer mortality rates among white women continued in younger age groups and birth cohorts in California, but the decline was slower or even reversed among women younger than 50 years of age and for women born after the 1950s in the remaining 22 states analyzed, especially in the South and Midwest.[11]

Europe

Worldwide, the estimated incidence of lung cancer among women is 516,000, of which 100,000 are diagnosed in the United States and 70,000 in Europe.[2,12] There are still differences when incidence rates from European cancer registries are compared with rates in the United States, suggesting that the lung cancer epidemic among women in Europe may not yet have reached the US rate from the 1990s (>25 lung cancers/100,000 women). Nevertheless, in the European Union (EU), the lung cancer mortality rate for women increased by 50% between the mid-1960s and the early 2000s and steady upward trends have been seen even in the youngest age groups in some southern European countries such as France and Spain up to the early 2000s.[13]

In the EU, lung cancer mortality rates for women increased during the past decade, from 11.3/100,000 to 12.7/100,000 (2.3% per year) for all ages (a further increase is predicted to reach 14/100,000 women in 2015) and from 18.6/100,000 to 21.5/100,000 (3.0% per year) for middle-age women (Fig. 5.3).[14]

Despite the reduction in breast cancer mortality, this disease is still the leading cause of cancer-related deaths among women across the EU, as well as specifically in France, Germany, Italy, and Spain. Lung cancer is the leading cause of cancer-related deaths in several countries in Northern and Eastern Europe, including Denmark, Hungary, the Netherlands, Poland, Sweden, and the United Kingdom.[14–17] The projected cancer mortality rate has increased among women in several European countries. In Serbia, colorectal cancer in men and lung cancer in women are estimated to have the most significant increase over time (2010 to 2014): 0.42/100,000 ($p = 0.036$) and 0.626/100,000 ($p < 0.001$) per year, respectively.[18] From 1996 to 2001, the National Health Service Breast Screening Programme in the United Kingdom recruited 1.3 million women into the Million Women Study.[16]

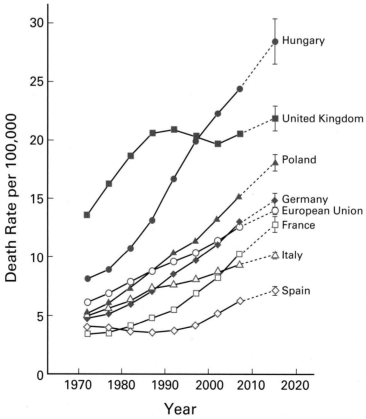

Fig. 5.3. Age-standardized (world population) death rates for lung cancer in women from major European countries and the European Union as a whole from 1970 and 2009, and predicted rates for 2015. *(Modified with permission from Bosetti C, Malvezzi M, Rosso T, et al. Lung cancer mortality in European women: trends and predictions.* Lung Cancer. *2012;78:171–178.)*

The women signed consent forms and completed a questionnaire about lifestyle, medical history, and sociodemographic factors and were resurveyed by mail about 3 years and 8 years later. Twenty-three of the 30 most common causes of death occurred more frequently in smokers; the rate ratio for lung cancer was 21.4 (19.7–23.2). The increased mortality among smokers compared with never-smokers was mainly from diseases such as lung cancer that can be attributed to tobacco smoking. Among former smokers who stopped smoking permanently between the ages of 25 years and 34 years or between the ages of 35 years and 44 years, the respective relative risks were 1.05 (95% CI, 1.00–1.11) and 1.20 (95% CI, 1.14–1.26) for all-cause mortality and 1.84 (95% CI, 1.45–2.34) and 3.34 (95% CI, 2.76–4.03) for lung cancer–specific mortality.[19]

In the EU in 2012, nearly 88,000 women died from breast cancer, corresponding to almost 16% of all cancer deaths among women. The projected lung cancer-related deaths for 2015 are 187,000 for men and 85,204 for women.[14–20] In a pooled analysis of 13,169 lung cancer cases and 16,010 controls from Europe and Canada, the most common histologic subtype was squamous cell carcinoma among men (4747 of 8891; 53.4%) and adenocarcinoma among women (1013 of 2017; 50.2%). No clear-cut evidence for gender preference was found among the major subtypes of small cell lung cancer (SCLC): 19.8% in men and 21.9% in women. Never-smoking status was reported for 220 (2.1%) men and 609 (24.2%) women; the most common subtype was adenocarcinoma (57.6% in men and 70.1% in women).[21]

Similar to US data, an epidemiologic study conducted in Poland showed that a higher proportion of women (23%) were diagnosed with lung cancer at a younger age (less than 50 years) compared with men (12%).[22]

Asia

In Asia, the lung cancer mortality rates for women are lower than in the United States and Europe. However, these rates are increasing across several Asian countries, including China, South Korea, and Japan.[23–25] Adenocarcinoma tends to be the most common histologic type in women in Asia, and this proportion continues to increase over time.[26–31] Although tobacco smoke is the most common cause of lung cancer in women throughout the rest of the world, the cause of lung cancer in Asian woman is considered more complex (Fig. 5.4). The proportion of women with lung cancer who are never-smokers ranges from 61% to 83%.[32,33] In fact, the smoking rate is higher than 10% only for Filipino and Japanese women.[34] Environmental tobacco smoke and indoor pollutants, including cooking oil fumes and burning coal, have been implicated in increasing the risk of lung cancer among nonsmoking Asian women.[35–46]

In China, cancer incidence and mortality data for 2009, including demographic information from 104 population-based cancer registries, were reported to the National Central Cancer Registry, a government organization for cancer surveillance.[46] After an evaluation procedure, data from 72 registries were deemed satisfactory and were then compiled for analysis. According to these data, lung cancer was the most common cancer in China overall and in its urban areas and the second most common cancer in its rural areas. There were 197,833 new cancer cases and 122,136 deaths. The crude cancer mortality was 184.67/100,000 overall, 228.14/100,000 for men and 140.48/100,000 for women. These findings indicate that lung cancer was the most common cancer for men in all areas, particularly urban areas, and second to breast cancer in women, especially in urban areas. Lung cancer was the leading cause of cancer-related deaths in all groups stratified by gender and area. Ages over 50 years were the high-risk age groups because of the increase in incidence and mortality rates that accompany increasing age.[46]

In India, over a 2-year period, 130 trained physicians independently assigned causes to 122,429 deaths in 6671 randomly selected small areas from the 1991 census and monitored all births and deaths in 1.1 million homes representative of all of India.[47] Among people 30 years to 69 years old, the three most common fatal cancers among men were oral (including lip and pharynx, 45,800 [22.9%]), gastric (25,200 [12.6%]), and lung (including trachea and larynx, 22,900 [11.4%]); among women, the three most common fatal cancers were cervical (33,400 [17.1%]), gastric (27,500 [14.1%]), and breast (19,900) [10.2%]). Tobacco-related cancers represented 42.0% (84,000) and 18.3% (35,700) of cancer-related deaths among men and women, respectively, and there were twice as many deaths caused by oral cancers compared with lung cancers.[47]

Data from the Korean National Cancer Incidence Database on 599,288 adult patients diagnosed with solid cancers between 2005 and 2009 were analyzed to identify possible gender differences.[45] For all solid cancer sites combined, the risk of death for women was 11% lower than that for men (relative excess risk 0.89; 95% CI, 0.88–0.90) after adjusting for year of follow-up, age, stage, and case mix. The relative excess risks for cancer of the lung, head/neck, esophagus, small intestine, liver, nasal cavities, bone/cartilage, soft tissue, brain and central nervous system, and thyroid and melanoma were significantly lower for women.[48]

SUSCEPTIBILITY

Never-Smokers

Never-smokers with lung cancer represent a unique subset of all people with lung cancer. Globally, an estimated 15% of lung cancer cases in men and 53% of cases in women are not attributable to tobacco smoking.[4] The risk of lung cancer is 2.5 times more common among female lifetime nonsmokers than among male lifetime nonsmokers.[4] One of the most relevant risk factors for nonsmoking women is environmental tobacco smoke exposure. A meta-analysis of 55 studies of spousal smoking on the risk of lung cancer for a nonsmoking spouse showed a pooled relative risk of 1.27 (95% CI, 1.17–1.37), with risk increasing monotonically with increasing exposure. This association has been replicated in different populations across Asia, Europe, and North America.[49]

Nevertheless, there remains a large fraction of lung cancers among never-smokers that cannot be definitively associated with established environmental risk factors, and limited data

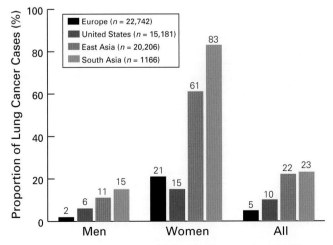

Fig. 5.4. Data from a review of published studies over the past 25 years showing geographic and gender variations in lung cancers in never-smokers. (*Modified with permission from Sun S, Schiller JH, Gazdar AF. Lung cancer in never smokers—a different disease. Nat Rev Cancer. 2007;7(10):778–790.*)

are available on the epidemiologic risk factors for lung cancer in never-smokers according to gender.[50] Although smoking prevalence has decreased, the incidence of lung cancer has increased steadily in Taiwan over the past several decades; only 9% to 10% of women with lung cancer and 79% to 86% of men with lung cancer are tobacco smokers. In a matched case–control study conducted between 2002 and 2009, several epidemiologic factors of lung cancer in never-smokers differed between men and women.[51] The risk for lung cancer was higher for people exposed to environmental tobacco smoke (odds ratio, 1.39; 95% CI, 1.17–1.67) with a history of pulmonary tuberculosis and with a family history of lung cancer in first-degree relatives (odds ratio, 2.44); people with a history of hormone-replacement therapy and who used fume extractors when cooking were protected. For men, only a family history of lung cancer in first-degree relatives was significantly associated with risk of lung cancer (odds ratio, 2.77).[51]

A case–control study in China included 399 lung cancer cases and 466 controls, of which 164 cases and 218 controls were female nonsmokers.[50] Among nonsmoking women, lung cancer was strongly associated with multiple sources of indoor air pollution, including heavy exposure to environmental tobacco smoke at work (adjusted odds ratio, 3.65), high frequency of cooking (adjusted odds ratio, 3.30), and use of solid fuel for cooking (adjusted odds ratio, 4.08) and heating (adjusted odds ratio for coal stove, 2.00). In addition, housing characteristics related to poor ventilation, including single story homes, less window area, absence of a separate kitchen, lack of a ventilator, and limited time with windows open, were associated with lung cancer.[52]

Smokers

A prospective evaluation of 50-year trends in smoking-related mortality in the United States demonstrated that the relative and absolute risks of death from smoking continue to increase among female smokers.[53] The relative risks of death from lung cancer, chronic obstructive pulmonary disease (COPD), ischemic heart disease, any type of stroke, and all causes are now nearly identical for female and male smokers. The risk of death from lung cancer among male smokers appears to have stabilized since the 1980s, whereas it continues to increase among female smokers. For women aged 60 years to 74 years old, the all-cause mortality rate is now at least three times as high among current smokers as among never-smokers.[53]

Currently, no conclusive data are available on the susceptibility of lung cancer among female smokers. Some studies have shown a greater risk of lung cancer for female smokers than for male smokers. Data generated by the American Health Foundation database indicate that the odds ratio for the major lung cancer types is consistently higher for women than for men at every level of exposure to cigarette smoke.[54] The dose–response odds ratios for lung cancer among women are 1.2-fold to 1.7-fold higher than among men. A Canadian case–control study of gender differences in lung cancer from 1981 to 1985 showed that with a 40-pack-year smoking history (compared with lifelong nonsmokers), the odds ratio for the development of lung cancer was 27.9 for women and 9.6 for men.[55] In both of these studies, the increase in lung cancer risk held for all major histologic types. In a pooled analysis that included 13,169 cases and 16,010 controls from Europe and Canada, the odds ratio for different histologies of lung cancer was assessed. For male current smokers (average of 30 cigarettes per day), the odds ratios were 103.5 (95% CI, 74.8–143.2) for squamous carcinoma, 111.3 (95% CI, 69.8–177.5) for SCLC, and 21.9 (95% CI, 16.6–29.0) for adenocarcinoma. For female current smokers, the corresponding odds ratios were 62.7 (95% CI, 31.5–124.6), 108.6 (95% CI, 50.7–232.8), and 16.8 (95% CI, 9.2–30.6).[21]

Other studies have shown comparable risks for men and women when controlling for smoking exposure.[56–60] A gender-smoking interaction in association with lung cancer risk within a population-based case–control study (Lombardy, Italy, 2002–2005) was evaluated in 2100 cases with incident lung cancer and 2120 controls.[61] Lung cancer odds ratios for pack-years (categorical) were higher for men than women, with a negative gender-smoking interaction for women ($p = 0.0009$). For medium (20–29 pack-years) and high (40 pack-years or more) categories, the risk of lung cancer was similar for men and women.[61]

GENETIC FACTORS

Polymorphisms of genes that encode for enzymes involved in the breakdown of tobacco-derived carcinogens may potentially play a role in the development of lung cancer in female smokers and never-smokers. Arylamine N-acetyltransferase (NAT2) is an enzyme involved in biotransformation of xenobiotics, mainly aromatic and heterocyclic amines and hydrazines. NAT2 activity can influence the risk of lung cancer as well as cytochrome P (CYP)450 CYP1A2 activity (see Chapter 6). In nonsmoking Chinese women, low NAT2 activity and fast CYP1A2 activity were associated with a higher risk for the development of lung cancer, with an adjusted odds ratio of 6.9 compared with high NAT2 activity and slow CYP1A2 activity.

CYP1A1 is associated with an increased risk of lung cancer in female nonsmokers (odds ratio, 3.97; 95% CI, 1.85–7.28). CYP1A1 plays a role in converting tobacco carcinogens into DNA-binding metabolites that are important in DNA adduct formation. Glutathione S-transferase (GSTM1) and GSTT1 are relevant for the detoxification of carcinogens. GSTM1 null genotype has been associated with an increased risk of lung cancer in some studies but not in others.[62–65] One study conducted among Japanese women demonstrated an association between GSTM1 null genotype and an increased risk of lung cancer, particularly among female never-smokers with the null genotype.[65] Additionally, an association was found between the GSTM1 null genotype and an increased risk of lung cancer in female never-smokers with the null genotype who had a substantial exposure to environmental tobacco smoke (odds ratio, 2.27; 95% CI, 1.13–2.7) compared with female never-smokers without the null genotype who did not have substantial exposure.[66] Similar to GSTM1, the null genotype of GSTT1 increases the risk for the development of lung cancer in never-smokers.[67]

To gain insights into the etiology of lung cancer in never-smoking women, the Female Lung Cancer Consortium in Asia (FLCCA), which includes mainland China, South Korea, Japan, Singapore, Taiwan, and Hong Kong, was founded. The FLCCA identified a distinct pattern of environmental risk factors causally linked to lung cancer in never-smoking Asian women, as well as a distinct molecular phenotype of lung cancer in never-smokers by the identification of three new susceptibility loci at 10q25.2, 6q22.2, and 6p21.32 (Fig. 5.5).[68]

In six Korean female never-smokers, novel genetic aberrations, which included 47 somatic mutations and 19 fusion transcripts, were identified. Most of the altered genes were responsible for disturbances in G2/M transition and mitotic progression, causally linked to tumorigenesis in these patients (Fig. 5.6).[69]

In a study of the genotype of 3026 lung adenocarcinomas, correlation of the major epidermal growth factor receptor (EGFR) mutations (exon 19 deletions and L858R) and V-Ki-ras2 Kirsten rat sarcoma viral oncogene homolog (KRAS) mutations (G12, G13) with demographic, clinical, and smoking history data indicated a higher frequency of KRAS G12C mutations in women, who were also younger at the time of diagnosis than men with the same mutation (median age, 65 years vs. 69 years; $p = 0.0008$) and less exposed to active smoking. These findings support an increased susceptibility to tobacco carcinogens.[70] Distinct

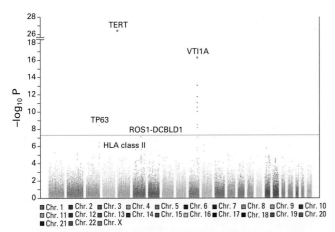

Fig. 5.5. Manhattan plot based on *p* values derived from 1-degree-of-freedom tests of genotype trend effect in unconditional logistic regression analysis adjusted for study, age, and three eigenvectors in a genome-wide association study of lung cancer in never-smoking Asian women (5510 with lung cancer and 4544 controls). The x-axis represents chromosome location, and the y-axis shows *p* values on a negative logarithmic scale. The red horizontal line represents the genome-wide significance threshold of $p = 5 \times 10^{-8}$. Labeled are two previously associated loci (TERT at 5p15.33 and TP63 at 3q28) together with three newly identified loci (VTI1A on chromosome 10 and ROS1-DCBLD1 and the HLA class II region on chromosome 6). *(Reprinted with permission from Lan Q, Hsiung CA, Matsuo K, et al. Genome-wide association analysis identifies new lung cancer susceptibility loci in never-smoking women in Asia. Nat Genetics. 2012;44:1330–1335.)*

differences in gender, age, and stage distribution were found for the two most common types of EGFR mutations.

FAMILY HISTORY

Nitadori et al.[71] evaluated the association between the incidence of lung cancer and family history in Japan. The authors concluded that, for women, the risk of lung cancer was higher if a first-degree relative was diagnosed with lung cancer (hazard ratio, 2.65, compared with 1.69 for men). However, this has not been a consistent finding. In a Taiwanese study, a family history of lung cancer in first-degree relatives was associated with a significantly increased risk of lung cancer for both men and women.[51] In another study, there was a 1.51-fold increase (95% CI, 1.39–1.63) in lung cancer risk for individuals who had a first-degree relative with lung cancer compared with individuals who had no family history of the disease, after adjustment for proband age, proband gender, ethnicity, education, smoking status of the proband, pack-years of smoking, and study number.[72] For ever-smoking individuals with a family history of lung cancer in a first-degree relative, the risk of lung cancer was increased 3.19-fold compared with never-smokers without a history of lung cancer in a first-degree relative. When stratified by relative type, the association was strongest for individuals who had a sibling with lung cancer (odds ratio, 1.82; 95% CI, 1.62–2.05), compared with a father (odds ratio, 1.25; 95% CI, 1.13–1.39) or mother (odds ratio, 1.37; 95% CI, 1.17–1.61). This pattern was similar in male and female probands (and for every histologic type examined), and the association was stronger among Asian individuals and those who were younger at the time of diagnosis (odds ratio, 1.83 and 1.45, respectively).[72]

VIRAL FACTORS

Human papillomavirus (HPV) may play a role in the development of lung cancer, especially in Asia. Some studies have shown that the prevalence of HPV-16 and HPV-18 infection is higher among never-smoking women older than 60 years of age with lung cancer compared with control patients (without cancer).[73,74] However, other studies have yielded different results.[75] In a retrospective evaluation of 223 lung cancer cases, HPV infection had no role in the pathogenesis of primary lung cancer, whereas HPV positivity was indicative of pulmonary metastasis from a primary HPV-associated cancer elsewhere in the body.[76] HPV has been associated with lung cancer in Asian populations, especially patients with EGFR activating mutations, who are often women. The prevalence of HPV infection among patients with lung cancer was 32% in a study from Taiwan; HPV infection and EGFR mutation were both found to be independently predictive of better survival.[77]

ENVIRONMENTAL EXPOSURES, DIET, AND PREEXISTING LUNG DISEASE

Environmental Exposures

The relationship between gender and the risk of lung cancer due to environmental exposures (asbestos, radiation, other chemicals, radon) and diet has not been extensively investigated. The risk for lung cancer has been higher among never-smoking women exposed to asbestos (odds ratio, 3.5; 95% CI, 1.2–10) and pesticides (odds ratio, 2.4; 95% CI, 1.1–5.6).[78] In a recent review, the burden of lung cancer in never-smokers attributable to previously identified risk factors was evaluated in different geographic regions. The population-attributable fractions of lung cancer related to the selected risk factors varied by geographic region. These risk factors appeared to be responsible for a substantial proportion of lung cancer in China, but accounted for a smaller proportion of cases in Europe and North America. In China, known risk factors accounted for a larger proportion of lung cancer cases in women than in men. For instance, increased levels of several carcinogens were found in the urine of nonsmoking Chinese women who reported frequent wok-style cooking.[50] Radiotherapy for breast cancer has been reported to increase the risk of lung cancer particularly in smokers. Among women who received adjuvant radiotherapy after mastectomy the risk of lung cancer was increased for women who smoked (odds ratio, 18.9; 95% CI, 7.9–45.4), but not for never-smokers.[79] According to data on 558,871 women with breast cancer in the Surveillance, Epidemiology and End Results (SEER) database who were followed for more than 20 years, the mortality rate was increased for women who had radiation therapy during 1973 to 1982 and 1983 to 1992, but not for women who had radiation therapy after 1993.[80]

Exposure to high levels of radon is also associated with an increased risk for the development of lung cancer, particularly in smokers or people exposed to secondhand smoke.[81] Bonner et al.[82] reported data on 66 women that were pooled from several case–control studies in which exposure to secondhand smoke and radon was assessed. Among women exposed to residential radon, the risk of lung cancer was threefold higher for women who had the *GSTM1* null genotype than for *GSTM1* carriers (odds ratio, 3.41; 95% CI, 1.10–10.61), even after adjusting for age, smoking status, and secondhand smoke exposure.[82]

In a Spanish study, the exposure to residential radon was evaluated in 69 never-smokers or light-smokers with lung cancer.[83] The median concentration of radon in men's homes was 199 Bq/m³, compared with 238 Bq/m³ in women's homes; the median concentration was 237 Bq/m³, a level higher than the reference level of 100 Bq/m³ recently recommended by WHO.[84] Higher radon concentrations were mainly associated with large cell and small cell histology. However, the study has some limitations, including the small cohort and the fact that residential radon concentrations among the participants were almost three times higher than that found in almost 2500 homes in the region studied.[83]

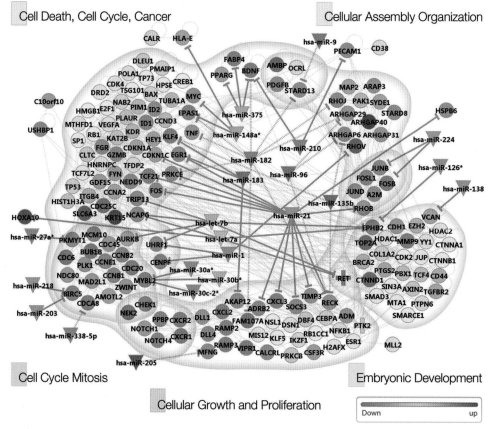

Fig. 5.6. Nonsmall cell lung cancer pathway modeling for female never-smokers. The pathway information was obtained from an ingenuity pathway analysis (IPA) using the 66 network module genes as an input list. The resulting genes were grouped into five functional categories as suggested by IPA. Validated and predicted microRNA-target relations are shown in solid and dotted lines, respectively. Changes in expression levels are indicated by node color (red for upregulation and blue for downregulation). For c-RET and PTK2, the "+" symbol is used to indicate that they are involved in a gene fusion event. *(Reprinted with permission from Kim SC, Jung Y, Park J, et al. A high-dimensional, deep-sequencing study of lung adenocarcinoma in female never-smokers.* PLoS One. *2013;8(2):e55596.)*

Diet

In case–control and cohort studies, high dietary intake of fruits and vegetables has reduced the risk of lung cancer.[85] Tomatoes and cruciferous consumption have also been associated with a decreased risk for lung cancer.[86–88] More than 71,000 Chinese women with no history of smoking or cancer at baseline were prospectively evaluated for their dietary intake with a follow-up time exceeding 11 years.[89] The main food contributors to riboflavin intake were rice, fresh milk, eggs, and bok choy; dietary riboflavin intake was inversely associated with lung cancer risk (hazard ratio, 0.62; 95% CI, 0.43–0.89; p = 0.03 for the highest quartile compared with the lowest).[89] In the same cohort, the intake of soy food before the diagnosis of lung cancer was associated with better overall survival.[90]

Preexisting Lung Disease

Preexisting lung diseases such as asthma and COPD can represent other potential risk factors for lung cancer. Several case–control studies have demonstrated an increased risk for the development of lung cancer in both men and women diagnosed with these nonneoplastic lung diseases.[91] Even after controlling for active and passive tobacco exposure, some studies have shown an increased risk for lung cancer.[92] Wu et al.[93] found that the risk for lung cancer was increased for nonsmoking women with

previous lung disease (adjusted odds ratio, 1.56; 95% CI, 1.2–2.0) and this finding was mainly driven by the prevalence of tuberculosis in this population.

STEROID HORMONES IN LUNG CANCER

Classical steroid hormone pathways have been successfully targeted in the treatment of breast and prostate cancer, where hormone-dependent growth has been well established. Steroid hormone receptors are known to be expressed in tissues outside the reproductive tract and to have biologic effects in tumors in nonreproductive sites. Some effects mediated by steroid receptors appear to be independent of steroid ligands and result from activation of steroid receptors by phosphorylation pathways. Steroid hormone receptors could thus have biologic activity via steroid-induced signaling or steroid-independent signaling. The findings of population studies and preclinical research suggest that steroid hormone pathways are involved in the biology of lung cancer, and the estrogen signaling pathway is a promising target for lung cancer therapy. The progesterone receptor (PR) may play a role in lung cancer biology as well.

Estrogen Receptors

The results of studies of gender differences in lung cancer risk and disease presentation suggest that estrogen may be involved

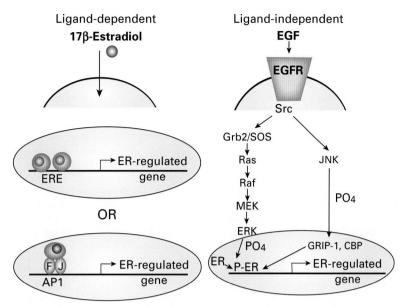

Fig. 5.7. Classic nuclear estrogenic effects in the lung. Nuclear estrogen receptors (ERs) can be activated in a ligand-dependent manner by 17-β-estradiol binding to nuclear ERs at either estrogen responsive elements (EREs) or activator protein 1 (AP1) sites utilizing the fos (F) and jun (J) transcription factors in the promoters of estrogen-regulated genes. Alternatively, nuclear ERs can be activated in a ligand-independent manner, such as through epidermal growth factor (EGF)-mediated ER receptor phosphorylation. EGF receptor (EGFR) activation is an example of such a pathway. *CBP*, calcium binding protein; *ERK*, extracellular regulated MAP kinase; *Grb2/SOS*, growth factor receptor bound protein 2/son of sevenless; *GRIP-1*, glutamate receptor interacting protein 1; *JNK*, c-jun N-terminal kinase; *MEK*, MAP kinase-ERK kinase; *P-ER*, phosphorylated estrogen receptor; *PO₄*, phosphate; *Raf*, cellular homolog of viral raf gene (v-raf); *Ras*, rat sarcoma; *Src*, Rous sarcoma oncogene. *(Reprinted with permission from Novello S, Brahmer JR, Stabile L, Siegfried JM. Gender-related differences in lung cancer. In: Pass HI, Carbone DP, Johnson DH, et al. (eds). Principles & Practice of Lung Cancer. The Official Reference Text of the IASLC, 4th ed. Copyright: Wolters Kluwer, Lippincott Williams & Wilkins; 2010.)*

in the etiology of this disease.[94] For example, women are more likely than men to have adenocarcinoma of the lung and to be never-smokers.[54] Also, the rate of diagnosis of lung cancer among never-smoking women is higher than among never-smoking men.[95] Estrogen receptors (ERs), members of the nuclear steroid receptor superfamily, mediate cellular response to estrogen. These proteins either function as ligand-activated transcription factors or can be activated by phosphorylation independent of ligand (Fig. 5.7).[96] Two forms of the ER have been identified, ERα and ERβ, which are encoded by separate genes and display different tissue distributions. In addition, multiple isoforms of ERα and ERβ exist, including at least five ERβ isoforms.[97–99]

The reports on the presence of ERs in lung tumors have been inconsistent. These differences could be due to interpretation of staining, antibodies and dilutions used, variability in the scoring assessment, or differences in patient cohort characteristics. With the identification of antibodies that distinguish between ERα and ERβ and more standard immunohistochemical procedures, it is now clear that ERβ is expressed and functional in most human nonsmall cell lung cancer (NSCLC) cell lines and is present in primary specimens of human NSCLCs from both men and women.[100–105] However, the frequency and function of the different ERβ isoforms in lung cancer are still not completely understood. There is less agreement about the expression of ERα in the lung. ERα was mainly found in the cytoplasm and membrane in immunohistochemical studies and was found to be composed of mostly alternatively spliced variants on immunoblot and RNA analysis.[100] This nonnuclear ERα pool may consist of a variant isoform that lacks the amino-terminal because it is differentially detected by antibodies that recognize the ERα amino- and carboxy-terminal.[100] ERβ, in contrast, is found in both the nucleus

and the cytoplasm and is composed of mainly full-length protein in addition to some variants.[100] ER-mediated RNA transcription and proliferation in lung tumor cell lines support the hypothesis that at least some forms of ER are functional.[100–106]

Several reports relating ER status to survival in NSCLC have shown nuclear localization of ERβ in 45.8% to 69% of lung cancer cases,[101–105] which was found to be a favorable prognostic indicator in some studies. In some reports, the prognostic significance was found only in men or was limited to a subset of patients with a particular mutation. However, most of these studies used antibodies to total ERβ that did not distinguish between the different ERβ isoforms. Recently, cytoplasmic ERβ-1 was identified as an independent negative prognostic factor for lung cancer.[105] This isoform specificity was confirmed in an additional study that showed that ERβ-1, but not ERβ-2, was linked to a worse prognosis in women with stage I lung cancer.[107] Nuclear ERβ-1 correlated with poor survival for patients with metastatic lung cancer but not in a cohort of patients with early-stage lung cancer.[108] Both ERβ-2 and ERβ-5 have been linked to better survival in lung cancer.[109]

Nuclear ERα expression is never or rarely detected in NSCLC tumors.[102–105] Prognostic significance of ERα was shown to have either no effect on survival or to correlate with poor prognosis.[101,102,105] Kawai et al.[101] reported that the presence of cytoplasmic ERα is associated with a worse prognosis among patients with NSCLC. Clearly, both nuclear and cytoplasmic ERs are important, and each component should be assessed separately and together when examining tissue specimens for clinical evaluation. In addition, further analysis on the various ERβ isoforms will be necessary to completely understand the role of ERβ in lung cancer. Standardized approaches should be developed and validated for screening of lung tumor ERs to validate the prognostic significance of these hormone markers. These markers may also be useful to identify patients who may have a response to hormone therapy for lung cancer.

Several studies have shown that women with advanced NSCLC live longer than men with advanced NSCLC.[110,111] A population study examining lung cancer presentation and survival in premenopausal and postmenopausal women demonstrated that more premenopausal women had advanced disease at the time of diagnosis, including poorly differentiated tumors with less favorable histologies.[112] However, in that study, survival for the two groups did not differ significantly. In a more recent study, women older than 60 years of age had a significant survival advantage over both men and younger women; the difference compared with younger women is potentially due to higher levels of circulating estrogen in the younger population.[113] Survival did not differ by age among men.

Exposure to exogenous estrogens through hormone replacement therapy (HRT) has a negative effect on lung cancer survival. Ganti et al.[114] evaluated nearly 500 women with lung cancer and found a significant association between both a lower median age at the time of lung cancer diagnosis and a shorter median survival time for women who used HRT around the time of diagnosis compared with women who did not. This effect was more pronounced in women who smoked than in women who did not, suggesting an interaction between estrogens and tobacco carcinogens. The Women's Health Initiative also reported a strong adverse effect on survival after a lung cancer diagnosis in women who received HRT.[115] In that randomized, placebo-controlled trial, more than 16,000 postmenopausal women received placebo or daily HRT for 5 years. The likelihood of dying from lung cancer was significantly greater in the HRT group, with a trend toward more lung cancer diagnoses compared with the placebo group. This increase in lung cancer incidence by HRT was also demonstrated in the Vitamins and Lifestyle Study, and the effect of HRT on lung cancer risk was duration dependent.[116] However, the findings of other studies have suggested that HRT use could actually protect women from the development of lung cancer, especially if they smoked.[117] An inverse relationship was also found between HRT use and NSCLC risk in postmenopausal women with ER-positive but not ER-negative lung tumors.[118] This finding may suggest different effects on the balance between induction of cell differentiation and cell proliferation by estrogen in normal lung epithelium compared with malignant epithelium. Because lung tumors are also known to produce aromatase (discussed later), it is possible that use of exogenous hormones reduced local estrogen production by inhibiting aromatase expression. Exact HRT used, duration of use, and timing of use is crucial information needed to elucidate the exact role of HRT on lung cancer risk and survival of women with lung cancer in future studies.

Retrospective population studies have recently demonstrated that antiestrogen use can influence survival in lung cancer. An observational study that included more than 6500 women with breast cancer showed significantly lower lung cancer mortality for women who received antiestrogen treatment.[119] Similarly, in the Manitoba Cancer Registry, in which 2320 women with or without exposure to antiestrogens were evaluated,[120] antiestrogen use both before and after lung cancer diagnosis was significantly associated with decreased mortality. Together, these studies on HRT and antiestrogen use support the idea of estrogen acting as a promoter of lung cancer aggressiveness and formation and perhaps having a key role not only in the biology but also the outcome of lung cancer.

Preclinical evidence also demonstrates that estrogen is a major driver of lung cancer. Estrogen acts to induce cell proliferation of NSCLC cells in vitro and in vivo and can modulate expression of genes in NSCLC cell lines that are important for inducing cell proliferation.[100,106] Genomic estrogen signaling has been demonstrated to occur mainly through ERβ in NSCLC

cells.[121,122] Furthermore, fulvestrant, an ER antagonist with no agonist effects, inhibits cell proliferation in vitro and lung tumor xenograft growth in severe combined immunodeficient mice by approximately 40%.[100] Thus, preclinical evidence strongly suggests that targeting the estrogen signaling pathway may have therapeutic value in the treatment or prevention of lung cancer.

Three strategies are currently available to target the estrogen signaling pathway in cancer cells: (1) antagonists of ER function through drugs such as tamoxifen and raloxifene; (2) downregulation of ER function through agents such as fulvestrant; and (3) reduction of estrogen levels through aromatase inhibitors, such as the reversible nonsteroidal agents letrozole and anastrozole and the irreversible steroidal inactivator exemestane.[123,124] Tamoxifen and raloxifene have partial agonist effects in certain tissues, such as endometrium. Tamoxifen has been shown to increase lung tumor xenograft growth and is not an appropriate choice of therapy for NSCLC.[121] Additionally, the National Surgical Adjuvant Breast and Bowel Project Breast Cancer Prevention Trial did not show any decreased risk of lung cancer.[125] Seventeen tumors of the lung, trachea, and bronchus were reported among the placebo group, and 20 were reported among the women in the tamoxifen group. Although not significant, these results suggest that tamoxifen could have some agonistic effects in the lung.

Aromatase

Lung cancer cells can also produce their own estrogen.[126] The aromatase enzyme, a member of the CYP450 family, catalyzes the conversion of the androgens androstenedione and testosterone to estrone and estradiol, respectively, and is expressed in the lung.[127,128] Preclinical work suggests that aromatase inhibitors are also potential inhibitors for lung cancer therapy. Aromatase protein was expressed in lung tumor cell lines and tumor tissue and was demonstrated to be functional.[126] Additionally, the growth of lung tumor xenografts decreased substantially when treated with anastrozole. Anastrozole was recently shown to prevent tobacco-induced lung carcinogenesis in female mice, and this effect was further enhanced when anastrozole was combined with fulvestrant.[129] Interestingly, in this animal model of lung cancer prevention, aromatase expression was confined almost exclusively to inflammatory cells that had infiltrated preneoplastic areas of the lungs, whereas the abnormal epithelial cells were mostly negative.[129] Thus, an important source of estrogen synthesis may be inflammatory cells that infiltrate the lungs in response to carcinogens, beginning early in carcinogenesis. This local production of estrogen may be part of the chronic inflammatory reaction occurring in lung tumors. Aromatase inhibitor therapy in lung cancer is further supported by Coombes et al.,[130] who reported a decreased incidence of primary lung cancer in women with breast cancer who were treated with exemestane after 2 years to 3 years of tamoxifen therapy (4 women) compared with continued tamoxifen treatment (12 women).

Mah et al.[131] identified aromatase as an early-stage predictive biomarker of lung cancer survival. Among women older than 65 years of age, lower levels of aromatase in tumor tissue predicted a greater chance of survival compared with women who had tumors with higher levels of aromatase expression. Furthermore, the prognostic value of aromatase expression was greatest for patients with stage I or II lung cancer. In this population of patients with low levels of circulating estrogen levels (because of decreased production by the ovaries), tumor cells could compensate for the loss by producing estrogen through aromatase. However, no general association between aromatase and lung cancer survival was found in a separate cohort unless aromatase expression was combined with that of other markers, such as ERβ, EGFR, and PR.[129] These results strongly suggest that aromatase inhibitors, which are already approved to treat breast cancer, may be of use to treat lung cancer in women with lung cancers that have high levels of aromatase. Aromatase expression may also be a new tool to predict survival at an early stage of disease, when more treatment options are available. A phase I clinical trial (NCT01664754) is currently underway to evaluate the side effects and best dose of the aromatase inhibitor exemestane in combination with pemetrexed and carboplatin to treat late-stage lung cancer. Other enzymes involved in intratumoral production and metabolism of estrogens are currently under investigation as potential targets for lung cancer therapy.[132]

Nongenomic Estrogen Signaling and Interactions With Growth Factor Receptor Signaling Pathways

In addition to the nuclear mechanisms of ER action, such as increased cell proliferation and gene transcription, estrogen can also rapidly activate signaling in seconds to minutes. These rapid signaling effects are referred to as nongenomic effects and occur via nonnuclear ERs located in the membrane or in the cytoplasm (Fig. 5.8). In human breast cancer cells, a membrane ER was identified as a G protein–coupled receptor called GPR30.[133,134] Expression of GPR30 has recently been demonstrated in lung cancer cells, but the function and regulation of GPR30 in the lung is still unknown.[135] In NSCLC cells, other extranuclear ERs have been identified in plasma membrane fractions and cytoplasmic fractions and have been shown to promote rapid stimulation of signaling pathways.[122,136] These effects can be inhibited by the addition of fulvestrant.

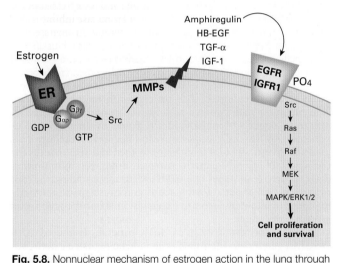

Fig. 5.8. Nonnuclear mechanism of estrogen action in the lung through rapid activation of growth factor receptors such as epidermal growth factor receptor (EGFR) and insulin growth factor receptor (IGFR1) in the cell membrane. Estrogen can bind to the estrogen receptor (ER) and activate G-proteins, which can activate Rous sarcoma oncogene (Src) and cause matrix metalloproteinases (MMPs) to cleave growth factor receptor ligands, such as amphiregulin, heparin-binding–epidermal growth factor (HB-EGF), tumor growth factor-α (TGF-α), and insulin-like growth factor-1 (IGF-1), to allow them to bind to EGFR. The ERK downstream signaling pathway is then activated, which ultimately leads to cell proliferation and survival. *GDP*, guanosine diphosphate; *GTP*, guanosine triphosphate; *MAPK/ERK1/2*, mitogen-activated kinase-like protein/elk-related tyrosine kinase; *MEK*, MAP kinase-ERK kinase; *PO₄*, phosphate; *Ras*, rat sarcoma; *Raf*, cellular homolog of viral raf gene (v-raf). *(Reprinted with permission from Novello S, Brahmer JR, Stabile L, Siegfried JM. Gender-related differences in lung cancer. In: Pass HI, Carbone DP, Johnson DH, et al. (eds). Principles & Practice of Lung Cancer. The Official Reference Text of the IASLC, 4th ed. Copyright: Wolters Kluwer, Lippincott Williams & Wilkins; 2010.)*

Nongenomic ER signaling acts in concert with growth factor signaling pathways, such as EGFR/HER-1 and the insulin-like growth factor 1 receptor (IGF-1R). EGFR is a member of the tyrosine kinase receptor family that also includes HER2, HER3, and HER4.[137] These receptors have been implicated in proliferation, cell motility, angiogenesis, cell survival, and differentiation.[138] Clinically, overexpression of EGFR correlates with poor prognosis in people with NSCLC.[101,139] Furthermore, combined overexpression of EGFR and ERα was demonstrated to be an independent indicator of poorer prognosis in lung cancer, consistent with cross-talk between these two pathways.[101] An interaction between ER and EGFR has been demonstrated in lung cancer cells.[121,140] In this regard, estrogen can rapidly activate EGFR in lung cancer cell lines (ligand-dependent signaling) and the combination of fulvestrant and gefitinib, an EGFR tyrosine kinase inhibitor (TKI), in NSCLC can maximally inhibit cell proliferation, induce apoptosis, and affect downstream signaling pathways both in vitro and in vivo.[121,141] The more clinically relevant EGFR TKI, erlotinib, also showed superior antitumor activity in NSCLC tumor xenograft experiments when used in combination with fulvestrant compared with single agent therapy as well as a multitargeted TKI, vandetanib.[141,142] A synergistic effect of gefitinib and the aromatase inhibitor anastrozole was found in lung cancer cell lines, further supporting a functional interaction between these pathways.[143] In addition, membrane ERs were found to be colocalized with EGFR in lung tumors.[136] Ligand-independent nongenomic signaling can also occur. EGF can directly phosphorylate ER at specific serine residues.[144] These residues were found to be phosphorylated in 87.5% of ER-positive lung tumors examined.[140]

A reciprocal control mechanism was also observed between ER and EGFR in lung cancer cells. EGFR protein expression was downregulated in response to estrogen and upregulated in response to fulvestrant in vitro, suggesting that the EGFR pathway is activated when estrogen is depleted.[121] Conversely, ERβ protein expression was downregulated in response to EGF and upregulated in response to gefitinib, providing a rationale to target these two pathways simultaneously.[121] Similar cross-talk has also recently been reported between the estrogen signaling pathway and the IGF-1R pathway in lung cancer. The IGF-1R signaling pathway has been implicated in lung cancer development. Estrogen has been shown to upregulate IGF-1R expression specifically through ERβ in lung cancer cells and tissues.[145] Furthermore, both aromatase and ERβ expression were positively correlated with IGF1 and IGF-1R expression. These pathways have also been demonstrated to act synergistically to promote the development of lung adenocarcinomas in mice.[146] Additionally, combined treatment with fulvestrant and an IGF-1R inhibitor showed maximum antitumor effects compared with single agent treatment in a carcinogen-induced lung cancer murine model.[146] Targeting EGFR through small molecule TKIs is of limited use in the absence of an EGFR mutation, which occurs in a minority of patients. Interestingly, the patients who have a response to EGFR TKIs are mainly women and never-smokers, which may relate to the bidirectional signaling between EGFR and ER in lung cancer.[147] Additionally, some studies have demonstrated a correlation between EGFR mutation and ER expression.[148,149] These observations have been translated to a phase I clinical trial using drugs that target these two signaling pathways to assess the toxicity of combined treatment with gefitinib and fulvestrant in 22 postmenopausal women.[150] Targeting both pathways was found to be safe and have antitumor activity in women with stage IIIB/IV NSCLC. Additionally, nuclear ERβ was correlated with improved patient survival. A phase II trial comparing the combination of erlotinib and fulvestrant with erlotinib alone showed that the combination treatment was well tolerated and progression-free survival was similar for the two treatments.[151] In patients with EGFR wild-type tumors, the clinical benefit rate was significantly higher among patients treated with the combination

(3 people who had a partial response) compared with erlotinib alone, with a trend toward improved survival. The findings of these clinical trials suggest that targeting the ER signaling pathway via both nuclear and extranuclear receptors in conjunction with the EGFR signaling pathway has increased beneficial antitumor effects in NSCLC, as has been observed in breast cancer cells,[152] particularly in patients whose tumors do not contain an EGFR mutation. The combination of antiestrogen therapy with an IGF-1R inhibitor also warrants clinical investigation.

Progesterone Receptors

Progesterone effects are mediated through the PR. There are two main isoforms of PR, PR-A and PR-B, which play different roles in modulating cellular responses to progesterone. In general, the presence of PR in breast cancer indicates a more differentiated tumor that is responsive to antiestrogen therapy, and PR is a known estrogen-responsive gene. The ratio of PR-A:PR-B is thought to affect the clinical outcome in breast cancer. Several studies have demonstrated the expression of total PR by primary NSCLC, although the reported frequency of expression has varied greatly.[104,105,153–158] Several studies found little or no PR in NSCLC,[104,155,158] whereas PR expression was lower in lung tumors than in matched normal lung tissue.[105] Two studies showed that PR is a strong protective factor for lung cancer.[105,156] The antibodies used in these lung cancer survival studies do not distinguish between the PR-A and PR-B isoforms, which could exert different functions. Enzymes capable of synthesizing progesterone were also detected in many NSCLCs, and a positive correlation was found between intratumoral levels of progesterone and the presence of three enzymes that participate in progesterone synthesis.[156] Progesterone treatment led to growth inhibition of tumor xenografts and concomitant induction of apoptosis, in agreement with clinical data suggesting that the presence of PR was correlated with longer overall survival in NSCLC.[156] In addition, progesterone has been shown to inhibit the migration and invasion of lung cancer cell lines.[159] In breast cancer, PR is known to signal through ligand-independent mechanisms due to phosphorylation by kinases.[160] One mechanism for low tumor PR expression in breast tumors is through increased growth factor signaling, which leads to a more aggressive tumor biology with faster progression.[161] Whether this same mechanism occurs in lung tumors is unknown and is currently being investigated.

Progesterone derivatives have been useful in the treatment of both endometrial cancer and breast cancer.[162,163] Agents such as medroxyprogesterone acetate, which can be given orally, have potential for treatment of lung cancer, perhaps in combination with agents that suppress either the ER pathway or act on growth factor pathways such as EGFR or c-Met, or other TKIs. Long-term progesterone treatment may even be feasible for chemoprevention of lung cancer.

Implications for Lung Cancer Therapy

Research on estrogen in lung cancer is likely to benefit both men and women. Because lung tumors from both men and women express ER and aromatase and cell lines derived from both men and women respond to estrogens, antiestrogens, and aromatase inhibitors, these types of treatments may be beneficial for both populations, not solely women. Preclinical evidence suggests that these hormone therapies are effective in male mice (Stabile and Siegfried, unpublished data). Further understanding of the role of estrogen, estrogen synthesis, and ERs in lung cancer will provide a rationale for future targeting of this pathway for therapy earlier in the course of disease and possibly for lung cancer prevention. Additional understanding of the role of nonnuclear versus nuclear ERs as well as PRs in lung cancer and which drugs affect which receptors will be important for designing new effective treatments and clinically exploitable strategies. As hormone therapies are currently being evaluated in the clinic for lung cancer, identification of patients most likely to benefit is warranted to guide the design of future clinical trials targeting this pathway. Biomarker identification will be key to selecting the best candidates for hormone therapy in lung cancer. Because antiestrogens are safe and can be given for long periods of time, there is tremendous potential to bring them to clinical use for lung cancer.

GENDER AS A PROGNOSTIC FACTOR IN EARLY-STAGE LUNG CANCER

Although several studies have addressed different aspects of gender and lung cancer, the causes of these differences are still not yet well-defined, and, consequently, gender differences are not currently accounted for in terms of public health or of diagnosis and treatment. Several authors have reported a more favorable prognosis of lung cancer in women than in men, regardless of a longer life expectancy or the influence of other factors (Fig. 5.9). For all cancer sites combined, studies have shown better survival for women than for men. In an observational analysis performed in Tyrol, after adjusting for staging distribution, investigators found that the risk of death was lower among women (compared with men) who had lung, stomach, or head and neck cancer, as well as for all cancer sites combined, after adjusting for case mix.[164] A study of 3742 people with lung cancer (26% women), showed a significant reduction of the relative excess risk (0.82; 95% CI, 0.75–0.90) for women compared with men.[164] In a large population-based analysis conducted in patients with early disease, more women had surgery (64% vs. 56%; $p = 0.001$), and more men received radiation therapy (23% vs. 18%; $p = 0.001$). A similar trend, although to a lesser extent, was also reported for patients with local-regional disease.[22] In a Polish cancer registry, information regarding 20,561 patients diagnosed from 1995 to 1998 was collected, and a univariate analysis demonstrated that the relative risk of death for women was significantly inferior ($p = 0.001$) to that for men.[22]

In a French cohort of 208 patients with lung cancer, after adjustment for stage, women with each stage of disease lived significantly longer.[165] Similarly, in a retrospective review of 7553 patients with NSCLC treated between 1974 and 1998, the overall median survival was 12.4 months for women and 10.3 months for men ($p = 0.001$), and again, the survival advantage was uniformly detected across all stages ($p = 0.001$).[166] In these studies, the lack of information about smoking status and cause-specific mortality does not allow any definitive conclusion about the prognostic influence of gender.

In a prospective cohort of 4618 patients diagnosed with NSCLC, gender was identified as an independent prognostic factor after adjusting for age at diagnosis, tumor histology and grade, stage, smoking history (in pack-years), and treatment (resection, radiation therapy, or chemotherapy).[167] Stage of disease at diagnosis and treatment did not differ between men and women. The estimated 1-year and 5-year survival rates were 51% (95% CI, 49%, 53%) and 15% (95% CI, 12%, 17%), respectively, for men, compared with 60% (95% CI, 58%, 62%) and 19% (95% CI, 16%, 22%) for women. Men were at a significantly increased risk for death compared with women (adjusted relative risk, 1.20; 95% CI, 1.11–1.30), especially for men with stage III/IV disease or adenocarcinoma.

Data on a cohort of 10,908 patients with NSCLC (6665 men and 4243 women) from the Manitoba Cancer Registry showed a significantly better survival rate for women, independent of treatment, age, year of diagnosis, and histology ($p < 0.001$).[168] The adjusted hazard ratio for death for men compared with women was 1.13 (95% CI, 1.04–1.23; $p = 0.004$). Gender modified the effect of surgical treatment (hazard ratio, 1.26; 95% CI, 1.13–1.40; $p < 0.001$) and adenocarcinoma histology (hazard ratio, 1.36; 95% CI, 1.24–1.50; $p < 0.001$) when treatment was taken into account.

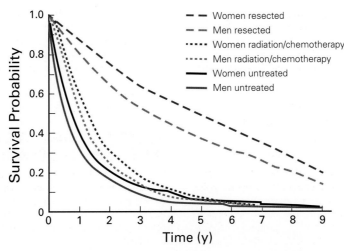

Fig. 5.9. Lung cancer–specific survival curves by gender and type of treatment. Women had a significant survival benefit compared with men, regardless of the type of treatment. *(Reprinted with permission from Novello S, Brahmer JR, Stabile L, Siegfried JM. Gender-related differences in lung cancer. In: Pass HI, Carbone DP, Johnson DH, et al. (eds).* Principles & Practice of Lung Cancer. The Official Reference Text of the IASLC, 4th ed. *Copyright: Wolters Kluwer, Lippincott Williams & Wilkins; 2010.)*

A retrospective analysis of data in a prospectively validated thoracic surgery database demonstrated superior survival for women with all disease stages (*p* = 0.0003).[169] Subset analysis by histologic type demonstrated that, among patients with adenocarcinoma, survival was superior for women (*p* < 0.001); no gender difference was found for squamous cell carcinoma (*p* = 0.2).

One potential explanation for such differences is telomere length in peripheral blood, which would have significant predictive value for risk of recurrence after curative resection in NSCLC. One prospective study including 473 patients with histologically confirmed early stage NSCLC who underwent curative resection between 1995 and 2008 suggests that long relative telomere length is associated with recurrence and that women and patients with adenocarcinoma appear to represent a subgroup in which telomere biology may play an important role.[170]

Researchers analyzing data from the SEER-Medicare database covering the period 2000 to 2005 identified patients who had had lobectomy for stage I NSCLC and evaluated the in-hospital postoperative complications (pulmonary, cardiac, infectious, noncardiopulmonary) that led to a longer hospital stay (>8 days). These complications were significantly associated with male gender, older age at diagnosis (75 years or older), higher comorbidity index, larger tumors, and treatment at nonteaching hospitals (*p* < 0.05).[171]

Some of these findings have been confirmed in prospective studies. Cerfolio et al.[169] analyzed a cohort of 1085 patients and detected an overall age-adjusted and stage-adjusted 5-year survival rate favoring women (60% vs. 50%; *p* = 0.001). Stage-specific 5-year survival rates were also better for women (Table 5.1). Women who received neoadjuvant chemotherapy were more likely than men to have a complete or partial response (*p* = 0.025). These findings were similar to those in a single institution study of patients with completely resected NSCLC, in which pathologic stage, female gender, and squamous cell histology were independent predictors of survival.[173] Women with pathologic stage I disease had a significant survival advantage compared with men (*p* = 0.01), and women with stage II and stage III disease had moderately better survival (*p* = 0.3). This survival benefit was also demonstrated in a small study (Table 5.1).[166] A similar survival trend according to stage, with a more pronounced survival difference for stage I and II, was also confirmed in two other studies, and the impact of gender on survival independent from smoking status was also reported in a large Japanese cohort of 12,703 patients with resected NSCLC.[174–176]

TABLE 5.1 Comparison of Five-Year Survival for Men and Women According to Stage of Lung Cancer in Three Studies

	5-Year Survival (%)	
	Women	**Men**
CERFOLIO ET AL.[172] (414 WOMEN, 671 MEN)		
Stage I	69	64
Stage II	60	50
Stage III	46	37
ALEXIOU ET AL.[173] (252 WOMEN, 581 MEN)		
Stage I	56	42
Stage II	41	32
Stage III	21	16
OUELLETTE ET AL.[165] (104 WOMEN, 104 MEN)		
Stage I	47.2	32.7
Stage II	63.1	51.5
Stage III	14.5	6.1

The survival advantage for women is also maintained among older patient populations. A population-based analysis of data from the SEER database focused on the cases of 18,967 patients aged 65 years or older with stage I or II NSCLC diagnosed between 1991 and 1999.[177] Patients were grouped into three categories according to treatment: surgery, radiation therapy or chemotherapy, or no treatment. Survival data were controlled for competing risks, including lung cancer–specific survival, overall survival adjusting for comorbidities, and relative survival. In all treatment groups, the lung cancer–specific, overall, and relative survival were better for women than for men (*p* = 0.0001), and this benefit was retained in multivariate analysis. Sensitivity analyses demonstrated that these survival differences were not related to different smoking behaviors. Gender differences were also found among untreated patients, and this may suggest that lung cancer has a different natural history in women.[177]

Findings from population-based studies have indicated that more women have earlier stage disease at the time of diagnosis. A higher rate of health-care access among women in ongoing early detection studies raises the issue of whether or not the survival advantage by gender may be attributable to more frequent medical consultation and radiographic assessment rather than to differences in genetic predisposition and natural history of the neoplastic disease.

TABLE 5.2 Survival Data for Men and Women With Advanced Nonsmall Cell Lung Cancer

Author	Treatment	Survival			
		Median (Mos.)		1 Year (%)	
Albain et al.[111] (1949 men, 582 women)	Platinum and nonplatinum-based (phase II/III)	5.7[a]	4.8	19	14
O'Connell et al.[110] (265 men, 113 women)	Cisplatin and vinca alkaloids	12.4[b]	8.8	NR	NR
Schiller et al.[183] (760 men, 447 women)	Cisplatin and paclitaxel Cisplatin and gemcitabine Cisplatin and docetaxel Carboplatin and paclitaxel	9.2[c]	7.3	38	31

[a] $p < 0.01$.

[b] $p = 0.001$.

[c] $p = 0.004$.
NR, not reported.

The Early Lung Cancer Action Program screening project gave insights into women and lung cancer.[178] In the International Early Lung Cancer Action Program, baseline computed tomography (CT) screening for lung cancer was done on 14,435 asymptomatic volunteers who were at least 40 years of age, had no history of cancer, were past or current cigarette smokers, and were fit to undergo thoracic surgery.[179] Lung cancer was diagnosed in 111 of 6296 women and 93 of 8139 men. In terms of prevalence, the women-to-men odds ratio was 1.6 ($p \leq 0.001$). Women who were diagnosed with lung cancer were of a comparable age to men (67 years vs. 68 years) but had a significantly reduced tobacco exposure (47 pack-years vs. 64 pack-years). Additionally, women were more frequently diagnosed with clinical stage I disease (89% vs. 80%), but the rate of resection for stage I disease was only slightly higher than that for men (90% vs. 88%). The proportion of adenocarcinoma subtype among women and men was 73% and 59%, respectively.[179]

According to the findings of this study, the hypothesis that women may be more susceptible to tobacco carcinogens appears biologically plausible. If lung cancer risk for women who smoke is indeed higher than the risk for men of the same age who smoke, antismoking efforts directed to girls and women should be even more aggressive than those directed to boys and men. Because early detection programs are conducted among smokers, female gender may call for screening at lower levels of tobacco exposure than the threshold for men.

Consistent findings were reported from NELSON, a European study of CT screening of 15,822 participants.[180] Women diagnosed with lung cancer were significantly younger (58 years vs. 62 years; $p = 0.03$), had a lower smoking load (36 pack-years vs. 43 pack-years; $p = 0.03$), and had a lower body mass index (23.8 vs. 25.9; $p = 0.03$) than men. However, the percentage of current smokers was similar (56.7% vs. 55.9%; $p = 0.93$). Histologic subtypes were evenly distributed between men and women. Significantly more women had an early stage of disease at the time of diagnosis ($p = 0.005$). This finding held true after correcting for gender differences in age, smoking load, and body mass index ($p = 0.028$).[180]

PROGNOSTIC/PREDICTIVE ROLE OF GENDER IN ADVANCED DISEASE

Insights From Therapeutic Trials: NSCLC

Chemotherapy

Gender may be potentially considered either prognostic or predictive of a higher effectiveness of chemotherapy. The findings of a retrospective population-based study of 15,185 Japanese and 13,332 white patients treated between 1991 and 2001 suggested that Japanese ethnicity ($p = 0.003$) and never-smoking status ($p = 0.010$) were independent favorable factors for overall survival in addition to female gender and other variables such as younger age, early stage, and treatment received.[181]

A large retrospective study was conducted to review 13 Southwestern Oncology Group (SWOG) trials in which 2531 women were enrolled in clinical trials between 1974 and 1987.[108] Women had a survival advantage, with a median survival of 5.7 months compared with 4.8 months for men, and 1-year survival rates of 19% and 14% ($p < 0.01$). This benefit, however, was not maintained in multivariate analysis. Similarly, a nonsignificant difference in survival by gender was reported in the setting of multimodality therapy for locally advanced disease (median survival, 21 months for women vs. 12 months for men).[182] Survival advantage according to gender was also demonstrated in a single institution study of 378 patients with advanced stage NSCLC treated with chemotherapy, in which female gender was one of four predictors of improved survival in a multivariate analysis, and in the Eastern Cooperative Oncology Group (ECOG) 1594 study (Table 5.2).[110,183,184]

The prognostic role of gender was extensively assessed in ECOG 1594 because of the lack of survival difference among four treatment arms.[183,184] The median survival for the 1207 enrolled patients was 8 months, and all the other efficacy outcomes were comparable among the four arms. Men were more likely to have weight loss (65% vs. 58%, $p = 0.02$) and to be slightly older (mean age, 61.9 years vs. 60.5 years, $p = 0.02$). Women were more likely to have adenocarcinoma histology (63% vs. 53%, $p = 0.003$). The overall response rate did not differ by gender (19% in both cohorts; $p = 0.15$). The median progression-free survival and median survival time differed by gender; the median progression-free survival was 3.8 months for women compared with 3.5 months for men ($p = 0.022$), and the median survival was 9.2 months for women and 7.3 months for men ($p = 0.004$). Survival was also better at 1, 2, and 3 years: 38%, 14%, and 7% for women, respectively, compared with 31%, 11%, and 5% for men. This survival difference remained significant after adjusting for performance status, weight loss of more than 10%, presence of brain metastases, and stage (IIIB vs. IV). In terms of toxicity, nausea, vomiting, alopecia, neurosensory deficits, and neuropsychiatric deficits tended to be common among women.

The European Lung Cancer Working Party retrospectively analyzed 1052 patients treated between 1980 and 1991 for locally advanced or metastatic NSCLC.[185] The statistical analysis included 23 pretreatment variables, and female gender was one of eight variables significantly associated with improved survival, with a relative risk of death of 0.7 ($p = 0.03$) in a multivariate analysis.

Gender-related differences in survival were not identified in a study by the North Central Cancer Treatment Group.[183] Nine trials (6 phase II and 3 phase III) conducted from 1985 to 2001 were retrospectively considered. The chemotherapy regimen was platinum-based in five of the trials. In the multivariate analysis, gender was not an independent prognostic factor for improved overall survival and time to progression. Similar to the ECOG 1594 study, a difference in toxicity was found: the rates of both grade 3 hematologic and nonhematologic toxicities were higher for women than men, with an odds ratio of 1.60 ($p = 0.0007$) and 1.71 ($p < 0.001$), respectively.[186]

The TAX 326 trial was a multinational, phase III study of docetaxel plus carboplatin or docetaxel plus cisplatin compared with a reference regimen of vinorelbine plus cisplatin.[184] Baseline characteristics were well-balanced across treatment groups. Approximately two-thirds of the patients in each treatment group had stage IV disease. Within each arm of the study, a trend favored a survival advantage for women.[187,188] Again, gender differences in toxicity were noted: women were more likely than men to have grade 3 nausea and vomiting and neurotoxicity across all three treatment arms, whereas the rate of hematologic and other nonhematologic toxicity was similar for both groups.

A large randomized clinical trial compared cisplatin plus gemcitabine to cisplatin plus pemetrexed in 1725 chemotherapy naive patients (515 women) with stage IIIB or IV NSCLC.[189] The study showed the superior activity (better response rate and overall survival) of cisplatin and pemetrexed in "nonsquamous" NSCLC. Factors that had a significant prognostic impact on survival (independent of treatment) included gender, race, performance status, disease stage, and histology.

As a consequence of the prognostic significance of gender, a hypothetical clinical trial of a new therapy that includes patients with lower stages of disease, performance status of 0 or 1, and a high percentage of women will yield favorable results based on these selection factors alone, independent of the efficacy of therapy.

One potential explanation for better survival among women is gender differences in DNA-repair capacities that make tumors in women more responsive to platinum-based chemotherapies. DNA-repair machinery has been shown to be more defective in women, making them more susceptible to respiratory carcinogens but also more sensitive to DNA-interfering agents. Wei et al.[190] showed an association between suboptimal DNA repair and an increased risk of lung cancer. These findings were subsequently confirmed in other studies, which identified pack-years smoked as an independent predictor of lung cancer risk and also found higher DNA repair in patients with a greater smoking history and lower DNA repair in women than in men.[190,191]

NSCLC is considered to be relatively refractory to chemotherapy, which has been associated with elevated nucleotide excision repair in tumor tissue. In a case–control study, 375 patients with newly diagnosed NSCLC were accrued, and nucleotide excision repair activity was estimated by the DNA repair capacity (DRC) measured in the patient's peripheral blood lymphocytes by the host cell reactivation assay.[192] For every unit of increase in DRC, there was a progressive increase in the relative risk of death. Of the 86 patients who received chemotherapy, patients in the top quartile of the DRC distribution were at twice the relative risk of death as patients in the lowest quartile (relative risk, 2.72; 95% CI, 1.24–5.95; $p = 0.01$), whereas effective DRC was not a risk factor for death among patients who did not receive chemotherapy. In univariate analysis of the relationship between DRC and clinical and demographic variables, DRC was significantly higher in men than in women (8.37% ± 2.92% vs. 7.13% ± 2.37%; $p < 0.001$) but was not related to stage of disease, histology, differentiation of the tumor, or self-reported weight loss.[192]

Targeted Therapies

From a molecular biology perspective, lung cancer in women should be considered a specific entity. For instance, EGFR mutation appears to occur more frequently in women than in men, leading to a better response rate to treatment with an EGFR TKI.[193] When primary lung tumor tissues from surgically treated patients (50 men, 50 women) were analyzed and compared for expression of some hormone receptors and EGFR and KRAS mutations, EGFR mutation was significantly more frequent in women than in men ($p = 0.05$).[194] In addition, a positive link between EGFR expression and both ERα ($p = 0.028$) and ERβ ($p = 0.047$) expression both in men and women was found. The frequency of KRAS mutation was similar for men and women (13%).

In the Biomarker-Integrated Approaches of Targeted Therapy for Lung Cancer Elimination trial, 255 patients with previously treated NSCLC were randomly assigned to four separate phase II targeted-therapy treatments (erlotinib, erlotinib and bexarotene, vandetanib, and sorafenib), guided by the analysis of 11 prespecified markers assessed in core tumor biopsies.[195] Tumor tissue biomarkers showed distinct differences by gender and age: women were more likely to have an EGFR mutation (9.8% vs. 5.6%, $p = 0.02$) and EGFR gene amplification (9.9% vs. 6.1%, $p = 0.04$), whereas men were more likely to have a BRAF or KRAS mutation. Nelson et al.[196] showed that, among smokers, female gender and the presence of KRAS mutation were significantly associated, and this association persisted after adjustment for carcinogen exposures (odds ratio, 3.3; 95% CI, 1.3–7.9).[196] These findings suggest a possible role of estrogen exposure in either the initiation or the selection of KRAS mutant clones in adenocarcinoma.

Data from several phase II and III clinical trials that evaluated the role of reversible EGFR TKIs, erlotinib and gefitinib, in the setting of second- and third-line treatment of NSCLC indicate a higher responsiveness to these agents among women. In the Iressa Dose Evaluation in Advanced Lung Cancer (IDEAL) 1 and 2 studies, female gender was associated with improved outcomes with gefitinib for treatment of advanced NSCLC that had been previously treated with one or two lines of chemotherapy (Table 5.3).[193,197] In the IDEAL 2 study, 50% of women had improvement in symptoms compared with 31% of men, and 82% of the partial responses occurred in women.[193]

In a randomized double-blind, placebo-controlled phase III trial in second- and third-line treatment of advanced NSCLC, the response rate for patients treated with daily erlotinib was 8.9%, with a median survival of 6.7 months; the median survival was 4.7 months for patients who received placebo, resulting in a 42% improvement in median survival associated with erlotinib.[198] The 1-year survival rate was 31% in the erlotinib arm and 21% in the placebo arm. The response rate was significantly superior in women (Table 5.3), but in the multivariate analysis, gender was not predictive of increased response to erlotinib.

In a large phase II study, 138 patients with a diagnosis of bronchoalveolar carcinoma received gefitinib as first- or second-line treatment. Superior activity was reported for women, and survival was significantly superior for previously untreated women compared with untreated men ($p = 0.04$).[199]

Deng et al.[200] conducted a prospective clinical study that enrolled 40 Chinese women (97.5% never-smokers) with locally advanced or metastatic NSCLC (mostly adenocarcinomas) that had not responded to at least one platinum-based chemotherapy regimen.[200] The women received gefitinib monotherapy (250 mg/day), and the overall response rate was 62.5%. The median overall survival was 20 months (95% CI, 11.9–28), with 70% of women surviving 1 year and 32.5% surviving 2 years. Survival for women who had clinical benefit (complete response, partial response, or stable disease) was significantly longer than that for women who had progressive disease ($p = 0.024$), and survival for

TABLE 5.3 Gender Differences in Patients With Nonsmall Cell Lung Cancer Treated With an Epidermal Growth Factor Receptor (EGFR) Inhibitor

Author	Treatment	Overall Response Rate (Men and Women) (%)	Gender Difference
Fukuoka et al.[197]	Gefitinib 250 mg (78 men, 26 women) Gefitinib 500 mg (70 men, 36 women)	18.4 19.0	Odds ratio, W:M: 2.6 (p = 0.017)
Kris et al.[193]	Gefitinib 250 mg (60 men, 42 women) Gefitinib 500 mg (63 men, 51 women)	12 10	Response rate: 10% (women) vs. 2% (men)
Shepherd et al.[198]	Erlotinib (315 men, 173 women) Placebo (160 men, 83 women)	8.9 <1	Response rate: 14.4% (women) vs. 6.0% (men)

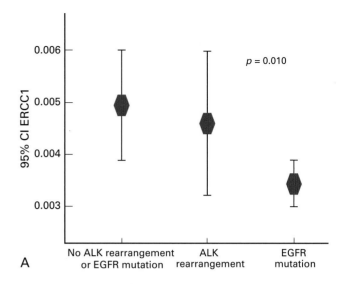

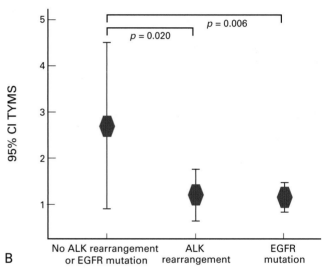

Fig. 5.10. (A) Bar plots illustrating the distribution of excision repair cross-complementing 1 (ERCC1) mRNA expression. (B) Bar plots illustrating the distribution of excision repair cross-complementing thymidylate synthetase (TYMS) mRNA expression. Expression of ERCC1 mRNA and of TYMS mRNA differed significantly among patients who had anaplastic lymphoma kinase (ALK) rearrangement, epidermal growth factor receptor (EGFR) mutation, or neither genetic abnormality. (Three-sided U test p values are given in A and two-sided t test p values are given in B.) *(Modified with permission from Ren S, Chen X, Kuang P, et al. Association of EGFR mutation or ALK rearrangement with expression of DNA repair and synthesis genes in never-smoker women with pulmonary adenocarcinoma. Cancer. 2012;118(22):5588–5594.)*

women with stable disease was not inferior to that for women with complete or partial response (p = 0.742). The median progression-free survival was 13 months (95% CI, 8.0–17.9).[200]

To date, none of the randomized trials addressing the role of EGFR TKIs as first-line treatment compared with platinum-based chemotherapy has shown gender differences in terms of efficacy or toxicity profile.

Published data indicate that the majority of lung adenocarcinomas from nonsmoking East Asian women can be molecularly characterized by targetable oncogenic mutant kinases, mainly EGFR mutation and anaplastic lymphoma kinase (ALK) rearrangement. Sun et al.[201] reported that the rate of EGFR mutation was as high as 82.9% in pulmonary adenocarcinoma samples from 41 Chinese women who were nonsmokers.[201] Furthermore, Wu et al.[202] documented a 34% rate of ALK rearrangement among Taiwanese patients with wild-type EGFR.[202] In another study, 104 Chinese never-smoking women with resected lung adenocarcinoma were analyzed for EGFR mutation; ALK rearrangement; and mRNA expression of the ERCC1, RRM1, TS, and BRCA1 genes. EGFR mutation was documented in 70.2% of the women and ALK rearrangement in 9.6%.[203] Specimens that harbored activating EGFR mutation were more likely to express low ERCC1 and TS mRNA levels, whereas specimens with ALK rearrangement were more likely to express low TS mRNA levels. These findings support the hypothesis that EGFR mutation and ALK rearrangement affect the efficacy of chemotherapy through the pathways of DNA repair and synthesis genes (Fig. 5.10).[203]

Vandetanib is an oral TKI with dual activity against both the vascular endothelial growth factor receptor and EGFR pathways that failed to demonstrate a survival improvement in NSCLC. However, across different trials, a trend for greater benefit was found among women who received vandetanib.[204,205]

The ECOG 4599 trial compared carboplatin and paclitaxel with or without bevacizumab in patients with advanced-stage NSCLC.[206] Bevacizumab improved all the efficacy outcomes including overall response rate, progression-free survival, and overall survival. However, an unplanned subset analysis did not show a survival benefit for women treated with bevacizumab. Women accounted for 46% (387) of the enrolled patients, with some unbalances in baseline characteristics that were well-balanced in men. Fewer women had liver involvement (11.7% vs. 23.2%, p = 0.003), compared with men in both arms of the study (20.6% and 20.0%, respectively), and this unbalance could be one of the reasons for the different outcomes. A slightly higher proportion of women who received the triplet combination had weight loss of 5% or more before therapy compared with women treated with the doublet

(32.4% vs. 24.4%, p = 0.09). Although the addition of bevacizumab improved both overall response rate and progression-free survival for men and women, the addition of bevacizumab had a different effect on overall survival. Overall survival was improved in both groups (12.3 months for the triplet vs. 10.3 months for the doublet), but the beneficial effect on survival was limited to men (11.7 vs. 8.7 months; hazard ratio, 0.70; 95% CI, 0.57–0.87; p ≥ 0.001). The outcomes for women were similar in both groups (13.3 vs. 13.1 months; hazard ratio, 0.98; 95% CI, 0.77–1.25; p = 0.87) (Table 5.4).[203]

In an attempt to explain the lack of survival benefit for women, researchers have already explored some variables, such as the

TABLE 5.4 Efficacy of Bevacizumab in Advanced Nonsmall Cell Lung Cancer, by Gender

	Paclitaxel and Carboplatin		Paclitaxel and Carboplatin and Bevacizumab	
	Women (*n* = 162)	Men (*n* = 230)	Women (*n* = 190)	Men (*n* = 191)
Response rate (%)	14.2	15.7	41.1	28.8
Progression-free survival (mo)	5.3	4.3	4.3	6.3
Overall survival (mo)	13.1	8.7	13.3	11.7

number of cycles and maintenance with bevacizumab, second-line therapies, and factors that affect clearance of bevacizumab (body mass index, albumin concentration, liver metastases), but whether the survival data are related to statistical chance or represent a true gender-based difference is still unclear. A difference in some toxicities was also noted: grade 5 neutropenia or infections with neutropenia were more common among women than among men who were treated with the triplet regimen. In addition, the rate of constipation was higher (4.7% vs. 1.4%, *p* = 0.05) and the rate of abdominal pain was higher (5.2% vs. 0.9%, *p* = 0.01). However, the potential unbalance in other prognostic factors, such as EGFR mutation, smoking status, or comorbidities, should also be assessed. Further analysis of this patient population showed a differential survival benefit from bevacizumab by age in women, but not men: women aged 60 years or older treated with chemotherapy lived longer than their male counterparts and younger women; in contrast, the survival benefit with bevacizumab was more pronounced in men of any age and in younger women.[113]

Insights From Therapeutic Trials: SCLC

Less information about gender-related differences in survival in SCLC is available. The analysis of four consecutive prospective trials showed a better overall survival favoring women.[207] A total of 2580 patients (from 10 SWOG trials) with limited disease and extensive disease were analyzed for prognostic factors. Female gender was a significant favorable independent predictor of survival only for limited disease (*p* ≤ 0.0001).[208]

Individual patient data from six randomized phase II/ III chemotherapy trials investigating chemotherapy regimens in limited stage or extensive stage SCLC, conducted by the Manchester Lung Group and the Medical Research Council from 1993 to 2005, were pooled for analysis: 1707 patients were included, 44% of whom were women.[209] Response rates were similar for women and men (77% vs. 76%, *p* = 0.64), but in univariate and multivariate analyses, female gender predicted longer survival. As in previous studies, grade 3 or grade 4 emesis was more common among women (18% vs. 9%, *p* < 0.0001), as was grade 3 or grade 4 mucositis (13% vs. 8%, *p* = 0.005); no gender differences were found in terms of hematologic toxicities in dose intensity, infections, transfusions, or treatment-related deaths.[209]

CONCLUSION

Although in recent years the mortality rates for lung cancer have reached a plateau, the number of women who will die from lung cancer remains alarmingly high. A better understanding of the genetic, metabolic, and hormonal factors that affect the way women react to carcinogens and lung cancer represents a research priority. This information could affect the way patients who smoke are screened and evaluated, as well as the way smoking cessation and lung cancer prevention programs are directed.

Evidence suggests that the development of lung cancer is different in women than in men. Adenocarcinoma of the lung is more likely to develop in female smokers than in male smokers. Among never-smokers, lung cancer is more likely to develop in women than in men. Women with lung cancer also live longer than men with lung cancer, regardless of therapy and stage, although this is also true of other types of cancer. Differences between men and women with regard to the etiology and clinical presentation of lung cancer are most likely caused by a complex interaction between differences in exposure to lung carcinogenesis as well as hormonal, genetic, and metabolic differences. The variations in response to EGFR inhibitors and antiangiogenesis drugs between men and women are intriguing but insufficient to allow the gender of the patient guide the choice of therapy. All large trials in lung cancer should stratify patients according to gender, and as we enter the era of more personalized medicine, an understanding of how lung cancer in men and women differs will be a crucial factor in therapeutic choice in the future.

KEY REFERENCES

11. Jemal A, Ma J, Rosenberg PS, et al. Increasing lung cancer death rates among young women in southern and midwestern states. *J Clin Oncol.* 2012;30(22):2739–2744.
14. Bosetti C, Malvezzi M, Rosso T, et al. Lung cancer mortality in European women: trends and predictions. *Lung Cancer.* 2012;78:171–178.
19. Pirie K, Peto R, Reeves GK, et al. The 21st century hazards of smoking and benefits of stopping: a prospective study of one million women in the UK. *Lancet.* 2013;381:133–141.
22. Radzikowska E, Glaz P, Roszkowski K. Lung cancer in women: age, smoking, histology, performance status, stage, initial treatment, and survival. Population-based study of 20,561 cases. *Ann Oncol.* 2002;13:1087–1093.
29. Lam KY, Fu KH, Wong MP, et al. Significant changes in the distribution of histologic types of lung cancer in Hong Kong. *Pathology.* 1993;25(2):103–105.
50. Sisti J, Boffetta P. What proportion of lung cancer in never smokers can be attributed to known risk factors? *Int J Cancer.* 2012;131(2):265–275.
64. Raimondi S, Boffetta P, Anttila S, et al. Metabolic gene polymorphisms and lung cancer risk in non-smokers. An update of the GSEC study. *Mutat Res.* 2005;592(1–2):45–57.
68. Lan QA, Hsiung CA, Matsuo K, et al. Genome-wide association analysis identifies new lung cancer susceptibility loci in never-smoking women in Asia. *Nature Genetics.* 2012;44(12):1330–1337.
94. Patel JD, Bach PB, Kris MG. Lung cancer in US women: a contemporary epidemic. *JAMA.* 2004;291(14):1763–1768.
100. Stabile LP, Davis AL, Gubish CT, et al. Human non-small cell lung tumors and cells derived from normal lung express both estrogen receptor alpha and beta and show biological responses to estrogen. *Cancer Res.* 2002;62(7):2141–2150.
105. Stabile LP, Dacic S, Land SR, et al. Combined analysis of estrogen receptor beta-1 and progesterone receptor expression identifies lung cancer patients with poor outcome. *Clin Cancer Res.* 2011;17(1):154–164.
149. Mazieres J, Rouquette I, Lepage B, et al. Specificities of lung adenocarcinoma in women who have never smoked. *J Thorac Oncol.* 2013;8(7):923–929.
150. Traynor AM, Schiller JH, Stabile LP, et al. Pilot study of gefitinib and fulvestrant in the treatment of post-menopausal women with advanced non-small cell lung cancer. *Lung Cancer.* 2009;64(1):51–59.
167. Visbal AL, Williams BA, Nichols III FC, et al. Gender differences in non-small-cell lung cancer survival: an analysis of 4,618 patients diagnosed between 1997 and 2002. *Ann Thorac Surg.* 2004;78:209–215.
201. Sun Y, Ren Y, Fang Z, et al. Lung adenocarcinoma from East Asian never-smokers is a disease largely defined by targetable oncogenic mutant kinases. *J Clin Oncol.* 2010;28:4616–4620.

See Expertconsult.com for full list of references.

6 Genetic Susceptibility to Lung Cancer

Ann G. Schwartz, Joan E. Bailey-Wilson, and Chris I. Amos

SUMMARY OF KEY POINTS

- While 85% to 90% of lung cancer is attributable to cigarette smoking, substantial evidence exists to support genetic susceptibility to this disease.
- A family history of lung cancer is associated with a 1.5 to 4-fold increased risk of lung cancer after adjustment for the clustering of smoking in families.
- A family-based linkage study has identified a region on chromosome 6q that segregates with lung cancer in high-risk lung cancer families. *PARK2* has been identified as one possible lung cancer susceptibility gene in this region.
- Genome-wide association studies have identified several regions associated with lung cancer risk. These include chromosome 15q25, containing *CHRNA3* and *CHRNA5*, chromosome 6p21, containing *BAT3* and *MSH5*, and chromosome 5p15, containing *TERT* and *CLPTM1L*.
- Challenges remain in better defining lung cancer susceptibility genes, with studies underway using whole genome and whole exome sequencing methods and considering other populations including African-Americans and never-smokers.

Lung cancer is the most common cause of cancer death in the United States, with an estimated 158,080 deaths in 2016 (accounting for 27% of all cancer deaths), and the second most frequent cancer diagnosed, behind breast cancer in women and prostate cancer in men, with an estimated 224,390 new diagnoses in 2016.[1] Both lung cancer incidence and mortality rates have decreased with the reduction in tobacco smoking; however, lung cancer continues to be the cause of substantial morbidity and mortality. Survival remains poor, with a 5-year survival rate of about 17%. The 5-year survival rate has changed little over time because lung cancers are still most often diagnosed at advanced stages when treatment is less effective.[2] Only recently has there been evidence that screening for lung cancer using low-dose computed tomography is an effective means of reducing mortality.[3] In 2013, the US Preventive Services Task Force issued a recommendation for lung cancer screening for high-risk individuals.[4] Advances in the treatment of lung cancer have also been slow. Since the early 2000s, treatment targeted to molecular signatures in lung tumors, such as epidermal growth factor receptor (*EGFR*) inhibitors, has resulted in improved survival in particular subgroups of patients.[5,6] Unfortunately, the development of drug-resistant mutations is a problem that affects overall survival for patients with lung cancer, and continued drug development is crucial. To better understand the profile of a high-risk individual and to aid in the development of chemopreventive agents and targeted treatments, it is essential to understand the genetics underlying lung cancer development.

Cancer of the lung has frequently been cited and is a well-established example of a malignancy that is solely determined by the environment,[7] with risks associated with cigarette smoking and certain occupations, such as mining, asbestos exposure, shipbuilding, and petroleum refining.[8–10] About 85% to 90% of lung cancer risk is attributable to cigarette smoking.[11–13] However, lung cancer develops in only 15% of smokers, suggesting a differential susceptibility to the effects of tobacco carcinogens. It is possible that variation in genetic profiles contributes to this differential susceptibility. In addition, 10% to 15% of lung cancers occur in never-smokers. Little is understood about risk in never-smokers, although exposure to secondhand cigarette smoke certainly contributes to the risk of lung cancer. Environmental tobacco smoke exposure has been associated with a 20% to 30% increased risk for the development of lung cancer among never-smokers.[14] In a meta-analysis of 22 studies, the authors reported that exposure to tobacco smoke in the workplace increased the risk of lung cancer by 24% and this increased risk was highly correlated with duration of exposure.[15]

There is overwhelming evidence of the carcinogenic effects of cigarette smoking and other environmental exposures and the occurrence of multiple somatic mutations in lung tumors. Known mutations and loss of heterozygosity in oncogenes and tumor suppressor genes involved in lung carcinogenesis accumulate in individual somatic cells during lung tumor initiation and progression.[16–19] In 2013, the systematic genetic analysis of alterations in lung tumors was described in several published reports. The Cancer Genome Atlas noted that the results of sequencing 178 squamous cell carcinomas demonstrated the complexity of lung tumors, with a mean of 360 exonic mutations, 165 genomic rearrangements, and 323 copy number alterations per tumor.[19] These observations highlight the genetic complexity of lung cancers compared with most other cancers. Recurrent mutations were identified in 11 genes. A total of 64% of cases carried a somatic alteration in a gene for which a targeted treatment could be proposed based on currently existing therapies (although many of these therapies are not currently indicated for lung cancer). Similarly, sequencing of 183 lung adenocarcinoma tumor/normal DNA pairs showed a mean exonic somatic mutation rate of 12 events per megabase.[20] Higher mutation rates were seen among smokers than among never-smokers, and the mutation signature varied with smoking. Several previously identified mutations were reported, including those in tumor protein p53 (*TP53*), Kirsten rat sarcoma (*KRAS*), *EGFR*, serine/threonine kinase 11 (*STK11*), and v-raf murine sarcoma viral oncogene homologB (*BRAF*). In addition, novel candidates were identified. In total, 25 genes were significantly mutated and often associated with smoking history, age, stage, and progression-free survival. Smaller numbers of small cell lung tumors have been sequenced. In another study of 53 tumor samples/normal tissue pairs, investigators identified 22 significantly mutated genes, including members of the sex determining region Y (SRY)-box (*SOX*) family of genes.[21] Susceptibility to selected mutations also varies according to host-specific factors. For example, mutations in *EGFR* are much more common in women, Asians, and never-smokers and individuals presenting with adenocarcinomas,[22] while mutations affecting *KRAS* are more common in men, individuals of European descent, smokers, and those with squamous histology.[23] Susceptibility to somatic mutations may be due to individual differences in risk associated with the inhalation of known carcinogens; i.e., individuals differ in their susceptibility to these environmental insults.[24–26] The potential role that inherited germline genetic variation plays in influencing lung cancer susceptibility is the topic of this chapter.

Evidence indicates that allelic variation at genetic loci affects inherited susceptibility to lung cancer. Epidemiologic evidence demonstrates familial aggregation of lung cancer after adjusting for familial clustering of cigarette smoking and other risk factors, and differential susceptibility to lung cancer is inherited in some families. Studies of inherited susceptibility to lung cancer, including major susceptibility loci and loci with less pronounced effects, are described in this chapter. Also discussed is how these genetic risks relate to well-known environmental factors, particularly cigarette smoking.

BIOLOGIC RISK FACTORS

When determining whether susceptibility to a complex disease or trait such as lung cancer has a genetic component, three questions are typically addressed in family-based studies.

1. Does the lung cancer cluster or aggregate in families? If risk of lung cancer is inherited, one would find more clustering of lung cancer beyond what would be expected by chance.
2. If lung cancer does aggregate in families, can it be explained by shared environmental/cultural risk factors? For lung cancer, one must assess whether familial aggregation of lung cancer is driven solely as a result of clustering of smoking behaviors or other environmental exposures within families.
3. If the excess familial clustering is not explained by measured environmental risk factors, is the pattern of lung cancers in families consistent with mendelian transmission of a major gene; i.e., transmission in some families of a rare, moderately high-penetrance risk allele, and can this gene(s) be localized and identified in the human genome?

In addition, inherited susceptibility may be acquired through a more common, low-penetrance risk allele that may interact with environmental exposures. Evidence in support of this type of inheritance of risk is most likely derived from case-controlled, and not family-based, studies.

EVIDENCE FOR FAMILIAL AGGREGATION OF LUNG CANCER

Twin Studies

For common diseases, investigators often perform twin studies as a first approach to estimating the impact of genetic factors in disease causation. In twin studies, investigators typically report the observed concordance rates for lung cancer among monozygotic (MZ) twins compared with the observed concordance rates for lung cancer among dizygotic (DZ) twins. Identifying enough twins to conduct a meaningful analysis of cancer risk has been challenging; the combination of data from the Swedish, Finnish, and Danish registries with national cancer registries allowed investigators to analyze data on 44,708 pairs.[27] The results of this analysis showed substantial increases in risk for cotwins, with relative risks of 7.7 and 6.7 for male MZ and DZ cotwins, respectively; for female MZ and DZ cotwins, the risks were 25.3 and 1.8, respectively. Furthermore, a biometrical analysis of these data was performed, and investigators estimated that 26% of variance in risk was attributable to heritable factors, 12% to shared environmental factors, and 62% to individual-specific risks. The estimated heritable proportions are comparable to estimates for breast and ovarian cancer but lower than estimates for colorectal or prostate cancers. Strong evidence against the so-called constitutional hypothesis, proposed by Sir Ronald Fisher, was found in studies of MZ twins discordant for smoking, and the same host factors predispose these individuals to both smoking and lung cancer; therefore smoking does not have any direct causal link to lung cancer risk.[28,29] However, a large US study showed a much lower relative risk when comparing smoking with nonsmoking MZ cotwins (5.5), and higher risk in DZ cotwins (11.0), which suggests a partial role of genetic factors in both smoking and lung cancer.[29]

Case–Control and Case–Family Cohort Studies

In 1963, Tokuhata and Lilienfeld[30,31] showed familial aggregation of lung cancer. After they accounted for personal smoking, the results suggested the possible interaction of genes, shared environment, and common lifestyle factors in the etiology of lung cancer. In their study of 270 people with lung cancer and 270 age-, sex-, race-, and location-matched controls and their relatives, the authors found a 2.0-fold to 2.5-fold increased lung cancer mortality among smoking relatives of people with lung cancer compared with smoking relatives of control participants. Nonsmoking relatives of people with lung cancer were also at higher risk than nonsmoking relatives of control participants. Smoking was a more important risk factor than family history of lung cancer for men, but family history was more important for women. The authors also noted a synergistic interaction between family history of lung cancer and smoking, with a much higher risk of lung cancer among smoking relatives of people with lung cancer than among either nonsmoking relatives of people with lung cancer or smoking relatives of control participants. Additionally, the authors found a substantial increase in mortality related to other respiratory diseases in relatives of people with lung cancer compared with relatives of control participants, suggesting that the relatives of people with lung cancer have a common susceptibility to respiratory diseases. No significant differences were noted between the spouses of people with lung cancer and control participants with respect to lung cancer mortality, mortality from other respiratory diseases, or smoking habits. One strength of this study was that risk factor data, including age and smoking status, were collected for the relatives; however a major weakness of the study was that smoking status alone, and not smoking intensity or duration, was used, so there was potential for residual confounding due to clustering of smoking habits in families.

Since this initial study, authors of several other studies have reported familial aggregation of lung cancer.[32-34] The best designed studies considered the number of relatives in the families and the risk factor profiles of each relative so that the effect of familial clustering of smoking habits could be taken into account, and the discussion focused on these types of studies. In southern Louisiana, authors of case-controlled studies reported an increased familial risk of lung cancer and other smoking-related cancers among relatives of lung cancer probands (the index case leading the family to be studied) after the effects of age, sex, occupation, and smoking history had been accounted for.[33-35] In these studies, investigators performed familial aggregation analyses on 337 lung cancer probands (cases), their spouses (controls), and the parents, siblings, half-siblings, and offspring of both the cases and controls. The probands were white men and women who died of lung cancer between 1976 and 1979 in a 10-parish (county) area of southern Louisiana. A strong excess risk of lung cancer was detected among first-degree relatives of probands compared with relatives of controls after adjustment for age, sex, smoking status, total duration of smoking, number of cigarette pack-years, and a cumulative index of occupational/industrial exposures. The risk of lung cancer for parents of probands was fourfold compared with parents of controls. Women older than age 40 years who were relatives of probands were at a nine times higher risk of lung cancer than similar female relatives of controls, even among nonsmokers without excessive exposure to hazardous occupational materials. Heavy-smoking female relatives of probands had a fourfold to sixfold increased lung cancer risk compared with heavy-smoking female relatives of controls. Overall, the lung cancer risk was greater for male relatives of probands than for their female counterparts. After controlling for the confounding effects of the measured environmental risk factors, the authors found that relationship to a lung cancer proband (i.e., having a family history of lung cancer) remained a determinant of lung cancer, associated with a 2.4-fold higher lung cancer risk.

This same set of families was evaluated to determine whether cancers other than lung cancer were associated with similar familial aggregation.[35] Proband families were 1.7 times more likely than control families to have one family member other than the proband with cancer, and 2.2 times more likely to have two family members with cancer. Comparing case relatives and control relatives, families that had three cancers or four or more cancers occurred with relative risks of 3.7 and 5.0, respectively. The most striking differences in cancer prevalence between case and control families were noted for cancers of the nasal cavity/sinus, mid-ear, and larynx (odds ratio, 4.6); trachea, bronchus, and lung (odds ratio, 3.0); skin (odds ratio, 2.8); and uterus, placenta, ovary, and other female organs (odds ratio, 2.1). After controlling for age, sex, cigarette smoking, and occupational/industrial exposures, the authors found that the risk of cancers other than lung cancer remained significantly increased for relatives of cases compared with relatives of controls ($p < 0.05$).

Etzel et al.[36] conducted a large case–control study in Texas that adjusted for smoking histories among relatives and discovered similar findings. The authors studied 806 lung cancer cases and 663 matched controls in the Houston area and reported familial aggregation of lung cancer and smoking-related cancers after adjustment for smoking histories of the cases and controls and their relatives. In this study, familial aggregation was not stronger in families of early-onset cases (defined as diagnosed at age 55 years or younger) or in families of never-smokers.

Familial aggregation of lung cancer in families of early-onset lung cancer cases was evaluated by Cote et al.[37] in a large study in metropolitan Detroit that enrolled 692 white and black individuals with early-onset lung cancer (defined as diagnosed before the age of 50 years), along with 773 frequency-matched population-based control participants. Data on risk factors, including smoking pack-years, age, sex, and a history of other lung diseases, were collected for each first-degree relative of the people with early-onset lung cancer and control participants. After adjustment for these risk factors, relatives of people with early-onset lung cancer were twice as likely to have lung cancer compared with relatives of control participants. The lung cancer risk associated with family history of lung cancer was highest in black families. Increased lung cancer risk in relatives of never-smoking individuals with lung cancer was not reported in this study, however the sample size was small. The authors of the study reported a 1.5-fold increased risk of tobacco-related cancers. This risk was even higher when the analysis included only black families.[38]

The largest study of familial aggregation involved the evaluation of people with lung cancer and control participants in Iceland.[39] The authors of the study used a population-based approach and obtained familial risks of 2.69 when parents of people with lung cancer were compared with parents of control participants, and this risk increased to 3.48 when parents of people younger than age 60 years (early-onset lung cancer) were compared with age-matched control participants. The risk to siblings was increased 2.02-fold in general but increased to 3.3-fold for siblings of people with early-onset lung cancer.

Studies of never-smokers with lung cancer are limited.[36,40–43] Schwartz et al.[41] found an increased risk of lung cancer among relatives of younger, population-based nonsmokers with lung cancer compared with relatives of younger control participants after adjustment for smoking, occupation, and medical history of each family member.[41] Mayne et al.[43] studied never-smokers and former smokers (cessation at least 10 years before they were interviewed) and reported that a positive family history of lung cancer was associated with increased lung cancer risk after adjustment for age and smoking status.

In addition to studies that include an analysis of risk factor data among relatives, a meta-analysis of 28 case–control studies and 17 cohort studies demonstrated fairly consistent findings, with an approximately twofold increased risk of lung cancer associated with family history across a range of study designs.[32] Risk was generally higher for relatives of people in whom lung cancer was diagnosed at a young age and when multiple family members were affected. A recent pooled analysis from the International Lung Cancer Consortium included data from approximately 24,000 lung cancer cases and 23,000 controls, making it the largest study to date.[33] The authors reported a 1.5-fold increased risk of lung cancer associated with a family history, after adjustment for smoking and other potential confounders in cases and controls, and a 1.25-fold increased risk for never-smokers. No variation in familial risk by histology was noted. When the analysis was limited to studies that included risk factor data for each family member, relative risks for lung cancer among relatives with a family history of lung cancer were 1.55 overall, 1.53 for white, 2.09 for black, and 1.97 for relatives of people with early-onset lung cancer (diagnosed before 50 years of age). The findings from these studies help to answer the first two questions posed at the beginning of this chapter: there is substantial evidence for familial aggregation of lung cancer and it remains after adjustment for clustering of cigarette smoking within family members.

HIGH-RISK SYNDROMES CONFERRING AN INCREASED RISK OF LUNG CANCER

Further evidence suggesting an inherited component to lung cancer is the occurrence of lung cancer in families with inherited, well-defined cancer syndromes. Leonard et al.[44] reported that survivors of familial retinoblastoma may be at increased risk for small cell lung cancer (SCLC).[44] The standard mortality ratio for SCLC estimates a 15-fold increased risk.[45,46] Kleinerman et al.[46] reported lung cancer developing among individuals with germline retinoblastoma mutations and a history of heavy smoking. Overall, retinoblastoma survivors tend to smoke less than the general population, suggesting that targeting counseling to avoid this risky behavior in this high-risk population may be effective.[47] The retinoblastoma gene is inactivated in 90% of SCLCs, indicating the biologic relevance of this gene in SCLC etiology.[48]

Germline mutations in the *p53* gene cause the inherited Li-Fraumeni syndrome. Individuals with this syndrome are at greater increased risk for many other cancers, including breast and lung cancers, sarcomas, leukemias and lymphomas, and adrenocortical tumors. The standard incidence ratio for lung cancer was estimated at 38 in a prospectively collected cohort of *p53* mutation carriers.[49] Cigarette smoking further increased an individual's risk by threefold.

Mutations in the *EGFR* gene are often found in adenocarcinomas of the lung arising in never-smoking women and in Asian populations.[50] One family with multiple lung adenocarcinomas was found to have segregation of an *EGFR* mutation, indicating that rarely inherited mutations of this locus can increase the risk of lung cancer.[51] However, in another study of 237 familial lung cancer cases from families with three or more affected relatives, including 45 bronchoalveolar cancers, investigators failed to find any germline *EGFR*-T790 mutations, suggesting that inheritable mutations in this gene are uncommon in the general US population.[52]

SEGREGATON ANALYSES OF LUNG AND OTHER TOBACCO-RELATED CANCERS

Given the evidence for familial aggregation of lung and other tobacco-related cancers, after adjustment for familial clustering of smoking habits, determining whether patterns of transmission within families is consistent with at least one major, high-penetrance genetic locus is the next step in answering the last question posed at the beginning of this chapter. Sellers et al.[53] performed genetic segregation analyses on the lung cancer proband families in the study by Ooi et al.[34] The trait was expressed as a dichotomy, affected or unaffected with lung cancer. These analyses used the general transmission probability model,[54] which allowed for variable age of onset of the lung cancers.[55–57] The likelihood of the models was calculated using a correction factor appropriate for single ascertainment,[58,59] that is, conditioning the likelihood of each pedigree of the probands being affected by their age at examination or death.

Age of onset of lung cancer was assumed to follow a logistic distribution that depended on pack-years of cigarette smoke exposure and its square, an age coefficient, and a baseline parameter. Results indicated compatibility of the data with mendelian codominant inheritance of a rare major autosomal gene that produces cancer at an earlier age of onset. Segregation at this putative locus may account for 69% and 47% of the cumulative incidence of lung cancer in individuals up to ages 50 and 60 years, respectively. The gene was predicted to be involved in 22% of all lung cancer in persons up to age 70 years, a reflection of an increasing proportion of noncarriers becoming affected by long-term exposure to tobacco.[54,60]

Gauderman et al.[61] reanalyzed these same data from Ooi's study using a Gibbs sampler method to examine gene by environment interactions and found evidence of a major dominant susceptibility locus that acts in conjunction with cigarette smoking to increase risk.[61] This analysis was very similar to the previous study results because the codominant mendelian models predicted very small numbers of homozygous susceptibility allele carriers.

Yang et al.[62] performed a complex segregation analysis on the families of never-smoking lung cancer probands in metropolitan Detroit from the study by Schwartz et al.[41] The authors found evidence of mendelian codominant inheritance with modifying effects of smoking and chronic bronchitis in families of never-smoking cases. The estimated risk allele frequency was 0.004. Although homozygous individuals with the risk allele were rare in the study population, penetrance was very high for early-onset lung cancer (85% in men and 74% in women by age 60). The probability of lung cancer developing by 60 years of age in individuals heterozygous for the rare allele was low in the absence of smoking and chronic bronchitis (7% in men and 4% in women), but in the presence of these risk factors it increased to 85% in men and 74% in women, which was the same level predicted for homozygotes. The attributable risk associated with the high-risk allele declined with age, when the role of tobacco smoking and chronic bronchitis become more important. Investigators conducted a small study in Taiwan that analyzed the families of 125 female never-smoking lung cancer probands and found evidence for effects from a dominant genetic locus.[63]

The Taiwan, Detroit, and Louisiana studies share remarkably similar results and provide substantial evidence for at least one major gene that acts in conjunction with smoking and possibly with chronic bronchitis to increase the risk of lung cancer in families. Segregation studies have some limitations. The studies did not include all potential risk factors for lung cancer, such as passive smoking or occupational exposures, in each relative, and only one study included history of other lung diseases in the models. Furthermore, segregation analyses are not sufficient to prove the existence of a major locus because only a subset of all possible models can be tested. Segregation analyses are useful, however, because they provide a model that can be used in family-based linkage studies aimed at the identification of a specific lung cancer gene. These analyses also provide insights into the best study design for identifying genes that confer a high risk of disease.

RARE, HIGH-PENETRANCE GENES: LINKAGE ANALYSIS OF LUNG CANCER

Linkage analysis is a statistical analysis of pedigree data that investigators use to look for evidence of cosegregation of alleles at a genetic "susceptibility" locus and some known genetic "marker" locus (usually a DNA polymorphism) through generations of families. This type of analysis is a powerful method for detecting genetic loci that are highly penetrant (after adjustment for environmental risk factors). Power is greatest to detect susceptibility alleles that are rare and highly penetrant; power decreases as susceptibility alleles become more common and less penetrant. Because cigarette smoking is an extremely strong risk factor for lung cancer, it is important to include this factor in all linkage studies of lung cancer.

Bailey-Wilson et al.[64] published the first evidence of linkage of a lung cancer susceptibility locus to a region on chromosome 6. Data were collected from multiple sites by the Genetic Epidemiology of Lung Cancer Consortium (GELCC). In the initial publication, the authors reported that 13.7% of the 26,108 people with lung cancer screened had at least one first-degree relative with lung cancer. For each family recruited, data regarding cancer status of all family members, birth dates, age at diagnosis, and vital status for affected family members and archival tissue and blood or saliva were collected. Cancers were verified by medical records, pathology reports, cancer registry records, or death certificates for 69% of the individuals affected with either lung or throat cancers and for another 31% through reporting by multiple family members. Initial genotyping of 392 microsatellite (short tandem repeat polymorphisms) marker loci was conducted in 52 families. The data were analyzed using both parametric and nonparametric linkage methods. Marker allele frequencies and linkage analyses were evaluated separately for white and black families, with the results combined in overall tests of linkage.

The primary analytical approach assumed a model with 10% penetrance in carriers and 1% penetrance in noncarriers, with weighting given only to affected individuals. This linkage model was used because of uncertainty about the strength of the relationship between smoking behavior and lung cancer risk in the high-risk families and because software was not available in any multipoint linkage analysis program to model complex gene–environment interactions. In addition, because about 90% of the affected family members smoked, weighting only the affected individuals in a simple dominant, low-penetrance model had the effect of jointly allowing for smoking status. Genetic heterogeneity (different families having different genetic causation) was allowed in the analysis. Secondary analyses used more complex models that included age and pack-years of cigarette smoking to modify the penetrance estimates. A genetic regressive model based on the segregation analysis by Sellers et al.[53] was used. Nonparametric analyses were also performed as secondary analyses with variance component models using Sequential Oligogenic Linkage Analysis Routines (SOLAR) (binary trait option) and mixed effects Cox regression models, in which time to onset of disease was modeled as a quantitative trait.

Multipoint parametric linkage under the simple dominant low-penetrance affected only model yielded a maximum heterogeneity logarithm of the odds (LOD [to the base 10]) (heterogeneity LOD score [HLOD]) score of 2.79 at 155 cM (marker D6S2436) on chromosome 6q23-25 in the 52 families, with 67% of the families estimated to be linked. Multipoint analysis of the subset of 38 families with four affected relatives yielded an HLOD of 3.47 at this same location, with 78% of the families estimated to be linked. For the 23 highest-risk families, i.e., those with five or more affected members in two or more generations, the multipoint HLOD was 4.26, with 94% of the families estimated to be linked to this region.[51] Nonparametric analyses and the two-point parametric analyses that used the model of Sellers et al.[35,53] all provided evidence in support of linkage in this region.

In an update to the GELCC linkage study, additional genotyping was conducted on a total of 93 high-risk lung cancer families.[65] Nearly 400 markers were again genotyped, and the primary analysis used the same model as specified previously. HLODs were calculated from output from SimWalk2 software (a statistical genetics computer application), with initial evidence for linkage estimated from each family separately, and analyses were performed separately within genotyping set and race, with results summed across study and race. Across the 6q linkage region in linked families, the investigators assigned haplotypes using SimWalk2 and visual inspection to assign carrier status. They performed Kaplan-Meier and Cox regression analyses, conditioned on carrier status and smoking behavior, to assess the relationship between smoking and lung cancer risk by carrier status. This extended analysis again identified a region on chromosome 6q, with a maximum HLOD of 4.67 in families with five or more affected individuals in two or more generations. Furthermore, lung cancer risk for putative carriers was higher than for noncarriers, even among never-smokers. Lung cancer risk for smoking noncarriers demonstrated the usual dose–response curves, with increasing risk associated with an increasing amount the individual smoked. Among smoking carriers, although risk was higher than that for noncarriers, the usual dose–response curves were not evident, suggesting that any level of tobacco exposure increased risk among those individuals with inherited lung cancer susceptibility. In this region, a germline mutation in *PARK2* was linked to lung cancer risk in one family with eight affected family members.[66] The authors found additional evidence of linkage for regions on chromosomes 12q, 5q, 14q, 16q, and 20p.[67] This study is ongoing, with additional families being genotyped with more than 6000 genome-wide single nucleotide polymorphism (SNP) markers.

COMMON, LOW-PENETRANCE GENES: GENOME-WIDE ASSOCIATION STUDIES

The GELCC linkage study was designed to identify rare, high-penetrance genes with large effects, but the search for genes contributing to lung cancer susceptibility also includes studies designed to identify more common, low-penetrance genes with more moderate effects. Initially, analyses were done to evaluate specific genetic polymorphisms in biologically plausible pathways, including metabolic genes, growth factors, growth factor receptors, DNA damage and repair genes, oncogenes, and tumor suppressor genes. These studies were typically small, focused on a very limited number of polymorphisms, and the findings have not been replicated. The authors of two reviews provided overviews of these studies.[68,69] With improved technology, the search for more common, low-penetrance genes with modest effects has been conducted in genome-wide association studies (GWAS), in which investigators rely on very large samples and more than 300,000 markers across the genome. The findings from these studies have provided highly significant and reproducible results.

In three articles published at the same time in *Nature* and *Nature Genetics*, researchers identified through GWAS the same region of chromosome 15q25.1 as being significantly associated with lung cancer.[70–72] The region that the authors identified included a neuronal nicotinic acetylcholine receptor gene cluster comprising cholinergic receptor nicotine alpha 3 (*CHRNA3*), *CHRNA5*, and *CHRNA4* subunits. Nicotinic receptors are composed of pentamers that include alpha and beta units and are ubiquitously expressed, but at higher levels in the brain. Thorgeirsson et al.[71] conducted GWAS on 14,000 individuals to identify the 15q region in association with smoking quantity and further explored the effect of the region on smoking dependence and lung cancer risk. The other two studies were lung cancer case–control studies with large sample sizes.[70,72] In all the studies, the authors identified the 15q25 region as being

associated with an approximately 1.29-fold increased risk of lung cancer among individuals carrying a heterozygous mutation (44.2% of controls for marker rs8034191) and about a 1.80-fold increase for individuals homozygous for the mutation (10.7% of controls). Because of the strong linkage disequilibrium among the markers studied and the strong link between smoking and lung cancer risk, the authors reported some disagreement between the studies as to the relevance of the region; i.e., was the region associated with smoking behavior and then indirectly to lung cancer or was the association directly with lung cancer. Thorgeirsson et al.[71] concluded that the region affected smoking behavior. Furthermore, Amos et al.[72] found stronger effects on lung cancer risk that remained highly significant ($p < 1 \times 10^{-17}$) after adjustment for smoking behavior, whereas Hung et al.[70] did not find any association of this region with smoking behavior.[70,72]

Since these initial studies, multiple investigations of the 15q region have been conducted. A meta-analysis in which smokers, people with lung cancer and lung cancer-free controls, and people with chronic obstructive pulmonary disease and controls (no chronic obstructive pulmonary disease) was conducted, and the authors reported that multiple loci within this region were associated with cigarettes smoked per day. One locus was associated with lung cancer independent of the amount the individual smoked.[73]

Findings from GWAS also prompted multiple reports of regions on chromosomes 6p21 and 5p15 being associated with lung cancer risk.[70–72,74,75] Human leukocyte antigen (HLA)-3 associated transcript 3 (*BAT3*) and MutS homolog 5 (*MSH5*) are located in the 6p21 region, but telomerase reverse transcriptase (*TERT*) and cleft lip and palate transmembrane 1-like (*CLPTM1L*) are located in the 5p15 region. Associations with lung cancer risk have been shown to vary by histologic type; however individual GWAS, even with large sample sizes, are limited in the context of lung cancer subtypes. In a large meta-analysis of 14,900 people with lung cancer and 29,485 control participants from 16 GWAS, all of whom were of European ancestry, additional support was provided for loci associated with increased lung cancer risk in the 5p15, 6p21, and 15q25 regions.[76] The 15q25 region associations for the two strongest SNPs were seen in smokers but not in never-smokers. Associations with SNPs in the 5p15 region varied by histologic type. Other than 5p15, 6p21, and 15q25, no SNP-lung cancer association was found to reach genome-wide significance. There were, however, other regions associated with squamous cell carcinomas: 12p13 (*RAD52*), 9p21 (cyclin-dependent kinase inhibitor 1B/antisense noncoding RNA in the INK4 locus [*CDKN1B/ANRIL*]), and 2q32. Authors of a GWAS conducted in the Han Chinese population also found evidence for lung cancer risk associations in the 5p15 region, along with regions not identified in individuals of European ancestry: the 3q28 (tumor protein 63 [*TP63*]), 13q12 (mitochondrial intermediate peptidase-tumor necrosis factor receptor superfamily, member 19 [*MIPEP-TNFRSF19*]), and 22q12 (myotubularin related protein 3–HORMA domain containing 2-leukemia inhibitory factor [*MTMR3–HORMAD2-LIF*]) regions.[77] With additional samples, Dong et al.[78] were able to identify more regions of interest in the 10p14, 5q32, and 20q13 regions. In the Japanese population, Shiraishi et al.[79] replicated the 5p15 and 3q28 findings reported in the Chinese population and the 6p21 findings in individuals with European ancestry. That study was restricted to adenocarcinomas.

Imputation analysis yielded several new loci influencing lung cancer risk in European descent populations.[80] Notably, an uncommon stop mutation, K3326X, in *BRCA2* occurring in a little less than 1% of Europeans was associated with a twofold overall increased risk for lung cancer and a 2.5-fold increased risk for squamous carcinomas. This increased risk of cancer development has also been noted in other smoking-related cancers including head and neck and esophageal cancers.[81] The variant was associated with decreased risk of ovarian cancer among *BRCA1* or *BRCA2* mutation carriers and only confers a 1.3-fold increased risk for breast cancer.[82,83] Imputation analysis also identified variants of *TP63* influencing lung cancer risk in European descent individuals and a previously identified rare *CHEK2* variant disruptive of protein dimerization that is associated with decreased lung cancer risk.[84]

Little work has been completed to identify susceptibility genes in European-descent never-smokers using a GWAS approach, in part because these individuals are not as common in the population making it more difficult to identify the numbers of participants needed for GWAS. In never-smoking women in Asia, Lan et al.[85] replicated the 6p21, 5p15, and 3q28 findings discussed previously and also reported regions of interest in 10q25 and 6q22. The authors found no association between lung cancer risk in never-smoking women and SNPs in the 15q25 region. In addition to this study, a large study is underway involving individuals of European ancestry, and results from several smaller studies have been published.[86,87] Even less has been studied in the black population. The associations between lung cancer risk and SNPs in the 15q25, 5p15, and 6p21 regions that have been identified in individuals of European ancestry have been replicated in black individuals.[88,89] A recent GWAS study of African-Americans from multiple US sites did not identify new loci specific to this population but did identify novel African-American specific variants in the *CHRNA5* region.[90]

CONCLUSION

The evidence presented clearly supports the notion of a genetic component to the risk of lung cancer, with multiple genetic loci influencing risk under investigation. The aggregation of lung cancer in families that remains after adjustment for smoking history of each relative suggests that a segment of the population is at risk due to an inherited mutation. The first and only lung cancer linkage study provided evidence of linkage to a region on chromosome 6q. If a susceptibility locus can be identified in this region, it will be of major public health importance because it will allow for the identification of a high-risk group that can be targeted for smoking prevention/cessation and for screening programs. It will also provide new understanding of the mechanism of carcinogenesis and may suggest to clinicians better methods of prevention and targeted treatment. The findings from GWAS of more common and lower penetrance SNPs associated with lung cancer risk will also contribute in the same way; however, the risk for this population may be lower than that found within high-risk families.

Challenges remain in the identification of lung cancer susceptibility genes. Once a region is identified, the actual genetic alteration driving the association has to be determined. Heterogeneity is also a problem that affects multiple points in the discovery process:

(1) at the level of histologic types of lung cancer; (2) at the level of exposure to various environmental risk factors; and (3) at the level of inherited susceptibility; i.e., the locus responsible for lung cancer in one family may not be the same as the locus in another family. The potential for gene–environment interactions and gene–gene interactions must also be considered. Given that lung cancer continues to be the leading cause of cancer death, and with the new potential for effective lung cancer screening, research into the genetic contribution to lung cancer susceptibility remains important.

Acknowledgments

This work was supported in part by the Intramural Research Program of the National Human Genome Research Institute, National Institutes of Health (NIH), and by funding from NIH R01CA148127 and P30CA022453.

KEY REFERENCES

10. Doll R, Peto R, Wheatley K, Gray R, Sutherland I. Mortality in relation to smoking: 40 years' observations on male British doctors. *BMJ*. 1994;309(6959):901–911.
13. Peto R, Darby S, Deo H, Silcocks P, Whitley E, Doll R. Smoking, smoking cessation, and lung cancer in the UK since 1950: combination of national statistics with two case–control studies. *BMJ*. 2000;321(7257):323–329.
33. Cote ML, Liu M, Bonassi S, et al. Increased risk of lung cancer in individuals with a family history of the disease: a pooled analysis from the International Lung Cancer Consortium. *Eur J Cancer*. 2012;48(13):1957–1968.
53. Sellers TA, Bailey-Wilson JE, Elston RC, et al. Evidence for mendelian inheritance in the pathogenesis of lung cancer. *J Natl Cancer Inst*. 1990;82(15):1272–1279.
64. Bailey-Wilson JE, Amos CI, Pinney SM, et al. A major lung cancer susceptibility locus maps to chromosome 6q23–25. *Am J Hum Genet*. 2004;75(3):460–474.
65. Amos CI, Pinney SM, Li Y, et al. A susceptibility locus on chromosome 6q greatly increases lung cancer risk among light and never smokers. *Cancer Res*. 2010;70(6):2359–2367.
70. Hung RJ, McKay JD, Gaborieau V, et al. A susceptibility locus for lung cancer maps to nicotinic acetylcholine receptor subunit genes on 15q25. *Nature*. 2008;452(7187):633–637.
71. Thorgeirsson TE, Geller F, Sulem P, et al. A variant associated with nicotine dependence, lung cancer and peripheral arterial disease. *Nature*. 2008;452(7187):638–642.
72. Amos CI, Wu X, Broderick P, et al. Genome-wide association scan of tag SNPs identifies a susceptibility locus for lung cancer at 15q25.1. *Nat Genet*. 2008;40(5):616–622.
76. Timofeeva MN, Hung RJ, Rafnar T, et al. Influence of common genetic variation on lung cancer risk: meta-analysis of 14,900 cases and 29,485 controls. *Hum Mol Genet*. 2012;21(22):4980–4995.
89. Walsh KM, Gorlov IP, Hansen HM, et al. Fine-mapping of the 5p15.33, 6p22.1-p21.31, and 15q25.1 regions identifies functional and histology-specific lung cancer susceptibility loci in African-Americans. *Cancer Epidemiol Biomarkers Prev*. 2013;22(2):251–260.

See Expertconsult.com for full list of references.

7 Screening for Lung Cancer

Annette McWilliams, Fraser Brims, Nanda Horeweg, Harry J. de Koning, and James R. Jett

SUMMARY OF KEY POINTS

- The National Lung Screening Trial has definitively shown a reduction in **lung cancer mortality** in a research setting but effective implementation of a lung cancer screening program needs to be evaluated in different health-care communities.
- **Selection** of high-risk participants for low-dose (radiation) computed tomography screening is improved by the use of multivariate risk prediction models.
- A range of **recruitment** strategies will be required based on available health infrastructure and the distribution of the high-risk population.
- Simplified management algorithms for **pulmonary nodules**, incorporating risk prediction models and image analysis techniques, will likely lead to reduction in downstream investigations and surgery for benign disease.
- **Overdiagnosis** represents an important potential harm for participants in any lung cancer screening program. Rates of overdiagnosis vary with histologic subtype of the screen-detected cancer and with the phenotype of the screened population.
- **Smoking cessation** is critical to the overall benefit and cost-effectiveness of a lung cancer screening program. The best strategy to optimize the intervention and integrate it into a program is not known.
- The precision and **cost-effectiveness** of a lung cancer screening program is likely to be improved with probabilistic risk modeling and protocol-driven nodule management. The cost-effectiveness of a program will likely be a key determinant in federal or national decision making to adopt a lung cancer screening program.
- **Biomarkers** have the potential to further refine a risk-based approach to screening through identification of high-risk phenotypes or following identification of an indeterminate nodule. At present, there are no molecular biomarkers approved for clinical practice in lung cancer screening.

Lung cancer is the most common cancer and the greatest cause of cancer death in our world.[1,2] According to GLOBOCAN, there were an estimated 1.8 million cases of lung cancer diagnosed in 2012 and there were 1.59 million lung cancer–related deaths.[2] The association between smoking and lung cancer was first described more than 50 years ago.[3] Worldwide, smoking accounts for 80% of lung cancers in men and for 50% in women. About 30% of the world population reaching adulthood will start smoking, and the majority will continue to smoke throughout their lives.[1] Although smoking rates are decreasing in most high-income countries, they are increasing or persistent in low- to middle-income countries.[1] In some high-income countries with lower current smoking rates, a greater proportion of lung cancer is occurring in former

smokers.[4,5] The excess risk of lung cancer in former smokers is influenced by the age of smoking cessation, where 90% of lung cancer risk can be avoided if cessation occurs before 40 years of age.[1,3,4]

The fatality rate (ratio of mortality to incidence) for lung cancer is high, estimated to be 0.87 in the GLOBOCAN report.[2] The 5-year survival rate is generally low at less than 15% with a relative lack of variability amongst different world regions.[1,2] Most patients have advanced and incurable disease at the time of diagnosis.[1] In the United States (US), 56% of patients have distant metastasis and 22% have regional spread of disease; 15% of lung cancers are localized at the time of initial diagnosis.[6] The reason for this low percentage of early-stage disease is that it is asymptomatic; most early-stage lung cancers are currently detected by chance imaging procedures performed for other reasons.[7]

Until recently, there has been no role for lung cancer screening. Screening trials in which chest radiography and sputum cytology were evaluated did not demonstrate a decrease in lung cancer–related mortality.[8–11] In the 1990s, single-arm screening trials with low-dose (radiation) computed tomography (LDCT) of the chest demonstrated an increase in sensitivity for detecting lung cancer compared with chest radiography.[12–14] Authors of the initial trials reported that 60% to 80% of detected lung cancers were stage I disease.[15–21] These studies led to a number of randomized screening trials to compare LDCT with either chest radiography or observation alone.

There are a number of European randomized control trials that include an LDCT screening arm and a control arm.[22–31] However, these trials are likely underpowered to detect a clinically plausible benefit in terms of lung cancer–related mortality.[32] Subsequently, two larger randomized studies have been undertaken, the National Lung Screening Trial (NLST) in the US and the Dutch-Belgian Randomised Lung Cancer Screening Trial (NELSON).[33–35] The NLST study has been published and determined that LDCT screening was associated with a 20% reduction in lung cancer mortality compared with chest radiography.[36] The NELSON study is nearing completion.

The NLST has definitively shown a reduction in all-cause and disease-specific mortality in a research setting but effective implementation of a lung cancer screening program needs to be clarified in different health-care communities. The International Association for the Study of Lung Cancer Strategic Screening Advisory Committee published position statements in 2012 and 2014 to inform the process of implementation of lung cancer screening. They have recommended incorporation of a multidisciplinary group of experts and identified a number of specific issues that need to be addressed for broader community implementation. These include identification of high-risk individuals, uniform radiology standards, standardized reporting and management of CT findings, and integration of smoking cessation programs.[37,38]

The US Preventive Services Task Force (USPSTF) published recommendations on LDCT screening for lung cancer in the US in 2014.[32,39,40] Following the final decision on February 5, 2015, by the Centers of Medicare and Medicaid Services to cover lung CT screening of Americans aged 55 years to 77 years who had smoked at least 30 pack-years, lung cancer screening is being implemented in the US health-care system.[39] Many other countries are evaluating the translation of LDCT screening into

TABLE 7.1 Eligibility Criteria for Lung Cancer Screening

	Age (y)	Smoking History
NLST[33]	55–74	≥30 pack-years; Quit <15 years
NELSON[35]	50–74	≥15 cigs/d for 25 years; ≥10 cigs/d for ≥30 years; Quit ≤10 years
USPSTF[46]	55–80	≥30 pack-years; Quit <15 years

cigs, cigarettes; NELSON, Dutch-Belgian Randomised Lung Cancer Screening Trial; NLST, National Lung Screening Trial; USPSTF, United States Preventive Services Task Force.

clinical practice and implementation of coordinated programs in their respective health systems.[40–43]

In this chapter, we summarize the current knowledge for lung cancer screening with LDCT and discuss the issues that require ongoing clarification.

PARTICIPANT SELECTION

Rather than a population-based strategy, as exists for breast and colorectal cancer, proposed lung cancer screening programs involve screening identified high-risk groups. A significant proportion of our community are current or former smokers who may be eligible for screening. There are an estimated 1.1 billion smokers worldwide.[1,44] To develop cost-effective lung cancer screening programs, an improved definition of a high-risk individual to target screening efforts is needed.

It is also important to consider comorbidities in participants who are potential candidates for screening. To achieve the benefits of screening, both at an individual and at a community level, participants must be able to undergo curative treatments and have a reasonable life expectancy. Smokers are at an increased risk of other comorbidities that may limit curative therapy or life span.[45] USPSTF guidelines for screening in the US recommend discontinuing screening if a person develops a health problem that substantially limits life expectancy or the ability or willingness to have curative lung surgery.[46]

Selection criteria for LDCT screening used in research trials have largely been based on age and smoking history, but lung cancer screening is most effective when applied to people at highest risk.[47] The identification of high-risk individuals using age and smoking criteria alone was used in the NLST and NELSON trials and is the basis of current eligibility criteria in the US (USPSTF criteria; Table 7.1).

Selection of individuals for lung cancer screening using risk prediction models is superior to selection using age and smoking criteria alone.[47–51] Multiple risk prediction models exist but one of the best studied is the prostate, lung, colorectal, and ovarian (PLCO) model that is based on prospectively collected data from the Prostate, Lung, Colorectal, and Ovarian Cancer Screening Trial.[11] The use of this model in analysis of NLST data showed improved performance compared with NLST enrollment criteria.[48] In 2014, Tammemagi and colleagues presented an evidence-based risk threshold based on the PLCO$_{m2012}$ model and NLST mortality outcomes.[49] At PLCO$_{m2012}$ risk of 1.51% or more over 6 years there was consistently lower lung cancer mortality in those NLST participants screened with LDCT compared with chest x-ray. This risk threshold performed better than USPSTF criteria. More lung cancers were detected and fewer were missed using the risk model. The number needed to screen to prevent one lung cancer death was 255 compared with 963 in the lower-risk category. Importantly, the use of USPSTF criteria alone resulted in the screening of a substantial number of low-risk individuals and exclusion of some high-risk individuals.[49]

External validation and comparison of four published risk prediction models were performed in 20,700 ever-smokers of the EPIC-Germany cohort (Bach model, Spitz model, Liverpool Lung Project, and PLCO$_{m2012}$). The results revealed that the PLCO$_{m2012}$ model showed the best performance. All of the models, except the Spitz model, showed better prediction and performance than screening trials eligibility criteria using age/smoking criteria alone.[50]

The use of multivariate risk prediction models to select participants who will most benefit from screening is likely to be the most cost-effective strategy. The IASLC High Risk Working Group has recommended the use of these prediction models in a coordinated program.[37,51]

Recruitment

The success of a screening program is dependent on uptake by the target population.[52,53] Recruitment research from other screening programs such as breast and colorectal cancers has shown that there are many different barriers to uptake of screening, particularly in some minority groups and deprived populations, and there is no universal approach.[52,54]

There is no disease-specific evidence available to advise on the best method of recruitment to a lung cancer screening program. Most published lung cancer screening trials used a combination of various media advertising, mailed invitations, and approach via general practitioners or primary practice databases to recruit participants. Analysis of eligible participants who declined LDCT screening in the trial setting revealed a variety of factors contributing to the decision. These included practical barriers (e.g., traveling, carer responsibilities, too difficult/too much effort), emotional barriers (e.g., fear of diagnosis, anxiety), fatalistic beliefs, avoidance, low perceived risk and/or benefits, knowledge barriers, and dislikes of health-care systems.[53,55,56]

In the community, current smokers generally have lower socioeconomic status and lower education levels compared with former smokers or never-smokers.[45,54,57] In the US they also were less likely to have a regular general practitioner and have reduced access to health care.[45] Respondents to lung cancer screening trials are more likely to be younger, former smokers, better educated, more health conscious, and have better access to medical care.[34–61]

Attitudes toward lung cancer screening vary in different cohorts. In the US, published surveys of different populations have highlighted some of these variations.[45,61–63] In one cross-sectional telephone survey of 2000 individuals from the general population, less than 25% of current smokers and 7.7% of former smokers believed they were at increased risk of lung cancer.[45] Current smokers were less willing to undergo surgery and had less perceived benefit of screening. Other cohorts have shown greater awareness of risk and willingness to undergo screening.[61,63] In a separate cross-sectional written survey of war veterans in the US, 80% of current smokers and 16% of former smokers believed they were at an increased risk of lung cancer.[61] The majority of participants were willing to take part in screening, have surgery, and had higher perceived benefits of screening. This cohort differed from the general population in that the majority had good access to health-care facilities.[61] In an ethnically diverse cohort recruited from a US primary care center uptake of screening was affected by fatalistic beliefs, sense of self-efficacy, understanding of impact of lung cancer, concerns about radiation effects, and mistrust of health-care workers.[62] Costs also play a role in screening uptake in health-care systems that are not fully publicly funded. It was noted in this cohort that a requirement to pay for a CT scan would be likely to reduce screening uptake.[45,62,63]

A cross-sectional survey in the United Kingdom specifically addressed smokers in socioeconomically deprived communities and also revealed complex attitudes to screening.[54] Participants

TABLE 7.2 Summary of Randomized LDCT Screening Studies

Trial	NLST[69,70]	NELSON[71,72]	ITALUNG[28,29]	MILD[25]	LUSI[30,31]	DANTE[22–24]	DLCST[26,27]	UKLS[64]
Country	United States	The Netherlands, Belgium	Italy	Italy	Germany	Italy	Denmark	Great Britain
ENROLLMENT								
Age (years)	55–74	50–75	55–69	49–75	50–69	60–74	50–70	50–75
Quit (years)	≤15	≤10	<10	<10	≤10	<10	<10	LLP risk
Pack-years	≥30	>15	≥20	≥20	≥15	≥20	≥20	≥5%
SCREENING								
Screen interval (y)	1	1, 2, 2.5	1	1 or 2	1	1	1	0
Rounds	3	4	4	5 or 10	5	5	5	1
Arms	LDCT vs. CXR	LDCT vs. usual care	LDCT vs. usual care	LDCT vs. usual care	LDCT vs. usual care	LDCT vs. usual care[a]	LDCT vs. usual care	LDCT vs. usual care
PARTICIPANTS								
Total number	53,454	15,822	3206	4099	4052	2450	4104	4055
LDCT arm	26,309	7582	1406	2376	2028	1264	2502	1994
Men (%)	59	84	65	68	65	100	55	75
Mean age (y)	61	59	61	59	NR	65	57	67
Mean pack-years	56	38	42	39	NR	47	NR	NR
Current smoker (%)	48	56	65	69	62	57	76	39
LDCT-DETECTED LUNG CANCER								
Detection of lung cancer (%)	2.6	2.6	2.7	2.1	2.9	5.2	2.7	2.1
Stage I (%)	59	71	66	65	72	64	68	67
Surgery for benign disease (%)	24	29	10	9	NR	19	NR	10

[a]All patients had baseline CXR and sputum cytology.

CXR, chest x-ray; *DANTE*, Discontinuation of Antihypertensive Treatment in Elderly People; *DLCST*, Danish Lung Cancer Screening Trial; *ITALUNG*, Italian Lung Cancer Screening Trial; *LDCT*, low-dose (radiation) computed tomography; *LLP*, Liverpool Lung Project; *LUSI*, German Lung Cancer Screening Intervention Trial; *MILD*, Multicentric Italian Lung Detection; *NELSON*, Dutch-Belgian Randomised Lung Cancer Screening Trial; *NLST*, National Lung Screening Trial; *NR*, not reported; *UKLS*, UK Lung Cancer Screening.

were positive in principle about screening, had high levels of fear of lung cancer but had low perceived benefits of screening, felt stigmatized, and held avoidant and fatalistic beliefs, particularly amongst current smokers.

These findings suggest that implementation of a lung cancer screening program in a general population may have some difficulty recruiting current smokers, would need to educate current and former smokers about their perceived risks of lung cancer and benefits of screening, and would need to design targeted education and recruitment strategies to allay fears and anxiety in certain community groups. CT costs likely need to be fully covered, and programs would preferably have multiple access points in the community (i.e., noncentralized LDCT access).[45,62]

A range of recruitment strategies will be required based on available health infrastructure and the distribution of the high-risk population in each country. National support and a centrally organized coordinated program are more likely to result in higher uptakes of screening. Approaches using invitations customized to the characteristics of the target group and involvement of the primary care team are also likely to have some benefit.[52] Therefore to target different high-risk populations in the community, to maximize uptake in a screening program, and to ultimately reduce lung cancer mortality, we face a variety of challenges both within and between countries.

SUMMARY OF RANDOMIZED SCREENING TRIALS

Published single-arm, observational screening trials since 1999 have established that lung cancer screening with LDCT is feasible.[13–21] The majority of cancers detected by LDCT are at an early stage, making them amenable to curative techniques. The NLST and the NELSON were established to assess the mortality benefit of lung cancer screening but had notable differences in design (Table 7.2). In addition, there are a number of smaller

randomized studies in Europe including the Discontinuation of Antihypertensive Treatment in Elderly People (DANTE),[22,24] Multicentric Italian Lung Detection (MILD),[25] Danish Lung Cancer Screening Trial (DLCST),[26,27] Italian Lung Cancer Screening Trial (ITALUNG),[28,29] UK Lung Cancer Screening (UKLS),[64] and German Lung Cancer Screening Intervention Trial (LUSI)[30,31] studies that are at varying degrees of follow-up and maturity (Table 7.2).[65–67] One particularly notable difference is that the NELSON and other randomized European studies have predominantly male participants compared with the NLST study (Table 7.2). This may influence the final mortality benefit, as subset analysis of the NLST data suggested greater mortality benefit for LDCT screening in women.[68]

The NLST was powered to show a mortality benefit of at least 20% and enrolled 53,456 participants with three annual screening scans (Fig. 7.1). The NELSON study was designed to show a mortality benefit of at least 25% but only enrolled about 15,822 participants with repeat screening scans at increasing intervals. The European CT screening trials collaborative group will pool the smaller randomized European studies with the NELSON study data for mortality evaluation (Table 7.2).[66,67]

Because the random assignment of eligible participants in the NELSON study took place from 2004 to 2006, 10 years of follow-up will be reached for all participants in 2016. To perform the mortality analyses, data linkages with national cancer and death registries must be undertaken and complete data will become available in early 2019. The final mortality analyses of NELSON and pooling of data with other trials within the European consortium will then be performed.[66]

PULMONARY NODULES

Screening LDCT scans in ever-smokers over 50 years of age frequently detects noncalcified pulmonary nodules.[65,73,74] A number

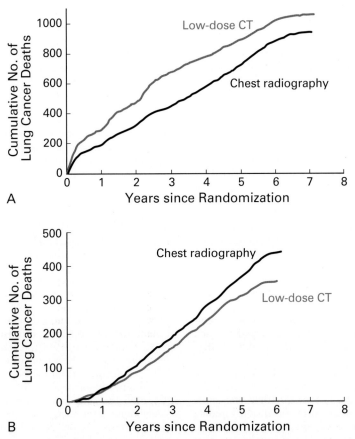

Fig. 7.1. Cumulative numbers of lung cancers and deaths from lung cancer in the National Lung Cancer Screening Trial. (A) The number of lung cancers includes lung cancers that were diagnosed from the date of randomization to December 31, 2009. (B) The number of deaths from lung cancer includes deaths that occurred from the date of randomization to January 15, 2009. *CT,* computed tomography. *(Reprinted with permission from National Lung Screening Trial Research Team, Aberle DR, Adams AM, et al. Reduced lung-cancer mortality with low-dose computed tomographic screening.* N Engl J Med. *2011;365(5):395–409.)*

of guidelines have been published to assist in the management of nodules found on the baseline LDCT and to minimize downstream investigations or unnecessary biopsy/surgery. The guidelines have used different nodule measurement techniques, action thresholds, and diagnostic algorithms and have become increasingly complex.[75–78]

In published studies, pulmonary nodules can be seen on the baseline LDCT in up to 70% of screened participants.[16,73,74] The majority of these nodules are in subcentimeters and only a small proportion will eventually be diagnosed as lung cancer, the remainder being benign. They require further surveillance or investigation because there is usually no prior imaging available to assist in nodule analysis and decision making. This may create additional work, further radiation exposure, investigations, anxiety for participants, and even unnecessary surgery.

The term "positive screen" and/or "indeterminate screen" has been used to define an action threshold that will prompt investigation before the next annual screening LDCT, that is, an "interval" assessment. The investigation may be only further radiologic follow-up at a short-term interval or could include positron emission tomography scan, biopsy, or surgery. The definition of a "positive or indeterminate screen" has varied between published studies but generally the definition uses nodule size or nodule volume thresholds and nodule appearance.[65,79] These varying definitions have caused some confusion in interpretation of different LDCT studies, and a "negative screen" did not necessarily mean an absence of pulmonary nodules. In the NLST and NELSON studies, a similar proportion of

participants had a baseline LDCT result that required a short-term interval repeat LDCT: about 19.6% and 19.2%, respectively; about 1.8% to 2.1% had biopsies, and 1.1% to 1.2% had surgery.[66,71,73,80] Surgery performed for benign disease varies between 10% and 29% with the NLST and NELSON results at the upper range of reported rates in the randomized studies (Table 7.2).

Baseline Probabilistic Nodule Risk Prediction

Although nodule size and type are important, in 20% of screening participants the largest nodule is not the malignant lesion.[80] A different approach to evaluation of pulmonary nodules detected on LDCT screening was described using the Pan-Canadian nodule prediction model.[80] This nodule risk prediction tool was based on prospectively collected longitudinal nodule data in a screened cohort of current or former smokers over 50 years of age and validated in a separate screened cohort. It utilizes both participant and nodule characteristics. The area under the curve was 0.97 and the performance persisted even when applied to nodules less than 10 mm in diameter.[80] Using this model, the number of participants with a "positive screen" requiring interval assessment after baseline LDCT can be reduced to 8% compared with 20% as seen in the NLST and NELSON trials.[79] This approach may assist in improved definition of low- and high-risk groups and simplifying the clinical decision algorithm when a nodule is detected on a baseline LDCT without the need for further imaging, investigation, or volumetric analysis.[79,80]

This risk model was subsequently validated in two independent cohorts and has been suggested to have superior performance to the American College of Radiology Lung Imaging Reporting and Data System (Lung-RADS) classification.[81–83] It has been recommended by the American College of Radiology Lung-RADS and the British Thoracic Society Guidelines. It is being prospectively evaluated in the International Lung Cancer Screening Study in Australia and Canada.[78,84]

The Lung-RADS (http://www.acr.org/Quality-Safety/Resources/LungRADS) was designed to facilitate uniform reporting of abnormalities seen on lung CT screening. The system has been validated using the NLST data and was reported to lower the false-positive rate from 27% for the NLST to 13% for Lung-RADS, and after baseline decreased to 5.1% for Lung-RADS compared with 21.8% for the NLST. A corresponding decrease in sensitivity for Lung-RADS was also noted.[85]

Prospective validation studies for this system, now that lung cancer screening is approved in the US, will help to define Lung-RADS's performance and possible integration with volumetric studies and nodule risk models.

Longitudinal Surveillance

For nodules that do not prompt immediate investigation, longitudinal assessment of behavior is the usual management, with growth or development of a solid component prompting intervention. Management of nodules detected at the baseline LDCT has been approached in different ways.[65,79,86] The majority have used maximum two-dimensional measurements and appearance of the lesion. More recently, the NELSON study and some other European studies have utilized three-dimensional nodule reconstruction, volumetric analysis of nodules, and calculation of tumor volume-doubling time (VDT) to evaluate the detection of nodule growth.[25,30,31,64] NELSON utilized a nodule protocol based on volumetric assessment, nodule growth (defined as a change in volume of ≥25%), and VDT.[87,88]

LDCT results were defined as follows: (1) negative, screened at next round (new nodules <50 mm^3 or previously detected nodule with growth <25% or growth ≥25% and VDT >600 days); (2) positive, referred to pulmonologist (new nodules >500 mm^3 or previously detected nodule with growth ≥25% and VDT <400 days); and (3) indeterminate, referred for a short-term follow-up CT (new nodules 50–500 mm^3 or previously detected nodule with VDT 400–600 days). The use of this nodule management strategy resulted in a higher positive predictive value (40.6% vs. 3.6%) and a substantially lower false-positive result (59.4% vs. 96.4%) than in the NLST.[86] The calculation of VDT, however, does require a second LDCT for comparison, and approximately 20% of NELSON participants therefore required further interval LDCT after a baseline LDCT using this algorithm. Volumetric analysis is currently limited to solid nodules and requires specific software.[89] The continued development of software systems to assist in nodule detection, automated risk calculation, or image analysis will likely significantly improve the workflow in an LDCT screening program.[90,91] Such programs are likely to include automated nodule risk assessment at baseline and volumetric analysis longitudinally in high-risk lesions (Figs. 7.1 and 7.2).

OVERDIAGNOSIS

Overdiagnosis refers to the detection of cancers that would not have led to death if untreated.[92] This includes patients who will die from another cause, for example, comorbidity or an unexpected event, even if the detected cancer becomes clinically significant.

The challenge for clinicians with overdiagnosis is that it can only be applied retrospectively and therefore it is very difficult to relate this population-based concept to an individual to assist with clinical decision making. It is important to note that overdiagnosis does not affect the known mortality benefit of LDCT screening for lung cancer, but does represent an important potential harm of screening, because it incurs additional cost, anxiety, and morbidity associated with (perhaps unnecessary) treatment.

Overdiagnosis is present in all screening programs, for any cancer type. The prevalence of overdiagnosed cancers in LDCT screening trials is certain, but the precise magnitude is not known. There are wide-ranging estimates of overdiagnosis from LDCT screening for lung cancer, dependent on statistical approach, the population being studied, accounting for lead time and length time bias, histopathologic cell type, the definition of a positive screen, and even the definition of overdiagnosis itself. Modeling studies by the Cancer Intervention and Surveillance Modeling Network estimate that 9.5% to 11.9% of screen-detected lung cancers are overdiagnosed.[46] Analysis of the 1089 lung cancers reported in the LDCT arm and 969 in the chest x-ray arm of the NLST suggested that the probability of overdiagnosis for any screen-detected lung cancer was 18.5% (95% confidence interval [CI], 5.4% to 30.6%).[93] Other modeling estimates with different approaches to account for length and lead time bias suggest that the proportion of overdiagnosed cases may be less than 10%.[94] For bronchioalveolar lung cancers (now considered in situ adenocarcinomas) in the NLST, this figure was estimated to be 78.9% (95% CI, 62.2% to 93.5%). Overdiagnosis may also relate to the phenotype of the screened population: after stratification of 18,475 individuals from the NLST by the presence, or absence, of spirometric-defined chronic obstructive pulmonary disease (COPD), the early-stage adenocarcinomas were almost exclusively found in the normal-spirometry group.[95] This suggests that overdiagnosis is more likely in individuals with no spirometric evidence of COPD.

From a clinical perspective, mitigating the possible harm of overdiagnosis requires careful use of terminology and perhaps even judicious use of terminology for a positive screen, for instance not regarding a lesion with long VDT of over 600 days, or a pure ground-glass opacity, as a true-positive screen.[96] Models developed from the NLST data suggest that only some lung cancers with low aggressive behavior (i.e., predominantly the in situ adenocarcinomas/atypical adenomatous hyperplasia) will become symptomatic, with 14% at 5 years and 27% at 10 years becoming clinically significant.[93,97] Similarly, long-term follow-up of pure ground-glass opacity lesions in a Japanese cohort indicated 16% demonstrating tumor growth after 3 years' follow-up.[98] Clinical decision making with consideration for the probability of a lesion becoming clinically relevant, in tandem with attention to age and comorbidities (with their associated risk), and personal preference, is required for individuals in whom such (possibly) indolent cancers are identified on LDCT.

SMOKING CESSATION

Aside from the clear impact of smoking cessation on all-cause mortality, the importance is highlighted following resection for lung cancer with a large systematic review reporting a 5-year survival rate of 77% in those able to quit and 33% in those continuing to smoke.[99,100] This study reported statistically significant increased hazard ratios for all-cause mortality, reoccurrence, and development of second primary with continued smoking after resection of early-stage nonsmall cell lung cancer.

Within lung cancer screening studies the proportion of current smokers has ranged from 47.3% to 76.1% at baseline.[22,26–28,30,36,101,102] Cessation rates of study participants have ranged from 6.6% to 29.0%,[27,103–111] which are likely to be higher than spontaneous quit rates in the general population (5% to 10%).[112,113] Increased numbers of quit attempts amongst participants likely lead to higher cessation rates in some, but not

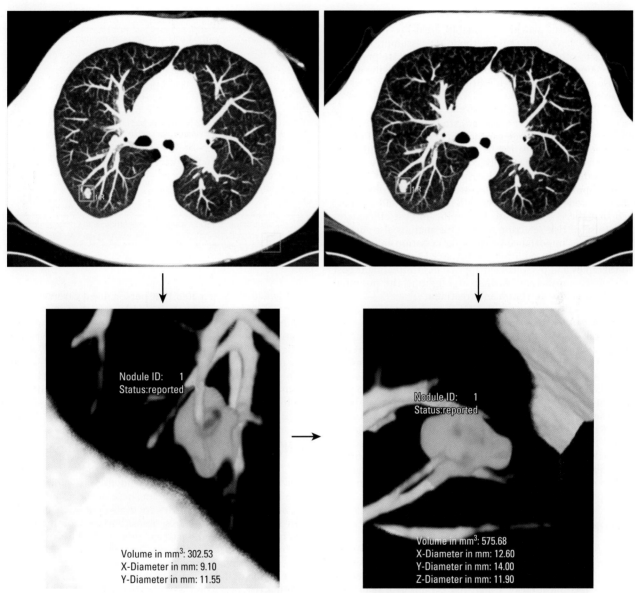

Fig. 7.2. Example of assessment of nodule size using volumetric software in the NELSON trial. Baseline low-dose computed tomography shows a nodule with a volume of 302 mm³ in the right upper lobe of a 66-year-old man. Three months later, the volume increased to 575 mm³; the volume-doubling time was 98 days. On diagnostic workup, a pT1 N0 Mx squamous cell carcinoma was diagnosed.

all, studies.[103,105–110] It is not known whether the higher quit and cessation rate is a result of selection bias, of increased health awareness due to participation in a cancer screening trial, of the accompanying smoking cessation interventions, or perhaps related to the CT scan result itself.

The number of quit attempts by participants with an abnormal result on LDCT screening is higher than that by participants with a normal result.[103,105–110] The positive relationship of an abnormal CT scan and smoking cessation is present for any abnormal CT finding, but is stronger for abnormalities suspicious for lung cancer, with persistent effect for up to 5 years.[114] This observation suggests that the finding of an abnormality on CT screening may be a teachable moment for current smokers.

Some studies have demonstrated an initial low uptake of optional smoking cessation services, hence the need to integrate smoking cessation both at enrollment and also with repeated interventions over multiple time points.[111,115,116] Most guidelines now recommend integrated smoking cessation within a lung cancer screening program, and integrated smoking cessation is a requirement for Medicare-funded screening in the US.[37,46,117–119] There are recent data supporting the cost-effectiveness,[120] additional mortality benefit,[121] and a high sustained quit rate with such an approach,[114] although the best strategy to optimize smoking cessation and long-term abstinence in the context of LDCT screening is not known.[111]

Cost-Effectiveness

The cost-effectiveness of any screening intervention is one of the major considerations for national or federal policy.[122] There has been a wide variance of cost-effectiveness from different (observational) studies, with varying methods, outcomes, assumptions, and data sources.[123–126] Randomized controlled trial data on cost-effectiveness from the NLST report $67,000 per quality-adjusted life year gained (95% CI, $52,000–186,000) and £8466 (95% CI, £5542–12,569) from the UKLS study.[64,127] As randomized controlled trial data, these reports provide invaluable "real-life" data, and these reports have different methodolgic assumptions and approaches to others (as well as differing health-care practices in the US compared with many other countries), making direct comparisons difficult and highlighting the continuing need for local data.

Cost-effectiveness modeling of the Pan-Canadian Early Detection of Lung Cancer (PanCan) study demonstrated that LDCT-detected early-stage cancers treated by surgical resection are cheaper than treating later-stage lung cancer and that the cost-effectiveness of any program is most sensitive to all-cause mortality and the annual costs of screening.[128] Importantly, the approach in the PanCan study utilized probabilistic prediction modeling (as did the UKLS study) and demonstrated that there are likely to be significant cost efficiencies from the use of risk-selection tools. This analysis also further highlighted the importance of smoking cessation influencing cost-effectiveness. In addition, in advanced lung cancer, targeted therapies and personalized approaches to treatment cost more than chemotherapy, further highlighting the potential importance of early detection and treatment.[129]

In the NLST, screening with LDCT was much more cost-effective in women than in men and among the groups with a higher risk of lung cancer, which demonstrates the importance of identifying high-risk groups and enhancing pretest probability.[127] Identifying the most appropriate means of recruitment of high-risk individuals,[130] the size of the potential population at risk,[128] development of an accurate risk prediction model,[48] nodule management algorithms minimizing repeat scans for false-positive nodules,[80] and effective smoking cessation interventions[131] are key factors in determining the cost of a lung cancer screening program. The challenge for policy makers is assessing unique federal or national conditions, health-care systems, and costs to judge if a lung cancer screening program will be cost-effective, and thus appropriate for local populations.

BIOMARKERS

Since the publication of the NLST data, there has been renewed interest in the development of biomarkers that might assist in improving pretest probability of a positive result for screening (i.e., better identification of a high-risk group, with reduction in number needed to treat) and/or to improving specificity for diagnosis following identification of an indeterminate nodule.

A molecular biomarker could come from a variety of sources including sources that are tissue based (dependent on accessibility) or biofluid based (including peripheral blood, urine, sputum, and breath). Such biofluid-based markers include circulating tumor cells, cell-free DNA and RNA, proteins, peptides, metabolites, microRNA, antibodies to tumor-associated antigens or tumor microenvironment, and exhaled breath condensate.[132] Despite hundreds of biomarkers reaching Food and Drug Administration phases I and II of development, few have reached phase III (the capacity of the biomarker to longitudinally detect preclinical disease) and currently four are in phase IV (prospective evaluation: summarized in Table 7.3). At present, no biomarkers are currently used in clinical practice.[133,134]

Arguably, the most informative biomarker available at this time is the measurement of spirometry (forced expiratory volume over 1 second and forced vital capacity), which in turn can identify individuals with airflow obstruction and COPD. The presence of COPD improves risk selection for lung cancer screening, including a subanalysis from the CT arm of the NLST, demonstrating that spirometric airflow limitation was associated with a doubling of lung cancer risk, no apparent overdiagnosis, and a more favorable stage shift.[48,95,135–137,139]

TABLE 7.3 Biomarkers Under Prospective Evaluation

Autoantibody signature[135]	The EarlyCDT-Lung test performs an assay for seven autoantibody signatures. Undergoing evaluation as a pre-CT screening tool.
Serum miRNA[136]	A 34-miRNA signature capable of stratifying risk in early and advanced NSCLC, benign lesions, and other tumor types. Evaluation as part of the COSMOS study.
Plasma miRNA[137]	A 24-miRNA signature for the detection of NSCLC with stratification of low, intermediate, and high risk. Evaluation as part of the MILD study.
Prosurfactant B[138]	The integration of plasma pro-SFTPB levels into a lung cancer risk prediction model (using phenotypic information) significantly improves lung cancer prediction in a high-risk cohort. Evaluated as part of the PanCan study.

CT, computed tomography; *MILD,* Multicentric Italian Lung Detection; *miRNA,* microRNA; *NSCLC,* nonsmall cell lung cancer; *SFTPB,* surfactant protein B.

It is widely anticipated that personalized care will increasingly influence clinical decision making in the future. As such, the drive to identify and develop biomarkers that can assist in discrimination of high or low risk of lung cancer, or benign or malignant tumor will continue. A future biomarker will need to gain sufficiently high sensitivity (to rule out disease), or high specificity (to rule in disease), or alter clinical decision making, as well as being acceptable to patients, and contribute to the cost-effectiveness of any lung cancer early detection program.

CONCLUSION

LDCT screening for lung cancer has produced a significant reduction in lung cancer–specific and all-cause mortality in the NLST study. Screening programs have now commenced in the US, and many other countries are evaluating implementation in their individual health-care systems. Further mortality outcome data from the NELSON trial and other pooled European studies will become available in the near future.

In the interim, we anticipate continued efforts to help improve the selection of individuals who will benefit most from screening by using risk prediction models to characterize the highest risk groups in our communities. In addition, further improvements in the management of screen-detected pulmonary nodules by utilizing prediction models, volumetric and CT image analysis, and incorporation of biomarkers are needed to reduce unnecessary investigations and surgery for benign disease and maximize cost-effectiveness.

The future implementation of lung cancer screening will require coordinated programs with multidisciplinary team management, integrated smoking cessation, quality assurance/accreditation, and standardized algorithms to maximize the benefits and minimize the harms of screening. It is paramount that these endeavors continue in parallel with efforts to reduce smoking prevalence.

KEY REFERENCES

37. Field J, Smith R, Aberle D, et al. International Association for the study of lung cancer computed tomography screening workshop 2011 report. *J Thorac Oncol.* 2012;7:10–19.
46. Moyer VA. Screening for lung cancer: US Preventive Services Task Force recommendation statement. *Ann Intern Med.* 2014;160:330–338.

See Expertconsult.com for full list of references.

8 Preclinical Biomarkers for the Early Detection of Lung Cancer

Jun-Chieh J. Tsay, Alissa K. Greenberg, William N. Rom, and Pierre P. Massion

SUMMARY OF KEY POINTS

- This chapter provides a review of some of the most promising recent studies of diagnostic biomarkers in lung cancer.
- We discuss the challenges and the importance of biomarker validation. Current guidelines recommend a study design to include prospective collections of specimens and retrospective blinded evaluation.
- A novel multiomics approach to biomarker discovery has greatly advanced the field of early lung cancer detection.
- Noninvasive biomarkers in the blood, sputum, airway epithelium, or exhaled breath can be combined with imaging to detect early stage lung cancer and improve mortality.

Lung cancer is the leading cause of cancer deaths in the United States and worldwide.[1] This statistic is largely due to the persistent poor survival of patients diagnosed with lung cancer. In the United States as of 2009, the overall 5-year survival for nonsmall cell lung cancer (NSCLC) remained at only 16.6%.[2] However, if the cancer is detected at an early stage, the 5-year survival exceeds 50%.[3] For this reason, in the last decade, the quest for an effective means of early diagnosis has intensified. In 2011, the results of the randomized multicenter National Lung Screening Trial (NLST) were published, confirming that early diagnosis of lung cancer can improve survival.[4] Screening for lung cancer in the high-risk group studied in the NLST now has the support of the US Preventive Services Task Force (grade B recommendation).[5] However, low-dose computed tomography (CT) of the chest for lung cancer screening has significant drawbacks, including cost, radiation exposure, high false-positive rates, and a risk of overdiagnosis of indolent cancers. Thus the results of NLST have sparked even greater interest in developing more practical and more specific means of early detection of lung cancer, using noninvasive biomarkers of early disease.

Biomarkers for lung cancer have several potential clinical uses in addition to early detection (Fig. 8.1). They may be used for risk stratification, optimal treatment selection, prognostication, and monitoring for recurrence. Markers of risk can help identify a population to be screened. At this preclinical stage, the marker identifies individuals without disease but with factors that may predispose them to lung cancer. Given the high false-positive rate with CT screening, a marker that could more clearly define the at-risk population could decrease the number of screening CT scans conducted and also improve the specificity of CT screening, thus decreasing patient anxiety and the need for repeated CT and invasive procedures induced by false-positive nodules.

Markers are currently used for treatment selection, prognostication, and monitoring for recurrence in patients with known disease. A variety of markers, reflecting the biology of lung cancer

progression from premalignant lesions to invasive lung cancer, may prove to be more useful for each of these roles. In this chapter, we focus on current and potential biomarkers for the early detection of lung cancer. Markers of risk and prognosis are not reviewed.

EARLY DETECTION

For the foreseeable future, CT will undoubtedly remain an important part of any program for the early detection of lung cancer. CT can detect the small noncalcified nodules that may represent early lung cancers. However, as a stand-alone screening tool, this technique is problematic. First, it has poor specificity because of the high prevalence of nonspecific benign pulmonary nodules.[4-6] Second, CT is costly, and the necessity for repeated CT to determine growth rates over time can expose patients to potentially harmful radiation.[7] Lastly, we cannot predict which early lung cancers will progress and which will remain indolent for prolonged periods.

The ultimate goal of lung cancer early detection biomarker research is to develop a marker that identifies early stage lung cancer (or even preneoplasia) and prompts a change in clinical practice that saves lives. A more obtainable target may be a marker that can be used in conjunction with chest CT to help distinguish malignant from benign nodules found on CT images or identify aggressive or indolent phenotypes of early lung cancers found by imaging.[8] Depending on the selected size cutoff, 15% to more than 50% of individuals in CT screening programs have nodules.[4,9-14] NLST demonstrated that more than 96% of the nodules identified were thought to be benign based on stability on follow-up CT. Of nodules that are ultimately surgically resected, up to 30% are found to have benign pathology.[15] In the NLST, 24% of patients who underwent an invasive diagnostic procedure were found to have nodules of benign etiology. To address the issue of large numbers of false-positive findings on CT, experts have suggested using a larger nodule size cutoff of 7 mm or 8 mm, which would decrease the number of positive CT results to 5% to 7%,[16] or narrowing the definition of high-risk individuals who would be eligible for screening.[17] An effective biomarker would also be an invaluable aid in the management of these indeterminate pulmonary nodules. Depending on their assay performance characteristics, biomarkers could guide the clinician toward reassurance, watchful waiting, or immediate biopsy or resection, and thus decrease the anxiety, cost, and uncertainty of lung cancer screening.

Lung cancer biomarkers may also reduce the problem of overdiagnosis in lung cancer screening. Although the NLST demonstrated that screening can decrease lung cancer mortality, a percentage of cancers diagnosed are likely indolent malignancies that may not progress if disregarded. At the New York University screening program, one-third of the cancers diagnosed were indolent adenocarcinomas, which were followed for a prolonged period before resection and were still stage I at the time of surgery.[14] A biomarker that could a priori identify these indolent cancers may spare older patients or patients with other medical problems unnecessary surgeries.

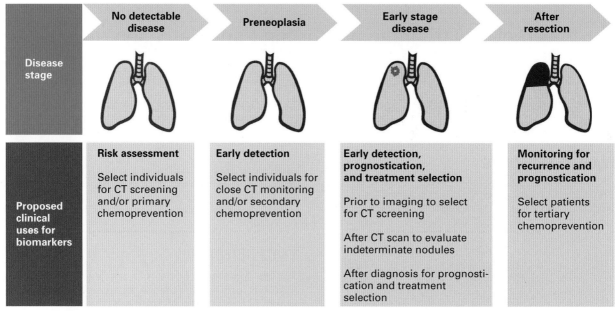

Fig. 8.1. Lung cancer biomarkers have many potential clinical uses, depending on the marker and the clinical stage. Four clinical contexts for biomarker use include the following: (1) During the period before lung cancer is detectable, markers may be used for risk assessment and to identify populations that may benefit from lung cancer screening or chemopreventive measures. (2) When lung cancer is in the preneoplastic stage, it is generally not clinically detectable. Biomarkers that identify preneoplasia would lead clinicians to recommend close monitoring and chemoprevention if available. (3) Early stage disease can be detected by thoracic imaging, but this technique is nonspecific, and indeterminate nodules are frequent. Lung cancer biomarkers may be used either to identify individuals who should undergo computed tomography (CT) screening or to differentiate benign from malignant nodules. At this stage, biomarkers may also be used for prognostication and treatment selection if they can distinguish indolent from aggressive disease. (4) After lung cancer has been treated, biomarkers may be useful for monitoring for recurrence or to determine prognosis and select patients for adjuvant chemotherapy or tertiary chemoprevention.

The Biology of Lung Carcinogenesis

Continued progress in understanding the sequence of molecular changes underlying the progression from preneoplasia to invasive lung cancer has galvanized research into discovery and validation of lung cancer biomarkers for early detection. It has also raised the possibility of personalizing lung cancer treatment using biomarker profiles. The World Health Organization defines the various preneoplastic lesions of the bronchial epithelium as squamous dysplasia and carcinoma in situ, which progresses to squamous cell carcinoma; atypical adenomatous hyperplasia, which may precede adenocarcinoma; and diffuse idiopathic pulmonary neuroendocrine cell hyperplasia, which may progress to carcinoid. Small cell lung cancer (SCLC) is believed to arise from extensively molecularly damaged epithelium without going through recognizable preneoplastic stages.[18–20]

Alterations in gene expression and chromosome structure known to be associated with malignant transformation have been demonstrated in these preneoplastic lesions, and the changes appear to be sequential; in particular, their frequency and number increase with increasing atypia. Some of the alterations found in preneoplastic lesions include hyperproliferation and loss of cell cycle control; abnormalities in the p53 pathway, the RAS genes, and genes in the genomic region of 3p14.2 and 3q26-29;[21] aberrant gene promoter methylation;[22] increased vascular growth; altered extracellular matrix; decreased retinoic acid and retinoid X receptor expression;[23] and many other genetic and epigenetic changes.[18,19]

Biomarker Validation

The validation of a biomarker for clinical use is challenging. Any biomarker considered for use in a clinical setting must satisfy a host of criteria related to ease of use and performance. The biomarker must be relatively noninvasive, require only small amounts of material needing a minimum of preparation, be quantifiable and reproducible in multiple populations and laboratories, have a proven clinical use with acceptable sensitivity and specificity for this use, be acceptable to the target population, and be cost-effective and reimbursed by health insurers.[24] No markers have yet made it through these rigorous requirements, although many are in the pipeline.[25] Appropriate study design will be crucial to bringing any of these markers to clinical use.

Guidelines for biomarker study design and statistical evaluation suggest that validation should be conducted using a prospective specimen collection retrospective blinded evaluation design.[26] In this approach, specimens are collected prospectively from a longitudinal cohort that represents the target population. After the outcome status is determined, a nested case–control study can be designed. Cases and controls are selected randomly for biomarker studies, with the investigators blinded to the case–control status. Random sampling of cases and controls from within a well-defined cohort provides validity to the case–control design. An important element of this study design is that the validation population must be representative of the population in which the biomarker will be used, to minimize false positives. In the case of lung cancer, this means that individuals with a history of tobacco use and its related morbidities, including chronic obstructive pulmonary disease, cardiovascular disease, and other malignancies, must be included in the validation cohort. Ideally, the biomarker can be tested in longitudinal samples to ensure its accuracy in detecting early, preclinical disease. Measures of validity include sensitivity, specificity, negative predictive value, and positive predictive value (which can be summarized with a receiver operating characteristic [ROC] curve).[27] The prevalence of the disease influences these measures, thus it is important that the biomarker validation process be applied to all possible populations in which the marker would be used. Lastly, when a potential marker has been validated as effective for early diagnosis, it should be evaluated in a screening trial with lung cancer mortality as the end point to prove that use of the biomarker decreases mortality and the validation studies were not hampered by problems of overdiagnosis, lead-time bias, or length bias. The Early Detection Research Network of the US National Cancer Institute has established guidelines for cancer biomarker development and validation.[28]

Advances in Techniques for Biomarker Discovery

Currently, we see a profusion of potential biomarkers for lung cancer. Different histologic types, different stages of disease, and a variety of molecular pathways to transformation contribute to making the process of biomarker discovery for lung cancer complex. New high-throughput technologies allow researchers to look for and validate multiple biomarkers simultaneously. Microarrays are used to evaluate thousands of potential markers concurrently.

For example, circulating DNA (cDNA) microarrays identify thousands of genes that are differentially expressed in lung cancers, preneoplasias, and normal lung; antibody arrays evaluate multiple antigens or antibodies at once; and methylation arrays identify methylation of many different gene promoters simultaneously. Proteomics is the study of protein profiles in tissues and body fluids. Matrix-assisted laser desorption/ionization time-of-flight mass spectrometry (MALDI-TOF MS) and surface-enhanced laser desorption/ionization have been used to describe protein profiles and to identify individual protein markers in lung cancer. The ability to accurately measure quantitative transcriptome in individual cells with relatively small number of sequencing read makes single-cell RNA sequencing a popular technology for biomarker discovery. In recent years, important advances in the development and validation of these and other high-throughput technologies have raised the potential for great strides in biomarker discovery.

Specimen Types

One of the most important criteria for a successful biomarker is that the testing material be easily accessible. Current markers use multiple biologic sources. Tissue-based assays are generally the most invasive, but may be acceptable in some circumstances. The concept of field cancerization supports the theory that surrogate tissues—such as bronchial, buccal, and nasal brushings; endobronchial biopsy specimens; or even exhaled breath—may be used as markers of increased risk for lung cancer. Genetic and epigenetic changes in the bronchial epithelium or perhaps the nasal or buccal epithelium may mirror changes in the lower respiratory tract and suggest that a lesion seen on CT images represents malignancy. Although obtaining the tissue may require bronchoscopy, pairing molecular markers obtained from the airways with a high-risk profile and a lesion on CT images may increase the specificity of lung cancer screening. The potential use of tissue-based biomarkers is highly dependent on the accessibility of the specimens and the robustness of the assay offered. It may take additional time to refine airway epithelium-based biomarkers because banked samples are not as readily available as they are for tumor tissues or blood. Blood-based assays are attractive due to the ease of acquisition. This simplicity aids in the discovery process, the validation process, and the acceptance into clinical practice. Altered or methylated DNA, overexpressed messenger RNA (mRNA), microRNA (miRNA), proteins, peptides, metabolites, and even circulating tumor cells (CTCs) can all be detected in the circulating blood; however, there are significant challenges as well. Blood is a dynamic medium, which reflects various physiologic and pathologic states that can overwhelm the detection of an early stage, preclinical cancer.

Other biofluids—exhaled breath condensate, sputum, and urine—are also easily accessible samples for biomarker analysis. Each type of sample has its own appeal and its challenges. Exhaled breath is easily and painlessly obtained, and large volumes can be collected without detriment to the patient. Theoretically, the use of exhaled breath analysis may allow for a more specific lung cancer diagnosis. However, only volatile compounds can be detected and genetic material is sparse or absent. Sputum has the advantage of perhaps giving results specific to lung cancer, as it contains both bronchial epithelial cells and other secretions reflecting the local milieu of the lung.[29,30] However, it is difficult to obtain adequate sputum samples from the lower airways, and samples are frequently exclusively saliva. Urine is an easily accessible biofluid, but it may be less specific to lung cancer. Lung cancer biomarker research using urine as the biologic sample is still in its infancy.

LUNG CANCER BIOMARKERS FOR EARLY DETECTION

Given the many different genetic and epigenetic changes involved in malignant transformation in lung cancer, it is not surprising that innumerable potential biomarkers exist. With progress in understanding the biology of lung carcinogenesis, the development of high-throughput techniques for biomarker discovery, and increased focus on early detection of lung cancer, the field of lung cancer biomarker research has expanded at a phenomenal rate. As yet, no biomarker has been shown to have adequate sensitivity, specificity, reproducibility, and ease of use to be validated as a biomarker for the early detection of lung cancer. However, many studies of biomarkers for the early diagnosis of lung cancer have shown promising results (Table 8.1).

Cytology

Sputum contains bronchial epithelial cells from the central airways and theoretically may provide a means to detect a central malignancy or changes reflecting field cancerization, which suggest a high risk that the lungs may harbor a malignancy. However, trying to detect early lung cancer by sputum cytology has not been particularly successful. Bronchial epithelial cells comprise less than 5% of sputum samples, and even after using techniques to enrich for these cells, detecting morphologic changes is subjective and therefore unreliable. Studies have shown that sputum cytology has very low sensitivity and specificity and is a particularly poor method for detecting adenocarcinoma.[35] However, when sputum cytology is combined with some other markers described here (including genetic abnormalities,[36] chromosomal aneusomy,[37,38] DNA methylation,[39,40] or miRNA[41,42]), sensitivity increases. Automated cytometry for more objective and quantitative cytopathologic assessment may also help address the issues of subjectivity and low sensitivity. In some reports, an automated system quantifying the DNA content improved the sensitivity of sputum cytology to the range of 75% to 80% in heavy smokers.[43,44]

Buccal epithelium is easily obtained, may be used as a surrogate for bronchial epithelium, and reflects the field cancerization effect. Backman et al.[45] reported the ability to detect abnormal nanostructure architecture in microscopically normal-appearing buccal

TABLE 8.1 Biomarkers Evaluated for Detection of Lung Cancers

Author (y)	Type of Marker	Type of Specimen	Marker(s)	No. of Markers	Platform	No. in Training Set	No. in Test Set	Sensitivity[a] (%)	Specificity[a] (%)	AUC[a]
CYTOLOGY										
Varella-Garcia et al. (2004)[37]	Chromosomal aneusomy and cytology	Sputum	Multitarget DNA FISH assay and cytology	2	FISH	33	NR	83	80	NR
Xin et al. (2005)[43]	Sputum cytometry	Sputum	DNA content and cytologic malignancy grade	2	Automated DNA image cytometry	2461	NR	80	93	0.87
Kemp et al. (2007)[44]	Sputum cytometry	Sputum	Lung sign: Cell nuclear features (DNA content, chromatin distribution)	13 features	Automated DNA image cytometry	1123	NR	40	91	0.69
Roy et al. (2010)[45]	Nanoarchitectural alterations	Buccal epithelium	Disorder strength of cell nanoarchitecture L (d)	1	Partial wave spectroscopic microscopy	207	46	78	78	0.84
NONCODING RNAs										
Xing et al. (2010)[42]	MicroRNA	Sputum	miR-205, miR-210, miR-708 (squamous)	3	qRT-PCR	96	122	73	96	0.87
Xie et al. (2010)[71]	MicroRNA	Sputum	miR-21	1	qRT-PCR	50	NR	70	100	0.90
Yu et al. (2010)[72]	MicroRNA	Sputum	miRNA signature for adenocarcinoma	7	qRT-PCR	72	122	81	92	0.90
Bianchi et al. (2011)[60]	MicroRNA	Serum	miRNA signature	34	qRT-PCR	64	64	71	90	0.89
Boeri et al. (2011)[59]	MicroRNA	Plasma	miRNA signature	15	miRNA array and qRT-PCR	20	15	80	90	0.85
Boeri et al. (2011)[59]	MicroRNA	Plasma	miRNA signature	13	miRNA array and qRT-PCR	19	16	75	100	0.88
Shen et al. (2011)[62]	MicroRNA	Plasma	miR-21, miR-126, miR-210, miR-486-5p	4	qRT-PCR	28	87	86	97	0.93
Shen et al. (2011)[63]	MicroRNA	Plasma	miR-21, miR-210, miR-486-5p	3	qRT-PCR	94	156	75	85	0.86
Chen et al. (2012)[179]	MicroRNA	Serum	miRNA signature	10	qRT-PCR	310	310	93	90	0.97
Hennessey (2012)[61]	MicroRNA	Serum	miR-15b and miR-27b	2	qRT-PCR	50	130	100	84	0.98
Patnaik et al. (2012)[69]	MicroRNA	Whole blood	miRNA signature	96	Locked nucleic acid microarrays	45	NR	88	89	0.94
Liao et al. (2010)[73]	Small nucleolar RNA	Plasma	snoRD33, snoRD66, and snoRD76	3	qRT-PCR	85	NR	81	96	0.88
GENETIC CHANGES AND GENE EXPRESSION										
Miura et al. (2006)[123]	mRNA	Serum	Human telomerase catalytic component and epidermal growth factor receptor	2	qRT-PCR	192	NR	89	73	NR
Li et al. (2007)[36]	Genetic deletions	Sputum	FHIT and HYAL2	2	FISH	74	NR	76	92	NR
Spira et al. (2007)[87]	mRNA	Airway epithelium	Gene expression signature	80	Affymetrix array (Santa Clara, CA, USA)	77	52	80	84	NR
Blomquist et al. (2009)[89]	Gene expression	Bronchial epithelium	Antioxidant, DNA repair, and transcription factor genes	14	Standardized RT-PCR	49	40	82	80	0.87
Showe et al. (2009)[90]	Gene expression	PBMC	Gene signature	29	Illumina human whole genome bead array	228	NR	91	80	NR
Zander et al. (2011)[64]	Gene expression	Whole blood	Gene expression profile	484	Illumina human whole genome bead array	77	156	97	89	0.97
DNA METHYLATION										
Palmisano et al. (2000)[39]	DNA methylation	Sputum	P16, O6-MGMT	2	PCR	144	NR	100	n/a	NR
Kim et al. (2004)[106]	DNA methylation	Bronchoalveolar lavage	p16, RARβ, H-cadherin, RASSF1A	4	MS-PCR	212	NR	68	NR	NR
Grote et al. (2004)[108]	DNA methylation	Bronchial aspirates	APC	1	qMS-PCR	222	NR	39	99	NR
Grote et al. (2005)[109]	DNA methylation	Bronchial aspirates	p16(INK4a), RARB2	2	qMS-PCR	139	NR	69	87	NR
Belinsky et al. (2006)[98]	DNA methylation	Sputum	p16, MGMT, DAPK, RASSF1A, PAX5β, GATA5	6	Nested MS-PCR	190	NR	64	64	NR
Grote et al. (2006)[107]	DNA methylation	Bronchial aspirates	RASSF1A	1	qMS-PCR	203	NR	46	100	NR
Ostrow et al. (2010)[104]	DNA methylation	Plasma	DCC, Kif1a, NISCH, Rarb	4	qRT-PCR	37	183	73	71	0.64
Schmidt et al. (2010)[180]	DNA methylation	Bronchial aspirates	SHOX2	1	PCR	n/a	523	68	95	0.86
Begum et al. (2011)[97]	DNA methylation	Serum	APC, CDH1, MGMT, DCC, RASSF1A, AIM	6	qPCR	401	106	84	57	NR
Kneip et al. (2011)[181]	DNA methylation	Plasma	SHOX2	1	qPCR	40	371	60	90	0.78
Richards et al. (2011)[182]	DNA methylation	Lung tissues	TCF21	1	PCR	42	63	76	98	NR
PROTEIN AND PROTEOMIC MARKERS										
Khan et al. (2004)[131]	Protein	Serum	Serum amyloid A	1	ELISA	50	NR	60	64	NR

8

Study	Sample	Biomarker class	Markers	No.	Technology	n1	n2	Sens.	Spec.	AUC
Rahman et al. (2005)[183]	Bronchial biopsies	Proteomic profile	TMLS4, ACBP, CSTA, cytoC, MIF, ubiquitin, ACBP, Des-ubiquitin	8	MALDI-MS	51	60	66	88	0.77
Patz et al. (2007)[132]	Serum	Protein panel	CEA, RBP, α1-antitrypsin, SCCA	4	ELISA	100	97	78	75	NR
Yildiz et al. (2007)[134]	Serum	Proteomic profile	Proteomic signature	7 features	MALDI-MS	185	106	58	86	0.82
Farlow et al. (2010)[151]	Serum	Protein panel	TNFα, CYFRA 21-1, IL-1ra, MMP-2, MCP-1, and sE selectin	6	Luminex (Austin, TX, USA) and ELISA	133	88	99	95	0.98
Gessner et al. (2010)[177]	Exhaled breath condensate	Proteins (cytokines)	VEGF, bFGF, angiogenin	3	Multiplex bead-based immunoassay	75	NR	100	95	0.99
Ostroff et al. (2010)[135]	Serum	Aptamers	Aptamer signature	12	Aptamers	985	341	89	83	0.90
Joseph et al. (2012)[120]	Plasma	Protein	Osteopontin velocity	1	ELISA	43	NR	80	88	0.88
Lee et al. (2012)[184]	Serum	Proteomics	AAT, CYFRA 21-1, IGF-1, RANTES, AFP	5	Luminex	347	49	80.3	99.3	0.99
Higgins et al. (2012)[121]	Plasma	Protein	Variant Ciz1	1	Western blot	170	160	95	74	0.90
Ajona et al. (2013)[129]	Plasma	Complement fragment	C4d	1	Immunocytochemistry	190	NR	NR	NR	0.73
Patz et al. (2013)[133]	Serum	Protein panel, clinical features	CEA, α1-antitrypsin, SCCA, nodule size	4	ELISA	509	399	80	89	NR
Li et al. (2013)[136]	Serum	Protein panel	Protein panel	13	Multiple reaction monitoring mass spectrometry	143	104	71	44	NR
AUTOANTIBODIES AND TUMOR-ASSOCIATED ANTIGENS										
Zhong et al. (2005)[147]	Plasma	Autoantibodies	Phage peptides	5	Fluorescent protein microarray	41	40	90	95	0.98
Zhong et al. (2006)[143]	Serum	Autoantibodies	Phage peptides	5	ELISA	46	56	91	91	0.99
Qiu et al. (2008)[150]	Serum	Autoantibodies	Annexin I, 14-3-3 theta, LAMR1	3	Protein array	NR	170	51	82	0.73
Rom et al. (2010)[152]	Serum	Tumor-associated antigens	Panel of tumor-associated antigens	10	ELISA	194	NR	81	97	0.90
Wu et al. (2010)[146]	Serum	Autoantibodies	Phage peptide clones	6	ELISA	20	180	92	92	0.96
Boyle et al. (2011)[155]	Serum	Autoantibodies	p53, NY-ESO-1, CAGE, GBU4-5, annexin 1, SOX2	6	ELISA	241	255	32	91	0.64
Lam et al. (2011)[158]	Serum	Autoantibodies	p53, NY-ESO-1, CAGE, GBU4-5, annexin 1, SOX2	6	ELISA	NR	1376	39	87	NR
Chapman et al. (2012)[159]	Serum	Autoantibodies	p53, NY-ESO-1, CAGE, GBU4-5, SOX2, HuD, and MAGE A4	7	ELISA	501	836	41	93	NR
Pedchenko et al. (2013)[148]	Serum	Autoantibodies	Single-chain fragment variable antibodies to IgM autoantibodies	6	Fluorometric microvolume and homogeneous bridging MESA SCALE DISCOVERY	30	43	80	87	0.88
VOLATILE ORGANIC COMPOUNDS										
Phillips et al. (1999)[168]	Exhaled breath	VOC	VOC profile	22	GC/MS	108	100	100	81	NR
Phillips et al. (2003)[74]	Exhaled breath	VOC	VOC profile	9	GC/MS	178	108	85	80	NR
Poli et al. (2005)[167]	Exhaled breath	VOC	VOC profile	13	GC/MS	146	72	72	93	NR
Mazzone et al. (2007)[172]	Exhaled breath	VOC	VOC pattern	36 sensors	Colorimetric sensor array	100	43	73	72	NR
Bajtarevic et al. (2009)[170]	Exhaled breath	VOC	VOC profile	21	Proton transfer reaction MS/solid-phase microextraction, GC/MS	96	NR	71	100	NR
Ligor et al. (2009)[171]	Exhaled breath	VOC	VOC profile	8	Solid-phase microextraction, GC/MS	96	NR	51	100	NR
Fuchs et al. (2010)[169]	Exhaled breath	VOC	Aldehydes: pentanal, hexanal, octanal, and nonanal	4	GC/MS	36	NR	75	96	NR

aWhen test set available, sensitivity, specificity, and AUC apply to the test set.

AFP, alpha-fetoprotein; AUC, area under the receiver operating characteristic curve; bFGF, basic fibroblast growth factor; CEA, carcinoembryonic antigen; ELISA, enzyme-linked immunosorbent assay; FISH, fluorescent in situ hybridization; GC/MS, gas chromatography/mass spectrometry; IGF, insulin-like growth factor; IgM, immunoglobulin M; IL, interleukin; MALDI-MS, matrix-assisted laser desorption/ionization mass spectrometry; miRNA, microRNA (miRNA); mRNA, messenger RNA; MS-PCR, methylation-specific PCR; NR, not reported; PBMC, peripheral blood mononuclear cell; qRT-PCR, quantitative reverse-transcriptase polymerase chain reaction; RBP, retinol binding protein; SCCA, squamous cell carcinoma antigen; TNF, tumor necrosis factor; VEGF, vascular endothelial growth factor; VOC, volatile organic compound.

epithelial cells, using partial wave spectroscopic microscopy. They evaluated 63 smokers with lung cancer and compared the findings with those for 72 individuals without lung cancer, including 50 smokers and 22 nonsmokers, and reported an area under the ROC curve (AUC) ranging from 0.81 to 0.88 depending on the control group used. Modification in the protocol with the introduction of low-coherence enhanced backscattering spectroscopy directly applied to the buccal mucosa also generated an excellent diagnostic tool with 94% sensitivity, 80% specificity, and 95% accuracy in distinguishing lung cancer patients from smoker controls.[46]

Circulating Tumor Cells and Circulating Tumor DNA

Liquid biopsy as a noninvasive method to detect tumors has generated excitement in the field of circulating biomarkers. CTCs are cells that originate from a malignancy and circulate in the peripheral blood. Research indicates that in patients with known malignancy, these cells may shed into the circulation and, even at early stages of cancer, can be detected. CTCs can be captured by immobilized antiepithelial cell adhesion molecule (EpCAM or tumor-associated calcium signal transducer 1 [TACSTD1]) antibodies, using a chip or bead platform.[31-34] The presence of "sentinel" CTCs detected by the International Symposium on Endovascular Therapy filtration-enrichment technique in combination with CT scan in chronic obstructive pulmonary disease patients has the potential for early detection of lung cancer.[47] This research is in its early stages but clearly holds appeal, as the test detects actual tumor cells rather than less-specific markers.

Circulating tumor DNA (ctDNA) is composed of small fragments of nucleic acid that are cell free (not associated with cells or cell fragments) and can be collected from different bodily sources. Levels of circulating cell-free DNA in plasma and serum are generally reported to be higher in patients with cancer than in healthy controls.[48-49] The circulating DNA in patients with lung cancer exhibits genetic and epigenetic changes typical of the tumor (chromosome loss, oncogene activation, and tumor-suppressor gene inactivation by methylation).[50,51] A novel ultrasensitive method for quantitating ctDNA using cancer personalized profiling by deep sequencing (CAPP-Seq) is a promising technique for the development of a ctDNA biomarker for early detection of lung cancer.[53] In NSCLC, CAPP-Seq was able to identify somatic alterations in over 95% of tumors, with ctDNA levels highly correlating with tumor volume. Measurement of ctDNA levels has the potential to monitor treatment response as well as for early lung cancer screening. When combined with integrated digital error suppression, CAPP-Seq was able to profile epidermal growth factor receptor (EGFR) mutations in NSCLC with 90% sensitivity and 96% specificity.[54]

Mitochondrial DNA

The mitochondrial genome has an increased mutation rate compared with that of the nuclear genome, and DNA repair is less efficient. Because mitochondrial DNA lacks introns, mutations are also more likely to accumulate in coding regions. Mutations in the mitochondrial genome—including point mutations, deletions, and admixtures—are associated with cancer and other disorders. Sequence variants in mitochondrial DNA can be rapidly detected using high-throughput resequencing microarrays.[52] Using this method, Jakupciak et al.[55] analyzed blood, tumor, and body fluids from 26 patients with early stage cancer (lung, bladder, kidney), compared the results with those for 12 smokers without cancer, and found that patients with cancer had a significantly higher incidence of mitochondrial DNA mutations.[55]

Noncoding RNAs

Noncoding RNAs (ncRNAs) are functional transcripts that do not code for proteins, but play an important role in regulating gene expression. Of these, several small ncRNAs have been studied for their roles in carcinogenesis and as possible biomarkers for cancer.[56] The most extensively studied so far are the microRNAs (miRNAs). These are small, ncRNA segments that are thought to regulate gene expression. miRNAs are abnormally expressed in several types of cancer,[57] but have tissue specificity as well,[55] making them ideal for biomarker research. Furthermore, miRNAs are generally stable and well preserved in formalin-fixed tissue. They are also present in the circulation, both intracellularly and extracellularly, where they can be detected by reverse transcription-polymerase chain reaction (RT-PCR), thus allowing for noninvasive testing. It is thought that extracellular miRNAs are released into the circulation by all cells in the body and therefore may reflect the body's systemic response to the presence of cancer, perhaps including changes in miRNA expression in circulating blood cells.

Changes in miRNA profiles have been identified in the blood of patients with lung cancer, and this is an active field of research, with multiple studies examining miRNA expression profiles as possible lung cancer biomarkers. As an example, a recent study of miRNA profiles in plasma from two independent cohorts of patients showed that a signature of 15 miRNAs in the blood identified patients at high risk for the development of lung cancer with 80% sensitivity and 90% specificity.[59] In another study, investigators described a panel of 34 serum miRNAs that could identify high-risk, asymptomatic patients with early stage NSCLCs with 80% accuracy.[60] Other investigators identified two miRNAs that distinguished early stage lung cancer from normal controls with 100% sensitivity and 84% specificity.[61] In patients with solitary pulmonary nodules on CT images, a panel of miRNAs was promising as a tool to distinguish benign from malignant nodules.[62,63] In another approach, miRNA profiles in whole blood were studied to capture intracellular miRNA.[69] This approach has had promising results.[61-66] A serum-based four-miRNA (miR-193b, miR-301, miR-141, and miR-200b) panel signature was able to discriminate lung cancer patients from noncancer individuals in an independent cohort with an AUC of 0.993 (95% confidence interval [CI], 0.979–1.000, $p < 0.001$).[70] miRNAs can also be detected in sputum samples, and several studies have demonstrated success in identifying both squamous cell and adenocarcinoma using a panel of miRNA markers in sputum samples.[42,67,68,71,72] Using quantitative RT-PCR, a panel of three sputum-based miRNA (miR-21, miR-31, and miR-210) was studied in patients with solitary pulmonary nodules; the sensitivity and specificity of the test for detecting lung cancer were 81% to 82% and 86% to 88%, respectively, in two independent cohorts.[74]

Another type of small ncRNA is small nucleolar RNA (snoRNA). Although snoRNAs are the largest group of ncRNAs, we are just beginning to understand the diverse functions of these molecules. Recent studies have indicated that snoRNAs may play a role in the development and progression of malignancy. One study of snoRNA expression signatures found that certain snoRNAs were significantly upregulated in both tumor tissue and plasma from patients with lung cancer compared with controls.[73] Like miRNA, snoRNA was shown to be stable and readily detectable in the plasma by quantitative RT-PCR.

Genetic Changes

Microsatellite instability (MSI) and loss of heterozygosity (LOH) are two allelic alterations that have been investigated as potential biomarkers for lung cancer. Microsatellites are segments of DNA in which a short motif is repeated multiple times.[75] These areas are prone to mutations during replication due to the transient split of the two helical strands and slippage of the DNA polymerase complex at reannealing, which generates an insertion or deletion loop. MSI occurs when these mutations result in a somatic change in length. MSI is associated with an impaired DNA repair mechanism. Changes in microsatellite repeats correlate with altered gene expression. LOH is the loss of one allele of a gene when the other allele is already inactivated, resulting in loss of function of the gene. LOH can be caused by numerous genetic mechanisms.

Numerous instances of LOH and MSI exist throughout the human genome. LOH and MSI at particular chromosomal regions seem to be more common in different tumor types. Losses of genetic material from chromosomes 3p and 9p are two of the earliest genetic changes occurring during bronchial carcinogenesis, and multiple lung cancer tumor suppressor genes are located on these chromosomes, including RBSP3, NPRL2, RASSF1A, and FHIT on 3p and CDKN2A and CDKN2B on 9p. Several studies have evaluated whether MSI and LOH in these regions could be found in circulating DNA69 or sputum of patients with lung cancer.[76–78] However, this technique can be problematic, because the proportion of circulating DNA derived from the cancer cells is likely to be low. In general, genetic alterations (LOH or MSI) were found in circulating DNA of 27% to 88% of patients with lung cancer.[79] When multiple markers are combined, the sensitivity can be increased, but often at the cost of specificity. Again, combining MSI or LOH with other markers, such as methylation and sputum cytology, may increase accuracy.[80,81]

Individual Genetic Mutations

We have long understood that lung carcinogenesis is associated with an accumulation of genetic mutations, and this was one of the first areas of focus for biomarker discovery. Mutations in the *KRAS* gene can result in constitutive activation. *KRAS* mutations occur in a limited number of hot spots, making mutations in this gene easier to detect through screening. *KRAS* mutations in circulating DNA are present in 20% to 30% of patients with lung cancer,[82,83] and *KRAS* mutations were found in bronchoalveolar lavage fluid in over 50% of patients with adenocarcinoma.[84,85] p53 mutations in circulating DNA have been found in 27% of patients with lung cancer.[82] EGFR is a receptor tyrosine kinase that is involved in cellular signaling in the mitogen-activated protein kinase (MAPK), phosphoinositide 3-kinase (PI3K), and signal transducers and activators of transcription (STAT) pathways. Mutations in the *EGFR* gene can result in constitutive activation and uncontrolled downstream signaling. *EGFR* mutations are more common in adenocarcinomas and in nonsmokers with lung cancer, and therefore this may be a more useful biomarker in nonsmokers.

Genomics

Genomic techniques allow for high-throughput detection of multiple mutant alleles simultaneously and the identification of gene expression profiles associated with the presence of malignancy.

Gene expression profiling in the sputum, bronchial epithelium, and peripheral blood is being studied as a method for early detection. Genomic techniques have been used to develop panels of genetic changes that could be used to screen sputum. In one study, the investigators identified a panel of six genes that could distinguish patients with early stage lung cancer from controls with 86.7% sensitivity and 93.9% specificity.[86]

Spira et al.[87] reported that an 80-gene microarray signature from the right main stem bronchial epithelium achieved 80% sensitivity and 84% specificity for distinguishing smokers with and without lung cancer. Bronchial-airway gene-expression classifier was validated in two multicenter prospective studies, AEGIS-1 and AEGIS-2, with an AUC of 0.78 (95% CI, 0.73–0.83) and 0.74 (95% CI, 0.68–0.80), respectively.[88] Another group developed a 14-antioxidant gene panel for the bronchial epithelium that achieved an AUC of 0.82 for discriminating patients with lung cancer from controls.[89]

Showe et al.[90] have proposed that gene expression profiling in peripheral blood mononuclear cells may be useful for early detection of lung cancer. They postulate that the immune response to the presence of malignant cells results in a change in the gene expression profile of circulating mononuclear cells. They initially analyzed gene expression in peripheral blood mononuclear cells in 137 patients with NSCLC compared with 91 controls with benign disease (including benign nodules) and found a 29-gene signature that identified patients with lung cancer with 91% sensitivity and 80% specificity.[90] In their validation set, they reported 78% accuracy. They also demonstrated that the gene signature was significantly reduced after tumor resection. In a subsequent study, they reported that resection of early lung tumors significantly changed the expression of more than 3000 genes. They also identified five miRNAs whose expression level decreased significantly after tumor removal.[91]

Gene Hypermethylation

Methylation of promoters in many different tumor suppressor genes occurs early in the development of lung cancer. DNA methylation involves the addition of a methyl group to the fifth position of the cytosine located 5′ to a guanosine in a CpG dinucleotide. A CpG island is a stretch of DNA that contains high CpG contents. Hypermethylation of CpG islands in gene promoter regions results in a conformational change of the chromatin, preventing RNA polymerase and other regulatory proteins from accessing the region, and thus silencing of gene transcription. Silencing by hypermethylation affects genes involved in all aspects of normal cell function and is a critical trigger for malignant transformation and progression. Methylation can be detected by methylation-specific PCR analysis. With this analysis, bisulfite is used to convert all unmethylated (but not methylated) cytosines to uracil. Amplification is then done with primers specific for methylated versus unmethylated DNA. In modified methylation-specific PCR, a two-step nested PCR improves the sensitivity of the assay.

Gene hypermethylation has become a very active area of research. In previous studies, aberrant methylation of p16INK4a, APC, TMS1, CDH1, RARβ-2 RASSF1, MGMT, DCC, AIM1, DAPK, and others has been reported in lung cancer.[92–97] Belinsky et al.[98] found that hypermethylation of the promoter region of many different genes in the blood and sputum is associated with lung cancer and may even precede the clinical diagnosis of lung cancer. Other lung cancer studies have demonstrated aberrant promoter methylation of PRSS3 (serine protease family member-trypsinogen IV, a putative tumor-suppressor gene),[99] human DAB2 interactive protein gene,[99] and apoptosis-associated speck-like protein containing a caspase and activation and recruitment domain (ASC).[101] Hypermethylation of p16 and FHIT genes may be associated with an increased risk of lung cancer recurrence after therapy.[102,103] In 2010, Ostrow et al.[104] used quantitative methylation-specific PCR to evaluate the frequency of promoter methylation of five candidate tumor-suppressor genes (kif1a, NISCH, RARβ, DCC, and B4GALT1) in the plasma of individuals with abnormal CT findings. They reported that 73% of patients with malignancy had methylation of at least one gene, whereas only 29% of controls had methylation. In a follow-up study, this group focused on the *NISCH* gene, a tumor suppressor located on chromosome 3p21 (frequently lost in lung cancer) that codes for the protein Nischarin.[105] Nischarin inhibits cell migration and possibly transformation. Hypermethylation of *NISCH* was found in 68% of heavy smokers without disease and 69% of light smokers with lung cancer and was absent in light smokers without disease. These data suggest that *NISCH* methylation may be a marker of risk for lung cancer.

Investigators have also evaluated methylation in other body fluids and tissues. In bronchoalveolar lavage, methylation of p16, RASSF1A, H-cadherin, and RARβ was associated with the presence of lung cancer, whereas FHIT methylation seemed to be related to tobacco exposure.[106] Using bronchial aspirates, RASSF1A promoter hypermethylation was found in 88% of patients with SCLC and in 28% of patients with NSCLC. No hypermethylation was found in patients with benign lung disease.[107] In other studies, this group found aberrant promoter methylation of APC,[108] p16, and RARβ2[109] in bronchoalveolar lavages from patients with lung cancer. They reported a sensitivity of 69% and specificity of 87% for the detection of lung cancer using this combination of genes.

A high-throughput global expression profiling approach has been used to identify new cancer-specific methylation markers. Using this technique, applied to multiple lung cancer cell lines, 132 genes that had been suppressed by methylation were identified. The investigators confirmed that these genes are expressed in normal lung,[110] but often not in companion primary lung cancers. They also found that seven of these loci were also commonly methylated in breast, colon, and prostate cancers. Ehrich et al.[111] reported the use of quantitative DNA methylation analysis technology to complete a large-scale cytosine methylation profiling study and thereby perhaps identify new methylation markers.[111] They analyzed methylation at 47 different gene promoter regions in lung tumor tissue and adjacent normal lung from 96 patients with lung cancer. Using a technique that combines MALDI-TOF MS of methylation-dependent sequence changes introduced by bisulfite treatment, they were able to identify six genes with significant differences in methylation in lung cancer tissues compared with normal tissues. These studies demonstrate that with the use of new techniques, high-throughput analysis of methylation status at multiple different promoter regions is possible.

Protein Markers

Protein markers have the advantage of reflecting phenotype rather than genotype and therefore theoretically may be more accurate than genetic markers as means for early detection of disease, rather than risk of disease. Several individual protein markers are currently used for monitoring or prognostication in lung cancer, and many of these have also been investigated as potential biomarkers for early detection, although none have adequate accuracy for this clinical use.[79] Carcinoembryonic antigen (CEA), CYFRA 21-1, and squamous cell carcinoma antigen (SCCA) have been evaluated for the diagnosis of squamous cell lung cancer.[112-114] Neuron-specific enolase, progastrin-releasing peptide, and neural cell adhesion molecule may have some utility in the detection of SCLC.[115–117]

Osteopontin is a ubiquitous extracellular phosphoprotein that interacts with cell-surface receptors to stimulate a variety of downstream processes. It is an important bone matrix protein and a mediator of immune cell recruitment, wound healing, and tissue remodeling, but has also been associated with tumor progression or cellular transformation. Overexpression of osteopontin has been found in both tissue and serum in lung cancer patients, but decreases after resection of the tumor and may be associated with more aggressive disease.[118,119] In an intriguing, small, case-controlled study, investigators evaluated osteopontin levels over time in longitudinal samples obtained from a lung cancer screening program.[120] They found that the rate of increase of osteopontin levels was significantly higher in patients in whom incidence lung cancers developed than in those in whom these did not. These data suggest that monitoring osteopontin levels may be useful in conjunction with CT to aid in distinguishing benign from malignant nodules.

Ciz1 is a nuclear matrix-associated DNA replication factor that promotes initiation of DNA replication and helps coordinate the sequential functions of cyclin E- and A-dependent protein kinases. It influences both DNA replication and cell proliferation. Normally Ciz1 is attached to the nuclear matrix. Recently, Higgins et al.[121] reported the identification of a stable Ciz1 variant, which lacks part of the C-terminal domain involved in nuclear matrix attachment and seems to be present only in tumor cells. Using a polyclonal antibody specific to this variant and Western blot analysis, the investigators were able to identify the presence of variant Ciz1 in the plasma of patients with lung cancer. In two independent sets, the presence of variant Ciz1 in the serum distinguished patients with cancer from controls with extremely high accuracy (AUC, 0.905–0.958). These results warrant the pursuit of further validation studies.

Many other proteins have been investigated as biomarkers for lung cancer. hnRNP B1, an RNA-binding protein involved in mRNA transportation and RNA mutation, is common in squamous cell carcinoma of the lung. Expression in the sputum has been correlated with risk of lung cancer development in certain populations, and the protein has been found to be overexpressed in early stage lung cancer.[122] Human telomeres function as a protective structure capping the ends of chromosomes. Dysfunction plays an important role in cancer initiation and progression. Human telomerase catalytic component is known to be elevated in cancers, and the copy number of human telomerase catalytic component mRNA in serum may correlate with lung cancer stage and risk of metastasis or recurrence.[123]

Some other proteins investigated, with variable results, include survivin, a protein that inhibits apoptosis and promotes mitosis;[124,125] Fas-associated death domain, which inactivates nuclear factor-kappaB, and is associated with overexpression of cyclins D1 and B1, thereby affecting the cell cycle;[126] and soluble e-cadherin, which plays a role in cell–cell adhesion.[128] Functional polymorphisms of matrix metalloproteinase 9 have been associated with risk of lung cancer and recurrence.[129]

A recent study indicates that a degradation product of complement activation, C4d, may serve as a biomarker for early diagnosis and prognosis of lung cancer.[129] This candidate biomarker was studied in the tumors, bronchoalveolar lavage, and blood of individuals with and without lung cancer, including patients diagnosed with preclinical disease in the context of a screening program. This biomarker had remarkable performance and deserves further validation.

It is unlikely that any single protein will serve as a biomarker for early detection of lung cancer, but perhaps a panel of proteins, identified through traditional or proteomic techniques, may achieve adequate sensitivity and specificity.

Proteomics

In the earliest clinical proteomics studies to identify markers for lung cancer, investigators used MALDI-TOF MS and identified proteins such as serum amyloid A and macrophage migration-inhibitory factor as being increased in lung cancer.[130] In a follow-up study, enzyme-linked immunosorbent assay (ELISA) analysis confirmed that serum amyloid A was increased in patients with lung cancer, but macrophage-inhibitory factor levels did not differentiate patients with lung cancer from those with other diseases.[131] Some of these investigators then used a combination of proteomics techniques and literature search for known tumor-associated proteins to establish a panel of serum protein markers: CEA, retinol binding protein, α1-antitrypsin, and SCCA.[132] Combining an assay of three of these proteins (CEA, α1-antitrypsin, and SCCA) with measurement of nodule size on CT images resulted in 80% sensitivity and 89% specificity for distinguishing malignant from benign nodules.[133]

Serum proteomic profiling has also identified peptide signatures that may be used to discriminate lung cancer from matched controls.[134] Investigators further evaluated the same MALDI MS signature in a population with indeterminate pulmonary nodules. They demonstrated that peptide signatures may add to the diagnostic accuracy of chest CT.[135] More recently, investigators used multiple reaction monitoring MS to measure the concentration of 13 candidate proteins identified in the literature and in freshly resected lung tumors and in plasma of patients with lung cancer and controls from three different sites. They reported a negative predictive value of 94% using this classifier. Importantly, the classifier score obtained was independent of other risk factors for malignancy, such as nodule size, smoking history, and age, indicating that this test may provide complementary information when evaluating pulmonary nodules.[136] In a follow-up study, the investigators performed a validation of the protein classifier that prioritizes sensitivity and negative predictive value to rule out patients with benign nodules. The result was a 90% negative predictive value at 92% sensitivity and 20% specificity.[137]

In one of the largest clinical proteomic biomarker studies to date, investigators used proteomic technology to analyze serum from 1326 tobacco-exposed individuals, including 291 lung cancer cases, from four different lung cancer screening trials.[136] In that study, the investigators used a highly automated technique that used DNA aptamers as extremely specific protein-binding reagents to measure levels of 813 different human proteins. In the training set, 44 candidate biomarkers were identified, and the most highly discriminatory proteins were used to create a 12-protein panel (cadherin-1, CD30 ligand, endostatin, HSP90α, LRIG3, MIP-4, pleiotrophin, PRKCI, RGM-C, SCF-sR, sL-selectin, and YES). In the validation step, this panel was able to discriminate NSCLC from controls with 89% sensitivity and 83% specificity. The proteins identified—six of which were upregulated and six of which were downregulated in the lung cancers—are known to play roles in cell movement and growth, cell–cell adhesion, inflammation, and immune monitoring. These investigators further analyzed the effect of variations in blood collection to improve reproducibility across populations. After adjusting for confounding proteins through sample mapping vectors, a seven-marker protein panel resulted in an AUC of 0.85, which was validated in two independent cohorts.[138]

Another proteomic technique is to use MS to identify protein markers in lung cancer tissues and then screen for these in patient serum, differentiating benign from malignant nodules.[136] MS can identify protein biomarkers that can then be screened in patient serum using ELISA.[137]

Autoantibodies and Tumor-Associated Antigens

As mentioned, the presence of malignant cells can activate the immune system, and cancer has been shown to induce autoimmunity to autologous cellular antigens.[140] Many of the target antigens are cellular proteins, whose deregulation, aberrant expression misfolding, truncation, or proteolysis could lead to or result from tumorigenesis. These changes may result in loss of immunologic tolerance. A systemic response to these tumor-specific antigens provides an opportunity to detect cancers at an early stage. Numerous immunogenic tumor-associated antigens have been identified in human sera using high-throughput analysis, such as recombinant cDNA expression libraries, phage display, and protein microarrays.[141,142] Autoantibodies to some of these antigens have been found in patients with lung cancers.[143,144] Several studies have identified autoantibody panels as markers of lung cancer. In some of these studies, protein microarray and phage display techniques were used.[145–148] In others, autoantibodies against known lung cancer–associated proteins (e.g., p53, c-Myc, HER2, Muc1, CAGE, GBU4-5, NY-ESO-1, annexin 1, PGP9.5 and 14-3-3 theta, LAMAR1, IMPDH, PGAM1, and ANXA2) were investigated.[149–152] Sensitivity and specificity approaching 90% have been reported, although validation studies are needed. In one study, the investigators used microarrays to identify autoantibodies in sera from patients prior to the clinical diagnosis of lung cancer and were able to show that levels of autoantibodies to annexin I, 14-3-3 theta, and LAMR1 were elevated prior to clinical diagnosis in patients in whom lung cancer subsequently developed compared with patients in whom it did not.[152] This same group has further developed a five-autoantibody classifier (tetratricopeptide repeat domain

14 [TTC14]; B-Raf proto-oncogene, serine/threonine kinase [BRAF]; actin-like 6B [ACTL6B]; MORC family CW-type zinc finger 2 [MORC2]; and cancer/testis antigen 1B [CTAG1B]) to differentiate lung cancers from smoker controls with a specificity as high as 89%.[153] The EarlyCDT-Lung test (Oncimmune LLC, De Soto, Kansas, USA) is the first clinically available biomarker test marketed for the early detection of lung cancer. The assay is an ELISA measuring autoantibody reactivity to a panel of six tumor-associated antigens (p53, NY-ESO-1, CAGE, GBU4–5, annexin 1, and SOX2). In 2010 and 2011, the technical feasibility and clinical utility of the test were reported,[154–156] and approximately 40% of lung cancers could be detected using the assay, with 90% specificity. The test is now available, and subsequent studies have confirmed these results in independent samples.[157] Adding additional autoantibodies to the panel may improve the assay.[159] Its performance in clinical practice was evaluated in 1600 patients. It had a sensitivity of 41%, with positive EarlyCDT-Lung test result associated with a 5.4-fold increase in lung cancer incident. Over 50% of positive results were of early stage lung cancer (stages I and II).[157]

Because of the heterogeneity of the immune system, as well as of lung cancer, it is unlikely that reactivity to any single tumor-associated antigen will identify all lung cancers. Microarray analysis allows for the evaluation of multiple different tumor-associated antigens simultaneously. The microarrays can be spotted with tumor proteins and then hybridized to the sera of patients with lung cancer. Using this technique, Qiu et al.[160] found reactivity patterns that may identify patients with lung cancer. Alternatively, the microarray can be spotted with antibodies to known tumor antigens and then hybridized to patients' sera to identify circulating tumor-associated antigens. Using this technique, Gao et al.[161] identified a distinctive serum protein profile in patients with lung cancer compared with controls.

Metabolomics

Metabolomics, measurements and quantification of end products of cellular metabolism, is a relatively new research area in oncology. It has the potential to be an attractive noninvasive biomarker, because metabolites in blood are end products of cellular processes in disease and cancer states. There are two common ways to measure metabolites: mass spectroscopy and nuclear magnetic resonance spectroscopy. In one study, investigators used gas chromatography TOF MS to analyze metabolome, including 462 lipid, carbohydrate, amino acid, organic acid, and nucleotide metabolites, in serum and plasma to develop classifiers to distinguish NSCLC from a control. Cancer-associated biochemical changes were identified as decrease in glucose levels, change in cellular redox, increase in nucleotide metabolites 5,6-dihydrouracil and xanthine, increase in de novo purine synthesis, and increase in protein glycosylation. A validated classifier using a multimetabolite model yielded an AUC of 0.885 with 92.3% sensitivity and 84.6% specificity.[162,163] Another group used proton nuclear magnetic resonance spectroscopy and was able to discriminate adenocarcinoma of the breast from adenocarcinoma of the lung with an AUC of 0.96.[164] Further, proton nuclear magnetic resonance was able to detect metabolic phenotype of blood plasma in 233 lung cancer patients and 226 controls. A validated classification model discriminated between the two groups with an AUC of 0.88.[165]

Volatile Organic Compounds

An intriguing idea is the use of markers in the exhaled breath to diagnose lung cancer. Studies have reported that dogs are able to distinguish breath samples from patients with lung cancer from healthy controls with great accuracy.[166] Tumor cell growth is accompanied by alterations of protein expression patterns, which lead to peroxidation of the cell membrane, and the emission of volatile organic compounds (VOCs). Studies have indicated that VOCs, mainly alkanes and aromatic compounds, are preferentially produced and exhaled by patients with lung cancer. Poli et al.[167] reported that the measurement of a combination of 13 VOCs in the exhaled breath allowed correct classification of lung cancer in 80% of cases. Several studies have used gas chromatography combined with mass spectrometric analysis of VOCs.[168–172] The colorimetric sensor array signature of exhaled breath volatile organic compounds was able to distinguish lung cancer patients from control with an AUC between 0.794 and 0.861.[173] In one study, Phillips et al.[174] measured the alveolar gradient of C4–C20 alkanes and monomethylated alkanes in patients with lung cancer compared with controls. They developed a model using nine VOCs to predict the presence of lung cancer and in their test set achieved a sensitivity of 85% and specificity of 81%. Subsequently, they reported similar sensitivity and specificity using a weighted digital analysis model that included 30 breath VOCs.[175] Other groups have designed nanosensors to detect changes in electrical resistance from the identified organic compounds in patients' exhaled breath.[176] These assays are sensitive to humidity and other environmental factors. In addition to VOCs, investigators have tried to identify volatile proteins and peptides in exhaled breath condensate that could be used for the early detection of lung cancer.[177,178] The lack of interinstitutional reproducibility in studies of exhaled breath biomarkers is troubling. Validation of a standardized exhaled breath collection device is needed if markers identified through these studies are to be useful.

CONCLUSION

The development of noninvasive lung cancer biomarkers for early detection could have a dramatic impact on lung cancer outcomes. The development of lung cancer biomarkers may allow us to identify populations that would benefit from CT screening, could distinguish individuals with benign pulmonary nodules from those with early malignancies, may differentiate patients with indolent versus aggressive tumors, and will allow for personalization of lung cancer treatment based on tumor characteristics. Significant advances in our understanding of the molecular and genetic changes involved in lung carcinogenesis have provided the basis for many investigations into possible lung cancer biomarkers. The development of new and improved high-throughput technologies raises the potential for great strides in biomarker discovery. Over the last few years, there has been a proliferation of research on lung cancer biomarkers, and a large number of potential diagnostic biomarkers have been identified. The slow progress through the validation pipeline can be attributed to many factors. First, current discovery methods are inefficient and lack reproducibility. In addition, many of the technologies have limited power to detect low-abundance cancer markers against a high background of high-abundance molecules in the complex matrices of biologic samples. Further, we have limited capacity to verify and validate candidate markers due to the novelty of the technology and the insufficient availability of biosamples from prospective studies and early stage disease. The reproducibility of biomarker data has also been flawed because of inconsistent study design, model overfitting, changing technologies, and lack of cross-validation and independent validation. Many studies report high sensitivity and specificity. However, these studies are often troubled by small size, a lack of reproducibility, or inconsistent controls between studies. All of the biomarkers identified so far must be validated in larger independent clinical cohorts.

The discovery of lung cancer biomarkers is progressing rapidly. A high volume of data from multiple high-throughput techniques has been accumulating at an exponential rate in the last few years, generating a large number of biomarker candidates. Standardization of validation studies and the development of high-quality longitudinal cohorts for testing of promising markers should usher in a new age of biomarker validation. A biofluids-based molecular test can improve the selection of individuals for CT screening, distinguish malignant from benign nodules, and differentiate indolent from more aggressive cancers. Low-dose CT screening for lung cancer can detect 18% to 33% indolent cancers that may be considered overdiagnosed.

Acknowledgment

This work was supported in part by NCI EDRN-sponsored Clinical Validation Center CA086137 (W.N.R.) and by NCI EDRN-sponsored Clinical Validation Center CA152662 (P.P.M.).

KEY REFERENCES

4. National Lung Screening Trial Research Team Aberle DR, Adams AM, et al. Reduced lung-cancer mortality with low-dose computed tomographic screening. *N Engl J Med*. 2011;365:395–409.
26. Pepe MS, Feng Z, Janes H, et al. Pivotal evaluation of the accuracy of a biomarker used for classification or prediction: standards for study design. *J Natl Cancer Inst*. 2008;100(20):1432–1438.
33. Nagrath S, Sequist LV, Maheswaran S, et al. Isolation of rare circulating tumour cells in cancer patients by microchip technology. *Nature*. 2007;450:1235–1239.
53. Newman AM, Bratman SV, To J, et al. An ultrasensitive method for quantitating circulating tumor DNA with broad patient coverage. *Nat Med*. 2014;20:548–554.
59. Boeri M, Verri C, Conte D, et al. Micro RNA signatures in tissues and plasma predict development and prognosis of computed tomography detected lung cancer. *Proc Natl Acad Sci U. S. A.* 2011;108:3713–3718.
70. Nadal E, Truini A, Nakata A, et al. A novel serum 4-microRNA signature for lung cancer detection. *Sci Rep*. 2015;5:12464.
74. Xing L, Su J, Guarnera MA, et al. Sputum microRNA biomarkers for identifying lung cancer in indeterminate solitary pulmonary nodules. *Clin Cancer Res*. 2015;21:484–489.
87. Spira A, Bean JF, Shah V, et al. Airway epithelial gene expression in the diagnostic evaluation of smokers with suspect lung cancer. *Nat Med*. 2007;13:361–366.
88. Silvestri GA, Vachani A, Whitney D, et al. A bronchial genomic classifier for the diagnostic evaluation of lung cancer. *N Engl J Med*. 2015;373:243–251.
90. Showe MK, Vachani A, Kossenkov AV, et al. Gene expression profiles in peripheral blood mononuclear cells can distinguish patients with non-small cell lung cancer from patients with nonmalignant lung disease. *Cancer Res*. 2009;24:9202–9210.
133. Patz Jr EF, Campa MJ, Gottlin EB, et al. Biomarkers to help guide management of patients with pulmonary nodules. *Am J Respir Crit Care Med*. 2013;188(4):461–465.
135. Ostroff RM, Bigbee WL, Franklin W, et al. Unlocking biomarker discovery: large scale application of aptamer proteomic technology for early detection of lung cancer. *PLoS One*. 2010;5(12):e15003.
137. Vachani A, Pass HI, Rom WN, et al. Validation of a multiprotein plasma classifier to identify benign lung nodules. *J Thorac Oncol*. 2015;10(4):629–637.
158. Lam S, Boyle P, Healey GF, et al. EarlyCDT-Lung: an immunobiomarker test as an aid to early detection of lung cancer. *Cancer Prev Res (Phila)*. 2011;4(7):1126–1134.
163. Wikoff WR, Grapov D, Fahrmann JF, et al. Metabolomic markers of altered nucleotide metabolism in early stage adenocarcinoma. *Cancer Prev Res (Phila)*. 2015;8:410–418.
173. Mazzone PJ, Wang XF, Lim S, et al. Progress in the development of volatile exhaled breath signatures of lung cancer. *Ann Am Thorac Soc*. 2015;12:752–757.

See Expertconsult.com for full list of references.

9 Chemoprevention of Lung Cancer and Management of Early Lung Cancer

Swati Gulati, James L. Mulshine, and Nico van Zandwijk

SUMMARY OF KEY POINTS

- Most chemoprevention research is focused on natural products and is not amenable to traditional pharmaceutical development.
- Robust research and development for lung cancer chemoprevention by the pharmaceutical industry is largely lacking.
- The traditional model of developing drugs for advanced disease and then backing successful agents into early disease application is not working.
- Safety is coequal to efficacy in developing a successful chemopreventive agent.
- Lung cancer screening with spiral computed tomography is being implemented, and as a result more stage I curative cases will be found.
- Individuals followed after successful management of their initial lung cancer will experience a high rate of metachronous second primary lung cancer (1% to 3% cumulative), and this will be a growing new cohort of patients that would benefit from successful chemoprevention management.
- Locoregional delivery of potential chemoprevention drugs by "aerosolized approaches" may reduce cost and improve safety.
- Systematic study of resected early-stage lung cancers and surrounding injured bronchial tissues may provide insight into the molecular drivers of (early) lung cancer using the precedent of Vogelstein and coworkers' mapping of colon carcinogenesis.

In a recent editorial published in the *Lancet*, advances in lung cancer treatment outcomes were reviewed and it was concluded that simple preventive measures, such as banning advertising, blank cigarette packaging, and increasing awareness of the harms of smoking, might result in more reductions in mortality than all new promising agents combined.[1] For the tens of millions of tobacco-exposed individuals, including former smokers, who will remain at increased risk of lung cancer for most of their remaining life, this is a grim message.[2] At the same time, there is clear progress in early detection of lung cancer and computed tomography (CT) screening, which has been endorsed and is being implemented in the United States, and endorsed in Canada and China with pilot screening evaluations being implemented in a number of other countries.[3] Screening will result in finding more early-stage cancers, which in many instances can be cured by surgery, but as outlined in the discussion of field carcinogenesis reviewed in this chapter, many of the surgically cured individuals at a frequency of 1% to 3% per year will manifest a second primary lung cancer.[4] The net effect of this lung cancer screening dynamic is that before too long, we will have tens of thousands of people in follow-up for metachronous primary lung cancer.

In a perfect world that would mean the pharmaceutical industry would be focusing on developing drugs that would target the mechanisms driving field carcinogenesis and short circuit the development of these metachronous lung cancers. A comprehensive recent review of chemoprevention relates that for lung cancer there are no new (approved) products and the studies that are being done in this space are generally small, investigator-driven studies of plant-derived agents with little prospect for evolution to a full-fledged pharmaceutical product.[5] Although many studies continue to demonstrate the importance of anti-inflammatory agents, the lung cancer prevention field is remarkably free of major pharmaceutical investment. In this most innovative time in the history of biomedicine, for the world's most lethal cancer, we have no lead compound and no obvious serious, commercially viable effort to find one. Publications have noted for decades that the incentives for major pharmaceutical involvement in the field of chemoprevention are inadequate, but no structure fix has been implemented.[6]

In a recent chemoprevention review it has been suggested that the process to develop chemopreventive agents mirrored the steps in developing drugs for advanced lung cancer. This position seems to reflect conventional wisdom, but is that really the optimal way to develop a drug to stop or delay the occurrence of early lung cancer? Late drug development failures are often the consequence of off-target drug effects.[7] In considering the application of chemoprevention drugs in asymptomatic target populations, the issue of off-target toxicity is vitally important and more an issue than off-target effects of drugs for symptomatic late-stage lung cancer. Chemopreventive agents have to be effective and safe at the same time. Further, target identification of potential drugs to arrest carcinogenesis of lung cancer has to be derived from tissue that is representative for early carcinogenesis. A model for this would be the comprehensive mapping that Vogelstein and colleagues[8] have conducted in mapping molecular events with colon carcinogenesis. Finally, lung cancer arises principally from the aerosolized delivery of tobacco combustion products to the airway. The epithelial lining of the airways represents a remarkably small volume of cells that can be targeted economically and safely using established methods. Many successfully approved aerosolized products exist for obstructive pulmonary and infectious disease.[9,10] Chemoprevention for lung cancer presents an exceptionally strategic opportunity for making a major impact in the War on Cancer and generating a new class of lung cancer drugs. It is time to get serious about bringing such tools into being.

Lung cancer is by far the leading cause of cancer-related deaths worldwide. In the United States alone, 158,080 deaths were projected for 2016, accounting for about 27% of all cancer deaths.[11] Median survival in all stages of disease has improved during the past decades, but the likelihood of obtaining a cure, even with optimal modern therapy, is low because most cases are detected after the development of symptoms from respiratory cancer, and these occur when the disease is in a regional or distant metastatic stage. Lung cancer is usually related to exposure to carcinogens that occurred over 10 years to 20 years and requires multiple molecular genetic changes before the development of invasive lung cancer.[12,13] Consequently, a strong rationale exists for detecting lung carcinogenesis before the development of invasive metastatic cancer. This detection includes prudent implementation of lung cancer screening as a high-quality service to identify early, curable lung cancer.

After an exhaustive review of the evidence, the US Preventive Services Task Force (USPSTF) endorsed low-dose lung cancer screening as an early-detection approach with the potential to significantly reduce deaths from lung cancer.[14] Prospective detection of lung cancer in high-risk cohorts in the absence of symptoms mandates a clinical management approach that differs significantly from the routine management of lung cancer detected on the basis of symptoms. As with other cancer screening services, this screening service must be delivered with high quality, low cost, and ready accessibility. This chapter reviews strategies that contribute to routinely achieving that level of proficiency, and this information may constitute a useful reference for clinicians communicating about the merits and limitations of this service to high-risk individuals who are considering participation in lung cancer screening. As early detection becomes more successful, more patients will survive lung cancer. As a by-product of this success, more patients with cured lung cancer, especially those with heavy exposure to tobacco products, will have a high risk of the development of new primary lung cancers. This outcome produces a strong demand for new tools to manage this earliest form of lung cancer. Chemoprevention is the term used for the process of implementing drugs to interfere with carcinogenesis.

Tobacco smoking is estimated to account for at least 80% of the attributable risk for lung cancer.[15] Smoking cessation, especially before middle age, is associated with significantly lower tobacco-attributable cancer risk.[15] Clearly, we must continue our efforts in tobacco control, which have substantially reduced smoking prevalence in several countries. However, 1.3 billion people worldwide still smoke, and the multinational tobacco companies continue to introduce cancer-causing products designed to entice teenagers into a lifetime of nicotine addiction. In addition, despite a significant reduction in the prevalence of smoking among US adults, from 42% to 19% between 1965 and 2011, lung cancer incidence has not decreased because of the growing number of aging people.[11,16] Despite smoking cessation, lung cancer risk remains elevated and never reaches the level of risk among nonsmokers.[15] A significant percentage of newly diagnosed lung cancer occurs in former smokers.[17] Thus in certain individuals, the carcinogenic process elicited by tobacco smoke continues to evolve despite smoking cessation. These observations underline why strategies to slow, halt, or even reverse carcinogenesis continue to gain great interest and why it is of interest to explore the evolution and progress of chemoprevention efforts.

In early chemoprevention studies, researchers evaluated vitamins or micronutrients in an attempt to reduce cancer incidence as the primary end point. A challenge with this approach was cost, because such studies required thousands of participants and many years of follow-up to detect a significant chemoprotective benefit. Interpreting results from these trials may also have been complicated by the comingling of study participants who continued to smoke with individuals who had stopped smoking.[18] More recently, study designs have focused on cancer incidence as the primary end point in populations who are at high risk for lung cancer. An example is to exclude individuals with a 20-pack/year history who do not have more than a 10% to 15% lifetime risk of lung cancer. Intermediate marker end points can be used to quickly designate risk strata to select trial populations in whom lung cancer is more likely to develop so that smaller trials can be more informative. Chemoprevention of lung carcinogenesis remains a highly attractive concept, especially in targeting trials on agents that are involved in downstream effects of multiple

carcinogens, tumor promoters, and inflammatory compounds in cigarette smoke.[19]

Lung cancer is strongly associated with direct consumption of tobacco products, and 87% of all lung cancers are detected in individuals who are active or former smokers. An additional 6% to 7% of lung cancer occurs in partners of smokers or their offspring. The second and third most common known causes of lung cancer are radon and asbestos, and epidemiologic evidence from the 2000s points to a clear association between lung cancer and air pollution.[20,21] Despite the high degree of certainty that a link exists between tobacco smoke and lung cancer, establishing the causal link between tobacco exposure and lung cancer took several decades. The discovery that tobacco smoke was capable of producing identical p53 mutations both in patients with lung cancer and in mice exposed to tobacco smoke added incontrovertible evidence for a strong epidemiologic association.[22]

The original description of so-called field of cancerization dates back to the pioneering work of Slaughter et al.,[23] who showed that multiple foci of epithelial hyperplasia, hyperkeratinization, atypia, dysplasia, and carcinoma in situ occurred in otherwise normal-appearing epithelium adjacent to cancers of the oral pharynx in smokers. This empiric evidence suggested that carcinogen exposure has widespread effects throughout the epithelial field subjected to carcinogen damage. Auerbach et al.[24] reported that the same pattern of heterogeneous, multifocal histologic changes occurred throughout the bronchial epithelium of smokers who had lung cancer, consistent with the concept of field of cancerization. Translated into contemporary biologic terms, field of cancerization means that areas of histologically normal-appearing tissue adjacent to neoplastic lesions display molecular abnormalities, some of which are the same as in the tumors.[24] Several studies have shown the field of injury created by cigarette smoke, and molecular studies support the stepwise model of lung carcinogenesis, with genetic and epigenetic alterations occurring in the cells.[25] Field carcinogenesis also forms the basis for the observation that among individuals who survive a first cancer, a second malignancy is likely to develop in the region of the tobacco-exposed epithelium.[26–29]

Among the earliest molecular findings in the aerodigestive tract of chronic smokers are loss of heterozygosity in chromosomes 3p, 9p, and 17p; p53 mutations; and changes in promoter methylation and in telomerase activity of noncancerous epithelial cells.[13,30–35] Loss of heterozygosity is a crucial event. For example, loss of the short arm of chromosome 3, which is often the earliest loss and is demonstrated occasionally even in early hyperplasia,[30] results in the loss of a region rich in tumor suppressor genes. Evidence also indicates loss of the short arms of chromosomes 9 and 17, resulting in loss of tumor suppressor genes in p16 and p53, both of which are important to the cell's ability to repair DNA damage elicited by tobacco smoke. Gene p53, in particular, acts as a transcription factor in the control of G_1 arrest and apoptosis, or programmed cell death, thereby allowing the cell to repair any existing DNA damage or induce apoptosis once the cell is too far damaged for repair. The gene p16, found on chromosome 9p, negatively controls cyclin-dependent kinase–cyclin activity by overexpression of cyclin-D1. Inhibiting cyclin-D1/cyclin-dependent kinase prevents the damaged cell from entering into mitosis and proliferating with damaged DNA. Studies have proved that methylation of the p16 gene in the oral epithelium induced by tobacco smoke is an independent risk factor for lung cancer in current and former smokers.[36]

The loss of these and other tumor suppressor genes in lung cancer seems to be augmented by the activation of several crucial proto-oncogenes. For example, Ras, myc, and the epidermal growth factor receptor (EGFR) are all tumor-promoting genes that are activated progressively during lung carcinogenesis. Mutations of Kirsten rat sarcoma (KRAS) are particularly common in adenocarcinomas of the lung; some studies have shown that 30% of lung adenocarcinomas in smokers contain KRAS mutations.[37]

Other mechanisms of lung carcinogenesis are also relevant, such as amplification of EGFR.[38] Mutations have been detected in the EGFR tyrosine kinase (TK) binding domain, which confer sensitivity to small-molecule EGFR TK inhibitors (TKIs).[39–41] Both KRAS mutations and EGFR mutations have been found in the airways of smokers and nonsmokers in regions distant from the primary tumor, suggesting that both play a role in field carcinogenesis.[37,42]

Gene mutations and rearrangements have also been mapped to specific histologic and clinical characteristics among the lung cancer subtypes. This discovery has led to the development of target-specific chemotherapeutic drugs, which have revolutionized the treatment of lung cancer.

Rearrangements of the anaplastic lymphoma kinase (ALK) gene, which result from an inversion in the short arm of chromosome 2, have been identified in a subset of patients with nonsmall cell lung cancer (NSCLC). This subset causes distinct clinical and pathologic features and usually affects younger patients with no history or a light history of smoking.[43,44] ALK TKIs such as crizotinib and alectinib have been shown to increase progression-free survival rates. Similarly, rearrangements of the c-ros oncogene 1 (ROS1) and ret proto-oncogene (RET) genes have been isolated in adenocarcinoma and in some subsets of advanced NSCLC. These patients, too, are mostly young with little or no history of smoking.[45–49]

Some mutations are mutually exclusive of each other, such as EGFR and KRAS mutations. Amplification of fibroblast growth factor receptor 1 is seen in patients with squamous cell lung cancer. This mutation is associated with cigarette smoking in a dose-dependent fashion and is an independent negative prognostic factor.[50]

Global messenger RNA and microRNA (miRNA) expression profiles have been described in the bronchial epithelium of so-called healthy smokers, and cancer-specific gene expression profiles have been reported in smokers with and without lung cancer.[51,52]

GENE SILENCING

Another mechanism of lung carcinogenesis is loss of function of tumor suppressor genes. A growing body of evidence suggests that gene silencing through epigenetic means is crucial in lung carcinogenesis. For example, the tumor suppressor gene in NSCLC known as RASSF1A, which is also located in the region of chromosome 3p rich in tumor suppressor genes, encodes a protein that heterodimerizes with Nore-1, an important RAS effector with a proapoptotic effect.[53] Evidence suggests that in NSCLC, RASSF1A can be inactivated by hypermethylation.[54,55]

Another important gene that can be inactivated by epigenetic means is the retinoic acid receptor-β (RAR-β), which also maps to chromosome 3p. RAR-β is a nuclear retinoid receptor with vitamin A–dependent transcriptional activity.[56] The RAR-β gene is gradually lost during lung carcinogenesis,[57] and this may be caused by loss or hypermethylation.[58,59] The maintenance of RAR-β in mature tumors is a risk factor for poor prognosis,[60] and the RAR-β gene is differentially regulated in current as opposed to former smokers. For example, a retrospective study on methylation status and the occurrence of second primary tumors (SPTs) in patients with completely resected NSCLC showed an association between RAR-β2 hypermethylation in the development of SPTs only in former smokers.[61] In current smokers, hypermethylation was associated with a protective effect, pointing to the value of context with regard to smoking status in understanding the biologic effects of retinoid receptors in lung cancer.[61,62]

The role of miRNAs may also prove to be crucial. These small noncoding RNA molecules have been recognized as important in epigenetic control by altering the translation of proteins from messenger RNAs. miRNAs are able to target a multitude of messenger RNAs and have emerged as key posttranscriptional regulators of gene expression involved in cell proliferation, apoptosis, and stress resistance. miRNAs are also located in cancer-associated genomic regions or in fragile sites, suggesting that differences in miRNA expression may be induced by genomic alterations and play either a tumor suppressor or oncogenic role.[63]

Cigarette smoke is a potent source of such molecular injury, and recent studies have shown that the components in cigarette smoke affect miRNA levels in the respiratory tract.[64,65] An emerging notion is that smoking may lead to downregulation of miRNAs in the airway. The mechanistic understanding of the link between these miRNA changes and early lung carcinogenesis is just beginning to emerge. The fact that miRNA dysregulation is an early event in lung carcinogenesis may offer opportunities for chemopreventive approaches (i.e., reversing aberrant miRNA expression induced by smoking).[66] For example, miRNA changes were found in biopsy specimens obtained in a phase II trial comparing iloprost (a prostacyclin analog) with placebo in high-risk patients, and these changes were related to histologic findings at baseline.[67] Proteomic analyses of preinvasive lesions in the bronchial tree have uncovered patterns clearly different from those in normal epithelium,[68] supporting the rationale for chemopreventive strategies.

SUSCEPTIBILITY TO LUNG CANCER AND BALANCING OF ANTAGONISTIC PATHWAYS

The risk of the development of lung cancer, even among the heaviest smokers, varies widely, perhaps because of genetic and even dietary factors. In fact, 85% of heavy smokers will not develop lung cancer, which suggests important differences among individuals in susceptibility to lung cancer. Several prediction models for lung cancer have been proposed. The Bach model uses variables related to age, smoking, and asbestos exposure in black populations, whereas the Spitz model and Liverpool Lung Project include family history and other occupational exposures in addition to age and smoking history in white populations.[69–71] Although these models are easy to administer and calculate, their discriminatory power is only moderate, which is not surprising because the models fail to account for many comorbidities and other epigenetic factors. In 2012, Hoggart et al.[72] proposed a prediction model that includes more variables, including biomarker exposure; socioeconomic status; comorbidities including pneumonia, chronic obstructive pulmonary disease (COPD), and emphysema; and body mass index for current smokers, former smokers, and nonsmokers.[72] Despite researchers' best attempts, a prediction model cannot assimilate all possible epigenetic and genetic factors to make consistently accurate predictions.

Accumulating evidence suggests that genetic and epigenetic factors are crucial in modulating individual susceptibility to lung cancer.[73] An example is the identification of a susceptibility locus for lung cancer at 15q25 in a large genome-wide association study.[74,75] Locus 15q25 contains nicotinic acetylcholine receptor subunit genes and seems to be involved in carcinogen metabolism. The two major carcinogens from cigarette smoke, benzo[a] pyrene and 4-(methylnitrosamino)-1-(3-pyridyl)-1-butanone, require metabolic activation before they can exert full carcinogenic effects.

Various activation pathways compete with detoxification pathways, and the balance between the two is crucial in modulating cancer risk. Cytochrome P450s serve as carcinogen-metabolizing enzymes, whereas glutathione transferases serve as detoxification enzymes. Both sets of these important genes are known to have significant polymorphisms that correlate with variations in lung cancer risk.[76–78] Gene polymorphisms in microsomal epoxide hydrolase and their patterns of expression in the respiratory epithelium also influence the activity of antioxidant enzymes, skewing the balance between the two redox pathways.[79]

Moreover, many researchers believe that DNA repair capacity may play an important role in susceptibility to lung cancer.[80] CYP1A1, an enzyme of the cytochrome P450 family, plays a role in the development of EGFR mutations, hence altering the risk profile of lung cancer among smokers.[81] Other modulators of risk in lung cancer include diet and gender. Dietary factors function as epigenetic modulators of lung cancer susceptibility. In several case–control studies, defective detoxification and defective repair of genetic damage were associated with increased individual susceptibility to lung cancer.[82,83] Food constituents, such as those found in fruits and specific vegetables, appear to afford marked protection to individuals with limitations in their detoxification capacity.[84] This relationship between diet and lung cancer has been explored extensively and is being used as a basis for the development of preventive approaches to lung cancer.

VITAMINS AND MICRONUTRIENTS

Specific micronutrients have been associated with a lower risk of lung cancer, including vitamin E, selenium, isothiocyanates, polyphenols, betaine, and choline. A number of large randomized trials have sought to delineate which compounds in the human diet may be responsible for the protective effects.[85–87] Among heavy smokers, a diet high in red meat consumption and with low adherence to the so-called Mediterranean diet has been found to be associated with increased risk of lung cancer.[84] Conversely, a diet high in vegetable fats and fiber was shown to reduce lung cancer incidence among heavy smokers.[88] The role of selenium has been investigated for preventing lung cancer among patients with selenium deficiency. A trial that sought to prevent SPTs after primary skin cancer in a selenium-poor population in Arizona showed a 34% reduction in lung cancer incidence,[86] and because of this success, the role of selenium as a chemoprotective agent was explored in other malignancies. The Selenium and Vitamin E Cancer Prevention Trial[89] was conducted to study the effect of selenium on prostate cancer incidence. In this trial, 32,400 men were randomly assigned to receive oral selenium, vitamin E, or selenium plus vitamin E as compared with placebo in a double-blind fashion and were monitored for a median of 5.46 years. The trial showed no benefit of selenium or vitamin E, or the combination, to confer any protection against prostate cancer. A phase III prevention study was published in 2013 by the Eastern Cooperative Oncology Group in which patients with resected stage I NSCLC were randomly assigned in a 2:1 ratio to receive selenium methionine at 200 µg/day or placebo. In this trial, selenium failed to demonstrate any objective benefit compared with placebo in protecting against the development of lung SPTs.[90]

However, the Eastern Cooperative Oncology Group study was initiated without preliminary studies, and the recommendation must be to continue to build biomarker-driven, targeted, phase II approaches that appropriately pursue modulation of a crucial biomarker, followed by confirmation, before proceeding with large-scale studies.

Initially, researchers found considerable epidemiologic evidence for the potency of carotenoids and retinoids in reducing cancer risk in general, and lung cancer risk in particular. In fact, the original definition of chemoprevention as "attempts to reverse, suppress, and prevent carcinogenic progression to overt cancer" was based on experimental work showing that vitamin A analogs were capable of reversing or preventing epithelial carcinogenesis in animal experiments.[91]

Early chemoprevention trials included broad populations of individuals who were at risk because of their exposure to tobacco and/or asbestos. Others trials focused on specific high-risk populations, such as uranium miners. Thus, with several decades of epidemiologic and dietary investigation augmented by various experimental systems, a number of compounds, including retinoids and carotenoids, were found to be capable of reversing cell damage. Considerable effort was invested in testing this approach in human populations. The trials focused on broad patient populations, including individuals at very high risk. In other words, studies included individuals with known premalignancy of the airway and patients who already had a primary tobacco-related cancer, because these cohorts were known to have extraordinary risk for developing an SPT and therefore offered a more efficient approach for evaluating candidate chemoprevention agents.

STATUS OF LUNG CANCER SCREENING AND ITS RELATIONSHIP TO CHEMOPREVENTION

After decades of disappointing results, a robust approach to detect and cure early lung cancer has finally emerged. The National Lung Screening Trial (NLST)—the most expensive screening trial ever conducted by the National Cancer Institute—found that the use of low-dose CT (LDCT) in at-risk populations was associated with a significant reduction in lung cancer mortality.[92] Based on this finding and related data, LDCT screening is now recommended by the USPSTF. Humphrey et al.[12] outlined the underpinnings of the USPSTF draft statement on lung cancer screening in individuals at high risk of lung cancer and summarized the benefits and potential harms of this new screening approach.[12] From a review of this synthesis, a number of evidence-based conclusions emerge that clarify important issues about this new public health service as we begin national dissemination of LDCT screening.

To begin, no strict definition of LDCT exists; it is typically considered to use 10% to 30% of the dose of radiation applied in a standard, noncontrast CT. LDCT has been demonstrated to be as accurate as standard-dose CT for detecting solid pulmonary nodules in most adults. In the NLST, acceptable chest CT screening was accomplished at an overall average effective dose of less than 2 millisievert (mSv), which is considerably less than the average effective dose of 7 mSv used for a typical standard-dose chest CT.[93]

The use of low-dose radiation for screening reflects the context of this imaging application. In a physician's office, an individual presenting with the appropriate history combined with signs or symptoms of lung cancer is much more likely to have lung cancer than is an asymptomatic individual participating in a lung cancer screening effort. With screening, the balance of risks and benefits is much narrower than in the standard setting of symptom-detected cancer, and so defining the optimal approach to the LDCT process with the greatest efficiency and quality while minimizing costs and harms is the fundamental challenge as we move toward national implementation of lung cancer screening.

The National Comprehensive Cancer Network (NCCN) has provided a useful source of information about how to approach this LDCT screening process.[94] An example of the management and follow-up for one set of findings after LDCT screening is shown in Fig. 9.1.

NCCN proposes that LDCT screening requires sophisticated multidetector CT scanners and analytic software, professional physicists and staff who can certify equipment and perform studies to a consistent standard at acceptable radiation exposures, qualified radiologists who use standardized terminology and standardized interpretation, appropriate guidelines, reliable communication with primary care physicians, medical environments that can absorb patients who require ongoing management, and the responsibility of tracking screened individuals and documenting outcomes.

NCCN has stratified risk groups that may be eligible for LDCT screening (Table 9.1).[94] The highest-risk group mirrors the eligibility criteria of the NLST, but the lower-risk strata still

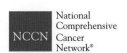

NCCN Guidelines Index
Table of Contents
Discussion

NCCN Guidelines Version 1.2017
Lung Cancer Screening

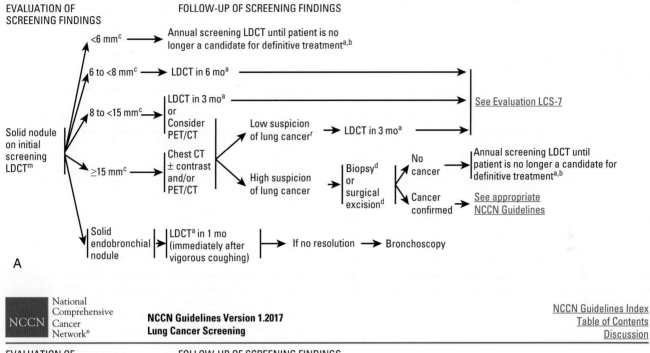

NCCN Guidelines Index
Table of Contents
Discussion

NCCN Guidelines Version 1.2017
Lung Cancer Screening

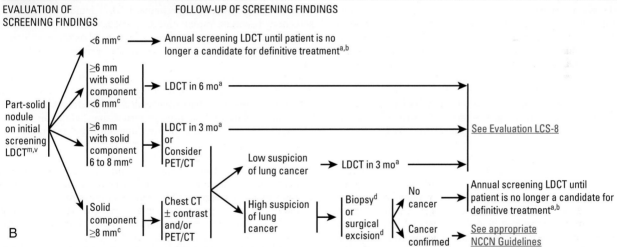

Fig. 9.1. Algorithm recommended by the NCCN for the management of solid (A) or part-solid nodules (B) detected by low-dose computed tomography (LDCT) screening. *CT,* computed tomography; *NCCN,* National Comprehensive Cancer Network; *PET,* positron emission tomography. All screening and follow-up CT scans should be performed at low dose (100 kVp to 120 kVp and 40 mAs to 60 mAs or less), unless evaluating mediastinal abnormalities or lymph nodes, where standard-dose CT with intravenous (IV) contrast might be appropriate (see Table 9.2). There should be a systematic process for appropriate follow-up. [a]There is uncertainty about the appropriate duration of screening and the age at which screening is no longer appropriate. [b]For nodules less than 15 mm: increase in mean diameter over 2 mm in any nodule or in the solid portion of a part-solid nodule compared with baseline scan. For nodules over 5 mm: increase in mean diameter of over 15% compared with baseline scan. [c]Rapid increase in size should raise suspicion of inflammatory etiology or malignancy other than nonsmall cell lung cancer. [d]Tissue samples need to be adequate for both histology and molecular testing. Travis WD, Brambilla E, Noguchi M, et al. Diagnosis of lung cancer in small biopsies and cytology: implications of the 2011 International Association for the Study of Lung Cancer/American Thoracic Society/European Respiratory Society Classification. *Arch Pathol Lab Med.* 2013;137:668–684. *Note:* All recommendations are category 2A unless otherwise indicated. *Clinical Trials:* NCCN believes that the best management of any cancer patient is in a clinical trial. Participation in clinical trials is especially encouraged. *(Adapted from the NCCN Guidelines for Lung Cancer Screening V.1.2017. 2014 National Comprehensive Cancer Network, Inc. All rights reserved. The NCCN Guidelines and illustrations herein may not be reproduced in any form for any purpose without the express written permission of the NCCN. To view the most recent and complete version of the NCCN Guidelines, go online to NCCN.org. NATIONAL COMPREHENSIVE CANCER NETWORK, NCCN, NCCN GUIDELINES, and all other NCCN Content are trademarks owned by the National Comprehensive Cancer Network, Inc.)*

TABLE 9.1 Guidelines of the NCCN on Eligibility for Low-Dose Computed Tomography Screening[a]

Risk Level			Risk Factors
High risk[b]	Age 55–74 years and 30-pack/year history of smoking and smoking cessation <15 years (category 1)[c]	or	20-pack/year history of smoking and one additional risk factor (including radon exposure, cancer history, family history of lung cancer, history of lung disease, and occupational exposure to lung carcinogens such as asbestos and diesel fumes; category 2B)[c]
Moderate risk[d]	Age 50 years and 20-pack/year history of smoking	or	Second-hand smoke exposure (no additional risk factors)[e]
Low risk[d]	Age <50 years	and/or	<20 pack/year history of smoking

[a]Moderate-risk and low-risk patients are not recommended for screening.
[b]Screening is recommended for the high-risk groups in the NCCN Guidelines for Lung Cancer Screening.
[c]Category 1: Based on high-level evidence, there is uniform NCCN consensus that the intervention is appropriate. Category 2B: Based on lower-level evidence, there is NCCN consensus that the intervention is appropriate.
[d]Screening with LDCT is not recommended for the moderate-risk and low-risk groups in the NCCN Guidelines for Lung Cancer Screening.
[e]Risk factors include radon exposure, cancer history, family history of lung cancer, history of lung disease, and occupational exposure to lung carcinogens (e.g., asbestos, diesel fumes).
Adapted with permission from the NCCN Clinical Practice Guidelines in Oncology (NCCN Guidelines) for Lung Cancer Screening V.2.2014. 2014 National Comprehensive Cancer Network, Inc. All rights reserved. The NCCN Guidelines and illustrations herein may not be reproduced in any form for any purpose without the express written permission of the NCCN. To view the most recent and complete version of the NCCN Guidelines, go online to NCCN.org. NATIONAL COMPREHENSIVE CANCER NETWORK, NCCN, NCCN GUIDELINES, and all other NCCN Content are trademarks owned by the National Comprehensive Cancer Network, Inc.
LDCT, low-dose computed tomography; NCCN, National Comprehensive Cancer Network.

include people who may develop lung cancer but in whom the cost-to-benefit ratio may be narrower. NCCN also has a patient summary for lung cancer screening, which is an excellent source of objective information for the clinician to guide discussions with potential screening candidates on topics such as who is an appropriate candidate for LDCT screening and what the likely risk is relative to benefit.[95]

An important topic that frequently arises when considering the benefits of screening is the concept of overdiagnosis. Overdiagnosis occurs when a cancer detected during screening does not behave in a lethal fashion, such that an individual may die with, not from, a screen-detected cancer. The USPSTF recently commented on the extent of overdiagnosis with chest x-ray screening in the Prostate, Lung, Colorectal, and Ovarian (PLCO) screening trial. Chest x-ray screening was the initial basis of concern for overdiagnosis in lung cancer screening.[96] In the PLCO trial, among participants at risk for lung cancer due to heavy tobacco exposure, the cumulative incidence of lung cancer after 6 years of follow-up was the same in both the chest x-ray and usual-care groups (606 per 100,000 person-years vs. 608 per 100,000 person-years, respectively; relative risk, 1.00; 95% confidence interval [CI], 0.88–1.13). These results indicate a very small influence of overdiagnosis in this setting, and the PLCO findings suggest that overdiagnosis is not a major confounder in evaluating the benefit of lung cancer screening.[97]

However, many other questions remain unanswered as we consider the implementation of LDCT screening because many misconceptions exist about this new service. One of the most important concepts is understanding the difference between providing screening care for a patient at risk for lung cancer and the more typical situation of treating a symptomatic patient suspected to have lung cancer. The risk–benefit considerations in these two settings are very different, and these differences mandate distinct management approaches.

Regarding other misconceptions, the core design assumption of the NLST, which evaluated more than 53,000 current or former smokers at a cost in excess of $250 million, was widely vetted. The consensus that emerged was that a target reduction in mortality of 20% with LDCT compared with chest x-ray outcomes would constitute compelling evidence of an objective screening benefit. An analysis of the full benefit of LDCT would have been much more expensive and require considerably more time to complete. Therefore it is not surprising that a more recent analysis of NLST outcomes with a rederived eligibility

risk model constructed from PLCO case outcomes resulted in a more efficient rate of lung cancer detection.[98] In that report, the mortality reduction was 30%, compared with the 20% benefit reported in the NLST.[98] This example demonstrates how the LDCT screening process can be improved, and the reanalysis of the NLST data set underscores how valuable this data resource is in allowing process improvement for LDCT screening. As screening becomes implemented, it will be essential to continue to build screening registries from the data of as many screening individuals as possible so that continuous process improvement can be sustained.[98]

LDCT screening does entail a range of possible harms. A 2012 review article from a joint society initiative communicated reservations about the balance of risks and benefits of lung cancer screening.[99] The investigators reported that "uncertainty exists about the potential harms of screening and the generalizability of results."[99] By contrast, a comprehensive synthesis of the issues with screening management was published by the USPSTF in 2013 and conveyed a more optimistic perspective regarding how refined management approaches have improved the process of lung cancer screening. The USPSTF provides an excellent resource for guiding discussions to inform potential screening individuals about risks and benefits of this service.[12,97]

Results of the NLST and Other Clinical Trials Are Not Equal

Although disparate views exist regarding the strength of the evidence supporting LDCT, data synthesis from the comprehensive USPSTF analysis helps clarify this dialogue with its clear support for the strengths of this new approach. At the time of publication, the NLST was the only completed, fully powered, randomized, lung cancer screening trial reported,[92] and no comparable, adequately powered trial was currently under consideration. Comparisons of the mortality reduction reported in the NLST relative to the results of two small, randomized, European trials are not helpful because the latter studies were not adequately powered to give a reliable assessment of the mortality reduction of LDCT.[99] Although ongoing trials will generate interesting and important cost-related and other data that are complementary to those of the NLST, no existing trials will have sufficient study power to supersede the positive conclusion of the NLST relative to the end point of mortality reduction. The largest of the ongoing trials is the Dutch-Belgian Randomized Lung Cancer Screening Trial

TABLE 9.2 Summary Results of Large Clinical Trials Relative to Cancer Detection and Frequency of Stage I Lung Cancer

Study	No. of Cancers/Total Screened (%)		Stage I/All Detected Cancers (%)	
	Round 1	Round 2	Round 1	Round 2
NLST	168/24,715 (0.67)	211/24,102 (0.87)	104/165 (63)	141/204 (69)
NELSON	40/7289 (0.5)	57/7289[a] (0.8)	42/57 (73.7)	—

[a]NELSON round 2/3 data were presented together, reflecting the study design.[100]

NLST, National Lung Screening Trial; *NELSON*, Dutch acronym for Dutch-Belgian Randomized Lung Cancer Screening Trial.[101]

(Dutch acronym NELSON), a study being conducted by a consortium of Dutch and Belgian investigators.[100] Preliminary data from NELSON can be compared with follow-up data from the NLST91 (Table 9.2). As shown, the cancer detection rates are comparable and the stage I detection rates are similar as well, so a major reduction in benefit with LDCT in the NELSON trial is not expected.

From the perspective of US national policy, the NLST data represent the standard criterion showing that LDCT screening can reduce mortality from lung cancer. In the wake of the additional NLST follow-up results, the most relevant contribution of the NELSON trial may be the quality of the ancillary studies, such as the eventual economic analysis. The NELSON investigators embedded more advanced clinical screening management provisions because this trial started several years after the start of the NLST.

Meeting or Exceeding the Favorable Outcomes Reported in the NLST

Going forward, a crucial issue is whether the reported benefits of LDCT screening can be met or exceeded when LDCT is implemented nationally as a routine clinical service. This is a complex issue involving a number of variables that are all crucial in determining the overall benefit of this approach. For example, the risk of lung cancer after heavy smoking persists, despite smoking cessation, and remains elevated as long as the former smoker lives.[2] Therefore ongoing screening beyond the two rounds evaluated in the NLST could further improve the mortality benefit of lung cancer screening beyond the 20% threshold.[92] Two reports have suggested that sustained annual screening may reduce mortality from lung cancer by 40% to 60% under different screening scenarios.[103,104] LDCT has several robust features that enhance its performance as a cancer screening tool. Indeed, the rapid refinement of CT image resolution has resulted in routine detection of progressively smaller primary lung cancers. This evolution improves patients' outcomes for two reasons. First, smaller tumors are associated with better cancer-specific outcomes.[105] Second, smaller tumors are likely to be amenable to treatment with minimally invasive thoracic surgery, a new surgical approach associated with a better quality of life, better compliance with adjuvant therapy, and fewer postoperative complications.[106,107]

In the NLST, surgical clinical care was not specified by any optimized protocol and was typically not delivered in a center selected for excellence in thoracic surgical care. At the time of the NLST, minimally invasive surgery was used in only a minority of the cancers detected during the study. For these reasons, thoughtful national implementation coupled with current best practice could mean that LDCT screening meets or even exceeds the favorable results reported in the NLST. Definitive data for the optimal approach to surgical management in the screening setting do not exist. However, many centers of excellence have

reported favorable surgical outcomes using minimally invasive approaches, generally with video-assisted thoracoscopic surgery.[106,107] A retrospective review of 347 thoracic resections performed in the setting of a lung cancer screening program demonstrated that long-term (10-year) results of sublobar resection were equivalent to those of lobectomy for clinical stage 1A lung cancers.[108] In addition to these excellent results, sublobar resection preserves greater amounts of well-functioning lung tissue.

The Lung Cancer Alliance, an advocacy group, has proposed the mechanism of the Lung Cancer Screening Framework, which encourages institutions providing screening services to employ best practices for screening, including minimally invasive surgical techniques, so that the quality of screening services is maintained at a high level. To validate that institutions are successful in their screening management services, the framework process also mandates that participating institutions routinely report relevant screening outcomes and complication rates, so that potential screening individuals can make informed decisions about where they choose to receive their screening care.[109]

SCREENING INTERVAL AND SELECTION OF CANDIDATES

Questions regarding the optimal interval for the frequency of LDCT screening have been cited as a justification for delaying national implementation. A more efficient approach for defining candidates for LDCT would address much of the uncertainty cited with regard to candidate selection while providing timely access for patients most likely to benefit from LDCT screening. Given the complexity of predicting lung cancer risk, it is unlikely that a one-size-fits-all screening recommendation would suffice moving forward; however, new risk-stratification tools have been shown to provide more robust discrimination of lung cancer risk.[110]

The context for lung cancer screening is unique because tobacco exposure is such a powerful determinant of risk. In 2012, a large British meta-analysis that included data from more than 250,000 individuals resulted in the development of a tool that was very robust in stratifying risk using only the patient's history of tobacco exposure.[111] This approach is consistent with a report by Tammemägi et al.[98] that modeled a better screening outcome when using a more refined tool for cohort identification. Although more comprehensive molecular or genetic models are being developed, the risk tool based on tobacco exposure history would be a logical candidate to use when starting the national screening process and evaluating the generalizable benefit of LDCT screening.[110] Professional societies have suggested that it would be logical to extend LDCT screening to other target cohorts whose level of risk is similar to that of the NLST target population.[112,113] For example, screening could be recommended for individuals based on age, history of tobacco exposure, and other factors as determined by that risk tool, all of which might define a screening cohort equivalent to the validated risk strata found among NLST participants. Perhaps further work with the PLCO risk model could prospectively classify risk of lung cancer relative to the risk strata studied in the NLST as a normative tool for comparing new risk-stratifying tools going forward.[98]

OPPORTUNITIES TO IMPROVE LDCT SCREENING

Since the start of the NLST in 2002, substantial improvements have been made in several areas, including the imaging resolution of LDCT, tools to discriminate high-risk populations, efficiency of diagnostic workup algorithms, and the morbidity of curative thoracic surgical procedures.[12,97] The dose of medical radiation required for LDCT has also decreased.[92]

The LDCT screening setting, which, for now, involves annual follow-up, provides an opportunity to manage tobacco cessation at each annual encounter. The intensity of the cessation strategy can be tailored for the persistent smoker, and this new screening management setting therefore offers a new platform for personalized efforts at smoking cessation. More effective integration of screening and smoking cessation could enhance the public health benefit of this new service. The strength of this growing body of information supporting the safety and effectiveness of LDCT screening, as well as the growing number of endorsements by professionals, has led insurers, such as WellPoint and Anthem, to provide LDCT as a covered service. Third-party coverage through Medicare in the United States was adapted in 2015.

IMPROVEMENTS IN THE APPROACH TO SCREENING AND LDCT IMAGING

Since the inception of the NLST a decade ago, the approach to lung cancer screening that was built into the NLST protocol has improved substantially, yet these improvements—which could facilitate LDCT implementation by reducing potential harms and costs—have not been considered in evaluating the efficacy of CT screening. For example, multidetector scanners were used in the NLST because they are faster than earlier scanners and allow full visualization of lung fields within a single breath hold. The use of such scanners results in fewer CT image artifacts and allows more comprehensive analysis of the lung than that achievable with chest x-rays. However, recently developed CT scanners offer faster image acquisition, which may translate into technically better-quality studies with less motion artifact, and the image quality has continued to improve. These improvements lower both the risks and costs of imaging. All of these factors are pertinent in the public health implementation of LDCT as a national screening resource.

CHANGES IN NODULE EVALUATION AND DIAGNOSTIC WORKUP

Awareness is variable on the importance of the new findings regarding the approach to nodule evaluation.[99] Published reports have outlined considerable refinement in the clinical management of the screening process since the initiation of the NLST, which did not mandate a specific approach to nodule evaluation. Yankelevitz et al.[114] were the first to report that clinically important lung nodules could be identified by restricting the diagnostic workup to suspicious nodules that showed significant growth over a defined period. This interval-growth approach to the diagnostic workup was incorporated into the design of the NELSON trial and resulted in a favorable workup rate of 12% for the diagnosis of invasive nodules, with a diagnostic sensitivity of 95% and a specificity of 99% for LDCT.[100] More recently, this interval-growth criterion for suspicious nodules was used prospectively in a cohort of 4700 patients undergoing screening at the Princess Margaret Hospital; only 3% of the patients were required to undergo an invasive workup, and the false-positive diagnostic rate was 0.42%.[115] The validity of these findings is supported by a recent retrospective analysis of baseline lung cancer cases accrued in the International Early Lung Cancer Action Project. In this analysis, changing the threshold of nodule size for a lung cancer diagnostic workup from 4–5 mm to 7–8 mm was associated with timely diagnosis of early-stage lung cancer while significantly reducing the frequency of false-positive results.[116] Implementation of this approach could improve the efficiency of LDCT screening by reducing the costs and harms of invasive diagnostic workups within the baseline screening process. The NCCN has been integrating the evolving research information into its management recommendations

for screening (see Fig. 9.1). This information will allow more consistent management of LDCT, with expectations of more favorable outcomes.

FURTHER OPPORTUNITIES ASSOCIATED WITH LDCT SCREENING

A crucial opportunity to optimize the benefit of screening is to integrate smoking cessation into lung cancer screening.[117,118] Although integration of LDCT screening into smoking cessation has been reported with mixed success, to date little research has been done to optimize smoking cessation within the setting of recurrent screening. Some authors have characterized the screening encounter as a so-called teachable moment for a dialogue about smoking cessation, and the cost efficiency of this integration is projected to be extremely favorable.[119,120] Furthermore, every subsequent annual LDCT screening for a persistent smoker is an opportunity to explore more personalized or intensive measures for smoking cessation. Increasing success with smoking cessation would not only improve the inherent cost efficiency of the LDCT screening process relative to lung cancer outcomes, but would also accrue to the other well-validated health and economic benefits related to smoking cessation. Through new mechanisms required by the Centers for Medicare and Medicaid Services, reimbursement for LDCT screening services could be linked to demonstrating compliance with national quality measures for these services, especially with regard to risk stratification and smoking cessation.[121]

A related consideration with LDCT is the unprecedented potential to evaluate the status of other tobacco-related diseases. For example, recent reports have shown that coronary calcium analysis can be derived from LDCT images and may be a useful stratification tool for the risk of coronary artery disease.[122,123] Furthermore, an LDCT assessment of lung injury could serve as a metric of risk for progression of COPD.[124,125] Indeed, patients with tobacco exposure participating in lung cancer screening are known to experience a significant comorbid risk of COPD and cardiovascular disease. With further research, the opportunity exists to simultaneously evaluate for the three major host consequences of tobacco exposure—coronary artery disease, COPD, and cardiovascular disease—with only LDCT. These diseases represent three of the leading causes of premature death in our society.[126] The emerging setting of LDCT screening can therefore provide a useful window into the preclinical phase of three major chronic diseases, so the time is ripe to explore this important opportunity.

CHEMOPREVENTION TRIALS

Risk categories differ across the spectrum of lung carcinogenesis, from individuals exposed to carcinogens, to individuals with known premalignant lesions, to individuals who have already had cancer as a result of tobacco smoke exposure. Reducing the frequency of cancer in these three categories of at-risk individuals (carcinogen-exposed individuals) is the focus of chemoprevention. Specific terms are used to describe the various approaches to cancer prevention. The first is known as primary cancer prevention. Primary prevention involves intervening in patient populations who have only an increased risk, such as with tobacco control measures, to reduce exposure to tobacco combustion products. The purpose of primary prevention is to reduce the incidence of and mortality from lung cancer.

Secondary prevention applies to individuals with evidence of lung premalignancy and involves attempts to prevent the progression of that premalignancy or, ideally, to reverse it to an earlier stage of carcinogenesis. Chemoprevention falls into this category. An efficient way to study the benefit of chemoprevention drugs is to evaluate populations at the highest risk for cancer, meaning

TABLE 9.3 Primary Randomized Trials of Chemoprevention in Lung Cancer

Study	Intervention	End Point	No. of Patients	Outcome
ATBC20	β-carotene, α-tocopherol	Lung cancer	29,133	Negative/harmful
CARET[129]	β-carotene, retinol	Lung cancer	18,314	Negative/harmful
Physician's Health Study[130]	β-carotene	Lung cancer	22,071	Negative
Women's Health Study[131]	β-carotene, aspirin, vitamin E	Lung cancer	39,876	Negative

ATBC, Alpha-Tocopherol, Beta-Carotene Cancer Prevention Study; *CARET,* Beta-Carotene and Retinol Efficacy Trial.

patients who have already had a first tobacco-related malignancy and have a very high risk of an SPT developing. Many of the early trials focused on using retinoids and carotenoids as chemoprevention agents because of the strong epidemiologic and experimental evidence for the activity of these compounds.

Primary Chemoprevention

Several large, randomized studies were conducted in populations deemed to be at increased risk of lung cancer because of exposure to tobacco smoke or asbestos, or their occupation as uranium miners. The hypothesis that dietary β-carotene could lower the incidence of epithelial cancers was first proposed by Peto et al.[127] Later, three major studies, the Alpha-Tocopherol, Beta-Carotene Cancer Prevention (ATBC) Study, the Beta-Carotene and Retinol Efficacy Trial (CARET), and the Physician's Health Study, were carried out using increasingly high doses of the carotenoid β-carotene (Table 9.3).[128–130]

None of the three studies showed significant reductions in lung cancer risk using these compounds. In fact, the secondary end point in two of these studies, ATBC and CARET, showed an increase in the incidence of lung cancer associated with β-carotene supplementation. Both of these trials, which were 2 × 2 factorial studies, also involved a second agent, as an intervention. In these cases, neither the second agent nor vitamin A itself was found to be associated with an increased risk of lung cancer, but neither were they protective against lung cancer. Both of these studies showed that the risk of lung cancer was increased only among smokers.

The ATBC was a randomized, 2 × 2 factorial, double-blind, placebo-controlled, primary prevention study in which 29,143 Finnish male smokers received α-tocopherol (50 mg/day alone), β-carotene (20 mg/day), both α-tocopherol and β-carotene, or a placebo.[128] The enrolled participants were 50 years to 69 years of age, and all of them smoked five or more cigarettes per day; they received follow-up observation for 5 years to 8 years. Although the incidence of lung cancer, the primary end point, was not modified by supplementation with α-tocopherol alone, both groups that received β-carotene supplementation, either alone or with α-tocopherol, had an 18% increase in the incidence of lung cancer and an 8% increase in lung cancer mortality. This study showed a stronger adverse effect from β-carotene in men who smoked more than 20 cigarettes per day and was the first to raise the concern that pharmacologic doses of β-carotene could be harmful in active smokers. However, a follow-up analysis suggested that the excess risk among β-carotene recipients was no longer evident after 4 years to 6 years, and a continued, slight excess in total mortality was attributable to cardiovascular diseases.[132]

The results of CARET were consistent with the results of the ATBC trial. This was also a randomized, double-blind,

placebo-controlled trial testing the combination of β-carotene (30 mg/day) and retinyl palmitate (25,000 IU) in 18,314 men and women aged 50 years to 69 years who were considered to have an increased risk of lung cancer. Most participants had a smoking history of 20 or more pack-years and were either current smokers or recent former smokers. Significant or extensive occupational exposure to asbestos was noted in 4060 men in this trial.[133] The trial was terminated prematurely because of concern about possible harm, consistent with the findings of the ATBC study. Lung cancer incidence, the primary end point, was increased by 28% in the active intervention group, and overall mortality was increased by 17% in this group.[129]

This finding was different from those of the Physician's Health Study,[130] a randomized, double-blind, placebo-controlled trial that included 22,071 healthy male physicians. Half of the participants received 50 mg/day of β-carotene on alternate days, and the other half received placebo; no adverse effect of β-carotene supplementation was noted. The use of supplemental β-carotene in this study, which included mostly nonsmokers, showed no adverse or beneficial effects on cancer incidence or overall mortality rate during a 12-year follow-up.[130] Similarly, the Women's Health Study evaluated the effect of β-carotene supplementation and found no evidence of either benefit or harm. However, only 13% of the women were smokers in both the treatment and placebo groups.[131]

Subsequent subgroup analyses of the ATBC and CARET studies indicated that an excess of cancers was found only in the β-carotene study arms including high-risk heavy smokers or individuals with previous exposure to asbestos.[134]

A recent metabolomic analysis has proposed that increased mortality in the ATBC study could be related to dysregulation of glycemic control induced by β-carotene and induction of cytochrome P450 enzymes, leading to interactions with cardiovascular drugs.[135] This hypothesis must be considered in light of the emerging understanding that a high percentage of smokers died prematurely from cardiovascular causes, and this confounding factor can play a major role in the increased overall mortality rate in these chemoprevention trials. Tobacco is known to upregulate cytochrome P450 enzymes, and this effect can accelerate the metabolism not only of chemopreventive drugs, but also of other classes of therapeutic drugs, such as cardiovascular drugs.

The role of inhaled steroids as possible chemopreventive agents has been reported. Inhaled budesonide was associated with a dose-dependent reduction in the risk of lung cancer in a cohort of patients with COPD.[136] A phase II trial from 2011 studied the effects of oral budesonide on the size of CT-detected pulmonary nodules in current and former smokers. Treatment for 1 year did not significantly affect the size of peripheral lung nodules, but a trend toward regression of nonsolid and partially solid nodules was noted.[137] At least some of these ground-glass nodules are suspected to be cancer precursor lesions. Epithelial-directed drug delivery may be advantageous because it could result in high drug concentrations in areas of high tobacco-related injury in the airways, yet achieve nontoxic drug levels in the systemic circulation. Oral administration of these agents may not result in sufficient drug concentrations at the bronchial epithelium. Experimental studies in animal models with aerosolized 13-*cis*-retinoic acid and retinyl palmitate have shown significant improvements in histologic changes in the bronchial epithelium.[138] This pharmacologic approach has a strong theoretic appeal, and the preliminary positive results require further research.

Secondary Chemoprevention

Although authorities disagree about which premalignant markers most consistently predict the development of cancer, the success in studying patients with premalignancy has been limited. To date, randomized trials have used various end points, including

TABLE 9.4 Secondary Randomized Trials of Chemoprevention in Lung Cancer

Study	Intervention	End Point	No. of Patients	Outcome
Lee et al.[142]	Isotretinoin	Metaplasia	40	Negative
Kurie et al.[143]	Fenretinide	Metaplasia	82	Negative
Arnold et al.[144]	Etretinate	Metaplasia	150	Negative
McLarty et al.[145]	β-Carotene, retinol	Sputum atypia	755	Negative
Heimburger et al.[141]	Vitamin B12, folic acid	Sputum atypia	73	Positive
van Poppel et al.[146]	β-Carotene	Micronuclei sputum	114	Positive
Kurie et al.[139]	9-cis-Retinoic acid	RAR-β expression, metaplasia	226	Positive
Mao et al.[147]	Celecoxib	Ki-67 expression	20	Positive
Van Schooten et al.[148]	N-Acetylcysteine	DNA adducts	41	Positive
Lam et al.[149]	ADT	Dysplasia	101	Positive
Soria et al.[140]	Fenretinide	hTERT expression	57	Positive
Lam et al.[150]	Budesonide	Dysplasia	112	Negative
van den Berg et al.[151]	Fluticasone	Dysplasia	108	Negative
Gray et al.[152]	Enzastaurin	Dysplasia, Ki-67 LI	40	Negative
Kelly et al.[153]	13-cis-Retinoic acid, α-tocopherol	Dysplasia, Ki-67 LI	86	Negative
Mao et al.[154]	Celecoxib in former smokers	Dysplasia, Ki-67 LI	137	Positive
Keith et al.[155]	Iloprost	Dysplasia	152	Positive
Limburg et al.[156]	Sulindac	Dysplasia, Ki-67 LI	61	Negative

ADT, anethole dithiolethione; *hTERT*, human telomerase reverse transcriptase; *Ki-67 LI*, Ki-67 labeling index; *RAR*, retinoic acid receptor.

reversal of sputum atypia, reduction in DNA micronuclei, and reversal of dysplasia or hyperplasia (Table 9.4). Some of these trials have used retinoids and have shown that in the absence of smoking cessation, retinoids are incapable of reversing premalignant lesions. By contrast, some biomarker-driven studies using pan-retinoids, such as 9-cis-retinoic acid, or atypical retinoids, such as fenretinide, have shown that these agents can modulate biomarkers such as RAR-β or expression of human telomerase reverse transcriptase, respectively.[139,140] Little evidence is available to suggest that any of the compounds listed in Table 9.4 are capable of consistently reversing premalignant lesions. To date, one of the most positive studies has been the one that used folate and vitamin B12, which showed some improvement in metaplasia of the bronchial epithelium in smokers.[141] Given the difficulty in validating end points, however, even these positive results must be viewed with caution. Larger trials using biologic end points are needed to confirm efficacy.

The findings of Lee et al.[142] are interesting because they indicated that retinoids could be effective in conjunction with smoking cessation. No evidence of benefit was found in active (continuing) smokers, but that raises the issue of accelerated drug metabolism in current smokers due to induction of metabolizing enzymes. However, more recent studies using novel retinoids have indicated the potential for significant benefit. Kurie et al.[139] reported the results of a randomized controlled trial in former smokers who received either 9-cis-retinoic acid or 13-cis-retinoic acid with α-tocopherol. The end point of this trial was

upregulation of RAR-β, which may inhibit the process of pulmonary carcinogenesis. Of 177 evaluable participants, patients treated with 9-cis-retinoic acid were found to have restoration of RAR-β expression ($p < 0.03$), and this finding also correlated with a reduction of bronchial metaplasia ($p < 0.01$).[139] No significant effect was found among patients receiving 13-cis-retinoic acid with α-tocopherol, so this group of investigators planned to move forward with 9-cis-retinoic acid, a pan-retinoid agonist, targeting former smokers.

Ki-67, a biomarker for cell proliferation, has been used as an end point for changes in bronchial dysplasia in various secondary chemoprevention trials. For example, a phase II trial was conducted to study the effects of enzastaurin, a serine/threonine kinase inhibitor, to reduce the Ki-67 labeling index in former smokers. The patients were randomly assigned to receive oral enzastaurin (500 mg/day) or placebo daily for 6 months. The results failed to show any significant difference in changes in the Ki-67 labeling index between the experimental and placebo arms. However, in a subgroup analysis restricted to metaplastic and dysplastic samples, almost one-fifth of the participants had a 50% reduction in Ki-67 expression in the experimental arm compared with none in the placebo arm.[152]

A phase III trial evaluated the effect of 13-cis-retinoic acid (50 mg/day) in high-risk patients as measured by changes in the Ki-67 labeling index of the bronchial epithelium. The study included patients with more than a 30-pack/year history of smoking, evidence of airflow obstruction, or surgically cured stage I or II NSCLC. Results after 12-month follow-up failed to show any change in the Ki-67 labeling index,[153] but dosage reductions in 13-cis-retinoic acid were frequent because of adverse drug effects.

Sulindac was studied as a potential chemopreventive agent in a randomized, placebo-controlled phase II trial. However, results from this trial of squamous cell lung cancer chemoprevention failed to demonstrate sufficient benefits from sulindac as documented by changes in the Ki-67 labeling index.[156]

This result raises the question of whether Ki-67 is the appropriate biomarker. Data are conflicting as to whether Ki-67 expression is related to smoking status and degree of dysplasia or whether it predicts the eventual development of lung cancer.[157–159]

Various other natural agents, including curcumin, deguelin, bovine lactoferrin, *myo*-inositol, and epigallocatechin gallate, have been studied in animal models as potential agents to block tumor carcinogenesis, but these agents are in the very early stages of evaluation.[160–163]

The cyclooxygenases (COXs) have been reported to be involved in carcinogenesis. Inhibition of this enzyme, particularly COX-2, is a potential chemopreventive approach. In population-based cohort studies, the use of nonsteroidal anti-inflammatory drugs for more than 1 year was associated with a reduction in the relative risk of lung cancer and conferred chemoprotective effects in smokers.[164–166] In a phase IIb study, celecoxib, another COX-2 inhibitor, significantly reduced the Ki-67 labeling index and other secondary end points in former smokers.[164] However, these agents can be used only in specific populations with a low cardiovascular risk, which limits their utility in terms of chemoprevention of smoking-associated diseases.

Iloprost is another agent that modulates the COX cascade and has effects similar to those of the COX-2 inhibitors. Oral iloprost was shown to significantly improve endobronchial dysplasia in the epithelia of former smokers in a phase II trial. Confirmatory trials linking the administration of these agents to improvements in clinical end points are required before recommending broader use of these agents.[155]

Neoadjuvant window-of-opportunity trials entail the administration of specific drugs to patients with newly diagnosed lung cancer just before (typically 2 weeks before) lung cancer resection. In this manner, the expression analysis can be evaluated in comparison with postdrug exposure to define the signaling pathways that are active and influenced by the drug exposure. This approach gives a more precise signature of actual drug impact than is possible with conventional drug-development approaches for lung cancer and potentially identifies useful intermediate markers of drug effect. This class of trial also allows direct evaluation of the respiratory epithelium for mapping the extent of carcinogenic injury along with the drug response at those sites. Three such trials have been conducted in patients with stage I NSCLC. Chemotherapy is administered during the preoperative window, and then disease is assessed for response in terms of tumor load reduction and biomarker profiling. The first of these trials was conducted to explore the use of gefitinib in patients with stage I NSCLC to assess response in terms of tumor burden and to identify predictors of response.[167] Thirty-six patients received gefitinib (250 mg/day) for up to 4 weeks before surgical resection in this single-arm study. Tumor shrinkage was more common among nonsmokers and women, and the strongest factor to predict response was EGFR mutation; this finding supports gefitinib as part of a neoadjuvant regimen for early-stage NSCLC in selected populations (with EGFR mutations). These trials also serve as biomarker trials by identifying markers that are predictive of response and their potential use to select a target population for chemopreventive and therapeutic approaches. Another phase II trial explored the use of pazopanib, an oral anti-angiogenesis agent that inhibits vascular endothelial growth factor, in early-stage NSCLC. These investigators also conducted extensive biomarker profiling of cytokines and angiogenic factors (CAFs) to investigate the relationship between CAFs and tumor shrinkage. Levels of 11 CAFs were found to be associated with tumor shrinkage, notably interleukin-12 and interleukin-4. The authors proposed the use of CAF profiling to select target populations for pretreatment with pazopanib.[168]

Another trial used a combination of bexarotene and erlotinib in early-stage NSCLC. This combination was found to be active in KRAS-driven lung cancer cells and also in clinically active, chemorefractory mutant KRAS cancers, which was interesting because the presence of KRAS mutations was hypothesized to be a marker of resistance to gefitinib treatment.[169]

Linkage Chemoprevention and Future Research

Patients with tobacco-related cancers remain at a substantially elevated risk for subsequent tumors in the tobacco-damaged epithelium.[27,28,170–174] Although treatment of the initial cancer can often be successful, these patients have a high risk of an SPT.[175] The lifetime risk of an SPT in the head and neck region is approximately 20%. Although estimates have varied between 3% and 7% per year, the evidence remains very strong that SPTs are the major cause of death after curative surgical procedures for head and neck cancer.[173–178]

Given the high likelihood of both recurrence and SPTs in patients with advanced oral, oropharyngeal, or laryngeal squamous cell cancers, Hong et al.[179] launched a randomized, placebo-controlled study of 103 patients with stages I–IV head and neck squamous cell cancer (Table 9.5). The patients were randomly assigned to receive either high-dose 13-*cis*-retinoic acid (100 mg/m²/day) or placebo for 1 year after definitive local therapy. The dosage of 13-*cis*-retinoic acid was reduced to 50 mg/m²/day after 13 of the first 44 patients experienced intolerable adverse effects. The primary end points were recurrence of the primary tumor and development of an SPT. No difference was found between the treatment arms in local recurrence or distant metastases. However, the patients treated with 13-*cis*-retinoic acid had a dramatically lower incidence of SPTs. Of the 103 patients followed for a median of 42 months, SPTs developed in 6% (3/49) in the 13-*cis*-retinoic acid arm compared with 28% (14/51) in the placebo arm.

TABLE 9.5 Prevention Studies on Lung and Aerodigestive Secondary Primary Tumors (Tertiary Chemoprevention)

Study	Intervention	End Point	No. of Patients	Outcome
Pastorino et al.[180]	Retinyl palmitate	SPT	40	Positive
EUROSCAN[181]	Retinyl palmitate, *N*-acetylcysteine	SPT	82	Negative
Lippman et al.[182]	13-*cis*-Retinoic acid	SPT	150	Negative
Khuri et al.[183]	13-*cis*-Retinoic acid	SPT	755	Negative
Hong et al.[179]	Isotretinoin	SPT	73	Positive

SPT, secondary primary tumor.

A large-scale follow-up to this trial using a much lower dose of 13-*cis*-retinoic acid was published in 2006. In this randomized, double-blind, placebo-controlled study, launched in 1991, more than 1382 patients were registered and 1192 were randomly assigned to either low-dose 13-*cis*-retinoic acid (30 mg/day) or placebo. These patients were definitively treated for stage I or II head and neck squamous cell cancer. After a median follow-up of 7 years, no effect was seen with the low-dose retinoid for reducing the incidence of SPT in the lung or aerodigestive tract.[183] No pharmacologic assessment was done in this trial to demonstrate the adequacy of retinoid delivery into the bronchial epithelial tissue despite the major dosage reductions due to adverse effects (skin dryness, cheilitis, hypertriglyceridemia, conjunctivitis, etc.) encountered in the trial by Hong et al.[179]

Several phase III trials have been launched in an attempt to prevent SPTs in patients with lung cancer. The first of these was a trial by Pastorino et al.,[180] who randomly assigned more than 300 patients with early-stage lung cancer to retinyl palmitate or placebo. This study showed a significant reduction in the development of lung SPTs in the retinyl palmitate arm. A subsequent study by Bolla et al.[184] using a different synthetic retinoid, etretinate, failed to show a reduction in SPTs.

Two large follow-up phase III trials reported in the past decade include the EUROSCAN study and the US Intergroup 91-0001 trial.[181,182] EUROSCAN, a randomized study of adjuvant chemoprevention from the European Organisation for Research and Treatment of Cancer, studied the effects of vitamin A (retinyl palmitate) and *N*-acetylcysteine in patients with early-stage head and neck and lung cancer.[181] In this trial, 2592 patients with cancers of the larynx (TIS-T3 and 0-N1), oral cavity (TIS-T2 and 0-N1), or NSCLC (T1-T2 and 0-N1) received retinyl palmitate 300,000 IU/day in year 1 and 150,000 IU/day in year 2, *N*-acetylcysteine 600 mg/day for 2 years, both drugs, or placebo. No significant differences were seen for the three active treatment arms compared with placebo in terms of recurrence rates, SPT development, or survival. Of note, more than 90% of the patients were current smokers, with 43 median pack-years of tobacco exposure.

The US Intergroup 91-0001 trial was a randomized, double-blind, placebo-controlled study of low-dose (30 mg) 13-*cis*-retinoic acid administered after complete resection of stage I NSCLC.[182] This trial completed accrual in 1997 after enrolling 1486 participants. The study objective was to evaluate the efficacy of low-dose 13-*cis*-retinoic acid for 3 years at 30 mg/day compared with placebo in the prevention of SPTs. Patients were required to have complete resection of primary stage I NSCLC (postoperative T1 or T2 and 0) and to be registered between 6 weeks and 3 years after completion of therapy. After a median follow-up of 3.5 years, no significant differences were seen between placebo and 13-*cis*-retinoic acid with respect to time to SPT development, recurrence rate, or mortality. Multivariate analyses showed that the rate of SPTs was not affected by any stratification factor, and the recurrence rate was affected only by treatment stage, with evidence for a treatment-by-smoking interaction (hazard ratio for treatment by current smoking vs. never-smoking status, 3.11; 95% CI, 1.00–9.71). Therefore low-dose 13-*cis*-retinoic acid was not shown to affect overall survival rates or SPTs, recurrence rates, or mortality in patients with stage I NSCLC. Subsequent subset analyses have indicated that 13-*cis*-retinoic acid was associated with a higher rate of metastatic progression among current smokers and a suggestion of benefit among never-smokers.

FUTURE STRATEGIES

After more than two decades of unsuccessful chemopreventive interventions for patients with NSCLC, the accumulated evidence suggests that approaches relying exclusively on the development of epidemiologic guidance for selection of compounds are not sufficient to identify effective interventions across broad and disparate populations. Although clues continue to emerge from the epidemiologic literature suggesting that dietary constituents or specific medications, such as green tea polyphenols, curcumin, statins, and metformin, significantly reduce lung cancer risk,[185,186] few experts have suggested moving prevention approaches forward without further testing of these concepts in well-designed, biomarker-driven trials.

To date, substantial evidence shows that overexpression of EGFR occurs throughout lung carcinogenesis.[38,187,188] Furthermore, mutations of the EGFR TK binding domain can be seen diffusely across the normal-appearing airway in patients with resected adenocarcinomas who are nonsmokers and whose primary tumor harbors this mutation. This discovery of EGFR TK mutations in apparently normal-appearing airways not damaged by tobacco exposure, despite the absence of an identifiable carcinogen leading to EGFR mutations, represents a new and as yet poorly understood type of field effect.[42] Chemoprevention approaches using the EGFR TKI in high-risk patient populations have been proposed, and so-called window-of-opportunity trials have been conducted with pazopanib, gefitinib, and erlotinib, as elaborated earlier.[158,189–191]

EGFR inhibitors have also been examined in pilot studies in combination with bexarotene.[169] The incidence of EGFR TK mutations in adenocarcinomas of the lung is most prominent among Asian nonsmoking women; however, the identification of individuals at greatest risk is the biggest challenge.

Important data also indicate a progressive upregulation of COX-2 in lung carcinogenesis, and trials of suppression of COX-2 with selective COX-2 inhibitors have shown promising preliminary results.[147,192] Another approach has been to upregulate prostacyclin, thereby downregulating prostaglandin E2, potentially the crucial downstream effector pathway for COX-2.[193] These COX-directed chemopreventive strategies merit further evaluation.

Another targeted approach is based on experiments in vitro and on epidemiologic data. Govindarajan et al.[194] showed that thiazolidinediones, which stimulate the peroxisome proliferator-activated receptor (PPAR), are able to induce cell cycle arrest. These investigators performed a large cohort study of 87,678 male veterans 40 years and older and showed a 33% reduction of lung cancer risk among the 11,289 thiazolidinedione users. One caveat, however, is that this study failed to account for variations by smoking status. PPAR expression has been found to be more prevalent in squamous cell cancers than in adenocarcinomas. In squamous cell cancer, it is associated with bcl and c-myc positivity, whereas in adenocarcinoma it is associated with size of the tumor. These findings suggest the potential of PPAR expression as a prognostic marker and may have implications for chemotherapy and treatment.[195] Other researchers have used corticosteroids, both inhaled and oral, or inhaled retinoids, all of which have shown promise. Two randomized phase II pilot studies in high-risk patients failed to show a trend in favor of inhalational corticoids, but these trials had methodologic limitations, such as a focus on central airway changes and sample sizes that were not large enough to allow definitive conclusions.[150,151] Larger studies using more efficient delivery devices to target deep respiratory epithelium, thereby mirroring the deposition of tobacco-containing products, seem warranted.

Notwithstanding the negative outcomes of several large comparative trials, a considerable number of epidemiologic, experimental, and clinical observations continue to provide evidence that antioxidants, anti-inflammatory agents, EGFR TKIs, and phytochemicals may block various modes of carcinogenesis. However, the modes of action of several of these agents at the level of gene transcription are not yet completely understood. Thanks to new molecular biologic techniques, this insight is rapidly increasing, and after many years with meager results of chemoprevention studies, we may have entered a more positive era in this area of research.

CONCLUSION

The expanding understanding of the pathologic and genetic basis of lung carcinogenesis provides a foundation for chemopreventive research. The emergence of lung cancer screening with more frequent detection of early-stage lung cancer also will provide impetus for defining effective chemopreventive agents. Increased numbers of potentially cured early-stage lung cancers will result in many patients being followed with concerns of field of cancerization resulting in the development of second primary lung cancers. Despite concerted efforts, no successful chemopreventive strategy has been validated to date. New trial designs such as those with small trial cohorts including only a very "high-risk population" defined with biomarkers may allow for more rapid and economically chemopreventive drug development. Candidate intermediate biomarkers have been identified and have been used in trials with preliminary positive results. In addition, neoadjuvant, window-of-opportunity trials may also provide a valuable tool for better defining the mode of chemoprevention drug action, and the tissue specimens obtained before and after drug exposure in these window trials may help identify candidate companion diagnostic or therapeutic biomarkers to assess the response of the drug for use in subsequent drug development trials. Considering the ever-increasing burden of lung cancer worldwide, it is imperative to continue our efforts to identify effective chemopreventive agents to arrest early lung carcinogenesis. With increasing insight into the molecular basis coupled with a better screening strategy, the road is paved for more successful studies in the at-risk population.

KEY REFERENCES

2. Vineis P, Alavanja M, Buffler P, et al. Tobacco and cancer: recent epidemiological evidence. *J Natl Cancer Inst.* 2004;96(2):99–106.
5. Maresso KC, Tsai KY, Brown PH, Szabo E, Lippman S, Hawk ET. Molecular cancer prevention: current status and future directions. *CA Cancer J Clin.* 2015;65(5):345–383.
8. Vogelstein B, Kinzler KW. The path to cancer—three strikes and you're out. *N Engl J Med.* 2015;373:1895–1898.
9. Mulshine JL, DeLuca LM, Dedrick RL, Tockman MS, Webster R, Placke M. Considerations in developing successful population-based molecular screening and prevention of lung cancer. *Cancer Suppl.* 2000;11:2465–2467.
17. Tong L, Spitz MR, Fueger JJ, Amos CA. Lung carcinoma in former smokers. *Cancer.* 1996;78(5):1004–1010.
23. Slaughter DP, Southwick HW, Smejkal W. Field cancerization in oral stratified squamous epithelium: clinical implications of multicentric origin. *Cancer.* 1953;6(5):963–968.
24. Auerbach O, Hammond EC, Garfinkel L. Changes in bronchial epithelium in relation to cigarette smoking, 1955–1960 vs. 1970–1977. *N Engl J Med.* 1979;300(8):381–385.
32. Wistuba II, Lam S, Behrens C, et al. Molecular damage in the bronchial epithelium of current and former smokers. *J Natl Cancer Inst.* 1997;89(18):1366–1373.

71. Cassidy A, Duffy SW, Myles JP, Liloglou T, Field JK. Lung cancer risk prediction: a tool for early detection. *Int J Cancer.* 2007;120(1):1–6.

91. Sporn MB, Dunlop NM, Newton DL, Smith JM. Prevention of chemical carcinogenesis by vitamin A and its synthetic analogs (retinoids). *Fed Proc.* 1976;35(6):1332–1338.

92. Aberle D, Adams A, Berg C, et al. Reduced lung-cancer mortality with low-dose computed tomographic screening. *N Engl J Med.* 2011;365(5):395–409.

97. Humphrey L, Deffebach M, Pappas M, et al. *Screening for Lung Cancer: Systematic Review to Update the US Preventive Services Task Force Recommendation.* Rockville, MD: Agency for Healthcare Research and Quality; 2013.

100. van Klaveren RJ, Oudkerk M, Prokop M, et al. Management of lung nodules detected by volume CT scanning. *N Engl J Med.* 2009;361(23):2221–2229.

104. Henschke CI, Boffetta P, Gorlova O, Yip R, Delancey JO, Foy M. Assessment of lung-cancer mortality reduction from CT screening. *Lung Cancer.* 2011;71(3):328–332.

106. Flores RM, Park BJ, Dycoco J, et al. Lobectomy by video-assisted thoracic surgery (VATS) versus thoracotomy for lung cancer. *J Thorac Cardiovasc Surg.* 2009;138(1):11–18.

107. Paul S, Altorki NK, Sheng S, et al. Thoracoscopic lobectomy is associated with lower morbidity than open lobectomy: a propensity-matched analysis from the STS database. *J Thorac Cardiovasc Surg.* 2010;139(2):366–378.

109. National Framework for Excellence in Lung Cancer Screening and Continuum of Care. *Lung Cancer Alliance* 2016. http://www.lung-canceralliance.org/get-information/am-i-at-risk/national-framework-for-lung-screening-excellence.html; 2016.

113. Jaklitsch MT, Jacobson FL, Austin JH, et al. The American Association for Thoracic Surgery guidelines for lung cancer screening using low-dose computed tomography scans for lung cancer survivors and other high-risk groups. *J Thorac Cardiovasc Surg.* 2012;144(1):33–38.

114. Yankelevitz DF, Reeves AP, Kostis WJ, Zhao B, Henschke CI. Small pulmonary nodules: volumetrically determined growth rates based on CT evaluation. *Radiology.* 2000;217(1):251–256.

117. Field JK, Smith RA, Aberle DR, et al. International Association for the Study of Lung Cancer Computed Tomography Screening Workshop 2011 report. *J Thorac Oncol.* 2012;7(1):10–19.

118. Mulshine JL, Sullivan DC. Clinical practice. Lung cancer screening. *N Engl J Med.* 2005;352(26):2714–2720.

120. Pyenson BS, Sander MS, Jiang Y, Kahn H, Mulshine JL. An actuarial analysis shows that offering lung cancer screening as an insurance benefit would save lives at relatively low cost. *Health Aff (Millwood).* 2012;31(4):770–779.

127. Peto R, Doll R, Buckley JD, Sporn MB. Can dietary beta-carotene materially reduce human cancer rates? *Nature.* 1981;290(5803):201–208.

136. Parimon T, Chien JW, Bryson CL, McDonnell MB, Udris EM, Au DH. Inhaled corticosteroids and risk of lung cancer among patients with chronic obstructive pulmonary disease. *Am J Respir Crit Care Med.* 2007;175(7):712–719.

138. Kohlhäufl M, Häussinger K, Stanzel F, et al. Inhalation of aerosolized vitamin A: reversibility of metaplasia and dysplasia of human respiratory epithelia—a prospective pilot study. *Eur J Med Res.* 2002;7(2):72–78.

155. Keith RL, Blatchford PJ, Kittelson J, et al. Oral iloprost improves endobronchial dysplasia in former smokers. *Cancer Prev Res (Phila).* 2011;4(6):793–802.

See Expertconsult.com for full list of references.

10 Copy Number Abnormalities and Gene Fusions in Lung Cancer: Present and Developing Technologies

Marileila Varella-Garcia and Byoung Chul Cho

SUMMARY OF KEY POINTS

- Lung cancers commonly have structural chromosome aberrations and aneuploidy, with many of them associated with carcinogenesis.
- Gene amplification is a common mechanism of oncogenic activation in nonsmall cell lung cancer (NSCLC) involving genes such as *MYC, EGFR, ERBB2, MET, PIK3CA,* and *FGFR1.* Gene amplification is also associated with resistance to drugs, for instance, to epidermal growth factor receptor (EGFR) tyrosine kinase inhibitors when the T790M *EGFR* allele or the *MET* gene is amplified.
- More recently, genes such as *ALK, ROS1, RET,* and *NTRK1* were found to be activated in NSCLC by fusions with gene partners subjected to constitutive transcription or carrying specific domains inducing phosphorylation.
- Novel therapeutics have been developed to target those specific molecular drivers, and several drugs have succeeded in substantially improving survival and quality of life of patients carrying such molecular changes.
- NSCLC tumor profiling is achieved by numerous technologies focusing on different levels such as DNA (e.g., sequencing, fluorescence in situ hybridization [FISH]), RNA (e.g., reverse transcription-polymerase chain reaction [RT-PCR]), and protein (e.g., immunohistochemistry [IHC]). Technologies using in situ (FISH, IHC) and extraction (PCR based, sequencing) platforms have distinct advantages and limitations.
- Single tests and test panels are available, with the latter being most effective due to the low incidence of the rearrangements in the overall NSCLC population, the lower cost per gene tested, and the scarcity of tumor tissue in patients with advanced stage disease. Molecular drivers have been detected more commonly in lung adenocarcinomas than in squamous cell carcinomas (SCCs) but a strong effort is ongoing to better define potential therapeutic targets in SCC. Very little is known regarding markers for therapy in small cell lung cancer.

Lung cancer is a group of diseases displaying a high level of genomic instability and complex molecular changes. This chapter reviews the impact of molecular events detectable by cytogenetic techniques, such as instability, at the DNA and chromosome levels in lung cancer patients. In addition, the chapter also examines two of the major molecular mechanisms leading to the nonviral activation of oncogenes: gene amplification and gene fusion. Overexpression of proteins in conditions in which they are normally absent is commonly driven by an increase in gene copy number or the release of a specific gene from the ligand binding control, thus having its active domain under the control of the promoter or of the active domain of a constitutively activated gene. Amplification of genes in lung cancer was discovered in the mid-1980s for v-myc avian myelocytomatosis viral oncogene homolog (*MYC*) and Kirsten rat sarcoma viral oncogene homolog (*KRAS*).[1,2] Conversely, fusion proteins are a much newer phenomenon in lung cancer. Despite being common and well-known in leukemia and lymphoma as causal factors and targets for therapy, gene fusions were not described in lung cancer research before the start of the 21st century. However, with the progress of genomic technology, the number of activated gene fusions discovered mainly in NSCLC has increased rapidly, as will be detailed here.

GENETIC INSTABILITY IN LUNG CANCER

Accumulation of multiple genetic abnormalities is known to be associated with lung cancer initiation and progression. Genetic instability, which may cause these abnormalities, is a general term that refers to both chromosomal instability (CIN) and microsatellite instability (MSI).[3] Instability involving whole or partial regions of chromosomes (CIN) includes deletion, duplication, insertion, and translocation. CIN may induce loss of heterozygosity (LOH) of tumor suppressor genes or DNA repair genes when deletions occur, and amplification of oncogenes by multiple duplications of focal chromosome regions. Consequently, compelling evidence has supported the role of CIN in the pathogenesis of lung cancer.[4-7] In addition to alterations at the chromosomal level, instability at the nucleotide level, frequently referred to as MSI, is usually connected to mismatch repair (MMR) defects.[8,9] MSI may cause missense mutations that facilitate the inactivation of tumor suppressor genes, such as *p53*, which may contribute to the development and progression of lung cancer.[10,11] Both phenomena—CIN and MSI—obviously contribute to the phenotype instability and versatility of cancer cells. Therefore an understanding of the molecular mechanisms leading to genetic instability holds promise for the development of novel therapeutic strategies in lung cancer.

Microsatellite Instability

Microsatellites, also known as simple sequence repeats, are tandem repeats of short (fewer than 10 bp) DNA sequences, which are useful markers for genetic mapping and LOH of defined chromosomal loci. The most common microsatellite in humans is a dinucleotide repeat of CA, which occurs tens of thousands of times across the genome. Although the length of these microsatellites is highly variable from person to person, each individual has microsatellites of a set length. MSI, a hallmark of genetic instability, generally occurs because of abnormalities of the MMR genes, such as *hMSH2* and *hMLH1*, impairing the correction of errors that spontaneously occur during DNA replication.[12] The loss of MMR function renders tumor cells susceptible to the acquisition of somatic mutations throughout the genome, and microsatellites are particularly susceptible to mutations in the absence of MMR. MSI was initially identified in colorectal cancer and was immediately clinically significant because of its association with hereditary nonpolyposis colon cancer (HNPCC).[13] In HNPCC, the MSI of MMR genes due to germline alterations is an essential molecular basis of its development. By contrast, in lung cancer, CIN plays a more important role in carcinogenesis, as homozygous and heterozygous deletions of certain chromosomal loci or amplification of oncogenes frequently occur, as will be described.[6,14,15]

There are conflicting data on the relevance of MSI in lung cancer. The frequency of MSI has been reported to range from 0% to 69% in NSCLC and from 0% to 76% in small cell lung cancer (SCLC).[8,10,14,16–19] Interestingly, several studies of NSCLC have demonstrated a higher frequency of MSI in tetranucleotide-repeating regions than in traditional mononucleotide-repeating or dinucleotide-repeating regions, and the term "elevated microsatellite alterations at selected tetranucleotide" (EMAST) has been proposed to designate the phenomenon.[8,10,16,20] Furthermore, EMAST was reported to be associated with SCC with lymph node metastasis.[16] The molecular mechanisms leading to EMAST, distinct from traditional MSI, were not associated with defects in MMR, but it was suggested that p53 alterations may be involved.[10,16,20]

Aneuploidy and CIN

Most cancer cells possess an abnormal number of chromosomes, often in the triploid or tetraploid range.[3] In addition to the altered number of chromosomes, cancer cells commonly have structural chromosome aberrations, such as inversions, deletions, duplications, and translocations. Aneuploidy, defined as numerical and structural abnormalities of chromosomes, commonly results from CIN.[21] Aneuploidy and CIN can mediate the evolution of cancer cell populations under selection pressure and are associated with poor prognosis and distinctive histopathologic features in many tumors. CIN plays an important role in lung carcinogenesis by accelerating homozygous and heterozygous deletions of tumor suppressor genes and effectively amplifying oncogenes.[6,14,22] Therefore a better understanding of the causes and effects of aneuploidy and CIN may lead to new therapeutic venues for solid malignancies, including lung cancer.[23]

Early studies have shown that lung cancer frequently exhibits marked LOH as a result of CIN when genome-wide or specific regions such as chromosomes 12p, 14q, and 17q were investigated.[4,5,24] Moreover, LOH at 3p loci containing genes associated with antioxidant defenses (e.g., glutathione peroxidase I) is not only associated with the development of lung cancer but also with higher responsiveness to DNA damaging agents (e.g., radiation).[25]

Multiple mechanisms during cell cycle progression have been implicated in the advent of CIN and aneuploidy in lung cancer. These include failure at the mitotic checkpoint, mutations and amplifications in the kinetochore (protein structure on chromatids where the spindle fibers attach during cell division) and centrosome components, and mutations in DNA repair genes.[23] The mitotic checkpoint, also called the spindle assembly checkpoint, is activated when the kinetochore is not attached to the spindle, lacks microtubules, or has poor or inadequate tension, thereby deregulating metaphase–anaphase progression.[26] Loss-of-function mutations, or reduced gene expression of the mitotic checkpoint genes (mitotic arrest deficient-like 1 [MAD1/MAD2] and mitotic checkpoint serine/threonine kinase [BUB1, BUBR1]), lead to chromosomal missegregation and contribute to aneuploidy.[27,28] Given that loss of mutations in mitotic checkpoint genes were rarely detected in lung cancers (less than 3%) in the recent comprehensive genome-wide sequencing data collection, development of lung cancer and CIN is more closely related to their

dysfunction due to phosphorylation or cytoplasmic location.[29–32] Interestingly, a study in MAD2[+/−]p53[+/−] and MAD1[+/−]MAD2[+/−]p53[+/−] mice suggested a cooperative role of MAD1/MAD2 and p53 genes in generating increased aneuploidy and tumorigenesis.[33] Furthermore, the mitotic checkpoint has also been linked to DNA-damage response, and a defective mitotic checkpoint confers cancer cells' resistance to certain DNA-damaging anticancer drugs.[23,34] The centrosomes are thought to maintain genomic stability through the establishment of bipolar spindles during cell division, ensuring equal segregation of replicated chromosomes to two daughter cells.[35] STK15, encoding aurora kinase A (AURKA), is amplified and overexpressed in diverse types of human tumors, leading to centrosome amplification, CIN, and tumorigenesis.[36] Aurora kinases are serine/threonine kinases that function as key regulators of the mitosis process. Their dysfunction interferes with cell cycle checkpoints and allows genetically aberrant cells to enter mitosis and undergo cell division. Overexpression of aurora kinases can lead to aneuploidy, resulting in the failure to maintain chromosomal integrity.[37]

In one study, AURKA was highly overexpressed in 50% of NSCLC, and its overexpression was significantly upregulated in tumor samples compared with matched lung tissue ($p < 0.01$), suggesting a role as a tumor marker.[38] Moreover, AURKA was principally upregulated in moderately and poorly differentiated lung cancers, as well as in SCCs and adenocarcinomas, compared with the noninvasive bronchioloalveolar subtype.[38] The frequency of AURKA amplification in NSCLC ranges from 1% to 6% and seems to be more common in lung adenocarcinomas than in lung SCCs.[29,30] In comparison, aurora kinase B (AURKB) plays a less clear role in tumorigenesis.[37] However, many studies now support an association between AURKB and malignant transformation, with the involvement of additional factors. Although AURKB overexpression alone did not transform rodent fibroblast cells, increased kinase activity did facilitate Harvey rat sarcoma viral oncogene homolog (HRAS)-induced transformation, which led to the production of aneuploid cells.[39] In an IHC analysis of 160 NSCLC samples, 78% of tumors were found to overexpress AURKB, and its overexpression was also associated with adverse tumor features and poor prognosis in lung adenocarcinomas.[40] Contrary to AURKA, the overexpression of which is associated with gene amplification,[41] AURKB overexpression was associated with aberrant transcriptional regulation in primary lung carcinoma.[42]

Therefore overexpression and amplification of aurora kinases have been associated with neoplastic transformation, serving as attractive targets for cancer therapy.[43] A growing number of inhibitors of aurora kinases have been developed and, at the time of publication, were being evaluated in clinical trials to assess the therapeutic potential of aurora-based targeted therapy. These inhibitors include AMG900 (Amgen, Thousand Oaks, CA, USA), AT9283 (Astex Therapeutics, Dublin, CA, USA), AZD1152 (Astra Zeneca, London, UK), and PF03814735 and BI811283 (Boehringer-Ingelheim, Ridgefield, CT, USA).[44] Some of these drugs have selective activity against one aurora kinase subtype, whereas others exhibit pan-inhibitory effects.

In addition to mitotic checkpoint proteins and centrosome components, CIN may be caused by defects in the DNA double-strand break repair genes—ataxia telangiectasia mutated (ATM), BRCA1, BRCA2, x-ray repair complementing defective repair in Chinese hamster cells (double-strand-break rejoining; XRCC5)—or DNA-damage response.[5,45–47] Interestingly, the chromosomal regions at 2q33–35 and 13q12.3, which included loci encoding the XRCC5 and BRCA2 genes, showed a high frequency of LOH in NSCLC.[5] More recently, it was reported that low messenger RNA and protein expressions in BRCA1/BRCA2 and XRCC5 genes occur in lung adenocarcinoma and SCC and that promoter hypermethylation is the predominant mechanism in deregulation of these genes.[45] Given that BRCA1/BRCA2 proteins are central to p53-dependent elimination of tetraploid or aneuploid (often preceded by tetraploid state) cells, it is not surprising that these proteins are frequently inactivated or downregulated in NSCLC, synergizing with p53 inactivation to establish an atmosphere of tolerance for a nondiploid state.[48] Although unrepaired or incorrectly repaired DNA lesions may give rise to cancer-initiating mutations, one way to efficiently tackle cancer is to take advantage of such biologic differences between cancer and normal cells and exploit the defects of tumor-associated DNA-damage response in smart therapeutic strategies.[46]

AMPLIFICATION AS A MECHANISM OF ONCOGENESIS

Gene amplification refers to the expansion of gene copy number in a restricted region of a chromosome arm. It is prevalent in some tumors and is often associated with overexpression of the amplified gene, causing cancer cells to grow or become resistant to anticancer drugs.[49] Often, although not necessarily, gene amplification is seen as karyotypic abnormalities including the extrachromosomal, acentric structure known as double minutes and the homogeneously staining regions (Fig. 10.1).[50] High-throughput genomic analyses of thousands of cancer specimens showed that the majority (approximately 75%) of the gene amplifications were focal in nature (50 kb to 300 kb) and targeted primarily oncogenes, encoding signaling proteins crucial for cellular proliferation and survival.[51] This finding strongly supports the notion that gene amplification promotes tumor formation, tumor maintenance, and drug resistance. The preponderance of focal amplification targeting oncogenes contrasts sharply with large genomic deletions, which are mostly passenger mutations with only a few exceptions, such as cyclin-dependent kinase inhibitor 2A/B (*CDKN2A/B*), retinoblastoma 1 (*RB1*), and FAT atypical cadherin 1 (*FAT1*) tumor suppressor genes.[51] The contributing factors to CIN, including common chromosomal fragile sites, errors in DNA replication, and telomere dysfunction, are causally linked to amplification and large genomic deletions.[49]

Gene amplification is a common mechanism of oncogenic activation in NSCLC and, on a whole genome scale, has a strong effect on the level of protein expression.[15] Given the potential role of gene amplification in lung tumorigenesis and tumor progression, this event is commonly associated with unique clinicopathologic features and aggressive tumor behavior. Not surprisingly, amplifications of the EGFR, v-erb-b2 avian erythroblastic leukemia viral oncogene homolog 2 (*ERBB2*), met proto-oncogene (*MET*), *MYC*, and fibroblast growth factor receptor 1 (*FGFR1*) genes have been reported to be significantly associated with poor prognosis in NSCLC (as will be discussed). In addition, amplification has been identified as a mechanism of resistance to therapy.[49,52]

Because the tumor can become dependent on overexpression of the oncogenes for its survival and proliferation, amplifications of oncogenes usually define unique subsets of lung cancer and support their use as therapeutic targets. As best illustrated by the example of the success of trastuzumab in ERBB2-amplified breast cancer, amplification of specific oncogenes may provide diagnostic utility based on their impact on therapeutic response and patient outcome. In lung cancer, however, although the results of several studies have clearly demonstrated the clinical usefulness of testing for EGFR mutations and anaplastic lymphoma kinase (ALK) fusions to guide treatment and improve patient outcomes, selection of therapy based on gene amplification is yet to be approved.[53]

This chapter focuses on the most relevant examples of gene amplifications that have shown diagnostic usefulness because of prognostic and predictive values.

EGFR Amplification

Determination of EGFR gene copy number by fluorescence in situ hybridization (FISH) has prognostic and diagnostic usefulness in NSCLC (Fig. 10.1A). Based on a retrospective study of patients with advanced NSCLC who were treated with gefitinib, tumors are considered to have a high *EGFR* gene copy number (EGFR FISH+) if they show a high copy number or amplification of the *EGFR* gene.[54] Overall, tumors with a high *EGFR* gene copy number represent approximately 30% of NSCLC. Unlike *EGFR* mutations, which are more frequently found in Asian, female, and never-smoking patients, and in patients with adenocarcinoma histology, the distribution of *EGFR* copy numbers is mostly independent of these clinicopathologic characteristics.[55,56] Lung cancers with a high *EGFR* gene copy number seem to be associated with a worse prognosis than cancers with a low *EGFR* gene copy number, in both early and advanced stages. EGFR amplification usually coexists with mutations in lung adenocarcinoma, suggesting that the mutation occurs first, then induces gene amplification during tumor progression and metastasis. This hypothesis was clearly illustrated in a biomarker analysis of Iressa Pan-Asia Study (IPASS) that showed a concordance between EGFR mutation and high gene copy number in almost 90% of patients.[57] Interestingly, in an analysis from the Iressa Survival Evaluation in Lung Cancer phase III study in which patients were predominantly of non-Asian origin, the concordance rate between these two biomarkers seemed much lower, suggesting that the mechanism of the genomic gain of EGFR may have ethnic differences.[58]

Although *EGFR* gene copy number has been evaluated as a predictive biomarker for sensitivity to *EGFR* tyrosine kinase inhibitors (TKIs) in several studies, its predictive role remains controversial. Early studies showed that patients with EGFR FISH+ tumors were most likely to benefit from treatment with EGFR TKIs. However, in IPASS, patients with tumors with a high *EGFR* gene copy number had significantly longer progression-free survival with the *EGFR* inhibitor gefitinib only in the presence of an *EGFR* mutation, whereas patients with an *EGFR* mutation had longer progression-free survival with gefitinib irrespective of the *EGFR* gene copy number.[57,59] These findings suggest that the predictive value of the *EGFR* amplification was driven by coexisting *EGFR* mutations. The robust predictive value of *EGFR* mutations has been confirmed in subsequent phase III studies comparing first-line *EGFR* TKIs with chemotherapy in advanced NSCLC with activating *EGFR* mutations.[60–63]

Nevertheless, similar to the case of *EGFR* mutations, amplification of the *EGFR* gene can fully activate EGFR tyrosine kinase and trigger downstream oncogenic pathways. Therefore it seems reasonable to assume a correlation between an abnormality in the *EGFR* copy number and *EGFR* TKI sensitivity. In support of this hypothesis, it was reported that a high *EGFR* gene copy number may be used as a predictive marker in patients with advanced squamous cell lung carcinoma, in which activating *EGFR* mutations are very rare.[64] In addition to its effect on the prognosis and response to *EGFR* TKIs, focal amplification of *EGFR* that preferentially involves the T790M-containing allele confers resistance to the irreversible *EGFR* TKIs (e.g., dacomitinib).[65]

ERBB2 Amplification

ERBB2 is also a member of the family of EGFR tyrosine kinases, but it is not activated by a known cognate ligand and instead serves as a preferred dimerization partner to other family members. Amplification of the *ERBB2* gene, mapped at 17q11.2–q12, was reported to occur in approximately 2% of unselected NSCLCs, with a rise in frequency to 11% in poorly differentiated adenocarcinomas.[29,30,66,67] It was also reported that approximately 40% of ERBB2-amplified tumors had concurrent amplification and/or mutation of EGFR.[68] Therefore it is not surprising that ERBB2 amplification (Fig. 10.1B) was more frequently associated with female gender and never-smoking status, characteristics that are associated with the presence of EGFR mutation and amplification. ERBB2 amplification correlates well with protein overexpression and is associated with higher tumor grade, higher disease stage, and shorter survival, all of which provide evidence

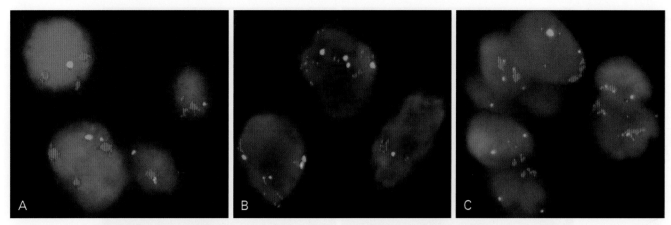

Fig. 10.1. Gene amplifications in lung adenocarcinomas. (A) EGFR *(red signal)* and centromere 7 *(green signal)*. (B) ERBB2 (HER2) and centromere 17. (C) MET *(red signal)* and centromere 7 *(green signal)*. Amplification of EGFR and MET occurred in large and tight clusters of gene signals while amplification of ERBB2 occurred in smaller and looser clusters. *EGFR,* epidermal growth factor receptor; *ERBB2,* Erb-B2 receptor tyrosine kinase 2.

supporting this receptor as a useful molecular target in the treatment of NSCLC.[69,70] Unfortunately, the addition of trastuzumab to gemcitabine and cisplatin did not appear to provide any benefit for patients with advanced NSCLC with ERBB2 overexpression or amplification.[71] However, because very few patients had ERBB2 3+/ amplification in this trial, further evaluation of trastuzumab in this specific subset of patients with lung cancer is desirable. Given the high intratumoral heterogeneity of ERBB2 amplification and discrepancies between primary tumors and their metastases, careful testing should be considered in the assessment of patients with NSCLC as candidates for ERBB2-targeted therapy.[66]

Of note, a high *ERBB2* gene copy number (ERBB2/FISH+) had a positive additive effect on the efficacy of *EGFR* TKI in the presence of EGFR mutation and/or amplifications, suggesting that testing of the ERBB2 gene copy number may have a complementary role for selection of patients who gain the greatest benefit from *EGFR* TKIs.[68] By contrast, ERBB2 amplification is an example of an acquired resistance mechanism to the EGFR inhibitor cetuximab. In the HCC827 NSCLC cell, aberrant ERBB2 activation leads to persistent extracellular signal-regulated kinase 1/2 signaling in the presence of cetuximab, thus preventing cetuximab-mediated growth inhibition.[72]

MET Amplification

MET, a proto-oncogene located on 7q31, encodes a transmembrane tyrosine kinase receptor for hepatocyte growth factor (HGF).[73] Binding of HGF to MET induces receptor dimerization and transphosphorylation, triggering conformational changes that activate MET tyrosine kinase activity. Preclinical findings also suggest that lung cancer cell lines harboring MET gene amplification are dependent on MET for growth and survival.[74] HGF stimulation of MET gene amplification leads to the activation of a number of signaling pathways, including phosphatidylinositol 3-kinase/v-akt murine thymoma (PI3K)/AKT, RAS/mitogen-activated protein kinase (MAPK), and phospholipase C-γ pathways.[73]

The frequency of MET amplification is rare and has been reported to be 1.4% to 7.3% among patients with NSCLC not previously treated with *EGFR* TKIs.[29,30,75–81] MET gene amplification, or MET FISH+ (Fig. 10.1C), has not been associated with gender, histology, or smoking status, but has been significantly associated with higher tumor grade and advanced stage.[77,78,82] Interestingly, albeit mutually exclusive with mutations in *EGFR, ERBB2,* and *KRAS* genes, MET FISH+ status was significantly associated with EGFR FISH+ status, likely because both genes are located in chromosome 7.[77,81,82] This finding may support the early preclinical demonstration of interaction between EGFR and MET signaling pathways.[83] For patients who had surgical resection, survival was shorter for those with MET FISH+ tumors (5 or more copies per cell) than for those with MET FISH− tumors.[77]

The rarity of MET amplification in NSCLC, particularly at the high levels found in *EGFR* TKI–resistant cell line models (MET gene copy number greater than 12), suggested that this event plays a limited role in primary resistance to *EGFR* TKIs.[78] Instead, HGF-stimulated MET signaling activation is more likely to be responsible for primary resistance to *EGFR* TKIs. Autocrine or paracrine secretion of HGF results in MET activation, reactivation of the MAPK, and PI3K/AKT signaling pathways and immediate resistance to EGFR inhibition.[84,85] Indeed, HGF and MET have been reported to participate in paracrine tumorigenic pathways in several other malignancies.[86]

By contrast, MET amplification is present in approximately 20% of tumors with acquired resistance to *EGFR* TKIs.[87] Engelman et al.[52] reported that NSCLC overcomes inhibition of *EGFR* TKIs by amplifying the MET oncogene to activate ERBB3, a member of the EGFR family, and the PI3K/AKT cell survival pathway. In another study, Bean et al.[79] showed MET amplification in 21% of patients with acquired resistance to gefitinib or erlotinib and in only 3% of untreated patients, confirming that MET could be a relevant therapeutic target for some individuals with acquired resistance to *EGFR* TKIs.[79]

PIK3CA Amplification

PI3K signaling is a major oncogenic pathway that functions in cancer cell growth, survival, motility, and metabolism.[88] Amplification of the phosphatidylinositol-4,5-bisphosphate 3-kinase, catalytic subunit alpha (*PIK3CA* gene), mapped at 3q26.3 and encoding the p110 catalytic subunit, was more frequently found in men, smokers, and patients with SCC.[89,90] Overall, the incidence of *PIK3CA* gene amplification has been reported to be 33.1% to 70% in squamous cell lung carcinoma and 1.6% to 19% in lung adenocarcinoma, suggesting that this genetic alteration mainly targets squamous cell lung carcinoma.[29,30,88,90–92] Furthermore, a high level of PIK3CA copy gain was present exclusively in SCCs.[92] Amplification of PIK3CA (Fig. 10.2A) occurs at higher frequencies than genomic mutations in lung cancer and they occur independently of each other, implying that either molecular event has equivalent oncogenic potential.[90–92]

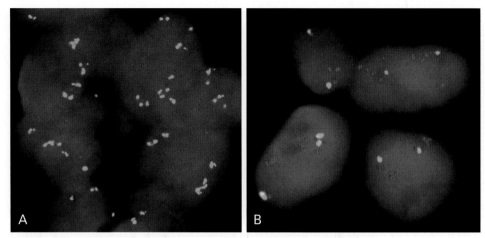

Fig. 10.2. Gene amplifications in squamous cell adenocarcinomas. (A) *PIK3CA (green signal)* and centromere 3 *(red signal)*. (B) *FGFR1 (red signal)* and centromere 8 *(green signal)*. Amplification of these genes occurred as numerous small clusters of gene signals diffusely spread. *FGFR1*, fibroblast growth factor receptor 1; *PIK3CA*, phosphatidylinositol-4,5-bisphosphate 3-kinase catalytic subunit alpha.

The functional importance of PIK3CA gene amplification is shown by increased PI3K activity and phosphorylated AKT.[92] Knockdown of PIK3CA inhibits anchorage-dependent and anchorage-independent growth in PIK3CA-amplified NSCLC cells, but has no effect in cells harboring wild-type PIK3CA.[92] Interestingly, coexistence of PIK3CA gene amplification and *EGFR* or *KRAS* mutation in a single tumor was less frequent in SCC than in adenocarcinoma. This finding suggests that PIK3CA copy gain may play a pivotal role in pathogenesis of lung SCCs, further providing a rationale for targeting the PI3K pathway in this disease. The significance of the PI3K pathway as a therapeutic target in squamous cell lung carcinomas has been highlighted in the most recent study by the Cancer Genome Atlas Research Network.[29] In that study, alterations in the PI3K/AKT pathway were found in 47% of tumors and, more important, approximately 38.2% of tumors (68 of 178) had PIK3CA amplifications. This finding is of particular interest because targeted agents have been successful for the treatment of only lung adenocarcinoma. The functional dependence of squamous cell lung carcinoma on the PI3K pathway should be validated by the successful treatment with targeted PI3K inhibitors, and such trials are underway.[80]

FGFR1 Amplification

The FGFR tyrosine kinase family comprises four kinases (FGFR 1–4) and plays a crucial role in cancer cell growth, survival, and resistance to chemotherapy.[80] Amplification of the FGFR1 locus at chromosome 8p12 has been described in several tumor types, particularly SCC of the lung (Fig. 10.2B) and SCLC.[93–100]

FGFR1 gene amplification is more commonly found in squamous cell lung carcinoma than lung adenocarcinoma, with a relatively high incidence of up to 24.8%, and has recently been reported to be a novel druggable target in this specific histologic subset.[94–100] Interestingly, Kim et al.[96] reported that the incidence of FGFR1 amplification was also associated with smoking status in a dose-dependent manner (current smoker, 28.9% vs. former smoker, 2.5% vs. nonsmoker, 0%; $p < 0.0001$), suggesting that FGFR1 gene amplification is an oncogenic aberration caused by cigarette smoking. FGFR1 gene amplification drives downstream activation of PI3K/AKT and RAS/MAPK signaling, and a selective FGFR inhibitor caused downstream inhibition and induction of apoptosis in FGFR1-amplified squamous cell lung carcinomas, strongly supporting the utility of FGFR1 gene amplification as a relevant therapeutic target in this disease.[100]

FGFR1 gene amplification also has been reported to hold a significant prognostic value. Kim et al.[96] found that FGFR1 amplification is a negative prognostic factor for patients with resected SCC of the lung, whereas Heist et al.[97] reported there was no significant difference in overall survival by FGFR1 amplification status. The conflicting results may be related to differences in method and cutoff values used to assess and define FGFR1 amplification.[99]

In one study, FGFR1 amplification was noted in 5.6% of SCLC, mostly at high levels and as homogeneous staining regions.[101] Furthermore, inhibition of FGFR has resulted in a blockade of tumor growth, suggesting an important role of the FGF–FGFR signaling pathway for SCLC growth, which indicates that FGFR1 amplification may also be a therapeutic target in SCLC.[102]

Standardized screening criteria have been proposed to reliably identify patients who have lung cancers with FGFR1 amplifications for clinical trials with FGFR inhibitors. According to these criteria, high-level FGFR1 amplification is defined as an FGFR1/centromere 8 ratio of 2.0 or higher, an average number of FGFR1 signals per tumor cell nucleus of six or more, or 10% or more tumor cells containing at least 15 FGFR1 signals or large clusters; low-level amplification is defined as five or more FGFR1 signals in at least 50% of tumor cells.[99] The utility of the proposed criteria should be validated by the clinical response data from clinical trials with FGFR inhibitors.

The identification of FGFR1 amplification holds promise for the development of novel molecularly targeted therapeutic agents in the treatment of squamous cell lung carcinoma and SCLC, and recently developed FGF/FGFR-targeting anticancer agents are being studied in clinical trials.[80]

STRUCTURAL CHANGES LEADING TO ONCOGENESIS BY GENE FUSIONS

ALK Fusion

In 2007, Soda et al.[103] discovered that oncogenic fusion genes consisting of echinoderm microtubule-associated protein like 4 (*EML4*) and *ALK* are present in a small subset of NSCLCs. The endogenous *ALK* gene is normally not expressed in most adult tissues, including the lung epithelium, but *EML4–ALK* fusion leads to both ectopic expression and constitutive activation of ALK and its downstream signaling pathways, resulting in uncontrolled cellular proliferation and survival (Fig. 10.3).[104] The prevalence of ALK

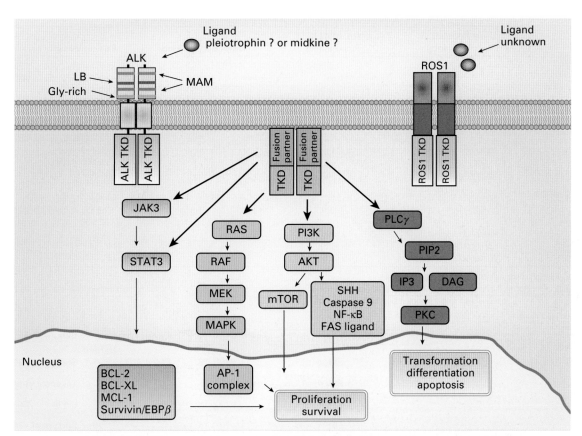

Fig. 10.3. *ALK* and *ROS1* signaling pathway. *ALK,* anaplastic lymphoma kinase; *DAG,* diacylglycerol; *IP3,* inositol triphosphate; *JAK3,* Janus kinase 3; *LB,* ligand banding; *MAM,* meprin/A5-protein/PTPmu; *MAPK,* mitogen-activated protein kinase; *mTOR,* mechanistic target of rapamycin; *NF-κB,* nuclear factor-κB; *PIP2,* phosphatidylinositol 4,5-bisphosphates; *PKC,* protein kinase C; *ROS1,* c-ros oncogene 1, receptor tyrosine kinase; *STAT3,* signal transducer and activator of transcription 3; *TKD,* tyrosine kinase domain.

fusions has been reported to be approximately 4% (range, 1.5% to 7.5%) in unselected NSCLC populations, representing potentially 40,000 new cases worldwide each year.[104,105] The frequency of ALK-positive tumors in NSCLC and methods to detect ALK have been evaluated in population studies (Table 10.1).[103,106–113] ALK-positive lung cancers are highly sensitive to ALK inhibitors, and an understanding of the resistance mechanisms to ALK inhibitors is crucial for the optimal therapy of ALK-positive NSCLC.[114]

ALK fusions result from various types of chromosomal rearrangements, all of which lead to aberrant activation of ALK.[115] *EML4–ALK* fusion, the most frequent ALK fusion in NSCLC, is the result of paracentric inversions (intrachromosomal rearrangement) involving the short arm of chromosome 2. Multiple studies have shown other, rare, fusion partners of *ALK,* such as kinesin family member 5B (*KIF5B;* 10p11.22), TRK-fused gene (*TFG;* 3q12.2), kinesin light chain 1 (*KLC1;* 14q32.3), and striatin, calmodulin binding protein (*STRN;* 2p22.2).[115–120] *ALK* fusion with *KIF5B, TFG,* or *KLC1* is the result of interchromosomal rearrangement, whereas *ALK* fusion with *STRN* is the result of intrachromosomal deletion.[120] Despite the diversity of fusion partners, most of them contain coiled-coil or leucine zipper domains that drive the dimerization or oligomerization of fusion kinase, which leads to ligand-independent activation of the tyrosine kinase.[115] To date, more than 20 *EML4–ALK* variants have been identified in NSCLC (Fig. 10.4).[103,106,109,116,117,119–127] Despite variable breakpoints of *EML4* (exons 2, 6, 13, 14, 15, 17, 18, 20, and 21), the genomic breakpoint within the *ALK* gene is conserved at exon 20 with few exceptions at exon 19.[127,128] Therefore all *EML4–ALK* fusion proteins involve the intracellular tyrosine kinase domain of ALK. All those rearrangements

are potentially detected by the break-apart FISH probe (Vysis ALK Break-Apart FISH Probe Kit, Abbott Molecular, Abbott Park, IL, USA; Fig. 10.5A). It is still unknown whether any particular *EML4–ALK* fusion variant may confer differential sensitivity to ALK inhibitors, which may underlie the heterogeneity in responses among patients with ALK-positive NSCLC. Heuckmann et al.[129] reported that *EML4–ALK* v2 had the shortest half-life and greatest sensitivity to crizotinib, whereas v1 and v3b had intermediate sensitivity and v3a had the least sensitivity.

ALK fusion has been associated with several distinct clinicopathologic features and treatment outcomes.[107,111–113,130] A strong association between *ALK* fusions and a never-smoking or light-smoking (fewer than 10 pack-years) history has been reported, with the frequency of *ALK* fusions in the never-smoking or light-smoking subgroup higher than in the unselected population and ranging from 8.3% to 39%.[107,111,112,130] A younger age at diagnosis and adenocarcinoma histology are other important features associated with *ALK*-positive lung cancers, and *ALK* fusions rarely overlap with other oncogenic drivers. Furthermore, *ALK*-positive tumors are substantially more likely to have abundant signet ring cells. Contrary to *EGFR*-mutant NSCLC, *ALK*-positive NSCLC has shown resistance to *EGFR* TKIs, and sensitivity of *ALK*-positive NSCLC to platinum-based chemotherapy has not differed from that of *ALK*-negative NSCLC.[112,113] The activity of pemetrexed-based chemotherapy in *ALK*-positive NSCLC is controversial and needs further validation.[112,131–133] According to guidelines from the National Comprehensive Cancer Network and from the College of American Pathologists/International Association for the Study of Lung Cancer/Association for Molecular Pathology, testing of *ALK* fusion and *EGFR* mutation

TABLE 10.1 The Frequency, Detection Methods, and Fusion Variants of ALK Fusions in Nonsmall Cell Lung Cancer

Study	Study Population (No. of patients)	No. of *ALK* Fusions (%)	Detection Method	Fusion Variants
Soda et al.[103]	Japanese (75)	5 (6.7)	RT-PCR	*EML4–ALK* (E13; A20, E20; A20)
Takeuchi et al.[106]	Japanese (364)	11 (3.0)	10RT-PCR	*EML4–ALK* (E13; A20, E20; A20)
Wong et al.[107]	Chinese (266)	13 (5.0)	RT-PCR Direct sequencing	*EML4–ALK* (E6; A20, E13; A20, E20; A20, E18; A20)
Inamura et al.[108]	Japanese (221)	5 (2.0)	RT-PCR	*EML4–ALK* (E20; A20)
Shinmura et al.[109]	Japanese (77)	2 (3.0)	RT-PCR	*EML4–ALK* (E13; A20, E20; A20)
Koivunen et al.[110]	Korean/U.S. (305)	8 (3.0)	RT-PCR	*EML4–ALK* (E13; A20, E20; A20, E6a/b; A20, E15; A20)
Shaw et al.[111]	Predominantly white (141)[a]	19 (13.0)	FISH	NA
Kim et al.[112]	Korean (229)[a]	19 (8.3)	FISH	NA
Gainor et al.[113]	White/Asian (1683)	75 (4.4)	FISH	NA

[a]Enriched population of never-smokers and light smokers.

ALK, anaplastic lymphoma receptor tyrosine kinase; *EML4*, echinoderm microtubule-associated protein like 4; *FISH*, fluorescence in situ hybridization; *NA*, not available; *RT-PCR*, reverse transcription-polymerase chain reaction.

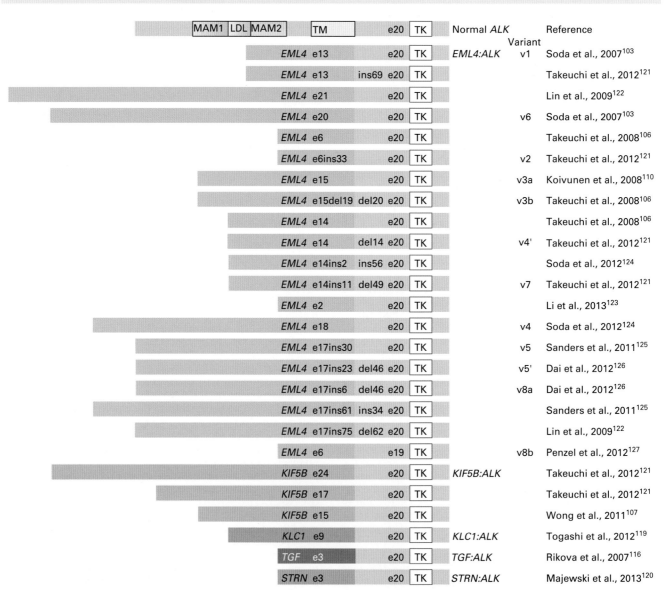

Fig. 10.4. ALK gene has been activated in lung cancer by numerous partners and multiple breakpoints and splicing forms have been identified. *ALK*, anaplastic lymphoma kinase; *EML4*, echinoderm microtubule-associated protein like 4; *KIF5B*, kinesin family member 5B; *KLC1*, kinesin light chain 1; *STRN*, striatin; *TGF*, transforming growth factor.

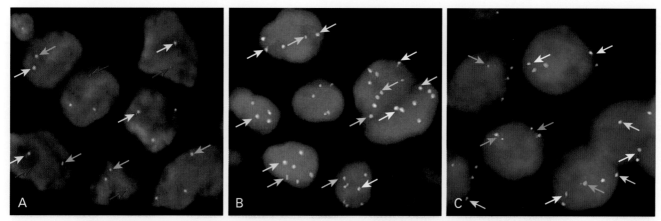

10

Fig. 10.5. Gene fusions in lung adenocarcinomas detected by break-apart FISH. (A) Two-target ALK FISH assay showing specimen positive for ALK rearrangement, represented by the split 3′ ALK and 5′ALK signals (red and green arrows, respectively); native copies of the *ALK* gene are represented by the fused *red/green* signals indicated by the *yellow arrows.* (B) Four-target FISH showing specimen positive for *ROS1* fusion. This assay combined two break-apart FISH probe sets, 3′-ALK *(red),* 5′-ALK *(green),* 3′-ROS1 *(aqua),* and 5′-ROS1 *(yellow).* Specimen was negative for ALK rearrangement with the fused 3′-ALK/5′-ALK signals indicated by the *yellow arrows,* and positive for *ROS1* rearrangement with single copies of 3′-ROS1 *(aqua)* indicated by the *turquoise arrows* and the native copies of native ROS1 *(fused aqua/yellow)* indicated by the *white arrows.* (C) Tritarget *RET–KIF5B* FISH assay *(red:* 3′-RET; *green:* 5′-RET; *yellow:* 5′-KIF5B) showing specimen positive for *KIF5B:RET* fusion. The native triplets (fused 3′-/3′-RET [red/green signals] and single 3′-KIF5B [yellow signal]) are indicated by the *pink arrows;* the abnormal triplet (fused 3′-RET:5′-KIF5B [red/yellow signals]) and single 5′-RET (green signal) are indicated by the *white arrows.* Specimen also has extra copies of single 5′-RET (green arrows) and 5′-KIF5B (yellow arrows). *ALK,* anaplastic lymphoma kinase; *FISH,* fluorescence in situ hybridization; *KIF5B,* kinesin family member 5B; *RET,* ret proto-oncogene; *ROS,* C-ros oncogene 1, receptor tyrosine kinase.

is now recommended for all patients with advanced nonsquamous NSCLC.[54,134] Therefore given the low frequency of this genetic alteration, efficient screening for *ALK* fusion is a crucial issue in clinical practice. Currently, reverse transcription (RT)-PCR, FISH, and IHC have been used to detect ALK fusion.[103,106,135–137] RT-PCR is a potentially rapid diagnostic method with high sensitivity. It provides direct evidence of the genomic fusion, but the difficulty in obtaining high-quality RNA limits the clinical utility of this method.[103,106] FISH is currently the standard criterion used in clinical trials for detection of *ALK* fusion, and it was the first Food and Drug Administration (FDA)-approved method (Vysis ALK Break-Apart FISH Probe Kit) for use of crizotinib in *ALK*-positive NSCLC.[138] Any type of *ALK* fusions could theoretically be detected using this method, but the main disadvantages are a relatively high cost and the specialized technical training required. Because normal adult tissue, except for neural tissue, does not express *ALK,* IHC has been reported to be quite effective at detecting *ALK* fusion in several studies.[118,123,135–137,139] The sensitivity of *ALK* IHC is highly dependent on the affinity of the primary antibody and the signal amplification system. Using high-affinity antibody clones and a sensitive detection system, the overall sensitivity and specificity of *ALK* IHC were 90% to 100% and 95.2% to 98.0%, respectively.[123,136,139] However, methodologic standardization and proof of clinical utility of the *ALK* IHC assay are still in progress.

Crizotinib has shown significant clinical benefit in *ALK*-positive NSCLC. During phase I (PROFILE 1001) and phase II (PROFILE 1005) studies of crizotinib, the objective response rate was approximately 60%.[115,138] The responses were often rapid and durable, and the median duration of response was 49.1 weeks; the median progression-free survival was 9.7 months in the most recent update of the phase I study.[140] Crizotinib has been well tolerated, with mild adverse events, including visual disturbance, nausea/vomiting, diarrhea, constipation, and peripheral edema. On the basis of clinical activity and tolerability demonstrated in phase I and phase II studies, crizotinib received accelerated FDA approval in August 2011 for the treatment of advanced *ALK*-positive NSCLC. This approval was conditioned on the results of randomized studies comparing crizotinib with standard chemotherapy (PROFILE 1007 and 1014). The results from the PROFILE 1007 phase III study were reported in 2013.[141] In this study, patients with advanced *ALK*-positive NSCLC were randomly assigned to receive either crizotinib or standard second-line chemotherapy (pemetrexed or docetaxel). Crizotinib was significantly superior to standard chemotherapy in terms of overall response (65% vs. 19%; $p < 0.001$) and progression-free survival (7.7 months vs. 3 months; $p < 0.001$). These results led to the regular approval by the US FDA in November 2013 for the treatment of advanced *ALK*-positive NSCLC.

Given the early success of crizotinib for the treatment of *ALK*-positive NSCLC, many next-generation *ALK* inhibitors are in development (Table 10.2). Some of these newer *ALK* inhibitors have shown activity against mutant forms of *ALK* that are resistant to crizotinib.

ROS1 Fusion

C-ros oncogene 1, receptor tyrosine kinase (*ROS1*) rearrangement has emerged as a new molecular subtype in NSCLC and now comprises a distinct molecular classification of NSCLC. *ROS1* rearrangements result in the formation of fusion proteins having constitutive tyrosine kinase activity, which subsequently stimulates downstream signaling (PI3K/AKT/mechanistic target of rapamycin [mTOR], RAS/MAPK, and signal transducer and activator of transcription 3 [acute-phase response factor], signal transducer and activator of transcription 3 [STAT3]), leading to enhanced cell growth, proliferation, and decreased apoptosis (Fig. 10.3).[142,143] The clinicopathologic characteristics of *ROS1* and *ALK* rearrangement overlap in patients with NSCLC, namely, younger age (median, approximately 50 years), history of never-smoking, and adenocarcinoma histology, suggesting that *ROS1* and *ALK* are evolutionarily related.[111,144,145]

TABLE 10.2 Clinical Trials of Drugs Targeting ALK Fusions

Drug	Sponsor[a]	Phase of Trial	Primary End Point	ClinicalTrials.gov Identifier
AP26113	Ariad	I/II	Overall response rate	01449461
CH5424802	Hoffmann-La Roche	I	Recommended phase II dose	01588028
		I/II (crizotinib-naive)	Overall response rate	01871805
		I/II (crizotinib-failed)		01801111
PF-06463922	Pfizer	I/II	Dose-limiting toxicity	01970865
			Overall response rate	
Ganetespib	Synta	II	Overall response rate	01562015
AUY922	Massachusetts General Hospital	II	Overall response rate	01752400
			Progression-free survival	
			Progression-free survival	
LDK378	Novartis	II (crizotinib-naive)	RT-PCR	01685138
		II (crizotinib-failed)		01685060
		III		01828099
		III		01828112
X-396	Xcovery	I	Maximum tolerated dose	01625234

[a]Ariad, Cambridge, MA, USA; Hoffmann-La Roche, Basel, Switzerland; Pfizer, New York, NY, USA; Synta, Lexington, MA, USA; Novartis, Basel, Switzerland; Xcovery, West Palm Beach, FL, USA.
ALK, Anaplastic lymphoma receptor tyrosine kinase; *RT-PCR*, reverse transcription-polymerase chain reaction.

TABLE 10.3 The Frequency, Detection Methods, and Fusion Variants of *ROS1* Fusions in Nonsmall Cell Lung Cancer

Study	Study Population (No. of patients)	No. of *ROS1* Fusions (%)	Method for Screening and Confirmation	Fusion Variants
Rikova et al.[116]	Chinese (150)	1 (0.7)	Phosphoproteomics RT-PCR	*CD74–ROS1* (C6;R34) *SLC34A2–ROS1* (S4;R32, S4;R34)
Bergethon et al.[144]	Total (1073) (Asian, 45; non-Asian, 942; ethnicity not available, 86)	18 (1.7) 5 (11.1) 13 (1.4) 0 (0)	FISH (break-apart) RT-PCR	*CD74–ROS1* (C6;R34) *SLC34A2–ROS1* (S4;R32)
Li et al.[156]	Chinese (202)[a]	2 (1.0)	RT-PCR Direct sequencing	*CD74–ROS1* (C6;R32, C6;R34)
Takeuchi et al.[121]	Japanese (1476)	13 (0.9)	FISH (break-apart) RT-PCR	*CD74–ROS1* (C6;R32, C6-R34) *SLC34A2–ROS1* (S4;R32, S4;R34) *EZR–ROS1* (E10;R34) *LRIG3–ROS1* (L16;R35) *SDC4–ROS1* (S2;R32, S2;R34) *TPM3–ROS1* (T8;R35)
Rimkunas et al.[148]	Chinese (556)	9 (1.6)	IHC screen RT-PCR	*FIG–ROS1* (F7;R35)
Cai et al.[146]	Chinese (392)	8 (2.0)	Multiplex RT-PCR Direct sequencing	*FIG–ROS1* (F7;R35)
Kim et al.[147]	Korean (208)[a]	7 (3.4)	FISH (break-apart) RT-PCR	*CD74–ROS1* (C6;R34)

[a]All patients were never-smokers.
CD74, CD74 molecule, major histocompatibility complex, class II invariant chain; *EZR*, ezrin; *FISH*, fluorescence in situ hybridization; *IHC*, immunohistochemistry; *LRIG3*, leucine-rich repeats and immunoglobulin-like domains protein 3; *ROS1*, c-ros oncogene 1, receptor tyrosine kinase; *RT-PCR*, reverse transcription-polymerase chain reaction; *SDC4*, syndecan 4; *SLC34A2*, solute carrier family 34 (type II sodium/phosphate contransporter), member 2; *TPM3*, tropomyosin 3.

Interestingly, the treatment outcome for *ROS1*-rearranged NSCLC has been similar to that for *ALK*-rearranged NSCLC, which also supports the biologic similarity of *ROS1* and *ALK*-rearranged NSCLC. Patients with *ROS1*-rearranged tumors have had poorer outcomes with *EGFR* TKIs and seemed to have had worse survival than patients with *ROS1*-negative tumors.[146,147] Of interest, *ROS1* rearrangement has been associated with significantly better overall response rate and median progression-free survival with pemetrexed than lack of *ROS1* rearrangement.[147] Similar to patients with *ALK*-rearranged tumors, patients with *ROS1*-rearranged lung adenocarcinomas and an HCC78 cell line seemed to have a low level of thymidylate synthase, supporting the clinical observation.[147]

ROS1 rearrangement may be detected by FISH (Fig. 10.5B) and other methods, and these screening methods, as well as the frequency of the rearrangement and its fusion variants, have been evaluated in population studies (Table 10.3). To date, nine *ROS1* fusion partners have been identified in lung adenocarcinomas (Fig. 10.6)—coiled-coil domain containing 6 (CCDC6)–ROS1; CD74 molecule, major histocompatibility complex, class II invariant chain (CD74)–ROS1; ezrin (EZR)–ROS1; Golgi-associated PDZ and coiled-coil motif containing protein (GOPC)–ROS1; KDEL (Lys–Asp–Glu–Leu) endoplasmic reticulum protein retention receptor 2 (KDELR2)–ROS1; leucine-rich repeats and immunoglobulin-like domains protein 3 (LRIG3)–ROS1; solute carrier family 34 (type II sodium/phosphate contransporter), member 2 (SLC34A2)–ROS1; syndecan 4 (SDC4)–ROS1; and tropomyosin 3

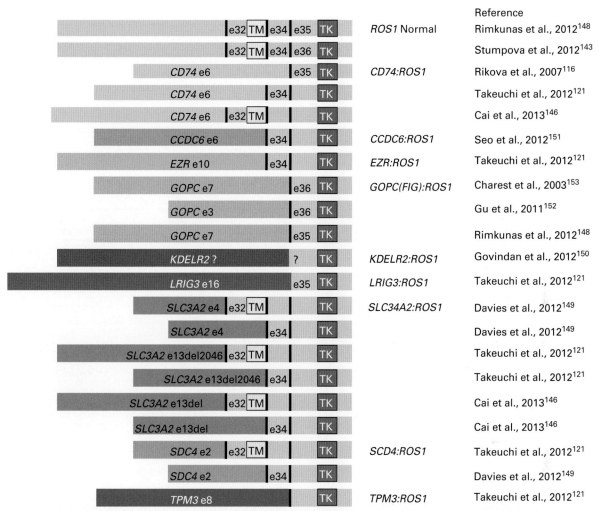

Fig. 10.6. *ROS1* gene fusion partners in lung cancer and schematic demonstration of breakpoints. *CCCD6,* Coiled-coil domain containing 6; *EZR,* ezrin; *GOPC,* Golgi-associated PDZ and coiled-coil motif containing protein; *KDELR2,* KDEL(Lys-Asp-Glu-Leu) endoplasmic reticulum retention receptor 2; *LRIG3,* leucine rich repeats and immunoglobulin-like domains protein 3; *ROS1,* c-ros oncogene 1, receptor tyrosine kinase; *SLC3A2,* solute carrier family 3 member 2; *SDC4,* syndecan 4; *TPM3,* tropomyosin 3.

(TPM3)–ROS1—all of which encode the same cytoplasmic portion of the ROS1 tyrosine kinase domain.[116,121,143,146,148–153] Of these fusion partners, CD74 is the most common ROS1 partner in NSCLC. The breakpoint of ROS1 in EZR and CCDC6 fusions is exon 34; in TPM3 fusion, the breakpoint is GOPC; in LRIG3 fusions, the breakpoint is exon 35; and in CD74, SDC4, and SLC34A2 fusions, the breakpoints are in exons 32 and 34.[154,155] The frequency of ROS1 rearrangement has ranged from 0.7% to 2.0% in unselected NSCLC populations.[116,121,144,146,148,149,156] However, enrichment of populations with never-smokers has resulted in a higher frequency (3.4%) of *ROS1* fusions, supporting that these fusions, together with EGFR mutations and ALK rearrangements, are the prevalent genetic alterations in never-smokers.[112,144,147] *ROS1* rearrangements rarely overlap with *EGFR* or *KRAS* mutations or *ALK* fusions, the three major recurrent oncogenic mutations in NSCLC.[144,147] The current knowledge defines *ROS1* rearrangement as a unique subset of lung cancer with a potentially targetable driver oncogene in populations enriched with never-smokers with EGFR/MET/ALK-negative (pan-negative) lung adenocarcinomas.[144,147,157]

Given that ALK and ROS1 share an approximately 49% amino acid sequence in the kinase domain, several ALK inhibitors have been shown to inhibit ROS1.[154] Using an automatic platform to examine the molecular basis of drug sensitivity, McDermott et al.[158] demonstrated that cell line HCC78 harboring *SLC34A2–ROS1* showed marked sensitivity to TAE684, a potent and selective ALK inhibitor. Subsequently, the transforming activity of the GOPC–ROS1 (FIG–ROS1) fusion transcripts found in cholangiocarcinoma was again successfully inhibited by TAE684 in vitro.[152] Crizotinib was reported to inhibit the growth of the HCC78 cell line and the phosphorylation of ROS1 in HEK293 cells transfected with CD74–ROS1 complementary DNA.[144] In addition, preliminary data from a phase I trial of crizotinib in the ROS1-positive NSCLC expansion cohort demonstrated an overall response rate of 61%.[159] Other clinical trials of second-generation ALK inhibitors targeting ROS1 rearrangement were ongoing at the time of publication (Table 10.4). A four-target, four-color ALK/ROS1 break-apart FISH probe has been developed for simultaneous testing of rearrangements in both genes (Fig. 10.5B) and will improve the efficiency of molecular testing in small specimens.

RET Fusion

The ret proto-oncogene (*RET*) encodes the tyrosine kinase receptor of growth factors belonging to the glial-derived neurotrophic factor family. *RET* rearrangement has been described

TABLE 10.4 Clinical Trials of Drugs Targeting *ROS1* Fusions

Drug	Sponsor[a]	Phase of Trial	Primary End Point	ClinicalTrials.gov NCT Identifier
Crizotinib	Pfizer	II	Overall response rate	01945021
LDK378	Yonsei Cancer Center, Severance Hospital	II	Overall response rate	01964157
AP26113	Ariad	I/II	Recommended phase II dose, overall response rate	01449461
ASP3026	Astellas	I	Safety and tolerability	01284192
AZD1480	AstraZeneca	I	Safety and tolerability	01219543
				01112397

[a]Pfizer, New York, NY, USA; Ariad, Cambridge, MA, USA; Astellas, Northbrook, IL, USA; and AstraZeneca, London, UK.
ROS1, c-ros oncogene 1, receptor tyrosine kinase.

TABLE 10.5 The Frequency, Detection Methods, and Fusion Variants of *RET* Fusions in Nonsmall Cell Lung Cancer

Study	Study Population (No. of patients)[a]	No. of *RET* Fusions (%)	Method for Screening and Confirmation	Fusion Variants
Lipson et al.[162]	Asian/U.S. (643)	12 (1.9)	IHC/qPCR Direct sequencing	*KIF5B–RET* (K15;R12, K16;R12, K22;R12, K15;R11)
Seo et al.[151]	Korean (200)	4 (1.5)	Transcriptome sequencing Direct sequencing	*KIF5B–RET* (K23;R12)
Takeuchi et al.[121]	Japanese (1482)	13 (0.9)	FISH (split) Fusion-specific RT-PCR	*KIF5B–RET* (K15;R12, K16;R12, K22;R12, K23;R12, K24;R11) *CCDC6–RET* (C1;R12)
Kohno et al.[161]	Japanese/U.S./ Norwegian (429)	7 (1.6)	Transcriptome sequencing/ RT-PCR Direct sequencing	*KIF5B–RET* (K15;R12, K16;R12, K23;R12, K24;R8)
Wang et al.[160]	Chinese (936)	13 (1.4%)	RT-PCR	*KIF5B–RET* (K15;R12)
Cai et al.[165]	Chinese (392)	6 (1.5%)	FISH Multiplex qPCR/Direct sequencing	*CCDC6–RET* (C1;R12) *NCOA4–RET* (N6;R12) *KIF5B–RET* (K15;R12, K22;R12)
Drilon et al.[164]	NA (31)[a]	5 (16%)	FISH RT-PCR	*TRIM33–RET* (T14;R12) *KIF5B–RET* (NA)

[a]Enriched population of never-smokers and patients with pan-negative tumors (absence of mutations in epidermal growth factor receptor [*EGFR*], Kirsten rat sarcoma viral oncogene homolog [*KRAS*], neuroblastoma RAS viral (v-ras) oncogene homolog [*NRAS*], v-raf murine sarcoma viral oncogene homolog B [*BRAF*], human epidermal growth factor receptor 2 [*HER2*], phosphatidylinositol-4,5-bisphosphate 3-kinase [*PIK3CA*], mitogen-activated protein kinase 1 [*MAP2K1*], and v-akt murine thymoma [*AKT*], and fusions of anaplastic lymphoma receptor tyrosine kinase [*ALK*] and c-ros oncogene 1 [*ROS1*]) in nonsquamous nonsmall cell lung cancers.
CCDC6, coiled-coil domain containing 6; *FISH*, fluorescence in situ hybridization; *IHC*, immunohistochemistry; *KIF5B*, kinesin family member 5B; *NA*, not available; *NCOA4*, nuclear receptor coactivator 4; *qPCR*, real-time polymerase chain reaction; *RET*, ret proto-oncogene; *RT-PCR*, reverse transcription-polymerase chain reaction; *TRIM33*, tripartite motif containing 33.

as a distinct molecular subset of NSCLC.[121,151,160–163] To date, four fusion partners for *RET*—KIF5B, CCDC6, tripartite motif containing 33 (TRIM33), and nuclear receptor coactivator 4 (*NCOA4*)—have been identified in lung adenocarcinoma. Expression of exogenous *KIF5B–RET* induced morphologic transformation and anchorage-independent growth of NIH3T3 fibroblasts.[161] *KIF5B–RET* is the most common type of fusion and is present in approximately 90% of fusions reported thus far.[164] The breakpoints are in exons 15 and 16 or 22–24 for *KIF5B* and in exons 8, 11, or 12 for *RET*.[121,151,160–165] All *KIF5B–RET* fusion variants contain the entire kinase domain of *RET*, but only the variant with fusion between exon 24 of *KIF5B* and exon 8 of *RET* (K24;R8) allows the resulting chimeric protein to harbor the transmembrane domain. All variants retain the coiled-coil domain necessary for homodimerization of the fusion proteins, contributing to aberrant activation of *RET* tyrosine kinase. Among all fusion variants, *KIF5B* exon 15 fused with *RET* exon 12 (K15;R12) was the most frequently found variant.[121,151,160,161,163,166–168]

The frequency of *RET*-positive NSCLCs and the screening methods used to detect the fusions have been reported in population studies (Table 10.5). The prevalence of *RET* fusions has been estimated to be approximately 0.9% to 1.9% in NSCLC and 1.2% to 2.0% in lung adenocarcinomas.[121,151,160–162,165] Kohno et al.[161] reported the identification of seven *KIF5B–RET* fusions in 429 lung adenocarcinomas. In a larger cohort of Japanese

patients, *KIF5B–RET* or *CCDC6–RET* fusions were identified in 13 (0.9%) of 1482 NSCLCs and in 13 (1.2%) of 1119 adenocarcinomas.[121] Of note, similar to the situation with *EML4–ALK* fusion, the frequency of *RET* fusion increases substantially (up to 10 [8.9%] of 112) among never-smokers with tumors lacking *EGFR* mutation.[160] In most studies, *RET* fusions have been found exclusively in lung adenocarcinomas. However, in more recent studies, *RET* fusions were found in SCCs and low-grade neuroendocrine tumors.[165,169]

Given the low incidence of *RET* fusion, identifying the enriched population of the fusion gene in NSCLC could contribute to improving the efficiency of future clinical screening. Among 936 Chinese patients with surgically resected NSCLC, patients with *RET*-positive lung adenocarcinomas tended to be younger and never-smokers, with more poorly differentiated tumors, tumors that displayed solid subtype, or smaller tumors with N2 disease.[160] *RET*-positive lung adenocarcinoma frequently shows signet ring cell pattern and mucinous cribriform pattern, which are distinctive histopathologic features of *EML4–ALK* fusion.[121,170] *RET* fusion has been mutually exclusive with other driver oncogenic mutations, such as *EGFR*, *ERBB2*, v-raf murine sarcoma viral oncogene homolog B (*BRAF*), or *KRAS* mutations or *EML4–ALK* fusion, indicating their role as driver mutations.[162,168] Of 70 *RET* fusions identified to date, 57 (81%) occurred in never-smokers or light smokers, suggesting a strong relationship of this genetic

TABLE 10.6 Clinical Trials of Drugs Targeting *RET* Fusions

Drug	Sponsor[a]	Phase of Trial	Primary End Point	ClinicalTrials.gov NCT Identifier
Lenvatinib	Eisai	II	Overall response rate	01877083
Cabozantinib	Memorial Sloan-Kettering Cancer Center	II	Overall response rate	01639508
Vandetanib	Seoul National University Hospital	II	Overall response rate	01823068
Ponatinib	Massachusetts General Hospital	II	Overall response rate	01813734
Ponatinib	University of Colorado	II	Overall response rate	01935336
Sunitinib	Dana-Farber Cancer Institute	II	Overall response rate	01829217
AUY922	National Taiwan University Hospital	II	Overall response rate	01922583

[a]Eisai, Woodcliff Lake, NJ, USA.
RET, ret proto-oncogene.

alteration with never-smoking history.[121,151,160–168] In a Chinese study, *KIF5B–RET* fusion-negative tumors were associated with a strong trend toward better overall survival than *KIF5B–RET* fusion-positive tumors.[165]

Various screening methods for *RET* fusion have been used, including RT-PCR, IHC, and FISH. The RT-PCR assay is highly sensitive, inexpensive, and easily available, but it can detect only known fusion gene variants.[165] The FISH assay allows the pathologist to perform a more reliable quantification of the genomic alteration, but presents challenges because several of the partner genes are mapped closely to *RET*. A customized three-target, three-color probe has been developed to assist with the interpretation (Fig. 10.5C). IHC staining has limited value in screening for *RET* fusion in NSCLC because there has been no substantial difference in *RET* staining between *RET*-positive and *RET*-negative tumors.[160]

RET fusions are potential targets for existing small molecule TKIs, including sorafenib, sunitinib, and vandetanib. These agents with *RET* inhibitory activity effectively inhibited *RET*-positive lung cancer cells in vitro.[121,161,162] Therefore *RET* kinase inhibitors should be tested in prospective clinical trials for therapeutic benefit in individuals with NSCLC with the *RET* fusion. Cabozantinib, an inhibitor of *MET*, *VEGFR*, and *RET*, has shown promising preliminary results (two confirmed partial responses and one prolonged stable disease) in patients with *RET*-positive advanced NSCLC.[164] Several clinical trials of *RET* inhibitors in NSCLC were ongoing at the time of publication (Table 10.6).

Other Fusions

Through targeted next-generation DNA sequencing and FISH assays, the new gene fusions involving the kinase domain of the neurotrophic tyrosine kinase, receptor, type 1 (*NTRK1*) gene that encodes the high-affinity nerve growth factor receptor (tropomyosin receptor kinase A [TRKA] protein) have been reported in 3 (3.3%) of 91 lung adenocarcinomas with no known oncogenic alterations.[171] The myosin phosphatase Rho interacting protein (*MPRIP*)–*NTRK1* and CD74–*NTRK1* fusions lead to constitutive *NTRK1* activity and are oncogenic. Treatment of cells expressing *NTRK1* fusions with TRKA inhibitors inhibited autophosphorylation of TRKA and cell growth.[171]

Although most oncogenic fusions have been found in lung adenocarcinomas, BCL2-associated athanogene 4 (BAG4)–FGFR1, FGFR2–KIAA1967, and transforming, acidic coiled-coil containing protein 3 (TACC3)–FGFR3 fusions have been newly identified in advanced SCCs of the lung through transcriptome sequencing.[120,172] All of these *FGFR* gene fusions expressed FGFR1–3 as a 5′ or 3′ fusion partner with intact kinase domains.

Like fusion partners for *RET*, all *FGFR* fusion partners have dimerization motifs, which suggests that oligomerization may serve as the common mechanism of activation of FGFR fusion proteins. Overexpression of FGFR fusion proteins induce cell proliferation, and cells harboring FGFR fusions have shown enhanced sensitivity to FGFR inhibitors.[172]

CONCLUSION

The first decade-and-a-half of the 21st century has brought new windows of opportunity for a better understanding of genomic and chromosomal factors and mechanisms causally related to lung cancer, mainly NSCLC. Importantly, the identification of driver genes and essential signaling pathways for lung oncogenesis has been supporting the discovery and development of novel targeted therapy agents, which are causing rapid, dramatic, and stable tumor shrinkage in many patients. This new scenario conveys a great deal of enthusiasm, not only for patients and their families, but also among a diversity of health-care professionals. Given this perspective, the role of molecular testing using cytogenetic strategies has reached an unprecedented clinical utility.

KEY REFERENCES

15. Lockwood WW, Chari R, Coe BP, et al. DNA amplification is a ubiquitous mechanism of oncogene activation in lung and other cancers. *Oncogene.* 2008;27(33):4615–4624.

29. Cancer Genome Atlas Research Network. Comprehensive genomic characterization of squamous cell lung cancers. *Nature.* 2012;489(7417):519–525.

30. Imielinski M, Berger AH, Hammerman PS, et al. Mapping the hallmarks of lung adenocarcinoma with massively parallel sequencing. *Cell.* 2012;150(6):1107–1120.

44. Kollareddy M, Zheleva D, Dzubak P, Brahmkshatriya PS, Lepsik M, Hajduch M. Aurora kinase inhibitors: progress towards the clinic. *Invest New Drugs.* 2012;30(6):2411–2432.

46. Curtin NJ. DNA repair dysregulation from cancer driver to therapeutic target. *Nat Rev Cancer.* 2012;12(12):801–817.

53. Lindeman NI, Cagle PT, Beaseley MB, et al. Molecular testing guideline for selection of lung cancer patients for EGFR and ALK tyrosine kinase inhibitors: guideline from the College of American Pathologists, International Association for the Study of Lung Cancer, and Association for Molecular Pathology. *Arch Pathol Lab Med.* 2013;137(6):828–860.

96. Kim HR, Kim DJ, Kang DR, et al. Fibroblast growth factor receptor 1 gene amplification is associated with poor survival and cigarette smoking dosage in patients with resected squamous cell lung cancer. *J Clin Oncol.* 2013;31(6):731–737.

103. Soda M, Choi YL, Enomoto M, et al. Identification of the transforming EML4-ALK fusion gene in non-small-cell lung cancer. *Nature.* 2007;448(7153):561–566.

104. Shaw AT, Engelman JA. ALK in lung cancer: past, present, and future. *J Clin Oncol.* 2013;31(8):1105–1111.
114. Doebele RC, Pilling AB, Aisner DL, et al. Mechanisms of resistance to crizotinibin patients with ALK gene rearranged non-small cell lung cancer. *Clin Cancer Res.* 2012;18(5):1472–1482.
115. Shaw AT, Hsu PP, Awad MM, Engelman JA. Tyrosine kinase gene rearrangements in epithelial malignancies. *Nat Rev Cancer.* 2013;13(11):772–787.
121. Takeuchi K, Soda M, Togashi Y, et al. RET, ROS1 and ALK fusions in lung cancer. *Nat Med.* 2012;18(3):378–381.
150. Govindan R, Ding L, Griffith M, et al. Genomic landscape of non-small cell lung cancer in smokers and never-smokers. *Cell.* 2012;150(6):1121–1134.
155. Davies KD, Doebele RC. Molecular pathways: ROS1 fusion proteins in cancer. *Clin Cancer Res.* 2013;19(15):4040–4045.
171. Vaishnavi A, Capelletti M, Le AT, et al. Oncogenic and drug-sensitive NTRK1 rearrangements in lung cancer. *Nat Med.* 2013;19(11):1469–1472.

See Expertconsult for full list of references.

11 Mutational Events in Lung Cancer: Present and Developing Technologies

Daniel Morgensztern, Siddhartha Devarakonda, Tetsuya Mitsudomi, Christopher Maher, and Ramaswamy Govindan

SUMMARY OF KEY POINTS

- Cancer genomes are characterized by the presence of a variety of alterations including base substitutions, copy-number alterations (amplifications or deletions), and structural rearrangements (translocations or chromosomal rearrangements).
- Among the early methods of DNA sequencing (now known as first-generation methods), the most successful has been the Sanger sequencing or chain termination reaction method. Despite its effectiveness, accuracy, and the substantial improvements since its original description, first-generation sequencing has been limited by high cost, labor intensity, and low throughput (amount of data generated per unit of time).
- Next-generation sequencing (NGS) is a broad term describing different technologies characterized by high-throughput, lower cost, and faster sequencing time compared with first-generation methods. NGS enhances the ability to comprehensively identify all alterations in the cancer genome, including mutations, copy-number alterations, and changes in gene expression, in a reasonable time frame.
- NGS studies in patients with lung cancer have allowed comprehensive characterization of the molecular alterations in lung adenocarcinomas, squamous cell carcinomas, and small cell carcinomas. These studies have also facilitated the study of the clonal architecture of lung cancer samples and its clinical implications.
- It is possible today, with newer technologies, to utilize circulating tumor DNA isolated from peripheral blood or other body fluids of patients for genetic testing. Such testing is less invasive and is becoming increasingly popular in the clinical setting.

The advent of targeted therapies has brought about a paradigm shift in the management of lung cancer. The majority of these drugs, however, only benefit a small subset of patients whose tumors are driven by specific aberrations in cell signaling pathways. Cancer cells demonstrate several types of genomic alterations including base substitutions, copy-number alterations (amplifications or deletions), and structural rearrangements (translocations or chromosomal rearrangements). Point mutations or single base substitutions (also known as single nucleotide variants [SNVs]) represent one of the most common types of DNA alteration. SNVs in protein-coding genes may result in a variety of effects in the resulting proteins. Synonymous mutations alter the DNA sequence of protein-coding genes in a way that the modified sequence at the mutated location still codes for the same amino acid. These mutations are therefore viewed as being "silent," although recent data suggest that some of these mutations could have important functional consequences.[3] By

contrast, missense and nonsense mutations are associated with the substitution of one amino acid for another or premature termination of protein synthesis, respectively. Mutations that arise from the insertion or deletion of one or more nucleotides are referred to as "Indels" (short for insertions and deletions). These mutations can result in frameshift mutations that alter the reading frame of a protein-coding gene. The reading frame of a coding sequence refers to groups of three bases (or codons) in the sequence of a gene, each of which codes for a specific amino acid. When the number of nucleotides inserted or deleted from a coding sequence is not a multiple of three, the reading frame of the coding sequence downstream of the mutation is shifted, resulting in missense or nonsense alterations and the production of an abnormal or nonfunctional protein.

The processing of precursor messenger RNA (mRNA) into mature form occurs through removal of introns and joining of exons in a process termed "splicing."[4] This process is regulated in cells through proteins that constitute a cell's splicing machinery. These proteins distinguish introns from exons based on characteristic base sequences within the intron, within the exon, and at intron–exon junctions. Splicing mutations alter these specific sites and deregulate splicing, leading to the abnormal inclusion or exclusion of introns or exons from the final mRNA. This can result in the production of aberrant and nonfunctional proteins. Copy-number alterations are changes in gene number from the two copies present in the normal diploid genome. Rearrangements occur when DNA from one segment is broken and rejoined to a DNA segment from elsewhere in the genome. Rearrangements occurring within the same chromosome or involving regions on different chromosomes are referred to as intrachromosomal or interchromosomal translocations, respectively.

Somatic mutations in cancer cells are identified by comparing the DNA sequence of cancer cells with that of noncancerous "normal" cells acquired from the same individual. Although these somatic mutations occur randomly throughout the genome of a cancer cell, a subset of somatic mutations occurs in a key set of genes that confer growth advantage to the cells harboring them. These "driver" mutations are positively selected during cancer evolution and implicated in oncogenesis.[5] One of the important objectives of cancer genomic studies is to distinguish these driver mutations from bystander "passenger" mutations that do not confer a survival advantage, in an unbiased fashion. This process entails the use of complex statistical algorithms.[2] Apart from offering an insight into the biology underlying malignant transformation, such analyses also facilitate the identification of novel therapeutic targets.

OVERVIEW OF GENOMIC TECHNOLOGIES

First-Generation Sequencing

Among the early methods of DNA sequencing (now known as first-generation methods), the most successful has been the Sanger sequencing or chain termination reaction method.[6] When a dideoxynucleotide triphosphate (ddNTP) is incorporated into a growing oligonucleotide DNA molecule instead of a deoxynucleotide (deoxynucleotide triphosphate [dNTP]), its lack of a 3′-hydroxyl group, which is required for the formation of a phosphodiester bond between two nucleotides, leads to the inhibition of DNA polymerase I and further strand elongation.[7] This chain termination forms the basis of Sanger sequencing. The first step in Sanger sequencing is the preparation of identical single-stranded DNA molecules with a short oligonucleotide annealed to each molecule. This short oligonucleotide helps prime DNA synthesis that is complementary to the single-stranded DNA (template) molecules. Both the DNA template and the primer are incubated with DNA polymerase in the presence of a mixture of the four dNTPs and a small amount of each of the four ddNTPs labeled with radioactive 32-P. Although DNA polymerase does not discriminate between dNTPs and ddNTPs, the considerably larger amount of dNTPs compared with ddNTPs allows the incorporation of several hundred nucleotides before a ddNTP is randomly incorporated into the nascent DNA. Because each reaction is performed with one subtype of ddNTP, the result is a group of nascent DNA molecules of different lengths, but with each ending in a ddNTP. The mixture with each of the ddNTPs is loaded into one of four parallel wells of polyacrylamide slab gel and the molecules are separated according to their molecular mass to allow a deduction of the DNA sequence by visualization of the bands by autoradiography. Because of the relatively easier process and reliability compared with the other technologies, autoradiography has become the method of choice for DNA sequencing. Advances in fluorescent technology allowed the tagging of either the primer or the terminating ddNTP with a specific fluorescent dye and the development of automated sequencing.[8–10] Four-color fluorescent dyes eventually replaced the radioactive labels and allowed the separation of molecules by capillary electrophoresis, which in turn replaced the slab gel method. One of the advantages of the capillary electrophoresis is that it allows all four reactions to be performed in a single tube.

Despite the effectiveness, high accuracy, and substantial improvements since its original description, first-generation sequencing has been limited by high cost, labor intensity, and time consumed due to the low throughput (defined as amount of data generated per unit of time). Using modern techniques, the automated chain-termination method can involve up to 96 sequencing reactions simultaneously. With each run capable of generating approximately 500 bases of sequence, the 96 sequencing reactions may produce, at most, approximately 48 kilobases (kb) every 2 hours. Although this technology was very useful for sequencing lower organisms,[11–13] it is not particularly suitable for sequencing the human genome, which is approximately 3 billion base pairs (bp) long.[14]

Next-Generation Sequencing

Next-generation sequencing (NGS) is a broad term describing different technologies characterized by high-throughput, lower cost, and faster sequencing time compared with first-generation methods. Although the Sanger sequencing method allowed the study of one modality of cancer genomic alterations at a time, NGS enhances the ability to comprehensively identify all alterations, including mutations, copy-number alterations, and changes in gene expression, in a reasonable time frame.[15] NGS is also referred to as massively parallel sequencing, because it allows for a substantial increase in the number of sequence reads simultaneously generated, facilitating higher throughput and leading to considerable cost reduction. Initially, the increased output was achieved with substantial sacrifices in length and accuracy of the individual reads compared with the Sanger sequencing method.[16] Nevertheless, to overcome the higher error rates, NGS platforms use a high level of redundancy or sequence coverage to increase the confidence in base calling. Sequence coverage or depth is the number of times a nucleotide mapped to a genome position is

read during the sequencing process, due to overlap of the reads generated during sequencing.[17] Physical coverage is the number of fragments that span a specific location in the genome. A common method to characterize the quality of sequencing reads is the combination of PHRED and PHRAP quality scores, which are algorithms used to evaluate the accuracy of base calling in the raw and assembled sequence, respectively.[18–20] Both scores correspond to an error probability of $10^{-x/10}$. Therefore, PHRED or PHRAP quality scores of 20 and 30 correspond to an accuracy of 99% and 99.9%, respectively.

The most common platforms used for NGS are the Roche 454 (Basel, Switzerland), Illumina (San Diego, CA, USA), and SOLiD (Sunnyvale, CA, USA). The Roche 454 was the first NGS platform available as a commercial product and uses pyrosequencing, an alternative method of DNA sequencing based on measuring inorganic pyrophosphate (PPi) generated during DNA synthesis.[21] In this method, the DNA fragment of interest is hybridized to a sequencing primer and incubated with DNA polymerase, adenosine triphosphate (ATP) sulfurylase, firefly luciferase, and a nucleotide-degrading enzyme.[22–24] Deoxynucleotides are added in repeated cycles and incorporated into the growing DNA strand at complementary sites of the template strand. During this process, PPi is released in equal molarity to the incorporated deoxynucleotide. ATP sulfurylase catalyzes the conversion of PPi and adenosine phosphosulfate into ATP and sulfate.[25] ATP provides the energy for the oxidation of luciferin into oxyluciferin by luciferase, generating light that can be estimated by a photodiode or charge-coupled device camera. The unincorporated deoxynucleotides are degraded between the cycles by a nucleotide-degrading enzyme, most commonly apyrase. The overall reaction from polymerization to light detection takes approximately 3 seconds to 4 seconds at room temperature. The Illumina platform uses a sequence-by-synthesis (SBS) approach where all four nucleotides, each carrying a base-unique fluorescent label, are added simultaneously to the flow channels together with DNA polymerase and reversible terminators. Each base incorporation step is followed by fluorescent imaging and chemical removal of the terminator. The unique feature of the SOLiD platform is the use of sequencing by ligation, which uses DNA ligase instead of DNA polymerase.[26,27] The Illumina platform is currently the most widely used platform for NGS.

APPLICATIONS OF NEXT-GENERATION SEQUENCING

Whole-Genome Sequencing

Whole-genome sequencing (WGS) is the analysis of the entire genomic DNA sequence of a cell at a single time, providing the most comprehensive characterization of the genome. WGS became available after the publication of the Human Genome Project, which generated the reference for human genome sequences.[14,28] With the use of matched noncancerous genomes, which are usually obtained from skin biopsies in patients with hematologic malignancies[26,29] and peripheral blood mononuclear cells or adjacent normal tissue in solid tumors for comparison,[30,31] WGS allows the detection of the full range of genomic alterations as well as noncoding somatic mutations in cancer cells.

The first whole cancer genome sequence was reported in 2008 in a patient with cytogenetically normal acute myeloid leukemia.[32] Using the patient's skin as the matched normal counterpart, the authors described 10 genes with acquired mutations, including two previously known and eight new mutations. Shortly after that, the initial studies on WGS in lung cancer and other solid tumors were reported.[33–35] Several tumor samples obtained from patients with various malignancies have been sequenced to date by independent groups and large-scale consortia such as The Cancer Genome Atlas (TCGA).[36,37]

Whole-Exome and Targeted Gene Sequencing

Whole-exome sequencing (WES) and targeted sequencing are alternatives to WGS that allow increased coverage of regions of interest at a lower cost. WES is a process used to evaluate the small percentage of the genome that encodes for proteins. Another approach is the use of cancer-specific gene panels through which only preselected genes are sequenced (Fig. 11.1). Targeted sequencing may be performed using multiplex polymerase chain reaction (PCR) or NGS. Multiplex PCR entails the simultaneous amplification of two or more DNA targets with unique label probes in a single reaction vessel.[38] Some of the benefits of multiplex PCR include the reduced sample requirements, decreased time, and lower cost compared with singleplex reactions. SNaPshot is one such multiplex PCR platform, in which multiplex PCR is followed by single-base extension reactions that generate allele-specific fluorescently labeled probes designed to test more than 50 hot-spot mutation sites in 14 key cancer genes.[39] With the advances in biotechnology and decreased cost of sequencing, NGS methods are quickly gaining popularity and being routinely employed for targeted sequencing, both in the research setting and in the clinical setting.[40]

Transcriptome

Transcriptome refers to the complete set of mRNA and noncoding RNA (ncRNA) transcripts produced by a cell. One method to characterize the transcriptome is the conversion of mRNA into complementary DNA (cDNA) followed by sequencing of the resulting cDNA library. The subsequent comparison between cDNA and genomic sequences enables the evaluation of actively transcribed regions. Although feasible, this approach with routine full-length cDNA was costly and had low coverage, limiting its use for the characterization of whole transcriptomes in multicellular species. The development of both expressed sequence tag and serial analysis of gene expression (SAGE) techniques allowed for substantial advances in transcriptome sequencing methodology.[41] Expressed sequence tags refer to single-pass sequencing reads from either the 3′ or 5′ end of a cDNA clone, which are then used to identify expressed genes.

These tags are short and, unlike full-length cDNA sequencing, do not cover the whole length of cDNA. SAGE represented the first sequencing-based method for high-throughput gene expression profiling. SAGE involves the generation of short sequence tags from 3′ ends of mRNA transcripts that are subsequently sequenced and measured to provide estimates of the transcript expression. With the development of NGS platforms, there has been a substantial increase in the throughput and the ability to identify sequence aberrations, alternative splice variants, and ncRNAs through RNA sequencing. ncRNAs are molecules transcribed from genomic DNA but not translated into proteins and include microRNAs, small interfering RNAs, and long ncRNAs. Transcriptome sequencing has also been shown to be a sensitive and efficient approach to detect intragenic fusions in solid tumors.[42,43]

Epigenome

Epigenome is the complete description of all the chemical modifications to DNA and histone proteins that regulate the expression of genes within the genome. These modifications occur without intrinsic changes in the primary DNA sequence and are necessary for key biologic processes, including differentiation, genomic imprinting of one of the two parental alleles of a gene to ensure monoallelic expression, and silencing of large chromosomal domains such as the X chromosome.[44] The most common mechanisms of epigenetic modification include DNA methylation, histone modifications, and transcription of small ncRNA. In humans, DNA methylation occurs in cytosines that precede guanines (dinucleotide CpGs). CpG-rich regions, also known as CpG islands, are present in approximately 50% to 70% of the 5′-gene promoter regions.[45] DNA methylation of the gene promoter at CpG islands is mediated by DNA methyltransferases, which leads to silencing by direct inhibition of transcription factor binding to their relative sites and recruitment of methyl-binding domain proteins.[46] Cancer cells frequently display global hypomethylation, which is found within the body of genes and regions flanking the genes, and CpG island promoter-specific hypermethylation. Whereas global hypomethylation accounts for the

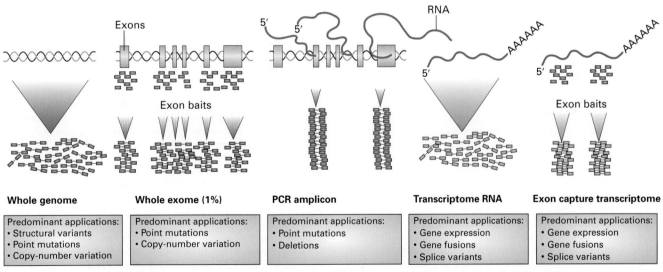

Whole genome

Predominant applications:
• Structural variants
• Point mutations
• Copy-number variation

Whole exome (1%)

Predominant applications:
• Point mutations
• Copy-number variation

PCR amplicon

Predominant applications:
• Point mutations
• Deletions

Transcriptome RNA

Predominant applications:
• Gene expression
• Gene fusions
• Splice variants

Exon capture transcriptome

Predominant applications:
• Gene expression
• Gene fusions
• Splice variants

Fig. 11.1. Applications of next-generation sequencing (NGS). Whole-genome sequencing and whole-exome sequencing evaluate the entire DNA sequence and the small percentage of the genome that encodes proteins, respectively. Targeted sequencing with multiplex evaluates two or more DNA targets in a single reaction vessel. Transcriptome evaluates the complete set of messenger RNA and noncoding RNA transcripts. *PCR,* polymerase chain reaction. *(Reprinted, with permission, from Simon R, Roychowdhury S. Implementing personalized cancer genomics in clinical trials.* Nat Rev Drug Discov. *2013;12(5):358–369.)*

activation of proto-oncogenes and loss of imprinting, promoter hypermethylation is associated with decreased gene expression, leading to an alternative way of silencing key tumor suppressor genes.[47] Epigenetic modifications have been implicated in conferring the second hit for cancer initiation by silencing the remaining active alleles of a previously mutated tumor suppressor gene. Posttranslational histone modifications occur mainly at the N-terminal tails of histones and are mediated by several enzymes, including histone methyltransferases and demethylases, which introduce and remove methyl groups, respectively, and acetyltransferases and deacetylases, which introduce and remove acetyl groups, respectively. The various combinations of modifications in specific genomic regions lead to changes in the chromatin structure with activation or repression of gene expression.[48]

The three most common techniques for the evaluation of DNA methylation are the digestion of genomic DNA with methyl-sensitive restriction enzymes, affinity-based enrichment of methylated DNA fragments, and chemical conversion methods.[49] The standard method for mapping DNA methylation is bisulfite sequencing, a chemical conversion method. Treatment of genomic DNA with sodium bisulfite chemically converts unmethylated cytosines to uracil. Assuming a near-complete bisulfite conversion, all unmethylated cytosines become thymidines after PCR and the remaining cytosines are the ones methylated at the fifth carbon or 5-methylcytosine.

COMPREHENSIVE GENOMIC STUDIES USING NGS IN LUNG CANCER

Nonsmall Cell Lung Cancer

Multiple independent groups and TCGA research network have together sequenced over a thousand lung cancer samples to date.[50–58] Data from these studies indicate that recurrent alterations in known receptor tyrosine kinase (RTK)-RAS (RAt sarcoma)-rapidly accelerated fibrosarcoma (RAF) pathway genes such as *EGFR*, *KRAS*, *BRAF*, *MET*, and *ALK* are observed in the majority of lung adenocarcinoma genomes. Nearly 76% of lung adenocarcinomas showed alterations in this pathway in a recent analysis including 660 tumor samples.[50] Although tumors obtained from both smokers and never-smokers show alterations in the RTK pathway genes, cancers arising in these populations differ in other aspects such as mutational burden and pattern of SNVs, and also show enrichment for alterations in specific genes.[51,53] The exonic mutation rates are significantly higher in smokers than in never-smokers (median, 9.8 vs. 1.7 per megabase [Mb], $p = 3 \times 10^{-9}$), with the predominant mutation patterns being C-to-T transitions and C-to-A transversions in never-smoker and smoker lung cancer genomes, respectively (Fig. 11.2).[51,54] In addition to mutations in RTK-RAS-RAF signaling, lung adenocarcinomas also show alterations in tumor suppressors such as *TP53*, *CDKN2A*, *STK11*, and *NF1*. Furthermore, adenocarcinomas also show recurrent alterations in genes involved in epigenetic or RNA deregulation such as *BRD3*, *SETD2*, and *ARID1A*, and genes that regulate splicing such as *U2AF1*, *RBM10*, and *SF3B1*. Alterations in these genes possibly drive malignant transformation by altering the splicing of oncogenes such as *CTNNB1*.[51] Because genes involved in epigenetic or RNA deregulation cannot be readily assigned to one of the 10 hallmarks of cancer that were originally described, these data suggest that such alterations could constitute the 11th hallmark (Fig. 11.3).[59,60]

In addition to the identification of recurrent pathway alterations, NGS also has the ability to identify potential targets for therapy.[53] For instance, TCGA investigators reported alterations in cellular pathways known to be potentially targetable, such as phosphatidylinositol-3-OH kinase (PI3K)/AKT and RTK-RAS-RAF, in nearly 75% of lung adenocarcinomas and 69% of

squamous cell carcinomas.[51,61] Targeted sequencing with a high-read coverage can also help in the estimation of variant allele frequencies, based on the distribution of which, it is possible to infer the number and size of clonal populations within each tumor sample. Using these techniques, several groups have described the clonal architecture of lung adenocarcinomas.[53,62–64] These analyses indicate that lung cancers show a considerable extent of intratumor heterogeneity (Fig. 11.4).[65]

Founder clone mutations refer to those mutations that are present ubiquitously within all tumors cells, implying that they are acquired early on in the course of disease evolution. In one analysis, Zhang et al.[64] observed that on average 76% of all mutations observed through multiregion sequencing of adenocarcinoma samples were present in all regions of the tumor. Alterations (mutations) in known cancer genes such as *TP53*, *EGFR*, and *KRAS* were ubiquitous, suggesting early acquisition. Understanding the clonal architecture of tumors has, in theory, the ability to guide therapy because treatments that target clonal alterations are more likely to succeed than those that target subclonal alterations.

TCGA investigators initially profiled tumor specimens from 178 patients with squamous cell lung cancer, along with peripheral blood (41 patients) or adjacent histologic normal tissues resected at the time of surgery (137 patients) as the matched noncancerous germline DNA.[61] Samples from all 178 patients were evaluated with WES, RNA sequencing, DNA methylation, and copy-number evaluation, whereas 18 paired samples were evaluated with WGS and 158 paired samples were evaluated with microRNA sequencing. WES and WGS were performed with the Illumina HiSeq platform. As observed in lung adenocarcinoma from smokers, the investigators identified a mean of 228 nonsilent exonic mutations per tumor (mean somatic mutation rate of 8.1 per Mb) in these tumors. Somatic alterations of potentially targetable genes were found in 114 (64%) samples. The most commonly altered pathways were the PI3K-RTK-RAS signaling (69%); squamous differentiation, including *SOX2*, *TP53*, *NOTCH1*, *NOTCH2*, *ASCL4*, and *FOXP1* (44%); and the oxidative stress response pathway consisting of *KEAP1*, *CUL3*, and *NFE2L2* (34%; Fig. 11.5). The *CDKN2A* tumor suppressor gene was inactivated in 72% of the cases by a variety of mechanisms, including homozygous deletion (29%), epigenetic silencing by methylation (21%), inactivating mutation (18%), and exon 1-beta skipping (4%).

However, unlike adenocarcinomas, mutations in RTK-RAS-RAF pathway genes such as *KRAS*, *EGFR*, and *BRAF* were infrequent in these tumors. In an updated analysis, TCGA investigators sequenced and compared mutational profiles of 660 adenocarcinomas and 484 squamous cell carcinomas.[50] Only a 12% overlap was observed between genes mutated at a statistically significant level between the two histologies. Interestingly, more similarity was observed among significantly mutated genes in squamous cell lung and other smoking-associated cancers such as head and neck squamous cell and bladder cancers, highlighting the molecularly distinct natures of the different subtypes of lung cancer, despite their identical anatomic site of origin.

Small Cell Lung Cancer

Unlike nonsmall cell lung cancers, small cell lung cancer (SCLC) samples rarely show mutations in RTK signaling pathways. However, almost all SCLCs show alterations in the tumor suppressors *TP53* and *RB1*.[55] Peifer et al.[56] sequenced 29 exomes, two genomes, and 15 transcriptomes from patients with SCLC using the Illumina HiSeq platform. Similar to other smoking-related tumors, the rate of the protein-changing mutations was 7.4 per Mb. Mutation and loss of *TP53* and *RB1* were noted in all patients, and preclinical studies have shown that conditional deletion of both genes in mice is associated with

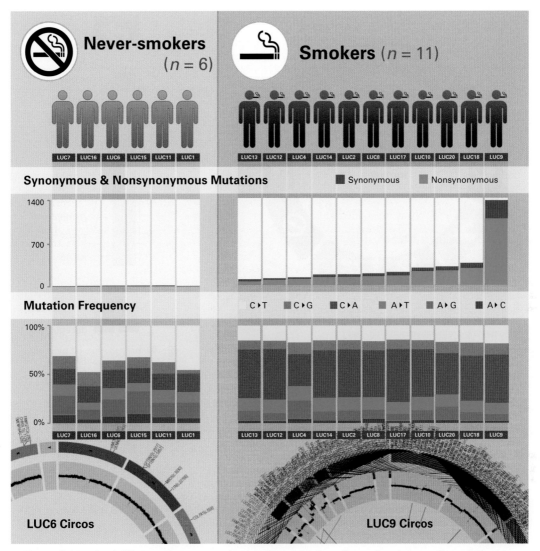

Fig. 11.2. Mutational differences between smokers and never-smokers. Comparison between the mutation rates and characteristics between smokers and never-smokers showed a significantly higher median number of point mutations among smokers. Among the point mutations, C-to-A transversions were the predominant type in smokers, whereas C-to-T transitions were the most common type in never-smokers. *(Reprinted, with permission, from Govindan R, Ding L, Griffith M, et al. Genomic landscape of non-small cell lung cancer in smokers and never-smokers.* Cell. *2012;150:1121–1134.)*

the development of SCLC.[66,67] Inactivation of cyclic adenosine monophosphate response element binding (CREB)-binding protein (*CREBBP*) and *EP300* are likely to play a substantial role in the development of SCLC as well, with mutations clustered around the sequence encoding the histone acetyltransferase domain of these genes occurring in 18% of patient samples and cell lines. The *MLL* gene, which codes for a histone-modifying enzyme, was mutated in 10% of the patient samples suggesting a substantial role for histone modifications in SCLC. Rudin et al.[57] evaluated the exome, transcriptome, and copy-number alterations in 80 SCLC samples using the Illumina HiSeq 2000 platform. The samples included 36 primary SCLC human tumors with adjacent normal sample pairs, 17 paired SCLC cell lines with matched lymphoblastoid cell lines, and four primary SCLC and 23 SCLC cell lines without matched controls. The investigators performed WGS in one SCLC tumor with a normal tissue pair and found an average of 175 nonsynonymous mutations per sample, with a mean of 5.5 mutations per Mb and a predominance of G-to-T transversions, which is the

smoking-related signature. Twenty-two genes were frequently mutated. The most commonly mutated genes from the combined initial and validation cohorts were *TP53* (77.4%), *RB1* (30.6%), *COL22A1* (25.8%), and *BCLAF1* (16.1%). Four of the 41 gene fusions identified in this analysis were recurrent, including the fusion between *RLF* and *MYCL1*, which was found in one primary SCLC tumor and four SCLC cell lines. The decreased proliferation of H1097 and CORL47 fusion-positive cell lines with the use of small interfering RNA targeting *MYCL1* supported *MYCL1*'s role as an oncogene in SCLC. Several of these findings were confirmed in a subsequent analysis of 110 SCLC samples by George et al.[55] In addition to recurrent *TP53* and *RB1* mutations, mutations in the tumor suppressors *TP73*, *PTEN*, *RBL1*, and *RBL2* were also observed in these samples. Mutations in the NOTCH family of genes were observed in 25% of the samples sequenced in this study. The NOTCH pathway plays an important role in regulating neuroendocrine differentiation, implying a crucial role for these alterations in the development and progression of SCLC.

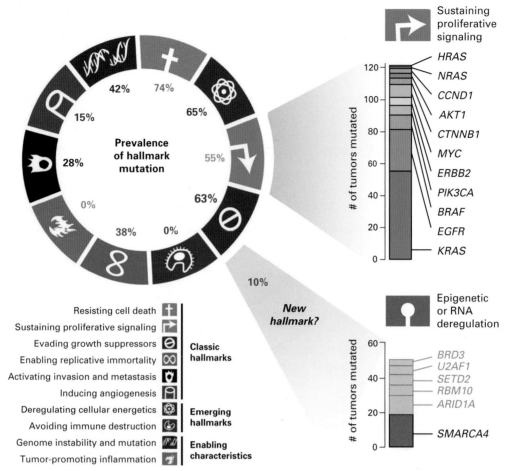

Fig. 11.3. Next-generation hallmark of lung adenocarcinomas. Prevalence of hallmark mutations in adenocarcinoma, genes in the sustained proliferative signaling, and the proposed 11th hallmark with genes involved in epigenetic and RNA deregulation. *(Reprinted, with permission, from Imielinski M, Berger AH, Hammerman PS, et al. Mapping the hallmarks of lung adenocarcinoma with massively parallel sequencing. Cell. 2012;150: 1107–1120.)*

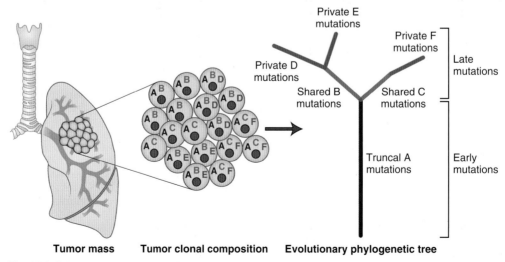

Fig. 11.4. Schematic representation of the clonal architecture and intratumoral heterogeneity of genetic alterations in lung cancer. *(Image adapted from Jamal-Hanjani M, Quezada SA, Larkin J, Swanton C. Translational implications of tumor heterogeneity. Clin Cancer Res. 2015;21:1258–1266.)*

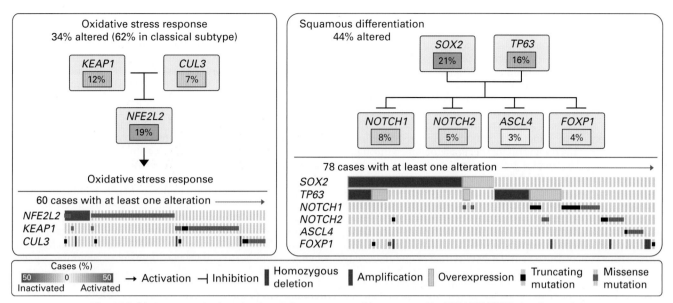

Fig. 11.5. Most commonly altered pathways in squamous cell lung cancer. The PI3K/RTK/RAS signaling pathway was altered in 69% of the samples, with multiple potential targets for therapy. The other two commonly affected pathways were the oxidative stress response and the genes involved in squamous differentiation. *PI3K*, phosphatidylinositol-3-OH kinase; *RAS*, RAt sarcoma; *RTK*, receptor tyrosine kinase. *(Reprinted, with permission, from Cancer Genome Atlas Research Network. Comprehensive genomic characterization of squamous cell lung cancers.* Nature. *2012;489:519–525.)*

EMERGING TECHNOLOGIES: THIRD-GENERATION SEQUENCING

Third-generation sequencing or single-molecule sequencing is the sequence analysis of individual molecules without prior cloning. This approach is associated with several potential benefits over NGS including overcoming the biases caused by PCR amplification and dephasing, leading to increased read lengths and a decrease in time to results. The increased read lengths may decrease the number of reads performed on each analysis as a necessary step to increase the coverage, possibly facilitating the bioinformatics analysis and improving the accuracy.[68,69] Another advantage of third-generation sequencing is the use of lower DNA input material, which could be particularly important in patients with unresected tumors, where the samples are often too small for NGS.

The two most advanced single-molecule sequencing platforms are the HeliScope and Pacific Biosciences platforms. Both platforms use SBS, in which laser excitation generates a fluorescent signal from the labeled nucleotides. Helicos Biosciences (Cambridge, MA, USA) introduced the first single-molecule DNA sequencer, HeliScope, which was based on labeled reversible chain-terminating nucleotides using an SBS method. This platform produces short reads of a maximal length of 55 bp and has not been widely adopted. PacBio RS from Pacific Biosciences (Menlo Park, CA, USA) is a platform based on the single-molecule real-time technology with nanostructures called zero-mode waveguides, each with a single DNA polymerase attached to it. The fluorescence of each nucleotide is detected in real time during its incorporation into the growing DNA strand. PacBio RS allows the simultaneous sequencing of 75,000 DNA molecules in parallel, and the read lengths are considerably longer than those with the HeliScope, averaging 1000 bp.[70]

An alternative approach is the use of sequencing with nanopores, which relies on the transit of single DNA molecules through nanoscale pores, with the bases detected by electric current or optic signal. Unlike all other sequencing methods, nanopore technologies usually do not require an exogenous label because they rely on the electronic or chemical structure of the different nucleotides for base calling.[68,71,72]

SEQUENCING IN SUBOPTIMAL SAMPLES

Formalin-Fixed Samples

Although fresh tissue from biopsy or surgery is the preferred specimen for most molecular tests, it is seldom available because of logistic issues related to the collection and storage of samples. Most specimens are formalin-fixed and paraffin-embedded (FFPE) tissue blocks, stored in the pathology laboratory. Formaldehyde from FFPE reacts with DNA and proteins with the formation of methylene, which crosslinks DNA to DNA, RNA, or proteins, resulting in sequence aberrations. Despite these challenges, studies comparing paired fresh-frozen and FFPE samples have shown the feasibility of NGS in FFPE samples.[73,74] In one such study, Spencer et al.[75] evaluated 27 cancer-related genes from 16 paired fresh-frozen and FFPE lung adenocarcinoma samples and observed no significant differences in the total number of reads, raw sequence error rate, or coverage of the target regions for the preselected genes. The agreement in base calling was greater than 99.99%. Nevertheless, because formalin promotes deamination of cytosine residues, there was an increase in C-to-T transitions in FFPE compared with fresh tissue.

Cytology Samples

Minimally invasive fine-needle aspiration (FNA) is a convenient method for establishing the diagnosis of solid tumors, with lower risks for complications compared with large-bore needle biopsies. However, although FNA is a standard modality for establishing morphologic diagnosis, the small tumor sample is often inadequate for NGS. Two studies have demonstrated the feasibility of FNA samples for NGS. Young et al.[76] evaluated FNA samples from 16 consecutive patients with pulmonary tumors and 26 with pancreatic tumors. NGS was performed with the Illumina HiSeq 2000 platform, and the tumor samples were evaluated for base substitutions, Indels, amplifications, homozygous deletions, and gene rearrangements. In this study, genomic profiles were successfully generated in 100% of patients with either pulmonary or pancreatic tumors. Kanagal-Shamanna et al.[77] evaluated 31 cytologic tumor specimens obtained through FNA, including 16 samples from patients with lung cancer. NGS was performed with the Torrent platform (V2.01; Life Technologies, Carlsbad, CA, USA) and the results were confirmed by at least one of three conventional platforms, including the Sanger sequencing, pyrosequencing, or MassARRAY system (Sequenom, San Diego, CA, USA). All tested samples underwent successful targeted sequencing of the selected panel of 46 genes, with a concordance of 100% between NGS and the conventional confirmatory platforms. Furthermore, NGS detected variants in 19 (61%) of 31 samples that were not detected by the traditional platforms. Therefore, the results of these two studies indicate that FNA may be an acceptable method to obtain samples for NGS.

Liquid Biopsies

Serial biopsies of patient tumors for treatment planning are becoming increasingly important with the development of therapies targeting resistance mechanisms in lung cancer patients progressing on tyrosine kinase inhibitors.[78–80] Because serial biopsies are invasive and associated with significant procedural risk, alternate methods of obtaining genomic DNA from circulating tumor cells, exosomes, or cell-free DNA (cfDNA) isolated from body fluids such as blood and urine (often referred to as "liquid biopsies") are gaining increasing popularity (Fig. 11.6).[81,82] Recent studies have shown the feasibility of these techniques in detecting targetable alterations without the need for invasive biopsy procedures.[83,84] In a recent analysis conducted by Wakelee et al.,[84] the ability to detect *EGFR* T790M mutations in patients enrolled into the phase 1/2 study TIGER-X was compared between assays based on cfDNA isolated from blood and urine, with DNA extracted from a matched tumor biopsy specimen. The agreements of T790M status between cfDNA obtained from blood and urine with matched tumor biopsy were 81.5% and 83.8%, respectively. Responses in T790M mutation-positive patients to rociletinib were comparable irrespective of the source of DNA.

Circulating tumor DNA assays are likely to contain DNA released from multiple tumor regions and can facilitate the

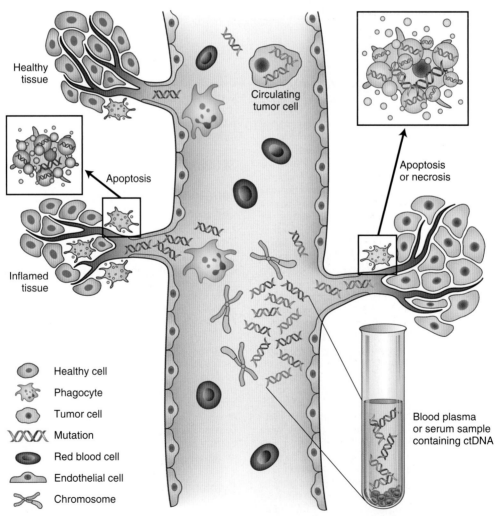

Fig. 11.6. Liquid biopsies for genotyping a tumor involve isolation of circulating free DNA that is released from dying cancer cells (through necrosis or apoptotic cell death), or DNA isolation from circulating tumor cells. *ctDNA*, circulating tumor DNA. *(Image adapted from Crowley E, Di Nicolantonio F, Loupakis F, Bardelli A. Liquid biopsy: monitoring cancer-genetics in the blood.* Nat Rev Clin Oncol. *2013;10:472–484.)*

identification of mutations missed on testing single-region tumor biopsies due to spatial heterogeneity in the clonal architecture of tumors. Seven patients in the study conducted by Wakelee et al.[84] who were negative for T790M mutations in the biopsy specimen, had detectable mutations through cfDNA testing and showed responses to rociletinib. These results demonstrate that circulating DNA testing could be complementary to traditional biopsy-based diagnostic testing for identifying targetable alterations in tumors and also facilitate the study of novel mechanisms underlying treatment resistance. Despite these advantages, these assays are limited by factors that affect the amount of DNA released by the tumor such as tumor size, disease burden, site of disease, and grade of the tumor.[85-87]

FUTURE DIRECTIONS

The use of NGS with integrated analyses of the genome, transcriptome, and epigenome of a large number (a few thousand) of tumor samples may allow a more comprehensive study of tumorigenesis, with the detection of low-frequency abnormalities that are unlikely to be found by first-generation unidimensional studies.[101] For example, the combined analysis of over 600 nonsmall cell lung cancer samples by TCGA highlighted the presence of low-frequency mutations in RTK-RAS-RAF pathway genes such as *VAV1*, *SOS1*, and *RASA1*, which were not mutated at a statistically significant level in previous studies owing to a sample size that was inadequate for their detection.

High tumor mutation burden has been shown to correlate with responses to immune checkpoint inhibitors.[102,103] In a recent analysis, McGranahan et al.[103] have also shown the clonality of neo-epitopes to play a predictive role in determining responses to immunotherapy, apart from the total mutation burden itself, with patients having a large fraction of clonal mutations showing durable responses compared with poor-responders whose tumors showed a large fraction of subclonal mutations. Determining the total mutation burden of a tumor sample and its clonal architecture therefore has important implications for therapy. The clonal architecture of a tumor can also serve as a prognostic biomarker and potentially guide adjuvant therapy in patients with early stage lung cancer, because patients with resected tumors with complex clonal architectures are more likely to relapse compared with those with less complex tumors.[64]

KEY REFERENCES

2. Stratton MR, Campbell PJ, Futreal PA. The cancer genome. *Nature.* 2009;458:719–724.
5. Vogelstein B, Papadopoulos N, Velculescu VE, Zhou S, Diaz LA, Kinzler KW. Cancer genome landscapes. *Science.* 2013;339:1546–1558.

12. Sanger F, Air GM, Barrell BG, et al. Nucleotide sequence of bacteriophage phi X174 DNA. *Nature.* 1977;265:687–695.
17. Meyerson M, Gabriel S, Getz G. Advances in understanding cancer genomes through second-generation sequencing. *Nat Rev Genet.* 2010;11:685–696.
50. Campbell JD, Alexandrov A, Kim J, et al. Distinct patterns of somatic genome alterations in lung adenocarcinomas and squamous cell carcinomas. *Nat Genet.* 2016;48(6):607–616.
51. Cancer Genome Atlas Research Network. Comprehensive molecular profiling of lung adenocarcinoma. *Nature.* 2014;511:543–550.
52. Cancer Genome Atlas Research Network. Comprehensive genomic characterization of squamous cell lung cancers. *Nature.* 2012;489:519–525.
53. Govindan R, Ding L, Griffith M, et al. Genomic landscape of non-small cell lung cancer in smokers and never-smokers. *Cell.* 2012;150:1121–1134.
54. Imielinski M, Berger AH, Hammerman PS, et al. Mapping the hallmarks of lung adenocarcinoma with massively parallel sequencing. *Cell.* 2012;150:1107–1120.
55. George J, Lim JS, Jang SJ, et al. Comprehensive genomic profiles of small cell lung cancer. *Nature.* 2015;524:47–53.
56. Peifer M, Fernández-Cuesta L, Sos ML, et al. Integrative genome analyses identify key somatic driver mutations of small-cell lung cancer. *Nat Genet.* 2012;44:1104–1110.
57. Rudin CM, Durinck S, Stawiski EW, et al. Comprehensive genomic analysis identifies SOX2 as a frequently amplified gene in small-cell lung cancer. *Nat Genet.* 2012;44:1111–1116.
58. Seo JS, Ju YS, Lee WC, et al. The transcriptional landscape and mutational profile of lung adenocarcinoma. *Genome Res.* 2012;22:2109–2119.
59. Hanahan D, Weinberg RA. Hallmarks of cancer: the next generation. *Cell.* 2011;144:646–674.
60. Hanahan D, Weinberg RA. The hallmarks of cancer. *Cell.* 2000;100:57–70.
61. Deleted in review.
62. McGranahan N, Favero F, de Bruin EC, Birkbak NJ, Szallasi Z, Swanton C. Clonal status of actionable driver events and the timing of mutational processes in cancer evolution. *Sci Transl Med.* 2015;7: 283ra54.
63. de Bruin EC, McGranahan N, Mitter R, et al. Spatial and temporal diversity in genomic instability processes defines lung cancer evolution. *Science.* 2014;346:251–256.
64. Zhang J, Fujimoto J, Wedge DC, et al. Intratumor heterogeneity in localized lung adenocarcinomas delineated by multiregion sequencing. *Science.* 2014;346:256–259.
65. Jamal-Hanjani M, Quezada SA, Larkin J, Swanton C. Translational implications of tumor heterogeneity. *Clin Cancer Res.* 2015;21:1258–1266.
102. Rizvi NA, Hellmann MD, Snyder A, et al. Cancer immunology. Mutational landscape determines sensitivity to PD-1 blockade in non-small cell lung cancer. *Science.* 2015;348:124–128.
103. McGranahan N, Furness AJ, Rosenthal R, et al. Clonal neoantigens elicit T cell immunoreactivity and sensitivity to immune checkpoint blockade. *Science.* 2016;351:1463–1469.

See Expertconsult.com for full list of references.

12 Epigenetic Events in Lung Cancer: Chromatin Remodeling and DNA Methylation

Ite A. Laird-Offringa and Montse Sanchez-Cespedes

SUMMARY OF KEY POINTS

- Distinct cellular phenotypes are based on differential gene expression, which is achieved through heritable epigenetic modifications that maintain active and inactive chromosomal regions.
- Epigenetic mechanisms include DNA methylation, histone modifications, regulatory DNA-binding proteins, regulatory RNAs, genome-organizing proteins, and chromatin remodeling complexes, all of which can be altered in lung cancer.
- Both *genetic* and *epigenetic* alterations can contribute to lung cancer and they can interact; genetic changes in epigenetic modifiers can affect the epigenome, and epigenetic silencing of genes involved in genome integrity can lead to genomic alterations.
- Numerous DNA methylation changes are seen in lung cancer, most commonly hypermethylation of promoter CpG-dense regions and loss of methylation in gene bodies, but only a fraction of DNA methylation alterations has functional consequences.
- DNA methylation alterations in a variety of bodily fluids can be used as biomarkers for the presence of lung cancer.
- Proteins involved in chromatin remodeling are commonly altered in lung cancer, with the ATPase BRG1 frequently mutated in non-small cell lung cancer tumors and cell lines.
- Epigenetic alterations are in principle reversible; epigenetic therapies thus offer opportunities for treatment by undoing cancer-driving epigenetic changes or by activating targets for therapy such as cancer/testis antigens and others.

The cells that make up the human body exhibit an incredible variety of phenotypes, despite the fact that they all carry the same genome, inherited from a single fertilized egg. This phenotypic diversity arises from the different gene expression profiles in each distinct cell type and is achieved by creating and maintaining specific activated and inactivated genomic regions as cells differentiate into their destined types. These distinct genomic regions are established through the layering of information, or so-called biomarks, on top of the genome. The study of these regions and marks is called epigenetics.

Epigenetic information can come in many forms (Fig. 12.1). One form is the direct chemical modification of DNA. The best studied chemical modification is DNA methylation,[1] but more recently, hydroxymethylation, formylation, and carboxylation have also been noted.[2] Chemical marks can also be deposited on the proteins that interact with DNA, the most prominent of which are the histones. Histones can be decorated with a wide variety of modifications, which can affect the accessibility of DNA to regulatory factors and thereby modulate the ability of genes to be expressed.[3,4] In addition to covalent modifications of the histone tails, chromatin structure is also regulated by movement of nucleosomes in an adenosine triphosphate (ATP)–dependent manner through the activity of chromatin remodeling complexes.[5–7] These complexes utilize ATP to disrupt nucleosome-DNA contacts and render DNA available to proteins requiring access to histones or DNA during distinct cellular processes. Besides histones and nucleosomes, other proteins can affect the epigenetic readout of the genome: numerous proteins or protein complexes bind directly or indirectly to the DNA and can either affect transcription through modulating the activity of enhancers or promoters, or can influence genomic organization and thereby gene activity. Lastly, regulatory RNAs, such as microRNAs (miRNAs) and long noncoding RNAs, exist that can epigenetically regulate gene expression.[6,8,9] Collectively, these biomarks on the DNA are referred to as the epigenome; they are inherited following cell division, allowing cell phenotypes to be passed on to daughter cells.

The importance of epigenetic marks in retaining proper cell phenotypes implies that their disruption would lead to disease. Indeed, it has become abundantly clear that epigenetic deregulation contributes very importantly to numerous diseases, including cancer.[8,10–13] Epigenetic alterations have been widely implicated in the development and progression of lung cancer.[14–19] Understanding the consequences of epigenetic changes can help dissect the molecular basis of lung cancer, providing insights into cancer development and progression, and thus new focal points for targeted therapies.[20] In addition, epigenetic alterations in lung cancer show potential as molecular markers that could be applied to early detection, tumor classification, risk assessment, prognostication, and monitoring of cancer recurrence.[14,21] Lastly, given that epigenetic information is layered on the genome without alteration of the DNA sequence, it is in principle reversible and is a prime target for the development and application of new therapies. Epigenetic drugs, such as histone deacetylase inhibitors and DNA methylation inhibitors, are in clinical trials for numerous cancers including those of the lung.[22,23] With the advent of ever more powerful tools for genome-wide assessment of epigenetic marks, our understanding of the lung cancer epigenome and its application to diagnosis and treatment promises to increase dramatically in the years to come.

In this chapter, we review the basic concepts of epigenetics and discuss the current knowledge concerning epigenetic alterations in lung cancer, including the types of changes identified and their pathologic and clinical implications. Given the large number of epigenetic alterations analyzed to date and the dramatic acceleration in acquired data, it is impossible to be comprehensive in one chapter. Therefore, we discuss the basic principles and focus in more detail on two specific areas: chromatin remodeling and DNA methylation. These two examples beautifully illustrate the importance of considering the interplay between genetic and epigenetic alterations in cancer. Due to space limitations, reviews are cited throughout as a source of more detailed information.

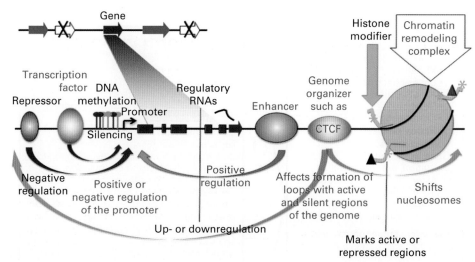

Fig. 12.1. Overview of epigenetic mechanisms. Gene expression can be affected by numerous epigenetic mechanisms, as indicated in the diagram. From left to right: Repressors can negatively regulate transcription; transcription factors can modulate transcription and aid in the response to environmental cues; DNA methylation, when present in promoter CpG islands (as seen in cancer) is commonly associated with gene silencing; regulatory RNAs include microRNAs and long noncoding RNAs that can upregulate or downregulate genes through a variety of mechanisms; enhancers can lie upstream or downstream of genes and can stimulate gene expression from a distance; genome organizers are proteins such as CCCTC-binding factor that create boundaries between genomic regions and aid in the higher order structuring of the genome; histone modifying enzymes affect the modifications of histone tails, which in turn can loosen or tighten chromatin, facilitating or decreasing gene expression; chromatin remodeling complexes organize the chromatin and can move the nucleosomes (consisting of an octamer of histones with approximately 150 nucleotides of DNA wound around them), modulating the access of other factors to the DNA.

GENETIC AND EPIGENETIC INTERACTIONS

Initial research into the molecular basis of lung cancer focused on genetic alterations, such as mutations, loss of heterozygosity, deletions, and gene amplification.[24,25] Well-known examples of genetic alterations in lung cancer include mutations in V-Ki-ras2 Kirsten rat sarcoma viral oncogene homolog *(KRAS)*, the epidermal growth factor receptor *(EFGR)*, and tumor protein 53 *(TP53)*.[26] However, it has become abundantly clear that epigenetic alterations contribute equally importantly to the development and progression of lung cancer.[14–19,27,28] Epigenetic alterations seen in lung cancer consist of changes in histone modifications, alterations in chromatin structure and chromatin-associated proteins, changes in regulatory RNAs such as microRNAs, and DNA methylation changes (both loss and gain of methylation).

The interaction between genetic and epigenetic hits in cancer cells further amplifies the consequences of these molecular alterations (Fig. 12.2).[10,29,30] For example, as discussed later, genetic alterations in the genes encoding components of the epigenetic machinery (such as histone (de)acetylases, chromatin remodeling complexes, and DNA methyltransferases) can affect the activity of these enzymes and thereby the transcriptional activity of many additional genes. Somatic changes in parts of the epigenetic machinery are found in numerous cancers, including lung cancer.[10,31] This potential for genetic alterations to affect epigenetics is further underscored by the reported link between genetic polymorphisms in several genes encoding epigenetic enzymes, and lung cancer risk.[31] Conversely, epigenetic alterations can lead to further genetic damage. For example, hypermethylation of DNA repair genes or genes encoding detoxification enzymes can affect the cell's susceptibility to mutagenesis and could result in the genetic (in)activation of additional genes.[32] DNA methylation of 6-O-methylguanine DNA methyltransferase *(MGMT)*, an enzyme involved in the repair of alkylated guanine, is commonly seen in lung cancer.[33] Inactivation of *MGMT* has been linked to

an increase in the frequency of *RAS* gene mutation.[34] In support of their potential to affect cancer development, polymorphisms in *MGMT* and other DNA repair genes have been linked to lung cancer risk in various populations.[35–37] These examples illustrate that genetic and epigenetic changes should not be seen as independent, but rather as components of a complex interactive network that is responsible for the development and progression of numerous cancers, including lung cancer. Combined analysis of both types of molecular changes will accelerate the elucidation of the molecular pathways affected in lung cancer and may be especially helpful in characterizing particular types of lung cancer (e.g., histologic subtypes or lung cancer from smokers compared with nonsmokers). This holistic view of epigenetic alterations is also highly relevant to the clinic, as the use of certain cytotoxic drugs may potentiate or inhibit the efficacy of epigenetic drugs and vice versa.[38–41]

HISTONE MODIFICATIONS AND THEIR ROLE IN LUNG CANCER

The nucleosomal core around which DNA is coiled is composed of two molecules each of histones 2A, 2B, 3, and 4. The lysine and arginine-rich *N*-terminal regions extend from the core and can be heavily decorated with mono-, di-, and trimethylation, acetylation, ubiquitination, phosphorylation, and other modifications.[3] These modifications do not exist in isolation; functional and physical crosstalk ensures a complex web of epigenetic signals, in which DNA methyltransferases, methyl-binding proteins, histone variants, histone modifying enzymes, and other chromatin and transcriptional components play a role (Fig. 12.3).[42] Many of the enzymes that modify histones recognize other modifications on the same or different histone tails or on DNA. For example, proteins that bind to methylated DNA frequently carry additional domains that interact directly or indirectly with histone-modifying proteins such as deacetylases.[43] Acetylation of histones on lysine promote active transcription. On one hand, this modification

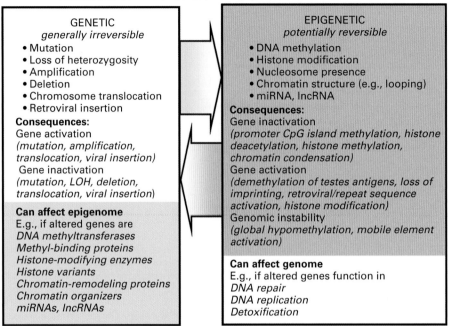

Fig. 12.2. Interaction between genetic and epigenetic alterations in cancer. Left panel: Genetic hits, which are generally irreversible and can result in activation or inactivation of the altered gene. If such a gene encodes a product involved in epigenetic regulation, like a histone methyltransferase, a DNA methyl-binding protein, a histone isoform, an enzyme that adds or removes histone modifications, or a protein that interacts with such modifications (transcriptional regulators, coactivators, or corepressors), this finding could result in epigenetic alterations. Right panel: Epigenetic hits are potentially reversible, and when they occur in genes that affect the integrity of the genome, such as DNA repair genes or genes encoding proteins involved in DNA replication or detoxification, they can increase the likelihood of acquisition of additional genetic alterations.

reduces a positive charge and minimizes the electrostatic attraction of the histone tails for the DNA phosphate backbone, thereby relaxing chromatin structure. On the other hand, acetylated histone N-terminal tails are landing pads for bromodomain-containing proteins, such as transcriptional coactivator p300/CBP associated factor and TAF1, a component of the transcription initiation complex.[4,44] Key acetylation marks are histone 3 lysine 27 acetylation (H3K27Ac), a mark found predominantly on active enhancers, and H3K9Ac, a mark found mainly on active promoters. Multiple enzymes that add or remove acetyl groups exist in the cell, and the deacetylases are particularly promising therapeutic targets in cancer.[45] In addition to acetylation, common histone tail modifications are methylation, ubiquitination, and phosphorylation.[46] Methylation does not affect histone tail charge, functioning instead by altering protein/protein interactions. One or two methyl groups can be added to arginine and up to three to lysine; the effects depend on the modified position and the number of added methyl groups. For example, histone 3 lysine 9 and lysine 27 trimethylation (H3K9me3, H3K27me3) are repressive marks, whereas H3K4me3 is found in transcribed regions.

As yet, relatively little is known about how histone modification is affected in lung cancer; molecular changes on the histone N-terminal regions are much more difficult to interrogate than DNA methylation changes. The most commonly used technique is chromatin immunoprecipitation (ChIP), in which formaldehyde crosslinking of cells is followed by specific immunoprecipitation of the proteins of interest (such as particular histone modifications) and local polymerase chain reaction (PCR)–based interrogation of specific regions. Due to advances in high-throughput sequencing technologies, ChIP can now be carried out genome-wide to gain global insights into the marks on or protein occupancy of the entire genome. In one study, researchers classified patients with

non-small cell lung cancer (NSCLC) into seven distinct groups based on differential histone modifications and noted differences in survival depending on histology and histone 3 modifications.[42] This early report hints at the potential use of this kind of epigenetic characterization to guide treatment. A key challenge in furthering these studies is the large amount of material needed for genome-wide interrogations, which limits current analyses largely to lung cancer cell lines. However, as the ability to extract epigenomic information from ever smaller quantities of material improves, the analysis of archival tumor specimens will become possible.

As alluded to previously, alterations in the enzymes that deposit or remove histone marks can lead to further epigenetic changes. A mutation of the histone acetyltransferase EP300 was found several years ago in a small cell lung cancer (SCLC) cell line.[47] More recently, genome-wide sequencing approaches have provided further evidence for alterations in numerous genes encoding enzymes involved in histone modification (Table 12.1). Mutations of the histone acetyltransferases CREBBP and EP300 and the histone methyltransferases MLL and MLL2 have now been detected in SCLC.[48] In NSCLC, mutations in multiple histone methyltransferases including ASH1L, MLL3, MLL4, WHSC1L1, and SETD2 have been noted.[49–51] Among these, one of the mutations in SETD2 was identified in a lung tumor from a never-smoker. More recently, amplification of the histone methyltransferase *SETDB1* gene was found in a subset of NSCLC and SCLC cell lines and primary tumors.[52] Depletion of SETDB1 expression in amplified cells was shown to reduce cancer growth in cell culture and in nude mice, whereas its overexpression increased tumor invasiveness. Mutations in histone demethylases and deacetylates have also been noted in NSCLC, further underlining the contributions of epigenetic deregulatory events in lung cancer.

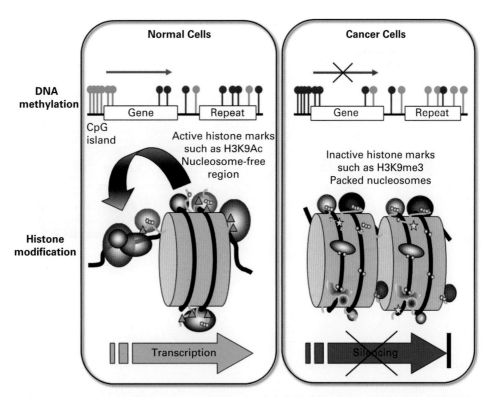

Fig. 12.3. Epigenetic abnormalities in cancer. In nontumor cells (left), CpG islands are generally unmethylated (green lollipops), whereas sporadic CpGs are usually methylated (red lollipops). In actively transcribed genes, the structure of chromatin is loose, allowing access of the transcriptional machinery to the promoter region. Acetylation of lysines (triangles) in the *N*-terminal tails of histones 3 and 4 reduces positive charge and relaxes the attraction to negatively charged DNA. Acetylation, mono-, di-, and trimethylation (balls), and other modifications such as phosphorylation and sumoylation (stars) of the histone tails can mediate interactions directly or indirectly with the transcriptional machinery and with enzymes that can add further posttranslational modifications. In cancer cells (right), a genome-wide loss of DNA methylation at sporadic CpGs and previously methylated sequences such as repeats is seen. (In certain cases this can lead to gene activation, not shown.) Simultaneously, many promoter CpG islands become hypermethylated, which can result in silencing of tumor suppressor genes. Methyl-binding proteins interacting with methylated cytosines can recruit histone deacetylases, which can in turn lead to reduced chromatin access and transcriptional silencing. This model is a simplification; methylation, histone modification, and transcription are not always concordant, not all methylated genes are silenced, nor are all silent genes methylated.

TABLE 12.1 Histone-Modifying Enzymes Altered in Lung Cancer[a]

Enzyme	Lung Cancer Type	Reference(s)
HISTONE DEMETHYLASES		
KDM6A	NSCLC	49
HISTONE METHYLTRANSFERASES		
ASH1L	NSCLC	49,51
MLL	NSCLC	49
MLL2	NSCLC	49
MLL3	NSCLC	51
MLL4	NSCLC	51
SETD2	NSCLC	50,51
SETDB1	NSCLC	52
WHSC1L1	NSCLC	51
MLL	SCLC	237
MLL2	SCLC	48
HISTONE ACETYLTRANSFERASES		
CREBBP	SCLC	237
EP300	SCLC	237
HISTONE DEACTYLASES		
HDAC9	NSCLC	49
HDAC9	NSCLC	49

[a]These data, obtained from high-throughput approaches, are preliminary, and validation in larger sets of well-characterized lung tumors is needed. *NSCLC*, Non-small cell lung cancer; *SCLC*, small cell lung cancer.

Abnormalities in genes encoding histone acetylases and deacetylases have also been found in noncancerous diseases of the lung, including chronic obstructive pulmonary disease (COPD), an irreversible and slowly progressive condition characterized by airflow limitation. Oxidative stress and inflammation are the major hallmarks of COPD, which, like lung cancer, has cigarette smoking as the major etiologic factor. In COPD, oxidative stress enhances inflammation by activating various kinase signaling pathways that lead to chromatin modifications (histone acetylation/deacetylation and histone methylation/demethylation). The activation of these pathways orchestrates several responses to stress, including proinflammatory and antioxidative responses. One of the main hurdles that precludes the clinical treatment of COPD is its resistance to antiinflammatory glucocorticoid (GC) treatment. GCs are not only involved in lung embryonic development and normal lung function but are also critical for lung cancer prevention.[53,54] In this regard, a failure to respond to GCs constitutes a risk factor for developing lung cancer, especially in smokers.[55] GC-mediated suppression of inflammation involves the recruitment by the GC receptor of histone deacetylase 2 (HDAC2) to the genes that mediate inflammation, resulting in histone deacetylation and reduced transcription.[56] The GC-resistance in patients with COPD appears to occur as the result of a marked reduction in the levels and activity of HDAC2 in the lung parenchyma, provoked by the chemicals in cigarette smoke and by oxidative stress.

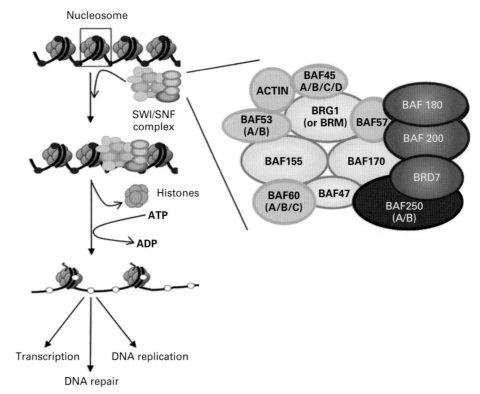

Fig. 12.4. The chromatin remodeling complex SWI/SNF. On the left, a schematic representation that depicts how the SWI/SNF complex alters the structure of the nearby nucleosomes, thereby permitting increased access of transcription factors, DNA polymerases, and other DNA-binding proteins, to the DNA. On the right, the different components of the SWI/SNF chromatin complex in humans are indicated. Light gray circles highlight the components that constitute the core members of the complex; the black-lined gray ovals show the noncore members that are common for both the BAF and the pBAF complexes; the purple and the blue ovals show the components that are unique to the BAF and the pBAF, respectively.

Taking into account that patients with bronchial obstructive changes, including COPD, are at increased risk for lung cancer,[55] and that lung cancer cells are refractory to GC,[57] it is interesting to speculate that the acquisition of resistance to GC may be among the factors that contribute to this increased lung cancer risk. However, there is as yet little evidence for decreased HDAC2 levels in lung cancer. One of the few reports examining the levels of HDACs in lung cancer specimens demonstrated a reduced expression of class II HDACs (HDACs 4–7, 9, and 10), especially HDAC10, and an association with poor prognosis.[58] In contrast, a different study reported that increased expression of HDAC1 in tumor cells was an independent predictor of poor prognosis in patients with lung adenocarcinoma.[59] Although the involvement of alterations in HDACs in lung cancer remains unclear, they should be considered as one of the possible mechanisms responsible for resistance to GC and similar compounds. Regardless of the possible involvement of alterations in HDACs, as discussed previously, loss of activity of chromatin remodeling complexes is among the most common causes of unresponsiveness to GC in lung cancer.[57]

CHROMATIN REMODELING COMPLEXES

Chromatin is controlled by multiprotein complexes that use the energy of ATP to disrupt histone–DNA contacts, thereby providing access to proteins that must contact DNA or histones during different cellular processes.[5,7] These processes include the establishment of transcriptional control during embryonic development, cell differentiation, and the reprogramming of somatic cells, as well as the formation of heterochromatin, the execution of DNA repair, and DNA replication.[7,60,61]

Four different families of chromatin remodeling complexes have been described: SWI/SNF, INO80, ISWI, and CHDs, distinguishable by the identity of their ATPase subunit.[7] Several chromatin remodeling complexes have been implicated in cancer initiation and progression, most prominently the "switch/sucrose not fermenting" (SWI/SNF) complex. Therefore, we focus mainly on the SWI/SNF complex. However, it is anticipated that other chromatin remodeling complexes may also be ultimately found to be relevant in carcinogenesis. The name SWI/SNF describes genes first identified in yeast screens for mutants affecting mating type switching and sucrose fermenting.[62,63] The SWI/SNF complex is powered by either of two ATPases that are highly homologous and have similar domains: ATP-dependent helicase SMARCA2 (BRM) or ATP-dependent helicase SMARCA4 (BRG1). In mammals, two different SWI/SNF multiprotein complexes have been described: BRG1 associated factors (BAF), also called SWI/SNF-α, and polybromo-BRG1 associated factors (PBAF), also known as SWI/SNF-β. The complexes contain a number of common proteins, such as BAF170, BAF155, BAF60a/b/c, BAF57, BAF53a/b, BAF47, BAF45a/b/c/d, and β-actin, but differ with respect to other components (Fig. 12.4).[7] The β complex contains up to three additional members: BAF180, BAF200, and BRD7. However, the main difference between the SWI/SNF complexes is the participating ATPase. In SWI/SNF-α the ATPase can be either BRG1 or BRM, but in SWI/SNF-β the ATPase is only BRG1. Numerous findings implicate subunits of these complexes in the development of lung cancer, as will be discussed. The nomenclature for involved factors is sometimes redundant (Table 12.2).

TABLE 12.2 Subunits of the Chromatin Remodeling Complex, SWI/SNF, and Mutations in Cancer

Name			Mutated in Cancer	Mutated in Lung Cancer	Characteristics of the Mutations in Lung Cancer
Official HNGC	**Other Common**	**Other Less Common**			
SMARCA4	BRG1	SNF2-like4, SNF2B, SNF2, SWI2, SNF2LB	Yes	Yes	More than 70% of truncating and nonsense mutations[66] Mutations preferentially in NSCLC[66] Mutations preferentially in smokers[68] Mutations mutually exclusive with amplification of MYC and mutations of EGFR[66]
ARID1A	SMARCF1, BAF250A	ELD, B120, OSA1, P270, hELD, BM029, MRD14 hOSA1,	Yes	Yes	About 50% of truncating and nonsense mutations[50] Mutations preferentially in NSCLC[50]
ARID2	BAF200	P200	Yes	Yes	About 50% of truncating and nonsense mutations[238] Mutations preferentially in NSCLC[51] Mutations in smokers and nonsmokers[238]
SMARCA2	BRM	SNF2, SWI2, NCBRS, Sth1p, BAF190, SNF2L2	Yes	NI	
SMARCB1	INI1, SNF5, BAF47	Snr1, MRD15, RTPS1, Sfh1p, hSNFS, SNF5L1	Yes	No	
SMARCC1	BAF155	Rsc8, SRG3, SWI3, CRACC1	Yes	NI	
ACTIN	ACTB		NI	NI	
ACTL6A	BAF53A	ACTL6A	NI	NI	
ACTL6B	BAF53B	ACTL6B,	NI	NI	
ARID1B	BAF250B	OSA2, 6A3–5, DAN15, MRD12, P250R, BRIGHT	Yes	NI	
BRD7		BP75; NAG4; CELTIX1	Yes	NI	
BRD9		PRO9856; LAVS3040	NI	NI	
PBRM1	BAF180	PB1	Yes	NI	
SMARCC2	BAF170	CRACC2, Rsc8	NI	NI	
SMARCD1	BAF60A	Rsc6p, CRACD1	Yes	NI	
SMARCD2	BAF60B	Rsc6p, CRACD2, PRO2451	NI	NI	
SMARCD3	BAF60C	Rsc6p, CRACD3	NI	NI	
SMARCE1	BAF57		Yes	NI	

HGNC, Human Genome Organization Gene Nomenclature Committee; *NI*, nonexhaustive information; *NSCLC*, non-small cell lung cancer.

Genetic Alterations at SWI/SNF Chromatin Remodeling Factors in Lung Cancer

The first observation that linked chromatin remodeling and cancer development was the presence of inactivating mutations at *SNF5* (also named *SMARCB1*) in rare cases of pediatric tumors, especially in malignant rhabdoid tumors.[64] Mutations at *SNF5* arise either somatically or in the germline, in the case of the germline conferring a cancer predisposition syndrome.[65] Although *SNF5* inactivation is infrequent in lung cancer, alterations at *BRG1* (also named *SMARCA4*) are a more common event. Inactivation of *BRG1* in lung cancer was first found by the detection of homozygous deletions of this gene in a small subset of cell lines of different tumor origins, including those from lung.[19] The restoration of *BRG1* in lung cancer cells induced growth arrest and a flattened phenotype.[19] A few years later, it was reported that alterations at *BRG1* occur in about one-third of NSCLC cell lines.[66] A role of *BRG1* loss in lung cancer has been verified in subsequent studies.[49,50] Taking into account our current genetic knowledge of lung cancer, *BRG1* can be considered among the five most commonly altered tumor suppressor genes in NSCLC, after *TP53*, *CDKN2A*, and *LKB1*.[50,67] In the vast majority of cases, the *BRG1* mutations detected in lung cancer cell lines are biallelic and the mechanisms for inactivation include loss of one allele in combination with deletion of the other allele or frameshifts, indels, and nonsense/missense mutations, most of them yielding a truncated protein.[17] The biallelic loss and inactivation mutations of *BRG1* leave little doubt that *BRG1* is a bona fide tumor suppressor gene, critical in the development of a large proportion of lung cancers. Mutations

at *BRG1* are more frequently detected in lung cancer cell lines as compared with lung primary tumors,[68,69] similar to the findings for other tumor suppressor genes, such as *TP53*, *CDKN2A*, and *LKB1*.[67] This finding could be attributed to technical difficulties related to the normal cell contamination often associated with the genetic analysis of primary tumors. In this regard, immunohistochemical evaluation of BRG1 levels in lung primary NSCLCs supports the absence of protein in 30% of the tumors.[70] In contrast to *BRG1*, genetic inactivation of BRM has not been reported in lung cancer.[57] Some lung cancer cell lines have no detectable BRM protein by Western blot, but the mechanisms underlying the apparent loss of *BRM* protein are still elusive.

To date there is little information about the clinical, pathologic, and molecular correlations with the loss of *BRG1* expression in lung cancer. Approximately one-third of NSCLC cell lines and 5% of SCLC cell lines have featured *BRG1* inactivation.[66] Moreover, these alterations seem to be associated with smoking and frequently coexist with mutations at other commonly altered genes in lung cancer, such as *TP53*, *KRAS*, and *LKB1*.[17] However, it was noted that mutations in *BRG1* were mutually exclusive with amplification of the V-Myc avian myelocytomatosis viral oncogene homolog *(MYC)* oncogenes.[57,71] Although these findings are still preliminary, they indicate that *MYC* and *BRG1* exert a similar biologic function during lung tumorigenesis, which is in agreement with functional observations demonstrating that the SWI/SNF complex is required for the *CMYC*-mediated gene transactivation and that recruitment of SWI/SNF to the promoters regulated by MYC depends on MYC-INI1 interaction.[72] In further support of the MYC-BRG1 functional relationship in lung cancer cells, it was found that wild-type BRG1 is required to decrease the levels of the MYC protein in response to differentiation agents.[57]

Immunohistochemical analysis of BRG1 in 41 primary lung adenocarcinomas and 19 primary lung squamous cell carcinomas showed that loss of nuclear expression of BRG1 and/or BRM was associated with worse survival in patients with NSCLC.[70] In another study, the levels of several core proteins involved in the chromatin remodeling machinery were determined in 150 lung adenocarcinomas and 150 squamous cell carcinomas, using immunohistochemistry.[73] Positive nuclear BRM staining correlated with a favorable prognosis in both patients with lung adenocarcinomas and primary lung squamous cell carcinomas with a 5-year survival rate of 53.5% compared with 32.3% for those whose tumors were negative for BRM ($p = 0.015$). Furthermore, patients whose tumors stained positive for both BRM and BRG1 had a significantly better 5-year survival (72% compared with 33.6% for those whose tumors were positive for either or negative for both markers) ($p = 0.013$). In another study, the authors found that loss of expression of BRG1 and BRM was found to be frequent in solid predominant lung adenocarcinomas and in tumors with low expression of lung transcription factor NKX2-1 (previously called thyroid transcription factor-1 or TTF-1) and low cytokeratins and E-cadherin.[74] The same study demonstrated that the loss of BRG1 protein was mutually exclusive with EGFR mutations, which is in agreement with the higher frequency of BRG1 mutations in lung cancers in smokers (Table 12.2).

In addition to mutations in *BRG1* and *BRM*, novel deep sequencing technologies of lung cancer samples have allowed the identification of inactivating mutations in numerous genes encoding core members of the SWI/SNF complex, including *ARID1A* and *ARID2* (Table 12.2).[75] Most of the data come from deep sequencing technologies applied to the whole genome or to exomes, a type of approach that leads to a certain number of false-negative results. It is anticipated that the rates of inactivation at each individual component of the SWI/SNF complex in the distinct types of tumors will become known in the coming years. Intriguingly, germline mutations of components of the SWI/SNF chromatin remodeling complex (i.e., *SMARCB1, BRG1/SMARCA4, SMARCE1, ARID1A, ARID1B,* and *BRM/ SMARCA2*) have also been noted and they have been linked to human syndromes. In particular, the very rare autosomal dominant syndromes Nicolaides–Baraitser and Coffin–Siris show several common clinical characteristics, including multiple congenital malformations, microcephaly, and intellectual disability.[75] To date, there is no information as to whether these syndromes confer a predisposition to lung cancer or any other type of cancer.

Although abnormal functioning of chromatin remodeling is now acknowledged to be involved in the development of lung cancer, our knowledge of the potential role of other epigenetic modifiers in lung cancer is still limited. As efforts to sequence the genomes of more tumors continue, more genes encoding chromatin modifiers are likely to emerge as mutated in lung cancer. However, functional analysis and validation in larger sets of well-characterized lung tumors will need to be undertaken to definitely determine the relevance of these different mutations in the development of lung cancer and to assess the precise frequency of alterations and the possible correlates with histopathology, etiology, and clinical parameters.

Functional Consequences of Abnormalities in Chromatin Remodelers and Other Epigenetic Modifiers in Lung Cancer Development

As previously mentioned, chromatin remodeling complexes function as transcriptional regulators of large sets of genes involved in multiple developmental pathways, including early embryonic development and tissue specification.[60,61,76] The control exerted by the SWI/SNF complex on some of these processes is related to its involvement in regulating hormone-responsive promoters. Specific components of the SWI/SNF complex bind to various nuclear receptors for estrogens, progesterone, corticoids, retinoic acid, and vitamin D3, leading to their recruitment to gene-specific promoters.[77–79] On the other hand, the ligands that bind specific nuclear receptors, such as retinoids and corticoids, are known to be critical for lung embryonic development as well as for normal lung differentiation and function.[53,54,80] Given the involvement of the SWI/SNF complex in tissue specification and in developmental programs, one of the processes that would be expected to be disrupted in cancer cells carrying inactivated SWI/SNF is the capability to sustain gene expression programs during cell differentiation. Indeed, restoration of BRG1 activity in lung cancer cells induces gene expression changes, increasing resemblance to normal lung gene expression signatures.[57] Furthermore, it was shown that lung cancer cells require wild-type BRG1 to respond to retinoic acid or GC treatment. Together, these findings support the notion that an inactive BRG1 confers resistance to retinoic acid and GCs, which prevent cancer cell differentiation. Given that BRG1 is part of the SWI/SNF complex, alterations in other members of the SWI/SNF complex may act through the same mechanism, although this hypothesis must be tested.

Several cancer-related proteins, such as P21, BRCA1, LKB1, SMADs, CFOS, CMYC, and FANCA, have been associated with BRG1 or other components of the SWI/SNF complex, supporting the participation of the SWI/SNF complex in other important cell processes, such as cell-cycle control, DNA repair, and the regulation of apoptosis in response to DNA damage.[17,81] However, how the SWI/SNF complex affects these processes in the development of lung cancer is still poorly understood. A mouse model that permits conditional biallelic knockout of *BRG1* in lung epithelial cells indicates that the loss of both *BRG1* alleles induces apoptosis, as determined by significant increase in Apo-BrdUrd and cleaved caspase-3 in nontransformed lung epithelial cells.[82] Furthermore, the homozygous loss of BRG1 in the lungs of the mice strongly potentiated the development of lung tumors after exposure to the carcinogen ethyl carbamate, which binds to DNA and generates DNA adducts. The observation of DNA adducts suggests that in the absence of a functional SWI/ SNF complex, timely DNA repair is not guaranteed and, consequently, cells are inadequately protected from the deleterious consequences of DNA damage.

DNA METHYLATION

Of the covalent epigenetic marks, DNA methylation has been the most widely studied. The methyl group is deposited at the 5-position of cytosine, in the context of a small inverted repeat: a CpG dinucleotide. The palindromic nature of methylation allows the propagation of this modification following DNA replication. In the normal mammalian genome, some areas are heavily methylated, such as sections of the X chromosomes in females, pericentromeric regions, and parentally imprinted genes. Indeed, DNA methylation is essential for proper development and viability.[83] Methylation in mammals is carried out by at least three enzymes: the maintenance DNA methyltransferase *DNMT1* (which methylates daughter strands following DNA replication) and de novo DNA methyltransferases *DNMT3A* and *3B*.[84] All three genes are essential, as illustrated by mouse knock-out experiments.[84] A large number of DNMT splice isoforms exist, a number of which appear to target particular genes or areas of the genome and some of which are implicated in cancer.[85,86] Overexpression of DNMTs and the associated factor UHRF1 has been linked to lung cancer.[87–91] CpG dinucleotides exist in two general environments in normal cells: sparsely distributed, and clustered (Fig. 12.3).[1] On the one hand, CpGs are sprinkled throughout the genome, and these CpGs are usually methylated. Spontaneous deamination of methyl-C results in thymine, which is less efficiently repaired than the uracil resulting from deamination of unmethylated cytosine. This has resulted in depletion over time of CpGs in areas that are usually methylated.[92] Thus, the remaining dense clusters of CpGs, called CpG islands,[93] are presumed to be normally unmethylated. It is estimated that about half of human genes contain such CpG islands in their promoter regions.[94]

In cancer, a profound disruption of DNA methylation is seen (Fig. 12.3).[1,10,95–98] Broadly stated, global hypomethylation occurs, in combination with local hypermethylation. Loss of DNA methylation has been thought to contribute to carcinogenesis in two possible ways: the transcriptional activation of previously methylated sequences and the loss of chromosome stability. In contrast, the local hypermethylation at promoter CpG islands has been assumed to contribute to carcinogenesis through gene inactivation, silencing a wide variety of growth control and tumor suppressor genes, such as genes involved in proliferation, adhesion, apoptosis, the cell cycle, differentiation, signaling, and transcription. Although these findings remain generally true, genome-wide assessment of DNA methylation has painted a more complex picture, in which gain of DNA methylation can be paired with increased gene expression, and DNA methylation loss can be associated with repression.[99] Genome-scale integration of DNA methylation and gene expression in lung cancer supports this observation.[28,100,101] Of key relevance is the location of the alteration with respect to neighboring genes (promoter, intron, coding region) or gene-distant regulatory elements (enhancer, genome organizer), and whether DNA methylation changes affect the binding of regulatory factors.[1]

One important reason for the extensive studies of DNA methylation to date is that relatively straightforward techniques exist to assess this modification.[102,103] Our ability to analyze DNA methylation patterns has increased dramatically, from studies of single genes at a time in the 1990s to current genome-wide approaches.[99,101,103] Given that methylation does not affect base pairing, and that DNA methylation information is lost following amplification by PCR, most DNA methylation assessing techniques employ a method to incorporate the DNA methylation information into the genomic sequence: bisulfite conversion. This process is a chemical treatment that converts unmethylated cytosines to uracil while methylated cytosines are protected;[104] it allows methylation information to be incorporated into the DNA sequence. Bisulfite-converted DNA can be analyzed by many methods.[103] Local bisulfite genomic sequencing, pyrosequencing, methylation-specific PCR, and its real-time version, MethyLight or its variation quantitative methyl-specific PCR, are still used to examine individual genes, but the development of increasingly powerful high-density bead arrays has provided a relatively low-cost way to interrogate hundreds of thousands of CpGs simultaneously.[105–107] Bisulfite genomic sequencing originally consisted of amplification followed by cloning and sequencing, providing information on the methylation status of all the Cs on the same DNA strand in the amplified area.[108] With the major advances in high-throughput sequencing, whole genome bisulfite sequencing has now become a reality, although it remains expensive and computationally challenging and, to our knowledge, has not yet been applied to entire lung cancer genomes.[99] It is anticipated that the application of genome-wide methods will continue to provide ever more detailed insight into DNA methylation alterations in lung cancer. This knowledge promises to change the way in which lung cancer is detected and treated. The biggest challenge that lies in our future is the analysis and interpretation of the wealth of information obtained from genomic methods. Just as with mutations in cancer, some DNA methylation changes are drivers of the cancer process, while others are passengers, occurring coincidentally as molecular changes accumulate in cancer cells. Thus, identifying common DNA methylation changes in lung cancer is only the very beginning; determining which of these changes are cancer drivers is the much bigger task, one for which we have barely scratched the surface.

DNA HYPOMETHYLATION IN LUNG CANCER

Because of the overall hypomethylation found in cancer cells, researchers originally assumed that the cancer-causing effect of methylation changes was based on loss of promoter CpG island methylation resulting in proto-oncogene activation.[109] Indeed, loss of methylation can promote the development of lung cancer in a murine model.[110] Although genes can be activated by hypomethylation,[100] they are not necessarily all considered canonical proto-oncogenes. One category of such genes is the parentally imprinted genes, genes for which either the maternally or paternally inherited allele is normally methylated. Hypomethylation can result in loss of imprinting, thereby contributing to cancer development; biallelic expression of the normally imprinted insulin-like growth factor 2, mesoderm-specific transcript, and H19 genes has been seen in lung cancer and is thought to contribute to the carcinogenic phenotype.[111,112] Another type of gene that can be activated by hypomethylation is the family of testis-specific antigens; these genes are usually methylated and silent in all somatic tissues but the testes.[113] Expression of testis-specific antigens has been noted in many tumor types including lung cancer, and these antigens are seen as potential immunotherapy targets.[113–116] Loss of methylation of transposable elements and repeats is also found in lung cancer[16,117] and can lead to mobility of such elements, causing further genetic damage.[97] In addition, read-through from such demethylated elements may result in the aberrant activation of neighboring genes. Hypomethylation might also play a role in the activation of microRNAs, many of which are deregulated in cancer.[8,118–120] For example, the normally methylated let-7a-3 microRNA was found to be hypomethylated in two of eight lung adenocarcinomas, and forced overexpression of this miRNA increased the oncogenic properties of lung cancer cell line A549.[121]

In addition to contributing to carcinogenesis through gene activation, a second consequence of hypomethylation is thought to be genomic instability. Mice genetically engineered to underexpress DNA methyltransferases show an increased frequency of loss of heterozygosity and an elevated incidence of hematopoietic malignancies.[122] Deletion of DNMT3A in a KRAS-dependent mouse of a lung cancer model was shown to promote tumor progression.[110] However, analysis of methylation of five human squamous cell lung carcinomas and normal matched tissue showed prominent hypomethylation of repetitive elements but little methylation loss in single-copy sequences.[117] This finding supports the notion that the effect of hypomethylation in lung cancer might be limited, which is important, because DNA methylation-blocking therapies are being widely explored, as will be discussed. These therapies appear to show promise in numerous cancers and are under investigation for lung cancer.[22] Importantly, leukemia-prone DNMT underexpressing mice show a lower incidence of intestinal cancer, pointing to a protective effect of hypomethylation in certain tumor types.[123] Indeed, treatment of a mouse xenograft model for human lung cancer with DNA methylation and histone deacetylation inhibitors suppressed tumor growth without apparent toxicity.[124] A similar treatment of a murine lung cancer model cut lung tumor development in half, emphasizing the potential of epigenetic drugs for lung cancer treatment.[125]

DNA Hypermethylation in Lung Cancer: Functional Implications

Although it would appear that the effects of hypomethylation in lung cancer are relatively modest, hypermethylation of promoter CpG islands is widely noted, with findings in lung cancer and

DNA methylation described in more than 1500 reports in Pub Med.[14,15,21,27,28,33,100,101,107,126–130] Hypermethylation can be associated with transcriptional shutdown.[83] This shutdown may happen directly, through steric interference of methylated cytosines with the binding sites for enhancer-binding proteins, transcription factors, cofactors, or chromatin organizers, or indirectly, through the attraction of methyl-binding proteins to the DNA, which in turn recruit histone deacetylase enzymes and other epigenetic modifiers (Figs. 12.1 and 12.3).[43]

Intensive investigation will be required to determine whether DNA methylation changes are driver or passenger events in the development and progression of cancer. For the purposes of prognostication or providing tailored therapies, it could be of great importance to know whether DNA methylation events have functional consequences. This idea is supported by the prognostic utility of expression arrays.[131] The first step in the approach to determine whether altered promoter CpG island methylation of a gene is functionally significant is the integration DNA methylation and gene expression information to identify genes showing concomitant changes in their DNA methylation and expression profiles (Fig. 12.5).[100,129,130] It has been frequently noted that only a minority of DNA methylation alterations show coincident changes in gene expression. This finding suggests that the rest are passenger events. However, there are other, as yet poorly explored, possibilities. For example, methylation changes may modulate binding of the chromatin organizer CTCF, thereby affecting alternative splicing events.[132] Changes in splicing may not immediately be obvious from gene expression analyses, depending on the platform used to examine expression. Another option is that some of these DNA methylation alterations affect the expression of distant genes by modifying regulatory elements such as enhancers. Proper investigation of these possibilities will require more detailed genome-wide knowledge concerning alternative splicing patterns and investigation of epigenetic regulatory elements in the different types of lung epithelial cells that constitute lung cancer precursors. The analysis of trans-effects of DNA methylation on distant genes is computationally and biostatistically challenging and is only just beginning.[133]

To obtain further circumstantial evidence that an epigenetically altered gene affected by cis-DNA methylation is a real target in cancer development and progression, it can be helpful to integrate other types of molecular profiles from cancer cells, such as copy number variation and mutational analyses;[28] a gene that is the target of numerous molecular changes is more likely to play a role in cancer. If lack of expression of a hypermethylated gene has been verified by mRNA and/ or protein analysis, DNMT inhibitors such as 5-azacytidine can be used to determine whether the gene can be reactivated in lung cancer cell lines. A potential caveat of such experiments is that reactivation could be the indirect consequence of demethylation of other genes. Next, reexpression of the gene in cancer cell lines in which the gene was silenced, and silencing of the gene in cells in which the gene is still expressed (e.g., through transfection of targeted inhibitory small hairpin RNAs), will help determine its role in cancer development and progression. In the silencing experiment, the choice of cells is important (primary, immortalized, transformed) and should be influenced by the perceived stage of cancer development at which the gene of interest is thought to play a role. Experiments such as these have implicated a variety of hypermethylated genes in lung cancer.[15,21,27,33,134,135] It should be noted that methylation of genes that were already silent in lung tissue may not be a functional event per se, but might still be informative, as it could provide hints to the origin of the cancer or the involvement of stem cells.[136]

Genes that appear to be silenced by methylation and that limit any aspect of the transformed phenotype when reactivated can be excellent targets for therapy but also could yield new tools for prognostication. Indeed, the testing of associations between

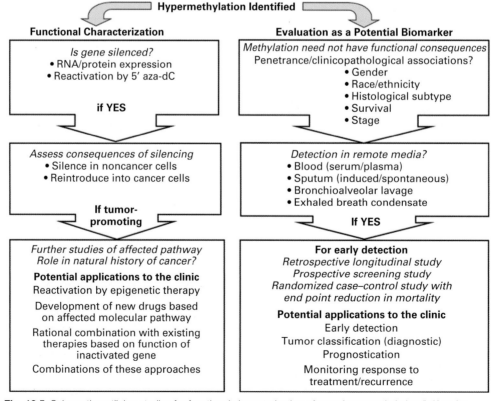

Fig. 12.5. Schematic outlining studies for functional characterization of gene hypermethylation (left) or for development of hypermethylated loci into lung cancer biomarkers (right).

clinical data and DNA methylation status in patient populations could provide markers for survival or response to therapy. An important caveat of studies of associations between DNA methylation and clinicopathologic variables is that a correction should be applied for multiple hypothesis testing when multiple new loci and clinical parameters are examined.[137]

Many genes/loci silenced in lung cancer by DNA methylation have been studied to date, but only a handful have been analyzed in depth. The most intensive focus has been on CDKN2A/p16, a gene encoding an inhibitor of cyclin-dependent kinases 4 and 6, which in turn bind to cyclin D1 and promote the phosphorylation and inactivation of the retinoblastoma gene product, RB. RB is a key cell cycle regulator that is frequently inactivated in SCLC.[25] In contrast, in NSCLC it is CDKN2A that is inactivated in the majority of tumors, and in many cases, this inactivation occurs through promoter hypermethylation.[14,33,138-140] Methylation of the CDKN2A promoter CpG island appears to be a very early change in the development of squamous cell lung cancer as well as adenocarinoma.[16,126,141,142] In a cohort of high-risk long-term smokers from whom sputum was examined for seven DNA methylation markers, hypermethylation of CDKN2A was most strongly associated with lung cancer risk.[143] Indeed, the results of a study published in 2013 confirm a modest association between CDKN2A methylation and smoking.[140] These findings mesh with the idea that disruption of cell cycle regulation is an important early event in the transition from normalcy to cancer, an observation that is emphasized by the fact that human bronchial epithelial cells can be immortalized through CDK4 activation in combination with overexpression of telomerase.[144] It is intriguing that in NSCLC the CDKN2A promoter CpG island appears to be the weak link in the regulatory pathway, and it is tempting to speculate that this might be linked to occupancy of this region by polycomb complexes in stem cells.[145] Methylation of the gene appears to become more pronounced during progression[142] and is associated with an unfavorable prognosis in lung adenocarcinoma and an increased risk of recurrence of stage I NSCLC.[146,147] In the latter study, a several-fold increased risk of recurrence was predicted based on CDKN2A hypermethylation detected in tumors or regional or mediastinal nodes. The prognostic implications of CDKN2A hypermethylation were confirmed in several studies that were included in two meta-analyses published in 2013.[148,149]

A second gene that has been extensively studied in DNA methylation analysis is MGMT.[14,33] Mentioned previously as a target of epigenetic regulation that could promote further genetic changes, this DNA repair gene appears to be another hot spot for early methylation, showing increasing methylation as cells progress from a field defect to hyperplasia and then to adenocarcinoma.[126,142] Interestingly, methylation was also found to be associated with tumor progression and poor survival rates.[150,151] Reports about the preferential methylation of MGMT in smokers compared with nonsmokers have conflicted.[150,152]

Another hypermethylated gene of interest is the retinoic acid receptor beta (RARB). As mentioned in the section on chromatin remodellers, retinoids, including vitamin A and its analogs, play important roles in development, differentiation, proliferation, and apoptosis and have been considered strong candidates for chemoprevention of lung cancer.[153] This idea appears to be supported by hypermethylation of RARB.[88,89,154-160] Unfortunately, the outcome of retinoid chemoprevention clinical trials was an increase rather than decrease in the risk of lung cancer.[161] Nevertheless, the results of in vitro experiments suggest that retinoic acid can prevent the oncogenic transformation of immortalized human bronchial epithelial cells.[162] Hypermethylation of RARB was linked with retinoic acid resistance in a human bronchial epithelial cell line, and treatment with DNA methylation inhibitor azacytidine restored the cells' ability to respond to retinoic acid.[163] As with methylation of MGMT, RARB hypermethylation appears to be an early event in the development of lung adenocarcinoma,

showing low but detectable levels in the adjacent lung, and increasing methylation in hyperplasia and adenocarcinoma.[142,164]

RASSF1, encoding a putative RAS effector protein, has been reported to be frequently methylated in human malignancies, including lung cancer.[14,16,33,142,165] The gene has alternative first exons, alpha and gamma, each with a CpG island. The upstream island (RASSF1A) is hypermethylated in lung cancer, and its methylation strongly correlates with expression of the delta subfamily of the DNA methyltranseferase 3B.[166] This DNMT3B subfamily consists of at least seven splice variants. Knockdown of DNMT3B4 in lung cancer cell lines resulted in reactivation of the RASSF1A but not the CDKN2A promoter, implying that DNMT3B isoforms could be involved in initiating promoter-specific DNA methylation. RASSF1A methylation is suggested to correlate with a poor prognosis, although this finding should be confirmed by an independent study.[167]

In addition to CDKN2A, MGMT, RARB, and RASSF1, many other genes may be of interest functionally or therapeutically. Genes worth mentioning briefly are OPCML, CHD13, and the HOX family.[16] OPCML, encoding an opioid-binding cell adhesion-like molecule, was suspected as a tumor suppressor gene many years ago by Minna et al.,[168] based on the apoptotic response of lung cancer cell lines to opioids, which antagonized the growth stimulatory effect of nicotine.[168] The frequent and high methylation of OPCML in both adenocarcinoma and squamous cell lung cancer also suggests that it might function as a pan-lung cancer marker.[169,170] Brock et al.[147] found that hypermethylation of CDH13, encoding the cell adhesion molecule heart cadherin, is associated with increased risk of recurrence of stage I NSCLC, and addition of CDH13 methylation to CDKN2A methylation further increased the odds ratio for recurrence, particularly when methylation was assessed in tumors. However, to our knowledge, these data have not yet been translated to the clinic. Of interest is that a genome-wide study with similar goals identified a five-marker prognostic panel that did not include CDKN2A in the top genes and did not yield odds ratios as high as the ratios in the study by Brock et al.[171] This finding points to possible differences when different platforms are used and suggests that further studies are required to validate markers and obtain consistent results. One of the markers included in the five-marker panel was HOXA9. Members of the HOX family of genes, which encode homeobox–containing transcription factors important in the embryonic body patterns, have been reported to be methylated in numerous cancer types, including lung cancer.[16,100,172] Numerous other genes hypermethylated in lung cancer are under investigation, and much further work is required before we have full insight into the most common DNA methylation cancer driver events.

In addition to methylation of genes, the hypermethylation of microRNAs is also of great interest.[8] The miR-29 family of three RNAs is an example of microRNAs that are silenced by hypermethylation in lung cancer (in contrast to the activated let-7a-3 mentioned earlier).[173] Expression of these RNAs is inversely correlated with DNMT3A and DNMT3B in lung cancer, which appears to be mediated by targeting of miR-29 to the 3' untranslated regions of the methyltransferase mRNAs. Reactivation of miR-29 could be one way in which methyltransferase expression and tumorigenic potential of lung cancer cells could be mitigated, as illustrated by the reduced tumor growth in nude mice of A549 lung cancer cells transfected with miR-29.[173] As with aberrantly methylated genes, much work remains to be done to fully characterize the role of epigenetically inactivated microRNAs in lung cancer.

From the data described previously, it is clear that progress is being made in understanding the functional consequences of changes in DNA methylation. Despite its promise, DNA methylation analysis has not yet become clinically implemented as a molecular assay applied to tumors. This finding may be related to the fact that analysis of DNA methylation requires an additional chemical step (bisulfite conversion), or it may be because more work must be done to independently verify findings before they can lead to clinical implementation. The general reversal of methylation is already a clinical target though, with numerous drugs that counteract DNA methylation under development and being evaluated in clinical trials.[22,38]

DNA Hypermethylation in Lung Cancer: Application to Marker Development

One of the driving forces behind DNA methylation research is the desire to identify DNA methylation markers for early lung cancer detection.[14,21,33] DNA hypermethylation analyses could yield powerful candidate markers for lung cancer because only a small region of each gene needs to be interrogated, and DNA is a PCR-amplifiable substance that can be detected in bodily fluids.[14,21,33,174,175] Successful development of markers for cancer is a long process that should culminate in a randomized case–control study that demonstrates a reduction in mortality (Fig. 12.3).[176]

The vast majority of DNA methylation studies in lung cancer have focused on NSCLC, which makes up about 85% of all lung cancers.[14,15,21,27,28,33,100,101,107,126,129,177] A comparison of methylation profiles of SCLC and NSCLC cell lines and tumors indicates that hypermethylation profiles are distinct for these two groups.[178–180] Studies in SCLC are few as yet;[127,128] it is a very aggressive cancer associated with poor survival, and surgery is infrequent, limiting the accessibility of samples for profiling. In addition, SCLC is considered by many to be an unsuitable candidate for the development of early detection molecular markers due to the rapid progression of the disease. In contrast, important benefits would be gained if NSCLC could be detected at an early stage, as these lung cancers, which include adenocarcinoma (approximately 40% of lung cancers), squamous cell carcinoma (approximately 30%), large cell carcinoma (approximately 10%), and miscellaneous other histologic subtypes, such as carcinoids and neuroendocrine cancers (approximately 5%), usually lead to death.[181,182] In particular, DNA methylation markers could be useful to complement low-dose spiral computed tomography (CT) screening. Low-dose CT was shown to sensitively detect early lung cancer when applied to long-term smokers, leading to a 20% reduction in mortality, but has a specificity of less than 4%.[183]

Not surprisingly, differences between hypermethylation profiles of NSCLC histologic subtypes have been reported,[16,28,33,100,107,129,169,170,179,184–186] meshing with other molecular and clinicopathologic differences found in these tumor types.[187–190] This finding suggests that a panel of DNA methylation markers would be optimal and that this panel should include pan-lung cancer markers as well as ones for distinct histologic subtypes.[107,169,170,177]

The first step in molecular marker development is the identification of promising candidate markers.[176] In the case of DNA methylation markers for lung cancer, it is of high priority to identify frequently methylated genes or loci (we refer to the CpG island section we are probing as a locus, because a given gene can be probed in multiple areas within a single or even multiple CpG islands). These loci should also show substantially increased methylation levels over those found in healthy tissues. Thus, the initial focus should be on penetrance and DNA methylation levels. Because even a noncancerous lung from a long-term smoker may have accumulated substantial methylation due to age and environmental exposure,[186,191–194] many labs (including ours) have chosen to compare cancer tissues to this type of "high background" control tissue (referred to as adjacent nontumor lung). This finding ensures that identified hypermethylation markers are indeed cancer-specific and not merely indicative of environmental exposure. Although smoking has been implicated in increased DNA methylation, it appears that some DNA methylation alterations are consistent between smokers and nonsmokers, which means it should be possible to develop broadly applicable biomarker panels.[100,177]

Many of the genes studied early on did not show high methylation frequencies,[33] but more recent efforts by numerous groups to examine much larger collections of genes have yielded a number of panels that may deliver high sensitivity and specificity, based on the examination of tissues.[100,101,117,169,170,184,195–204] Some of these panels contain genes that were identified early on (such as CDKN2A/p16, MGMT, and RASSF1),[170,184,197,204] but many new loci have been added to the repertoire, including homeotic genes involved in development, such as members of the HOX and PAX families.[100,101,117,169,170,199,201,204] Whether the hypermethylation of potential DNA methylation markers is functional or not (i.e., leads to transcriptional silencing) is not relevant, as long as penetrance is high and hypermethylation is associated with the presence of cancer. Many of the marker panels must still be validated on independent tumor sets, and their ability to identify lung cancer independently of gender, histologic subtype, racial/ethnic group, and/or stages of cancer must be further scrutinized (Fig. 12.3, right panel). Once that is accomplished, the marker panels can be taken to the next phase of marker development: clinical assay validation.[176] In order for these panels to function in early lung cancer detection, they must be detectable in patient remote media: body fluids that could carry methylated DNA molecules from the cancer and that could be sampled relatively noninvasively.

Detection of DNA Methylation Markers in Body Fluids

Potential remote media for lung cancer detection are blood (plasma or serum[205]), coughed-up sputum (spontaneously collected from smokers or induced in never-smokers or ex-smokers), bronchioalveolar lavage ([BAL], a saline rinse that can be collected during bronchoscopy), bronchial brushings, and exhaled breath condensate (collected as condensation from breath using a cooling device).[21] DNA methylation markers have been detected in plasma, serum, sputum, and BAL, and data from an ever-growing number of studies are reported. One problem that authors report with many studies is the lack of control participants, which makes results difficult to interpret. In addition, authors of some studies cite frequencies based on the number of methylation-positive remote samples found in patients in which the tumor is positive. This finding is helpful to determine the experimental sensitivity of the test, but it does not provide a good estimate of clinical sensitivity.

There are two published reports of detection of DNA methylation markers in exhaled breath condensate.[206,207] Although sensitivity is low, these studies do show feasibility and may be further developed. The use of sputum as a source for DNA methylation has been more deeply investigated and has been reviewed.[174] A review of results to date indicates that sensitivity and specificity still need to be improved, variability in methodology between studies makes comparisons difficult, and that there is a need for further studies. One noted concern is frequent signal in the negative controls, perhaps related to the many amplification cycles.[143] In addition, sputum is considered to favor the detection of centrally located tumors.

Blood (plasma or serum) would be the easiest body fluid to obtain for screening, but analyses to date indicate this medium too lacks sensitivity. In addition, DNA methylation signatures may arise from anywhere in the body. However, the new high-throughput DNA methylation profiling technologies might make it feasible to identify lung cancer–specific DNA methylation signatures. This would require the profiling of DNA methylation in all other common types of cancer, a process that is ongoing in different laboratories and in The Cancer Genome Atlas Project.[208] Preliminary analyses reported by investigators at the Laird-Offringa lab indicate that the markers with the highest sensitivity are not lung cancer–specific. Whether or not the signal should be unique to lung cancer will perhaps depend on how a resulting test is leveraged. If it is geared toward supplementary evaluation of a lesion detected by low-dose spiral CT, it may be less of an issue than when no other assays are available. It remains a question what size the tumor must be in order to shed sufficient DNA into the blood for remote detection. To date, the hunt for a blood-based marker panel with high sensitivity and specificity is ongoing.

Of the remote media tested, BAL appears the most promising, showing sensitivities for individual loci approaching 50% or higher. The combination of markers into panels will help increase sensitivity, as exemplified by studies of Grote et al.[157,209,210] The finding that combined methylation analysis of *CDKN2A* and *RARB* detects cases of lung cancer with a sensitivity of 69% and a specificity of 87% is highly encouraging.[157] The combination of *APC*, *CDKN2A*, and *RASSF1* also showed promise, detecting 63% of central cancers and 44% of peripheral cancers and exhibiting a very low background in one of 102 cases with benign lung disease.[210] Based on the detection of methylation in BAL from patients without cancer in a number of studies, it would be important to use quantitative measurements and to set a cut-off value for positive methylation.[157,209–212] The fact that the collection of lavage fluid can be directed to a particular area of the lung makes it especially suited to be combined with imaging approaches. This, in addition to the promising results obtained to date, suggests that analysis of DNA methylation in BAL might be the key to early detection of lung cancer.

In addition to their use for early detection, DNA methylation markers identified in body fluids could be applied to risk assessment and monitoring of recurrence. In the case of quantitative markers, cutoff values could be stratified to distinguish between methylation detected in normal tissue from nonsmokers, histologically normal tissue of cases prior to diagnosis, lung cancer, or recurring lung cancer. The authors of several studies have shown that methylation can be detectable long before the cancer becomes clinically apparent.[141,213,214] However, as noted previously, the sensitivity of the least invasive approaches (sputum, blood) have not been high, and use of BAL would require bronchoscopy.

EPIGENETIC THERAPY FOR LUNG CANCER

The cumulative role that DNA methylation, histone modifications, chromatin remodeling, and other epigenetic events play in the development of lung cancer has prompted investigations into targeting these changes therapeutically. Various strategies have been attempted or are ongoing to improve the treatment of patients with lung cancer by applying epigenetic approaches.

The ability to inhibit DNA methyltransferases and histone deacetylases gave rise to a flurry of drug development and preclinical studies, including ones using lung cancer cell lines.[38,215] The first identified epigenetic drug, 5-azacytidine, blocks DNA methylation. The DNA methyltransferase normally forms a covalent intermediate as it prepares to methylate cytosines, but when 5-azacytidine has been incorporated at that position, the 5 position is blocked and the methyltransferase becomes trapped and inactivated. In model systems, 5-azacytidine demonstrates intriguing antitumor activity. For example, in the H1299 lung cancer cell line implanted into nude mice, treatment with 5-azacytidine restored the expression of some hypermethylated genes and suppressed tumor growth.[124] However, although the 5-azacytidine derivative, decitabine (or 5-aza-2'-deoxycytidine), is used to treat myelodysplastic syndromes and acute myeloid leukemia,[216] clinical studies using hypomethylating agents alone for patients with lung cancer have been somewhat disappointing.

Histone deacetylase inhibitors are also currently used to treat hematologic malignancies.[217] However, clinical evaluations of HDAC inhibitors in patients with solid tumors have, in general, been only modestly successful. In NSCLC cell lines, several HDAC inhibitors were shown to induce cell death.[22] At least three different clinical trials have been undertaken with these inhibitors in NSCLC.[22] Although no major responses occurred in any of the patients, the major findings were stabilization of the disease in a subset of patients for a few months (Table 12.3). In this regard, the presence of alterations in genes encoding histone deacetylases (*HDAC1*, *HDAC2*, *HDAC6*, and *HDAC9*) in NSCLC is potentially of interest;[51] mutations in HDACs may determine the resistance or sensitivity to HDAC inhibitors. Of additional interest is the profiling of lung cancer cells to identify genes that modulate sensitivity to HDAC inhibitors.[218]

The modest success of clinical trials with either DNA methyltransferases or HDAC inhibitors as single agents has prompted their use in combination, either together or with other compounds. In a phase I/II trial of combined azacytidine and entinostat, an HDAC inhibitor, conducted in pretreated patients with recurrent metastatic NSCLC, the median survival for the entire cohort was significantly higher than that for existing therapeutic options. Among the patients who had a response to this combination treatment, one

TABLE 12.3 Clinical Trials Involving Epigenetic Agents in Lung Cancer[a]

Phase of Trial	Agent(s) (Type of Drug)	No. of Patients	Disease Characteristics	Effects
SINGLE AGENT				
I[239]	Decitabine (DNA-demethylating)	20	Stage III–IV NSCLC, refractory to standard therapies	Establishment of maximum tolerated doses; no objective responses
II[240]	Vorinostat (HDAC inhibitor)	14	Stage IIIB–IV NSCLC, progressive disease after traditional chemotherapy	No objective responses; stable disease in 57% of patients
II[241]	Romidepsin (HDAC inhibitor)	16	Recurrent SCLC, after platinum-based therapy	No objective responses; stable disease in 19% of patients
COMBINATIONS				
II (two randomized arms)[227]	Vorinostat/carboplatin/ paclitaxel (HDAC inhibitor/chemotherapy)	62 versus 32	Stage IIIB–IV NSCLC	Trend toward vorinostat enhancing the efficacy of chemotherapy
II (two randomized arms)[228]	Entinostat/erlotinib (HDAC inhibitor/tyrosine kinase inhibitor)	67 versus 66	Stage IIIB–IV NSCLC	Erlotinib and entinostat did not improve patient outcomes
I/II[219]	5-aza/entinostat (DNA demethylating/HDAC inhibitor)	45	Progressive, metastatic NSCLC	Objective responses in 4% of patients; antitumor activity was impressive in two patients

[a]Only trials that enrolled more than 14 patients with lung cancer are included.
HDAC, Histone deacetylase; *NSCLC*, non–small cell lung cancer; *SCLC*, small cell lung cancer.

patient had no evidence of disease for 1 year and another had stable disease for about 22 months and complete resolution of liver metastases, which remained undetectable more than 2 years after completion of therapy. This analysis also demonstrated the demethylation of four genes known to be associated with lung cancer, detectable in serial blood samples in these patients, which was associated with significantly improved progression-free and overall survival.[219] These promising results have given rise to other phase I and II clinical trials, and the excitement in the field is reflected by reviews published in 2013.[22,23] The combination of epigenetic therapies with other anticancer agents has also been investigated. HDAC inhibitors have been shown to be synergistic with cytotoxic agents, such as taxanes and platinum,[220,221] although in some cases it is not clear whether this is an effect of the HDAC inhibitor on histone tails or on other proteins that are acetylated, such as heat shock protein 90 (*HSP90*).[222] The HDAC inhibitor LBH589 increased HSP90 acetylation in lung cancer cells, thereby decreasing HSP90 protein chaperone ability, an activity that helps EGFR-mutant proteins maintain functionality.[223] These findings served as the rationale for the combination of inhibitors of EGFR signaling with HDAC inhibitors, an approach that showed promise in several studies using cancer cell lines.[224–226] Clinically, however, the combination of these agents has had little impact on patients' survival or response to treatment. A phase II study in advanced NSCLC suggested an improvement in response after the addition of the HDAC inhibitor, vorinostat, to a regimen of carboplatin and paclitaxel.[227] However, in another study, the combination of entinostat and erlotinib was not superior to erlotinib alone in an unselected NSCLC population.[228]

Another exciting combinatorial prospect is epigenetic therapy combined with immunotherapy, prompted by the finding that 5-azacytidine bolsters the expression of some immune modulators in lung cancer cell lines.[229] The combination of other standard therapies such as radiotherapy with HDAC inhibitors has also shown promise in preclinical models[230] and should be explored in clinical settings.

Lastly, a generation of novel drugs has been developed against bromodomains. Among these are the group of small molecule inhibitors of the bromo and extra terminal (BET) family of chromatin adaptors, which target the so-called BET proteins (e.g., *BRD2*, *BRD3*, *BRD4*, and *BRDT*). JQ1 is a BET inhibitor that suppresses cell growth in a variety of leukemia and lymphoma cell lines in the context of an activated MYC, either through chromosomal translocation or gene amplification.[231,232] In lung cancer, JQ1 has been tested only in lung adenocarcinoma cell lines, causing growth inhibition in about one-third of the cells. The exact mechanism for this inhibition is still not well understood, although it appears to be independent of MYC and may involve FOSL1.[233] The inhibitors of bromodomains may also have therapeutic applicability in the context of the SWI/SNF complex, depending on the genetic background of the cancer cell. Studies using interference RNAs have demonstrated that the inhibition of *BRM* in cells lacking functional *BRG1* causes cell death.[234,235] Likewise, the inhibition of *BRG1* is lethal in lung cancer cells, especially SCLC-carrying inactivation of the MYC-associated factor X gene, *MAX*.[236] These findings raise the possibility of using *BRM* or *BRG1* as targeted therapeutics in lung cancers carrying genetic inactivation of *BRG1* or *MAX*, respectively.[237] The coming years will witness the development of a variety of bromodomain inhibitors and other epigenetic-related drugs as well as the clinical trials that will test them. We anticipate that some of these new drugs will become valuable tools in the growing arsenal to treat patients with lung cancer.

CONCLUSION

Powerful tools are being honed for the epigenomic analysis of lung cancer, and these tools will continue to increase our understanding of the molecular underpinnings of the development and progression of lung cancer. In addition, they will provide molecular markers for detection, diagnosis, prognostication, and monitoring of recurrence. A key area that will require rapid development to make the most of these technologies is bioinformatics, because the staggering amount of data generated must be analyzed and interpreted. The combination of new epigenetic knowledge with novel epigenetic drugs, and insight into how these and other drugs function, has generated an aura of hope and excitement in the field of lung cancer. The possibility to build on existing therapies, such as EGFR inhibitors or radiotherapy, by combining them with inhibitors of HDACs and DNA methylation opens many new therapeutic avenues. With progress looming on the fronts of early detection as well as treatment, it can truly be said that epigenetics has given new breath to the fight against lung cancer.

Acknowledgments

DNA methylation research support for the Laird-Offringa lab comes from NIH/NCI grants R21 102247, R01 CA120689, R01 CA119029, the Canary Foundation, the Thomas G. Labrecque Foundation, the Whittier Foundation, and the Tobacco Disease-Related Research Program. Research support for chromatin remodeling in the Sanchez-Cespedes lab comes from the Spanish Ministry Economía y Competitividad (Spanish Grants SAF2011-22897 and RD12/0036/0045) and the European Community's Seventh Framework Programme (FP7/2007-13), under grant agreement n°HEALTH-F2-2010-258677–CURELUNG. Neither the Laird-Offringa or the Sanchez-Cespedes laboratories accept any money from the tobacco industry. The content of this chapter is solely the responsibility of the authors and does not necessarily represent the official views of the funding agencies.

KEY REFERENCES

7. Hargreaves DC, Crabtree GR. ATP-dependent chromatin remodeling: genetics, genomics and mechanisms. *Cell Res*. 2011;21(3):396–420.
10. Shen H, Laird PW. Interplay between the cancer genome and epigenome. 2013;153(1):38–55.
14. Belinsky SA. Gene-promoter hypermethylation as a biomarker in lung cancer. *Nat Rev Cancer*. 2004;4(9):707–717.
15. Risch A, Plass C. Lung cancer epigenetics and genetics. *Int J Cancer*. 2008;123(1):1–7.
17. Rodriguez-Nieto S, Sanchez-Cespedes M. BRG1 and LKB1: tales of two tumor suppressor genes on chromosome 19p and lung cancer. *Carcinogenesis*. 2009;30(4):547–554.
22. Liu SV, Fabbri M, Gitlitz BJ, Laird-Offringa IA. Epigenetic therapy in lung cancer. *Front Oncol*. 2013;3:135.
23. Jakopovic M, Thomas A, Balasubramaniam S, Schrump D, Giaccone G, Bates SE. Targeting the epigenome in lung cancer: expanding approaches to epigenetic therapy. *Front Oncol*. 2013;3:261.
42. Adcock IM, Ford P, Ito K, Barnes PJ. Epigenetics and airways disease. *Respir Res*. 2006;7:21.
45. Dokmanovic M, Clarke C, Marks PA. Histone deacetylase inhibitors: overview and perspectives. *Mol Cancer Res*. 2007;5(10):981–989.
49. Liu J, Lee W, Jiang Z, et al. Genome and transcriptome sequencing of lung cancers reveal diverse mutational and splicing events. *Genome Res*. 2012;22(12):2315–2327.
50. Imielinski M, Berger AH, Hammerman PS, et al. Mapping the hallmarks of lung adenocarcinoma with massively parallel sequencing. *Cell*. 2012;150(6):1107–1120.
51. Govindan R, Ding L, Griffith M, et al. Genomic landscape of non-small cell lung cancer in smokers and never-smokers. *Cell*. 2012;150(6):1121–1134.
75. Romero OA, Sanchez-Cespedes M. The SWI/SNF genetic blockade: effects in cell differentiation, cancer and developmental diseases. *Oncogene*. 2014;33(21):2681–2689.
100. Selamat SA, Chung BS, Girard L, et al. Genome-scale analysis of DNA methylation in lung adenocarcinoma and integration with mRNA expression. *Genome Res*. 2012;22(7):1197–1211.
229. Wrangle J, Wang W, Koch A, et al. Alterations of immune response of non-small cell lung cancer with azacytidine. *Oncotarget*. 2013;4(11):2067–2079.

See Expertconsult.com for full list of references.

13 Stem Cells and Lung Cancer: In Vitro and In Vivo Studies

Dean A. Fennell and David M. Jablons

SUMMARY OF KEY POINTS

- The use of mouse models to study the initiation and evolution of lung cancers has been crucial in advancing the field through the identification of putative stem cell niches within the lung.
- Bronchoalveolar stem cells (BASCs) are the putative cell of origin for lung adenocarcinoma.
- The tumor suppressor gene phosphatase and tensin homolog (PTEN) exerts a brake on BASC transformation to adenocarcinoma.
- Basal cells of the trachea are the putative cell of origin for squamous lung cancer.
- In small cell lung cancer (SCLC), a common neuroendocrine cell of origin may undergo RAS-driven transformation to a CD44-expressing non-neuroendocrine clone.
- Hedgehog (Hh) signaling persists in SCLC and is required for tumor growth in mouse xenograft models.

The cancer stem cell hypothesis, when applied to lung cancers, is underpinned by the concept of a cellular hierarchy in which a relatively rare somatic stem cell population with self-renewal capability, differentiation, and innate drug resistance gives rise to the bulk of the cancer.[1] Evidence of this concept has been reported in studies on hematologic malignancies and solid cancers.[2-5] Lung cancers, like other cancers, are heterogeneous with respect to histology and are spatially associated with the cellular origin of initiation.[6] With the advent of large-scale DNA sequencing, heterogeneity at the genetic level has been observed within these histologic subclasses, especially in adenocarcinomas.[7-11] This heterogeneity in adenocarcinomas indicates complexity in the mechanisms underlying cellular initiation and evolution of lung cancers as a result of specific mutational processes.[12] This chapter focuses on the evidence supporting the existence of spatially restricted initiator cell populations in lung cancer (cells of origin), including evidence for specific pathways involved in their maintenance, as well as the less well-supported evidence for cancer stem cells.

NORMAL LUNG

Over time, a model has been developed in which the lung is subdivided into regions associated with their own stem cell population capable of rapidly responding to lung injury, thus enabling cellular repopulation.[13] Accordingly, the trachea, bronchus, bronchioles, and alveolus exhibit their own complement of cells capable of repopulation following lung injury.

For the trachea and bronchus, these repopulating cells are the basal mucous secretory cells. Evidence supports the existence of a cellular compartment in the human airway surface epithelium that can restore the full repertoire of epithelial lining cells in a xenograft model in severe combined immunodeficiency mice.[14]

By contrast, the basal/parabasal origin of tracheal stem cells has been proposed based on data showing that a cytokeratin 5 (CK5), CK14-, and mindbomb E3 ubiquitin protein ligase 1-positive cell population comprising only 0.87% of lung cells accounts for 48% of proliferating cells with basal localization.[15] Tracheal gland ductal cells that express CK14 and CK18 have been shown to retain sulfur dioxide labeling up to 4 weeks after inhalation damage in adult mice and can repopulate the tracheal surface after injury.[16]

In the bronchioles and alveoli, the club cell (formally known as the Clara cell) and type II pneumocyte have been implicated in repopulation. Accordingly, specific depletion of club cells in rodent models by either intraperitoneal naphthalene or activation of the suicide substrate ganciclovir by Clara cell secretory protein (CCSP)-promoter-driven herpes simplex virus thymidine kinase in transgenic mice is sufficient to cause irreversible, fatal lung injury.[17] In rodent fetal lung, the existence of a possible bipolar stem cell (M3E3/C3) capable of differentiating into club or type II pneumocytes when grown in different media is supported by data from Finkelstein et al.[18] Bleomycin causes specific alveolar type I (AT1) cell injury, and it has been proposed that AT2 cells can repopulate and repair the alveolar epithelium.[19] A unique, naphthalene-resistant stem cell population has been identified at the bronchoalveolar junction and can repopulate the terminal bronchioles after club cell depletion injury. These cells express CCSP and are independent of the neuroepithelial body microenvironment, implicating a distinct stem cell niche.[20] Similarly, a so-called side population of cells (i.e., a rare cellular subset enriched for stem cell activity) exhibiting typical breast cancer-resistant protein-mediated Hoechst dye efflux has been identified in 0.03% to 0.07% of total lung cells.[21,22]

NONSMALL CELL LUNG CANCER

Adenocarcinoma and the Cells of Origin

Nonsmall cell lung cancer (NSCLC) can be subdivided into two distinct subtypes that reflect the histologic characteristics of distinct regions within the lung: 80% are adenocarcinomas and 20% are squamous cell carcinomas.[23] The adenocarcinoma subtype and adenoma precursors exhibit club and AT2 cell markers consistent with a peripheral or endobronchial origin,[24,25] whereas squamous cell carcinomas exhibit mature epithelial cell characteristics consistent with trachea and proximal airways origin. The AT2-specific marker surfactant protein has been shown to be expressed in lung adenocarcinoma and squamous cell carcinomas. Accordingly, Ten Have-Opbroek et al.[26] postulated that the AT2 cell may be the pluripotential cell for NSCLC in humans.

Isolation of a CD133-Positive Stem-Like Population in Lung Cancer

Rare populations of cells (<1.5%) have been shown to form colonies in soft agar and recapitulate features of the original lung cancer in athymic mice.[27] In a study that was aimed to isolate rare populations of cells from primary lung cancer specimens expressing the marker CD133, an undifferentiated cell population was identified, capable of indefinitely growing as tumor spheres in serum-free medium containing epidermal growth factor and basic fibroblast growth factor.[28] This approach had previously been used to isolate a putative hemopoietic cell of origin in human acute myeloid leukemia.[29] These putative lung cancer stem cells were able to acquire specific lineage markers in tumor xenografts (which were identical to the original tumor) and differentiated to lose tumorigenic potential and CD133 expression. In association with aldehyde dehydrogenase 1A1, a marker of the stem cell phenotype, CD133 has been shown to be associated with a poor prognosis—related to shorter recurrence-free survival—for patients with lung cancer.[30,31]

In previous studies, CD133-positive cells have been isolated from cell lines. In one study, CD133-positive cells were found to coexpress octamer-binding transcription factor 4 (OCT-4), NANOG, alpha-integrin, and C-X-C chemokine receptor type 4, and these cells were found to be resistant to cisplatin.[32] In another study, following chemotherapy, cells with CD133 were isolated and then enriched in the surviving populations with CD133 positivity.[33] Consistent with the observation that isolated CD133-positive cells are resistant to cisplatin, selecting cells specifically for resistance to cisplatin over several months through long-term treatment led to enrichment of a CD133-positive/CD44-positive/aldehyde dehydrogenase-active clone that expresses NANOG/OCT-4/sex determining region Y-box 2 (SOX2).[34] However, isolation of CD133-positive cells from the A549 cell lines has also been shown to result in high potential for liver metastases,[35] and tumor growth factor-beta has been shown to increase the migratory capacity of these CD133-positive A549 cells in association with induction of epithelial to mesenchymal transition.[36]

The Cell of Origin in Conditional Oncogene-Driven Adenocarcinoma

Activating mutations of Kirsten rat sarcoma (KRAS) are identified in approximately 25% of adenocarcinomas. A Lox-Stop-Lox KRAS conditional mouse strain (LSL K-ras G12D) harboring an oncogenic KRAS under control of a removable transcriptional termination stop element by adeno-CRE infection has been reported as a model for monitoring the initiation of tumor formation over time through different stages of progression.[37,38] Three distinct types of lesions have been identified: atypical adenomatous hyperplasia (AAH), epithelial hyperplasia of the bronchioles, and adenomas. AAH is an atypical epithelial cell proliferation that grows along the alveolar septa but is noninvasive; it has been proposed by Kerr to be an adenoma-like precursor of adenocarcinoma.[39] Immunohistochemical analysis has shown negativity for the Clara cell-specific marker Clara cell antigen (CCA) and positivity for AT2 cell-specific marker prosurfactant apoprotein-C (pulmonary surfactant apoprotein C [SP-C]) consistent with AT2 cell origin. By contrast, epithelial hyperplasia lesions exhibit CCA positivity and SP-C negativity consistent with club cell origin. Importantly, endothelial hyperplasia lesions contiguous with AAH lesions exhibit double CCA/SP-C expression at the single-cell level, demonstrating a unique double-positive population that exhibits properties of both club and AT2 cells.[37] Monitoring progression following KRAS activation over time has demonstrated formation of adenomas (outnumbering AAH lesions) at 12 weeks after adeno-CRE infection, and adenocarcinomas that form at 16 weeks in the absence of AAH lesions suggest a precursor origin of these cancers.[37]

SP-C/CCA double-positive cells have been subsequently shown to be the putative cell of adenocarcinoma origin in the LSL-K-ras G12D model.[40] Such double-positive cells, which express markers of both AT2 and club cells, have been previously identified in mice.[41] In normal adult lungs, double immunofluorescence has been used to identify a subpopulation of cells that are positive for CCA and SP-C and that are restricted through localization to the bronchoalveolar duct junction; CCA is distributed in the columnar bronchial epithelium and SP-C in the AT2 cells. These double-positive cells respond to both naphthalene- and bleomycin-induced lung injury by proliferating, while club cell or AT1 cell loss occurs as a result of specific toxicities.[40]

Isolation of these double-positive cells has shown a putative stem cell population—termed BASCs—that reside at the bronchoalveolar duct junction and repopulate the bronchiolar or alveolar epithelium following damage. BASCs constitute 0.4% of the total lung cell population and exhibit an immunophenotype that is negative for platelet endothelial cell adhesion molecule (Pecam), CD45, and CD34 and positive for stem cell antigen 1 (Sca1). These cells are clonal, as evidenced by single-cell culture.[40] BASCs exhibit multipotent lineage potential and can give rise to AT2-like or club-like cells while undergoing self-renewal during culture.

During tumorigenesis in the LSL-K-ras G12D model, infection with adeno-CRE leads to an expansion of the BASC pool, coincident with the formation of AAH. The amount of BASC expansion correlates with the titer of adeno-CRE used to infect the LSL-K-ras G12D transgenic mice.

Loss of PTEN Expands the BASC Pool

BASCs require PTEN to prevent formation of lung adenocarcinomas.[42] PTEN is a tumor suppressor that inhibits the phosphoinositide 3 kinase (PI3K)/AKT survival pathway by dephosphorylating phosphatidylinositol-3,4,5-trisphosphate at the cell membrane, and it is required for maintenance of other organ-specific stem cells.[43] Loss of PTEN is a frequent occurrence in lung adenocarcinoma.[44–46] To study the effects of PTEN, bronchoalveolar epithelium-specific, PTEN-deficient mice were established. These mice had impaired lung morphogenesis, impaired alveolar epithelial cell differentiation, defective expression of the molecular markers (increased sprouty gene 2 [Spry2] and sonic hedgehog [Shh]), and bronchoalveolar epithelial hyperplasia.[42] Furthermore, loss of PTEN led to an increase in the numbers of BASCs and was sufficient to induce spontaneous adenocarcinomas, of which 33% were shown to exhibit secondary codon 61 KRAS mutations. By contrast, PI3K has been shown to mediate BASC expansion in oncogenic KRAS-induced lung cancer, demonstrating a critical role for this pathway in regulating the stem cell pool during formation of adenocarcinomas.[47] As with the PI3K pathway, Gata6-wingless-related integration site (wnt) signaling and B lymphoma Moloney murine leukemia virus insertion region 1 homolog (Bmi1) have been identified as regulators of BASC expansion.[48,49]

Maintenance of Stem Cell Populations: Notch and Wnt Signaling

Asymmetric cell division is a characteristic of stem cells that is regulated by the highly conserved notch signaling pathway, which, in turn, is mediated by cell–cell interactions. This pathway is involved in normal lung development, as evidenced by knockout of the downstream notch target hairy and enhancer of split 1 (Hes1), which is expressed in neuroendocrine cells and is associated with their expansion.[50] In RAS-transformed cells, RAS increases the level and activity of the notch pathway by increasing the levels of intracellular notch-1, and upregulating notch ligand delta-1 and p38 pathway-dependent processing of presenilin-1. This notch activation is essential for maintaining the neoplastic phenotype in vitro and in vivo.[51] Recently, it has been shown that Notch3 signaling in KRAS-driven adenocarcinoma is dependent on the oncogene protein kinase C iota (PKCiota), and simultaneous pharmacologic inhibition of both Notch and PKCiota exhibits synergistic antagonism of KRAS-driven lung adenocarcinoma in vitro and in vivo.[52] The Wnt pathway activation is essential for maintaining the cancer stem cell phenotype and, although not commonly mutated in NSCLC, is constitutively activated. It has recently been shown that Wnt signaling is enhanced by microRNA 582-3p-mediated suppression of Wnt inhibitors axis inhibition protein 2, Dickkopf WNT signaling pathway inhibitor 3, and secreted frizzled-related protein 1. Inhibition of MiR582-3p results in suppression of Wnt and inhibition of both tumor initiation and in vivo xenograft progression, suggesting its potential as a therapeutic target.[53]

Squamous Cell Lung Carcinoma

Basal cells of the trachea have been implicated as possible cells of origin of squamous cell lung carcinoma. In mouse models, squamous cell lung carcinomas exhibit similar expression patterns of p63, CK5, and CK14, as well as spatial localization to intracartilaginous boundaries and mucosal junctions.[16,52] CK5-positive basal cells have self-renewal properties and are under the control of SOX2;[54] in squamous cell lung carcinomas, the *SOX2* gene is frequently amplified at chromosome 3q26.33.[55]

SMALL CELL LUNG CANCER

Neuroendocrine Airway Epithelia and the Origin of Small Cell Lung Cancers

SCLC arises from cells residing in the epithelial lining of the bronchi and exhibits a neuroendocrine phenotype.[56] Approximately 90% of SCLCs exhibit inactivating mutations in both p53 and retinoblastoma 1 (Rb1) tumor suppressor genes.[57–59] Accordingly, a transgenic mouse model has been established with use of Cre-Lox-mediated, epithelial-specific deletion of both Rb1 and p53.[60] Coincidental loss of these tumor suppressor genes leads to the formation of neoplastic lesions following intratracheal intubation. These lesions exhibit neuroendocrine differentiation, as evidenced by expression of synaptophysin (Syp) and neural cell adhesion molecule (Ncam1, also known as CD56), consistent with germline mutation of these genes in mice.[61] No proliferation of club or AT2 cells has been reported, despite these cells harboring p53/Rb1 mutations in the transgenic model, which suggests a specific genotype–phenotype interaction in the neuroendocrine cell pool. Similar to humans, transgenic mice harboring SCLC can express anti-Hu antibodies (14% compared with 16% of humans).[62]

Restricting the targeting Rb1/p53 loss to specific lung epithelial cell subsets has demonstrated that targeting of either neuroendocrine or AT2 cells can lead to the formation of SCLC (the latter with lower efficiency). By contrast, however, club cells are resistant to this path of transformation. This technique has enabled identification of the cell type of origin in pancreatic and prostate cancers.[63,64] The finding that club cells are resistant to neuroendocrine cells with respect to transformation by conditional p53/Rb1 loss implies that neuroendocrine cells are the predominant cell of origin associated with SCLC, although AT2 cells also have the capacity to transform.[65]

Neuroendocrine Hedgehog Signaling Mediates Airway Repair and SCLC

A naphthalene-induced acute lung injury model leads to loss of club cells approximately 24 hours after administration, with epithelial regeneration occurring within 72 hours, as well as an expansion of rare neuroendocrine cells.[66,67] During this regeneration phase, there is activation of widespread Hh pathway signaling, evidenced by upregulation of Hh signaling (Shh ligand and GLI protein). However, GLI is lost following neuroendocrine differentiation by day 4 after naphthalene-induced injury in nascent calcitonin gene-related peptide-positive epithelial cells.[68] Using a transgenic model to monitor Hh signaling by replacing one allele of Ptch (a transcriptional target of GLI proteins) with beta-galactosidase, it has been possible to show that during normal development, this pathway is activated in the airway epithelial compartment.[68]

Hh signaling persists in SCLC, as evidenced by GLI and Shh expression in 50% of primary SCLC specimens (in contrast to 23% in NSCLC).[66] SCLC cells and xenografts are dependent on Hh signaling for growth, as evidenced by sensitivity to cyclopamine and, conversely, their rescue by ectopic expression of GLI1, similar to medulloblastoma.[69] SCLC cells do not exhibit mutations in Ptch, but rather exhibit juxtacrine Hh signaling similar to that seen in development and airway repair.

Tumor Heterogeneity and SCLC

One of the unique clinical features of SCLC is initial sensitivity to chemotherapy, followed by recurrence and a marked acquisition of resistance, occasionally associated with a transformation to the NSCLC phenotype.[70] This behavior of SCLC probably reflects underlying tumor heterogeneity, with initial selection for a culture of clones that are resistant to chemotherapy. SCLC cell cultures derived from primary SCLC specimens grow as suspensions of small cellular aggregates, with some that attach to plastic dishes. This activity has also been noted for cells derived from disaggregation of tumors from Rb1/p53 transgenic mice harboring SCLCs.[71,72] In the latter model, attaching cells exhibit a large cell phenotype without expressing the neuroendocrine markers achaete-scute homolog 1 (Ash1) or Syp, in contrast to paired suspension cells from each tumor. Gene expression profiling data obtained from these paired cell lines have been analyzed by principal component analysis and demonstrated two groups: small cell clones (neuroendocrine) and large cell clones (non-neuroendocrine).[72] Only the neuroendocrine cell type is capable of generating SCLC tumors when injected into BALB/c NU/NU nude mice, whereas the large cell tumors generated by subcutaneous injection exhibit a mesenchymal phenotype expressing CD44. Neither cell type can regenerate the heterogeneity seen in the primary tumor; however, they exhibit a clonal relationship evidenced by spectral karyotyping and comparative genomic hybridization.[72]

H-Ras signaling has been shown to drive transition of SCLC to a dedifferentiated phenotype characterized by downregulation of neuroendocrine markers.[73,74] When neuroendocrine cells from SCLC cell lines obtained from Rb1/p53 transgenic mice are retrovirally transduced with RAS^{V12}, they undergo a transition to an adherent phenotype with downregulation of neuroendocrine markers Syp and Ash1 and expression of CD44, and a shift in gene expression, with clustering of non-neuroendocrine cells on principal component analysis. Mixing neuroendocrine and non-neuroendocrine clones leads to cell–cell crosstalk that confers metastatic potential. Together, these data suggest that a common neuroendocrine cell of origin may undergo RAS-driven transformation to a CD44-expressing non-neuroendocrine clone.

CONCLUSION

The use of mouse models to study the initiation and evolution of lung cancers has been crucial in advancing the field through the identification of putative stem cell niches within the lung. In addition, these models have increased our understanding of the pathways that regulate tumor evolution following conditional oncogene activation. Based on the genomic complexity associated with multiple putative driver mutations, the processes governing cancer initiation are still relatively unclear. Furthermore, knowledge of the processes that drive genomic instability following tumor initiation, which lead to both spatial and temporal genomic complexity in lung cancer, will be essential for developing novel, more effective treatment paradigms, particularly in advanced disease.

KEY REFERENCES

6. Burrell RA, McGranahan N, Bartek J, Swanton C. The causes and consequences of genetic heterogeneity in cancer evolution. *Nature*. 2013;501(7467):338–345.
27. Carney DN, Gazdar AF, Bunn Jr PA, Guccion JG. Demonstration of the stem cell nature of clonogenic tumor cells from lung cancer patients. *Stem Cells*. 1982;1(3):149–164.
32. Bertolini G, Roz L, Perego P, et al. Highly tumorigenic lung cancer CD133+ cells display stem-like features and are spared by cisplatin treatment. *Proc Natl Acad Sci USA*. 2009;106(38):16281–16286.
37. Jackson EL, Willis N, Mercer K, et al. Analysis of lung tumor initiation and progression using conditional expression of oncogenic K-ras. *Genes Dev*. 2001;15(24):3243–3248.
52. Ali SA, Justilien V, Jamieson, Murray NR, Fields AP. Protein kinase Cι drives a NOTCH3-dependent stem-like phenotype in mutant KRAS lung adenocarcinoma. *Cancer Cell*. 2016;29:367–378.
53. Fang L, Cai J, Chen B, et al. Aberrantly expressed miR-582-3p maintains lung cancer stem cell-like traits by activating Wnt/β-catenin signalling. *Nat Commun*. 2015;6:8640.
60. Meuwissen R, Linn SC, Linnoila RI, Zevenhoven J, Mooi WJ, Berns A. Induction of small cell lung cancer by somatic inactivation of both Trp53 and Rb1 in a conditional mouse model. *Cancer Cell*. 2003;4(3):181–189.
65. Sutherland KD, Proost N, Brouns I, Adriaensen D, Song JY, Berns A. Cell of origin of small cell lung cancer: inactivation of Trp53 and Rb1 in distinct cell types of adult mouse lung. *Cancer Cell*. 2011;19(6):754–764.
68. Watkins DN, Berman DM, Burkholder SG, Wang B, Beachy PA, Baylin SB. Hedgehog signalling within airway epithelial progenitors and in small-cell lung cancer. *Nature*. 2003;422(6929):313–317.
72. Calbo J, van Montfort E, Proost N, et al. A functional role for tumor cell heterogeneity in a mouse model of small cell lung cancer. *Cancer Cell*. 2011;19(2):244–256.

See Expertconsult.com for full list of references.

14 Microenvironment and Lung Cancer

Tonya C. Walser, Elvira L. Liclican, Kenneth J. O'Byrne, William C.S. Cho, and Steven M. Dubinett

SUMMARY OF KEY POINTS

- There is untapped potential for targeted lung cancer prevention and therapy that requires, as a first step, a more clear delineation of the biology underlying the lung carcinogenesis process.

- The pulmonary microenvironment represents a unique milieu in which lung carcinogenesis proceeds in complicity with the four main components of the tumor microenvironment (TME): the field, cellular, soluble, and structural components.

- The literature now suggests that the adjacent histologically normal-appearing epithelium is a participant in the dynamic process of lung tumor initiation and carcinogenesis.

- Evidence continues to mount in support of the stromal compartment of the TME as an active participant in carcinogenesis, often driving the aggressiveness of tumors via its impact on the tumor cell secretome.

- Molecular signatures composed mainly of immune- and inflammation-related cytokines characterizing the cellular and soluble components of the TME correlate with important clinical parameters.

- The developing lung TME is populated by diverse cell types with both immune-protective and immune-suppressive potential—it is the balance of these effectors and their secretory products, along with their spatial and temporal context (i.e., the immune contexture), that often dictates clinical outcomes.

- One of the consequences of the inflammatory TME is suppression of antitumor immunity, thus recent strategies have been designed to specifically target the immune system.

- Dendritic cells are one of the cellular components of the TME that can be successfully utilized to redistribute soluble components of the TME (e.g., CCL21), ultimately redirecting the trafficking of immune cells into the tumor and enhancing immune activation.

- Two families of drugs directed at the immune system include pattern recognition receptor agonists (PRRago) and immunostimulatory monoclonal antibodies (immune checkpoint inhibitors).

Many questions central to a discussion of the influence of the lung tumor microenvironment (TME) on tumorigenesis and progression persist: the cells of origin for cancers arising in the proximal versus distal airways; the identities of key driver versus passenger mutations distinguishing histologically diverse tumors; the critical mass or combination of molecular and environmental events tipping the balance in favor of malignant conversion of the airway; and the order of events characterizing tumor initiation and systematic progression. Regardless of the answers to these questions, there is undoubtedly untapped potential for targeted lung cancer prevention and therapy that requires, as a first step, a clearer delineation of the biology underlying the lung carcinogenesis process. Perhaps no clinical approach holds more potential than targeting the molecular underpinnings of the interplay between premalignant lesions and the developing lung TME. The opportunities for combination approaches that target multiple components of the TME simultaneously also abound and are extremely promising clinically. Past and present attempts to molecularly delineate lung carcinogenesis and to target the epithelial-TME interface are discussed in this chapter.

LUNG CARCINOGENESIS

The link between premalignancy and subsequent development of cancer is well established for some organ systems, but not for the lung.[1] For example, removal of premalignant lesions is the standard of care and has been shown to decrease cancer incidence and mortality in the case of cervical dysplasia and colorectal polyps. However, it has been difficult to demonstrate the link between premalignant histologic airway abnormalities and subsequent development of lung cancer.[2] Uncertainties about the clinical behavior of a premalignant lung lesion can lead to either inappropriate inaction or inappropriate aggressive treatment, both of which can result in harm to the patient.

The seminal autopsy studies of Auerbach et al.[3] from the early 1960s demonstrated multiple histologic abnormalities in nonmalignant bronchial epithelia of smokers with and without lung cancer. Because progressive sputum abnormalities have been shown to precede the development of lung cancer,[4] it has been suggested that the development of lung cancer proceeds in an orderly fashion through increasing grades of histologic abnormalities that culminate in metastatic carcinoma, as in cervical and colorectal cancer. Recent molecular findings support this stepwise lung tumor initiation model in which injury or inflammation leads to dysregulated repair by stem cells.[2] Tobacco smoking is a leading source of chronic injury and inflammation; thus, the majority of heavy smokers bear regions of airway epithelial dysplasia that are classified as premalignant lesions.[5] Additional genetic and epigenetic alterations prevent normal differentiation of cells in these lesions and facilitate proliferation and expansion of the field, gradually displacing the normal epithelium and giving rise to full-blown malignancy and metastatic behavior. The initiation and expansion of this premalignant field (i.e., field cancerization) appear to be critical steps in lung carcinogenesis that can persist even after smoking cessation.[6,7]

The originally proposed and still prevailing model of lung cancer progression, termed the linear progression model, places the focus on the fully malignant primary tumor and its size, and metastatic dissemination is conditional on both.[8,9] Conversely, the more recently posited parallel progression model proposes that metastases may also arise from the early dissemination of premalignant epithelial cells before their full malignant conversion or collective growth into a large primary tumor.[8,9] Cell invasion and metastasis are hallmarks of cancer that are mediated by epithelial-to-mesenchymal transition (EMT) and typically are associated with late-stage disease.[9–11] As per the linear progression model, EMT only occurs in rare cells at the leading invasive edge of advanced cancers, facilitating the final step (i.e., metastasis) in tumor progression. However, many groups have now demonstrated that EMT also drives malignant transformation and early dissemination of epithelial malignancies, including tobacco-related cancers.[9,12,13] In addition, consistent with the parallel progression model, it was recently proposed that EMT promotes dissemination of lung epithelial cells prior to, or concomitant with, their malignant conversion. These alternate models of tumor initiation and progression were highlighted by Sanchez-Garcia[9] in 2009, because they represented paradigm shifts in terms of our understanding of the protracted process of epithelial cell conversion from normal to cancer. Importantly, the parallel progression model may represent a more accurate model of lung cancer progression, given the clinical observation that 30% of patients with early-stage lung cancer who have surgery subsequently have metastatic disease, an indication that undetected micrometastatic disease may have already been present at the time of surgery.[14]

THE DEVELOPING LUNG TUMOR MICROENVIRONMENT

In the not-so-distant past, malignant epithelial cells were considered the tumor, and the adjacent histologically normal appearing epithelium, immune effector cells, inflammatory mediators, and the stroma were all considered irrelevant bystanders. Although genetic changes are critical for the malignant transformation of epithelial cells, we now understand that all components of the developing lung TME are active participants in the events precipitating lung cancer development. In fact, most tumors arise within, and are dependent on, a cellular microenvironment characterized by suppressed host immunity, dysregulated inflammation, and increased production of cellular growth and survival factors that induce angiogenesis and inhibit apoptosis. The pulmonary microenvironment, in particular, represents a unique milieu in which lung carcinogenesis proceeds in complicity with each of what we consider the four main components of the TME: the field, cellular, soluble, and structural components.

TME Field Component: Adjacent Histologically Normal-Appearing Epithelium

Slaughter et al.[15] initially coined the term "field cancerization" in 1953 to describe the histologically normal-appearing tissue adjacent to a neoplastic lesion that displays molecular abnormalities often identical to those in the tumor. The concept was seemingly rediscovered more than four decades later, when investigators renewed the effort to define the molecular mechanisms precipitating the development of an array of epithelial malignancies, including lung cancer.[2,16–18] In contrast to other common epithelial malignancies, there is not yet a clinical rationale to evaluate potential premalignant lesions in people at risk for lung cancer. Thus, carefully designed clinical investigations are required to harvest these clinical specimens that would not otherwise be collected from these individuals. Although knowledge regarding the molecular changes that occur in the airway in the setting of lung carcinogenesis is only fragmentary at present, it is generally accepted that there are alterations in the airway epithelium that mirror many of the changes seen in the primary lung tumor.

For example, in lung cancer, mutations in the Kirsten rat sarcoma viral oncogene homolog (KRAS) gene were described in nonmalignant histologically normal-appearing lung tissue adjacent to lung tumor.[16,19] Moreover, loss of heterozygosity events were frequent in cells obtained from bronchial brushings of normal and abnormal lungs from patients undergoing diagnostic bronchoscopy and were detected in cells from the ipsilateral and contralateral lungs.[20] Likewise, mutations in the epidermal growth factor receptor (EGFR) oncogene were reported in normal-appearing tissue adjacent to EGFR-mutant

lung adenocarcinoma and also occurred at a higher frequency at sites more proximal to the adenocarcinomas than at more distant regions.[21,22] Global mRNA and microRNA expression profiles were also described in the normal-appearing bronchial epithelium of healthy smokers,[23,24] and a cancer-specific gene expression biomarker was developed from the mainstem bronchus that can distinguish smokers with and without lung cancer.[25,26] In addition, modulation of global gene expression in the normal bronchial epithelium in healthy smokers was similar in the large and small airways, and the smoking-induced alterations were mirrored in the epithelia of the mainstem bronchus and the buccal and nasal cavities.[17,27,28]

Kadara et al.[29,30] advanced the field in 2013 with their investigation of the spatial and temporal molecular field of injury in individuals with early-stage nonsmall cell lung cancer (NSCLC), as determined by expression profiling of the large airways after definitive surgery. The normal airway epithelia were collected by endoscopic bronchoscopy brushings 12 months after surgical removal of the tumors, then every 12 months thereafter for up to 36 months. Although the study had key limitations, gene networks mediated by the phosphoinositide 3-kinase (PI3K) and ERK gene networks were upregulated in the airways adjacent to the resected tumor, suggesting that PI3K pathway dysregulation in the field of cancerization represents an early event in lung carcinogenesis that may persist even after resection of the primary tumor. In a follow-up study, the same researchers performed expression profiling of multiple normal-appearing airways various distances from tumors in conjunction with paired NSCLC tumors and normal lung tissues that were still in situ at the time of airway epithelial cell collection.[31] Site-independent profiles, as well as gradient and localized airway expression patterns, characterized the adjacent airway field of cancerization, suggesting they may be useful for distinguishing the large airways of people with lung cancer from those of cancer-free smokers. Such studies of the field of cancerization enrich our understanding of the molecular pathogenesis of lung cancer and have transformative clinical potential. Biomarker signatures within the field could be used for risk assessment, diagnosis, monitoring progression of disease during active surveillance, and predicting the efficacy of adjuvant therapies following surgery.

TME Cellular and Soluble Components: Immune Effector Cells and Cell-Secreted Inflammatory Mediators

Since the early 2000s, the authors of gene expression profiling studies of several tumor types have described molecular signatures associated with carcinogenesis and progression. The molecular signatures that emerged from the original gene sets were composed mainly of cytokine genes involved in immune and inflammatory responses. In a seminal study by Bhattacharjee et al.[32] in 2001, microarray-based expression profiling of resected tumor specimens allowed the investigators to discriminate between biologically distinct subclasses of adenocarcinomas, as well as primary lung adenocarcinomas and metastases of nonlung origin. Soon thereafter, Beer et al.[33] used expression profiling to predict survival among patients with early-stage lung adenocarcinomas. Likewise, an mRNA expression profile developed by Potti et al.[34] identified a subset of patients with early-stage NSCLC at high risk of recurrence. More recently, to inquire whether gene expression changes in the noncancerous tissue surrounding tumors could be used as a biomarker to predict cancer progression and prognosis, Seike et al.[35] conducted a molecular profiling study of paired noncancerous and tumor tissues from patients with adenocarcinoma. Many of the genes identified were part of an immune and inflammatory response signature previously reported in other cancers, but a unique subset of the genes was also predictive of lymph node status and disease prognosis among patients with NSCLC.[36] Together, these studies provided the earliest indication of the potential for expression profiling and clear evidence that molecular signatures composed mainly of immune- and inflammation-related cytokines characterizing the cellular and soluble components of the TME correlate with important clinical parameters.

TME Structural Component: Stroma

As mentioned previously, the stroma was long thought to be the inert framework of the lung and irrelevant to the carcinogenesis process. Farmer et al.[37] were the first to report a major contribution of stromal genes to drug sensitivity, although not in the lung, in the context of a randomized clinical trial. These researchers used tumor biopsy specimens from individuals in the European Organization for Research and Treatment of Cancer 10994/BIG 00-01 trial with estrogen receptor-negative breast cancer treated with 5-fluorouracil, epirubicin, and cyclophosphamide and described a stromal gene signature that predicted resistance to preoperative chemotherapy. This study expanded the clinical significance of the identification of TME stroma-associated gene signatures, and it encouraged the development of antistromal agents as a new approach to overcome chemotherapy resistance.

An important translational study by Zhong et al.[38] also defined tumor cell and stromal cell interactions that inform the course of NSCLC progression. By coculturing a *KRAS*-mutant lung adenocarcinoma cell line with one of three lung stromal cells lines (macrophage, endothelial, or fibroblast) and subsequently profiling the secreted proteins, the group developed an in vitro model for evaluating the mechanisms by which stromal cells regulate the biologic properties of lung cancer cells. By two different proteomic approaches, the investigators concluded that stromal cells in the TME alter the tumor cell secretome, including proteins required for tumor growth and dissemination. Furthermore, they confirmed that the in vitro model robustly recapitulated many of the features of their *KRAS*-mutant murine model and human NSCLC specimens, suggesting its usefulness as a model of the lung TME.

Still more recently, Li et al.[39] demonstrated that mesenchymal stem cells (MSCs) recruited to the tumor stroma influence the phenotype of the tumor cells. Specifically, tumor cell-derived interleukin (IL)-1 induces prostaglandin E_2 (PGE_2) secretion by MSCs recruited to the tumor-associated stroma, which then acts in an autocrine manner to induce cytokine expression by the MSCs. The MSC-derived cytokines and PGE2 subsequently elicit a mesenchymal or stem cell–like phenotype in the tumor cells through activation of β-catenin signaling. Collectively, the results of these studies suggest that the stromal compartment of the TME is an active participant in carcinogenesis, often driving the aggressiveness of tumors via its impact on the tumor cell secretome. By extension, inhibition of specific interactions between tumor cells and the tumor-adjacent stroma holds significant potential in our search for novel lung cancer preventives and therapeutics.

PROTOTYPICAL CELL TYPES COMPRISING THE CELLULAR COMPONENT OF THE DEVELOPING LUNG TUMOR MICROENVIRONMENT

The developing lung TME is a unique and ever-changing milieu populated by diverse cell types with both immune-protective and immune-suppressive potential. The cell types are too numerous to describe in detail in the pages that follow. Thus, we discuss the induction, targeting, and potential pitfalls associated with attempting to harness three prototypical cell types characterizing the cellular component of the developing lung TME: cytotoxic and helper T cells, T regulatory cells (T regs), and dendritic cells.

Cytotoxic and Helper T Cells

The presence of tumor-infiltrating lymphocytes (TILs) has long been considered a manifestation of antitumor immunity. However, the prognostic significance of TILs was only appreciated after the development of markers that define the individual subsets of TILs.[40,41] Traditionally identified as a component of the cellular immune response to bacterial and viral infections, the integral role of cytotoxic CD8+ T cells (CTLs) in cell-mediated antitumor immune responses is now recognized. The reduced infiltration of CTLs, along with their reduced proliferation rate, increased susceptibility to spontaneous apoptosis, and impaired cytolytic activity against tumor cells, contributes to the immunosuppressive milieu that characterizes the developing lung TME.[42,43] Accordingly, a high infiltration of CTLs expressing granzyme B, the classic effector of CTL cytolytic activity, as well as the location of TILs in tumor cell nests, is associated with a good clinical outcome in several types of cancer, including colorectal cancer, ovarian cancer, and lung cancer.[44–50] Several reports have demonstrated that CTLs are associated with prolonged survival in lung cancer and positively correlated with favorable prognosis in patients with lung cancer.[43,46,51,52] However, more important than the number of CTLs present is the ratio of effector to regulatory TILs. In recent studies of patients with hepatocellular and ovarian cancer, it was shown that the ratio of CD8+ TIL:T regs was an independent prognostic factor, whereas the numbers of T regs and CD8+ TILs by themselves had lower or no predictive value, respectively.[53,54]

It is becoming increasingly clear that CD4+ helper T cells are also a critical determinant of effective antitumor immune responses. On stimulation, naïve CD4+ T cells differentiate into effector cells known as T helper (Th) cells, of which there are four subsets: Th1, Th2, Th17, and T regs. While T regs dampen antitumor immunity (discussed later), Th1 cells, characterized by production of interferon gamma and tumor necrosis factor-alpha, often lead to enhanced activation of CTLs, dendritic cells, and macrophages and beneficial downstream antitumor effects. In addition to assisting with the activation of other innate and adaptive immune cells, CD4+ helper T cells can induce apoptosis in tumor cells through Fas cell surface death receptor (FAS)- or tumor necrosis factor-related apoptosis-inducing ligand-dependent pathways.[55,56] Accumulating evidence also suggests that CD4+ helper T cells can acquire cytolytic activity.[57,58] As with CTLs, tumor-driven aberrant CD4+ T-cell differentiation and apoptosis, as well as Th dysfunction characterized by increased expression of the immune checkpoint molecule programmed death-1 (PD-1), contribute to the tolerogenic nature of the developing lung TME.[59] In this regard, immunotherapy strategies that aim to enhance the infiltration and/or activity of both CTLs and CD4+ helper T cells are found to have a synergistic effect in boosting antitumor immunity.

T Regulatory Cells

One major impediment to our efforts in both the prevention and treatment of lung cancer is our inadequate understanding of how lung cancer cells escape immune surveillance and inhibit antitumor immunity. Thus, identification of T regs in patients with cancer was a finding of great clinical importance. June et al.[60,61] were the first to document increased CD4+CD25+ T reg populations at the tumor site in patients with lung cancer. A subsequent examination of normal and tumor tissue from patients with NSCLC also indicated that tumor tissues have significantly higher expression of *FOXP3* mRNA than normal tissues, rendering CD4+CD25+FOXP3+ the more specific phenotypic marker of functional T regs at the time.[62] Next, investigators began to note increased numbers of T regs in the peripheral blood of patients with lung cancer relative to healthy volunteers and even patients with breast cancer.[63] Zhang et al.[64] made another key finding when they discovered that among patients with NSCLC receiving paclitaxel-based chemotherapy, the mitotic inhibitor selectively decreased the size of the T reg cell population in the peripheral blood, but not the size of the effector T cell subsets. They went on to determine that the effect was mediated by the upregulation of the cell death receptor Fas (CD95) and selective induction of apoptosis of T regs. Although T reg cell function was significantly impaired, production of Th1 cytokines and expression of the CD44 activation marker were intact and even elevated within the helper and effector T cell subsets after treatment with paclitaxel. In addition to these studies in lung cancer, there are numerous reports of increased T regs in the peripheral blood coincident with increased TILs in the tumor bed in other malignant diseases.[65–68] These seminal findings are consistent with studies in murine models demonstrating that depletion of T regs can significantly augment the efficacy of cancer vaccination.[69] Together, these data suggest that T regs are selectively recruited to developing lung tumors, where they contribute to the immunosuppressive microenvironment that facilitates progression and metastasis. Likewise, the data suggest that T reg status can serve as an indicator of responsiveness to certain therapeutic regimens.

One of the first studies to link T reg cell recruitment and prognosis, although not for lung cancer, came from Curiel et al.,[70] who discovered that an increase in the number of tumor T regs was a significant predictor of increased risk for death and reduced survival in those with ovarian cancer. They also discovered that tumor cells and tumor-adjacent macrophages were contributors of the CCL22 chemokine that mediated trafficking of the T regs to the tumor. This was the first report of functional CCL22 within the lung TME and the earliest indication that blocking CCL22 in vivo reduces human T reg cell tumor trafficking. This report paved the way for those that followed seeking to develop novel immune-boosting strategies based on eradication of the T reg cell population in patients with cancer.

Lastly, our group reported on the phenomenon of cycloxygenase-2 (COX-2) and PGE_2 inhibition of immune responses in lung cancer via promotion of T reg activity. Numerous studies have now demonstrated that PGE_2 enhances the in vitro inhibitory function of T regs and induces a regulatory phenotype in T helper cells.[71–73] These and other basic and translational research investigations have informed our understanding of the role of CD4+CD25+ T regs in the developing lung TME, collectively suggesting that the development of clinical strategies to reduce the suppressive effects of these T regs in lung cancer is warranted. Efforts directed at ablating the suppressive activities of T regs have included clinical trials that use total lymphodepletion.[74–76] Others have evaluated immunotoxins to specifically ablate the T reg population,[77] and ongoing clinical investigations are assessing the role of celecoxib in controlling T reg numbers, activity, and differentiation in human NSCLC. While lymphodepletion or therapy with T reg immunotoxins may prove beneficial, COX-2/ PGE_2 inhibition has additional potential benefits in the setting of NSCLC. In addition to the potential capacity to clinically decrease T reg cell function, COX-2 inhibition has been found to limit angiogenesis, decrease tumor invasiveness, and decrease tumor resistance to apoptosis in NSCLC.[78–80] These pathways and malignant phenotypes may be inhibited by several different agents in the class of nonsteroidal anti-inflammatory drugs.[81] Therefore, trials are evaluating COX inhibition in combination with other therapies.[80] Such studies will help further define the required interventions in this pathway and lead to more specifically targeted agents to diminish T reg cell activities in cancer. These agents could then be combined with other immune-based clinical therapies in an informed manner.

Dendritic Cells

In a seminal publication, Dieu-Nosjean et al.[46,82,83] identified ectopic lymph nodes or tertiary lymphoid structures within human NSCLC specimens and correlated their cellular content with clinical outcome. Specifically, the density of mature dendritic cells within these structures was a predictor of long-term survival in patients with lung cancer.[46] These findings were the first to suggest that ectopic lymph nodes participate in the host's antitumor immune response and are consistent with now abundant preclinical and clinical data.[84–88] For example, in murine tumor models, dendritic cells genetically modified to secrete CCL21 were reported to produce lymphoid cell aggregates and prime naïve T cells extranodally within a tumor mass, resulting in the generation of tumor-specific T cells and subsequent tumor regression.[85,89] Thus, the intratumoral approach may achieve tumor antigen presentation by utilizing the tumor as an in vivo source of antigen for the dendritic cells. In contrast to in vitro immunization with purified peptide antigen(s), autologous tumor has the capacity to provide the activated dendritic cells administered at the tumor site access to the entire repertoire of available antigens in situ. This may increase the likelihood of a response and reduce the potential for tumor resistance due to phenotypic modulation.

Dendritic cells are the most potent antigen-presenting cell capable of inducing primary immune responses.[90] Dendritic cells express high levels of major histocompatibility complex and costimulatory molecules, such as CD40, CD80, and CD86. Dendritic cells also release high levels of cytokines and chemokines into the TME that attract antigen-specific T cells in vivo. These properties, combined with efficient capture of antigens by immature dendritic cells, allow them to efficiently present antigenic peptides and costimulate antigen-specific naïve T cells.[90] Presentation of tumor-associated antigens by dendritic cells and their recognition by CTLs play an important role in the eradication of tumor cells.[91] Based on the importance of dendritic cells in tumor immunity, a variety of strategies have been used to exploit this cell type in cancer immunotherapy.[92–94] Advances in the isolation and in vitro propagation of dendritic cells, combined with identification of specific tumor antigens, have facilitated the start of clinical trials to evaluate dendritic cell-based vaccines,[92–94] and dendritic cell transfer has since been demonstrated to be a safe approach for clinical evaluation.[95–100]

Strategies involving the use of dendritic cells in immunotherapy have included pulsing isolated dendritic cells with tumor antigen peptides, apoptotic tumor cells, or tumor lysates ex vivo.[101–103] Dendritic cells have also been genetically modified with genes encoding tumor antigens or immunomodulatory proteins.[104–106] There is evidence that dendritic cells transduced with adenoviral vectors (AdV) have prolonged survival and resistance to spontaneous and Fas-mediated cell death, suggesting their utility in delivering immunotherapy more efficiently and robustly.[107] AdV transduction itself can also augment the capacity of dendritic cells to induce protective antitumor immunity.[108] In addition, enhanced local and systemic antitumor effects have been demonstrated when AdV-transduced dendritic cells expressing cytokine genes have been injected intratumorally.[109] AdVs are often used to transduce dendritic cells, because they efficiently induce strong heterologous gene expression in these cells.[108,109]

C-C motif chemokine ligand 21 (CCL21) is a cysteine-cysteine motif (CC) chemokine that belongs to a family of proteins involved in leukocyte chemotaxis and activation. Expressed in high endothelial venules and T cell zones of the spleen and lymph nodes, CCL21 exerts potent attraction of naïve T cells and mature dendritic cells, promoting their colocalization in secondary lymphoid organs and promoting cognate T cell activation.[110] Potent antitumor properties of CCL21 in murine cancer models have been reported.[111–113] CCL21 has also shown antiangiogenic activities in mice, thus strengthening its immunotherapeutic potential in cancer.[114,115] Based on the so-called ectopic lymph node concept posited by Dieu-Nosjean et al.[46] and the body of dendritic cell (DC)-CCL21 preclinical data available at the time, our group initiated a phase I clinical trial at the University of California, Los Angeles in patients with advanced stage NSCLC. The trial consisted of intratumoral administration of autologous DCs transduced with a replication deficient adenoviral vector to express the CCL21.[116] In situ vaccination with DC-CCL21 was well tolerated and induced systemic tumor antigen-specific immune responses and enhanced CD8+ T cell infiltration of the primary tumor. This study is one clinically relevant approach by which to harness the cellular component of the TME and manipulate the soluble component of the TME to the advantage of patients.

PROTOTYPICAL CELL-SECRETED PRODUCTS COMPRISING THE SOLUBLE COMPONENT OF THE DEVELOPING LUNG TUMOR MICROENVIRONMENT

Chronic or dysregulated inflammation in the pulmonary microenvironment characterizes pulmonary diseases associated with the greatest risk for the development of lung cancer, such as emphysema, chronic obstructive pulmonary disease, and pulmonary fibrosis.[117–119] Here, we will discuss the induction, targeting, and potential/pitfalls associated with manipulating the following prototypical inflammatory mediators found in the developing lung TME: IL-2, IL-6, and transforming growth factor-beta (TGF-β).[120]

Interleukin-2

IL-2, produced by T cells during an immune response,[121] is necessary for the growth, proliferation, and differentiation of naïve T cells into effector T cells. The use of IL-2 is approved by the US Food and Drug Administration (FDA) for cancer immunotherapy, and it is currently in clinical trials for the treatment of chronic viral infection.[122] Combination treatment with IL-2 and anti-IL-2 monoclonal antibodies protects against tumor metastases in the lung,[123] and although pulmonary edema was a side effect, high-dose IL-2 led to an antitumor response against pulmonary tumor nodules.[124] IL-2 with a D20T mutation retains the antimetastatic activity of IL-2 via its interaction with the high-affinity IL-2 receptor, but it has a lower toxicity profile.[125] Of interest is a recent study demonstrating that acupoint stimulation elicited a pronounced immunomodulatory effect among patients with lung cancer, as shown by increased production of IL-2.[126] Collectively, these studies support the potential of harnessing IL-2 production for the benefit of patients.

Interleukin-6

IL-6 is a multifunctional cytokine that can act as both a proinflammatory and an anti-inflammatory mediator. It is secreted by T cells and macrophages to stimulate immune responses, and increased levels of IL-6 have been associated with trauma, infection, and elevated cancer risk. IL-6 function is mediated primarily through the Janus kinase-signal transducer and activator of transcription-zinc finger protein 1–2 signaling pathway, and an elevated level of IL-6 has been shown to increase the production of collagen and alpha-actin, which together induce interstitial lung disease. High levels of IL-6 are also responsible for enhanced neoangiogenesis, inhibition of cancer cell apoptosis, and dysregulation of other control mechanisms in the TME.[127] IL-6 has also been implicated in acquired resistance to EGFR inhibitors in patients with lung cancer. Furthermore, IL-6 is associated with poor prognosis and many of the debilitating symptoms that often affect patients with late-stage lung cancer, such as fatigue, thromboembolism, cachexia, and anemia. Consequently, a monoclonal antibody targeting IL-6 (ALD518) was recently developed to treat these

IL-6-dependent morbidities. In preclinical, phase I, and phase II trials in advanced stage NSCLC, ALD518 appears to be well tolerated and to effectively ameliorate anemia and cachexia.[128]

Transforming Growth Factor-β

TGF-β is a cytokine that controls proliferation, cellular differentiation, and other functions in most cells. Secreted by many cell types, including macrophages, it plays a role in immunity and carcinogenesis. When a cell is transformed into a cancer cell, parts of the TGF-β signaling pathway are mutated, resulting in proliferation of the cancer cells and surrounding stromal cells (fibroblasts). Additionally, both cell types increase their production of TGF-β, which then acts on the surrounding stromal, immune, endothelial, and smooth-muscle cells to induce immunosuppression and angiogenesis and to make the cancer more invasive.[129] TME-derived TGF-β induces malignant phenotypes, such as epithelial mesenchymal transition (EMT) and aberrant cell motility, in lung cancer. TGF-β-induced translocation of β-catenin from E-cadherin complexes into the cytoplasm is involved in the transcription of EMT target genes.[130] Many studies have indicated that high levels of TGF-β characterize most tumor tissues, primarily released from tumor cells to maintain their metastatic potential and the protumorigenic TME.[131]

A TME enriched in TGF-β is broadly immunosuppressive, in part, due to its inhibition of natural killer cell function. Several studies have shown that miR-183-dependent repression of DNA polymerase III subunit tau (DNAX) activating protein 12 kDa (*DAP12*) transcription and translation in NSCLC is mediated by TGF-β.[132,133] TGF-β also converts effector T cells into T regs. Of interest, IL-6 enhances epithelial cell EMT and stimulates tumor progression by enhancing TGF-β signaling. Thus, IL-6 and TGF-β may play a contributing role in the maintenance of a paracrine loop between fibroblasts and NSCLC cells that facilitates tumor progression.[134] Like IL-6, TGF-β is a pleiotropic inflammatory mediator that interacts with premalignant lesions and the developing tumor in ways that are malleable and potentially manipulatable for the advantage of patients.

RECENT ATTEMPTS TO MOLECULARLY DEFINE THE FIELD COMPONENT OF THE LUNG TUMOR MICROENVIRONMENT

In our review of the recent translational research, several studies highlight the field's renewed appreciation for the urgent need to better define the key events driving lung carcinogenesis, if we are to ever achieve effective targeted lung cancer prevention. In the first of these studies, Ooi et al.[135] identified molecular alterations that characterize premalignant lesions and carcinogenesis in lung squamous cell carcinoma using a novel approach. In this first report of a gene expression profiling study of airway premalignant lesions and patient-matched normal tissue and squamous cell carcinoma samples, the authors discovered transcriptomic changes and identified genomic pathways altered with initiation and progression of squamous cell carcinoma within individual patients. Additionally, their analysis identified coordinate changes in the activity of upstream regulators and the expression of downstream genes within the same patient during early- and late-stage carcinogenesis, enhancing our understanding of the stepwise carcinogenesis of squamous cell carcinoma. In another study, by Perdomo et al.,[136] next-generation sequencing of small RNA from human bronchial airway epithelium identified miR-4423 as a regulator of airway epithelium differentiation and a repressor of lung carcinogenesis. Expression of miR-4423 is downregulated in the cytologically normal bronchial airway epithelium of smokers with lung cancer, which suggests that expression of miR-4423 and/or other miRNAs may be influenced by a field cancerization effect and could be useful for the early detection of lung cancer in the relatively accessible proximal airway. Inflammation-induced upregulation of the zinc-finger transcription factor Snail has also been demonstrated to contribute to diverse aspects of lung carcinogenesis and progression, including EMT and angiogenesis.[137,138] Snail was previously shown to be upregulated in human NSCLC tissues, to be associated with poor prognosis in patients, and to have promoted cancer cell growth and progression in vivo.[138] More recently, we discovered that one mechanism by which Snail acts is via upregulation of secreted protein, acidic and rich in cysteine (*SPARC*), which drives SPARC-dependent invasion in a model of human lung premalignancy.[139]

The literature now suggests that the adjacent histologically normal-appearing epithelium is a participant in the dynamic process of lung tumor initiation and carcinogenesis. Work to define the interconnectedness of the field of cancerization to the other components of the TME and the developing or established primary tumor may be a rich source for biomarkers of initiation, progression, and targets for prevention and therapy. Development of more accurate in vitro and in vivo models of human premalignancy and lung carcinogenesis will further advance these efforts.

RECENT ATTEMPTS TO MANIPULATE THE CELLULAR (IMMUNITY) AND SOLUBLE (INFLAMMATION) COMPONENTS OF THE TUMOR MICROENVIRONMENT FOR LUNG CANCER CHEMOPREVENTION AND THERAPY

One of the consequences of the inflammatory TME is suppression of antitumor immunity, thus recent strategies have been designed to specifically target the immune system. As mentioned briefly, one approach to enhance immune responses is DC-based vaccines, in which DCs are used as a vehicle to intratumorally deliver chemokines and subsequently redirect the trafficking of immune cells into the tumor and enhance their activation.[82,116] Using two murine models of lung cancer, we demonstrated for the first time that intratumoral administration of recombinant CCL21 could lead to potent immune-dependent antitumor responses and, consequently, reduce tumor growth.[140] Importantly, CCL21-mediated antitumor responses were lymphocyte-dependent. Therapy did not alter tumor growth in severe combined immunodeficiency mice, whereas intratumoral injection of CCL21 led to a significant increase in CD4+ and CD8+ T lymphocytes and DCs infiltrating both the tumor and draining lymph nodes in immunocompetent mice. Further studies in *CD4* and *CD8* gene knockout mice determined that both CD4+ and CD8+ T cell subsets accounted for the CCL21-mediated tumor regression.[140] Intratumoral administration of CCL21 gene-modified DCs was also shown to generate systemic antitumor responses and confer tumor immunity via recruitment and activation of T effector cells in a transplantable and a spontaneous bronchoalveolar cell carcinoma model of lung cancer.[141,142] These studies additionally demonstrated that elaboration of CCL21 in the tumors by DCs promotes the CXCR3/CXCR3 ligand efferent arm of the immune response for the modulation of antitumor activity; i.e., neutralization of the CXCR3 ligands CXCL9 or CXCL10 inhibited the antitumor responses.[82,141]

As the number of circulating competent DCs is decreased in patients with lung cancer,[143] injecting DCs within the lung tumor site may be a particularly effective approach. In fact, there is a relationship between tumor-infiltrating DC aggregation and apoptosis in situ in human NSCLC.[144] To this end, intratumoral administration of clinical grade CCL21-transduced DCs was evaluated in a phase I clinical trial for late-stage NSCLC.[116] Patients with stage IIIB/IV NSCLC with a tumor accessible by computed tomography–guided or bronchoscopic intervention and disease refractory to standard therapy were selected. The objectives of the trial were to (1) determine the safety and

maximum tolerated dose of CCL21 gene-modified DCs (Ad-CCL21-DC) when administered into the primary lung cancer of patients with advanced NSCLC and (2) determine the local and systemic biologic activity of AD-CCL21 DC. Intratumoral vaccination with Ad-CCL21-DC was well tolerated and resulted in (1) induction of systemic tumor antigen-specific immune responses and (2) enhanced tumor CD8+ T cell infiltration accompanied by increased *PD-L1* expression.[82,116] Thus, DCs are a cellular component of the TME that can be utilized to redistribute soluble components of the TME (e.g., CCL21), ultimately redirecting trafficking of the immune cells into the tumor and enhancing specific immune activation. DC-CCL21 in situ vaccination will next be evaluated in combination with checkpoint inhibitor therapy.

Intratumoral immunization represents another avenue for reversing cancer-induced immunotolerance, allowing an antitumor response to occur.[145–147] This strategy has recently been supported by the positive results of clinical trials in metastatic melanoma, renal cell carcinoma, and NSCLC, cancers with low sensitivity to conventional cytotoxic therapies.[146] Two families of drugs that are currently directed at the immune system and in clinical development include pattern recognition receptor agonists (PRRago) and immunostimulatory monoclonal antibodies (immune checkpoint inhibitors). In contrast to conventional anticancer drugs, these immunostimulatory drugs can be directly delivered into the tumor and generate a systemic antitumor immune response. Furthermore, intratumoral delivery can potentially trigger more potent antitumor immune responses while causing less autoimmune toxicity.

PRRs constitute a growing family of receptors that recognize pathogen-associated molecular patterns, such as viral DNA or bacterial cell wall molecules, and damage-associated molecular patterns (DAMP) that are released upon cell death, stress, or tissue injury. PRRs are typically known for their role in the activation of immune responses against infectious pathogens, and evidence now suggests that activation of PRRs, such as toll-like receptors (TLRs) expressed by immune cells, also plays a role in immune responses against tumor cells.[146] In this regard, it has been demonstrated that TLR stimulation of antigen-presenting cells within mice and in the human TME modifies their phenotype from tolerogenic to immunogenic, with an upregulation of class II major histocompatibility complex, CD80, and CD86.[148,149] TLRs can also be expressed by tumor cells, and the direct activation of these TLRs can result in the death of the targeted tumor cell and/or upregulate antigen-presentation molecules.[150,151] Furthermore, with chemotherapy or tumor-targeted therapy, tumor cells can release DAMPs, which can then stimulate the immune cells surrounding the tumor cells. This is exemplified by high mobility group protein B1, an intracellular protein released in the TME upon tumor cell death that is subsequently recognized by TLR-4 expressed on tumor-infiltrating immune cells. Although the mechanism of the therapeutic effect of intratumoral PRRago is multifactorial, depending on the tumor cell type, the TME, and the PRRago used, a common feature is stimulation of tumor-infiltrating antigen-presenting cells, including B cells, DCs, tumor-associated macrophages, and other myeloid-derived suppressor cells. It should be noted, however, that although activation of tumor-infiltrating antigen-presenting cells is a prerequisite for mounting an efficient adaptive antitumor immune response against tumor-associated antigens, it does not address immunosuppressive tumor-infiltrating T regs and exhausted tumor-infiltrating CTLs.

Immunostimulatory monoclonal antibodies are designed to reverse tumor immunotolerance and stimulate antitumor immune responses by targeting checkpoints for T cell activation. Of the checkpoint inhibitors in clinical development, the anti-CTL antigen-4 (CTLA-4) monoclonal antibody ipilimumab has already been approved for metastatic melanoma.[146,147] CTLA-4 is a cell surface receptor constitutively expressed by FOXP3+ CD4+ T regs, and it is a critical negative immune checkpoint that limits the induction of potent CTL responses. In two randomized phase III clinical trials, systemic intravenous therapy with ipilimumab generated long-lasting tumor responses in up to 20% of patients with refractory/relapsing melanoma.[152,153] However, this therapy was associated with major autoimmune toxicities requiring high-dose corticosteroids in about 60% of patients treated. The efficacy of anti-CTLA-4 has thus far been attributed to its ability to block the inhibitory interaction of CTLA-4 expressed on effector T cells with CD80/86 expressed by tolerogenic tumor antigen-presenting cells and, more recently, to intratumoral depletion of T regs rather than an interaction with CD4+ effector T cells.[146,147,152,153] Intratumoral tumor-specific T regs express high levels of CTLA-4, which can be depleted by therapy with anti-CTLA-4 via FcγR+ tumor-infiltrating cells.[146] Although no biomarkers exist to definitively predict which patients will benefit from anti-CTLA-4 therapy, there is a pattern in which a pretreatment gene signature demonstrating CD8 T cell infiltrates and CD8-attracting chemokines is, at least to some degree, positively correlated with benefit.[154] Current use of anti-CTLA-4 agents in NSCLC is still limited to phase I–III trials.

Based on the positive results of anti-CTLA-4 monoclonal antibodies, a second negative immune checkpoint mediated through interactions of PD-1 with its ligands PD-L1 and PD-L2 has been investigated as a target for cancer immunotherapy.[145–147] Monoclonal antibodies targeting the PD-1/PD-L1 axis have demonstrated strong and encouraging clinical activity in patients with metastatic melanoma, renal cell carcinoma, and NSCLC.[155,156] Late-phase clinical trials of these anti-PD-1 agents in patients with advanced lung cancers translated into improved clinical outcomes compared with standard-of-care chemotherapy.[157–161] Thus, two of the agents, nivolumab and pembrolizumab, are now FDA-approved for NSCLC in the second-line setting.[157,158] FDA approval for these agents as first-line therapy for NSCLC is anticipated. Importantly, preclinical models have demonstrated that the efficacy of immunostimulatory monoclonal antibodies may be potentiated when used in combination. Indeed, in murine models of melanoma, the combination of anti-PD-1 and anti-CTLA-4 monoclonal antibodies may be more effective than either agent alone, due to the complementary functional roles of these two negative immune checkpoints. Intratumoral injection of immunostimulatory agents is also postulated to have a potentiating effect. Local delivery, rather than systemic, allows concentration of the agent in the TME, limiting the toxicity of the monoclonal antibodies and increasing the efficacy of PRRago. This strategy relies on accessibility of the tumor site for injection, however, which can be an issue if repeated injections are needed.

As with anti-CTLA-4 therapy, no definitive predictive biomarkers exist for monoclonal antibodies targeting the PD-1/PD-L1 axis. However, transcriptomic profiling and whole-exome sequencing of melanoma from patients treated with anti-PD-1, a subset of whom had received prior mitogen-activated protein kinase inhibitor treatment, has given us insight into the relevance of transcriptomic changes and tumor mutations to therapeutic responsiveness.[162] Description of an innate anti-PD-1 resistance signature (IPRES) consisting of a set of coenriched genes in nonresponders is an important first step toward the identification of better biomarkers of response. With the approval of nivolumab and pembrolizumab for NSCLC, similar advances may soon be brought to bear against lung cancer as well. In addition to their report of a melanoma IPRES, Hugo et al.[162] also described a correlation between tumor mutational load and improved patient survival, but no statistically significant association between high mutational load and response to anti-PD-1 therapy was observed. Conversely, a number of other groups have reported a positive correlation between overall mutational load and both anti-CTLA-4 and anti-PD-1 treatment responsiveness.[162–166] There are still other preclinical reports suggesting that it is not mutational load in general that predicts response, but rather key driver mutations specifically upregulate PD-L1 for the purpose of immune evasion, thereby linking those specific mutations to anti-PD-1 treatment responsiveness.[145,167,168] For example, Akbay

et al.[145] suggest that EGFR-driven tumors may be characterized by host T cell exhaustion via upregulation of the PD-1/PD-L1 axis. Using a mouse model of EGFR-driven lung cancer, the authors demonstrated that administration of anti-PD-1 monoclonal antibodies reduced tumor growth and improved survival by enhancing T cell effector function and reducing the levels of tumor-promoting cytokines. Preclinical investigations of *KRAS* and *MYC* driver mutations also identify upregulation of PD-L1 by these oncogenic drivers, along with a concomitant increase in other key tumorigenic phenotypes.[167,168] Perhaps in alignment with these preclinical observations, Rizvi et al.[158,169] found that mutations in *KRAS* were evident in 7 of 14 tumors from NSCLC patients with partial or stable response >6 months compared with 1 of 17 in those that had no durable benefit from pembrolizumab. However, this finding may be explained by the association between *KRAS* mutations in NSCLC with smoking, given that smokers often harbor a substantially greater mutational load with each mutation serving as a potential source of neoantigens.[169,170]

CONCLUSION

Although the epithelial compartment remains central, investigators now understand that lung carcinogenesis proceeds in complicity with each of the four main components of the TME—the field, cellular, soluble, and stromal components. The epithelial and field compartments are definitively interconnected, but a more complete understanding of the molecular pathogenesis of lung cancer is required for the development of biomarker signatures, noninvasively obtained from the field, that are useful for risk assessment, diagnosis, disease monitoring, and predicting adjuvant therapy efficacy following surgery. Numerous cell types and cell-secreted products comprise the developing lung TME, and there are both advantages and disadvantages associated with attempting to harness each for the benefit of patients. Our review of the most recent translational and clinical literature highlights the field's evolving approach to the manipulation of these two particular TME components, including the rise of immunotherapeutics targeting the tumor-TME interface. On the whole, targeting the interplay between the epithelial compartment and the developing lung TME as a lung cancer prevention and therapy strategy has clear clinical potential that finally appears to be approaching fruition.

KEY REFERENCES

2. Gomperts BN, Spira A, Massion PP, et al. Evolving concepts in lung carcinogenesis. *Semin Respir Crit Care Med.* 2011;32(1):32–44.
6. Wistuba II. Genetics of preneoplasia: lessons from lung cancer. *Curr Mol Med.* 2007;7(1):3–14.
8. Klein CA. Parallel progression of primary tumours and metastases. *Nat Rev Cancer.* 2009;9(4):302–312.
9. Sanchez-Garcia I. The crossroads of oncogenesis and metastasis. *N Engl J Med.* 2009;360(3):297–299.
15. Slaughter DP, Southwick HW, Smejkal W. Field cancerization in oral stratified squamous epithelium; clinical implications of multicentric origin. *Cancer.* 1953;6(5):963–968.
17. Steiling K, Ryan J, Brody JS, Spira A. The field of tissue injury in the lung and airway. *Cancer Prev Res (Phila).* 2008;1(6):396–403.
29. Kadara H, Shen L, Fujimoto J, et al. Characterizing the molecular spatial and temporal field of injury in early-stage smoker non-small cell lung cancer patients after definitive surgery by expression profiling. *Cancer Prev Res (Phila).* 2013;6(1):8–17.
30. Gomperts BN, Walser TC, Spira A, Dubinett SM. Enriching the molecular definition of the airway "field of cancerization:" establishing new paradigms for the patient at risk for lung cancer. *Cancer Prev Res (Phila).* 2013;6(1):4–7.
32. Bhattacharjee A, Richards WG, Staunton J, et al. Classification of human lung carcinomas by mRNA expression profiling reveals distinct adenocarcinoma subclasses. *Proc Natl Acad Sci USA.* 2001;98(24):13790–13795.
33. Beer DG, Kardia SL, Huang CC, et al. Gene-expression profiles predict survival of patients with lung adenocarcinoma. *Nat Med.* 2002;8(8):816–824.

38. Zhong L, Roybal J, Chaerkady R, et al. Identification of secreted proteins that mediate cell-cell interactions in an in vitro model of the lung cancer microenvironment. *Cancer Res.* 2008;68(17):7237–7245.

46. Dieu-Nosjean MC, Antoine M, Danel C, et al. Long-term survival for patients with non-small-cell lung cancer with intratumoral lymphoid structures. *J Clin Oncol.* 2008;26(27):4410–4417.

116. Lee JM, Lee MH, Garon EB, et al. *Society for Immunotherapy of Cancer (SITC) Annual Meeting.* Maryland: National Harbor; 2016.

118. Heinrich EL, Walser TC, Krysan K, et al. The inflammatory tumor microenvironment, epithelial mesenchymal transition and lung carcinogenesis. *Cancer Microenviron.* 2012;5(1):5–18.

135. Ooi AT, Gower AC, Zhang KX, et al. Molecular profiling of premalignant lesions in lung squamous cell carcinomas identifies mechanisms involved in stepwise carcinogenesis. *Cancer Prev Res (Phila).* 2014;7(5):487–495.

136. Perdomo C, Campbell JD, Gerrein J, et al. MicroRNA 4423 is a primate-specific regulator of airway epithelial cell differentiation and lung carcinogenesis. *Proc Natl Acad Sci USA.* 2013;110(47):18946–18951.

139. Grant JL, Fishbein MC, Hong LS, et al. A novel molecular pathway for snail-dependent, SPARC-mediated invasion in non-small cell lung cancer pathogenesis. *Cancer Prev Res (Phila).* 2014;7(1):150–160.

151. Brody JD, Ai WZ, Czerwinski DK, et al. In situ vaccination with a TLR9 agonist induces systemic lymphoma regression: a phase I/II study. *J Clin Oncol.* 2010;28(28):4324–4332.

152. Hodi FS, O'Day SJ, McDermott DF, et al. Improved survival with ipilimumab in patients with metastatic melanoma. *N Engl J Med.* 2010;363(8):711–723.

157. Brahmer J, Reckamp KL, Baas P, Crino L, Eberhardt WE, Poddubskaya E, et al. Nivolumab versus docetaxel in advanced squamous-cell non-small-cell lung cancer. *N Engl J Med.* 2015;373:123–135.

158. Garon EB, Rizvi NA, Hui R, Leighl N, Balmanoukian AS, Eder JP, et al. Pembrolizumab for the treatment of non-small-cell lung cancer. *N Engl J Med.* 2015;372:2018–2028.

162. Hugo W, Zaretsky JM, Sun L, et al. Genomic and transcriptomic features of response to anti-PD-1 therapy in metastatic nelanoma. *Cell.* 2016;165:35–44.

169. Rizvi NA, Hellmann MD, Snyder A, et al. Mutational landscape determines sensitivity to PD-1 blockade in non-small cell lung cancer. *Science.* 2015;348:124–128.

See Expertconsult.com for full list of references.

15 MicroRNAs as Biomarkers for Lung Cancer

William C.S. Cho

SUMMARY OF KEY POINTS

- The biologic roles of microRNAs (miRNAs) in lung cancer indicate their correlation with disease status, prognosis, and therapeutic outcome. The discovery of miRNAs has opened a new avenue for individualized disease diagnosis and treatment.

- Dysfunctions of miRNAs are frequently found in lung cancer. These noncoding RNAs have been recognized as some of the main regulatory gatekeepers of coding genes in the human genome.

- Owing to their high stability during storage and handling, miRNAs are optimal biomarkers presenting in blood, urine, and other body fluids.

- Early detection is a key to improve the survival of patients with lung cancer. Recent studies have suggested that circulating miRNAs may become promising biomarkers for risk assessment and diagnosis of lung cancer in blood and sputum.

- Some single nucleotide polymorphisms (SNPs) are significantly associated with an increased risk of nonsmall cell lung cancer (NSCLC) and its prognosis.

- Identification of specific miRNAs may provide accurate subclassification of NSCLC.

- Recent studies have demonstrated that miRNAs may serve as predictive biomarkers for the chemoresistance of lung cancer among patients treated with systemic chemotherapy and/or targeted therapies.

- Large prospective cohort studies and cross-validation are needed to consolidate the significant findings demonstrated by studies of miRNA profiling.

- In conjunction with genetic and proteomic signatures and other screening approaches, miRNA biomarkers may represent a new milestone in lung cancer theranostics.

miRNAs are a class of evolutionarily conserved, endogenous, small noncoding RNAs of about 21 to 23 nucleotides in length that participate in diverse biologic pathways and function as posttranscriptional gene regulators during tumorigenesis. These small molecules mainly bind imperfectly to the 3′ untranslated region (UTR) of target messenger RNAs (mRNAs). They are encoded in the genome and are generally transcribed by RNA polymerase II. miRNAs work via RNA-induced silencing complexes to target mRNAs in a sequence-specific manner, resulting in mRNA deadenylation followed by exonucleolytic decay, mRNA endonucleolytic cleavage, or translational inhibition. Deregulation of miRNAs is associated with epigenetic and genetic alterations, such as aberrant DNA methylation, amplification, deletion, and point mutation.[1] More than 1000 miRNAs exist in the human genome, and each one can potentially regulate hundreds of mRNAs. miRNAs therefore play an important role in many cellular processes, including apoptosis, differentiation, proliferation, and the stress response.[2]

Lung cancer is the leading cause of cancer mortality worldwide, yet few molecular markers are available for risk screening, subclassification, early diagnosis, survival prognosis, and prediction of treatment response. Researchers have suggested that aberrant miRNA expression profiles may act as oncogenes or tumor suppressors in many types of cancer, including lung cancer. The biologic roles of miRNAs in lung cancer indicate a correlation with disease status, prognosis, and therapeutic outcome. The discovery of miRNAs has opened a new avenue for individualized disease diagnosis and treatment.[3]

THE IMPORTANCE OF MICRORNAS IN LUNG CANCER

Implications of miRNAs in the Diagnosis of Lung Cancer

Identifying patients with early-stage lung cancer who will benefit the most from effective therapies may reduce the mortality of this deadly disease. Early detection is thus a key to improving the survival of patients with lung cancer. The results of investigational studies suggest that miRNAs may become promising biomarkers for risk assessment and diagnosis of lung cancer (Tables 15.1 and 15.2).

The let-7 family is a global genetic regulator important in controlling the expression of lung cancer oncogenes. Chin et al.[4] sequenced the let-7 complementary sites (LCS) in the Kirsten rat sarcoma (*KRAS*) 3′ UTR from 74 cases of NSCLC and identified a SNP at LCS6 significantly associated with an increased risk for NSCLC among moderate smokers (odds ratio, 2.3; 95% CI, 1.1–4.6). The LCS6 variant allele showed a 2.3-fold increase in risk for NSCLC among patients who smoked the equivalent of less than 40 pack-years.

A survey has reported that the SNP rs11614913 in miR-196a2 may affect mature miR-196a expression and target mRNA-binding activity and is significantly associated with survival from NSCLC. In a case–control study of 1058 patients with incident lung cancer and 1035 cancer-free controls in a Chinese population, Tian et al.[5] found that miR-196a2 rs11614913 variant homozygote CC was associated with a significant increase of approximately 25% (odds ratio, 1.25; 95% CI, 1.01–1.54) in the risk of lung cancer compared with the wild-type homozygote TT and heterozygote TC. To further determine whether any association exists between four common SNPs (miR-196a2 C>T, rs11614913; miR-146a G>C, rs2910164; miR-499 A>G, rs3746444; and miR-149 C>T, rs2292832) and the risk for lung cancer, He et al.[6] performed a meta-analysis of 40 published case–control studies. Their results demonstrated that the rs11614913 TT genotype was significantly associated with a decreased risk of lung cancer for an Asian population subgroup (TT vs. CC: odds ratio, 0.7; 95% CI, 0.57–0.85; *p* = 0.284). Squamous cell carcinoma is one major subtype of lung cancer for which biomarkers are urgently needed to aid patient management. Measuring the miRNA expression in cancerous and noncancerous tissue pairs collected from 60 Chinese patients with squamous cell carcinoma (stages I–III), Tan et al.[7] identified a panel of five miRNAs (miR-30a, miR-140-3p, miR-182, miR-210, and miR-486-5p) that distinguished squamous cell carcinoma from normal lung tissues with an accuracy of 94%. They also showed that high expression

TABLE 15.1 Single MicroRNAs (miRNAs) as Diagnostic Biomarkers for Lung Cancer

miRNAs	Deregulation in Cancer	Materials	Descriptions	References
let-7	Downregulated	Tissue/TTNA tissue	A SNP in a let-7 complementary site in the *KRAS* 3' untranslated region increases NSCLC risk Profiling the let-7 family is a promising method for differentiating adenocarcinoma from squamous cell carcinoma, even in small specimens, such as those obtained with TTNA	4,9
let-7a	Downregulated	Serum	Expression levels show 0.74-fold change in cases vs. controls	14
miR-10b	Upregulated	Serum	High serum miR-10b value is associated with elevated level of tissue polypeptide antigen	18
miR-17-5p	Downregulated	Serum	Expression levels show 0.82-fold change in cases vs. controls	14
miR-25	Upregulated	Serum	The copy numbers of miR-25 are much higher in lung cancer than in healthy control samples	16
miR-27a	Downregulated	Serum	Expression levels show 0.87-fold change in cases vs. controls	14
miR-29c	Upregulated	Serum	The increased expression levels may reflect an increased systemic concentration of miR-29c in response to cancer processes	14
miR-106a	Downregulated	Serum	Expression levels show 0.87-fold change in cases vs. controls	14
miR-141	Upregulated	Serum	High serum miR-141 value is associated with elevated level of urokinase plasminogen activator	18
miR-145*	Downregulated	FFPE tissue	miR-145* inhibits cell invasion and metastasis	22
miR-146b	Downregulated	Serum	miR-146b is significantly decreased in lung cancer regardless of stage or histology	14
miR-155	Downregulated	Serum	Expression levels show 0.77-fold change in cases vs. controls	14
miR-196a2	Upregulated	Blood	Functional SNP rs11614913 in miR-196a2 can contribute to lung cancer susceptibility The rs11614913 TT genotype is associated with a significantly decreased risk of lung cancer for an Asian subgroup	5,6
miR-198	Downregulated	PE	Cell-free miR-198 from patients with lung adenocarcinoma may have diagnostic potential for differentiating malignant PE from benign PE	19
miR-205	Downregulated	FFPE tissue/TTNA tissue	miR-205 provides highly accurate subclassification of squamous cell carcinoma in NSCLC Profiling miR-205 is a promising method for differentiating adenocarcinoma from squamous cell carcinoma, even in small specimens such as those obtained with TTNA	8,9
miR-221	Downregulated	Serum	miR-221 is significantly decreased in lung cancer regardless of stage or histology	14
miR-223	Upregulated	Serum	The copy numbers of miR-223 are much higher in lung cancer than in healthy control samples	16
miR-328	Upregulated	FFPE tissue	miR-328 has a role in conferring migratory potential to NSCLC cells working in part through *PRKCA*	21

FFPE, formalin-fixed, paraffin-embedded; *NSCLC*, nonsmall cell lung cancer; *PE*, pleural effusion; *PRKCA*, protein kinase C, alpha; *SNP*, single nucleotide polymorphism; *TTNA*, transthoracic needle aspiration.

of miR-31 was associated with poor survival among patients with squamous cell carcinoma.

Recent advances in the treatment of lung cancer require greater accuracy in the subclassification of NSCLC. Using a high-throughput microarray to measure the miRNA expression levels in 122 samples of adenocarcinoma and squamous cell carcinoma, Lebanony et al.[8] identified miR-205 as a highly specific marker (96% sensitivity and 90% specificity) for squamous cell carcinoma. This standardized diagnostic assay may provide accurate subclassification of NSCLC. Fassina et al.[9] investigated the accuracy of miRNAs in differentiating squamous cell carcinoma from adenocarcinoma within scant and distorted specimens obtained by transthoracic needle aspiration. Quantification of the let-7 family and miR-205 expression levels in 18 adenocarcinoma and 13 squamous cell carcinoma specimens by quantitative reverse transcription-polymerase chain reaction (RT-PCR) showed a significant upregulation of the let-7 family and a significant downregulation of miR-205 in adenocarcinoma specimens (all, $p < 0.05$). Xing et al.[10] profiled miRNA expression signatures in 15 samples of lung squamous cell carcinoma and matched normal lung samples with an miRNA array (GeneChip; Affymetrix, Santa Clara, CA, USA). They identified three miRNAs (miR-205, miR-210, and miR-708) that distinguished the sputum samples of patients with stage I lung squamous cell carcinoma from

those of healthy individuals with 73% sensitivity and 96% specificity. Early detection is also the key to improving the survival of patients with lung adenocarcinoma. Using miRNA profiling on 20 paired samples of adenocarcinoma and normal lung tissue, Yu et al.[11] identified four miRNAs (miR-21, miR-200b, miR-375, and miR-486) that distinguished the sputum samples of patients with stage I lung adenocarcinoma from those of healthy individuals with 81% sensitivity and 92% specificity.

Other studies were designed to identify serum-based miRNAs with the ability to diagnose NSCLC at an early stage. Owing to their high stability during storage and handling, miRNAs are optimal biomarkers present in the blood, urine, and other body fluids.[12] Foss et al.[13] performed miRNA profiling on total RNA extracted from serum obtained from 11 patients with early-stage NSCLC and 11 controls. The authors found that the expression of miR-574-5p and miR-1254 was significantly increased in the samples of early-stage NSCLC with respect to the controls ($p = 0.0277$). Receiver operating characteristic curves plotting these two miRNAs were able to discriminate early-stage NSCLC from control samples with 82% sensitivity and 77% specificity. Using quantitative RT-PCR to measure the circulating levels of miRNAs in paired serum and plasma samples from 220 patients with early-stage NSCLC and 220 matched controls, Heegaard et al.[14] also demonstrated that the expression levels of let-7a,

TABLE 15.2 Combinations of MicroRNAs (miRNAs) as Diagnostic Biomarkers for Lung Cancer

miRNAs	Deregulation in Cancer	Materials	Descriptions	References
miR-20a	Upregulated	Serum	This 10-miRNA panel is correlated with the stage of NSCLC, especially in younger patients and patients who are current smokers	15
miR-24	Upregulated			
miR-145	Upregulated			
miR-152	Upregulated			
miR-199a-5p	Upregulated			
miR-221	Upregulated			
miR-222	Upregulated			
miR-223	Upregulated			
miR-320	Upregulated			
miR-21	Upregulated	Sputum	The combination of these four markers may improve the early detection of lung adenocarcinoma	11
miR-200b	Upregulated			
miR-375	Upregulated			
miR-486	Downregulated			
miR-28-3p	Downregulated	Plasma	These miRNAs in plasma may have a role as molecular predictors of lung cancer development and aggressiveness	20
miR-30c	Downregulated			
miR-92a	Upregulated			
miR-140-5p	Downregulated			
miR-451	Upregulated			
miR-660	Upregulated			
miR-30a	Downregulated	Tissue	This five-miRNA signature may be a new diagnostic classifier for squamous cell carcinoma among Chinese patients	7
miR-140-3p	Downregulated			
miR-182	Upregulated			
miR-210	Upregulated			
miR-486-5p	Downregulated			
miR-30a-30p	Upregulated	Plasma	This six-miRNA diagnostic test can discriminate between lung adenocarcinoma and granuloma	17
miR-100	Upregulated			
miR-151a-5p	Upregulated			
miR-154-3p	Upregulated			
miR-200b-5p	Upregulated			
miR-629	Upregulated			
miR-139-5p	Upregulated	Plasma	This four-miRNA screening test is useful to divide nodule and nonnodule groups	17
miR-200b-5p	Upregulated			
miR-378a	Upregulated			
miR-379	Upregulated			
miR-205	Upregulated	Sputum	The combination of these three markers may improve the early detection of lung squamous cell carcinoma	10
miR-210	Upregulated			
miR-708	Upregulated			
miR-574-5p	Upregulated	Serum	These two markers may be used as minimally invasive screening and triage tools for early-stage NSCLC	13
miR-1254	Upregulated			

NSCLC, nonsmall cell lung cancer.

miR-17-5p, miR-27a, miR-106a, miR-146b, miR-155, and miR-221 were significantly reduced in the serum of patients with NSCLC, whereas miR-29c was significantly increased (all, $p < 0.05$). Performing risk–score analysis to evaluate the diagnostic values of serum miRNA profiling among 400 patients with NSCLC and 200 controls, Chen et al.[15] showed that a panel of 10 serum miRNAs (miR-20a, miR-24, miR-25, miR-145, miR-152, miR-199a-5p, miR-221, miR-222, miR-223, and miR-320) accurately distinguished patients with NSCLC from controls even up to 33 months before the clinical diagnosis of NSCLC.

The levels of miRNAs in serum are stable, reproducible, and consistent among individuals of the same species. Chen et al.[16] used Solexa sequencing on serum miRNAs of human participants and obtained two miRNAs (miR-25 and miR-223) specific for NSCLC. The study conducted expression profiles of serum miRNAs in 21 healthy human patients and 11 NSCLC patients. Their results were validated in an independent cohort of 152 lung cancer patients and 75 healthy controls. The results of these analyses suggest that the copy numbers of these two serum miRNAs may serve as biomarkers for the detection of NSCLC. Cazzoli et al.[17] used exosome-based techniques to analyze the miRNAs of 30 plasma samples (10 lung adenocarcinomas, 10 lung granulomas, and 10 healthy smokers) and subsequently validated them on an independent group of 105 specimens. The results showed that a screening test of four miRNAs (miR-139-5p, miR-200b-5p,

miR-378a, and miR-379) was useful to divide the nodule and nonnodule groups (97.5% sensitivity, 72% specificity, and 90.8% area under the receiver operating characteristic curve [AUC]). The authors also developed a diagnostic test of six miRNAs (miR-30a-3p, miR-100, miR-151a-5p, miR-154-3p, miR-200b-5p, and miR-629) to discriminate between lung adenocarcinoma and granuloma (96% sensitivity, 60% specificity, and 76% AUC).

To examine whether circulating miRNAs have the potential to become suitable blood-based markers for the diagnosis and progression of lung cancer, Roth et al.[18] measured the concentrations of four miRNAs in the serum of 35 patients with lung cancer and seven patients with benign lung tumors. The levels of miR-10b ($p = 0.002$) and miR-141 ($p = 0.0001$) were significantly higher in patients with lung cancer than in patients with benign disease. High serum concentrations of miR-10b were also found to be associated with lymph node metastasis among patients with lung cancer. Circulating cell-free miRNAs in pleural effusion are also potential biomarkers for cancer. Using microarrays to screen miRNAs in 10 malignant pleural effusions associated with lung adenocarcinoma and 10 benign pleural effusions, Han et al.[19] showed that miR-198 was significantly downregulated in malignant pleural effusion compared with benign pleural effusion ($p = 0.002$). The results of miRNA microarray analysis were confirmed by quantitative RT-PCR using a validation set comprising 45 malignant pleural effusions associated with lung adenocarcinoma and 42 benign pleural effusions. The AUC for miR-198 was 0.887.

Although early detection using chest x-ray and spiral computed tomography (CT) has resulted in a marked increase in the number of lung cancer diagnoses, these efforts may also lead to unnecessary treatments, and this possibility indicates the need for biomarkers of aggressive disease. Boeri et al.[20] explored the miRNA expression profiles of 74 plasma samples collected during the 5-year screening plan and identified 12 of 15 samples collected before lung cancer detection by spiral CT, with sensitivity of 80% and specificity of 90%. The 5-year screening plan was a longitudinal analysis of 3246 current or former smokers screened for lung cancer beginning in 1998 either in the United States or in Italy to assess whether CT screening might increase the frequency of lung cancer diagnosis. The median amount of follow-up from the initial CT evaluation to the mortality end point was nearly 5 years. The most frequently deregulated miRNAs were miR-28-3p, miR-30c, miR-92a, miR-140-5p, miR-451, and miR-660.

Brain metastasis affects approximately 25% of patients with NSCLC during their lifetime. Arora et al.[21] performed miRNA microarray profiling on samples from seven patients with NSCLC with brain metastasis and six without brain metastasis, and confirmed that the expression of miR-328 was able to correctly classify patients with and without brain metastasis. This miRNA may be incorporated into clinical treatment decision making to stratify patients with NSCLC who have a higher risk for brain metastasis. Profiling miRNAs extracted from 527 stage I NSCLCs on the human miRNA expression profiling panel, Lu et al.[22] found that miR-145* was associated with brain metastasis by virtue of inhibiting cell invasion and metastasis. This miRNA holds potential as a target for preventing and treating brain metastasis among patients with stage I NSCLC.

MicroRNAs as Prognostic Biomarkers for Lung Cancer

Despite the availability of effective treatments, recurrence is common even for early-stage lung cancer. Prognostic biomarkers that can predict tumor progression and survival are required to provide better guidance on postoperative surveillance and therapeutic decisions for patients with lung cancer. Recent evidence suggests that specific miRNAs with altered expression levels have great potential to serve as prognostic biomarkers for lung cancer (Tables 15.3 and 15.4).

Takamizawa et al.[23] reported that the expression of let-7 was able to classify 143 cases of human NSCLC into two major groups. Reduced expression of let-7 was significantly associated ($p = 0.0003$) with shorter postoperative survival, suggesting the potential prognostic impact of this miRNA alteration. Yanaihara et al.[24] also found that low expression of let-7a-2 and high expression of miR-155 correlated with poor survival of 65 patients with lung adenocarcinoma.

Evaluating the miRNA expression levels in 48 pairs of NSCLC tissue specimens by looped real-time RT-PCR, Markou et al.[25] detected a significant correlation ($p = 0.027$) between miR-21 overexpression and overall survival of patients with NSCLC. These results indicate that miRNA expression profiles may be prognostic markers of lung cancer. Saito et al.[26] also tested the expression of specific miRNAs by quantitative RT-PCR in tissues from 317 patients with lung adenocarcinoma. Elevated miR-21 was associated with worse cancer-specific mortality and worse relapse-free survival independent of other clinical factors in patients with stage I disease; these findings suggest that expression of miR-21 may contribute to lung carcinogenesis and serve as an early-stage prognostic biomarker for lung adenocarcinoma. Evaluating a combination four-gene panel (breast cancer 1 [BRCA1], hypoxia inducible factor 1, alpha [HIF1A], deleted in liver cancer 1 [DLC1], and exportin 1 [XPO1]) with miR-21

expression from 148 patients with stage I lung adenocarcinoma, Akagi et al.[27] found that the combination improved the association with prognosis. To synthesize the evidence of miR-21 as a prognostic biomarker in lung cancer, Yang et al.[28] conducted a meta-analysis for miR-21 with a median study size of 88 patients. The pooled hazard ratio suggested that high expression of miR-21 has a negative impact on relapse-free survival in lung adenocarcinoma and on overall survival in NSCLC. Their results also indicated that miR-21 can predict recurrence and poor survival in NSCLC.

Profiling 61 lung squamous cell carcinoma samples on miRNA bioarrays, Raponi et al.[29] showed that miR-146b and miR-155 have prognostic value in squamous cell carcinomas. Used alone, miR-146b had the strongest prediction accuracy, at approximately 78%, for stratifying prognostic groups in lung squamous cell carcinoma. Analyzing 140 pairs of NSCLC paraffin-embedded specimens and their corresponding adjacent noncancerous tissues, Cai et al.[30] discovered a uniform decrease in miR-186 expression correlating with poor survival, with median overall survival time of 63.0 or 21.5 months among patients with high or low levels of miR-186, respectively. Enforced overexpression of miR-186 in NSCLC cells inhibits proliferation by inducing G1-S checkpoint arrest. Their findings establish a tumor-suppressive role for miR-186 in the progression of NSCLC.

Profiling miRNA expression in 103 pairs of matched lung adenocarcinoma samples from never-smokers, Jang et al.[31] found that a high expression level of miR-708 in the tumors was strongly associated with an increased risk of death after adjustment for all clinically significant factors including age, gender, and tumor stage. This miRNA acts as an oncogene contributing to tumor growth and disease progression by directly downregulating TMEM88, a negative regulator of the Wnt signaling pathway in lung cancer. Meng et al.[32] conducted genome-wide miRNA sequencing in primary cancer tissue from patients with lung adenocarcinoma and found that miR-31 was upregulated among patients with lymph node metastases compared with patients without lymph node metastases. This marker was validated in an external cohort of 233 cases of lung adenocarcinoma in The Cancer Genome Atlas (https://wiki.nci.nih.gov/display/TCGA/miRNASeq). Exploratory in-silico analysis showed that low expression of miR-31 was associated with excellent survival for T2 N0 patients.

Discovering prognostic markers that can predict relapse is a key part of cancer research. Campayo et al.[33] assessed miRNA expression in 70 resected NSCLC samples (TaqMan miRNA assays; Life Technologies, Carlsbad, CA, USA) and found that the mean time to relapse was 18.4 months for patients who had tumors with low levels of miR-145 and 28.2 months for patients who had tumors with high levels. The mean time to relapse was 29.1 months for tumors with low levels of miR-367 and 23.4 months for tumors with high levels. The expression levels of these miRNAs can be potential markers for relapse in surgically treated NSCLC.

The miR-34 family is part of the p53 network, and its expression is directly induced by p53 in response to DNA damage or oncogenic stress. In a study using stem-loop RT-PCR to analyze the expression of the miR-34 family in tumor tissues from 70 patients with surgically resected NSCLC, Gallardo et al.[34] found that low levels of miR-34a expression were correlated with a high probability of relapse. Patients with both *p53* mutations and low miR-34a levels had the highest probability of relapse. Nadal et al.[35] assessed the aberrant methylation and expression of miR-34b/c in 15 lung adenocarcinoma cell lines and a cohort of 140 patients with early-stage, surgically resected lung adenocarcinoma. They found that expression of miR-34b/c was significantly reduced ($p = 0.001$) in all methylated cell lines and primary tumors, especially in those harboring a *TP53* mutation. Patients who had tumors with high levels of miR-34b/c methylation had

TABLE 15.3 Single MicroRNAs (miRNAs) as Prognostic Biomarkers for Lung Cancer

miRNAs	Deregulation in Cancer	Materials	Descriptions	References
let-7	Downregulated	Tissue	Overexpression of let-7 in NSCLC cells inhibits cell growth in vitro	23
let-7a-2	Downregulated	Tissue	Low expression of let-7a-2 correlates with poor survival of patients with lung adenocarcinoma	24
let-7f	Upregulated	Plasma	Expression level of let-7f is associated with overall survival in NSCLC	42
miR-16	Downregulated	Serum	High expression of miR-16 is associated with significantly better survival in patients with advanced NSCLC	44
miR-21	Upregulated	Tissue	Overexpression of miR-21 is an independent negative prognostic factor for overall survival in NSCLC	25,26,28
			Inhibition of miR-21 inhibits cell growth in vitro and inhibits tumor growth in xenograft mouse models of lung adenocarcinoma	
			High expression of miR-21 has a negative impact on relapse-free survival in lung adenocarcinoma and overall survival in NSCLC	
miR-30c-1	Downregulated	Tissue	The expression of the host nuclear transcription factor Y gene is correlated with pri-miR-30c-1, but not with rs928508 genotypes among patients with NSCLC	40
miR-30e-3p	Downregulated	Plasma	The expression level of miR-30e-3p is associated with short disease-free survival in NSCLC	42
miR-31	Upregulated	Tissue	miR-31 represses DICER1 activity but not PPP2R2A or LATS2 in lung squamous cell carcinoma	7,32
			In vitro functional assays show that miR-31 increases cell migration, invasion, and proliferation in an ERK1/2 signaling-dependent manner in lung adenocarcinoma	
miR-34a	Downregulated	Tissue	A relation has been found between *MIRN34A* methylation and miR-34a expression in NSCLC	34
miR-34b	Downregulated	Tissue	Overexpression of miR-34b decreases the expression of *c-Met* in NSCLC cells	36
miR-34b/c	Downregulated	Tissue	Ectopic expression of miR-34b/c in lung adenocarcinoma cells decreases cell proliferation, migration, and invasion	35
miR-145	Downregulated	Tissue	miR-145 regulates *SOX2* and *OCT4* translation, and *p53* regulates miR-145 expression	33
miR-146b	Upregulated	Tissue	High expression of miR-146b correlates with poor overall survival for patients with lung squamous cell carcinoma	29
miR-149	Downregulated	Tissue	miR-149 may be involved in the pathogenesis of NSCLC	41
miR-155	Upregulated	Tissue	High expression of miR-155 correlates with poor survival of patients with lung adenocarcinoma	24,29
			High expression of miR-155 correlates with poor overall survival for patients with lung squamous cell carcinoma	
miR-186	Downregulated	Cell line	*Cyclin D1, CDK2,* and *CDK6* are each directly inhibited by miR-186, and restoring their expression levels reverses miR-186-mediated inhibition of cell cycle progression	30
miR-196a	Upregulated	Tissue	miR-196a may be involved in the pathogenesis of NSCLC	41
miR-196a2	Upregulated	Tissue	rs11614913 CC is associated with a significant increase in mature miR-196a expression, but not with changes in levels of the precursor for NSCLC	39
miR-367	Upregulated	Tissue	SOX2 and OCT4 transcription factors regulate the expression of miR-367	33
miR-651	Downregulated	Blood	The FAS:rs2234978 G allele is significantly associated with survival in early-stage NSCLC, and the *FAS* single nucleotide polymorphism created a miR-651 functional binding site	45
miR-708	Upregulated	Tissue	Forced miR-708 expression reduces *TMEM88* transcript levels and increases the rate of cell proliferation, invasion, and migration in culture	31

DICER1, dicer 1, ribonuclease type III; *FAS*, Fas cell surface death receptor; *LATS2*, large tumor suppressor kinase 2; *NSCLC*, nonsmall cell lung cancer; *OCT4*, octamer-binding transcription factor 4; *PPP2R2A*, protein phosphatase 2, regulatory subunit B, alpha; *SOX2*, SRY (sex determining region Y)-box 2; *TMEM88,* transmembrane protein 88.

TABLE 15.4 Combinations of MicroRNAs (miRNAs) as Prognostic Biomarkers for Lung Cancer

miRNAs	Deregulation in Cancer	Materials	Descriptions	References
let-7a	Downregulated	FFPE tissue	Low expression of these five miRNAs is associated with up to fourfold excess mortality for male smokers with early-stage squamous cell carcinoma	38
miR-25	Downregulated			
miR-34a	Downregulated			
miR-34c-5p	Downregulated			
miR-191	Downregulated			
let-7a	Downregulated	Tissue	Patients with NSCLC and a high risk score for this five-miRNA signature have increased risk of cancer relapse and shortened survival	37
miR-137	Upregulated			
miR-182*	Upregulated			
miR-221	Downregulated			
miR-372	Upregulated			
miR-1	Downregulated	Serum	Patients with NSCLC carrying two or more of these high-risk miRNAs have significantly increased probability of cancer death in a dose-dependent manner compared with patients carrying zero or one high-risk miRNA	43
miR-30d	Upregulated			
miR-486	Upregulated			
miR-499	Downregulated			

FFPE, formalin-fixed, paraffin-embedded; *NSCLC*, nonsmall cell lung cancer.

significantly shorter disease-free survival ($p = 0.016$) and overall survival ($p = 0.027$) compared with patients who had tumors with unmethylated miR-34b/c or a low level of miR-34b/c methylation. Patients who had tumors with high levels of miR-34b/c methylation had significantly shorter disease-free survival and overall survival compared with patients who had tumors with unmethylated miR-34b/c or a low level of miR-34b/c methylation. Their results suggest that epigenetic inactivation of miR-34b/c by DNA methylation has independent prognostic value in early-stage lung adenocarcinoma. Mapping human miRNAs on autosomal chromosomes and selecting 55 miRNAs in silico, Watanabe et al.[36] found that miR-34b was silenced by the DNA methylation of its own promoter. The 5-aza-2'-deoxycytidine treatment of NSCLC cells resulted in increased miR-34b expression and decreased c-Met protein. The DNA methylation status of miR-34b was analyzed in 99 patients with primary NSCLC, and multivariate analysis showed that both miR-34b methylation ($p = 0.007$) and c-Met expression ($p = 0.005$) were significantly associated with lymphatic invasion. These results suggest that the DNA methylation of miR-34b may be used as a biomarker for an invasive phenotype of NSCLC.

Using real-time RT-PCR, Yu et al.[37] identified a five-miRNA signature (let-7a, miR-137, miR-182*, miR-221, and miR-372) that was associated with relapse and survival in 112 patients with NSCLC. Patients with a high-risk score for this five-miRNA signature in their tumor specimens had faster cancer relapse and shorter survival. These results suggest that miRNAs may play an important role in the clinical progression and prognosis of NSCLC. Landi et al.[38] analyzed miRNA expression in 125 tissue samples of squamous cell carcinoma from the Environment and Genetics in Lung Cancer Etiology study using a custom oligo array. This group also found that lower expression of five miRNAs (let-7e, miR-25, miR-34a, miR-34c-5p, and miR-191) strongly predicted poor survival for male smokers with stage I–IIIA squamous cell carcinomas. These miRNAs may have important implications for prognosis and treatment of this histologic subgroup of lung cancer.

SNPs in pre-miRNAs may alter miRNA processing, expression, and binding to target mRNA. In a systematic survey of common pre-miRNA SNPs among 893 patients with NSCLC, Hu et al.[39] found that SNP rs11614913 in miR-196a2 was associated with survival. Survival was significantly decreased for individuals who were homozygous CC at SNP rs11614913, indicating that the rs11614913 SNP in miR-196a2 may be a prognostic biomarker for NSCLC ($p = 0.033$). Hu et al.[40] further conducted a two-stage study to examine the impact of SNPs on the overall survival of 923 patients with NSCLC in China. They found that miR-30c-1 rs928508 was consistently a predictor of survival in NSCLC, and the protective role of rs928508 AG/GG genotypes was more pronounced among patients with stage I–II disease and patients treated with surgical procedures. Their data indicate that genetic polymorphisms in the pre-miRNA flanking region may be prognostic biomarkers of NSCLC. Using a PCR–restriction fragment length polymorphism assay, Hong et al.[41] evaluated the effects of four SNPs in pre-miRNAs of 363 patients with surgically resected early-stage NSCLC. The pre-miR-149 rs2292832 TC or CC genotype portended a significantly better overall survival (adjusted hazard ratio, 0.66; 95% CI, 0.47–0.92) and disease-free survival (adjusted hazard ratio, 0.64; 95% CI, 0.48–0.87) than the TT genotype, and the pre-miR-196a rs11614913 CT or TT genotype was associated with a significantly better overall survival (adjusted hazard ratio, 0.70; 95% CI, 0.49–0.99) and disease-free survival (adjusted hazard ratio, 0.66; 95% CI, 0.48–0.90) than the CC genotype. Their results suggest that miR-149 rs2292832 and miR-196a rs11614913 may be used as prognostic markers for patients with surgically resected early-stage NSCLC.

Human blood contains stably expressed miRNAs that may have great potential to predict survival. To identify tumor biomarkers using noninvasive procedures, Silva et al.[42] analyzed the plasma from 28 patients with NSCLC by low-density arrays (Taqman) and validated selected miRNAs by real-time PCR in the plasma from 78 samples of NSCLC. The plasma level of let-7f was associated with overall survival, and the plasma level of miR-30e-3p was associated with short disease-free survival. These two plasma vesicle-related miRNAs may serve as circulating tumor biomarkers with prognostic value. Using genome-wide miRNA expression analysis to test the levels of serum miRNAs among 243 patients with NSCLC, Hu et al.[43] also found four miRNAs (miR-1, miR-30d, miR-486, and miR-499) in the serum to be significantly associated with overall survival ($p \leq 0.001$). This four-miRNA signature may serve as a noninvasive predictor for the prognosis of NSCLC. Wang et al.[44] used quantitative RT-PCR to assay 35 miRNAs that have binding sites within the 3' UTRs of 11 genes in the transforming growth factor-β signaling pathway to determine their associations with survival; the serum samples were from 383 patients with advanced NSCLC. The authors identified 17 miRNAs that were significantly associated with 2-year survival. Among them, high expression of miR-16 exhibited the most highly significant association with better survival (adjusted hazard ratio, 0.4; 95% CI, 0.3–0.5). A combined 17-miRNA risk score was created and showed that patients with a high risk score had a 2.5-fold increased risk of death compared with patients with a low risk score. Genotyping 240 miRNA-related SNPs in the blood of 535 patients with stage I and II NSCLC, Pu et al.[45] determined that the FAS (Fas cell surface death receptor:rs2234978) G allele was significantly associated with survival in early-stage NSCLC (hazard ratio, 0.59; 95% CI, 0.44–0.77). Luciferase assays showed that the FAS SNP created a miR-651 functional binding site. Their results indicate that miRNA-related polymorphisms may be associated with clinical outcomes among patients with NSCLC through altered miRNA regulation of target genes.

The Role of miRNAs in the Response to Treatment

Although most patients with lung cancer have a response to initial chemotherapy, chemoresistance can develop, leading to inferior outcomes. Predictive biomarkers are needed to aid researchers in designing clinical trials that better stratify patients and in identifying new treatments for specific subpopulations. Recent studies have demonstrated that miRNAs may serve as predictive biomarkers for chemoresistance of lung cancer among patients treated with systemic chemotherapy and/or targeted therapies (Table 15.5).

Platinum-based chemotherapy is the backbone of current combination strategies for the treatment of small cell lung cancer (SCLC). However, more than 95% of patients with SCLC eventually die of cancer. Ranade et al.[46] performed miRNA microarray profiling on 34 diagnostic SCLC tumor samples and analysis by a data integration and discovery tool (XenoBase; Van Andel Research Institute, Grand Rapids, MI, USA) showing that higher levels of miR-92a-2* in the tumors were associated with chemoresistance. This miRNA may have an application in screening patients with SCLC at risk for de novo chemoresistance in an effort to design more tailored clinical trials for SCLC.

Researchers have also hypothesized a role of miRNAs in the resistance to platinum-based chemotherapy for NSCLC. Investigating the expression profiles of serum miRNAs in 260 patients with inoperable, advanced NSCLC treated with cisplatin-based chemotherapy, Cui et al.[47] showed that miR-125b was significantly associated with therapeutic response, with higher expression levels in the tumors of patients who did not have a response to treatment ($p = 0.003$). These results suggest that miR-125b is a potential predictive biomarker for NSCLC and may aid in the development of targeted therapeutics to overcome chemotherapeutic resistance in NSCLC. Employing a

TABLE 15.5 Single MicroRNAs (miRNAs) as Predictive Biomarkers for Treatment Response in Lung Cancer

miRNAs	Deregulation in Cancer	Materials	Descriptions	References
miR-10a	Downregulated	Cell line	Genes with significantly altered expression and putatively mediated by the expression-changed miRNAs are mainly enriched in chromatin assembly, antiapoptosis, protein kinase, and small GTPase-mediated signal transduction	50
miR-21	Upregulated	Tissue/plasma	Transfection of NSCLC cells with anti-miR-21 increases the expression of *PTEN* and decreases *Bcl-2*	48
miR-22	Upregulated	Blood	Significantly higher miR-22 expression is found in patients who have progressive NSCLC	49
miR-24-2	Downregulated	Serum	Genes with significantly altered expression and putatively mediated by the expression-changed miRNAs are mainly enriched in chromatin assembly, antiapoptosis, protein kinase, and small GTPase-mediated signal transduction	50
miR-25*	Upregulated	Cell line	Genes with significantly altered expression and putatively mediated by the expression-changed miRNAs are mainly enriched in chromatin assembly, antiapoptosis, protein kinase, and small GTPase-mediated signal transduction	50
miR-30a	Downregulated	Cell line	Genes with significantly altered expression and putatively mediated by the expression-changed miRNAs are mainly enriched in chromatin assembly, antiapoptosis, protein kinase, and small GTPase-mediated signal transduction	50
miR-30c-2*	Downregulated	Cell line	Genes with significantly altered expression and putatively mediated by the expression-changed miRNAs are mainly enriched in chromatin assembly, antiapoptosis, protein kinase, and small GTPase-mediated signal transduction	50
miR-92a-2*	Upregulated	FFPE tissue	Higher tumor levels of miR-92a-2* are associated with chemoresistance and with decreased survival in patients with small cell lung cancer	46
miR-125b	Upregulated	Serum	High level of miR-125b is significantly correlated with poor therapeutic response in patients with inoperable, advanced NSCLC treated with cisplatin–based chemotherapy	47
miR-155	Downregulated	Cell line	Genes with significantly altered expression and putatively mediated by the expression-changed miRNAs are mainly enriched in chromatin assembly, antiapoptosis, protein kinase, and small GTPase-mediated signal transduction	50
miR-195	Downregulated	Cell line	Genes with significantly altered expression and putatively mediated by the expression-changed miRNAs are mainly enriched in chromatin assembly, antiapoptosis, protein kinase, and small GTPase-mediated signal transduction	50
miR-200c	Downregulated	Cell line	Genes with significantly altered expression and putatively mediated by the expression-changed miRNAs are mainly enriched in chromatin assembly, antiapoptosis, protein kinase, and small GTPase-mediated signal transduction. Treatment with TGFβ1 changes the expression of miR-200c and proteins involved in the epithelial-to-mesenchymal transition and modulates migration in lung cancer cells	50,54
miR-203	Upregulated	Cell line	Genes with significantly altered expression and putatively mediated by the expression-changed miRNAs are mainly enriched in chromatin assembly, antiapoptosis, protein kinase, and small GTPase-mediated signal transduction	50
miR-221	Upregulated	Cell line	High expression level of miR-221 is needed to maintain the TRAIL-resistant phenotype in NSCLC	51
miR-222	Upregulated	Cell line	High expression level of miR-222 is needed to maintain the TRAIL-resistant phenotype in NSCLC	51
miR-885-5p	Upregulated	Cell line	Genes with significantly altered expression and putatively mediated by the expression-changed miRNAs are mainly enriched in chromatin assembly, antiapoptosis, protein kinase, and small GTPase-mediated signal transduction	50

FFPE, formalin-fixed, paraffin-embedded; *GTP*, guanosine triphosphate; *NSCLC*, nonsmall cell lung cancer; *PTEN*, phosphatase and tensin homolog; *TGF*, transforming growth factor; *TRAIL*, tumor necrosis factor-related apoptosis-inducing ligand.

microarray to compare the expression levels of miRNAs, Gao et al.[48] found that increased expression of miR-21 also significantly increased the resistance of NSCLC cells to platinum, whereas reduced expression of miR-21 decreased the resistance of NSCLC cells ($p = 0.007$). This finding was further validated in the tissue samples of 58 patients and matched plasma samples. These data suggest that the expression level of miR-21 in tumor tissue and plasma may be used as a biomarker to predict the response to adjuvant platinum-based chemotherapy in patients with NSCLC.

Pemetrexed has been widely used in patients with advanced NSCLC. Franchina et al.[49] evaluated the expression levels of circulating miRNAs possibly involved in the folate pathway in 22 patients with NSCLC treated with pemetrexed. They found a correlation between high expression of miR-22 in whole blood and a lack of response in these patients. Their results indicate that miR-22 may represent a predictive biomarker for pemetrexed-based treatment.

Gemcitabine is also one of the most widely used drugs for the treatment of advanced NSCLC. Applying miRNA expression chips to determine biomarkers for gemcitabine sensitivity, Zhang et al.[50] found that miR-10a, miR-24-2*, miR-30a, miR-30c-2*, and miR-155 were upregulated in sensitive cells, whereas miR-25*, miR-195, miR-200c, miR-203, and miR-885-5p were increased in resistant cells. Their results may provide potential biomarkers for the prediction of gemcitabine sensitivity and putative targets to overcome gemcitabine resistance in patients with NSCLC.

NSCLC cells show differential sensitivity to therapy with tumor necrosis factor-related apoptosis-inducing ligand (TRAIL). Performing genome-wide expression profiling of miRNAs, Garofalo et al.[51] showed that high expression levels of miR-221 and miR-222 were needed to maintain the TRAIL-resistant phenotype in NSCLC. These miRNAs may thus be used as diagnostic tools for TRAIL resistance in NSCLC. In addition, miRNAs have been reported to have significant associations with epidermal growth factor receptor (*EGFR; p* < 0.05), and epithelial-to-mesenchymal transition may predict resistance to EGFR inhibitors and metastatic behavior.[52,53] Using a model system for an NSCLC cell line, Bryant et al.[54] found that ectopic expression of miR-200c altered the expression of proteins responsible for the epithelial-to-mesenchymal transition, sensitivity to erlotinib, and migration in lung cancer cells. Their data suggest that the tumor microenvironment may stimulate miR-200c, which then induces resistance to anti-EGFR therapy and drives lung tumor cells to the epithelial-to-mesenchymal transition, invasion, and metastasis.

FUTURE PERSPECTIVES

Dysfunctions of miRNAs are frequently found in lung cancer.[55] These noncoding RNAs have been recognized as some of the main regulatory gatekeepers of coding genes in the human genome. For the most part, miRNAs silence gene expression by binding imperfectly matched sequences in the 3′ UTR of target mRNAs.[56] By targeting and controlling the expression of mRNAs, miRNAs may control highly complex signal transduction pathways and other biologic pathways.[57] Rapid advances in platform technologies, such as SNP analysis, genome-wide transcriptional profiling, miRNA microarrays, next-generation sequencing, and other so-called omics technologies, offer the potential for revolutionary developments in the study of miRNAs in lung cancer.[58]

Studies since the early 2000s have shown the oncogenic and tumor suppressive characteristics of miRNAs and have inspired researchers to begin elucidating the specific roles of miRNAs as potential biomarkers for the diagnosis and prognosis of lung cancer.[59] Numerous studies have documented the implications of miRNAs in nearly every carcinogenic process of lung cancer, including tumor growth and apoptosis, progression and metastasis, and resistance to anticancer agents.[60–64] These small molecules are produced in a tissue-specific manner, yet they are also found to be stable in human blood. By exploiting the unique characteristics of miRNAs in solid tumors and circulating samples, including their tissue specificity, stability, ease of detection, and ready manipulation, clinicians come ever closer to achieving the goal of personalized cancer therapy.[65,66] Furthermore, using circulating miRNAs in blood and/or sputum as noninvasive diagnostic biomarkers may create a breakthrough in the early detection of lung cancer.[67]

Early detection and swift treatment can significantly affect the prognosis of patients with lung cancer. However, massive screening may lead to overdiagnosis and eventually overtreatment. A number of studies have reported that specific miRNAs are able to differentiate benign from malignant lung lesions. Combining these molecular biomarkers with massive screening may reduce the risk of overdiagnosis in lung cancer.[68] On the other hand, the utility of some protein-encoding gene biomarkers has already been exploited in routine clinical practice. The translational study of miRNAs may provide complementary or superior information to these existing biomarkers to enhance the diagnostic, prognostic, and predictive power of molecular characterization of lung cancer.[69] Indeed, an emerging trend is to combine several miRNAs into a panel biomarker to improve sensitivity and specificity. Similarly, the combination of miRNA biomarkers with other molecular markers (such as SNPs and methylation signatures) may also help to better diagnose or predict the treatment outcomes of individual patients.[70]

Although the identification of miRNA-based signatures in lung cancer has shown promising results in recent years, no single biomarker has made the transition into the clinic. Further efforts are essential to fully realize and define common procedures, standards, and controls so as to translate valuable laboratory findings into clinically relevant procedures for patients with lung cancer.[71] Large prospective cohorts and cross-validation are needed to consolidate the significant findings demonstrated by studies of miRNA profiling. Over time, in conjunction with genetic and proteomic signatures and other screening approaches, miRNA biomarkers may represent a new milestone in lung cancer theranostics.[72]

KEY REFERENCES

1. Cho WC. OncomiRs: the discovery and progress of microRNAs in cancers. *Mol Cancer*. 2007;6:60.
8. Lebanony D, Benjamin H, Gilad S, et al. Diagnostic assay based on hsa-miR-205 expression distinguishes squamous from non-squamous nonsmall-cell lung carcinoma. *J Clin Oncol*. 2009;27(12):2030–2037.
12. Schwarzenbach H, Nishida N, Calin GA, Pantel K. Clinical relevance of circulating cell-free microRNAs in cancer. *Nat Rev Clin Oncol*. 2014;11(3):145–156.
20. Boeri M, Verri C, Conte D, et al. MicroRNA signatures in tissues and plasma predict development and prognosis of computed tomography detected lung cancer. *Proc Natl Acad Sci U S A*. 2011;108(9): 3713–3718.
23. Takamizawa J, Konishi H, Yanagisawa K, et al. Reduced expression of the let-7 microRNAs in human lung cancers in association with shortened postoperative survival. *Cancer Res*. 2004;64(11):3753–3756.
35. Nadal E, Chen G, Gallegos M, et al. Epigenetic inactivation of microRNA-34b/c predicts poor disease-free survival in early stage lung adenocarcinoma. *Clin Cancer Res*. 2013;19(24):6842–6852.
37. Yu SL, Chen HY, Chang GC, et al. MicroRNA signature predicts survival and relapse in lung cancer. *Cancer Cell*. 2008;13(1):48–57.
39. Hu Z, Chen J, Tian T, et al. Genetic variants of miRNA sequences and non-small cell lung cancer survival. *J Clin Invest*. 2008;118(7):2600– 2608.
43. Hu Z, Chen X, Zhao Y, et al. Serum microRNA signatures identified in a genome-wide serum microRNA expression profiling predict survival of nonsmall-cell lung cancer. *J Clin Oncol*. 2010;28(10):1721– 1726.
45. Pu X, Roth JA, Hildebrandt MA, et al. MicroRNA-related genetic variants associated with clinical outcomes in early-stage non-small cell lung cancer patients. *Cancer Res*. 2013;73(6):1867–1875.
53. Cho WC, Chow AS, Au JS. MiR-145 inhibits cell proliferation of human lung adenocarcinoma by targeting EGFR and NUDT1. *RNA Biol*. 2011;8(1):125–131.
66. Yu HW, Cho WC. The emerging role of miRNAs in combined cancer therapy. *Expert Opin Biol Ther*. 2015;15(7):923–925.

See Expertconsult.com for full list of references.

16 Humoral and Cellular Immune Dysregulation and Lung Cancer

Anish Thomas, Julie R. Brahmer, and Giuseppe Giaccone

SUMMARY OF KEY POINTS

- Humoral and cellular immune dysregulation in the tumor microenvironment contributes to immune evasion, a key hallmark of lung cancer.
- Immunosuppressive mechanisms observed in lung cancer include defective antigen presentation, secretion of immunosuppressive tumor-derived soluble factors, and immunosuppressive cells infiltrating the tumors.
- Suppression of antigen-presenting machinery in lung cancer results from several mechanisms including deficiencies in expression of antigen-processing genes and haplotype loss of human leukocyte antigen (HLA) class I antigens.
- Immune inhibitory cytokines secreted by the tumor cells impair T-cell survival and help avoid T cell-mediated immune responses.
- Immune checkpoints expressed on the surface of T lymphocytes modulate the immune response to antigens via inhibitory or stimulatory signaling to T cells.
- Tobacco smoke markedly influences the immune microenvironment in lung cancer.

Advances in the understanding of cellular immunology and tumor–host immune interactions have led to the development of promising immunotherapies in lung cancer.[1] This chapter provides a review of the current understanding of the basic immunologic abnormalities in lung cancer. Clinical trials of immunotherapy in lung cancer are discussed in Chapter 50.

Although lung cancer was traditionally thought to be a nonimmunogenic tumor unlike melanoma or renal cell cancer,[2] accumulating evidence suggests both cellular (T lymphocyte-mediated) and humoral (antibody-mediated) immune antitumor responses even in patients with advanced lung cancer.[3,4] Despite the immune responses, spontaneous tumor regressions rarely occur, indicating the ability of the tumor cells to escape an immune response. In fact, lung cancer is among the many tumors that are known to promote immune tolerance and escape host immune surveillance. It is thought that the immune system actively inhibits the formation and progression of transformed cells and ultimately "shapes" nascent tumors by forcing the selective evolution of tumor cells that can evade the immune response, a phenomenon called tumor immunoediting.[5] Tumors also utilize numerous other pathways to inhibit immune responses, including local immune suppression, induction of tolerance, and systemic dysfunction in T-cell signaling.[6–9] Although these immunosuppressive mechanisms are categorized discretely, the clinically observed deficits are interrelated (Fig. 16.1).

SUPPRESSION OF THE ANTIGEN-PRESENTING MACHINERY

An adaptive immune response requires two signals between the antigen-presenting cells (APCs) and the effector T cell. The first signal is mediated by the T-cell receptor and the specific antigenic peptide presented in the context of major histocompatibility complex (MHC) class I or class II molecules expressed on the APC surface. The second signal is mediated through constitutively expressed costimulatory molecules on the T cell (CD28) and the APC (B7-1/CD80 or B7-2/CD86; Fig. 16.1). The presence of both signals trigger intracellular events resulting in the activation and interleukin-2 (IL-2)-dependent clonal proliferation of T cells.

The MHC class I molecules are essential components of the adaptive immune system and are crucial to the immune recognition of tumor cells. MHC class I molecules report on cellular transformation to CD8+ cytotoxic T lymphocytes (CTLs) through a multistep process of antigenic peptide acquisition, tagging them for destruction by ubiquitylation, proteolysis, delivery of peptides from cytosol to the endoplasmic reticulum via the heterodimeric transporter associated with antigen processing (TAP) 1 and TAP2 subunits, binding of peptides to MHC class I molecules, and displaying of peptide–MHC class I complexes on the cell surface.[10]

Under physiologic conditions, the components of MHC class I antigen-processing machinery (APM) are constitutively expressed in all adult nucleated cells (except immune privileged tissue). Their expression is regulated by cytokines that can alter the surface expression of MHC class I molecules. Aberrant MHC class I expression has been conclusively demonstrated as an important immune escape mechanism in cancers. MHC class I abnormalities have been frequently found in a variety of human cancers, are associated with unfavorable prognoses in some tumor types, and have a negative impact on the outcome of T cell-based immunotherapy.[11–13] Marked deficiency or lack of expression of MHC class I molecules has been demonstrated in lung cancer.[14,15]

The molecular mechanisms of MHC class I expression loss are diverse and include structural alterations or dysregulations of genes encoding the classical MHC class I antigens and/or components of the MHC class I APM. The dysregulation of APM components may occur at the epigenetic, transcriptional, or posttranscriptional level.[11] Mechanisms underlying the aberrant expression of MHC class I antigens in lung cancer include deficiencies in the expression of antigen-processing genes (e.g., genes that encode proteasome subunits and the peptide transporters), which result in defective peptide transport to the cell surface from the endoplasmic reticulum.[15–18] Haplotype loss of HLA class I antigens is another mechanism of abnormal HLA expression in lung cancer and has been demonstrated in about 40% of lung cancer cell lines.[19–21] Structural alterations such as β2-microglobulin gene abnormalities resulting from loss of messenger RNA and

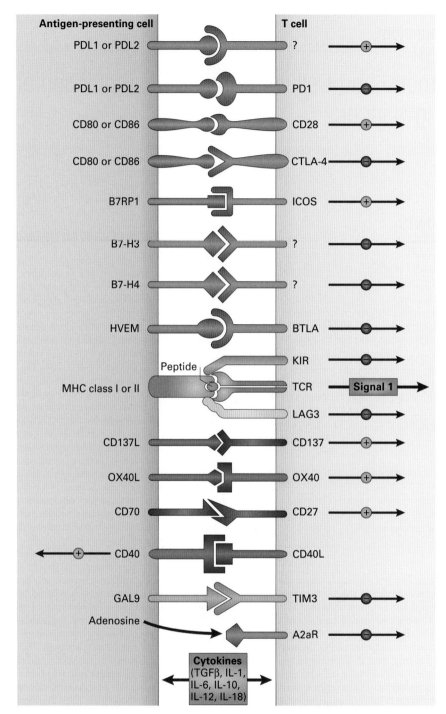

Nature Reviews | Cancer

Fig. 16.1. Multiple costimulatory and inhibitory interactions regulate T-cell responses. *BTLA,* B and T lymphocyte attenuator; *CTLA-4,* cytotoxic T lymphocyte-associated antigen; *HVEM,* herpes virus entry mediator; *ICOS,* inducible costimulatory; *IL,* interleukin; *KIR,* killer cell immunoglobulin like receptors; *Lag3,* Lymphocyte activating gene 3; *MHC,* major histocompatibility complex; *PD-1,* programmed cell death 1; *PDL,* programmed death ligand; *TCR,* T-cell receptor; *TGF,* transforming growth factor; *TIM3,* T cell immunoglobulin and mucin domain. *(Reprinted with permission from Pardoll DM. The blockade of immune checkpoints in cancer immunotherapy.* Nat Rev Cancer. *2012;12(4):252–264.)*

point mutations are less common mechanisms of altered MHC class I expression in lung cancer.[19,22]

Studies in which lung cancer cell lines with haplotype loss of HLA class I antigens are used indicate that tumor cells with a normal HLA class I expression may be killed by CTLs at an early stage of carcinogenesis, and only immunoselected tumor cells that lack HLA class I expression can escape this immune attack and develop into cancer.[23] Furthermore, some defects in MHC class I expression in lung cancer, for example, deficiencies in expression of antigen-processing genes and not β2-microglobulin gene abnormalities, may be reversible with cytokines. Interferon-γ (*IFN-γ*) gene transfection into HLA-deficient small cell lung

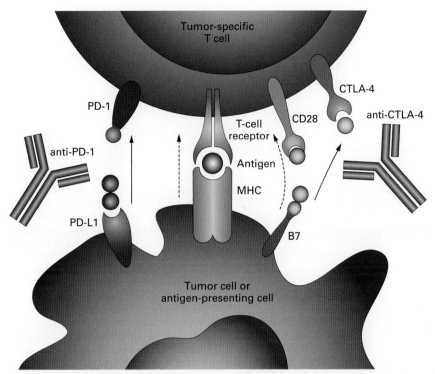

Fig. 16.2. Immune checkpoint blockade. *CTLA-4,* cytotoxic T lymphocyte-associated antigen; *MHC,* major histocompatibility complex; *PD-1,* programmed cell death 1. *(Reprinted with permission from Drake CG, Lipson EJ, Brahmer JR. Breathing new life into immunotherapy: review of melanoma, lung and kidney cancer. Nat Rev Clin Oncol. 2014;11(1):24–37.)*

cancer (SCLC) was able to restore its ability to present endogenous tumor antigens to CTL with a concomitant increase in cell-surface expression of class I molecules.[15,18,24]

The results of immunohistochemical studies of surgically resected samples with monoclonal antibodies against a common framework determinant of HLA class I antigens have shown deficient expression in HLA class I antigens in 25% to 33% of nonsmall cell lung cancer (NSCLC).[25–28] As evident from studies of transfected tumor cells lacking expression of these antigens, MHC class I molecules are required for presentation of antigens on tumor cells to the CTL. Thus tumor cells that have lost MHC class I antigens have the advantage of being able to escape lysis by CTL.[29] In lung cancers, the absence of expression of HLA class I molecules has been associated with poor differentiation and aneuploidy, suggesting that lung cancers with abnormal HLA expression may be biologically more aggressive.[25–27] Taken together, these findings may suggest that tumors with aberrant expression of HLA class I molecules are associated with a poorer prognosis. However, the prognostic implications of HLA class I antigen downregulation in NSCLC are not clear.[25–27,30]

Despite expressing antigens recognizable by the host immune system, tumors are very poor at initiating effective immune responses. However, antigen presentation alone is insufficient to activate T cells. In addition to T-cell receptor engagement of an antigenic peptide bound to MHC molecules, additional costimulatory signals are necessary for T-cell activation. The most important of these costimulatory signals is provided by the interaction of CD28 on T cells with its primary ligands B7-1 (CD80) and B7-2 (CD86) on the surface of APCs.[31]

Cytotoxic T lymphocyte-associated antigen 4 (CTLA-4), a member of the immunoglobulin super family and homolog of CD28, binds members of the B7 family with a much higher affinity than CD28. In effect, CTLA-4 competes with CD28 for binding to the B7 family. Upregulation of surface CTLA-4 follows clonal expansion of T cells and regulates the immune response by inducing inhibitory signals in effector T cells that lead to the dampening of the effector T-cell response.[32] CTLA-4 is thus one of the endogenous immune checkpoints that normally terminate immune responses after antigen activation. These T cells are eventually eliminated via apoptosis. CTLA-4 may also contribute to the immune-suppressive function of T-regulatory cells. Upregulation of CTLA-4 on the surface of T-regulatory cells results in suppression of activation and expansion of effector cells specific for both normal self-antigens and tumor antigens.[33,34] CTLA-4 is constitutively expressed in NSCLC cell lines, where it induces apoptotic cell death on engagement with soluble B7-1 and B7-2 recombinant ligands.[35] Furthermore, CTLA-4 expression in resected early-stage NSCLC was shown to be a good prognostic indicator in a retrospective analysis that was limited by a small number of patients.[36]

Programmed cell death 1 (PD-1) is another key immune checkpoint receptor that is structurally similar to CTLA-4, but with distinct biologic functions and ligand specificity that is expressed by activated T cells and mediates immunosuppression. PD-1 functions primarily in peripheral tissues, where T cells may encounter the immunosuppressive PD-1 ligands PD-L1 (B7-H1) and PD-L2 (B7-DC), which are expressed by tumor cells, stromal cells, or both (Fig. 16.2).[37] The immune inhibitory signals mediated by CTLA-4 and PD-1 are different, as evidenced by the early mortality of CTLA-4 knockout mice compared with modest late-onset strain-specific and organ-specific autoimmunity of PD-1 knockout mice.[38]

Most lung cancer samples, but not samples with normal alveolar cells, express high levels of PD-L1, which is limited to the tumor plasma membrane or cytoplasm.[39] Dendritic cells (DCs) isolated from tumoral and nontumoral lung tissues express low, although significantly higher, levels of B7-1 and B7-2 molecules compared with blood DCs.[40] In surgically resected NSCLC, no relationship was found between the expression of PD-L1 or PD-L2 and clinicopathologic variables, such as histology, stage, or postoperative survival.[41] In a limited subset of patients, fewer tumor-infiltrating lymphocytes (TILs) were identified in PD-L1-positive tumor regions than in PD-L1-negative tumor regions. Tumor-infiltrating and circulating CD8+ T cells from patients with NSCLC showed increased PD-1 expression compared with peripheral blood mononuclear cells from normal volunteers, but showed impaired immune function, including reduced cytokine production capability and impaired capacity to proliferate.[42] Blocking the PD-1 and PD-L1 pathway by anti-PD-L1 antibodies increased cytokine production and proliferation of PD-1+ tumor-infiltrating CD8+ T cells.[42]

TUMOR-DERIVED SOLUBLE FACTORS

Tumor cells avoid lymphocyte-mediated immune responses by secreting immune inhibitory cytokines in the tumor milieu. In addition to secreting immune-suppressive mediators, tumor cells may also signal surrounding inflammatory cells to release immune-suppressive mediators, augment the trafficking of suppressor cells to the tumor site, and promote the differentiation of effector lymphocytes to a T-regulatory phenotype.[43,44] Tumor-derived soluble factors also impair T-cell survival. NSCLC cell line supernatants contribute to enhanced activation-induced T-cell apoptosis in the tumor environment. The increased T-cell apoptosis after mitogen stimulation is due to the inhibition of nuclear factor-κB activation in the tumor milieu.[45]

Interleukin-10

Human bronchial epithelial cells constitutively produce IL-10, which regulates the local immune response in normal lungs.[46] Although the precise role of IL-10 in carcinogenesis remains controversial,[47] results of several studies suggest that IL-10 is a potent immunosuppressive molecule that may promote lung cancer growth by suppressing T-cell and macrophage function and enabling tumors to escape immune detection.[48–50] In vitro, human lung tumors produce greater amounts of IL-10 than normal lung tissue.[51,52] Tumor cells also induce T lymphocyte-derived IL-10 via a prostaglandin E_2 (PGE_2)-mediated pathway.[50] In vivo, lung carcinoma cells grow more rapidly in IL-10 transgenic mice compared with controls.[53] IL-10 transgenic mice also demonstrate a reduced capacity for antigen presentation, CTL generation, and type 1 cytokine production, reflecting defects in both T-cell and APC function.[48] Increased IL-10 expression of tumor-associated macrophages in patients with NSCLC correlates with late-stage disease and other adverse prognostic features, suggesting its potential role in the progression of NSCLC.[54,55] Furthermore, in patients with advanced-stage NSCLC receiving platinum-based chemotherapy, an elevated baseline serum IL-10 level was an independent predictor of poorer survival.[56] In patients with early-stage NSCLC, an elevated IL-10 messenger RNA level was associated with worse survival.[57]

However, preclinical and clinical models suggest that IL-10 possesses an immunostimulating property that favors immune-mediated rejection of cancer.[47] In patients with NSCLC, the percentage of CD8+ cells expressing IL-10 was higher in cancerous tissue than in cancer-free tissue and correlated with both early-stage tumors and better survival rates.[58] In clinical studies, lack of tumor IL-10 expression was associated with a worse disease-specific survival rate in patients with early-stage NSCLC.[59,60]

Conflicting evidence on the immune regulatory function of IL-10 likely reflects its pleiotropic ability to positively or negatively influence the function of innate and adaptive immunity, resulting in immunostimulation or immunosuppression depending on its source (tumor compared with tumor-infiltrating immune cells) and on the interactions with factors found in the tumor microenvironment.[47,61]

Transforming Growth Factor-β

Transforming growth factor-β (TGF-β) is a member of a family of multifunctional proteins that through complex cell signaling pathways regulate cell proliferation, differentiation, and angiogenesis.[62] Three highly conserved and tissue-specific TGF-β isoforms, namely, TGF-β1, TGF-β2, and TGF-β3, signal through heteromeric complexes of three cell-surface receptors, that is, the type III TGF-β receptors: TβRIII, TβRII, and TβRI.[63] TGF-β ligands initiate signaling by binding to and bringing together TβRI and TβRII receptor serine and threonine kinases on the cell surface. This process allows TβRII to phosphorylate the TβRI kinase domain, which propagates the signal through phosphorylation of the small mothers against decapentaplegic (SMAD) proteins, which then translocate into the nucleus and interact in a cell-specific manner with transcription factors to regulate specifically the transcription of a multitude of TGF-β-responsive genes. While TGF-β acts as a tumor suppressor via its effects on proliferation, replication potential, and apoptosis, it also acts as a tumor promoter via its effects on migration, invasion, angiogenesis, and the immune system.[64] TGF-β enables tumors to evade immune surveillance and kill through various mechanisms, most of which converge on the impairment of tumor cell killing by immune effector cells.[65]

Normal bronchial epithelial cells have high-affinity receptors for TGF-β. TGF-β inhibits proliferation and induces differentiation of normal bronchial epithelial cells.[66] TGF-β secreted by tumor cells mediates conversion of CD4+CD25− T cells to regulatory T (T-reg) cells. Neutralization of TGF-β abrogates this conversion both in vitro and in vivo.[67] Cigarette smoking promotes tumorigenicity partly by abrogating TGF-β-mediated growth inhibition and apoptosis by reducing expression of SMAD3.[68] Both SCLC and NSCLC overexpress TGF-β, and high levels of TGF-β are also detected in the serum of patients with lung cancer compared with normal individuals.[69,70] Elevated plasma levels of TGF-β confer a poorer prognosis for patients with lung cancer.[71]

A variety of other tumor-derived soluble factors contribute to the immunosuppressive milieu including vascular endothelial growth factor, PGE_2, soluble phosphatidylserine, soluble Fas, soluble Fas-L, and soluble MHC class I–related chain A proteins.[72] Although deposited at the primary tumor site, these factors can extend immunosuppressive effects to local lymph nodes and the spleen, thereby promoting invasion and metastasis.[73]

TUMOR-INFILTRATING T LYMPHOCYTES

The lymphocyte population that infiltrates the tumor is quite heterogeneous and consists of many different clones of lymphocytes that contain a variety of cell surface markers. The protumor and antitumor effects of interactions between tumor and immune cells in the tumor microenvironment are influenced not just by the type of immune cells (CD8+, CD4+, CD20+, and forkhead box P3 [FoxP3+]), but also by their density and location within the tumors.[74] In NSCLC, tumor stroma inflammatory cells are mainly lymphocytes (approximately two-thirds, and among them 20% B cells and 80% T cells) and tumor-associated macrophages (approximately one-third), with a low percentage of DCs and a very low percentage of natural killer (NK) cells.[75] Although the cell surface markers and distribution among various lymphocyte subtypes are similar, TILs are functionally different from lymphocytes that are found in regional lymph nodes and peripheral blood. TILs are markedly suppressed in their functional capacity based on assessments of their proliferative and cytotoxic activities. In addition, tumor-infiltrating NK cells have markedly diminished activity compared with peripheral blood lymphocytes.[76]

Using genetically engineered mouse lung adenocarcinoma into which exogenous antigens were introduced to mimic tumor neoantigens, DuPage et al.[77] showed that endogenous T cells responded to and infiltrated tumors early during tumor development, substantially delaying malignant progression. However, despite continued antigen expression, T-cell infiltration did not persist and tumors ultimately escaped immune attack. Moreover, very few tumor-reactive T cells in the lungs were functional, as evidenced by their limited capacity to produce both IFN-γ and tumor necrosis factor-alpha (TNF-α). Immunohistochemical analysis in patients with NSCLC demonstrated significantly higher CD8+ T-cell counts within the tumor when compared with the invasive margin.[78] However, the number of peritumoral CD8+ T cells correlated with the IFN-γ production, whereas this association was not observed intratumorally, suggesting that CD8+ T cells are able to infiltrate the tumor, but they are not able to mount a robust antitumor response once within the tumor nest.

Although TILs are associated with a favorable prognosis in many malignancies,[79] the association between CD8+ T-cell infiltration and prognosis is controversial in lung cancer.[80] However, high numbers of CD4+ T cells within cancer cell nests positively correlated with a favorable prognosis, suggesting that CD4+ T cells may be required for initiating and maintaining antitumor immune responses, as without CD4+ T-cell help, the resultant CD4-unhelped CD8+ T cells do not differentiate into sustainable memory cells.[81]

Although TILs accumulate in lung cancer tissues, they fail to mount an immune response to tumor cells,[82] in part because high proportions of NSCLC TILs are T-reg cells.[83] TILs that are CD4+CD25+, the activated phenotype of T-reg cells, inhibit T-cell proliferation and prevent the host from mounting an immune response to tumor antigens.[84] A preponderance of these T-reg cells could lead to a failure of tumor immunosurveillance or to enhanced tumor growth. In patients with NSCLC, T cells derived from the tumor show considerably increased proportions of CD4+CD25+ T cells that produce TGF-β.[85] These cells uniformly express high levels of CTLA-4 on their cell surface. In addition, CD4+CD25+ T cells isolated from tumors mediate potent inhibition of the proliferation of autologous peripheral blood T cells stimulated by anti-CD3 or anti-CD3 and anti-CD28.[83] An increased pool of CD4+CD25+ T-reg cells with potent immunosuppressive features also exists in the peripheral blood of patients with NSCLC.[86]

Although the activation of T-reg cells is considered antigen specific, their immunosuppressive function is nonspecific and results from inhibition of multiple phases and events in the immune response from antigen presentation to effector functions.[87] Secretion of immunosuppressive cytokines such as TGF-β may play a role in the immune-suppressive function of T-reg cells.[88] However, TGF-β may not be required for inhibition of proliferation of T-reg cells in patients with lung cancer: TGF-β neutralization did not abrogate the suppressive effect of CD4+CD25+ T cells on autologous T-cell proliferation.[83]

FoxP3, a forkhead transcription factor family member encoded on the X chromosome, is a critical control gene for the development and function of natural CD4+CD25+ T-reg cells. In lung cancer cells, tumor-derived cyclooxygenase-2 (COX-2)/PGE$_2$ induced expression of *FoxP3* and increased T-reg cell activity.[89] In vivo, inhibition of COX-2 reduced T-reg activity, attenuated *FoxP3* expression in TILs, and decreased tumor burden. In stage I to III NSCLC, tumor-infiltrating FoxP3+ T-regs

correlated with COX-2 expression and an increased tumor recurrence.[90]

MYELOID-DERIVED SUPPRESSOR CELLS

Myeloid-derived suppressor cells (MDSCs) are a phenotypically heterogeneous population of cells of myeloid origin that expand during cancer, inflammation, and infection, characterized by their immature state and ability to suppress T-cell responses.[91,92] Unlike the physiologic state where immature myeloid cells generated in bone marrow quickly differentiate into mature granulocytes, macrophages, or DCs, in cancer, a partial block in the differentiation of immature myeloid cells into mature myeloid cells results in an expansion of MDSCs. MDSCs express the common myeloid marker CD33, but lack the expression of markers of mature myeloid and lymphoid cells and the MHC class-II molecule HLA-DR11.[91] Two main subsets of MDSCs that suppress antigen-specific T-cell proliferation to an equal extent, despite their different mechanisms of action, have been identified: a granulocytic subset and a monocytic subset.[93] The MDSC population is influenced by several different factors. The factors that are known to induce MDSC expansion in lung cancer include granulocyte-macrophage colony-stimulating factor,[94] granulocyte colony-stimulating factor,[95] and prostaglandins.[96] The signaling pathways in MDSCs that are triggered by most of these factors converge on Janus kinase protein family members and signal transducer and activator of transcription 3 (STAT3), which are involved in cell survival, proliferation, differentiation, and apoptosis.[91]

The immune-suppressive activity of MDSC is thought to be a result of several mechanisms including upregulated expression of immune-suppressive factors, such as arginase and inducible nitric oxide synthase, and an increase in the production of NO and reactive oxygen species.[91] Arginase, which metabolizes L-arginine to L-ornithine, plays an important role in T-cell suppression through depletion of arginine, which is required for T-cell proliferation and cytokine production.[97] Using the 3LL mouse lung carcinoma model, Rodriguez et al.[98] showed that arginine depletion in the microenvironment by arginase I–producing MDSCs inhibited T-cell receptor CD3 expression and blocked T-cell functions. Arginase I in MDSC was induced by COX-2, and inhibition of COX-2 blocked arginase I induction in vitro and in vivo.[96] Furthermore, blocking arginase I expression using COX-2 inhibitors elicited a lymphocyte-mediated antitumor response.[96]

Further evidence supporting the immunosuppressive effect of MDSCs is derived from experiments of antibody-mediated depletion of MDSC in 3LL tumor-bearing mice. MDSC depletion increased APC activity and augmented the frequency and activity of NK and T-cell effectors that led to reduced tumor growth, enhanced therapeutic vaccination responses, and conferred immunologic memory.[99] MDSC numbers are increased in the peripheral blood of patients with NSCLC compared with healthy volunteers and these cells are capable of directly inhibiting antigen-specific T-cell responses.[100–105] As with many other cancers, MDSC levels correlate with clinical cancer stage and response to therapy in NSCLC.[102,105] In patients with advanced NSCLC, higher peripheral blood MDSC numbers were associated with poor response to cisplatin-based chemotherapy and predicted shorter progression-free survival.[100,105] In patients with early-stage NSCLC, peripheral blood MDSC numbers declined after removal of the tumor.[105] A negative association existed between the population of circulating MDSCs and the frequency of CD8+ T lymphocytes.[105] In a small study of patients with advanced NSCLC who received erlotinib, circulating MDSCs were substantially decreased in patients who had a partial response compared with patients who had progressive disease, and there was a negative correlation between the progression-free survival and MDSC numbers.[106] The prognostic significance of MDSCs in the tumor microenvironment of patient samples in lung cancer is not clear.

MDSC gene expression varies in different tumor types, and an understanding of its clinical significance requires the full characterization of these cells. Despite the lack of consensus over the definition and phenotype of MDSCs, and considerable heterogeneity in how they are defined clinically, their immunosuppressive properties are clear in NSCLC. The mechanisms by which MDSC functions are regulated within the tumor microenvironment, and how they differ from MDSCs that operate at peripheral sites, remain unclear.

CIGARETTE SMOKING AND IMMUNE DYSFUNCTION

Tobacco smoke has been shown to exert proinflammatory effects. For example, smoking increases production of several proinflammatory cytokines, such as TNF-α, IL-1, IL-6, and IL-8, and decreases anti-inflammatory cytokines such as IL-10. DC maturation is inhibited by cigarette smoking, as demonstrated by reduced cell-surface expression of MHC class II and the costimulatory molecules CD80 and CD86. Consequently, DCs from cigarette smoke–exposed animals show reduced capacity to stimulate and activate antigen-specific T cells in vitro. Reduced antigen-specific T-cell proliferation is also found in smoke-exposed mice.[107] Activation of CD8[+] T cells is also impaired in the presence of cigarette smoke in mouse models.[108,109] CD8[+] T-cell predominance is a characteristic of smoking-related chronic obstructive pulmonary disease and has been implicated in the progression of emphysema.[110,111]

CONCLUSION

Although traditionally thought to be a nonimmunogenic tumor, both cellular and humoral immune antitumor immune responses are found in lung cancer. Despite this finding, spontaneous tumor regressions rarely occur, indicating the ability of the tumor cells to escape the immune response. Immune dysregulation at multiple levels has been noted in experimental lung cancer models. These include defective antigen presentation, secretion of immunosuppressive tumor derived-soluble factors, and immunosuppressive cells infiltrating the tumors. Immune evasion mechanisms in other solid tumors may not play a major role in lung cancer as a result of the proinflammatory and immunosuppressive effects of tobacco smoke,[112] the major risk factor for lung cancer. In this context, it is important to consider that findings in a particular cancer model may not be broadly applicable to all immune–tumor interactions because immune response and tumor response are likely to vary greatly depending on the originating tissue and the genetic pathology

of the disease. An understanding of the complex issues surrounding cancer immunosurveillance, immunoediting, the role of host cellular networks in lung tumorigenesis, and tumor-mediated immunosuppression will offer additional therapeutic opportunities in lung cancers.

KEY REFERENCES

5. Dunn GP, Bruce AT, Ikeda H, Old LJ, Schreiber RD. Cancer immunoediting: from immunosurveillance to tumor escape. *Nat Immunol.* 2002;3(11):991–998.
14. Doyle A, Martin WJ, Funa K, et al. Markedly decreased expression of class I histocompatibility antigens, protein, and mRNA in human small-cell lung cancer. *J Exp Med.* 1985;161(5):1135–1151.
16. Chen HL, Gabrilovich D, Tampe R, Girgis KR, Nadaf S, Carbone DP. A functionally defective allele of TAP1 results in loss of MHC class I antigen presentation in a human lung cancer. *Nat Genet.* 1996;13(2):210–213.
32. Brunet JF, Denizot F, Luciani MF, et al. A new member of the immunoglobulin superfamily-Ctla-4. *Nature.* 1987;328(6127):267–270.
39. Dong HD, Strome SE, Salomao DR, et al. Tumor-associated B7-H1 promotes T-cell apoptosis: a potential mechanism of immune evasion. *Nat Med.* 2002;8(8):793–800.
48. Sharma S, Stolina M, Lin Y, et al. T cell-derived IL-10 promotes lung cancer growth by suppressing both T cell and APC function. *J Immunol.* 1999;163(9):5020–5028.
73. Kim R, Emi M, Tanabe K, Arihiro K. Tumor-driven evolution of immunosuppressive networks during malignant progression. *Cancer Res.* 2006;66(11):5527–5536.
77. DuPage M, Cheung AF, Mazumdar C, et al. Endogenous T cell responses to antigens expressed in lung adenocarcinomas delay malignant tumor progression. *Cancer Cell.* 2011;19(1):72–85.
80. Suzuki K, Kachala SS, Kadota K, et al. Prognostic immune markers in non-small cell lung cancer. *Clin Cancer Res.* 2011;17(16):5247–5256.
83. Woo EY, Yeh H, Chu CS, et al. Cutting edge: regulatory T cells from lung cancer patients directly inhibit autologous T cell proliferation. *J Immunol.* 2002;168(9):4272–4276.
87. Von Boehmer H. Mechanisms of suppression by suppressor T cells. *Nat Immunol.* 2005;6(4):338–344.
92. Gabrilovich DI, Ostrand-Rosenberg S, Bronte V. Coordinated regulation of myeloid cells by tumours. *Nat Rev Immunol.* 2012;12(4):253–268.
101. Almand B, Clark JI, Nikitina E, et al. Increased production of immature myeloid cells in cancer patients: a mechanism of immunosuppression in cancer. *J Immunol.* 2001;166(1):678–689.
109. Kalra R, Singh SP, Savage SM, Finch GL, Sopori ML. Effects of cigarette smoke on immune response: chronic exposure to cigarette smoke impairs antigen-mediated signaling in T cells and depletes IP3-sensitive Ca[2+] stores. *J Pharmacol Exp Ther.* 2000;293(1):166–171.

See Expertconsult.com for full list of references.

17 Classic Anatomic Pathology and Lung Cancer

Ignacio I. Wistuba, Elisabeth Brambilla, and Masayuki Noguchi

SUMMARY OF KEY POINTS

- A clinically relevant pathologic classification of lung cancer is essential for accurate diagnosis and for patients to receive appropriate therapy.
- Although classification of the majority of lung cancers is straightforward, areas of controversy and diagnostic challenges remain.
- The current lung cancer classification is applicable to surgically resected tumors and small biopsy specimens.
- Pathologists play a critical role in properly handling tissue and cytology specimens for molecular testing of lung cancer.
- The recently developed classification and approaches for lung cancer diagnosis are aligned with current clinical practice and open new avenues for research.

Lung cancer continues to be the most common and deadly malignancy worldwide.[1] The main challenge to improve the poor survival rate (5-year survival approximately 15%) of this disease is to develop better strategies for stratifying high-risk populations for early diagnosis and for selecting adequate treatment for different subsets of lung cancer. The mortality associated with this disease is high primarily because most lung cancers are diagnosed at advanced stages, when options for treatment are mostly palliative. Accurate pathologic classification and diagnosis of lung cancer are essential for patients to receive appropriate therapy.[2] Although classification of the vast majority of lung cancers is straightforward, areas of controversy and diagnostic challenges remain.

From pathologic and biologic perspectives, lung cancer is a highly complex neoplasm with several histologic types.[3] Although most lung cancers are associated with smoking, a significant proportion of them (approximately 15%) occur among never-smokers, mostly with adenocarcinoma tumor histology. Lung tumors are the result of a multistep process in which normal lung cells accumulate multiple genetic and epigenetic abnormalities and evolve into cells with malignant biologic capabilities.[3] Recent advances in understanding the complex biology of nonsmall cell lung carcinoma (NSCLC), particularly activation of oncogenes by mutation, translocation, and amplification, have provided new treatment targets and allowed the identification of subsets of NSCLC tumors with unique molecular profiles that can predict response to therapy in this disease.[4] The identification of a specific genetic and molecular abnormality using tumor tissue specimens, followed by administration of a specific inhibitor to the target, is the basis of personalized cancer treatment. In this new paradigm for lung cancer, making a precise pathologic diagnosis and properly handling tissue and cytology samples for molecular testing are becoming increasingly important. These changes in the paradigms of lung cancer diagnosis and treatment have posed multiple new challenges for pathologists to adequately integrate both routine histopathologic analysis and molecular testing into

the clinical examination for tumor diagnosis and subsequent selection of the most appropriate therapy.

In this chapter we describe the pathologic features of the major types of lung cancer and the diagnostic tools available for their diagnosis, with special emphasis on the challenges involved in classifying lung cancer using small tissue biopsies and cytology specimens. In Table 17.1 we summarize the current approach for the histologic classification of surgically resected tumors in lung cancer as described in the new lung cancer classifications from the World Health Organization.[5]

NONSMALL CELL LUNG CARCINOMA

The generally denominated NSCLCs are by far the most common type (representing approximately 85%) of lung cancer. Although NSCLC displays numerous histologic patterns, most tumors can be grouped into three main categories: squamous cell carcinoma (30%), adenocarcinoma (40%), and large cell carcinoma (3–9%).[6] Traditionally, the NSCLC designation was used for tumors that had histologic and cytologic features different than small cell carcinoma (SCLC). However, more recently, with the use of new therapeutic strategies and molecular diagnostic testing, it has become imperative to provide a more specific diagnosis of lung cancer, and the histologic subtypes must be part of the pathology report. As explained later, pathologists are more often required to perform a panel of immunohistochemical staining in biopsy and cytology specimens when the histologic subtype is not clear.

Adenocarcinoma

Adenocarcinoma is a malignant epithelial tumor with glandular differentiation or mucin production, showing various growth patterns, with expression of either mucin or thyroid transcription factor-1 (TTF-1). A significant change in pathologic classification of lung cancer occurred in 2011 with the publication of the revised classification of lung adenocarcinoma under the sponsorship of the International Association for the Study of Lung Cancer (IASLC), the American Thoracic Society (ATS), and the European Respiratory Society (ERS). This new classification of adenocarcinoma outlined many paradigm shifts that affect clinical diagnosis and management and open new avenues for research.[7] A major point in this classification was the concept that personalized medicine for patients with advanced lung cancer is determined by histology and genetics and that strategic tissue management of small biopsy specimens is critical for pathologic and molecular diagnosis. This publication was a multidisciplinary effort rather than one primarily addressed by pathologists; clinicians, radiologists, molecular biologists, and surgeons were involved. This collaboration led to an emphasis on correlations between pathology and clinical, radiologic, and molecular characteristics. In addition, the experts recognized that 70% of patients with lung cancer present with advanced-stage disease, which is usually diagnosed based on small biopsy and cytology specimens. Because the previous (2004) classifications from the WHO focused on lung cancer diagnosis in resection specimens, which are obtained in only 30% of cases, a major new effort was

TABLE 17.1 Current Classification of Lung Cancer

Category	Description

Adenocarcinoma	• Preinvasive lesions
	  – Atypical adenomatous hyperplasia
	  – Adenocarcinoma in situ
	• Minimally invasive adenocarcinoma
	• Invasive adenocarcinoma
	• Variants of invasive adenocarcinoma

Squamous cell carcinoma	• Preinvasive lesions
	  – Dysplasia
	  – Carcinoma in situ
	• Keratinizing
	• Nonkeratinizing
	• Basaloid carcinoma

LARGE CELL CARCINOMA	

Neuroendocrine tumors	• Preinvasive lesion
	  – DIPNECH
	• Carcinoid tumors
	  – Typical carcinoid
	  – Atypical carcinoid
	• Large cell neuroendocrine carcinoma
	• Small cell carcinoma

ADENOSQUAMOUS CARCINOMA	
Sarcomatoid carcinoma	• Pleomorphic • Spindle cell • Giant cell carcinoma • Carcinosarcoma • Pulmonary blastoma
Other and unclassified carcinomas	• Lymphoepithelioma-like carcinoma • NUT carcinoma
Salivary gland tumors	• Mucoepidermoid carcinoma • Adenoid cystic carcinoma • Epithelial–myoepithelial carcinoma • Pleomorphic adenoma
Papillomas	• Squamous cell papilloma • Glandular papilloma • Mixed squamous cell and glandular papilloma
Adenomas	• Sclerosing pneumocytoma • Alveolar adenoma • Papillary adenoma • Mucinous cystadenoma • Pneumocytic adenomyoepithelioma • Mucous gland adenoma
Mesenchymal tumors Lymphohistiocytic tumors Tumors of ectopic origin Metastatic tumors	

DIPNECH, diffuse idiopathic pulmonary neuroendocrine cell hyperplasia.

TABLE 17.2 Classification of Lung Adenocarcinomas in Resection Specimens[a]

Category	Description

Preinvasive lesions	• Atypical adenomatous hyperplasia
	• Adenocarcinoma in situ (≤3 cm, formerly solitary BAC)
	  – Nonmucinous
	  – Mucinous
	  – Mixed mucinous/nonmucinous

Minimally invasive adenocarcinoma (≤3-cm lepidic predominant tumor with ≤5-mm invasion)	• Nonmucinous • Mucinous • Mixed mucinous/nonmucinous
Invasive adenocarcinoma	• Lepidic predominant (formerly nonmucinous BAC pattern with >5 mm invasion) • Acinar predominant • Papillary predominant • Micropapillary predominant • Solid predominant
Variants of invasive adenocarcinoma	• Mucinous adenocarcinoma (including formerly mucinous BAC) • Colloid • Fetal (low-grade and high-grade) • Enteric

[a]Classification of the International Association for the Study of Lung Cancer, American Thoracic Society, and European Respiratory Society (IASLC/ATS/ERS).[6]
BAC, bronchioloalveolar carcinoma.

made in this new classification to define terminology and criteria to be used in small biopsies and cytology specimens.[8,9] Therefore, this classification is divided into two sections based on the diagnostic modalities of lung cancer (Table 17.2). These changes have been reflected in the recently released 2015 WHO Classification of Lung Cancer.[5] Resection specimens apply for patients with early-stage disease who are eligible for surgical resection, and small biopsy and cytology specimens for patients with advanced-stage lung cancer.

Several important modifications were made to the 2004 WHO classification concerning specimens in the 2011 IASLC/ATS/ERS and 2015 WHO classifications. The most significant change is the discontinuation of the term bronchiolo–alveolar cell carcinoma (BAC). This term had been used for at least five different entities with disparate clinical and molecular properties, leading to great confusion in routine clinical care and research.[7,8] To address two of these entities, the concepts of adenocarcinoma in situ (AIS) and minimally invasive adenocarcinoma (MIA) were proposed for small (no more than 3 cm), solitary adenocarcinomas with a

lepidic pattern that either lack invasion (AIS) or only show small foci of invasion measuring no more than 0.5 cm (MIA). AIS and MIA should define patients with either 100% or near 100% 5-year disease-free survival if the tumor is completely resected. The term mixed subtype was discontinued, and invasive adenocarcinomas were classified according to their predominant subtype. Using this approach, the proportions of each of the histologic subtypes should be estimated in a semiquantitative manner and a predominant pattern designated. The term lepidic predominant adenocarcinoma was proposed for nonmucinous tumors classified formerly as mixed subtype where the predominant subtype consists of the former nonmucinous BAC. Micropapillary adenocarcinoma was introduced as a major histologic subtype as multiple studies have shown that patients with such tumors have a poor prognosis.[10–13] The tumors formerly classified as mucinous BAC are now reclassified as mucinous AIS or MIA or invasive mucinous adenocarcinoma; these tumors on computed tomography (CT) scan frequently show nodules of consolidation with air bronchograms and a multinodular and multilobar distribution. Finally, clear cell and signet ring adenocarcinomas were discontinued as major subtypes because they represent cytologic features that can occur in multiple histologic patterns of adenocarcinoma; however, now these features can be recorded when any amount is present.[7,14]

In the new classification, tumors formerly regarded as BAC included a wide spectrum of entities with varied clinical behavior such as AIS, MIA, lepidic predominant adenocarcinoma, overtly invasive adenocarcinoma with a lepidic component, and invasive mucinous adenocarcinoma. AIS should not be equated with tumors previously classified as BAC, particularly in registry databases such as Surveillance, Epidemiology, and End Results Program (SEER).[15] Such data could be misleading as AIS is the rarest lung adenocarcinoma, representing only 0.2% to 3% of cases in white populations and up to 5% in a Japanese series.[16–18] Most cases previously classified as BAC represent tumors with invasive components. Since the publication of the 2011 IASLC/ETS/ERS classification, a series of studies validated various aspects of the classification in resection specimens. Studies from Australia,[17] Europe,[19] Asia,[18] and North America have demonstrated that the proposed subtyping has prognostic value.[16,20]

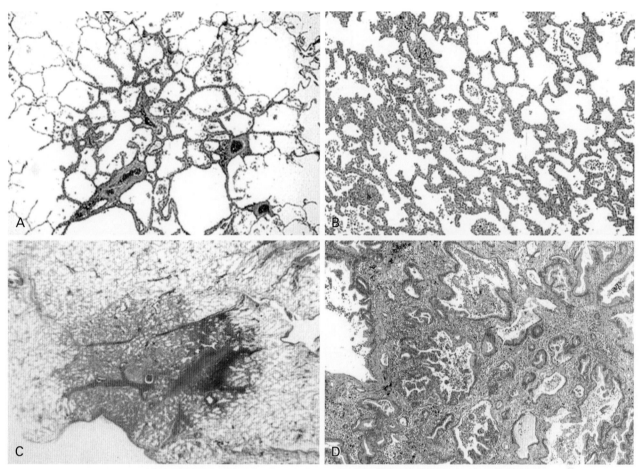

Fig. 17.1. Early lesions of lung adenocarcinoma. (A) Atypical adenomatous hyperplasia (*AAH*), (B) adenocarcinoma in situ (*AIS*), (C) microinvasive carcinoma (*MIA*), and (D) acinar growth pattern of the invasive component in the scar of a MIA (H&E stain).

Atypical Adenomatous Hyperplasia

Atypical adenomatous hyperplasia (AAH) is considered to be a precursor of adenocarcinoma.[21,22] AAH is a discrete parenchymal lesion in the alveoli close to terminal and respiratory bronchioles. Because of their size, AAH cells are usually incidental histologic findings, but they may be detected grossly, especially if they are 0.5 cm or larger. The increasing use of high-resolution CT scans for screening purposes has led to an increasing awareness of AAH, which remains one of the most important differential diagnoses of air-filled peripheral lesions (so-called ground-glass opacities). AAH maintains an alveolar structure lined by rounded, cuboidal, or low columnar cells (Fig. 17.1A). The postulated progression of AAH to adenocarcinoma with predominant lepidic growth features, apparent from the increasingly atypical morphology, is supported by the results of morphometric, cytofluorometric, and molecular studies.[22,23] The origin of AAH is still unknown, but the differentiation phenotype derived from immunohistochemical and ultrastructural features suggests an origin from the progenitor cells of the peripheral airways, such Clara cells and type II pneumocytes.[24,25]

Adenocarcinoma in Situ

AIS was added to the group of preinvasive lesions along with AAH (Table 17.2).[7,8,14] AIS is defined as a localized, small (no more than 3 cm) adenocarcinoma consisting of neoplastic pneumocytes growing along preexisting alveolar structures (lepidic growth), lacking stromal, vascular, or pleural invasion (Fig. 17.1B). No papillary or micropapillary patterns should be present, and intra-alveolar tumor cells are absent. AIS is typically nonmucinous, consisting of type II pneumocytes and/or Clara cells, but rare cases of mucinous AIS do occur. The concept of AIS was proposed with the intention of defining lesions that should correlate with a 100% disease-free survival if completely resected. This proposal was supported by retrospective observational studies in tumors measuring either 2 cm or less or 3 cm or less.[7] In the setting of multiple tumors, the criteria for AIS as well as MIA should be applied only if the other tumors are regarded as synchronous primaries rather than intrapulmonary metastases.

Minimally Invasive Carcinoma

MIA is defined as a small (no more than 3 cm), solitary adenocarcinoma with a predominantly lepidic pattern and invasion of no more than 5 mm in greatest dimension (Fig. 17.1C–D).[26,27] MIA is usually nonmucinous, but it may rarely be mucinous.[16] Measurement of the invasive component of MIA should include the following: (1) histologic subtypes other than a lepidic pattern (i.e., acinar, papillary, micropapillary, and/or solid) or (2) tumor cells infiltrating myofibroblastic stroma. MIA should not be diagnosed if the tumor invades lymphatics, blood vessels, or pleura or contains tumor necrosis. More details about measuring invasive size are explained elsewhere.[7,9] The concept of MIA was introduced to define a population of patients who should have a 100% or near 100% 5-year disease-free survival rate if the lesion is completely resected. Although less evidence was found to support the concept of MIA compared with AIS,[26,27] all published cases using these criteria have shown a 5-year disease-free survival rate of 100%.[16–18,20]

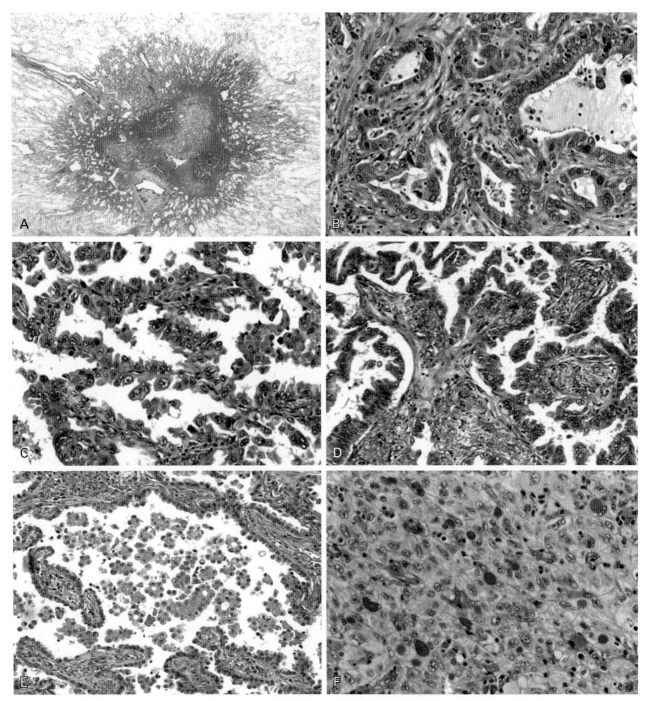

Fig. 17.2. Invasive adenocarcinoma. (A) Invasive lung adenocarcinoma with mixed patterns, including central acinar and peripheral lepidic components. Examples of invasive lung adenocarcinoma patterns: (B) acinar; (C) lepidic; (D) papillary; (E) micropapillary; and (F) solid with mucin. (A–C, E, H&E stain; D–F, mucin stain.)

The diagnosis of AIS or MIA requires that the tumor be completely sampled histologically (i.e., the patient has undergone a surgical resection). Both lesions should also have a discrete circumscribed border without miliary spread of small foci of tumor into adjacent lung parenchyma and/or with lobar consolidation. Review of CT scans may be helpful in evaluating pathologic specimens because the extent of ground-glass (usually lepidic) and solid (usually invasive) patterns can guide pathologists in assessing whether the lesion has been properly measured and/or sampled. For lesions suspected to be AIS or MIA larger than 3 cm, the term lepidic predominant adenocarcinoma is best applied, along with a comment that an invasive component cannot be excluded,

because the data are insufficient to show that such patients will have 100% 5-year disease-free survival.

Invasive Adenocarcinoma

Because of the rarity of AIS and MIA, overtly invasive adenocarcinomas represent more than 70% to 90% of surgically resected lung adenocarcinomas. These tumors typically consist of a complex, heterogeneous mixture of histologic patterns, thus explaining the former category of adenocarcinoma, mixed subtype (Fig. 17.2). The major subtypes of invasive adenocarcinoma are now classified according to the predominant component, after performing comprehensive histologic subtyping (Fig. 17.2B–F, and Table 17.2). Comprehensive histologic subtyping is performed by making a semiquantitative estimation of each of the patterns in 5% increments. It is useful to record in diagnostic reports each adenocarcinoma subtype that is present with the respective percentages. This approach may also provide a basis for architectural grading of lung adenocarcinomas.[16,28,29] Since the 2011 classification was initially published, a growing number of studies of resected lung adenocarcinomas have demonstrated its utility in identifying significant prognostic subsets and molecular correlations according to the predominant patterns.[17–19,28,30–32]

Lepidic Predominant Invasive Adenocarcinoma. This subtype consists of a proliferation of bland type II or Clara cells growing along the surface of alveolar walls, similar to the morphology defined in the earlier section on AIS and MIA (Fig. 17.2C). Invasive adenocarcinoma is present in at least one focus measuring more than 5 mm in greatest dimension. Invasion is defined as follows: (1) histologic subtypes other than a lepidic pattern (i.e., acinar, papillary, micropapillary, and/or solid); (2) myofibroblastic stroma associated with invasive tumor cells; (3) vascular or pleural invasion; and (4) spread through alveolar spaces (STAS).[33–35] Lepid predominant adenocarcinoma is diagnosed rather than MIA if the cancer invades lymphatics, blood vessels, or pleura or contains tumor necrosis. Several recent studies of early-stage adenocarcinomas published since 2011 have demonstrated that lepidic predominant tumors have a favorable prognosis, with 5-year disease-free survival rates of 86% to 90%.[17–19] The term adenocarcinoma with lepidic pattern corresponds to some cases previously referred to as adenocarcinoma with BAC features. The term lepidic predominant adenocarcinoma should not be used in the context of invasive mucinous adenocarcinoma with predominant lepidic growth; these tumors should be classified as mucinous adenocarcinomas.

Acinar Predominant Invasive Adenocarcinoma. This subtype shows a major component of glands that are round to oval with a central luminal space surrounded by tumor cells (Fig. 17.2B).[6] The neoplastic cells and/or glandular spaces may contain mucin. Cribriform structures can be found in the acinar pattern, are considered to be high grade, and are associated with poor prognosis.[36] Tumor cells may form aggregates of polarized cell without clear lumen, which is still recognized as an acinar pattern.

Papillary Predominant Adenocarcinoma. This subtype shows a major component of a growth of glandular cells along central fibrovascular cores (Fig. 17.2D).[6] If a tumor has lepidic growth, but the alveolar spaces are filled with papillary or micropapillary structures, the tumor is classified as papillary or micropapillary adenocarcinoma, respectively.

Micropapillary Predominant Adenocarcinoma. This subtype has tumor cells growing in papillary tufts or florets that lack fibrovascular cores (Fig. 17.2E).[6] These may appear detached and/or connected to the alveolar walls. The tumor cells are usually small and cuboidal with minimal nuclear atypia. STAS is a newly suggested pattern of invasion, often seen with the micropapillary pattern; it can occur with micropapillary clusters, solid nests, or single cells. STAS probably contributes to the high recurrence rate for patients with small stage I adenocarcinomas who undergo limited surgical resections and the poor prognosis observed by others.[12,33]

Solid Predominant Invasive Adenocarcinoma. The solid subtype with mucin production consists of a major component of polygonal tumor cells forming sheets but without any clear acinar, papillary, micropapillary, or lepidic growth (Fig. 17.2F).[6] If the tumor is 100% solid, intracellular mucin should be present in at least five tumor cells in each of two high-power fields, confirmed with histochemical stains for mucin.[6,9] Tumors formerly classified as large cell carcinomas that have immunohistochemical expression of TTF-1 and/or napsin A, even if mucin is not identified, are now classified as solid adenocarcinomas. Solid adenocarcinomas must be distinguished from nonkeratinizing squamous cell carcinomas and large cell carcinomas, both of which may show rare cells with intracellular mucin. Neuroendocrine markers, such as neural cell adhesion molecule (NCAM)/CD56, dense core granule associated protein chromogranin A, and synaptic vesicle protein synaptophysin should be performed only if neuroendocrine morphology is present, to allow the diagnosis of large cell neuroendocrine carcinoma (LCNEC).

Variants of Invasive Adenocarcinoma

Four variants of clinically relevant invasive lung adenocarcinomas are recognized: (1) invasive mucinous adenocarcinoma, with tumor cells that have a goblet or columnar cell morphology with abundant intracytoplasmic mucin (Fig. 17.3A); (2) colloid adenocarcinoma, with abundant mucin pools filling alveolar spaces; (3) fetal adenocarcinoma, resembling fetal lung; and, (4) enteric adenocarcinoma, an adenocarcinoma of the lung resembling enteric adenocarcinoma.

Invasive Mucinous Adenocarcinoma. Multiple studies have shown major differences in clinical, radiologic, pathologic, and genetic features between invasive mucinous adenocarcinomas and the tumors formerly classified as nonmucinous BAC.[37–42] Invasive mucinous adenocarcinomas have tumor cells with a goblet or columnar cell morphology with abundant intracytoplasmic mucin and aligned, basally located nucleoli (Fig. 17.3A). This pathognomonic cellular feature can be recognized in small lung samples. Similar to nonmucinous tumors, invasive mucinous adenocarcinomas may show the same heterogeneous mixture of lepidic, acinar, papillary, micropapillary, and solid growth, which will not be described in detail and quantified for this specific subtype. Although invasive mucinous adenocarcinomas frequently show lepidic predominant growth, extensive sampling usually shows invasive foci. Therefore, reports on biopsy specimens should include a remark such as mucinous adenocarcinoma with lepidic pattern. However, if a resection specimen of the mucinous tumor fulfills the diagnostic criteria of AIS or MIA, the tumor should be diagnosed as mucinous AIS or MIA, respectively, although such tumors are extremely rare. In some cases, mucinous adenocarcinoma appears in CT scans and pathology specimens with a pseudo-pneumonia growth pattern (Fig. 17.3B–C).

Colloid Adenocarcinoma. This subtype shows abundant extracellular mucin in pools, which distend the alveolar spaces and destroy their walls, showing an overtly invasive growth pattern into the alveolar spaces. Mucin deposits enlarge and dissect the lung parenchyma, creating pools of mucin-rich matrix, while tumor elements consist of foci of tall columnar cells with goblet-like features growing in a lepidic fashion. Tumor glands often float into the mucoid material, becoming poorly recognizable and then requiring extensive tumor sampling.

Fetal Adenocarcinoma. This subtype consists of complex glandular structures composed of glycogen-rich, nonciliated cells resembling a developing epithelium in the pseudoglandular phase of the fetal lung, with low nuclear atypia and morule formation.[43]

Primary Pulmonary Adenocarcinoma With Enteric Differentiation. This term is used to indicate a primary lung cancer resembling colorectal adenocarcinoma metastatic to the lung.[44–46]

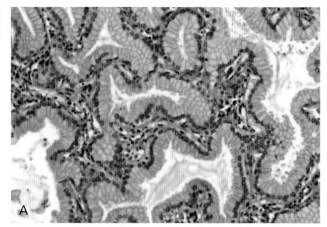

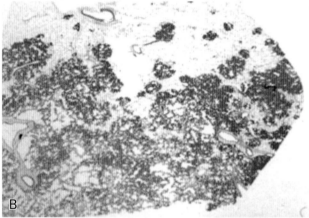

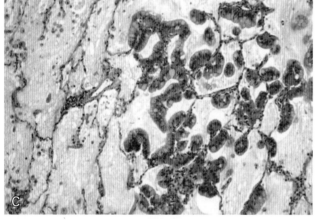

Fig. 17.3. Variants of invasive adenocarcinoma with mucinous histology. (A) Mucinous invasive adenocarcinoma, (B) mucinous invasive adenocarcinoma with pseudopneumonic alveolar pattern, and (C) higher magnification of a mucinous growth with lepidic features. (A–C, H&E stain.)

Its histologic characteristics include eosinophilic tall columnar cells with brush border, vesicular nuclei, central geographic or dotted necrosis, occasional central scar and pleural indentation, and papillo–tubular (or gland-like) structure. The histologic resemblance to colorectal cancer is a hallmark of this tumor. Although some tumors have enteric differentiation with positive immunohistochemical expression of CDX-2 (which encodes for an intestine-specific transcription factor) and cytokeratin (CK) 20, and negative expression of CK7, others have only enteric morphology.

Immunohistochemistry of Adenocarcinomas

The immunohistochemical expression of lung adenocarcinomas varies somewhat based on the subtype and degree of differentiation. TTF-1 and napsin A are nearly specific markers for lung adenocarcinoma, except that thyroid cancer expresses TTF-1 and renal cell carcinoma expresses napsin A. Approximately 75% of invasive adenocarcinomas are positive for TTF-1 (Fig. 17.4), and none of the squamous cell carcinomas express TTF-1. Among the adenocarcinoma subtypes, most lepidic and papillary predominant tumors are positive for TTF-1, as are the lepidic components of AIS and MIA, whereas positive frequency is lower in cases of solid predominant cancer.[32,47] The sensitivity of napsin A is comparable to that of TTF-1, but its specificity is far lower.[48] CK7 is another marker for lung adenocarcinoma, and its sensitivity, but not its specificity, is higher than that of TTF-1 and napsin A. Furthermore, tumor protein p63, which has been used as a marker for a squamous cell carcinoma, is also positive in some lung adenocarcinoma (up to 38%),[49] and a portion of these adenocarcinomas are positive for anaplastic lymphoma kinase (*ALK*) gene rearrangement.[50–52] In contrast, protein p40, an isoform of p63,[50] is never positive in adenocarcinomas except for those contained in adenosquamous carcinomas. Some adenocarcinomas may show a squamous appearance. In these cases, phenotyping with a limited panel of immunomarkers (including p40, and TTF-1) and mucin stain is necessary.[7,49,53,54]

Histologic and Molecular Correlations

Despite the discovery of multiple molecular abnormalities in lung adenocarcinoma, no significant, specific histologic and molecular correlations have been found. A number of driver gene alterations are now known to exist in lung adenocarcinomas including mutations of EGFR, KRAS, BRAF, and ERBB2/HER2, and rearrangements of ALK, RET, ROS1, NTRK1, and NRG1.[55–61] Among these mutations, EGFR and ALK are clinically relevant because molecular targeted drugs can be used in patients whose tumors have these molecular abnormalities. Adenocarcinomas with BRAF, HER2, ROS1, and NTRK1 abnormalities share clinicopathologic features with the EGFR-mutant and ALK-rearranged tumors in terms of involvement that is nearly specific to adenocarcinoma in lung cancer, particularly frequent in TTF-1–positive expression, and preferentially present in never-smokers and in women. The frequent finding of KRAS mutation and consistent lack of EGFR mutation in invasive mucinous adenocarcinoma is the strongest histologic and molecular correlation found in lung cancer. Most histologic subtypes of adenocarcinoma harbor EGFR and KRAS mutations, as well as ALK rearrangement. EGFR mutations are encountered most frequently in nonmucinous adenocarcinomas with a lepidic or papillary predominant pattern, whereas KRAS mutations tend to be found in solid predominant adenocarcinomas. ALK rearrangement has mostly been associated with an acinar pattern including a cribriform morphology and with signet-ring cell features, particularly in those tumors with TTF-1 and p63 coexpression.[51,62,63]

Impact of the New Classification on Tumor, Node, Metastasis Staging

The 2011 IASLC/ATS/ERS classification of adenocarcinoma can affect tumor, node, metastasis (TNM) staging in several ways. First, it may help in comparing histologic characteristics of multiple lung adenocarcinomas to determine whether they are intrapulmonary metastases or separate primaries. Using comprehensive histologic subtyping along with other histologic characteristics has been shown to correlate well with molecular analyses and clinical behavior.[64,65] Second, it may be more meaningful clinically to measure tumor size in lung adenocarcinomas that

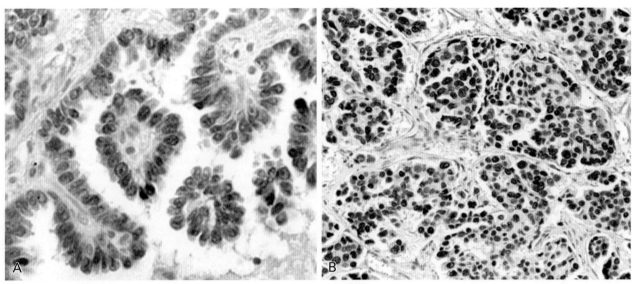

Fig. 17.4. Immunohistochemical markers of lung adenocarcinoma. Nuclear expression of thyroid transcription factor-1 (*TTF-1*) in adenocarcinomas with (A) papillary and (B) solid patterns.

TABLE 17.3 Specific Terminology and Criteria for Histologic Diagnosis of Nonsmall Cell Lung Cancer in Small Biopsy and Cytology Specimens[a]

2004 WHO Classification Including Updated 2011 IASLC/ATS/ERS Terminology	Morphology/Stains	IASLC/ATS/ERS Terminology for Small Biopsy and Cytology Specimens
Adenocarcinoma Mixed subtype Acinar Papillary Solid	Morphologic adenocarcinoma patterns clearly present	Adenocarcinoma (describe identifiable patterns)
Lepidic (nonmucinous)		Adenocarcinoma with lepidic pattern (if pure, add note: an invasive component cannot be excluded)
Lepidic (mucinous)		Invasive mucinous adenocarcinoma (describe patterns present; use term mucinous adenocarcinoma with lepidic pattern if pure lepidic pattern)
No 2004 WHO counterpart; most will be solid adenocarcinomas	Morphologic adenocarcinoma patterns not present (supported by special stains, i.e., positive TTF-1)	NSCLC, favor adenocarcinoma
Squamous cell carcinoma	Morphologic squamous cell patterns clearly present	Squamous cell carcinoma
No 2004 WHO counterpart	Morphologic squamous cell patterns not present (supported by special stains, i.e., positive p40)	NSCLC, favor squamous cell carcinoma
Large cell carcinoma	No clear adenocarcinoma, squamous, or neuroendocrine morphology or staining pattern	NSCLC-NOS[b]

[a]From Travis et al,[8] with permission: Travis WD, Brambilla E, Noguchi M, et al. Diagnosis of lung cancer in small biopsies and cytology: implications of the 2011 International Association for the Study of Lung Cancer/American Thoracic Society/European Respiratory Society classification. *Arch Pathol Lab Med.* 2013;137(5):668–684.

[b]*IASLC/ATS/ERS*, International Association for the Study of Lung Cancer, American Thoracic Society, and European Respiratory Society; *NSCLC-NOS*, nonsmall cell lung cancer, not otherwise specified. Pattern can be seen not only in large cell carcinomas, but also when the solid, poorly differentiated component of adenocarcinomas or squamous cell carcinomas does not express immunohistochemical markers or mucin; *TTF-1*, thyroid transcription factor-1; *WHO*, World Health Organization.

have a lepidic component by using the invasive size rather than total size to determine the final size of the tumor for TNM staging. It is possible that in the next edition of the TNM, AIS may be regarded as tumor carcinoma in situ (Tis) and MIA may be regarded as tumor microinvasive (Tmi).

Small Biopsy and Cytology Samples

In the past, NSCLCs were lumped together without attention to more specific histologic typing (e.g., adenocarcinoma, squamous cell carcinoma, etc.).[8] One of the major new proposals in the IASLC/ATS/ERS classification was the development of standardized criteria and terminology for the pathologic diagnosis of lung cancer in small biopsy and cytology specimens (Table 17.3).[8,9]

In addition to the criteria and terminology, two paradigm shifts have emerged for pathologists in terms of tumor classification and management of specimens. The first is the need to perform immunohistochemistry to further classify tumors formerly diagnosed as NSCLC not otherwise specified (NOS). Because the distinction between histologic types of lung cancer, particularly adenocarcinoma and squamous cell carcinoma, is so important, the new classification recommends that pathologists use special stains to try to further subtype carcinomas that are difficult to classify by light microscopic evaluation of histologic sections alone.

For tumors with classic morphologic features the diagnostic terms adenocarcinomas and squamous cell carcinomas can be used (Table 17.3). The morphologic features of these tumors are described in detail elsewhere.[6,7,9] If an NSCLC does not show clear glandular or squamous morphology in a small biopsy or cytology specimen, it is classified as NSCLC-NOS.[7,66] Tumors with this morphologic appearance should be studied with a limited special stain workup in an attempt to classify them further. It is recommended to use a single adenocarcinoma marker (e.g., TTF-1), a single squamous marker (e.g., p40), and/or mucin stain.[66,67] Tumors that are positive for an adenocarcinoma marker or mucin are classified as NSCLC, favor adenocarcinoma. Tumors that are positive for a squamous cell carcinoma immunohistochemical marker with negative adenocarcinoma markers are classified as NSCLC, favor squamous cell carcinoma. Cytology is a powerful diagnostic tool that can accurately subtype NSCLC in most cases,[66] and immunohistochemistry is readily available when cell blocks are prepared for the cytology samples.[68]

Squamous Cell Carcinoma

Squamous cell carcinoma is thought to arise from the airway epithelium and is characterized histologically by keratinization and/or intercellular bridges. If these morphologic hallmarks are absent, a diagnosis can be established only by positive immunohistochemical staining for markers such as p40 and CK5/6.

Squamous cell carcinoma usually arises in a main or lobar bronchus, but more peripheral locations are not uncommon. The centrally located hilar-type occasionally shows intraepithelial spread that may extend to the cut end of the resected bronchus; therefore, frozen sections of the mucosa at the resected end must be examined during surgical procedures. In comparison with adenocarcinoma, many peripherally located squamous cell carcinomas are only locally invasive, and pleural carcinomatosis is rare. The spread of squamous cell carcinoma is similar to that of other NSCLCs. Staging of squamous cell carcinoma, as for other malignant epithelial tumors of the lung, is performed according to the TNM system. Uncommonly, squamous cell carcinoma manifests as a superficial spreading tumor on the bronchial mucosa. Squamous cell carcinoma tends to be locally aggressive, involving adjacent structures through direct invasion.

Preinvasive Lesions

The histopathologic sequence of preinvasive lesions of squamous cell carcinoma has been identified and is characterized for different degrees of squamous dysplasia and carcinoma in situ (Fig. 17.5).[69] The criteria for squamous dysplasia and carcinoma in situ are similar to those for lesions occurring in the uterine cervix and oral cavity. However, the histologic appearance of these lesions is not uniform, because bronchial dysplasia originates from pseudostratified columnar epithelium and is not deeply associated with human papilloma virus (HPV) infection.

In a dysplastic lesion, the ciliated respiratory epithelium is replaced by thick, stratified squamous epithelium with moderate nuclear atypia, but still retaining the capacity for squamous differentiation. Angiogenic squamous dysplasia is a specific phenotype of dysplasia characterized by proliferation of small blood vessels in the submucosa; this subtype shows high proliferative activity and is associated with high-risk smokers.[70] Carcinoma in situ is composed of stratified epithelium (more than 10 cells thick) with an increased nuclear-to-cytoplasmic ratio and severe nuclear atypia, but it does not show invasive growth.

Early Invasive Squamous Cell Carcinoma

Centrally located (hilar-type) early invasive squamous cell carcinoma is defined as a tumor that arises in areas up to the subsegmental bronchus, is confined to the bronchial wall, and shows no lymph node metastasis. Early invasive squamous cell carcinoma is associated with a 5-year survival rate of more than 90% and

can be divided into the following subtypes: (1) polypoid type, frequently arising at the bronchial spar; (2) nodular type, arising at any bronchus and having a tendency to form a localized tumor showing vertical invasive growth; and, (3) superficially infiltrating type, showing in situ and microinvasive growths, often involving a wide area but exhibiting little tendency to produce bronchial stenosis and obstruction.

In comparison with the hilar-type, little is known about the peripheral type of squamous cell carcinoma. A unique subtype of squamous cell carcinoma with alveolar space filling (ASF) has been proposed.[71,72] Peripheral-type squamous cell carcinoma can be divided into two distinctive subtypes, the ASF-type and the expanding or destructive-type, based on the condition of the elastic fiber framework. The ASF-type shows growth that fills the alveolar space without destruction of the existing alveolar structure or elastic fiber network (Fig. 17.6A). It has been suggested that ASF growth represents an in situ lesion with an extremely favorable prognosis.

Invasive Squamous Cell Carcinoma

Invasive squamous cell carcinoma arises in both the major (main to segmental) bronchus and the peripheral parenchyma. The former type shows both endobronchial and invasive growth into the peribronchial soft tissue, lung parenchyma, and nearby lymph nodes. Squamous cell carcinoma growing in the endobronchial region sometimes blocks the bronchus, resulting in secondary changes to the distal lung, such as collapse, lipid pneumonia, and bronchopneumonia. On the other hand, squamous cell carcinoma arising in the peripheral region shows two different tumor growth types: the ASF-type and the compression-type. In comparison with the hilar-type, the peripheral squamous cell carcinoma frequently possesses mucin-containing cells and shows glandular cell charactertistics. Therefore, many tumors diagnosed as peripheral-type squamous cell carcinomas are actually adenosquamous cell carcinomas in the strict sense.

Invasive squamous cell carcinomas are grouped in three major histologic types, including the common types keratinizing and nonkeratinizing, and the basaloid type.

Keratinizing and Nonkeratinizing Squamous Cell Carcinoma. Most invasive squamous cell carcinomas are moderately or poorly differentiated. The well-differentiated carcinoma is not common in comparison with squamous cell carcinoma of stratified squamous epithelial origin, such as that of the oral cavity, pharynx, and esophagus. Squamous cell carcinoma arising from a major bronchus frequently shows an intraepithelial, in situ type of extension along the bronchus. Histologically, invasive squamous cell carcinoma shows geographic nests composed of polygonal cells with intercellular bridges and keratinization (Fig. 17.6B–C). As stated, the common type of squamous cell carcinoma is divided into two classes: keratinizing and nonkeratinizing. The keratinizing type is well to moderately differentiated and easy to diagnose as squamous cell carcinoma, whereas the nonkeratinizing type is sometimes difficult to diagnose if it does not contain intercellular bridges (Fig. 17.6D).

Keratinization and intercellular bridges are the hallmarks for the differential diagnosis of squamous cell carcinoma from other NSCLCs. However, if a tumor is poorly differentiated and differentiation is unclear, immunohistochemical analysis using a limited panel of markers and mucin staining is necessary. The most important diagnostic immunohistochemical marker of squamous cell carcinoma is p40 (Fig. 17.6F), which is more specific than p63 (Fig. 17.6E).[73,74] These markers are positive in the tumor cell nuclei and are fundamental markers for basal cells of the bronchial mucosa. CK5/6 is a less reliable marker of squamous cell carcinoma.[75] TTF-1, which is a very specific marker for adenocarcinoma, should be negative.[76] If

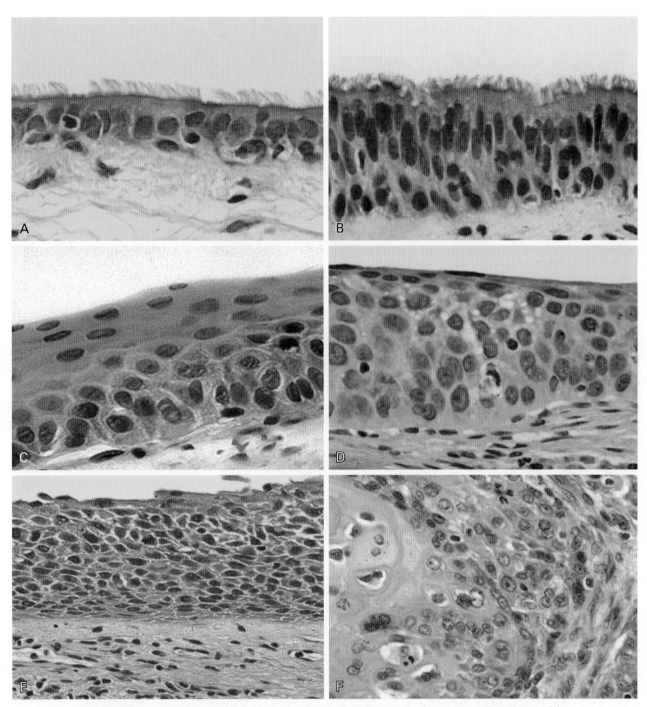

Fig. 17.5. Histopathologic sequential changes involved in the pathogenesis of squamous cell carcinoma of the lung. (A) Normal bronchial epithelium; (B) basal cell hyperplasia; (C) squamous metaplasia of bronchial epithelium; (D) moderate dysplasia; (E) carcinoma in situ; and (F) invasive squamous cell carcinoma. (A–F, H&E stain.)

the immunostaining profile is the only evidence for a diagnosis of squamous cell carcinoma, such cases should be diagnosed as tumor with squamous cell carcinoma nonkeratinizing type. It is sometimes difficult to differentiate pulmonary squamous cell carcinoma from metastatic squamous cell carcinoma of other sites, such as the head and neck, esophagus, or cervix. Genotypic fingerprinting for *TP53* mutation, loss of heterozygosity, or HPV genotyping has been reported to be useful for the differential diagnosis.[77] Despite the discovery of multiple molecular abnormalities in squamous cell carcinoma,[78,79] no significant, specific histologic and molecular correlations have been found in this tumor type.

Immunohistochemistry of Squamous Cell Carcinoma. Squamous cell carcinoma has traditionally been defined as a tumor that shows keratinization, pearl formation, and/or intercellular bridges. Immunohistochemistry is not needed in these tumors. As intercellular bridging may be scarce in nonkeratinizing squamous cell carcinoma, immunohistochemistry is needed to distinguish theses tumors from large cell carcinoma with a null immunophenotype in surgical resections, and NSCLCs with adenocarcinoma or NSCLC-NOS phenotype on small biopsies. For such tumors, diffuse positive staining with p40, p63, and/or CK5 or CK5/6 confirms their squamous phenotype and classification as a nonkeratinizing squamous cell carcinoma.

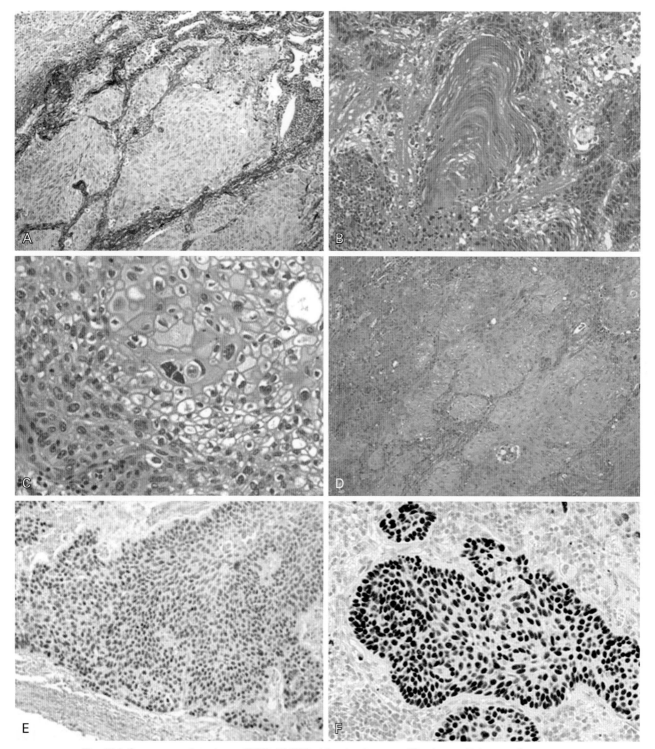

Fig. 17.6. Squamous cell carcinoma (SCC). (A) SCC of the alveolar space filling-type, with tumor cells preserving the elastic fiber framework; (B) SCC of the keratinizing type showing keratinization; (C) SCC of the keratinizing type showing cellular keratinization at higher magnification; (D) SCC of the nonkeratinizing type; (E) p63 immunohistochemical expression; and (F) p40 immunohistochemical expression. (A, elastic stain; B–D, H&E stain).

Both TTF-1 and mucin stains should be negative or only focally positive (for TTF-1, less than 10% of cells with faint staining).

Basaloid Carcinoma. Basaloid carcinoma is a variant of squamous cell carcinoma (Fig. 17.7). This is a poorly differentiated tumor that displays lobular architecture and peripheral palisading of nuclei at the edge of tumor nests and lacks squamous differentiation. The

tumor cells are relatively small with scanty cytoplasm and absent or focal nucleoli. The mitotic rate is high (15–50 per 2 mm²) and the proliferation index is high as assessed by Ki-67 (approximately 50–80%). In the 2004 WHO classification, this tumor was classified as the basaloid variant of large cell carcinoma; however, as it is usually positive for p40 immunohistochemical expression, recently it has been reclassified as a variant of squamous cell carcinoma (Fig.

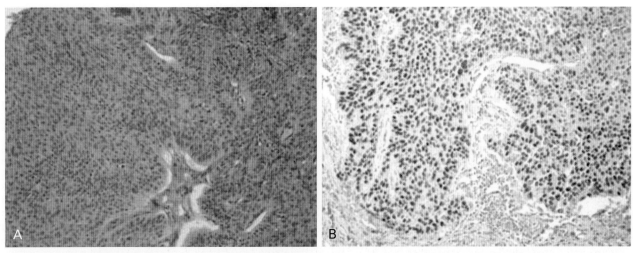

Fig. 17.7. Basaloid carcinoma. (A) Histology (H&E stain) and (B) p40 immunohistochemical staining.

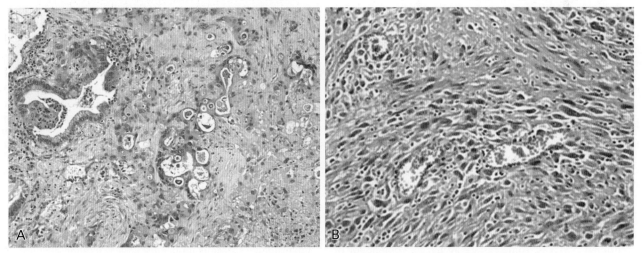

Fig. 17.8. (A) Adenosquamous carcinoma and (B) sarcomatoid carcinoma, spindle cell. (A and B, H&E stain.)

17.7B).[80] Tumors with keratinizing or nonkeratinizing squamous cell carcinoma features that have more than 50% basaloid component are classified as basaloid carcinoma. These changes were introduced to the new 2015 WHO classification.[5] Tumor spread and staging of basaloid carcinoma are similar to those of other squamous cell carcinomas of the lung.

Immunohistochemistry of Basaloid Carcinoma. Basaloid carcinoma is a specific subtype of nonkeratinizing squamous cell carcinoma that requires differential diagnosis with SCLC and LCNEC, with which it might be confused in the case of crushed artifact due to small cell size or the presence of rosettes and palisading with centrolobular necrosis. Basaloid carcinoma consistently shows diffuse and strong expression of p63 and its isoform p40 (Fig. 17.7B). CK5/6 and the cytokeratins included in the antibody 34βE12 (CKs 1, 5, 10, and 14) are also expressed in all cases, sometimes in a less diffuse fashion. TTF-1 is never expressed.[50,81] Neuroendocrine markers (NCAM/CD56, chromogranin A, and synaptophysin) are usually negative.

Adenosquamous Carcinoma

This tumor is characterized by the presence of both squamous cell and adenocarcinoma differentiations. A carcinoma showing histologic characteristics of each component in at least 10% of the tumor should be categorized as adenosquamous carcinoma (Fig. 17.8A). However, a situation where less than 10% of each histologic differentiation is present should be reported because recent molecular analyses have suggested that tumors with mixed features can reflect the genetic status of either component regardless of their proportion in the tumor.[82] The frequency of adenosquamous carcinoma is estimated at 0.4% to 4% of lung cancers.[6] Typically, adenosquamous carcinomas are located in the peripheral pulmonary parenchyma, but they have also been reported to arise centrally.[83] The clinical characteristics are similar to those of other NSCLCs. The outcome of adenosquamous carcinoma is significantly poorer than that of adenocarcinoma and squamous cell carcinoma, particularly in stages I and II.[84] The amount of each component does not affect the survival rate.

Immunohistochemistry of Adenosquamous Carcinoma

Although adenosquamous carcinoma is diagnosed on the basis of morphologic features, immunohistochemistry is sometimes useful for distinguishing the relatively poorly differentiated components, including solid adenocarcinoma and nonkeratinizing squamous cell carcinoma. TTF-1 (a hallmark of adenocarcinoma differentiation) and p40 (a hallmark of squamous cell carcinoma differentiation) are the two best markers for immunohistochemical analysis.[74] Only uniformly, diffusely, and clearly stained areas should be judged as positive immunostaining for p40.

Sarcomatoid Carcinoma

This category encompasses a heterogeneous group of uncommon tumors, including pleomorphic, spindle, and giant cell carcinomas, as well as carcinosarcomas and pulmonary blastomas.

Pleomorphic, Spindle, and Giant Cell Carcinomas

These tumors represent poorly differentiated NSCLCs, namely adenocarcinoma, squamous cell carcinoma, or large cell carcinoma containing at least 10% spindle cells (Fig. 17.8B) and/or giant cells.[85,86] A specific and definite diagnosis may be made only on a resected tumor. The specific histologic components should be mentioned in the diagnosis. In small biopsy specimens, the sarcomatoid elements should be described. Pure spindle cell carcinoma and giant cell carcinoma are very rare. The most common presentation is a large peripheral mass, usually in an upper lobe.[87] These are aggressive tumors with spread similar to that of other NSCLCs, and distant metastases are commonly found. Tumors are staged according to the TNM classification.

Immunohistochemistry is useful for highlighting the differentiation characteristics of the tumor cells. Evidence of keratin expression in the spindle or giant cell components is not required if carcinoma is clearly present. Various kinds of genetic alterations have been reported, but no specific mutations, rearrangements, and amplifications are found in this type of tumor.[86]

Carcinosarcoma

Carcinosarcoma is a malignant tumor consisting of a mixture of carcinoma and sarcoma containing heterologous elements such as rhabdomyosarcoma, chondrosarcoma, and osteosarcoma.[47] Carcinosarcoma arises either in the major bronchi or in the peripheral lung. The diagnosis of carcinosarcoma is difficult using small biopsy samples, and immunohistochemistry may be helpful for confirming clear epithelial and sarcomatous differentiation. Although most carcinosarcomas contain conventional NSCLC, some cases may have a component of high-grade fetal adenocarcinoma. This type of tumor may be referred to as the blastomatoid variant of carcinosarcoma. However, carcinosarcoma lacks the component of low-grade fetal adenocarcinoma and the primitive stroma of pulmonary blastoma.

Pulmonary Blastoma

Pulmonary blastoma is a biphasic tumor composed of low-grade fetal adenocarcinoma and primitive mesenchymal cells showing various degrees of differentiation. Foci of specific mesenchymal differentiation (e.g., immature cartilage) may exist, but they are not required for diagnosis. Pulmonary blastoma and well-differentiated fetal adenocarcinoma contain missense mutations in exon 3 of the beta-catenin gene, which result in activation of the Wnt pathway and aberrant nuclear localization of beta-catenin. Therefore, nuclear localization of beta-catenin is a unique diagnostic marker of pulmonary blastoma.[83,84] Because pulmonary blastoma is a biphasic tumor, it expresses both epithelial and mesenchymal immunomarkers.

Immunohistochemistry of Sarcomatoid Carcinoma

Although these tumors are diagnosed by morphologic features, immunohistochemistry may highlight the different cell components. The differentiated epithelial elements show the expected immunophenotypes. Cytokeratin expression is not required in the spindle or giant cell component if carcinoma is clearly present. The pleomorphic, spindle, or giant cell components express vimentin and fascin.[85,88–90] Cytokeratins and differentiation-associated markers such as napsin A,[91,92] TTF-1, p63, and CK5/6 are variably expressed in sarcomatoid elements.[88,93]

Large Cell Carcinoma

Large cell carcinoma is defined as an undifferentiated NSCLC that lacks the cytologic, architectural and immunohistochemical features of adenocarcinoma or squamous cell carcinoma. The diagnosis requires a thoroughly sampled resected tumor and can be made only on resected specimens and not in small biopsy specimens or cytology samples. Even if squamous or adenocarcinoma differentiation cannot be detected in biopsy material both morphologically and immunohistochemically, a diagnosis of large cell carcinoma cannot be made, because the tumor may contain squamous cell carcinoma and/or adenocarcinoma with a large cell component. Therefore, in that event, the tumor should be diagnosed NSCLC-NOS (Table 17.3). Many tumors previously classified as large cell carcinoma according to the 2004 WHO classification are now reclassified as per the 2015 WHO classification as adenocarcinoma, solid subtype (positive for TTF-1, napsin A, or mucin) or squamous cell carcinoma, nonkeratinizing subtype (positive for p40 or p63) based on use of immunohistochemistry and mucin stains.[5]

Historically, large cell carcinoma has accounted for about 10% of all lung carcinomas.[94] However, recent data from the SEER database in the United States have shown that the frequency has decreased from 9.4% to 2.3%. This change is explained by the more precise diagnosis of NSCLC subtypes using immunohistochemical staining. The average patient age at diagnosis is around the 7th decade, and the male-to-female ratio is 4:1 or 5:1, which lies between the ratios for squamous cell carcinoma and adenocarcinoma.[69] Large cell carcinoma arises more frequently in the periphery of the lung. It usually forms a spherical tumor with well-defined borders, and it has a bulging, fleshy, homogeneous, rather sarcomatous appearance. Necrosis is often found, but cavitation is rare. Some large cell carcinomas resemble poorly differentiated adenocarcinoma or squamous cell carcinoma grossly. On histological examination, most large cell carcinomas are composed of solid nests of polygonal cells with vesicular nuclei, prominent nucleoli, moderately abundant cytoplasm, well-defined cell borders, and a scant fibrovascular stroma (Fig. 17.9A). These histologic features suggest a poorly differentiated carcinoma in which differentiation to squamous cell carcinoma or adenocarcinoma cannot be confirmed.

The 2004 WHO classification listed five histologic variants of large cell carcinoma: LCNEC, basaloid carcinoma, lymphoepithelioma-like carcinoma, clear cell carcinoma, and large cell carcinoma with rhabdoid phenotype.[6] However, in the recently released 2015 WHO classification, LCNEC will be reclassified into the new category of neuroendocrine tumor, and basaloid carcinoma is included as a variant of squamous cell carcinoma (Table 17.1).[5] Pure large cell carcinomas with clear cells or rhabdoid phenotypes are quite rare, and they are not considered a variant of cell carcinoma. If these components are detected in a large cell carcinoma, their presence should be added in the histologic description.

Immunohistochemistry of Large Cell Carcinoma

Large cell carcinoma is an undifferentiated carcinoma from the aspects of both morphology and immunohistochemistry. Therefore, if a resected tumor cannot be diagnosed as adenocarcinoma or squamous cell carcinoma morphologically, immunohistochemical analysis should be performed.[75,76] Many immunohistochemical differentiation markers have been reported, but based on analyses of sensitivity and

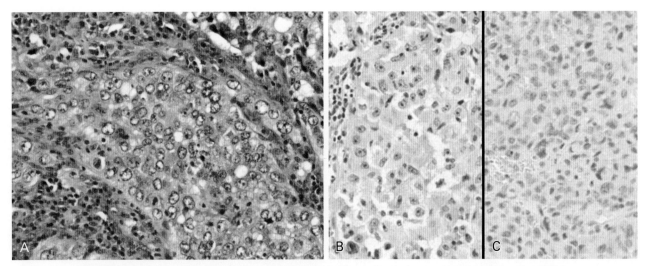

Fig. 17.9. Large cell carcinoma. (A) Histology (H&E stain); (B) negative for immunohistochemical marker TTF-1; and (C) negative for immunohistochemical marker p40.

specificity, the most useful are p40 and CK5/6 for identifying squamous differentiation, and TTF-1 and napsin A for identifying adenocarcinoma differentiation. Practically, if no morphologic differentiation can be detected in the resected specimen, immunohistochemical analysis should be done, and if squamous markers (p40 and/or CK5/6) are positive and adenocarcinoma markers (TTF-1 and/or napsin A) are negative, the tumor should be diagnosed as nonkeratinizing squamous cell carcinoma. On the other hand, if adenocarcinoma markers (TTF-1 and/or napsin A) are positive and squamous markers (p40 and/or CK5/6) are negative, the diagnosis should be of adenocarcinoma, solid subtype. A tumor that is negative for both adenocarcinoma and squamous cell carcinoma markers can be finally diagnosed as large cell carcinoma (Fig. 17.9B–C). However, if immunohistochemistry is not applicable, a comment should be included in the pathology report, such as diagnosed without immunohistochemical analysis or diagnosed by histology only.

NEUROENDOCRINE TUMORS

Neuroendocrine tumors account for approximately 15% of lung cancers. Neuroendocrine neoplasms of the lung are ubiquitous tumors composed of malignant cells showing neuroendocrine differentiation and representing a wide spectrum of clinical, biologic, and histopathologic features. Four major types of neuroendocrine tumors of the lung are recognized: typical and atypical carcinoids, considered low- and intermediate-grade tumors, respectively; and LCNEC and SCLC, considered high-grade malignancies.[95]

The precursor lesions for the most common type of neuroendocrine carcinoma of the lung, SCLC, are unknown.[21,23] However, a rare lesion called diffuse idiopathic pulmonary neuroendocrine cell hyperplasia (DIPNECH) has been associated with the development of typical and atypical carcinoids.[21,96,97] DIPNECH lesions include local extraluminal proliferations in the form of tumorlets. Carcinoid tumors are arbitrarily separated from tumorlets if the neuroendocrine proliferation is 0.5 cm or larger. The findings of more widespread and more extensive genetic damage in normal and hyperplastic bronchial epithelium among patients with SCLC, as compared with NSCLC, suggest that SCLC may arise directly from histologically normal or mildly abnormal epithelium without passing through a more complex histologic sequence.[98]

Carcinoid Tumors

Carcinoid tumors are thought to be derived from neuroendocrine cells known to exist in normal airways. However, in contrast to most other lung cancers, these tumors have no relationship to smoke exposure.[95] Compared with typical carcinoids, atypical carcinoids are larger and have a higher rate of metastases, and survival of patients with this type of tumor is significantly reduced.[99] The 5-year survival rates for metastatic typical and atypical carcinoids are approximately 90% and 60%, respectively; rates are higher for resectable tumors.[99]

Carcinoids are located centrally and peripherally in the lung.[100] When the tumor is centrally located, it commonly shows bronchial involvement, has a sessile and pedunculated shape, and often fills the bronchial lumen. An endobronchial component is found more frequently in typical than in atypical carcinoids. For staging, the current edition of the TNM classification is used. As with other types of lung cancer, tumor spread through lymphatics or the bloodstream may occur with metastasis in mediastinal lymph nodes, liver, and bones; as stated earlier, metastases are more common in atypical than in typical carcinoids.

Histologically, carcinoid tumors are characterized by an organoid growth pattern, uniform cytologic features, and immunohistochemical expression of neuroendocrine markers, such as chromogranin A, synaptophysin, and NCAM/CD56.[101] Recent molecular data support the notion that carcinoids are genetically and phenotypically independent neuroendocrine tumors and they are not early progenitors of high-grade neuroendocrine tumors, such as SCLC and LCNEC tumors.[102]

Typical carcinoids are characterized by growth patterns suggesting neuroendocrine differentiation (Fig. 17.10A). Several growth patterns and a variety of cell features have been described, including, among others, spindle, mucinous, and clear cells. The tumor cells are usually uniform in appearance with polygonal shape, finely granular nuclear chromatin, inconspicuous nucleoli, and scant to moderately abundant eosinophilic cytoplasm. In general, atypical carcinoids show the same histologic patterns as typical carcinoids. By definition, atypical carcinoids have 2 to 10 mitoses per 2 mm^2 and/or foci of necrosis (often punctuate), whereas typical carcinoids show fewer than 2 mitoses per 2 mm^2 and lack necrosis (Fig. 17.10B).[103] The findings may be focally distributed, so careful examination of a resected tumor is necessary for accurate diagnosis.

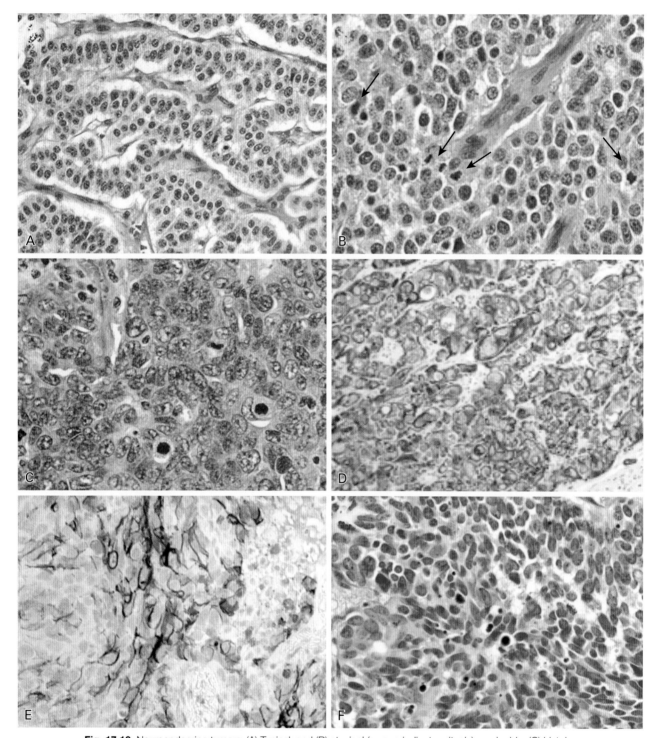

Fig. 17.10. Neuroendocrine tumors. (A) Typical, and (B) atypical (arrows indicate mitosis) carcinoids; (C) histology of large cell neuroendocrine carcinoma; (D) immunohistochemical expression of cytoplasmic chromogranin A; (E) membranous NCAM/CD56; and (F) histology of SCLC. (A–C and F, H&E.)

Although no immunohistochemical marker is available to subtype carcinoids, the finding of a low Ki-67 (approximately 10–20%) labeling index is valuable in small biopsy or cytology samples, particularly with crush artifact, to avoid misdiagnosing carcinoid tumors as high-grade neuroendocrine carcinomas.[104] However, the role of Ki-67 in discriminating between typical and atypical carcinoids has not been completely validated.[105]

Immunohistochemistry of Carcinoid Tumors

Immunohistochemical staining may be required to confirm neuroendocrine and epithelial differentiation, especially in small biopsy or cytology samples. An antibody panel approach including chromogranin A and synaptophysin (both with cytoplasmic expression) is recommended. NCAM/CD56 is mostly expressed in the cell membrane.[101,103] Most carcinoids are also reactive for low-molecular-weight cytokeratins, with negative cases mostly limited to a few peripheral tumors.[106] Pulmonary carcinoids may express several types of polypeptides such as calcitonin, gastrin-related peptide/bombesin, and adrenocorticotropic hormone similar to neuroendocrine tumors of the digestive tract.

Large Cell Neuroendocrine Carcinoma

LCNEC is a malignant epithelial tumor composed of large cells showing histologic features of neuroendocrine differentiation and immunohistochemical expression of neuroendocrine markers. In the 2004 WHO classification of lung tumors, LCNEC was considered a variant of large cell carcinoma.[6] However, the new 2015 WHO classification indicates that it should be categorized as a neuroendocrine carcinoma.[5]

Clinically, LCNEC is considered to be a high-grade neuroendocrine tumor. This tumor is commonly located in the periphery of the lung, but a central location occurs in approximately 20% of cases.[107] LCNEC harbors the potential to spread to many sites, mainly the thoracic lymph nodes, contralateral lung, liver, brain, and bones. Staging is similar to that of other NSCLCs. The tumor often invades the pleura, chest wall, and adjacent structures.[107]

Histologically, LCNEC shows neuroendocrine histologic patterns and is composed of large cells with moderate to abundant cytoplasm and often prominent nucleoli (Fig. 17.10C). Mitotic counts should be greater than 10 (average of 75) per 2 mm^2, and the count is rarely less than 30 per 2 mm^2. The Ki-67 proliferation index ranges from 40% to 80%. Necrosis usually consists of large zones, but it may be punctate. Rarely, these tumors look like atypical carcinoid, but if the mitotic rate exceeds 10 per 2 mm^2 they are classified as LCNEC. The diagnosis is difficult in small biopsy specimens unless all morphologic and immunohistochemical criteria are met; in this setting, the suggested diagnosis is NSCLC, suspect LCNEC.[108]

The neuroendocrine differentiation separates LCNEC from poorly differentiated NSCLC.[108] However, about 10% to 20% of typical lung squamous cell carcinomas, adenocarcinomas, and large cell carcinomas demonstrate neuroendocrine differentiation upon immunohistochemistry and/or electron microscopy analysis. These tumors are referred to as NSCLC with neuroendocrine differentiation on small biopsy specimens, or the specific subtype of NSCLC with neuroendocrine phenotype on resection samples. The clinical implications of this tumor category for response to therapy or survival are still unclear, so these subtypes are not here recognized as specific entities.

A LCNEC associated with components of adenocarcinoma, squamous cell carcinoma, and sarcomatoid carcinoma features is categorized as combined LCNEC. Combinations with SCLC also occur, but such tumors are classified as combined SCLC.

Immunohistochemistry of LCNEC

The diagnosis of LCNEC requires immunohistochemistry for confirmation of neuroendocrine differentiation.[109] In decreasing order of frequency, NCAM/CD56 stains 92% to 100% of LCNEC cases, followed by chromogranin A in 80% to 85%, and synaptophysin in 50% to 60% (Fig. 17.10 D–E).[110] Chromogranin A and synaptophysin are the most reliable stains for diagnostic accuracy in separating LCNEC from nonneuroendocrine tumors, and one positive marker is enough if the staining is clear.[110,111] About half of LCNEC tumors express TTF-1, a figure that is generally lower than that of SCLC,[49,110–112] but all LCNECs demonstrate reactivity to low-molecular-weight cytokeratin or CK7.[110] More than 70% of LCNEC also express CD117 (KIT protein) immunoreactivity,[113,114] which may be associated with reduced survival and increased recurrence rate.[114]

Small Cell Lung Cancer

SCLC is commonly located centrally in the major airways but may occur peripherally in the lungs in about 5% of cases. SCLCs are typically situated in a peribronchial location with infiltration of the bronchial submucosa and peribronchial tissue.[115] The tumors are large masses with extensive necrosis. SCLC can present as a solitary pulmonary nodule in less than 5% of cases.[116] Extensive lymph node metastases are common.[117] Staging is based on the TNM classification, which parallels the anatomic extent of the disease. The tendency toward widespread dissemination at presentation has sometimes led to the staging of SCLCs as limited or extensive disease rather than using the TNM system. However, the TNM classification is preferred because it separates different prognostic groups lumped together as limited disease.

On histologic examination, SCLC is characterized by small epithelial tumor cells with scant cytoplasm, round nuclei with finely granular chromatin, and absent or inconspicuous nucleoli (Fig. 17.10F).[115] Single cell necrosis is frequent and extensive, and the mitotic count is high (usually more than 10 per 2 mm^2). Although no precise upper limit of size has been specified for a cell to be defined as a small cell, it has been suggested that cells should measure approximately the diameter of two or three small mature lymphocytes.[118] In some areas, the histology is that of spindle cell with oval nucleoli. The diagnosis of SCLC is often more evident on cytology specimens than in biopsy specimens. Small biopsy samples are characterized by crush artifact and few viable cells. In larger specimens, the cell size may be larger with more abundant cytoplasm and scant pleomorphic malignant cells. Fewer than 10% of SCLCs demonstrate a mixture of other histologic types, usually adenocarcinoma, squamous cell carcinoma, large cell carcinoma, LCNEC, and, less commonly, spindle cell carcinoma or giant cell carcinoma; these tumors are referred to as combined SCLCs.[115,119] Interestingly, SCLC differentiation has been detected in tumors with acquired resistant to EGFR tyrosine kinase inhibitors therapy, and that before therapy exhibited adenocarcinoma histology and harbored an EGFR TKI sensitizing mutation.[120]

The diagnosis of SCLC is usually based on routine histologic and cytologic features; however, immunohistochemistry may be required to confirm the neuroendocrine nature of the tumor cells. Immunohistochemical expression of neuroendocrine markers, including NCAM/CD56, chromogranin A, and synaptophysin, is regularly present in SCLCs;[118,121] however, less than 10% of SCLCs are negative or focally positive for neuroendocrine markers, probably because of the lack of overt neuroendocrine differentiation.

In small biopsy specimens, the differential diagnosis of SCLC includes LCNEC, typical and atypical carcinoids, lymphoid infiltrates, the Ewing sarcoma family of tumors, and metastatic carcinomas. If examination shows marked expression of a neuroendocrine marker or a high proliferation index determined by Ki-67 immunohistochemical expression, the possibility of a lower-grade neuroendocrine carcinoma as an alternative for SCLC should be carefully excluded.[104]

Immunohistochemistry of SCLC

As stated earlier, SCLC can be diagnosed reliably on routine histologic and cytologic preparations, but immunohistochemistry may be required to confirm the neuroendocrine nature of the tumor cells. Broad reactivity to cytokeratin antibody mixtures is detected in essentially all cases of SCLC.[118] The high-molecular-weight cytokeratin cocktail (clone 34ßE12, recognizing types 1, 5, 10, and 14) is always negative in pure SCLC.[122] A panel of neuroendocrine markers is useful, including NCAM/CD56 (mostly decorating cell membrane),[101] chromogranin A, and synaptophysin (both with cytoplasmic labeling), which are regularly expressed in SCLC.[118,123] NCAM/CD56 is the most sensitive marker, but it is also less specific and should be interpreted in the appropriate morphologic context. Although synaptophysin and NCAM/CD56 stain SCLC diffusely and strongly, chromogranin A staining can be more focal and weak. Less than 10% of SCLCs, however, are completely unreactive or only very focally stainable for neuroendocrine markers, probably because of a lack of overt neuroendocrine differentiation or artifacts of preservation.[124] SCLC is also positive for TTF-1 in up to 75% to 85% of cases,[111] especially when using the less specific clone SPT24,[125,126] whereas napsin A, a marker of adenocarcinoma differentiation, is consistently unreactive. Markers of squamous cell carcinoma such as p63 may be found in pure forms of SCLC, raising concerns about the differential diagnosis, whereas p40 is negative.[53] More than 60% of SCLCs express CD11 also in a phosphorylated form.[127] Whenever possible, particularly in small biopsy specimens, the proliferation activity of SCLC as assessed by Ki-67 antigen immunostaining can be useful to avoid misdiagnosing carcinoid tumors in the presence of crush artifact. In SCLC, Ki-67 ranges from 64.5% to 77.5% and may reach 100%.[105]

OTHER UNCLASSIFIED TUMORS

Lymphoepithelioma-Like Carcinoma

Lymphoepithelioma-like carcinoma (LELC) is a rare type of lung carcinoma characterized by a poorly differentiated morphology admixed with marked lymphocyte infiltration and expression of Epstein-Barr virus in the nuclei of the neoplastic cells.[5] The tumors are usually solitary, circumscribed, and round to ovoid. LELCs are usually located in the peripheral lung. On histologic examination, the tumor has anastomosing smooth-contoured borders with irregular islands or diffuse sheets of cells. Focal squamous differentiation can occur. The accompanying lymphoid infiltration contains a mixture of CD3-positive T cells and CD20-positive B cells. Sometimes, Epstein-Barr virus is detected in the tumor nuclei. The tumor cells are usually positive for cytokeratin cocktails (AE1/AE3), CK5/6, p40, p63 and the B-cell lymphoma-2 (Bcl-2) marker, which suggests that LELC has squamous differentiation. No specific genetic abnormalities of LELC have been reported.

NUT Carcinoma

This uncommon tumor is usually referred to as nuclear protein in testis (NUT) midline carcinoma. This tumor occurs mainly in the sinonasal region and the upper respiratory or digestive tract. The hallmark of this carcinoma is a specific translocation between the NUT gene (NUT1) on chromosome 15q14 (100%) and other genes, including BRD4 on chromosome 19p13.1 (70%), BRD3 on chromosome 9q34.2 (6%), or unknown partner genes (22%). Histologically, NUT carcinoma is an undifferentiated carcinoma and sometimes contains foci of squamous differentiation. On immunohistochemical analysis, NUT carcinoma shows speckled nuclear positivity for NUT protein in more than 50% of the tumor cells, as demonstrated using a highly specific monoclonal anti-NUT antibody.[5]

SALIVARY GLAND–TYPE TUMORS

Because the upper respiratory tract is related to the oral cavity, salivary gland–type tumors can sometimes occur in the lung. These tumors are divided into four subtypes: mucoepidermoid carcinoma, adenoid cystic carcinoma, epithelial–myoepithelial carcinoma, and pleomorphic adenoma. These tumors arise from, or differentiate to, bronchial glands. Their clinicopathologic and immunohistochemical characteristics are similar to those of tumors arising from the salivary gland.

USE OF IMMUNOHISTOCHEMISTRY FOR LUNG CANCER DIAGNOSIS

One of the major new proposals in the IASLC/ATS/ERS classification is the development of standardized criteria and terminology for the pathologic diagnosis of lung cancer in small biopsy and cytology specimens (Table 17.3).[7,128] In addition to the criteria and terminology, the new classification creates two paradigm shifts for pathologists in terms of tumor classification and management of specimens. The first is the need to perform immunohistochemistry to further classify tumors formerly diagnosed as NSCLC-NOS. Because the distinction between histologic types of lung cancer, particularly adenocarcinoma and squamous cell carcinoma, is so important, the new classification recommends that pathologists use special stains to try to further subtype carcinomas that are difficult to classify by light microscopic evaluation of hematoxylin and eosin (H&E) sections alone. These advances have now made it essential for pathologists to make every effort to identify a specific histologic type for tumors formerly classified as NSCLC.

With all the new therapeutic targets recognized during the past decade, an urgent need arose to create a classification for nonresection specimens, in particular small biopsy and cytology samples. Furthermore, therapeutic targets are increasingly being recognized outside of adenocarcinoma, so that a firm diagnosis of squamous cell carcinoma may become just as important. Accordingly, tissue samples are no longer used just for diagnosis, but also for immunohistochemical staining and molecular testing (Fig. 17.11). This methodology is particularly important for small biopsy and cytology specimens because approximately 70% of lung cancers are unresectable, with presentation at an advanced stage, and targeted therapies that require molecular testing are mostly applied to patients with advanced NSCLC. Therefore, strategic tissue management is crucial for ancillary analyses, as well as histologic diagnosis.[129] Although there are many different approaches to manage these small specimens that vary greatly depending between laboratories, a minimum consensus for good clinical practice of small biopsies and cytology preparations is provided, based on multidisciplinary consensus (Table 17.3).[7] However, the guidelines emphasize that ancillary techniques are not always necessary. Many studies have reported that adenocarcinoma or squamous cell carcinoma can be diagnosed with biopsy or cytology specimens in 50% to 70% of patients based on morphology alone. Nevertheless, the application of immunohistochemistry refines the diagnosis so that the designation of NSCLC-NOS can be avoided in up to 90% of cases.[54,130] Indeed, the guidelines strongly recommend that the term NSCLC-NOS be used as little as possible, and only when a more specific diagnosis is not possible by morphology and/or special stains.[7,9]

Not all laboratories worldwide will have access to immunohistochemistry, or even a mucin stain, but the current classification must encompass scientific advances wherever relevant. Accepted markers for identifying differentiation toward adenocarcinoma are TTF-1[53,74,130] and napsin A,[131,132] both of which are approximately 80% sensitive. In relation to squamous differentiation, the markers CK5/6 and p63 have been advocated as both sensitive and specific,[49,130,131] although data from 2012 have suggested that p63 is less specific than first thought and the p63 isoform p40 has been reported as a more specific antibody in this setting.[53,73,74,133] Expression of p63 can occur in up to one-third of adenocarcinomas.[49,130,134] Therefore, among tumors that lack squamous cell morphology, virtually all tumors that show coexpression of p63 and TTF-1 are preferably classified as adenocarcinomas. Some investigators have also used CK7 as a marker of adenocarcinoma differentiation although this marker is not universally accepted.[134] Less commonly used markers for squamous differentiation include desmocollin-3 and desmoglein.[135,136] A reasonable recommendation is that, when immunohistochemistry is deemed

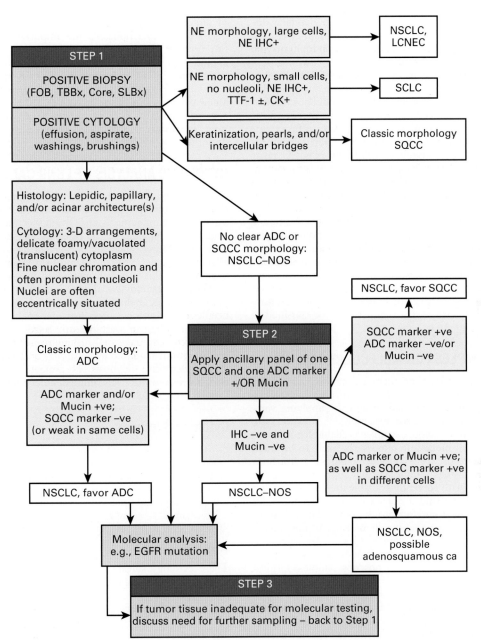

Fig. 17.11. Algorithm for the diagnosis of adenocarcinoma in small biopsy and/or cytology specimens. Step 1: When positive biopsy specimens (fiberoptic bronchoscopy [*FOB*], transbronchial [*TBBx*], core, or surgical lung biopsy [*SLBx*]) or cytology specimens (effusion, aspirate, washings, and brushings) show clear adenocarcinoma (*ADC*) or squamous cell carcinoma (*SQCC*) morphology, the diagnosis can be firmly established. If neuroendocrine morphology is detected, the tumor may be classified as small cell lung cancer (*SCLC*) or nonsmall cell lung cancer (*NSCLC*), probably large cell neuroendocrine carcinoma (LCNEC), according to standard criteria (+ve = positive; –ve = negative). If ADC or SQCC morphology is not clear, the tumor is regarded as NSCLC-not otherwise specified (*NOS*). Step 2: NSCLC-NOS can be further classified based on immunohistochemical stains, mucin stains (diastase–periodic acid Schiff [*DPAS*] or mucicarmine), or molecular data. If the stains all favor ADC with positive ADC marker(s) (i.e., positive for thyroid transcription factor-1 [*TTF-1*] and/or mucin) with negative SQCC markers, then the tumor is classified as NSCLC, favor ADC. If SQCC markers (i.e., p63 and/or CK5/6) are positive with negative ADC markers, the tumor is classified as NSCLC, favor SQCC. If the ADC and SQCC markers are both strongly positive in different populations of tumor cells, the tumor is classified as NSCLC-NOS, with a comment that it may represent adenosquamous carcinoma. If all markers are negative, the tumor is classified as NSCLC-NOS. See text for recommendations on NSCLCs with marked pleomorphic and overlapping ADC/SQCC morphology. †Mutation testing for epidermal growth factor receptor (*EGFR*) should be performed in classic ADC; NSCLC, favor ADC; NSCLC-NOS; and NSCLC-NOS, possible adenosquamous carcinoma. Step 3: If clinical management requires a more specific diagnosis than NSCLC-NOS, additional biopsies may be indicated. *IHC,* immunohistochemistry; *NE,* neuroendocrine; *CD,* cluster designation; *CK,* cytokeratin. (*Reprinted with permission from: Travis WD, Brambilla E, Noguchi M, et al. International Association for the Study of Lung Cancer/American Thoracic Society/European Respiratory Society international multidisciplinary classification of lung adenocarcinoma. J Thorac Oncol. 2011;6(2):244–285.*)

necessary, at least one antibody for squamous and glandular differentiation, but no more than two antibodies, should be used in each case.[131,134] Thus, a simple panel of TTF-1 and p40 may be able to classify most cases of NSCLC-NOS.

In small biopsy specimens, tumors that are positive for an adenocarcinoma marker (e.g., TTF-1) and/or mucin and are negative for a squamous marker (e.g., p40 or p63) should be classified as NSCLC, favor adenocarcinoma. Those tumors that are positive for a squamous marker, with at least moderate, diffuse staining, and negative for an adenocarcinoma immunohistochemistry marker and/or mucin stain, should be classified as NSCLC, favor nonkeratinizing squamous cell carcinoma, with a comment in the pathology report specifying whether the differentiation was detected by light microscopy and/or by special stains. These two markers, TTF-1 and p40, are generally mutually exclusive. If an adenocarcinoma marker such as TTF-1 is positive, the tumor should be classified as NSCLC, favor adenocarcinoma, despite any expression of squamous markers. If one population of tumor cells is reactive for TTF-1 and another population is positive for squamous markers, this may raise the possibility of adenosquamous carcinoma, although this diagnosis can be made only on a resection specimen. If no clear staining is found for adenocarcinoma or squamous markers, the tumor should be classified as NSCLC-NOS.

PATHOLOGY SAMPLES FOR MOLECULAR TESTING

The recent advances in targeted therapy for NSCLC require the analysis of a panel of molecular abnormalities, including gene mutations, amplifications, and fusions, by applying various methodologies to tumor tissue specimens.[137] However, the tissue (biopsy) and cell (cytology) samples available for molecular testing in advanced metastatic tumors are likely to be small specimens, including those from core-needle biopsy and/or fine-needle aspiration, and small sample size may limit the molecular and genomic analysis with currently available methodologies and technologies. The current and the newly emerging technologies must be adapted and incorporated into the molecular analysis of small tissue specimens from core-needle biopsy and fine-needle aspiration obtained from patients with NSCLC.

In pathology laboratories, the diagnostic tumor tissue specimens (e.g., core-needle biopsy, bronchoscopy samples, surgical resections, etc.) are fixed in formalin and embedded in paraffin for histologic processing. Both formalin fixation and paraffin embedding compromise the integrity of proteins and nucleic acids (RNA, DNA) for molecular testing, particularly when non-buffered formalin is used and the specimens are fixed in formalin for more than 24 hours. The cytology specimens (e.g., sputum, bronchial brushes, bronchoalveolar lavages, pleural fluids, and fine-needle aspiration) are usually fixed in alcohol, which is optimal for preservation of nucleic acids. When the cytology specimen has abundant material, the sample can be fixed in formalin and processed as a tissue specimen (cell block) to obtain histologic sections.[68] Although tissue specimens are preferable for molecular testing, most cytology samples with abundant malignant cells can be successfully used for molecular testing.

The handling of the biopsy and cytology specimens for histologic analysis and subsequent molecular testing requires thoughtful prioritization of sample use to prevent the loss of tissue in less important analysis when molecular testing is required for selection of therapy. Also, the pathologist should determine whether the amount of malignant cells available in the specimen is adequate for extraction of DNA and also for molecular tests based on histologic sections (e.g., fluorescence in situ hybridization and immunohistochemistry) (Fig. 17.11).

On the other hand, our growing understanding of the biology of NSCLC, particularly the molecular evolution of tumors during local progression and metastasis, and the identification of molecular abnormalities developing after resistance to targeted therapies emphasize the importance of characterizing the molecular abnormalities of the disease at every stage of its evolution. Tumor sampling and molecular testing of advanced metastatic NSCLC are important at each time point of clinical decision making.[138,139] Therefore, it is recommended to obtain a new tissue specimen for molecular testing in lung tumors that acquired resistance to a given targeted therapy to better determine the molecular resistance mechanisms and next therapy options.

CYTOLOGIC ANALYSIS OF LUNG CANCER

Cytology is a useful tool for diagnosis of lung cancer. The use of cytologic sampling approaches in lung cancer includes: (1) screening for lung carcinoma using sputum specimens; (2) presumptive diagnosis of lung cancer by brushing or scraping cytology; (3) diagnosis of lung cancer by fine-needle aspiration cytology; and (4) intraoperative cytologic diagnosis using the resected end of a bronchus or the resection margin in lung parenchyma.[94,140,142] Materials for cytologic diagnosis include sputum smears; smears prepared by bronchial scraping, brushing, or washing; fine-needle aspiration via a bronchoscope or through the chest wall; and pleural fluid or washing samples.[143–145,146,147–149] Materials obtained by curettage or brushing are usually scanty and must be fixed immediately to avoid drying artifacts, which may result in a false-positive diagnosis. To evaluate the surgical margin of wedge-resected materials, immediate cytologic diagnosis is performed using touch smears.

Cytologic Methods

Sputum Smears

Sputum cytology is a routine examination and/or screening method for detection of central-type lung carcinomas (squamous cell carcinoma and small cell carcinoma).

Smears Prepared by Bronchial Scraping, Brushing, or Washing

These cytology smears are obtained using bronchoscopy. For washing cytology, the lesion is washed with 20–40 mL of saline.[150]

Fine-Needle Aspiration Samples

Transbronchial lung biopsy or transcutaneous fine-needle aspiration cytology are two basic methods for collecting cytology samples from a tumor located in the periphery of the lung. Transcutaneous needle aspiration cytology is usually supported by CT examination.[151]

Pleural Fluid or Washing Materials

Normally, the pleural space contains little fluid, but exudative fluid may accumulate when lung cancer irritates the visceral pleural membrane.[152] Malignant pleural fluid that contains lung cancer cells may be detected by chest x-ray when the amount exceeds 200–300 mL. Pleural fluid is usually collected by percutaneous thoracocentesis.

Liquid-Based Cytology

This is a thin-layer or monolayer technique for slide preparation that has been introduced as a potential solution for improving the sensitivity and specificity of cytologic assessment.[153,154] Liquid-based cytology has gained favor over conventional smear and cytospin techniques and has been shown to yield equivalent or better diagnostic accuracy, particularly in specimens containing abundant mucus and/or blood. Liquid-based cytology is also more suitable for immunocytochemistry and for further investigations such as molecular analysis.

Special Staining and Immunocytochemistry of Cytology Specimens

After collection, the cytology slides should be fixed immediately in 95% ethyl alcohol for Papanicolaou staining, and the remaining slides should be air-dried and fixed in 100% methanol for May-Giemsa staining. For immunocytochemistry, the slides should be fixed in 15% formalin. The clinical applications of immunocytochemistry have been expanding because of the increasing need for differential diagnosis between squamous cell carcinoma and adenocarcinoma.[155] If the tumor is poorly differentiated, it is sometimes difficult to differentiate each histologic subtype by Papanicolaou staining. In those cases, staining for TTF-1 and p40 is very useful for establishing tumor differentiation and proper diagnosis.[156–158] However, cytologists should estimate antigenicity for TTF-1 carefully, because it is delicate and easily lost during long storage periods of the cytology smears. Cell blocks prepared from cytology specimens are useful tools for immunohistochemical analysis.

Molecular Analysis of Cytology Specimens

Cytologic specimens are very useful for DNA analysis, because they are fixed with alcohol or by dehydration.[159] Nucleic acids are well preserved in alcohol, in comparison with formalin. Therefore, pathologists should be encouraged to prepare a cell block for molecular testing.[160–162]

Cytologic Characteristics of Each Histologic Type of Lung Cancer

Because histologic heterogeneity is one of the characteristics of lung carcinoma, each specific histologic subtype shows specific cytologic features. The cytologic characteristics of several typical subtypes are introduced in the following text.

Adenocarcinoma

In addition to the histologic heterogeneity of lung adenocarcinoma, the cytologic features of these tumors are highly variable. The usual mixed type of adenocarcinoma shows an accumulated mass of tumor cells (Fig. 17.12A). The nuclei tend to be located in the periphery of the cytoplasm and to have vesicular chromatin with prominent nucleoli. The cytoplasm is usually finely vacuolated, and cytoplasmic mucin may be present. The glandular morphology may be detected as various arrangements of cells in organized units, including columnar cells lining up as so-called "pegshaped" cells arranged like a flat honeycomb, and cells organized as three-dimensional cell balls or branching groups with a smooth luminal border ("community border"). Poorly differentiated adenocarcinomas have nondescript overtly malignant cells, usually in cohesive groups, which may be impossible to distinguish from nonkeratinizing squamous cell carcinoma in the absence of ancillary studies such as immunocytochemistry.

AAH is unlikely to be sampled by cytologic techniques, but materials resected from stumps show cytomorphologic features similar to those of AIS with less nuclear atypia.[163] In nonmucinous AIS, the tumor cells are arranged in a flat monolayer. The nuclei include fine chromatin, inconspicuous pinpoint nucleoli, nuclear grooves, and nuclear pseudoinclusions. A specific diagnosis of AIS cannot be made from cytologic specimens because the possibility of an invasive component not present in the sample cannot be excluded.

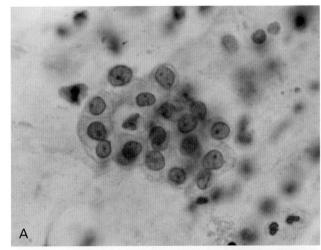

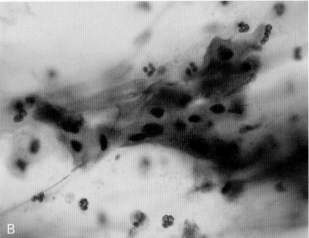

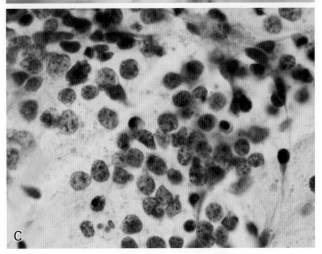

Fig. 17.12. Cytology of lung cancer. (A) Adenocarcinoma showing tumor cell cluster with tubular formation and cells with conspicuous nucleoli; (B) squamous cell carcinoma with atypical keratotic cell clusters; and (C) SCLC showing carcinoma cells with very high nuclear-to-cytoplasmic ratio and finely stippled chromatin. (A–C, sputum, Papanicolaou stain, ×1000.)

It is not possible to differentiate MIA from AIS cytologically because invasive tumor cells may not be included in the sample. Although no studies are available on the cytologic features of MIA, one would expect a mixture of frankly invasive carcinoma and AIS. If the tumor is located in the periphery and shows pure ground-glass opacity, and accumulated high-grade tumor cells are detected, then MIA may be included in the differential diagnosis.

Squamous Cell Carcinoma

The cytologic features of pulmonary squamous cell carcinoma are similar to those of squamous cell carcinoma at other sites and depend on the grade of the tumor. Well-differentiated squamous cell carcinomas show obvious keratinization, manifested as dense retractile cytoplasm showing red, orange, yellow, or light blue Papanicolaou staining (Fig. 17.12B). Unlike squamous cell carcinomas of the head and neck, pulmonary squamous tumors develop from metaplastic cells, and in most cases evidence of cytoplasmic keratinization is only focal. Typical nuclei of well-differentiated squamous cell carcinomas have dark nontransparent chromatin without obvious nuclear detail or prominent nucleoli. Spindle cell shapes are common. Necrosis and an inflammatory reaction are also common. Cells are usually present both singly and in large multilayered sheets. Poorly differentiated squamous cell carcinoma is difficult to differentiate from poorly differentiated adenocarcinoma because cytoplasmic keratinization is absent or unapparent, and the nuclei may have open chromatin with prominent nucleoli. In such cases, immunocytochemistry is sometimes effective for differentiating adenocarcinoma.

Cells derived from the precursor lesions of squamous cell carcinoma are much more likely to appear in exfoliative specimens than in aspiration biopsy samples.[169] The degree of dysplasia of cells in sputum specimens ranges from mild to severe according to the degree of cytocohesiveness, thickness of the cytoplasm, nucleus-to-cytoplasm ratio, roundness of the nucleus, and the pattern and distribution of chromatin. As the severity of dysplasia increases, the enlarged nuclei have more irregularities in the membrane contour, more darkly stained chromatin, and more coarsely granular and irregularly distributed chromatin granules or a homogeneous (pyknotic) appearance. Cytoplasmic keratinization may be present, especially in more severe lesions, and associated Papanicolaou staining has a brilliant, dense orange hue. The nuclear-to-cytoplasmic ratio also increases progressively. The dysplastic cells in scraped material are usually larger than those in sputum smears. The chromatin pattern is smoother and more finely granular than in sputum specimens because of the better degree of preservation.

Small Cell Lung Cancer

The cytologic characteristics of small cell carcinoma are very specific and pathognomonic. The individual tumor cells are small with round, oval, or spindle-shaped nuclei in which the chromatin is uniformly and finely divided and the nucleoli are not prominent, although chromocenters are sometimes visible (Fig. 17.12C). The accepted nuclear diameter is usually no greater than three lymphocytes. The nucleus-to-cytoplasm ratio is very high and the cytoplasm surrounding the nuclei is very scanty; nuclear molding is prominent. Chromatin streaking is a very specific feature of small cell carcinoma. Mitotic figures are not as common as might be expected.

CONCLUSION

A clinically relevant pathologic classification of lung cancer is essential for accurate diagnosis and for patients to receive appropriate therapy. Although classification of the vast majority of lung cancers is straightforward, areas of controversy and diagnostic challenges remain. Pathologists play a critical role in lung cancer therapy by providing a precise pathologic diagnosis and by properly handling tissue and cytology samples for molecular testing of lung cancer. The 2011 IASLC/ATS/ERS revised lung adenocarcinoma classification and the recently released 2015 WHO classification of lung cancers are applicable to surgically resected as well as small biopsy and cytologic specimens,[5] and they address the new therapeutic challenges in treating this disease. The recently developed classification and approaches for lung cancer diagnosis are aligned with current clinical practice and open new avenues for research.

KEY REFERENCES

5. Travis WD, Brambilla E, Burke AP, Marx A, Nicholson AG. WHO classification of tumours of the lung, pleura, thymus and heart. *WHO Classification of Tumours*. Vol 7. Lyon, France: International Agency for Research on Cancer (IARC); 2015.
7. Travis WD, Brambilla E, Noguchi M, et al. International Association for the Study of Lung Cancer/American Thoracic Society/European Respiratory Society international multidisciplinary classification of lung adenocarcinoma. *J Thorac Oncol.* 2011;6(2):244–285.
11. Miyoshi T, Satoh Y, Okumura S, et al. Early-stage lung adenocarcinomas with a micropapillary pattern, a distinct pathologic marker for a significantly poor prognosis. *Am J Surg Pathol.* Jan 2003;27(1):101–109.
17. Russell PA, Wainer Z, Wright GM, Daniels M, Conron M, Williams RA. Does lung adenocarcinoma subtype predict patient survival? A clinicopathologic study based on the new International Association for the Study of Lung Cancer, American Thoracic Society, European Respiratory Society international multidisciplinary lung adenocarcinoma classification. *J Thorac Oncol.* 2011;6(9):1496–1504.
19. Warth A, Muley T, Meister M, et al. The novel histologic International Association for the Study of Lung Cancer, American Thoracic Society, European Respiratory Society classification system of lung adenocarcinoma is a stage-independent predictor of survival. *J Clin Oncol.* 2012;30(13):1438–1446.
23. Kerr KM. Pulmonary preinvasive neoplasia. *J Clin Pathol.* 2001;54:257–271.
29. Kadota K, Villena-Vargas J, Yoshizawa A, et al. Prognostic significance of adenocarcinoma in situ, minimally invasive adenocarcinoma, and nonmucinous lepidic predominant invasive adenocarcinoma of the lung in patients with stage I disease. *Am J Surg Pathol.* 2014;38(4):448–460.
31. Sterlacci W, Savic S, Schmid T, et al. Tissue-sparing application of the newly proposed IASLC/ATS/ERS classification of adenocarcinoma of the lung shows practical diagnostic and prognostic impact. *Am J Clin Pathol.* 2012;137(6):946–956.
49. Rekhtman N, Ang DC, Sima CS, Travis WD, Moreira AL. Immunohistochemical algorithm for differentiation of lung adenocarcinoma and squamous cell carcinoma based on large series of whole-tissue sections with validation in small specimens. *Mod Pathol.* 2011;24(10):1348–1359.
53. Pelosi G, Rossi G, Cavazza A, et al. DeltaNp63 (p40) distribution inside lung cancer: a driver biomarker approach to tumor characterization. *Int J Surg Pathol.* 2013;21(3):229–239.
63. Inamura K, Takeuchi K, Togashi Y, et al. EML4-ALK fusion is linked to histological characteristics in a subset of lung cancers. *J Thorac Oncol.* 2008;3(1):13–17.
64. Girard N, Ostrovnaya I, Lau C, et al. Genomic and mutational profiling to assess clonal relationships between multiple non-small cell lung cancers. *Clin Cancer Res.* 2009;15(16):5184–5190.
66. Rekhtman N, Brandt SM, Sigel CS, et al. Suitability of thoracic cytology for new therapeutic paradigms in non-small cell lung carcinoma: high accuracy of tumor subtyping and feasibility of EGFR and KRAS molecular testing. *J Thorac Oncol.* 2011;6(3):451–458.
90. Pelosi G, Sonzogni A, De Pas T, et al. Review article: pulmonary sarcomatoid carcinomas: a practical overview. *Int J Surg Pathol.* 2010;18(2):103–120.
103. Rekhtman N. Neuroendocrine tumors of the lung: an update. *Arch Pathol Lab Med.* 2010;134(11):1628–1638.
104. Pelosi G, Rodriguez J, Viale G, Rosai J. Typical and atypical pulmonary carcinoid tumor overdiagnosed as small-cell carcinoma on biopsy specimens: a major pitfall in the management of lung cancer patients. *Am J Surg Pathol.* 2005;29(2):179–187.
128. Hirsch FR, Wynes MW, Gandara DR, Bunn Jr PA. The tissue is the issue: personalized medicine for non-small cell lung cancer. *Clin Cancer Res.* 2010;16(20):4909–4911.

139. Kim ES, Herbst RS, Wistuba II, et al. The BATTLE trial: personalizing therapy for lung cancer. *Cancer Discovery*. 2011;1:44–53.

143. Kondo H, Asamura H, Suemasu K, et al. Prognostic significance of pleural lavage cytology immediately after thoracotomy in patients with lung cancer. *J Thorac Cardiovasc Surg*. 1993;106(6):1092–1097.

147. Truong LD, Underwood RD, Greenberg SD, McLarty JW. Diagnosis and typing of lung carcinomas by cytopathologic methods. A review of 108 cases. *Acta Cytol*. 1985;29(3):379–384.

155. Kimbrell HZ, Gustafson KS, Huang M, Ehya H. Subclassification of non-small cell lung cancer by cytologic sampling: a logical approach with selective use of immunocytochemistry. *Acta Cytol*. 2012;56(4):419–424.

162. Moreira AL, Hasanovic A. Molecular characterization by immunocytochemistry of lung adenocarcinoma on cytology specimens. *Acta Cytol*. 2012;56(6):603–610.

163. Dacic S. Pulmonary preneoplasia. *Arch Pathol Lab Med*. 2008;132(7): 1073–1078.

See Expertconsult.com for full list of references.

Molecular Testing in Lung Cancer

Celine Mascaux, Ming-Sound Tsao, and Fred R. Hirsch

SUMMARY OF KEY POINTS

- Of key importance is whether a prognostic marker is also a predictive marker for therapeutic benefit.

- As predictive biomarkers become integral in the use of targeted therapies to treat lung cancer, multidisciplinary and evidence-based guidelines for molecular testing are needed; the College of American Pathologists, the International Association for the Study of Lung Cancer, and the Association of Molecular Pathologists have published a multidisciplinary and evidence-based guideline for molecular testing in lung cancer.

- Immunohistochemistry (IHC) is considered to be an easy and inexpensive clinically applicable assay.

- The method for detecting mutations needs to take into account the tumor content available, the possibility of detecting all mutations, the timing required for testing, and the urgency to start the patient's treatment.

- Mutation testing should be performed on formalin-fixed paraffin-embedded, frozen, or alcohol-fixed tissue specimens.

- The advantage of IHC and fluorescence in situ hybridization is that the evaluation of the protein expression level or genomic aberration can be analyzed more specifically on individual tumor cells.

- The choice of the biomarkers to be tested must be based on evidence of their clinical relevance for therapeutic decision.

- Epidermal growth factor receptor (EGFR) testing should be done for any mutation located in exons 18 to 21 with over 1% prevalence.

- Currently, EGFR mutation is detected by classic molecular tests.

- In addition to EGFR, the other approved targetable biomarker used in the treatment of patients with advanced lung cancer is anaplastic lymphoma kinase (ALK) gene rearrangement, which should be done on the same patient population as tested for EGFR mutations.

- Aside from EGFR mutations and ALK rearrangements, several other biomarkers have also been tested for their ability to predict lung cancer response to treatment, but none have shown sufficient evidence for current use in clinical practice.

- Tests for EGFR mutations, ALK, and ROS gene rearrangements to predict response to EGFR tyrosine kinase inhibitors (TKIs) and ALK/ROS1 TKIs, respectively, are currently the only biomarker tests recommended in clinical practice.

Biomarker research in lung cancer aims to characterize prognostic factors and to determine predictive markers of benefit, usually in terms of response rate or outcome from local treatment (e.g., radiation) or systemic treatment (e.g., chemotherapy, targeted therapy, and immunotherapy). These biomarkers can be used to select the patient groups who will most likely derive differential benefit from the treatments and can help to avoid the toxicities associated with ineffective therapies. It is important to distinguish between prognosis and prediction.[1] Prognostic factors are patient- and tumor-related factors that predict patient outcome (usually survival) and are independent of treatment administered. Predictive factors are clinical, cellular, and molecular markers that predict response of the tumor to treatment (either in terms of tumor shrinkage or a survival benefit from treatment). Therefore prognostic factors define the effects of tumor characteristics on the patient, whereas predictive factors define the effect of treatment on the tumor. Those measures are not always similar, as tumor response may not necessarily translate into greater survival benefit.[2]

Many candidate prognostic biomarkers have been reported to be associated with earlier stages of nonsmall cell lung cancer (NSCLC) in patients who are treated primarily by surgical resection. However, it should be emphasized that not all prognostic classifiers that may predict survival will be associated with the benefit of adjuvant chemotherapy. For this reason, it is important to demonstrate if a prognostic marker is also a predictive marker for therapeutic benefit. In this chapter, we mainly focus on clinical recommendations for the use of molecular testing as predictive biomarkers for response and outcome to systemic therapy, as there has been strong evidence for implementation of routine molecular testing in standard clinical practice. We also discuss the research data on prognostic biomarkers.

GENETIC ABNORMALITIES IN LUNG CANCER

The epidermal growth factor receptor (EGFR) mutation is the first molecular abnormality in lung cancer that has been associated with marked sensitivity to a tyrosine kinase inhibitor (TKI) with specificity for the EGFR.[3] This discovery revolutionized the diagnosis and treatment of lung cancer and established the paradigm for subsequent research to identify oncogenic driver mutations that could represent additional targets for the treatment of lung cancer. Shortly after the discovery of *EGFR* mutations, gene rearrangement involving the *anaplastic lymphoma kinase* (*ALK*) was identified as a potent oncogene in NSCLC and has become a predictor of very high rates of response and good outcomes with crizotinib, which inhibits hepatocyte growth factor receptor and ALK.[4] By direct and next-generation high-throughput sequencing, other mutations have subsequently been identified in different histologic types of lung cancers. First in lung adenocarcinoma, Ding et al.[5] reported on a set of 26 genes with significant mutations selected on the basis of statistic models, including known tumor suppressor genes (tumor protein 53 [P53], serine/threonine kinase 11 [STK11], neurofibromatosis 1 [NF1], ataxia telangiectasia mutated [ATM], adenomatous polyposis coli [APC], cyclin-dependent kinase inhibitor [CDKN2A], retinoblastoma 1 [RB1], inhibin beta A [INHBA]); known oncogenes (Kirsten rat sarcoma [KRAS], neuroblastoma RAS viral (v-ras) oncogene homolog [NRAS]); putative oncogenic tyrosine kinase receptors (EGFR, v-erb-b2 avian erythroblastic leukemia viral oncogene homolog [ERBB] 4, fibroblast growth factor receptor 4 [FGFR4], ephrin (EPH) receptor A3 [EPHA3], EPH receptor A5 [EPHA5], neurotrophic tyrosine kinase, receptor, type 1], kinase insert domain receptor [KDR], neurotrophic tyrosine kinase, receptor, type 3 [NTRK3], platelet-derived growth factor receptor, alpha polypeptide [PDGFRA], leukocyte receptor tyrosine kinase [LTK], p21 protein [Cdc42/Rac]-activated kinase 3 [PAK3]); and other genes with undetermined roles (low-density lipoprotein receptor-related protein 1B [LRP1B], protein tyrosine phosphatase, receptor type, D [PTPRD], GNAS complex locus [GNAS], zinc finger, MYND-type containing 10 [ZMYND10/ BLU], and solute carrier family 38, member 3 [SLC38A3]). Other studies using DNA and RNA next-generation sequencing (NGS) reported additional potentially actionable oncogene driver mutations, including ERBB2; v-akt murine thymoma viral oncogene homolog 1 (AKT1); met proto-oncogene (MET); lemur tyrosine kinase 2 (LMTK2); catenin (cadherin-associated protein), beta 1, 88 kDa (CTNNB1); neurogenic locus notch homolog protein 2 (NOTCH2); SWI/SNF-related, matrix-associated, actin-dependent regulator of chromatin, subfamily a, member 4 (SMARCA4); kelch-like epoxycyclohexanone (ECH)-associated protein 1 (KEAP1), AT-rich interactive domain 1A (SWI-like; ARID1A); U2 small nuclear RNA auxiliary factor 1 (U2AF1); and RNA binding motif protein 10 (RBM10), as well as gene fusions, including c-ROS oncogene 1, receptor tyrosine kinase (ROS1), ret proto-oncogene (RET), fibroblast growth factor receptor 2 (FGFR2), AXL receptor tyrosine kinase (AXL), microtubule-associated protein 4 (MAP4/3K3); and platelet-derived growth factor receptor, beta polypeptide (PDGFR1).[6-10] More recently, putative targetable mutations/amplifications were identified in lung squamous cell carcinoma, including phosphatidylinositol-4,5-bisphosphate 3-kinase, catalytic subunit alpha (PI3KCA); phosphatase and tensin homolog (PTEN); AKT1–3; FGFR1–3; EGFR; ERBB2; v-raf murine sarcoma viral oncogene homolog B (BRAF); NOTCH; RAS; TP53; cyclin-dependent kinase inhibitor 2A (CDK2N2A [p16INK4A])/Rb; KEAP1; cullin 3 (CUL3); nuclear factor, erythroid 2-like 2 (NFE2L2); SRY (sex determining region Y)-box 2 (SOX2); tumor protein p63 (TP63); NOTCH1/2; achaete–scute family bHLH transcription factor 4 (ASCL4); and Forkhead box P1 (FOXP1).[11-14] Much less data are available in small cell lung cancer (SCLC) because of the rarity of resected specimens. However, gene amplification has been detected with the use of array-comparative genomic hybridization in Janus kinase 2 (JAK2), FGFR1; and SOX2; and cyclin E1 and MYC family members.[15] Gene mutations have also been reported in SCLC in TP53, RB, PTEN, slit homolog 2 (SLIT2), and EPH7, and in genes playing a role in epigenetic gene regulations as CREB-binding protein (CREBBP), E1A-binding protein p300 (EP300), and myeloid/lymphoid or mixed-lineage leukemia (MLL) genes.[16-18]

Because EGFR mutations and ALK rearrangement have been found to predict therapeutic benefit with their respective targeted drugs, biomarker testing has been implemented and integrated into therapeutic decision making for patients with advanced NSCLC. As predictive biomarkers are becoming integral in the use of targeted therapies to treat patients with lung cancer, there is a need to establish a multidisciplinary and evidence-based guideline for molecular testing. In 2013, the College of American Pathologists (CAP), the International Association for the Study of Lung Cancer (IASLC), and the Association of Molecular Pathologists (AMP) published such guidelines for molecular testing in lung cancer.[19] Following a systematic review of the literature and consensus meetings as well as public consultation, an expert panel developed 37 guideline items addressing 14 subjects and made 15 recommendations, ranging from tissue acquisition and processing to assay interpretations. Several other guidelines for biomarker testing have been published by other organizations, including the National Consensus of the Spanish Society of Medical Oncology, the Spanish Society of Pathology, and the European Society of Medical Oncology.[20,21] In addition, specific recommendations for EGFR testing have been published in the Canadian National Consensus Statement, and recommendations for ALK testing have been made by the Italian Association of Medical Oncology/Italian Society of Pathology and Cytopathology and other international groups of authors.[22-26]

ASSAY PLATFORMS IN MOLECULAR TESTING

Protein Expression

Immunohistochemistry (IHC) is most commonly used for protein expression assessment in the clinical context. IHC is a process that is easily performed by investigators because of the short time needed to complete testing and low cost, and due to its applicability to formalin-fixed paraffin-embedded (FFPE) rather than fresh frozen tissue. In addition, IHC may help investigators assess protein expression at the cellular level, thus allowing them to evaluate cellular localization (e.g., membranous, nuclear, or cytoplasmic), topography (e.g., tumor or stromal cells), and heterogeneity of expression and is also applicable to very small specimens, including cytologic samples. However, many preanalytic and analytic factors may influence IHC reactions, resulting in potentially variable staining that may affect the interpretation of the results. Therefore optimizing and standardizing the protocols and conditions are required for each marker tested. Interpreting the results is also observer dependent and may vary between observers, thus requiring standardization of protocols and conditions. Lastly, the scores for defining positive or negative IHC results for their prognostic or predictive value of specific biomarkers need to be well defined and validated in multiple independent cohorts/institutions and clinical trial samples. However, despite the mentioned limitations, IHC is considered to be an easy and inexpensive clinically applicable assay, which already is available in most pathology departments.

Gene Mutations

The technologies available for mutation analyses are associated with different sensitivity. Analytic sensitivity is defined as the lowest percentage of tumor cells or tumor cell DNA concentration in which a mutation is detectable with confidence within replicate assays.[19] The standard method for detecting mutations has been direct sequencing by the Sanger method. This method allows the detection of a minimum of 25% of mutated allele frequency from tissue containing 50% cancer cells cellularity, if the mutation is heterozygous and in the absence of gene amplification. However, mutated driver oncogenes, such as EGFR and KRAS, are commonly amplified implying that a lower number of tumor cellularity in the sample may yield 25% mutated alleles. Bidirectional sequencing and confirmation by repeat sequencing on independently amplified polymerase chain reaction (PCR) products should be performed especially on FFPE tissue (see later). The impact of the lower sensitivity of the Sanger sequencing method resulting in a substantial false-negative response rate (approximately 30%) in the detection of EGFR mutations has been documented.[27]

To overcome the generally lower sensitivity of the Sanger sequencing method, various technologies are available that allow mutation detection at significantly higher sensitivity with a tumor cellularity of as low as 1% to 5% or mutated allele. These more sensitive technologies involve a mutated allele-enriching strategy, including the peptide nucleic acid/locked nucleic acid amplification, the coamplification at lower denaturation temperature-PCR, or the enzymatic digestion of wild-type sequences.[19] The US Food and Drug Administration (FDA) has approved two assays for the detection of EGFR mutation analyses in advanced NSCLC: the Scorpion-amplification refractory mutation system (ARMS) and cobas technologies (Roche Molecular Diagnostics, Pleasanton, CA, USA). Several other methods may be used to detect EGFR mutations (Table 18.1). The Scorpion-ARMS technology is available as a commercial kit that allows investigators to test for 29 EGFR mutations and has a sensitivity of at least 5%. The cobas EGFR mutation test is a reverse transcription-PCR-based (RT-PCR) test for the qualitative detection of exon 19 deletion and exon 21 L858R mutations of EGFR in DNA

TABLE 18.1 Commonly Used Methods for EGFR Mutation Detection[30,31]

Method	Tumor DNA Required (%)	Targeted or Screening Method	EGFR Mutations Detected	Detection of Deletions and Insertions
Sanger direct sequencing	25	Screening	Known and new	Yes
Real time/TaqMan PCR	10	Targeted	Known only	No
High-resolution melting analysis	5–10	Screening	Known and new	Yes
Cobas	5–10	Targeted	Known only	Yes
Pyrosequencing	5–10	Screening	Known only	Yes
SNaPshot PCR	1–10	Targeted	Known only	Yes
MALDI-TOF MS-based genotyping	5	Targeted	Known only	No
Cycleave PCR	5	Targeted	Known only	Yes
Fragment length and RFLP analysis	5	Screening/targeted	Known only	Yes
Allelic-specific PCR/Scorpion ARMS	1	Targeted	Known only	No
MassARRAY	1	Targeted	Known only	Yes
PNA–LNA PCR clamp	1	Targeted	Known only	No
Denaturing HPLC	1	Screening	Known and new	Yes
Massively parallel/NGS	0.1	Screening	Known and new	Yes
Digital droplet PCR	0.01	Targeted	Known only	Yes

ARMS, amplification refractory mutation system; *EGFR*, epidermal growth factor receptor; *HPLC*, high-performance liquid chromatography; *MALDI-TOF*, matrix-assisted laser desorption/ionization time-of-flight; *MS*, mass spectrometry; *NGS*, next-generation sequencing; *PCR*, polymerase chain reaction; *PNA–LNA*, peptide nucleic acid-locked nucleic acid; *RFLP*, restriction fragment length polymorphism.

extracted from FFPE tissue and was used by the investigators in the European Randomized Trial of Tarceva versus Chemotherapy (EURTAC) and LUX-Lung 3 trials.[28,29]

Several other available assays are based on different technologies. Their sensitivities vary, and only certain techniques have the ability to detect new mutations and/or insertions and deletions. In contrast to the Sanger method that lacks sensitivity for samples with fewer tumor cells, the more sensitive methods might give rise to false-positive results and a lower specificity. Therefore it is crucial that the appropriate positive and negative controls always be included in the assay. Of note, the Sanger method detects any mutation including previously unidentified mutations in the sequenced exons, but other assays are designed for specific mutation testing, as in the case of the digital droplet PCR that has a very high sensitivity. Another option could be a two-step procedure, starting with a highly sensitive detection of the presence of a mutation and the subsequent characterization of the mutation. When finding a mutation that has not or has rarely been reported, the results should not be considered as errors until the replicate test confirms or denies it. However, testing all mutations can require more time and might not be suitable for the clinical situation when treatment must be initiated without delay. In such cases, another approach can be used that tests the most common mutations first and then completes the screening of less frequent mutation.

The recent and rapid development of NGS accomplishes massive parallel gene mutation analyses and discovery and requires a small amount of tissue, preferably fresh frozen. This technology uses miniaturized and parallelized platforms for sequencing of millions of short nucleotides (50–400 bases). The different platforms all have in common a technical paradigm of massively parallel sequencing via clonally amplified, spatially separated DNA templates or single DNA molecules in a flow cell. Currently, NGS is used for research purposes rather than to test specific biomarkers. However, with the expansion of the use of molecular biomarkers and the rapidly growing targeted therapies available, using NGS to have a full molecular profiling of the tumor or at least multiplex mutation testing of a panel of biomarkers of interest might become preferable in the future in order to spare time and tissue. In addition, in a recent study, even for individual gene mutation analyses, NGS has been shown to have better sensitivity, as it detected all relevant *EGFR* mutations for prediction of response to EGFR TKIs in 24 tumors, compared with the Sanger method and pyro-sequencing, which resulted in four and two false-negative results, respectively.[32]

Nevertheless, the clinician's chosen approach needs to take into account the tumor content available, the possibility of detecting all mutations, the timing required for testing, and the urgency to start the patient's treatment. Usually a laboratory investigator will decide to choose a specific method based on equipment availability and cost and will conduct an assay optimization and standardization exercise and test for assay sensitivity and specificity.[19,20]

Changes in Gene Structure and Copy Number

Fluorescence in situ hybridization (FISH) is the standard method for assessing changes in gene structure and copy number. Similar to IHC, FISH can be performed on FFPE tissue but requires standardized protocols (Fig. 18.1). Interpreting and reading FISH specimens is observer dependent and requires a dark room and a specific microscope, and the reader needs specific training and expertise in order to achieve reproducible results. Of note is that the tissue structure is not well visualized, and this factor necessitates the preselection of areas to assess in order to discriminate tumor cells from nonmalignant cells. Furthermore, the fluorescence probes are unstable and fade over a short period, which can limit the possibility of revisiting the specimens. Therefore imaging the specimens in a short time frame is important. By using probes against multiple targets labeled with different fluorescent dyes, it is possible to assess multiple markers on the same sections. In addition to detecting the gene copy number, FISH is used to assess structural changes including fusions between genes. The example of ALK fusion is detailed later in this chapter.

Several alternative techniques to FISH have been developed, including chromogenic in situ hybridization and silver in situ hybridization. These techniques are used primarily in research and give results comparable with FISH; however, they are not commonly used in routine clinical testing in lung cancer. Silver in situ hybridization is now FDA approved for human epidermal growth factor receptor-2 (HER2) determination in breast cancer and is widely used for that indication. Multicolor assays are in development. Finally, gene copy number can be assessed by array-comparative genomic hybridization technique. However, comparative genomic hybridization is used mainly to probe for a large number of markers in exploratory discovery research, rather than to assess specific markers for clinical applications.

Another assay that is used for assessing gene copy number is PCR, which is a very sensitive method that requires specific primers and probes as are used in gene rearrangement in the ALK gene.[33] More recently, computational algorithms have also been developed to derive gene copy number estimate using high coverage NGS data.

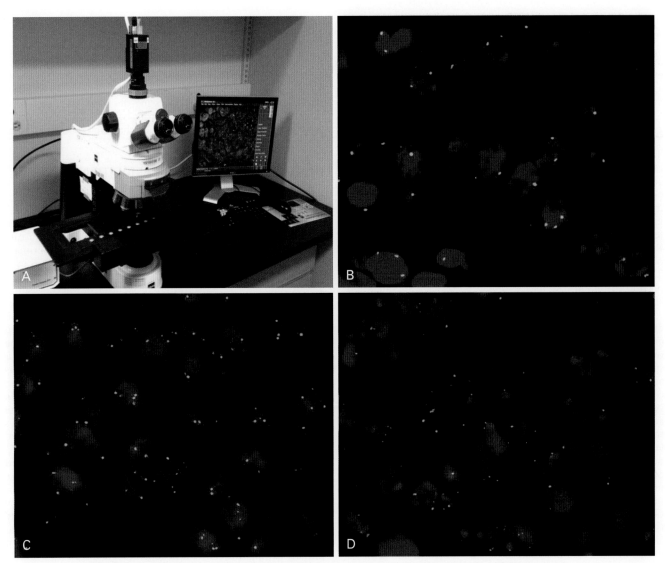

Fig. 18.1. Fluorescence in situ hybridization (FISH) to detect gene copy number changes. (A) FISH microscope. (B–D) Tumors that were hybridized to the EGFR (red signal) and chromosome 7 centromeric or CEP7 (green signal) probes, with cells showing two copies of each probe, consistent with disomy (B); high polysomy, as indicated by an increased number of green and red probes (C); or clusters of red probes, consistent with high amplification of the *epidermal growth factor receptor (EGFR)* gene.

TISSUE REQUIREMENTS FOR MOLECULAR TESTING

Preanalytic Factors

Based on expert consensus opinion mutation testing should be performed on FFPE, frozen, or alcohol-fixed tissue specimens.[19,20] The main advantage of using FFPE tissue is that it is the most commonly used method to process tissue for routine histology. FFPE also allows for a better evaluation of tumor cell content, which is also possible with fresh tissue, but is less convenient and requires cutting and staining of frozen sections adjacent to the section used for DNA extraction. The results of mutation testing with alcohol-fixed tissue specimens are also excellent. This fixation method is often used on cytologic specimens, which are then suitable for mutation testing. DNA isolated from fresh or frozen tissues may yield fragments of 1000 base pairs (bp) and longer. Fixation of tissue in formalin induces crosslinks between DNA, RNA and proteins, and DNA fragmentation that results in DNA fragments of 300 bp or less. Formalin fixation also creates random nucleotide base exchange, resulting in

false-positive results. This type of problem mostly occurs with low DNA yield and/or with ultrasensitive assays.[19] Tissue treated with acidic or heavy-metal fixatives, including lead, cobalt, chromium, silver, mercury, and sometimes even uranium and decalcifying solutions, may reduce the success rate of mutation testing and should be avoided when alternate FFPE specimens are available. In molecular biology, heavy-metal fixatives inhibit the DNA polymerases used in PCR testing. Acidic solutions, including the decalcifying solutions that are used to process samples obtained from bone metastasis, can induce a high rate of DNA fragmentation. For these types of specimens that are obtained specifically for molecular testing, nonacidic methods of decalcification, such as nonacidic chelating decalcifying solutions, should be used in the sample-processing step.

IHC and FISH should be performed on FFPE tissue, ideally on cut sections that have been stored for fewer than 6 weeks, to avoid the oxidation process that occurs over time. Whatever the method used, standardizing the fixation procedure and storage conditions is required. The fixation should be performed within hours after the sample has been obtained. Fixation duration should be controlled and not exceed 12 hours for small biopsy specimens and 18 hours to 24 hours for resected specimens.[19,20]

Data have shown that molecular testing (i.e., mutation testing or FISH) can be performed on liquid biopsies (circulating DNA extracted from plasma or circulating tumor cells).[34–38] These assays are still experimental and need to be reproduced and standardized before any clinical application.

Sample Processing and Analysis

Tumor tissue is heterogeneously composed of a mixture of tumor cells and host cells. Host cells include inflammatory cells and vascular endothelial and stromal fibroblasts and their abundance is highly variable but may have a substantial impact on the sensitivity of mutation testing (Fig. 18.2). The proportion of tumor cells in the specimen, as compared with normal tissue and inflammatory cells, may affect the result of the mutation analyses, mainly with less sensitive methods for mutation detection, as a low copy number of the DNA template generates artifacts in the results. To avoid false-negative results, specimens with a minimum proportion of tumor cells ideally should be selected for mutation analyses.[19]

Routinely, DNA is extracted from five to ten scratched unstained sections, depending on the size of tissue sample. However, in some cases, a very low amount of DNA is obtained. To overcome the low amount of DNA extracted from small tissue specimens, different techniques can be used. Whole-genome amplification has been developed and is used in research; however, this technique has not been implemented in clinical testing yet, as it may introduce bias. Performing the assay in duplicate, and ideally in triplicate, may ensure the accurate interpretation of the results, but these methods may not be practical in a clinical laboratory because of the lack of tissue and the time and labor needed to duplicate (or triplicate) testing. Different methods of tissue enrichment can be used for tissue with heterogeneity in areas with tumor cells, including gross macrodissection, coring areas with tumor cells out of an FFPE block, microdissection from the glass, flow sorting, or laser capture microdissection (LCM).[19,20] Macrodissection is used for clinical testing, but LCM is not routinely used because it is labor intensive and because the effects of a laser on mutation testing are unknown and must be evaluated. In addition, even if LCM produces a very pure sample of tumor cells, it also provides a very low DNA yield.

The advantage of IHC and FISH is that the evaluation of the protein expression level or genomic aberration can be analyzed more specifically on individual tumor cells. In IHC and FISH, cells are analyzed individually. Therefore the tumor cell's content is less crucial than for mutation testing. However, focusing the analysis on tumor-rich areas is important in FISH. Thus a corresponding hematoxylin and eosin (H&E)-stained section should be used to select areas for analysis. When using IHC, a larger sample size provides a better evaluation of the tumor heterogeneity and percentage of cells expressing the biomarker. However, obtaining larger samples is not easily controlled, as the sample size depends on the type of specimen that can be obtained from the tumor.[19]

SAMPLE AVAILABILITY AND PRIORITIZATION OF BIOMARKERS FOR TESTING

Three types of tissue samples can be used for molecular testing. A first approach is used for patients who originally presented with early-stage disease and had subsequent recurrence, a case in which large amounts of the initially resected archival primary tumor should be available for testing. A second approach is used for patients who presented with advanced-stage disease, for whom limited tissue in the form of bronchial, core-needle aspiration biopsy samples of the primary or metastatic tumor, or pleural effusion specimens are suitable for testing. In some instances, if the archival biopsy materials are no longer available or have been exhausted, a new biopsy for molecular testing purposes will be necessary. In all instances, histologic assessment of a freshly cut H&E-stained section of the tissue block should be performed, as part of the preanalytic quality control of the sample. However, in the case of repeat biopsy for testing purposes, there should be a clear indication to the pathologist about the purpose of the biopsy, such that unnecessary ancillary diagnostic IHC studies can be avoided to maximize samples for molecular testing.

Although biopsy tissue samples from patients with advanced-stage disease may be very limited, the tested biomarkers should be prioritized on the basis of their clinical relevance, and the methods used to test them should have a fast turnaround time for therapeutic decisions. In the initial diagnostic workup of biopsy materials, the biomarkers should be rationally and judiciously selected. Because each repeat facing of paraffin blocks results in tissue loss, cutting additional slides for molecular testing, when initially cutting the slides for histopathologic diagnosis, will help if further testing is necessary. However, this option is not always practical as it can increase the laboratory space needed for storing unstained sections, and more importantly, unstained sections stored at room air are no longer optimal for IHC or molecular studies beyond a few weeks or months. The more practical

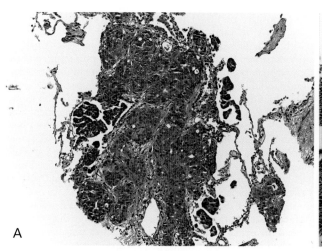
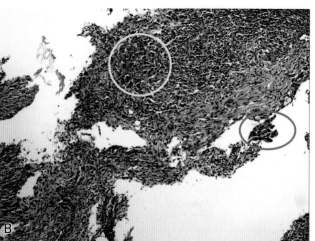

A

B

Fig. 18.2. Tumor cellularity in biopsy specimen. (A) Sample with more than 80% high cellularity. (B) Sample with less than 10% low cellularity, with circled areas showing small clusters of tumor cells.

approach is to order and perform all necessary biomarker testing simultaneously or use multiplex techniques. A third approach that is gaining more acceptance is to perform reflex testing, which is automatically initiated by the pathologist at the time of initial diagnosis. This approach provides the most rapid turnaround time and greatest saving of tissue for future additional studies that may be required for new biomarkers or participation in clinical trials.

Although mutation testing is ideally reported in histology samples, in many cases for patients with advanced disease, the only diagnostic material is based on fine-needle aspiration or cytologic samples. Despite the fact that some molecular/protein analyses can be performed on cytology smear specimens, mutation testing has been better performed on cell blocks prepared from these cells. Therefore cell block preparation is recommended in processing cytologic specimens.

The choice of the biomarkers to be tested must be based on evidence of their clinical relevance for therapeutic decision. To obtain consistent and dependable results, molecular testing should be performed in laboratories that are certified by regional or national regulatory bodies and by well-trained personnel using well-maintained equipment. When determining the methodologic and technical strategy for molecular testing, the main concerns include the sensitivity and specificity of the test, the amount of materials required for successful testing, equipment availability, turnaround time, and cost of the test.[19]

CURRENTLY RECOMMENDED PREDICTIVE BIOMARKERS IN LUNG CANCER

EGFR Mutations for EGFR TKI Therapy

The *EGFR* gene is located on chromosome 7. EGFR TK domain mutations are more frequent in East Asian (40% to 50%) than in white (10% to 20%) patients.[18] EGFR mutations are also found more often in never-smokers than in smokers, and in more women than in men. The mutations are mostly found in adenocarcinomas (around 50% in Asian patients and 25% in non-Asian patients), including adenosquamous carcinomas, but they are uncommon in squamous cell carcinomas (5%; Tables 18.2 and 18.3).[19]

In patients with advanced NSCLCs that harbor an *EGFR* activating mutation, the response rate to EGFR TKIs is 68% and the progression-free survival is 12 months, whereas in patients with unselected advanced NSCLC, the response rate and progression-free survival are 8% to 9% and 2.2 months to 3.0 months, respectively.[28,29,39–42] The discovery of this difference prompted investigators to conduct studies comparing chemotherapy with EGFR TKIs in NSCLC patients with an activating mutation. The Iressa Pan-Asia Study (IPASS) was the first randomized trial in which results showed an advantage for EGFR TKIs as compared with chemotherapy for first-line treatment of stage IIIB/IV disease in never-smoker East Asian patients with a tumor harboring an *EGFR* mutation (hazard ratio for progression-free survival, 0.48; $p < 0.001$).[1,40] Subsequently, in several other randomized trials, results showed the superiority of treatment with EGFR TKIs for patients with *EGFR*-mutated NSCLC tumors (Table 18.4).[28,29,39–42]

EGFR Mutations to Be Tested

Ninety percent of the activating somatic *EGFR* mutations are short in-frame deletions in exon 19 (most frequently, delE746-A750) and a point mutation in exon 21 (L858R; see Fig. 18.1).[43,44] These two mutations have been largely associated with sensitivity to EGFR TKIs. However, the other 10% of *EGFR* mutations are of interest for therapeutic decisions as well. The most frequent in-frame deletions in exon 19 are 15-bp and 19-bp deletions, involving three to seven codons centered on the uniformly deleted codons 747 to 749 (Leu–Arg–Glu sequence). However, 9-bp, 12-bp, 24-bp, and 27-bp deletions are also found, as well as 15-bp and 18-bp insertions.[45] Other, less frequent, *EGFR* activating mutations that have been identified are in exon 18 (E709 and G719X) and in exon 21 (T854 and L861X).[44] All of these

TABLE 18.2 Prevalence of EGFR Mutation in Lung Adenocarcinomas Among Different Patient Populations[18]

	No. of Studies	No. of Patients	EGFR+ No. of Patients	Prevalence (%)
Asian/Pacific Islander	31	3452	1547	45
White	10	3534	853	24
Black	3	97	19	29
Hispanic	4	372	65	17
Asian/Indian	1	220	114	52

EGFR, epidermal growth factor receptor.
Modified from Lindeman NI, Cagle PT, Beasley MB, et al. Molecular testing guideline for selection of lung cancer patients for EGFR and ALK tyrosine kinase inhibitors: guideline from the College of American Pathologists, International Association for the Study of Lung Cancer, and Association for Molecular Pathology. J Thorac Oncol. 2013;8(7):823–859.

TABLE 18.3 Clinical–Pathologic Characteristics in Relation to *EGFR* Mutation Status

	Asian Patients				Non-Asian Patients			
	No. of Studies	No. of Patients	No. of *EGFR*+	Prevalence of Mutation (%)	No. of Studies	No. of Patients	No. of *EGFR*+	Prevalence of Mutation (%)
GENDER								
Women	27	1760	1027	58	19	3098	859	28
Men	26	1418	456	32	19	2165	397	18
SMOKING STATUS								
Never	22	1442	843	58	18	1471	666	45
Ever	22	1032	265	26	18	3723	569	15
HISTOLOGY								
Adenocarcinoma	25	2534	1278	50	19	5184	1266	24
Squamous cell	8	168	8	5	9	110	6	5
Adenosquamous	2	6	4	67	2	8	1	13
Large cell	4	15	1	7	6	39	2	5

EGFR, epidermal growth factor receptor.
Modified from Lindeman NI, Cagle PT, Beasley MB, et al. Molecular testing guideline for selection of lung cancer patients for EGFR and ALK tyrosine kinase inhibitors: guideline from the College of American Pathologists, International Association for the Study of Lung Cancer, and Association for Molecular Pathology. J Thorac Oncol. 2013;8(7):823–859.

mutations result in an EGFR that is constitutively active and may be sensitive to EGFR TKIs.[46]

Both primary and acquired resistance to EGFR TKIs have been reported. After initial response or disease stabilization for several months, a great majority of EGFR mutation-positive tumors eventually become resistant to EGFR TKIs. Another EGFR mutation, the T790M mutation of exon 20, was found to be a resistance mechanism that is acquired secondarily to treatment with EGFR TKIs in almost 50% of cases.[47] Although the T790M mutation is usually acquired, rare cases of NSCLC harbor T790M-mutated cells, with or without an activating mutation, before treatment with EGFR TKIs and, based on preliminary data, the T790M mutation seems to initially confirm resistance to EGFR TKIs.[48–50] Inherited T790M germline mutations have also been identified in some families with lung cancer.[51]

Some other mutations in exon 20 include S768 and insertions and are associated with initial resistance to EGFR TKIs.[52,53] As more sensitive mutation assays are available and as more rare mutations are detected, studies are needed to establish the clinical and therapeutic roles of these rare mutations. More recently, a germline point mutation in exon 21 at codon 843 (vv8431) has been reported as the cause of familial lung adenocarcinoma with resistance to EGFR TKIs.[54,55]

The EGFR in-frame truncated variant (EGFR vIII), resulting from a deletion of exons 2–7 and consequently of a truncation of 801 bp in the extracellular domain, has been rarely reported in NSCLC.[56] The response of a tumor with the EGFR vIII mutation to EGFR TKIs is not known.

In conclusion, EGFR testing should be performed for any mutation located in exons 18–21 with over 1% prevalence.

Assays Used for Testing

Currently, the EGFR mutation is detected by classic molecular tests. Based on expert consensus opinion,[19] as for any other molecular testing, EGFR mutation testing should be performed on FFPE, frozen, or alcohol-fixed tissue specimens. The largest and best available quality tumor specimen should be used, even if the techniques can be adapted, and include tissue enrichment steps for cases where a low amount of DNA is obtained. The different methods for mutation testing have been described earlier in this chapter. The Sanger sequencing method, ideally used by performing bidirectional sequencing and by confirming with additional sequencing, can be used. However, using Sanger sequencing can result in missing approximately 30% of sensitizing

mutation because of the relative low sensitivity of this technique.[57] Therefore when using Sanger sequencing, the cellularity limit needs to be higher, at least 20%, and/or it should be used in combination with a more sensitive mutated allele-enriching strategy or both methods (standard and high sensitivity). When choosing the test, the clinician should take into account the clinical situation and the available tumor content. As mentioned earlier, EGFR mutation testing should be performed in a certified laboratory. The method used should test any mutations in exons 18–21 and be highly sensitive to detect any mutation with a prevalence over 1%. Data have shown the feasibility of detecting EGFR mutations in circulating DNA as well as in circulating tumor cells in patients with NSCLC.[34,38] The sensitivity of EGFR detection in circulating DNA, with the EGFR mutation detected on a tumor considered as the standard, is approximately 70%.[34–36] Thus circulating DNA could be used for screening in the first-line treatment setting, but further mutation tumor testing would be required on specimens that test negatively. Besides first-line testing, an increased interest has been shown for using liquid biopsies for monitoring molecular abnormalities and, particularly, to detect EGFR T790M mutations at the time of acquired resistance to first-line EGFR TKIs. The third-generation EGFR TKIs have shown very high response rates in patients whose tumor harbors T790M mutation that is resistant to first-line EGFR TKIs.[58] Therefore molecular testing at resistance is required but rebiopsy in a clinical practice may be challenging and the success rate is limited in advanced NSCLC patients.[59] Therefore T790M detection in the circulating DNA has been performed and showed a sensitivity between 40% and 70% according to the technique that was used.[60] Hence, testing the EGFR mutation with blood samples is a promising and attractive alternative, particularly in second and later lines of treatment, because it does not require an invasive procedure (biopsy), but stronger evidence is needed before it can be recommended as first-line testing. Currently, circulating DNA may be used for EGFR testing for first-line treatment in specific clinical settings in which tissue is absent or limited for molecular testing. Circulating DNA may be used to detect EGFR T790M mutations in NSCLC patients with progression or acquired resistance to first-line EGFR TKIs. However, as the sensitivity is modest, any negative results in the blood should be followed by EGFR testing in the tumor sample.

Specific antibodies for the detection of EGFR mutations by IHC have been assessed, and the authors of several studies have consistently reported good sensitivity and specificity for the detection of the exon 21 L858R mutations as well as the EGFR

TABLE 18.4 Select Randomized Phase III Trials Comparing EGFR TKI Therapy With Chemotherapy as First-Line Therapy for Patients With EGFR-Positive NSCLC

Study	Ethnicity	No. of Patients With EGFR Mutation	EGFR TKI	Chemotherapy	Outcomes: EGFR TKIs/Chemotherapy	
					Response Rate (%)	Progression-Free Survival (months)
IPASS[1,40]	Asian	261	Gefitinib (n = 132)	Carboplatin/paclitaxel (n = 129)	71/47	9.5/6.3 HR = 0.48; p < 0.0001
WJTOG3405[38]	Asian	117	Gefitinib (n = 58)	Cisplatin/docetaxel (n = 59)	62/32	9.2/6.3 HR = 0.49; p = 0.0001
NEJ002[39]	Asian	228	Gefitinib (n = 114)	Carboplatin/paclitaxel (n = 114)	74/31	10.8/5.4 HR = 0.30; p = 0.001
OPTIMAL[41]	Asian	154	Erlotinib (n = 82)	Carboplatin/gemcitabine (n = 72)	83/36	13.1/4.6 HR = 0.37; p = 0.0001
EURTAC[27]	White	173	Erlotinib (n = 86)	Platinum doublets (n = 87)	71/47	9.5/5.2 HR = 0.37; p = 0.0001
Ensure PMID:26105600	Asian	217	Erlotinib (n = 110)	Cisplatin/gemcitabine (n = 107)	63/34	11.0/5.5 HR = 0.34; (0.22–0.51)
LUX-Lung 3[28]	Any	345	Afatinib (n = 230)	Cisplatin/pemetrexed (n = 115)	56/23	11.1/6.9 HR = 0.58; p = 0.001
LUX-Lung 6 PMID:24439929	Asian	364	Afatinib (n = 242)	Cisplatin/gemcitabine (n = 122)	67/23	11.0/5.6 HR = 0.28; (0.20–0.39)

EGFR, epidermal growth factor receptor; *EURTAC*, European Randomized Trial of Tarceva versus Chemotherapy; *HR*, hazard ratio; *IPASS*, Iressa Pan-Asia Study; *n*, number; *NSCLC*, nonsmall cell lung cancer; *TKIs*, tyrosine kinase inhibitors.

exon 19 15-bp deletions.[61–64] Unfortunately, the sensitivity is lower for the detection of EGFR exon 19 deletion of other sizes.[62,63,65,66] After validation and standardization, IHC using mutation-specific antibodies could be an option for initial screening for patients with samples with low cellularity that otherwise would not be adequate for mutation testing. Tumors that test negatively by IHC would still need mutation testing. However, this option needs stronger evidence to be recommended for the selection of patients for EGFR TKI therapy.[19]

Proteomic profile using mass spectrometry has also been shown to predict response to EGFR TKIs. From an analysis of serum samples taken from 139 patients with NSCLC before treatment with gefitinib, investigators developed a proteomic signature that was used retrospectively to classify patients according to response, both in the first- and second-line treatment settings.[67] A significant difference in overall survival was found according to the outcome predicted by the proteomic signatures in gefitinib and erlotinib validation cohorts. The proteomic classifier has since been commercialized as VeriStrat (Biodesix, CO, USA). Testing with VeriStrat predicted survival outcome in the Eastern Cooperative Oncology Group 3503 phase II trial of erlotinib as first-line therapy in NSCLC.[68] However, in a retrospective analysis of patients treated in the National Cancer Institute Canada (NCIC) BR-21 study, testing with VeriStrat was found to be prognostic for both overall survival and progression-free survival and was predictive for response but was not able to predict for differential survival benefit for erlotinib.[69] The proteomic classifier, which is unrelated to EGFR mutation status, is currently being validated in several prospective studies. In PROSE (Randomized Proteomic Stratified Phase III Study of Second Line Erlotinib versus Chemotherapy in Patients with Inoperable Non-Small Cell Lung Cancer), investigators prospectively validated the VeriStrat classifier for second-line therapy in patients with advanced NSCLC.[70] Patients were classified as poor or good according to VeriStrat analysis, and the analysis clearly distinguished patients who would benefit from chemotherapy versus EGFR TKI.

Other Potential Biomarkers for EGFR TKI Sensitivity

Other biomarkers have been assessed for their potential association with sensitivity to EGFR TKI, including EGFR gene copy number and EGFR expression.

Tumors that are EGFR positive on FISH (including high polysomy and gene amplification using the Colorado scoring system[71]) have been found in 22% to 76% of patients with NSCLC and are associated with a 30% rate of response to EGFR TKIs.[27,72–78] However, the EGFR gene copy number is not recommended for prediction of response to EGFR TKIs for several reasons. The response rate of 30% among patients with an increased EGFR gene copy number remains much lower than the response rate of 68% in patients with activating EGFR mutations. In addition, there is a strong association between EGFR mutations and gene amplification and the higher response rate with gene amplification is a consequence of the association with EGFR activating mutations.[79,80] Some studies, including IPASS, have involved both EGFR gene copy number and EGFR mutation analysis. The response rate for patients with tumors harboring the EGFR mutation but with no increase in gene copy number remains at 68%.[2,41,79,80] For patients with an EGFR mutation-negative tumor, the response rate was low, irrespective of whether the EGFR gene copy number was high or normal. Lastly, in IPASS, the outcome with EGFR TKIs was better for patients with NSCLC who were selected on the basis of the presence of an EGFR mutation than it was for patients who were selected on the basis of the EGFR copy number.[2,41] Therefore EGFR copy number should not be used to select patients for EGFR TKI treatment. It is not well established whether EGFR gene copy number has a predictive value for response to EGFR TKIs in selected patients with EGFR

wild-type tumors. FISH-determined EGFR is currently being evaluated as a predictive biomarker for EGFR TKI therapy (i.e., cetuximab, necitumumab) in prospective studies.

EGFR protein expression by IHC has been assessed to predict response and outcome to EGFR TKIs. Total EGFR expression has not been shown to be associated with a better outcome to EGFR TKIs or with EGFR mutation.[79–81] In a retrospective analysis, the use of a specific antibody targeting the intracellular domain of EGFR has been shown to improve the prediction of response to EGFR TKIs compared with antibodies targeting the external domain.[82] Still, this method needs to be validated and does not appear to provide a better prediction than EGFR mutations can provide. Therefore total EGFR expression cannot currently be recommended to select patients for EGFR TKI therapy. However, high EGFR protein expression has been shown to predict response to anti-EGFR monoclonal antibody therapy (cetuximab).[83,84] The American Society of Clinical Oncology guidelines include cetuximab plus chemotherapy as an option for first-line treatment of patients with tumors positive for EGFR expression by IHC based on the results of the First-Line ErbituX in lung cancer (FLEX) study.[85] In the FLEX study update, there was a survival benefit for patients who had tumors with higher EGFR expression, when the score used considered the percentage of cells stained and the intensity of the staining (H score).[86] Further evidence and validation in independent clinical trials are warranted to recommend the use of EGFR expression in select patients for therapy with an anti-EGFR monoclonal antibody.

Other Biomarkers of Resistance to EGFR TKIs

In addition to EGFR mutations, other biomarkers have been indicated as potentially associated with primary resistance to EGFR TKIs. KRAS mutations with constitutive activation of the downstream pathways are seen in 30% of people with lung adenocarcinomas and have been associated with poor prognosis.[87] Based on retrospective analyses in trials of patients receiving EGFR TKIs as second- and third-line treatment, the presence of KRAS mutation is associated with lower response rates in patients taking EGFR TKIs (0% to 3%);[27,42,49,79,80,88–93] however, there is no substantial effect on outcome. Because KRAS and EGFR mutations are considered mutually exclusive, KRAS testing is sometimes used as a screening assay and only KRAS wild-type tumors are tested for the EGFR mutation. This approach has not been validated and implies that enough material is available for successive testing of KRAS and EGFR mutations and would not delay the results. Therefore more data are required and KRAS mutation testing cannot be recommended to exclude patients for EGFR TKI therapy.[19] Furthermore, although subtyping of KRAS mutations has been shown to have clinical relevance in colorectal cancer, no studies in lung cancer have established a clinically relevant difference between subtypes of KRAS mutations.

Mesenchymal–epithelial transition is another potential mechanism for resistance to EGFR TKIs. MET gene amplification has been associated with 10% to 20% of acquired resistance to EGFR TKIs.[94–96] More recently, HER2 has been associated with acquired resistance to EGFR TKIs.[97] High expression of insulin-like growth factor receptor 1 (IGF1R) has also been shown to be associated with resistance to EGFR TKIs.[98–100] Recently, BCL2 interacting protein (BIM) polymorphism has been shown to potentially induce EGFR TKI resistance in patients with NSCLC harboring EGFR mutations.[101] Currently, none of these biomarkers (MET, HER2, or IGF1R amplification) can be used for negative selection of patients for EGFR TKI treatment.

Patients Who Should Have Testing

Based on currently available published data, the EGFR sensitizing mutation is the only biomarker recommended as the predictive biomarker for testing of patients to receive EGFR TKI therapy. Although *EGFR* mutations are more frequent in tumors in patients who are Asian, female, or never-smokers, they also occur in other patients.[2,39,72,102] Therefore clinical characteristics are not recommended for selecting or excluding patients for EGFR mutation testing.

EGFR mutations are most frequently found in people with adenocarcinomas and are very uncommon in people with pure lung squamous cell carcinomas and in pure small cell carcinomas (such as SCLC).[103–107] However, mutations have been found in patients with other mixed carcinomas with an adenocarcinoma component, such as adenosquamous carcinomas or combined small cell carcinoma with an adenocarcinoma component. Consequently, in the absence of IHC evidence for the presence of an adenocarcinoma component, *EGFR* mutation testing is not recommended for patients with squamous cell carcinomas and SCLC carcinomas.[19] In patients with marginally sufficient lung cancer specimens, including samples from biopsy, fine-needle aspiration, and cytologic samples from pleural effusions, the diagnosis of adenosquamous or poorly differentiated adenocarcinoma may be challenging, and an adenocarcinoma component should not be entirely excluded.[19] This exclusion may explain why, in a few studies involving small specimens for EGFR mutation testing, *EGFR* mutations have been reported in rare cases of squamous cell carcinomas.[103] In addition, in order to alleviate misclassification of squamous cell carcinoma versus adenocarcinoma of the lung on small specimens, the optimal IHC diagnostic algorithm should be used.[108] The suitability of thoracic cytology for EGFR molecular testing has been confirmed, but IHC was used for histologic subtyping of the patients.[109] Thus in cases of limited lung cancer specimens that may not exclude definitively an adenocarcinoma component, *EGFR* mutation testing should be performed in all patients, including those with squamous cell and small cell carcinomas. However, *EGFR* mutations have been identified in patients with proven squamous cell carcinoma of the lung.[110,111] Therefore as recommended in the European Society for Medical Oncology guidelines and the CAP/IASLC/AMP guidelines, molecular testing could be performed in patients with squamous cell carcinoma of the lung who are never-smokers and former light-smokers (fewer than 15 pack-years).[19,112] *EGFR* mutation testing should also be performed for patients with tumors that are classified as NSCLC not otherwise specified (NOS), if possible.

When Testing Should Be Done

Evidence for the use of EGFR mutation testing in selecting patients for EGFR TKI therapy is available only for those with advanced NSCLC.[2,39,40,72] By contrast, evidence for its use to select patients for adjuvant TKI therapy in early-stage and surgically treated disease is currently not available.[113,114] The test is not useful for many of these patients who will have surgery with or without adjuvant chemotherapy. However, for 50% of patients who are expected to have relapse, no initial testing on the resected specimen may mean that the test must be done at the time of disease progression, with delayed availability of the result, lack of a readily available sample, and even the necessity of repeating biopsy. Thus clinicians must balance the cost of performing unnecessary tests in cured patients with delaying therapy in others because results are not readily available.[19] At the time of relapse, it is also relevant to consider the value of *EGFR* mutation on the diagnostic sample and the possibility of resistant mutations present in the metastatic relapse sites but not in the primary tumor.

Tumor Site to Be Used for Testing

The type of samples used for EGFR testing is largely determined by the convenience of sample availability. Currently, testing of the primary tumor or metastatic lesions is equally acceptable before initial EGFR TKI treatment. However, there is some debate with regard to sample choice for testing because of tumor heterogeneity. In some studies, *EGFR* mutation testing has been shown to be very consistent between the primary lung tumor and metastatic lesions.[69,115] However, other investigators have reported heterogeneity of the *EGFR* mutation status between the primary lung tumor and the metastasis.[116,117] Overall, the quality of the tissue should be the primary factor for choosing the sample for a patient with metastatic lung cancer. Nevertheless, as previously discussed, metastatic bone lesions might not be optimal for testing if the biopsy specimen has been processed in acidic decalcifying solutions. For patients with multiple primary sites, it seems rational to test each tumor separately, as the detection of different mutations in different primary tumors has been reported.[118]

Clinical Recommendations for EGFR Testing

The guideline by CAP/IASLC/AMP recommends that, at diagnosis, any patient with advanced NSCLC with an adenocarcinoma, a large cell carcinoma, or a carcinoma with an adenocarcinoma component should be tested for the *EGFR* mutation, using the most accessible tissue (primary tumor or metastasis). If the specimen is not large enough to exclude an adenocarcinoma component, other histologies, such as squamous cell carcinomas and small cell carcinoma, should be considered for EGFR mutation testing as well. For patients with early-stage NSCLC, *EGFR* mutation testing at the time of diagnosis is debatable, but seems reasonable and should be done if possible.[19]

ALK Rearrangement: A Predictor of Response to ALK Inhibitors

The other approved targetable biomarker used in the treatment of patients with advanced lung cancer is *ALK* gene rearrangement. The discovery in 2007 of the *ALK* gene rearrangement in lung cancer has been quickly translated into a therapeutic target.[4] The most frequent *ALK* rearrangement is an inversion on the short arm of chromosome 2 resulting in a fusion gene, *echinoderm microtubule-associated protein like 4 (EML4)–ALK*, of which the fusion protein product demonstrates a constitutive tyrosine kinase activity. In addition, other fusion partners of ALK have been reported in lung cancer, including kinesin family member 5B (KIF5B)–ALK and TRK-fused gene (TFG)–ALK, which are rare fusions involving a translocation with a chromosome segment other than 2p (Fig. 18.3). The prevalence of ALK fusion ranges from 2% to 7% of patients with NSCLC (Table 18.5). ALK rearrangements appear more frequently in never-smokers and, potentially, in younger people, and occur more often in adenocarcinomas than in other NSCLC histologic types. However, *ALK* rearrangements seem not to be associated with gender or ethnicity, in contrast to EGFR mutations.[119–131]

Crizotinib, a small-molecule inhibitor of the tyrosine kinase of ALK fusion protein, has been tested in patients with NSCLCs that harbor an *ALK* rearrangement. The response rate for this selected population was 57%.[123] In a more recent study, crizotinib was compared with chemotherapy in patients with advanced NSCLC with *ALK* rearrangements, and crizotinib was found to be associated with a significantly greater response rate (65% vs. 20%; $p < 0.001$) and progression-free survival (7.7 months vs. 3.0 months; hazard ratio, 0.49; $p < 0.001$).[131] Testing for *ALK* rearrangement to select patients for treatment with ALK inhibitors such as crizotinib is now generally recommended.

Despite reports of encouraging results from treatment with crizotinib, clinical resistance has emerged. Several secondary mutations occurring in *ALK* and conferring acquired resistance to crizotinib have been reported, including L1152R, C1156Y, F1174L, L1196M, L1198P, D1203N, and G1269A.[132–137] Several molecules have been developed to target these resistant ALK mutations and show high response rate.[138] However, there is

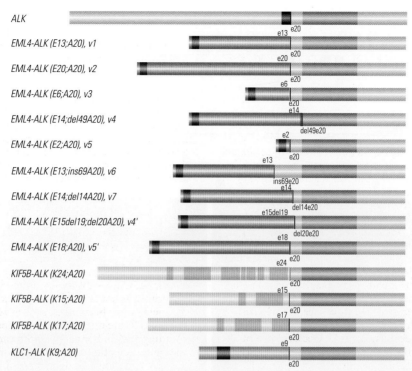

ALK

EML4-ALK (E13;A20), v1

EML4-ALK (E20;A20), v2

EML4-ALK (E6;A20), v3

EML4-ALK (E14;del49A20), v4

EML4-ALK (E2;A20), v5

EML4-ALK (E13;ins69A20), v6

EML4-ALK (E14;del14A20), v7

EML4-ALK (E15del19;del20A20), v4'

EML4-ALK (E18;A20), v5'

KIF5B-ALK (K24;A20)

KIF5B-ALK (K15;A20)

KIF5B-ALK (K17;A20)

KLC1-ALK (K9;A20)

Fig. 18.3. Wild-type and various types of anaplastic lymphoma kinase (ALK) fusions in lung cancer. *EML4,* echinoderm microtubule-associated protein like 4. *(Reprinted with permission from Tsao MS, Hirsch FR, Yatabe Y, eds.* IASLC Atlas of ALK Testing in Lung Cancer. *Aurora, CO: IASLC Press Office; 2013.)*

TABLE 18.5 Incidence of ALK Rearrangement in NSCLC[32]

Ethnicity	No. of Studies	No. of Patients	No. of ALK+	Prevalence of ALK+ (%)
UNSELECTED STUDIES				
Asia	21	5739	274	4.8
Europe	4	767	48	6.3
United States	6	4198	194	4.6
Mixed	2	908	24	2.7
Total	33	11,612	540	4.7
SELECTED FOR NEVER-/LIGHT-SMOKERS STUDIES				
Asia	4	619	65	10.5
United States	3	542	63	11.6
Total	7	1161	128	11.0
Overall Total	40	12,773	668	5.2

ALK, anaplastic lymphoma kinase; NSCLC, nonsmall cell lung cancer.
Modified from Tsao MS, Hirsch FR, Yatabe Y. IASLC Atlas of ALK Testing in Lung Cancer. *2013. Copyright International Association for the Study of Lung Cancer.*

currently insufficient evidence for recommending testing of these mutations in clinical practice. Resistance to ALK inhibitors may also involve activations of other pathways and development of other mutations, such as *EGFR* and *KRAS* mutations.[118,136]

Assays Used for Testing

In the United States, the FDA approved crizotinib for the treatment of patients with NSCLC that harbors an *ALK* rearrangement that can be detected using a commercial ALK break-apart assay (Vysis LSI ALK Break Apart FISH Probe Kit; Abbott Molecular, Abbott Park, IL, USA). This assay was used to detect *ALK* rearrangements in the clinical trials showing a clinical benefit with crizotinib in patients with NSCLC.[121,123,131,139] The assay involves hybridizing a telomeric 3′ probe labeled with Spectrum Orange (orange/red

signal) and a centromeric 5′ probe labeled with Spectrum Green (green signal) to FFPE tissue sections. In the absence of rearrangement, the probes are fused and the signal is yellow (Fig. 18.4). The inversion results typically in a separation of the probes that gives individual orange and green signals.

A tumor is considered positive for *ALK* rearrangement if at least 15% of 50 nuclei of tumor cells assessed harbor the typically described split signals of *ALK* rearrangement.[139] However, other FISH abnormalities may occur with an atypical FISH pattern.[33,112] Interpreting the results of the FISH assay require special training and expertise and need to be performed or supervised by a pathologist.

Because of cost and convenience, IHC as a first-line screening assay for *ALK* rearrangement has been considered and adopted worldwide. In several studies, the detection of the protein product of the ALK fusion gene has been reported to reach a sensitivity and specificity of nearly 100%.[33,140] A crucial consideration in the application of an ALK-IHC assay is the use of the signal amplification step.[33] Several antibodies have been tested. A special IHC assay (Ventana Medical Systems, Tucson, AZ, USA) using the D5F3 antibody has been studied for interobserver reproducibility and comparability to the ALK-FISH assay.[116] The assay was highly reproducible and the results were strongly correlated with those of the ALK-FISH assay. In the centers using IHC to screen for *ALK* rearrangement, FISH is still being performed subsequently to confirm the positivity of the tumor for *ALK* rearrangement.[19] Although positive findings on ALK-FISH are strongly associated with response and outcome with crizotinib, an increasing number of reports have noted that some NSCLCs that are ALK negative on FISH (using the FDA-approved criteria) are ALK positive on IHC.[141] More recently, an ALK-IHC companion diagnostics assay has received approval by the FDA and in several other countries for use as a stand-alone ALK assay to diagnose and treat ALK-rearranged lung cancer patients.

ALK testing with IHC and FISH are currently performed on FFPE tumor sections. FISH is a robust technique that might

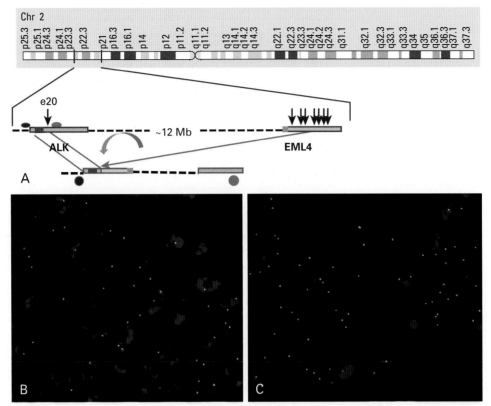

Fig. 18.4. Anaplastic lymphoma kinase (ALK) break-apart fluorescent in situ hybridization (FISH) assays. (A) Schematic diagram showing the location of *ALK* and *echinoderm microtubule-associated protein like 4 (EML4)* genes on chromosome 2p, and the location of the break-apart probes in relation to the inversion breakpoint with *ALK* gene rearrangement. Tumors were probed by the break-apart ALK probes. (B) Tumor showing close approximation of the green and orange/red (artificially colored red) signals, indicating normal ALK gene structure. (C) Separation of the green and red signals indicates an inversion-type ALK gene rearrangement.

technically also be applicable to cytologic specimens, such as direct smears, cytospins, or liquid-based preparations.[33] However, the criteria for ALK-FISH analyses are the same as the criteria used for histology. Cell blocks or cytologic specimens may not contain enough tumor cells in many cases. Although FISH analysis on cytologic preparations is not recommended for predictive ALK testing, cell blocks might be acceptable.[33]

ALK rearrangements have been detected in circulating tumor cells with a sensitivity and specificity of 100% compared with testing of the primary tumor as the standard.[37] The circulating tumor cells were collected with a filter-based technology that does not eliminate the cells in epithelial–mesenchymal transition, while the FDA-approved epithelial cell adhesion molecule-based technology would not retain these cells. Interestingly, new ALK rearrangement patterns were found in circulating tumor cells. In one study, the 15% cutoff could not be used because of a low number of tumor cells. In the case of circulating tumor cells, a cutoff of four or more circulating tumor cells with ALK rearrangement per 1 mL of blood was chosen based on a receiver operating characteristic curve that resulted in the optimal prediction of *ALK* rearrangement in tumors.[37]

PCR methods can also be used to detect *ALK* rearrangement. The method is highly sensitive, but requires probes for identified fusion partners. Studies comparing the advantages and disadvantages of ALK testing with FISH, IHC, and RT-PCR are ongoing.[33]

Patients Who Should Have Testing

ALK testing should be done on the same patient population tested for EGFR mutations. As mentioned previously, although *ALK* rearrangements are more frequent in never-smokers and younger people, they are also found in people with other clinical features. Therefore as with EGFR, clinical characteristics, except squamous cell carcinoma histology, should not be used to exclude patients with NSCLC from ALK testing.[119–130] *ALK* rearrangements are most common in adenocarcinomas and have been described in other lung cancers with adenocarcinoma components, but they are extremely uncommon in pure lung squamous cell carcinomas.[126,142–144] Because of this, as with EGFR testing, ALK testing should be done if IHC indicates that there is an adenocarcinoma component in a lung cancer specimen.[19] However, if a young never-smoker has a tumor with squamous cell histology, ALK testing should be recommended.

When Testing Should Be Done

The clinical results from different trials with crizotinib and preliminary results from studies of other ALK inhibitors have established the crucial role for *ALK* rearrangement testing in patients with advanced NSCLC.[123,131] For patients with curable early-stage disease, there are no data to support reflex testing at the time of diagnosis,[19] but the same argument can be made as for EGFR mutation testing, as previously discussed.

Tumor Site to Be Tested

For *ALK* rearrangements, no data are available regarding whether to test the primary tumor or metastatic lesions. However, because *ALK* rearrangements are driver oncogenes similar to *EGFR* mutations, consistency of results is expected between the primary lung tumor and metastatic lesions. Thus the quality of the tissue and the feasibility for obtaining it should be the primary factors for choosing the sample to be tested. Similar to the case with EGFR mutations, there are no data on patients with several primary tumors, but it seems rational to test every tumor separately.[19]

Clinical Recommendations for ALK Testing

The CAP/IASLC/AMP guidelines recommend that testing for *ALK* rearrangement should be performed at the time of diagnosis for any patient with an advanced NSCLC that is an adenocarcinoma or has an adenocarcinoma component, with testing done on the most accessible tissue (primary tumor or metastasis).[19] If the specimen is not large enough to exclude an adenocarcinoma component, tumors with other histologies, such as squamous cell carcinomas and small cell carcinoma, as well as NSCLC NOS, should also be considered for *ALK* mutation testing. Testing of early-stage tumors is debatable, but appears reasonable and should be done, if possible.

POTENTIAL NEW MOLECULAR MARKERS FOR THE FUTURE

Prognostic Markers

A very large number of individual biomarkers have been studied for their prognostic role in NSCLC, but to date, there is no evidence to recommend any of them in clinical practice. Most of the markers are IHC markers that have been studied by many investigators, but the results of different studies are discordant.[145] Some biomarkers have been studied in meta-analyses (KRAS, EGFR, P53, HER2, cyclooxygenase-2 [COX-2], Ki-67, and Bcl2), and several had a significant, but weak, impact on overall survival.[87,146–151] Six markers (overexpression of cyclin E and vascular endothelial growth factor A, and loss of p16INK4A, p27kip1, B-catenin, and E-cadherin) showed a consistent prognostic impact in more than half of the studies.[145] The absence of clinically relevant prognostic biomarkers and the discordant results are partially due to the lack of homogeneity of study cohorts and of standardization of the techniques used in different laboratories for each marker. A more pragmatic approach to biomarker study and validation is needed and could be achieved through a multiphase approach similar to that used in clinical trials.[145] Translational researchers from the NCIC Clinical Trials Group, the International Adjuvant Lung Cancer Trial Biologic Program (IALT-Bio), and the Lung Adjuvant Cisplatin Evaluation Biologic Program (LACE-Bio) have investigated the prognostic value of several biomarkers in large phase III randomized trials, which offer the advantage of more uniform and better defined patient populations and allow testing if the markers predict benefit from adjuvant chemotherapy. The studies performed by these groups might then provide more clinically relevant biomarkers. The LACE-Bio group pooled the analysis of the prognostic and predictive effects of *KRAS* mutation in patients with early-stage resected NSCLC in four trials of adjuvant chemotherapy. Among 1543 patients, of which 300 had *KRAS* mutations, the presence of *KRAS* mutation, either at codon 12 or 13, was not found to be a prognostic factor for overall survival.[150] In addition, the LACE-Bio group has reported that *TP53* mutation is also not a prognostic factor but is marginally predictive of poorer survival in patients who received adjuvant chemotherapy.[152] More recently, the investigators have also reported that intratumoral lymphocytic infiltrate and histologic subtype of lung adenocarcinoma are significant prognostic markers.[153,154]

Panels of biomarkers or signatures may be used to predict prognoses and could have greater power than individual biomarkers to discriminate patients with different prognoses. Many studies of prognostic gene signatures in patients with NSCLC have been published. Since 2005, the studies include validation in independent cohorts, in most cases based on publicly available gene expression data sets. However, the prospective validation of these signatures has been missing and very difficult to conduct, thus the clinical applicability of signatures with a large number of genes has been challenging. Zhu et al.[155] identified a 15-gene signature derived from patients participating in the JBR.10 study that discriminated patients at high- and low-risk in the observation arm. In addition, high-risk patients derived significant benefit from chemotherapy, but low-risk patients did not. Tang et al.[156] reported on another signature of 12 genes that predicted for survival benefit with adjuvant chemotherapy, identified in a cohort of 442 stage I–III NSCLC specimens and further validated in two independent data sets of 90 (University of Texas cohort) and 176 patients (JBR.10), respectively. In both cohorts, the groups that were predicted to benefit from adjuvant chemotherapy had an improved survival rate with adjuvant chemotherapy, and the groups that were predicted not to benefit from adjuvant chemotherapy did not have any survival benefit after adjuvant chemotherapy.[155] Kratz et al.[157] reported on a 14-gene signature, based on quantitative PCR assays of FFPE tissue samples in a testing cohort of 361 patients and two validation cohorts of 433 and 1006 patients, respectively. This signature identified patients at high risk of mortality after surgical resection of an early-stage NSCLC. To date, however, all signatures lack sufficient validation to be implemented in clinical practice.

Other Predictive Biomarkers

Aside from *EGFR* mutations and *ALK* rearrangements, several other biomarkers have also been tested for their ability to predict lung cancer response to treatment, but none have shown sufficient evidence for current use in clinical practice. Part of the reason is that predictive biomarkers are relevant only for therapies that show clinical efficacy, and to date, few targeted therapies have been approved for patients with NSCLC. Initial biomarker research has focused on prediction of outcome with systemic therapy in advanced NSCLC. More recently, however, the predictive biomarker research has focused on the adjuvant setting.

Biomarkers are commonly investigated for both prognostic value and for prediction of response to chemotherapy. To date, preliminary evidence from studies in NSCLC suggests that DNA repair markers may be prognostic and predictive for treatment with cisplatin (excision repair cross-complementing rodent repair deficiency, complementation group 1 [ERCC1] and MutS homolog 2 [MSH2]), gemcitabine (ribonucleotide reductase M1 [RRM1]), taxanes (breast cancer 1 [BRCA1]), and pemetrexed (thymidylate synthetase).[158–163] Class III beta-tubulin (TUBB3), a block for microtubules, is potentially predictive for outcome to agents targeting the microtubules, such as taxanes and vinca alkaloids.[164] The roles of other genes or proteins involved in the cell cycle (p27) or apoptosis (Bax) or multiple critical cell functions (P53, KRAS) have also been studied as potential predictive biomarkers.[165–167] Controversial results have been published on the prognostic role of p27 by the IALT-Bio and LACE-Bio programs.[165,168] In a pooled analysis of data from IALT-Bio and JBR.10, IHC protein expression of Bax significantly predicted survival benefit with adjuvant chemotherapy.[166] In the LACE-Bio study of *KRAS* mutation, no significant benefit of adjuvant chemotherapy was found in patients with wild-type or *KRAS* mutations in codon 12, but a deleterious effect with adjuvant chemotherapy was noted in patients with *KRAS* mutations in codon 13 (interaction $p = 0.002$).[169] This finding requires further validation. The LACE-Bio group assessed the role of *KRAS* in 426 patients with *EGFR* wild-type adenocarcinomas and found that the double *P53/KRAS* mutation status was not of prognostic value. However, compared with patients with double *P53/KRAS* wild-type tumors, patients with the double *P53/KRAS* mutations in the tumor had a detrimental effect of chemotherapy (compared with observation), with a comparative hazard ratio of 3.03 ($p = 0.01$).[170]

There has been a resurgence of interest in immunotherapy in lung cancer, with several drugs currently being evaluated in clinical trials. Immunotherapy covers three categories of treatments: (1) vaccines such as the antigen-specific melanoma-associated antigen 3 (MAGE-A3) vaccine (MAGE-A3 ASCI)[171] and the liposomal BLP25 vaccine (L-BLP25) targeting MUC1136; (2) checkpoint targets, including T-cell-modulating agents such as the monoclonal antibodies against program death-1 (PD1) and MPDL3280A against the ligand of PD1 (PDL1); and (3) T-cell antigens such as ipilimumab against the cytotoxic T lymphocyte-associated antigen-4.[172] Investigators are searching for biomarkers for prediction of response to these therapies and some biomarkers have been studied, but none is currently validated or recommended for clinical practice. For the vaccines, the MAGE-A3 messenger RNA level of expression is assessed for the prediction of response to the MAGE-A3 immune vaccine. As an example of gene expression signature, an 84-gene signature has been recently reported to be associated with clinical response to MAGE-A3 immunotherapy in metastatic melanoma, and this association has been confirmed in resected NSCLC.[173] Different biomarkers are also currently assessed for the checkpoint therapy; the PD1 and PDL1 expression are assessed by IHC as potential predictors of response to nivolumab and other checkpoint targeting agents. Variable and discordant results have been published for the predictive value of PDL1 expression with various PD1 and PDL1 inhibitors.[174,175] In nonsquamous carcinomas, a greater benefit of nivolumab was seen when PDL1 was chosen as the cutoff value and the amplitude of the benefit increased when a higher level of PDL1 expression was present,[176] but PDL1 expression was not predictive for the benefit of the same drug, nivolumab, in lung squamous carcinoma.[177] In addition, different methodologies, including different antibodies, variable cutoff values, and assessment of the staining in different cells' compartment, that is, tumor versus inflammatory cells, have been used in the different trials assessing the checkpoint inhibitors.[178] A coordinative study, the BLUEPRINT project, is currently comparing the different testing methods for PDL1 expression. Many other biomarkers are currently tested for their predictive value with checkpoint inhibitors including the high mutation load that seems to predict a better sensitivity.[179] Thus no biomarker can be currently recommended to predict sensitivity to checkpoint inhibitors. The PDL1 expression showed some positive results but the tested methods must be defined and standardized and a panel of other biomarkers may be useful alone or in combination.

Other targetable oncogenic drivers that have been identified more recently include RET[5] and ROS fusions,[1,5,180] phosphatidylinositol 3-kinase subunits (PIK3C),[181,182] BRAF,[183] HER2,[184] and exon 14 Met splice junction mutations.[185-191] Several new gene fusions have been discovered with use of NGS, including metabolic enzymes.[9,192] As new therapies are being developed and tested to target these new oncogenic drivers as well as drivers that have been difficult to target (e.g., *KRAS* mutant tumors), corresponding predictive biomarkers are being investigated as possible companion diagnostics in parallel with the clinical development of these drugs. The presence of the oncogenic drivers is expected to predict response to the targeted therapy, but it might not always be the case, thus requiring extensive preclinical as well as clinical validation studies. A consistent benefit has been shown when treating patients whose tumor harbors *ROS1* rearrangement with treatment by crizotinib in several trials, and crizotinib was approved by the FDA in *ROS1*-rearranged NSCLC patients.[193,194] Therefore ROS1 testing should be conducted for all patients with negative results for EGFR and ALK testing, and possibly in parallel when there is no concern about tissue availability. BRAF, RET, HER2, KRAS, and MET testing are not indicated in routine testing in first-line treatment yet. They may be tested in first-line treatment in the context of clinical trials or they may be part of a panel testing when routing EGFR, ALK, and ROS1 testing are negative. More recently, accumulating evidence suggests that lung cancer patients with *MET* exon 14 skipping mutation may experience dramatic clinical response to MET TKIs such as crizotinib.[195-197] This splice-site mutation results in the loss of exon 14 and Cbl-binding site on the MET receptor protein, resulting in its decreased degradation and high receptor expression level.[198,199]

Worldwide efforts are ongoing for extensive molecular testing on large cohorts of patients. In France, routine testing of *EGFR, KRAS, HER2, BRAF,* and *PIK3CA* mutations as well as *ALK* gene rearrangement is being performed in 28 centers. The results of testing in a very large cohort of more than 18,000 patients with NSCLC were published.[200,201] A known target was identified in around 50% of the samples, 51% of the patients received biomarker-guided treatment, and the presence of a genetic alteration was associated with an improved prognosis. In the United States, the Lung Cancer Mutation Consortium assessed the frequency of 10 oncogenic drivers in advanced lung adenocarcinomas and provided results to clinicians to select treatments or clinical trials based on testing results. Among 1007 patients, 64% had a known oncogenic driver and 28% of patients received targeted therapy.[202] Patients with oncogenic drivers in the tumor who received targeted therapy had a better outcome than patients who did not have targeted therapy.[202]

Strong clinical evidence of the predictive value of the biomarker and standardizing the assay are mandatory for clinical use. The publication of a report on a technical issue regarding ERCC1 testing highlights the importance of standardizing and validating the assays.[203] In this study, ERCC1 immunostaining was reassessed in a validation cohort (494 samples) from two independent phase III trials (JBR.10 and CALGB-9633) using 16 commercial ERCC1 antibodies. In addition, 589 samples of the IALT-Bio cohort were restained. The results of the previously studied IALT-Bio samples with the 8F1 antibody could not be validated, indicating a batch-to-batch variation of the antibodies. More important, however, none of the 16 antibodies could distinguish the four ERCC1 protein isoforms, although only one isoform was functional in terms of nucleotide excision repair and resistance to treatment with cisplatin.[203]

CONCLUSION

Many biomarkers have been or are being assessed for prediction of prognosis and of benefit from different types of systemic therapies. Tests for *EGFR* mutations, *ALK* and *ROS1* rearrangements to predict response to EGFR TKIs and ALK/ROS1 TKIs, respectively, are currently the only biomarker tests recommended in clinical practice. Both tests should be performed at the time of diagnosis, especially for patients who have advanced NSCLC adenocarcinoma or a carcinoma with an adenocarcinoma component, and the most accessible tissue (primary tumor or metastasis) should be used. EGFR and ALK testing at the time of diagnosis is debatable for patients with early-stage NSCLC, but seems reasonable and should be done if possible. Standardized methods proven to be associated with clinical benefit must be used to test these biomarkers in certified laboratories.

KEY REFERENCES

1. Shepherd FA, Tsao MS. Unraveling the mystery of prognostic and predictive factors in epidermal growth factor receptor therapy. *J Clin Oncol*. 2006;24(7):1219–1220.
10. Govindan R, Ding L, Griffith M, et al. Genomic landscape of non-small cell lung cancer in smokers and never-smokers. *Cell*. 2012;150(6):1121–1134.

14. Cancer Genome Atlas Research Network. Comprehensive genomic characterization of squamous cell lung cancers. *Nature*. 2012;489(7417):519–525.

19. Lindeman NI, Cagle PT, Beasley MB, et al. Molecular testing guideline for selection of lung cancer patients for EGFR and ALK tyrosine kinase inhibitors: guideline from the College of American Pathologists, International Association for the Study of Lung Cancer, and Association for Molecular Pathology. *J Thorac Oncol*. 2013;8(7):823–859.

20. Garrido P, de Castro J, Concha A, et al. Guidelines for biomarker testing in advanced non-small-cell lung cancer. A national consensus of the Spanish Society of Medical Oncology (SEOM) and the Spanish Society of Pathology (SEAP). *Clin Transl Oncol*. 2012;14(5):338–349.

21. Felip E, Gridelli C, Baas P, et al. Metastatic non-small-cell lung cancer: consensus on pathology and molecular tests, first-line, second-line, and third-line therapy: 1st ESMO Consensus Conference in Lung Cancer; Lugano 2010. *Ann Oncol*. 2011;22(7):1507–1519.

22. Ellis PM, Morzycki W, Melosky B, et al. The role of the epidermal growth factor receptor tyrosine kinase inhibitors as therapy for advanced, metastatic, and recurrent non-small-cell lung cancer: a Canadian national consensus statement. *Curr Oncol*. 2009;16(1):27–48.

23. Marchetti A, Ardizzoni A, Papotti M, et al. Recommendations for the analysis of ALK gene rearrangements in non-small-cell lung cancer: a consensus of the Italian Association of Medical Oncology and the Italian Society of Pathology and Cytopathology. *J Thorac Oncol*. 2013;8(3):352–358.

29. Sequist LV, Yang JC, Yamamoto N, et al. Phase III study of afatinib or cisplatin plus pemetrexed in patients with metastatic lung adenocarcinoma with EGFR mutations. *J Clin Oncol*. 2013;31(27):3327–3334.

34. Goto K, Ichinose Y, Ohe Y, et al. Epidermal growth factor receptor mutation status in circulating free DNA in serum: from IPASS, a phase III study of gefitinib or carboplatin/paclitaxel in non-small cell lung cancer. *J Thorac Oncol*. 2012;7(1):115–121.

41. Fukuoka M, Wu YL, Thongprasert S, et al. Biomarker analyses and final overall survival results from a phase III, randomized, open-label, first-line study of gefitinib versus carboplatin/paclitaxel in clinically selected patients with advanced non-small-cell lung cancer in Asia (IPASS). *J Clin Oncol*. 2011;29(21):2866–2874.

57. Zhu CQ, da Cunha Santos G, Ding K, et al. Role of KRAS and EGFR as biomarkers of response to erlotinib in National Cancer Institute of Canada Clinical Trials Group Study BR.21. *J Clin Oncol*. 2008;26:4268–4275.

59. Paleiron N, Bylicki O, André M, Rivière E, Grassin F, Robinet G, Chouaïd C. Targeted therapy for localized non-small-cell lung cancer: a review. *Onco Targets Ther*. 2016 Jul 5;9:4099–4104.

71. Hirsch FR, Varella-Garcia M, McCoy J, et al. Increased epidermal growth factor receptor gene copy number detected by fluorescence in situ hybridization associates with increased sensitivity to gefitinib in patients with bronchioloalveolar carcinoma subtypes: a Southwest Oncology Group Study. *J Clin Oncol*. 2005;23(28):6838–6845.

72. Douillard JY, Shepherd FA, Hirsh V, et al. Molecular predictors of outcome with gefitinib and docetaxel in previously treated non-small-cell lung cancer: data from the randomized phase III INTEREST trial. *J Clin Oncol*. 2010;28(5):744–752.

84. Azzoli CG, Baker Jr S, Temin S, et al. American Society of Clinical Oncology Clinical Practice Guideline update on chemotherapy for stage IV non-small-cell lung cancer. *J Clin Oncol*. 2009;27(36):6251–6266.

85. Pirker R, Pereira JR, Szczesna A, et al. Cetuximab plus chemotherapy in patients with advanced non-small-cell lung cancer (FLEX): an open-label randomised phase III trial. *Lancet*. 2009;373(9674):1525–1531.

86. Pirker R, Pereira JR, von Pawel J, et al. EGFR expression as a predictor of survival for first-line chemotherapy plus cetuximab in patients with advanced non-small-cell lung cancer: analysis of data from the phase 3 FLEX study. *Lancet Oncol*. 2012;13(1):33–42.

87. Mascaux C, Iannino N, Martin B, et al. The role of RAS oncogene in survival of patients with lung cancer: a systematic review of the literature with meta-analysis. *Br J Cancer*. 2005;92(1):131–139.

93. Zer A, Ding K, Lee SM, et al. Pooled analysis of the prognostic and predictive value of KRAS mutation status and mutation subtype in patients with non-small cell lung cancer treated with epidermal growth factor receptor tyrosine kinase inhibitors. *J Thorac Oncol*. 2016;11(3):312–323.

114. Kelly K, Altorki NK, Eberhardt WE, et al. Adjuvant erlotinib versus placebo in patients with stage IB–IIIA non-small-cell lung cancer (RADIANT): a randomized, double-blind, phase III trial. *J Clin Oncol*. 2015;33(34):4007–4014.

169. Shepherd FA, Domerg C, Hainaut P, et al. Pooled analysis of the prognostic and predictive effects of KRAS mutation status and KRAS mutation subtype in early-stage resected non-small-cell lung cancer in four trials of adjuvant chemotherapy. *J Clin Oncol*. 2013;31(17):2173–2181.

175. Chae YK, Pan A, Davis AA, et al. Biomarkers for PD-1/PD-L1 blockade therapy in non-small-cell lung cancer: is PD-L1 expression a good marker for patient selection? *Clin. Lung Cancer*. 17(5):350–361.

178. Patel SP, Kurzrock R. PD-L1 expression as a predictive biomarker in cancer immunotherapy. *Mol Cancer Ther*. 2015;14(4):847–856.

200. Barlesi F, Mazieres J, Merlio JP, et al. Routine molecular profiling of patients with advanced non-small-cell lung cancer: results of a 1-year nationwide programme of the French Cooperative Thoracic Intergroup (IFCT). *Lancet*. 2016;387(10026):1415–1426.

See Expertconsult.com for full list of references.

19 Management of Small Histologic and Cytologic Specimens in the Molecular Era

Anjali Saqi and David F. Yankelevitz

SUMMARY OF KEY POINTS

- Techniques for the optimal triage and preparation of small specimens for diagnosis and ancillary studies are provided.
- For optimal results, a standardized protocol and algorithm should be implemented in the laboratory.
- Various factors determine the decision to perform a core-needle biopsy or fine-needle aspiration, including operator and pathologist preference, availability of rapid onsite evaluation, risk of complications such as pneumothorax or hemorrhage, the possibility of tumor cell seeding, the type of lesion (epithelial or spindle cell), and the lesion's location and size.
- Optimal use of a specimen requires appropriate handling and triage, with attention to both the quantity and quality of the specimen.
- Several measures can ensure that there is sufficient material in cores and cell blocks and that the tissue is not exhausted; the interventionalist should perform a gross examination of the specimen.
- In 2011, changes were made to the classification of adenocarcinoma to emphasize the interrelation of the tumor's clinical, radiographic, and molecular characteristics.
- Cytologic preparations are important; each preparation is unique, and taken together, they offer complementary information that can be valuable in rendering a diagnosis.
- Smearing requires technical skill that is not always available or optimal.
- Cell blocks have been recommended instead of smears for use in ancillary tests by the College of American Pathologists/International Association for the Study of Lung Cancer/Association for Molecular Pathology (CAAP/IASLC/AMP) guidelines; yet despite the usefulness of cell blocks, there is no standardized procedure for processing them.
- Methods for the management of small biopsy samples in patients with lung cancer will improve in the future in order to maximize the use of material for diagnosis.

Lung cancer is the leading cause of cancer-related deaths worldwide, despite knowledge of the primary etiologic factor (tobacco use) and advances in identifying underlying mechanisms, detecting mutations, and developing new treatments.[1] At one time, treatment selection depended on distinguishing small cell lung cancer (SCLC) from nonsmall cell lung cancer (NSCLC), but histologic subtyping of NSCLC has become increasingly important for selecting therapy. The addition of targeted therapies to the armamentarium for lung cancer necessitates testing for the presence of particular key driver mutations in lung adenocarcinomas to determine if a patient is eligible for a targeted therapy.

Small histologic and cytologic specimens obtained by core-needle biopsy and fine-needle aspiration are increasingly common.[2,3] Use of computed tomography (CT), endobronchial ultrasound (EBUS), endoscopic ultrasound, and electromagnetic navigational bronchoscopy has enabled the collection of small specimens for more patients through minimally invasive procedures, replacing traditional methods for obtaining specimens, such as mediastinoscopy, video-assisted thoracoscopic surgery, and thoracotomy. Less invasive small specimen collection is especially useful for patients with advanced-stage cancer, nonsurgical diseases such as granuloma, or fibrosis after previous surgery, as well as for patients who are poor surgical candidates or who are undergoing restaging.[4] In some cases, only small specimens are obtainable.

Small samples present a challenge: although the quantity of sample tissue being obtained is much smaller, the information required from the sample has increased substantially. In the past, little importance was placed on triaging small biopsy or cytologic specimens; however, now that treatment decisions are based on the histologic subtype and molecular profile of NSCLC, triaging the small specimens that comprise most or all of the diagnostic tissue has become crucial.[5] A poorly managed specimen may preclude an accurate diagnosis. For patients with NSCLC, it is necessary to have sufficient tissue for ancillary studies, such as immunohistochemistry (IHC) and/or molecular tests, to determine treatment. Appropriate management is also necessary for cases that are not NSCLC.

The shift to using small specimens for diagnosis has created a practice gap, because limited guidance is available for the management of small specimens (Fig. 19.1).[6,7] An optimal algorithm would define the steps for appropriate triage and processing of tissue to select a course of treatment. It would provide for a tissue reserve for identifying novel predictive biomarkers and suggest personalized therapies. Testing for mutations is likely to increase, and access to sufficient tissue will be crucial.

Specimens obtained by surgical biopsy are typically placed in formalin at the time of acquisition and then processed in the laboratory; this procedure rarely varies, and formalin fixation and hematoxylin and eosin staining are standard. The handling of cytologic specimens, especially fine-needle aspirates, is much less standardized. A number of methods are available to prepare and fix fine-needle aspirates after the collection procedure and in the laboratory. Several stains (Diff-Quik, Papanicolaou, hematoxylin and eosin, and ultra-fast Papanicolaou stains), slide preparations (smear, cytospin, ThinPrep, and SurePath), cell block processing methods (at least 10 homebrews and automated processing), and fixatives (saline, alcohol-based, formalin, Roswell Park Memorial Institute [RPMI] culture medium, and CytoRich) are used.[8] Furthermore, specimens are not triaged uniformly according to a protocol. Together, these factors produce inconsistent results across laboratories.

For optimal results, a standardized protocol and algorithm should be implemented in the laboratory. Along with improvements in tissue preservation, triaging the sample at the time of the procedure is increasingly important. In an ideal scenario, an interventionalist would collect a specimen according to a well-defined protocol. A cytologist—preferably someone onsite—would immediately assess the specimen's adequacy, confirming the presence of diagnostic material and determining if there is enough material for any necessary ancillary studies. The interventionalist

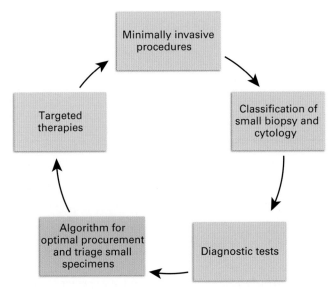

Fig. 19.1. The absence of a standardized algorithm for optimal procurement, processing, and triaging of small specimens has created a practice gap.

and the cytologist should communicate with each other at the time of the procedure, and the objectives of the sampling procedure should be specified to the extent possible. For example, if the initial small sample is needed only to confirm a diagnosis of malignant disease before definitive removal of the tumor, it is unnecessary to obtain additional samples because samples needed for advanced diagnostic studies could be obtained later during the surgical resection.

Techniques for the optimal triage and preparation of small specimens for diagnosis and ancillary studies are outlined in this chapter.

CORE-NEEDLE BIOPSY VERSUS FINE-NEEDLE ASPIRATION

The decision to perform a core-needle biopsy or fine-needle aspiration depends on various factors, including operator and pathologist preference, availability of rapid onsite evaluation (ROSE), risk of complications such as pneumothorax or hemorrhage, the possibility of tumor cell seeding, the type of lesion (epithelial or spindle cell), and the lesion's location and size.[9] To date, there has been no consensus on the preferred method. Critics of fine-needle aspiration question whether it is possible to obtain sufficient material for molecular diagnosis with this technique.[10,11] In contrast, proponents of cytologic specimens cite evidence that sampling different areas of a neoplasm with fine-needle aspiration is superior to using core-needle biopsy to obtain a specimen from a single area.[12,13] In a study published in 2012, it was reported that fine-needle aspiration and core-needle biopsy performed with ROSE provide equivalent results in terms of diagnosing a specific malignancy and obtaining sufficient material for ancillary studies (e.g., IHC and molecular testing) to guide tumor-specific treatment.[14] Lastly, molecular testing results showed 100% concordance between cytologic samples obtained by fine-needle aspiration and histologic resections obtained by core-needle biopsy.[15]

Some pathologists advocate a sequential approach to obtaining small specimens, namely, initial use of fine-needle aspiration followed by core-needle biopsy, if additional tissue is necessary.[13] Improved results have been demonstrated in studies in which fine-needle aspiration and core-needle biopsy are used together compared with either procedure alone.[16–18] A combined approach may be feasible for transthoracic CT-guided biopsy with use of a coaxial needle, which permits acquisition of either type of specimen while minimizing the number of punctures.[3]

The two methods of obtaining small specimens may provide complementary information. For this reason, reviewing cases with paired cytologic and histologic specimens can be useful in rendering a specific and concordant diagnosis and minimizing the number of diagnoses of NSCLC not otherwise specified that can result from having samples with poor differentiation or scant cellularity.[12,19,20]

Navigational Bronchoscopy for Sample Collection

With navigational bronchoscopy, a sample can be collected with either aspiration or core-needle biopsy forceps. Little has been published comparing the cellular yield of each method. In one study, it was reported that catheter aspiration was associated with a higher diagnostic yield than biopsy.[21] The authors hypothesized that the back-and-forth motion of the catheter and the aspiration enabled access to target cells that may not be accessible by forceps biopsy. When both sampling procedures are going to be performed, experience has shown that it is better to conduct the aspiration first because doing so produces a less bloody sample without diluting the cells of interest.

RAPID ONSITE EVALUATION

Advantages

One of the most effective ways to ensure appropriate management of fine-needle aspiration is with ROSE, which involves working with an experienced cytopathologist or cytotechnologist in an adjacent room at the time of the procedure.[3] Several studies have demonstrated the usefulness of ROSE in optimizing the yield and efficiency of fine-needle aspiration and increasing its diagnostic accuracy.[22–27]

Onsite assessment has many advantages. First, it is an integrated approach to diagnosis. The cytologist obtains the pertinent history and can correlate the morphologic features with clinical findings and imaging study results. A preliminary evaluation and diagnosis is valuable in patient management. For instance, when treatment is urgent or patients have travelled far for care, processing can be initiated when the sample arrives in the laboratory.[7] Appointments with clinicians involved in treatment can be scheduled, and additional imaging studies or laboratory tests can be performed without delay.

By providing real-time feedback, ROSE decreases the number of false-negative diagnoses, which usually result from sampling error by the interventionalist.[3,19] Well-defined sampling protocols for obtaining specimens may minimize false-negative results; an example is requiring documentation of the needle tip in the lesion. Sparse cellularity obscured by blood, inflammation, or foreign material in a cytologic specimen can contribute to false-negative results.[19] When an onsite cytologist determines that the specimen is inadequate, a second sample can be obtained during the same session rather than having the patient return for another procedure.

Although imaging provides guidance and confirmation of the needle's placement in the target, the needle may inadvertently catch nonneoplastic cells or elements as it traverses through other tissues. Many times a specimen obtained by EBUS biopsy appears grossly diagnostic but consists of bronchial cells, macrophages, mucus, cartilage, or blood clot.[7] With CT-guided sampling of pleural-based lesions, mesothelial cells may be the main cellular component. A core may consist mostly of necrotic tissue or clotted blood. In the absence of ROSE, these samples may be misinterpreted as diagnostic specimens.

ROSE confirms the presence of adequate viable, nonnecrotic tissue. In a setting without ROSE, additional dedicated passes are

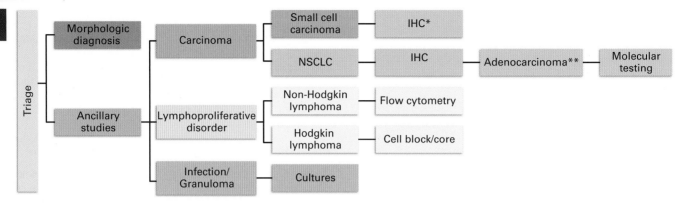

Fig. 19.2. Small specimens can be triaged for ancillary studies using this algorithm. *Perform IHC to confirm diagnosis, if necessary. **Perform molecular testing on carcinomas with adenocarcinoma or when a component of adenocarcinoma cannot entirely be excluded. *IHC*, immunohistochemistry; *NSCLC*, nonsmall cell lung cancer.

needed to increase the likelihood of a definitive diagnosis. Relative to a protocol that requires a fixed number of passes, immediate assessment with ROSE may mean fewer passes are necessary. Avoiding unnecessary passes decreases the duration of anesthesia or sedation and reduces potential morbidity. Benefits of shorter biopsy time include rapid turnover of the procedure room and imaging facilities and fewer repeat procedures, resulting in cost savings.[28–30]

With ROSE, the cytologist also is involved in the adequate preparation and triage of specimens. Based on the preliminary assessment, the specimen can be allocated for IHC or molecular testing for carcinomas, microbiologic cultures in cases of inflammation or granulomas, or flow cytometry for lymphoma assessment (Fig. 19.2).[31]

A biopsy or aspiration may be performed to determine whether a lymph node is negative for carcinoma, infection, or lymphoma; this scenario is common during EBUS staging procedures. With ROSE, a cytologist is able to assess whether the specimen is representative of a lymph node and whether a sufficient number of lymphocytes have been included to prevent a false-negative diagnosis and increase the negative predictive value.[24,32,33]

A well-prepared specimen expedites final examination by limiting the number of intradepartmental second opinions, consults, and deliberation necessitated by sparse cellularity, poor preparation, or artifacts; instead, cytologists can focus their attention on diagnostic dilemmas. When ROSE and the final interpretation are performed by the same cytologist, less time is required overall because a portion of the specimen has already been previewed.[7]

Disadvantages

Experience and training are necessary to prepare smears, assess a sample, and triage the specimen, and not all institutions have the resources or personnel to provide ROSE. ROSE can be time consuming: in addition to the procedure time, travel time to and from the procedure site can be substantial for large institutions or offsite practices. Given the time required for ROSE, reimbursement is low, and a pathologist can generate greater revenue and relative value units by examining slides under a microscope in his or her office.

Algorithm for Processing Small Samples

No standardized algorithm exists for processing small specimens, and few methods have been outlined.[6,34] The goal of processing small specimens is to preserve as much material as possible for molecular testing, especially for patients with advanced lung adeno cancer.[19,35] Ideally, each institution should engage a

multidisciplinary team and determine best practices for managing small specimens.[19] An algorithm and ROSE were used together to obtain sufficient cytologic material by EBUS-guided transbronchial needle aspiration for reflex molecular testing in 93% of patients with adenocarcinoma (Fig. 19.3 and Box 19.1).[6,36]

MANAGING SMALL SAMPLES WITHOUT RAPID ONSITE EVALUATION

When ROSE is not possible, there are some strategies to facilitate good management of samples obtained with fine-needle aspiration, although no standardized protocols exist. Interventionalists can prepare slides for the pathologist's review, either at the time of the procedure or afterward.[3] Telepathology, in which a pathologist views prepared slides from a remote location, may be an alternative to ROSE.[37] As technology improves, the role of telepathology is likely to increase, although additional studies are needed to determine best practices. Neither of these approaches ensures that an adequate specimen has been procured for ancillary testing or that the specimen will be triaged appropriately, however.

Performing a fixed number of aspirates per site (e.g., three) and a dedicated pass for cell block preparation or ancillary studies can enhance the cellular yield.[38,39] However, additional samples cannot always be obtained, especially when doing so poses an increased risk to the patient. To minimize suboptimal smearing and specimen use, the specimen can be placed directly into a fixative for liquid-based cytologic examination, or a cell block can be prepared; the usefulness of this technique has not been formally studied, though. Above all, it is essential to define a process for handling specimens in coordination with the cytopathology laboratory.

OPTIMIZATION AND TRIAGE

Optimal use of a specimen requires appropriate handling and triage, with attention to both the quantity and quality of the specimen.[3] Even in the presence of abundant tissue, poor preparation and allocation can preclude definitive diagnosis and ancillary studies.

Optimization

Slide Preparation for Fine-Needle Aspirate

It is necessary to prepare only enough smears to make a diagnosis; the preparation of excessive smears can leave insufficient tissue for ancillary studies.[36] Ideally for ROSE, only two smears should be prepared per pass: one air-dried for Diff-Quik staining and the

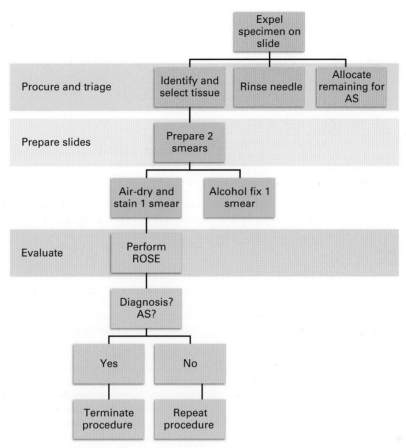

Fig. 19.3. The algorithm for optimizing samples obtained using fine-needle aspiration with rapid onsite evaluation is divided into three stages: (1) specimen procurement and triage, (2) slide preparation, and (3) tissue evaluation for diagnosis and assessment of sample adequacy for ancillary studies, if necessary. *AS,* ancillary studies; *ROSE,* rapid onsite evaluation.

BOX 19.1 Steps for Processing Fine-Needle Aspirate

1. For each pass of the needle, expel the specimen onto a single slide with a syringe. (Fig. 19.3).
   a. If clotting prevents the material from being expelled, use a stylet to dislodge the specimen.
2. Identify diagnostic tissue particles, often tan or white specks but may vary depending on the nature of the lesion (e.g., mucoid material in cases of a mucinous carcinoma), and select them with the corner of a second slide (Fig. 19.5).
   a. When there is significant clot formation, gently press the specimen in between two slides to identify tissue particles.
   b. A scant sample may allow for preparation of only one or two smears.
3. For each pass, prepare two smears from the selected tissue particles (Fig. 19.5).
   a. Air-dry one smear and stain with Diff-Quik, or similar method, for ROSE.
   b. Fix one smear in alcohol for Papanicolaou staining in the laboratory.
4. Flush the needle and/or syringe to remove any remaining cells.
   a. For CT-guided aspirations, rinse the needle and syringe in CytoLyt (or another preservative used by the laboratory).
   b. For EBUS and/or EUS fine-needle aspiration, pass approximately 0.5 cc to 1 cc of saline through the needle into CytoLyt (or other preservative used by the laboratory).
5. Place the remaining specimen in media appropriate for ancillary studies and/or cell block preparation.
   a. Cell blocks can be made by allowing the specimen to clot on the expelled slide for a few minutes and then placing it into formalin. (Partial) clotting simplifies cell block processing.
   b. Separate diagnostic material or more cellular elements from nondiagnostic ones (e.g., passes containing mostly blood) to prevent specimen dilution and improve the cellular yield of cell blocks.
6. Perform ROSE.
   a. Is there sufficient material for diagnosis?
      i. If not, repeat steps 1–5.
      ii. If yes, and ancillary studies are needed, determine whether the specimen includes sufficient material.
      iii. If no, perform dedicated passes for ancillary studies.
      iv. If yes, end the procedure.

CT, computed tomography; *EBUS,* endobronchial ultrasound; *EUS,* endoscopic ultrasound; *ROSE,* rapid onsite evaluation.

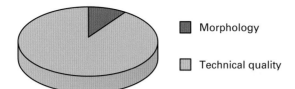

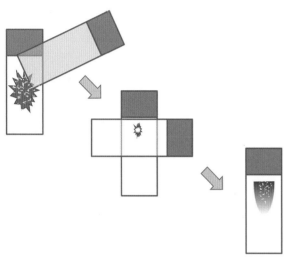

Fig. 19.4. Optimal tissue use involves preparing smears of selected tissue particles, which are stained with Diff-Quik and Papanicolaou stains, and then placing excess material in media for ancillary studies, if needed. With suboptimal preparation, slides are thick and bloody and contain clots, and the specimen is spread across almost the entire slide surface. Suboptimal preparation obscures cellular detail, hinders accurate interpretation of slides, and may leave inadequate material for ancillary studies.

Fig. 19.5. To prepare a smear, select a tissue particle with the corner of a slide. Place the tissue on a clean slide and smear, holding the second slide perpendicularly.

second fixed in alcohol for Papanicolaou staining. Any remaining material can be allocated for cell block preparation or other ancillary studies (Fig. 19.4). It is preferable to avoid thick smears. Not only do thin, even smears minimize tissue expenditure, they also allow for better visualization of diagnostic cells. Excess material and clots can be placed in a fixative or medium, which may obviate the need for additional passes for ancillary studies.

Use of excessive pressure when making the smears can create artifacts that hinder interpretation and lead to misdiagnosis. Slides should be placed perpendicular, rather than parallel, to each other to create smears with a concentration of specimen at the top and thin distribution below for easy visualization (Fig. 19.5).

Touch Preparation for Core-Needle Biopsy Specimens

The value of touch preparation for specimens obtained by core-needle biopsy is the subject of ongoing debate. Proponents argue that onsite touch preparation of CT-guided core biopsy specimens has been associated with greater diagnostic accuracy, because it guides the radiologist in obtaining additional cores needed for diagnosis and, possibly, molecular testing.[3,31] Critics note that the lesional cells may be transferred to the touch preparation, leaving only normal tissue on the histologic sections of the core.[31]

Gentle handling of the core can prevent cellular loss.[31] Typically, cores are thin and delicate. They dry rapidly and substantial

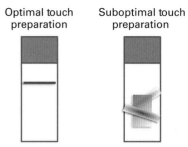

Fig. 19.6. For optimal touch preparation, gently touch the core to the slide once or twice. If the core adheres to the slide, lift it with a needle and place it in the appropriate medium for fixation or transport. A smear can be prepared from a touch preparation with excessive tissue or liquid. In suboptimal touch preparations, the core is smeared or rubbed onto a slide, which can result in crush artifact and the transfer of a significant portion of lesional cells onto the slide, hindering final interpretation and compromising the core.

manipulation can cause them to fragment. Touching the core on a slide once or twice while it is still in the sheath yields the best results (Fig. 19.6). If excessive material is transferred to the slide, it can be smeared with a second slide to distribute the cells thinly.

Preparing a touch preparation for Papanicolaou stain can be challenging. Even if the slide is touched rapidly and immediately placed in alcohol, the slide may have air-drying artifacts. Artifacts can be minimized by hydrating the slide with a few drops of normal saline, which is available in syringes, for a few minutes. Placing a slide hydrated in this manner in alcohol salvages the nuclear features. This technique can also be applied to fine-needle aspirate smears when there is a delay in alcohol fixation.

Processing Core-Needle Biopsy Specimens and Cell Blocks

Several measures can ensure that there is sufficient material in cores and cell blocks and that the tissue is not exhausted. For example, the interventionalist should perform a gross examination of the specimen. It is important to determine whether the core represents a solid piece of tan-white tissue, which is typical of neoplasms. Sometimes the specimen consists mainly of red blood cell clot, mucus, liquefied necrotic inflammatory tissue, or bronchial cell contamination.[36] In this case, additional tissue is likely necessary.

Obtaining more cores increases the likelihood of having sufficient tissue for ancillary testing. At the time of publication, no guidelines are available to suggest a minimum number of cores. However, if feasible and accessible without substantial risk to the patient, one to four cores from 18- to 20-gauge core needles can yield sufficient tissue for mutational analysis.[40–42] Placing no more than three fragments or a single core in a single histology cassette hedges against inadvertent trimming of one block by leaving others available for ancillary testing if necessary (Fig. 19.7).[19] The consequences of excessive facing of the block should also be communicated to the histotechnologists cutting the blocks.

Tissue is lost during routine trimming processes in histology laboratories. To minimize this loss, 10 to 20 blank slides can be cut for core biopsy specimens and cell blocks at the onset.[19] Although this practice may reduce the risk of having insufficient tissue, some of the cut slides may go unused.[35]

Immunohistochemistry

When using IHC to distinguish between adenocarcinoma and squamous cell carcinoma, a limited panel should be performed in a stepwise fashion. For example, in case of a suspected primary

- Create >1 block when possible
  - Core biopsies
    - Divide cores/fragments into multiple cassettes
  - Cell blocks
    - Exfoliative and FNA specimens
      - Divide excess tissue into multiple cassettes
    - FNAs with ROSE
      - Separate passes with scant diagnostic tissue from those with abundant blood lacking lesional tissue
- Minimize loss of tissue while trimming/facing paraffin block
  - ROSE
    - Order blank slides for ancillary studies up front
  - No ROSE
    - Cut blanks and/or save intervening levels up front
    - Following H&E evaluation and at time of IHC order, request blanks
- Limit one section per slide*

Fig. 19.7. Core biopsy and cell block management in the laboratory. Whenever possible, create more than one tissue block for core biopsies and cells blocks. If one tissue block is exhausted, an additional one(s) is available for ancillary studies. In cases of FNAs, separating passes with scant diagnostic tissue or mostly blood from those with diagnostic tissue can prevent dilution of the cell block. Limit trimming and facing of the paraffin blocks to avoid inadvertent loss of tissue. In cases with ROSE, blank slides can be ordered up front. By limiting one section to a slide, greater numbers of slides are available, as when a broader immunohistochemical panel is required in case of an unknown primary or metastasis. *FNAs*, Fine needle aspirations; *H&E*, hematoxylin and eosin; *IHC*, immunohistochemical; *ROSE,* rapid onsite evaluation.

lung carcinoma, a combination of p40 and thyroid transcription factor-1 may be sufficient to distinguish between squamous cell carcinoma and lung adenocarcinoma, respectively. This approach helps to ensure that tissue remains for molecular diagnosis in cases of lung adenocarcinoma.[43,44]

Molecular Testing

For patients with stage IV adenocarcinomas for whom therapy is suitable, testing for mutation of the epidermal growth factor receptor (*EGFR*) gene or rearrangement of the anaplastic lymphoma kinase (*ALK*) gene is the standard of care and should be ordered at the time of diagnosis.[35] More recently, the US Food and Drug Administration approved Ventana anti-ALK(D5F3) IHC, which is 90.9% and 99.8% sensitive and specific, respectively.[45] Even in the presence of an *EGFR* mutation or *ALK* rearrangement—for which targeted therapies are available—life expectancy is relatively short, and it is important to obtain sufficient tissue during the initial collection procedure and triage it appropriately to avoid repeat procedures.[35] Similarly, when EBUS is performed to stage and diagnose NSCLC simultaneously, the sample should be managed especially carefully. Dedicated passes improve the yield of the specimen.[46] Making an additional pass can be difficult for a number of reasons, including the inability of the patient to tolerate the procedure, risk of a pneumothorax, difficulty reaching the target, or lack of time or willingness.[46]

The number of cells necessary for *EGFR* molecular testing depends on a few factors, including the absolute number of cells, the proportion of tumor cells to nonneoplastic cells, the sensitivity of the methodology, and sample enrichment with microdissection. Per published guidelines, the method should be sufficiently sensitive to detect *EGFR* mutation in a sample with 50% tumor content; however, a method that can identify a mutation in a

sample with 10% neoplastic cells is ideal.[35] The minimum number of cells needed for EGFR molecular testing ranges from 50 to 400, with variation due to the sensitivity of the method and usage of microdissection to isolate neoplastic cells from others.[47,48]

Guidelines published in 2013 recommend that results of molecular testing be available within 10 days after the specimen is received in the molecular pathology laboratory.[35] Reflex testing is one way to expedite molecular testing results, but there are disadvantages. The drawbacks include performing additional fine-needle aspirations or core-needle biopsies, testing patients who have earlier stage localized cancer at the time of diagnosis, testing patients who may not be candidates for tyrosine kinase inhibitors (for example, because the cancer is advanced and the patient desires only palliative care), and conducting molecular testing when a larger resection is expected.[35]

In staging procedures for adenocarcinomas that have been previously diagnosed with IHC and molecular testing, the presence of tumor cells in a single sample is sufficient for molecular testing, especially if a patient cannot tolerate additional procedures to obtain biopsy specimens or aspirations.[7]

Adding Radiography for Evaluation of Adenocarcinomas

In 2011, changes were made to the classification of adenocarcinoma to emphasize the interrelation of the tumor's clinical, radiographic, and molecular characteristics. Given this evolution in adenocarcinoma classification, information from imaging studies often is used in conjunction with histologic evidence for the most accurate diagnosis.

Two of the new classifications are adenocarcinoma in situ (AIS; defined as localized adenocarcinoma 3 cm or less, with a pure lepidic pattern and without stromal, vascular, or pleural invasion) and minimally invasive carcinoma (MIA; defined as adenocarcinoma 3 cm or less, with a predominant lepidic pattern and invasion that is 5 mm or less, and without necrosis or lymph node, blood vessel, or pleural invasion).[2] Nonsolid and solid areas on a CT image correlate with lepidic and invasive (e.g., acinar) patterns, respectively, on histologic examination. Correlating a lepidic growth pattern on specimens collected using core-needle biopsy with the CT images may facilitate better assessment of the tumor. Aspirates taken from adenocarcinomas with a predominantly lepidic pattern have sheets of relatively bland-appearing cells, which may be accompanied by intranuclear grooves and invaginations.

When it is not possible to determine whether the cytologic sample shows hyperplasia or early cancer in a lepidic pattern, cross-referencing the image can be helpful. Larger lesion size and the presence of a solid component in the lesion outside of the area that may have been sampled virtually rule out hyperplasia.[49] A lepidic pattern may be recognized more easily on cell block sections, in which bland-appearing cells are seen as strips of cells.[22] The evaluation of the cell block is helpful because cells from MIA or AIS can be misinterpreted as benign.[14]

Triage
Carcinomas

In the case of carcinomas, smears should have enough material to render a diagnosis of SCLC or NSCLC. Any remaining material should be allocated for cell block preparation to be used in subclassification. A limited number of IHC stains can establish histologic subtype, especially in cases of poorly differentiated NSCLC.[12,49] For NSCLC, particularly in advanced stages, if adenocarcinoma is present or cannot entirely be excluded, an effort should be made to preserve as much tissue as possible for molecular analysis.[5]

Lymphoproliferative Disorders

Use of fine-needle aspirates to diagnose lymphoma is controversial.[7] Arguably, it can be difficult to obtain tissue from patients with nodular sclerosing Hodgkin lymphoma.[50] Although it is not possible to assess cell architecture in specimens obtained by fine-needle aspiration, aspirates can confirm recurrence in patients with a history of lymphoma.[50] They can also provide tissue to determine the cause of the underlying lymphadenopathy, obviating the need for an invasive procedure in the absence of a neoplastic process.

If clinical or morphologic evidence leads to suspicion of non-Hodgkin lymphoma, material should be obtained for flow cytometry. The sample should be placed into RPMI culture medium or saline. Some institutions routinely place samples in these media, especially in the absence of ROSE, so that flow cytometry can be performed, if necessary. Flow cytometry cannot be performed on alcohol- or formalin-fixed tissues.

Two or three dedicated passes for flow cytometry are recommended when lymphoma is suspected or ROSE is not available.[50] Adequacy of the sample can be ascertained by examining the saline or RPMI culture medium for clarity or cloudiness. In the absence of a bloody specimen, cloudiness indicates cellularity. Specimens obtained by core-needle biopsy and placed in RPMI culture medium or saline can be assessed the same way. A sample placed in RPMI culture medium can be sent for culture if further review of the slides leads the pathologist to suspect infection.

Infectious Processes and Granulomas

Small histologic specimens and aspirates play an important role in diagnosing nonneoplastic processes, including granulomas and infections. In fact, EBUS biopsy is used frequently for diagnosing sarcoidosis.[49] For patients with a disease of confirmed or suspected infectious etiology or a granuloma, a sample should be sent for microbiologic cultures to exclude the presence of organisms.[51,52] Material also should be reserved to perform special stains in the laboratory. Depending on the amount of material available, the syringe can be capped and sent directly to the lab, or the material can be expelled into sterile saline and then transported. Within each institution, a standardized approach to managing these samples should be developed jointly by pathologists and microbiologists.

CYTOLOGIC PREPARATIONS

Familiarity with the various cytologic preparations is important. Each preparation is unique; taken together they offer complementary information that can be valuable in rendering a diagnosis.

Diff-Quik Stain

The Diff-Quik stain is ideal for ROSE because it can be performed rapidly on smears and uses only three solutions. For diagnostic tissue, it enables assessment of the origin of cells—lymphoid (mostly single cells) or epithelial (mostly cohesive clusters)—and subtyping of the epithelial cells as either squamous or glandular based on cytoplasmic characteristics. Keratinizing squamous cells typically have dense, blue, and homogeneous cytoplasm, whereas the cytoplasm of glandular cells is often vacuolated or foamy. In addition, Diff-Quik stain highlights mucus and metachromatic stroma, which are key features associated with certain neoplasms, such as mucinous or colloid carcinomas and hamartomas, respectively.[53]

Allowing the tissue to dry completely is a crucial step in preparing a Diff-Quik smear. Staining a partially dried slide masks cellular detail, limits the evaluation of sample adequacy, and possibly leads to misinterpretation.

Papanicolaou Stain

A Papanicolaou stain is typically performed in the laboratory on alcohol-fixed slides. This stain reveals nuclear details—membrane irregularities, chromatin pattern, and intranuclear invaginations—important for establishing a diagnosis of malignancy, especially well-differentiated neoplasms that lack significant pleomorphism. The stain also shows the speckled—or so-called salt and pepper—chromatin pattern associated with neuroendocrine differentiation. Most important, the Papanicolaou stain highlights keratinizing squamous cells, which have orange or pink cytoplasm. This finding is specific for squamous cells and precludes the need for immunostaining to distinguish between cells of squamous and glandular origin.[20]

Unlike a Diff-Quik slide that has to be dried completely before staining, a slide for Papanicolaou staining must be placed in alcohol immediately. Any delay in fixation results in air-drying artifacts (e.g., cellular enlargement and loss of nuclear detail) that create challenges in interpretation and possibly prevent a definitive diagnosis. Air-drying artifacts can also lead to misdiagnosis because the cells may take on an orange hue, mimicking squamous differentiation. Spray fixation is an alternative to placing the slide in a jar of alcohol, although the spray has a tendency to aggregate cells in distinct colonies rather than maintain the even distribution of the smear.

Liquid-Based Preparations

A combination of well-prepared and properly fixed Diff-Quik–stained and Papanicolaou-stained smears are used most commonly to evaluate cytologic specimens. However, smearing requires technical skill that is not always available or optimal. For these reasons—and to limit obstruction from blood, inflammation, and debris—liquid-based preparations are a standardized alternative for slide preparation.

The two most frequently used methods are ThinPrep (Hologic, Inc., Bedford, MA, USA) and SurePath (BD [Becton, Dickinson and Company] Diagnostics, Franklin Lakes, NJ, USA). At the time of collection, the specimen is placed in an alcohol-based solution (e.g., CytoLyt [Hologic] or SurePath vial), which serves as a fixative and transport medium. This fixative can be used for fine-needle aspirates and other exfoliative specimens, including fluids, brushings, and lavages. In the laboratory, an automated processor homogenizes the specimen and prepares a slide with uniform cell distribution and no cell loss, while minimizing background blood, inflammation, mucus, and debris that could obscure the cells of interest. The slides are then stained with Papanicolaou stain. Provided that the sample is sufficient, additional slides with similar content can be prepared for ancillary studies.

Liquid-based preparations have several drawbacks. The equipment and supplies needed to use liquid-based preparations are additional costs. Because these specimens are fixed in alcohol rather than formalin—the preservative typically used for histologic specimens—a laboratory may need to conduct tests to validate the results of ancillary studies, particularly IHC. The automated processing of liquid-based preparations precludes their use for ROSE. Because the slide preparation technique differs from the preparation of conventional smears, there is a learning curve for interpreting liquid-based cytologic specimens. In particular, SCLC and granulomas often pose diagnostic challenges when liquid-based preparation is used. SCLC appears as dyshesive cells with subtle nuclear molding. Granulomas may also have disassociated cells.

Fixation and Considerations for Ancillary Testing

Several fixatives and transport media are available for cytology specimens, including saline, RPMI culture medium, CytoLyt, SurePath medium, and formalin, each of which has benefits and drawbacks. For instance, flow cytometry analysis only can be conducted on a specimen placed in saline or RPMI culture medium. Formalin is the standard fixative for histologic specimens, and it is the medium on which most laboratory tests are validated.

In their joint guidelines, the College of American Pathologists, International Association for the Study of Lung Cancer, and the Association for Molecular Pathology (CAP/IASLC/AMP) recommend using formalin-fixed (10% neutral buffered), alcohol-fixed (70% ethanol), fresh, or frozen specimens after validation for *EGFR* mutation testing.[35] The advantage of using formalin- or alcohol-fixed tissues embedded in paraffin is that the tumor content and proportion can be assessed. Alcohol fixation may be problematic for fluorescence in situ hybridization testing.[35] Cytologic specimens initially placed in other solutions (i.e., saline or RPMI culture medium) can subsequently be placed in formalin or alcohol. Fixation for 6 to 12 hours is recommended for small specimens.[35]

Other media, such as heavy metal fixatives (e.g., B5, acid zinc formalin, Zenker, B plus) and acidic solutions (e.g., decalcifying solution, Bouin solution), interfere with testing and should be avoided.[35] When sampling bone, performing a fine-needle aspiration instead of a core-needle biopsy is advantageous: fine-needle aspiration extracts the neoplastic cells without collecting bone, which typically would require decalcification that interferes with molecular testing.

Cell Blocks

Cell blocks serve as adjuncts to smears and liquid-based preparations. A cell block is a cohesive pellet formed from dyshesive cells or small tissue fragments that are present in a cytologic specimen. These particles are centrifuged and congealed together into a pellet with agents such as agar, plasma-thrombin, or gelatin.[7] This process requires technical expertise and can be challenging. Following coalescence, the cell blocks are embedded in paraffin and processed like a specimen obtained by biopsy.

Although they do not provide the cytomorphologic details of Papanicolaou-stained slides,[46] cell blocks complement smears and liquid-based preparations. For instance, they show architectural detail of the tissue fragments similar to what is seen in histologic specimens. Most important, they provide material for IHC stains and molecular testing. Cell blocks have been recommended instead of smears for use in ancillary tests by the CAP/IASLC/AMP guidelines. Recent studies have shown that smears provide an alternative source of cells for molecular testing; this is especially useful to minimize repeat procedures.[58,59]

Yet despite the usefulness of cell blocks, there is no standardized procedure for processing them. In a survey, 95 respondents named more than 10 different methods for preparing cell blocks.[8] Forty-four percent of respondents were either unsatisfied or sometimes satisfied with the quality of their cell blocks. Low cellular yield was the leading cause of dissatisfaction. Scant cellularity leads to inconclusive or nondiagnostic results, and a repeat sampling procedure may be necessary.[54] Although no protocols specify the optimal cell block processing technique, some preparations result in greater yield than others.[55,56]

When tissue is abundant, the technique used to prepare the cell block may not play a substantial role in optimizing the sample. However, when tissue is scant, it is crucial to minimize cellular loss during cell block preparation, retaining as much cellular content as possible for ancillary studies. As use of minimally invasive procedures expands in the future and testing for multiple biomarkers in small specimens becomes the standard of care, optimizing cell block preparation will become increasingly relevant.[7,57]

Cell blocks also should be prepared for nonaspirate cytology specimens from patients with suspected lung adenocarcinoma, including pleural effusions, bronchoalveolar lavages, and bronchial brushings.[19]

CONCLUSION

There is no doubt that our methods for the management of small biopsy samples in patients with lung cancer will improve in the future in order to maximize the use of material for diagnosis. In the meantime, all pulmonologists, thoracic surgeons, pathologists, and medical oncologists should be familiar with the limitations of processing at this time and should be able to triage for maximum benefit to their patients. Consensus reports, as described in this chapter, as well as the information provided, will at least establish a standardized method that international community-based as well as academic institutions can follow.

KEY REFERENCES

5. Cagle PT, Allen TC, Dacic S, et al. Revolution in lung cancer: new challenges for the surgical pathologist. *Arch Pathol Lab Med*. 2011;135(1):110–116.
6. Bulman W, Saqi A, Powell CA. Acquisition and processing of endobronchial ultrasound-guided transbronchial needle aspiration specimens in the era of targeted lung cancer chemotherapy. *Am J Respir Crit Care Med*. 2012;185(6):606–611.
8. Crapanzano JP, Heymann JJ, Monaco S, Nassar A, Saqi A. The state of cell block variation and satisfaction in the era of molecular diagnostics and personalized medicine. *Cytojournal*. 2014;11:7.
12. Rekhtman N, Brandt SM, Sigel CS, et al. Suitability of thoracic cytology for new therapeutic paradigms in non-small cell lung carcinoma: high accuracy of tumor subtyping and feasibility of EGFR and KRAS molecular testing. *J Thorac Oncol*. 2011;6(3):451–458.
20. Sigel CS, Moreira AL, Travis WD, et al. Subtyping of non-small cell lung carcinoma: a comparison of small biopsy and cytology specimens. *J Thorac Oncol*. 2011;6(11):1849–1856.
35. Lindeman NI, Cagle PT, Beasley MB, et al. Molecular testing guideline for selection of lung cancer patients for EGFR and ALK tyrosine kinase inhibitors: guideline from the College of American Pathologists, International Association for the Study of Lung Cancer, and Association for Molecular Pathology. *Arch Pathol Lab Med*. 2013;137(6):828–860.
44. Zhang K, Deng H, Cagle PT. Utility of immunohistochemistry in diagnosis of pleuropulmonary and mediastinal cancers: a review and update. *Arch Pathol Lab Med*. 2014;138(12):1611–1628.
45. Marchetti A, Di Lorito A, Pace MV, et al. ALK protein analysis by IHC staining after recent regulatory changes: a comparison of two widely used approaches, revision of the literature, and a new testing algorithm. *J Thorac Oncol*. 2016;11(4):487–495.
56. Balassanian R, Wood GD, Ono JC, Olejnik-Nave J, et al. A superior method for cell block preparation for fine needle aspiration biopsies. *Cancer Cytopathol*. 2016;124:508–518.
58. Knoepp SM, Roh MH. Ancillary techniques on direct-smear aspirate slides: a significant evolution for cytopathology techniques. *Cancer Cytopathol*. 2013;121:120–128.
59. Roy-Chowdhuri S, Goswami RS, Chen H, et al. Factors affecting the success of next-generation sequencing in cytology specimens. *Cancer Cytopathol*. 2015;123:659–668.

See ExpertConsult.com for full list of references.

20 Clinical Presentation and Prognostic Factors in Lung Cancer

Kristiaan Nackaerts, Keunchil Park, Jong-Mu Sun, and Kwun Fong

SUMMARY OF KEY POINTS

- Most people with lung cancer are symptomatic at the time of initial presentation; however, between 5% and 15% of people may be asymptomatic.
- Alarming symptoms for lung cancer like cough, hemoptysis, dyspnea, chest pain and weight loss should be timely recognized.
- No specific clinical manifestations exist to guide and help the physician distinguish between specific histologic subtypes.
- Increased awareness of cough, one of the most common lung cancer symptoms, may help in the earlier detection of lung cancer.
- Hemoptysis is the only symptom that typically causes people to be prompt in reporting to their primary care physician.
- Lung cancer is one of the most common etiologies for a malignant pleural effusion.
- Lung cancer is the cause of superior vena cava syndrome in about 50% of cases.
- Lung cancer is the most common cause of brain metastases.
- Paraneoplastic syndromes are not uncommon in lung cancer and may be the first clinical manifestation of the disease.
- Certain clinical as well as molecular factors may have a potential prognostic and/or predictive role for guiding lung cancer patients' personalized care.

Most people with lung cancer are symptomatic at the time of initial presentation; however, between 5% and 15% of people will be asymptomatic at the time of diagnosis.[1,2] Patients who do have symptoms at the time of diagnosis often have advanced disease and therefore have a poorer prognosis, with an overall 5-year survival rate of 15% or less.[3] In order to improve lung cancer survival, early detection with a screening method should be considered for asymptomatic people at highest risk.[4] Indeed, screening of asymptomatic high-risk individuals (defined as current or former smokers who are aged 55 to 74 years old, with a smoking history of a minimum of 30 pack-years) with use of low-dose computed tomography (CT) has been shown to be efficient not only for diagnosing lung cancer at an early stage but also for substantially reducing lung cancer–specific mortality.[6]

In contrast, people in whom lung cancer is detected during screening trials will usually be asymptomatic because these tumors are usually very small and peripherally located. Outside of screening programs, lung cancer in most asymptomatic people will be diagnosed coincidentally (e.g., on a chest x-ray for other indications or for a preoperative examination). It is of utmost importance for every clinician to be aware of all possible lung cancer symptoms at the time of initial presentation, and not just the so-called alarming symptoms. These alarming symptoms—cough, hemoptysis, dyspnea, chest pain, and weight loss—are mostly a result of local intrathoracic tumor growth, but may be further triggered by local–regional intrathoracic invasive growth and also by the development of extrathoracic metastases (Table 20.1). Timely recognition of alarming symptoms can be difficult because they often develop in older patients (aged 60 years or older) who are current or former smokers and who may also have comorbidities such as chronic obstructive pulmonary disease (COPD) or cardiac disease (e.g., heart failure, angina pectoris).[5] In certain cases of lung cancer, symptoms at presentation may be linked to specific paraneoplastic manifestations that, if unrecognized, may cause diagnostic dilemmas and further delay the diagnosis of lung cancer. The more common symptoms that occur at initial presentation of a person with lung cancer will be further described later in the chapter. Unfortunately, there are no specific clinical manifestations to guide and help the physician distinguish between specific histologic subtypes of lung cancer.[7] Physicians should also consider that as a result of a lung cancer diagnosis, other symptoms may arise that are not addressed in this chapter, including those caused by iatrogenic complications of surgery, systemic treatment or radiotherapy, or other symptoms that may only occur specifically during the end-of-life care of patients with lung cancer. Also addressed are a variety of clinical and molecular factors with potential use for early diagnosis and management of lung cancer, as well as for prognostication.

SYMPTOMS AND SIGNS OF LOCAL TUMOR GROWTH

Cough

One of the most common symptoms related to lung cancer is cough, which is reported in up to 60% to 70% of people at the time of diagnosis.[1,5,8] Increased awareness of cough may help in the earlier detection of lung cancer, resulting in better outcomes, as was demonstrated in a recent United Kingdom Cough Awareness Campaign.[9] Cough is most often caused by larger, centrally located bronchial mucosa invading lung tumors, but may also be present in smaller, peripheral lung tumors. A copious production of thin, colorless sputum (bronchorrhea) may be found in some patients with lung adenocarcinoma with a predominant lepidic growth pattern, but this is rare. Smaller but predominantly endobronchially located lung tumors may also cause cough. This cough may be either dry or nonproductive, but may be productive if respiratory infections occur as a consequence of the obstruction. Because cough is also a predominant symptom in other lung diseases such as COPD, it is sometimes difficult to recognize cough as a presenting symptom of lung cancer. When recording the medical history of the patient, special attention should be given to the changing cough pattern that may occur

TABLE 20.1 Clinical Presenting Symptoms and Signs in Lung Cancer

Asymptomatic
Symptoms caused by local tumor growth
  Cough
  Hemoptysis
  Chest pain
  Dyspnea/stridor
Symptoms caused by local–regional (intrathoracic) invasive growth
  Pleural effusion
  Pericardial effusion
  Hoarseness
  Superior vena cava syndrome
  Dysphagia
  Shoulder pain (Pancoast syndrome)
  Diaphragmatic paralysis
Symptoms due to extrathoracic or metastatic spread
  Metastatic sites in bone, brain, spinal cord, liver, adrenal gland, and
    others
Paraneoplastic symptoms
  Musculoskeletal
  Hematologic
  Vascular
  Endocrinologic
  Neurologic
  Cutaneous
  Miscellaneous

in patients with COPD or active smokers in whom lung cancer develops. The failure of an acute COPD exacerbation to resolve with adequate therapy should raise suspicion of an underlying respiratory malignancy.[10]

Hemoptysis

Hemoptysis is not only a common symptom in up to one-third of people at the time of lung cancer diagnosis, but is also the only symptom that typically causes people to be prompt in reporting to their primary care physician.[1,8,11,12] Approximately 20% of all cases of hemoptysis are associated with lung cancer; therefore, the occurrence of hemoptysis in a patient presenting to a primary care physician should always lead to further investigation, starting with chest x-rays.[7,11] Hemoptysis usually results from tumor necrosis, growth of new blood vessels in and around the tumor (neovascularization), and bronchial mucosa ulceration with erosion and invasion of bronchopulmonary vessels. It may also be caused by an obstructive pneumonia or by paraneoplastic pulmonary embolism. At presentation, hemoptysis may vary from mild (blood-streaked sputum) to moderate and severe blood loss. Fortunately, severe or massive hemoptysis (more than 200 mL of blood expectorated at once or over the course of 24 hours or 5–10 mL/h of blood expectorated over 24 hours) occurs rarely at initial presentation, but it may become an increasingly life-threatening problem during the palliative treatment phase of an advanced lung cancer. Treatment of massive hemoptysis at the time of diagnosis of lung cancer of an unknown stage or of a potentially curable, newly diagnosed lung cancer will require prompt securing of the airways by endotracheal intubation and maintaining of optimal oxygenation before more definitive alleviation of the hemoptysis by either endobronchial therapy or by urgent surgical intervention can be offered.[13] Moderate hemoptysis caused by tumors that cannot be reached by bronchoscope can be treated with bronchial artery embolization. For all other cases of endobronchial tumors causing hemoptysis, several endobronchial therapeutic modalities exist, ranging from photocoagulation with neodymium:yttrium aluminum garnet (Nd:YAG) laser to electrocautery to argon plasma coagulation. For distal or parenchymal-situated unresectable lung tumors, external-beam radiotherapy may be recommended.[14] Endobronchial brachytherapy has been used for the palliative treatment of hemoptysis

caused by endobronchially visible tumors, and the combination of high-dose-rate brachytherapy with external-beam radiotherapy demonstrated better symptom control than with external-beam radiotherapy alone.[15] In a recent Cochrane meta-analysis, external-beam radiotherapy alone was found to be more efficient for palliation compared with endobronchial brachytherapy alone, although there was insufficient evidence to support the superiority of the two modalities combined for palliative symptom relief compared with external-beam radiotherapy alone.[16]

Chest Pain

People with early-stage lung cancer may note vague, persistent chest pain or chest discomfort, even though no invasion of the chest wall, mediastinum, or pleura can be found.[7] The true origin of this pain sensation is not completely understood, as no pain fibers are present in the lung parenchyma. Peribronchial autonomic nerves are able to transmit sensations of discomfort via the vagus nerve, which may also cause rare craniofacial pain sensations in nonmetastatic lung cancers.[17] When further tumor growth occurs with local-regional invasion, such as in the pleura, mediastinum, or chest wall, more severe local pain symptoms may occur, requiring adequate analgesic treatment in combination with tumor-directed therapy.

Dyspnea, Stridor, Wheezing

Dyspnea is a common presenting symptom of lung cancer, occurring in up to 60% of people.[5] The causes of dyspnea are often multifactorial, related to the increasing tumor volume, endobronchial tumor obstruction causing parenchymal atelectasis, lymphangitic tumor spread in a lobe or the entire lung, or pulmonary artery embolism. When lung cancer starts its local–regional invasion into the trachea, pericardium, and pleura, dyspnea may become more severe. Besides the tumor-related causes of dyspnea, there may be other potential aggravating causes, particularly in people with lung cancer who have COPD or cardiac conditions. When a tumor occludes the lower trachea or a major central airway, an acute feeling of breathlessness can occur along with the typical sound of stridor (in cases of severe occlusion of the airway or trachea) or unilateral monophonic wheeze (in cases of left- or right-sided main airway subocclusion).[8,10] Standard treatment of the underlying cancer in people with early-stage or locally or regionally advanced disease will treat the dyspnea as well. For people with more advanced and symptomatic lung cancer, early palliative treatment of dyspnea (home oxygen therapy for hypoxemia, opioids, or inhaled furosemide) should be considered.[18]

SYMPTOMS AND SIGNS OF INVASIVE LOCAL–REGIONAL OR INTRATHORACIC SPREAD

Hoarseness

The left vocal cord is stimulated by the left recurrent laryngeal nerve, which passes deep into the left thoracic cavity and under the aortic arch before again climbing up to the left vocal cord. Enlarged lymph nodes in the aortic pulmonary window or a large, invasive tumor to the left of the aortic branch may cause left recurrent nerve entrapment, resulting in nerve palsy and vocal cord paralysis. This vocal cord paralysis—occurring in fewer than 10% of people with lung cancer—results in hoarseness and sometimes also cough and aspiration.[5] On a combination ^{18}F-2-deoxy-D-glucose (FDG)-positron emission tomography (PET)-CT, the internal laryngeal muscles on the opposite side of the entrapped recurrent laryngeal nerve (usually the left one) may present with false-positive increased FDG uptake because of the compensatory laryngeal muscle activation caused by the contralateral paralyzed vocal cord.[19] Entrapment of the right

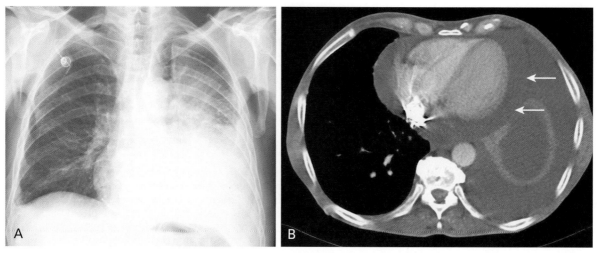

Fig. 20.1. Chest radiography (A) and chest computed tomography image (B) of a nonsmall cell lung cancer, showing a left-sided pleural effusion as well as a pericardial effusion *(white arrows)* in the same patient, caused by a lung adenocarcinoma of the left upper lobe.

recurrent laryngeal nerve by lung tumor tissue occurs much less frequently because this nerve does not extensively run through the right side of the chest.

Pleural Effusion

Lung cancer is one of the most common etiologies for a malignant pleural effusion.[20] Malignant pleural fluid accumulation will eventually develop in 7% to 23% of people with lung cancer, but not all of them will be symptomatic at the time of diagnosis.[21] Patients with a pleural fluid accumulation will generally report dyspnea, cough, chest pain, fatigue, and weight loss. The accumulation of malignant pleural fluid may be by direct invasion of the tumor into the pleura or by metastasis into the pleura (Fig. 20.1). Pleural fluid accumulation may also have other causes in people with lung cancer, and these causes should be excluded: chylothorax by lymphatic obstruction or nonmalignant causes such as heart failure, pleuropulmonary infection, pulmonary infarction, and cirrhosis.[22] Diagnostic thoracocentesis is therefore necessary to document the presence of malignant cells. In 40% to 50% of cases, the results of cytology examination will be false-negative and diagnostic medical thoracoscopy should be done to obtain a new sampling of pleural fluid combined with pleural biopsy to be examined.[23,24] When the pleural effusion is confirmed as malignant, the lung cancer should be classified as stage IV (M1a), which is associated with a poor prognosis.[25] Besides systemic therapy (chemotherapy, targeted therapy), treatment of malignant pleural effusion consists of fluid drainage and pleurodesis. Optimal treatment depends on an individual patient's symptoms, performance status, and prognosis.[26–28] For patients with a very poor prognosis (less than 3 months), repeated thoracenteses may be performed to alleviate dyspnea and pain. However, for most patients with lung cancer, a more definitive therapy for the malignant pleural effusion should be planned, either by talc slurry instillation via chest tube, thoracoscopy, or by insertion of an indwelling pleural catheter. The latter procedure is necessary in the event of lung entrapment by widespread pleural involvement.

Pericardial Effusion

Pericardial effusion occurs in 5% to 10% of people with lung cancer (Fig. 20.1). Pericardial invasion by malignant cells occurs either by direct tumor invasion or by hematogenous or lymphatic spread of cancer cells.[5] Patients who have pericardial effusion at presentation will either be asymptomatic (with only

radiographic documentation of the presence of pericardial fluid) or they will report symptoms such as increasing dyspnea (up to grade 3/4), orthopnea, anxiety, palpitations, and retrosternal pain. On physical examination, specific signs of right-sided heart failure, arrhythmias (atrial fibrillation), and pericardial tamponade (pulsus paradoxus) may be found. Cardiac tamponade should be regarded as a life-threatening condition requiring immediate intervention.[13,29] A suspected diagnosis of severe pericardial effusion should prompt investigation by echocardiography to document this effusion. When a right-sided ventricular collapse is found, urgent pericardiocentesis should be performed to provide relief. Following initial puncture, a pericardial catheter may be inserted for further fluid drainage. Recurrence of fluid accumulation after pericardial drainage has been performed may occur in one-third of patients.[30] After recurrence, a new pericardial puncture may be performed together with the instillation of a sclerosing agent (e.g., cisplatin, mitoxantrone).[29,31] Another treatment approach for patients with a better prognosis and a refractory pericardial effusion may be video-assisted surgical thoracoscopy with a pericardiotomy (pericardial window).[29]

Superior Vena Cava Syndrome

Obstruction or compression of the venous return from the head via the superior vena cava is a common complication of lung cancer. However, superior vena cava syndrome (SVCS) is rarely present (fewer than 5% of cases) at the time of initial lung cancer diagnosis. Lung cancer is the cause of SVCS in about 50% of cases, but other intrathoracic malignancies such as lymphoma, primary mediastinal tumors, and metastatic tumor in the mediastinum should be excluded as the cause.[32–34] SVCS results from a growing right upper lobe lung tumor that extends centrally to the superior vena cava or by growing, malignant right paratracheal lymph nodes. An intraluminal thrombus may also form.[7] Nonsmall cell lung cancer (NSCLC) causes SVCS more frequently than small cell lung cancer (SCLC).[32–34] The clinical presentation of SVCS typically involves swelling of the head and neck, edema of the eyelids, distention of the veins in the neck and on the chest wall, cough, breast swelling, dizziness, headache, blurred vision, dyspnea, dysphagia, and chest pain. When tumor growth is aggressive, symptoms may appear more rapidly because of lack of time for collateral circulation to develop proximal to the venous obstruction, particularly when the obstruction is situated above the level of the junction with the azygos vein.[5,7,8,10] Diagnosis of SVCS can be easily documented by chest CT

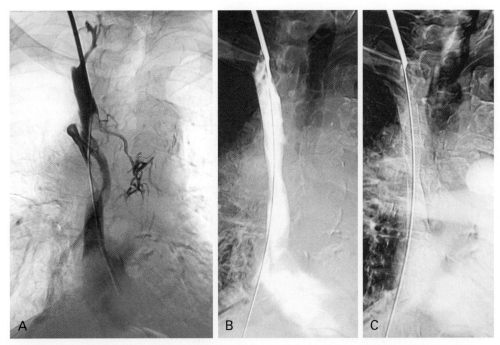

Fig. 20.2. (A) Subocclusion of the superior vena cava by a centrally located invasive lung cancer, resulting in clinical superior vena cava syndrome. (B–C) Reconstituted superior vena cava after percutaneous balloon dilatation and placement of endovascular stent. *(Figure courtesy of Hearns Charles MD, NYU Interventional Radiology Department).*

(Fig. 20.2), but a histologic diagnosis of the underlying cancer is mandatory before treatment can be initiated. Treatment of SVCS consists of alleviating symptoms as well as treating the underlying lung cancer.[35] In the case of a local–regionally advanced lung cancer, chemoradiation therapy can be initiated. For an advanced lung cancer (especially for a SCLC), chemotherapy may begin immediately.[34,35] When the patient is highly symptomatic, more rapid symptom relief can be achieved by placement of an endovascular stent than by chemoradiation therapy. Patients who present with stridor as a result of central airway obstruction or severe laryngeal edema, as well as patients who are in a coma caused by cerebral edema, should be immediately treated with endovascular stenting.[35] This procedure can be performed with use of different types of stents (e.g., stainless steel stents such as Gianturco, Wallstent, or Palmaz); however, nitinol stents currently appear to be more suitable for the safe and efficient endovascular management of SVCS.[36–38] Success rates associated with first stenting have ranged from 80% to 95%. Although the average risk of SVCS recurrence after stenting is 10% to 14%, recurrence can almost always be resolved by a new stenting procedure.

Pancoast Syndrome

A lung cancer that grows in the apex of the upper lobe toward the superior sulcus, ribs, and vertebrae will cause pain in the shoulder, scapula, and chest wall. Invasion of the brachial plexus (specifically the lower nerve roots of the ulnar nerve) will result in radiating pain and muscle wasting in the arm and hand. Horner syndrome, by invasion of the sympathetic chain and stellate ganglion, results in ptosis, miosis, and hemifacial anhidrosis, and may be part of the so-called Pancoast syndrome.[39] Typically, patients with Pancoast syndrome will have consulted other specialists before a final diagnosis of lung cancer is made, sometimes with a delay as long as 1 year from the time pain first occurred. Most people with lung cancer who present with Pancoast syndrome have NSCLC. Pancoast syndrome as an initial clinical presentation of lung cancer occurs in about 4% of cases.[7]

Dysphagia

Dysphagia may occur when the esophagus becomes obstructed by enlarged mediastinal lymph nodes or by a lung tumor invading the esophagus. Recurrent laryngeal nerve palsy may also cause dysphagia because of dysfunction of the laryngeal swallowing mechanism. Patients will typically note increasing difficulty swallowing and may subsequently become incapable of swallowing.[40] Therapy consists of treatment of the underlying local–regionally invasive lung cancer and temporary parenteral feeding, if necessary. Occasionally, palliative esophageal stenting is needed.

Diaphragmatic Paralysis

When the phrenic nerve gets trapped by a growing primary tumor or by bulky lymph nodes (typically originating from the aortic–pulmonary window lymph nodes), the diaphragm may become paralyzed, resulting in an increase in dyspnea.[7] Lung cancer invading the phrenic nerve is therefore an indication of locally advanced disease and should be staged as a cT3 tumor according to the International Association for the Study of Lung Cancer (IASLC) tumor, node, metastasis (TNM) classification eighth edition.[25]

SYMPTOMS AND SIGNS OF METASTATIC SPREAD

Bone Metastases

Bone metastases develop in approximately 30% to 40% of people with advanced NSCLC, with metastases either present at the time of diagnosis or developing during the course of the neoplastic disease.[41] Compared with bone scans, PET has similar sensitivity (at least 90%), but a higher specificity (at least 98%) and accuracy (at least 96%), and is therefore considered superior for detecting bone metastases.[42–44] Therefore, if no abnormality in bones is found on a PET scan of a patient who has no signs or symptoms suggestive of bone metastases, a bone scan is not needed.[45] Lung cancer metastases to bone are predominantly lytic.

Bone metastases cause significant pain and morbidity and are characterized by various skeletal-related events, including pathologic fractures, spinal cord compression, the need for radiation or surgery of the bone, and hypercalcemia of malignancy. Periosteal inflammation and elevation is the mechanism that most frequently causes pain from bone metastases. Pain that cannot be controlled with nonsteroidal anti-inflammatory drugs should be managed with narcotic analgesics. Most patients with symptomatic bone metastases achieve some pain relief with a low-dose, brief course of radiation therapy, as demonstrated in a trial from the Radiation Therapy Oncology Group (RTOG 97-14), which included patients with breast cancer or prostate cancer. In this trial, the efficacy of 8 Gy in a single fraction was comparable to that of the standard treatment course of 30 Gy delivered in 10 treatment fractions over 2 weeks in terms of response rates and the incidence of subsequent pathologic fractures. However, the retreatment rate was significantly higher in the 8-Gy arm (18% vs. 9%; $p < 0.001$).[46] Stereotactic ablative radiotherapy (SABR) has emerged as a new treatment for bone metastases, and several randomized trials have shown promising results.[47–49] In particular, the focal nature of SABR provides an otherwise unavailable noninvasive treatment option for previously radiated spinal metastases. For select patients with weight-bearing bone metastases at special risk of pathologic fracture, surgical operation may be considered. Vertebral augmentation procedures (kyphoplasty and vertebroplasty) are also important modalities when treating symptomatic vertebral compression fractures. In addition to the immediate pain relief, these procedures have several advantages, including applicability in previously radiated sites, the possibility of outpatient care, and obtaining of tissue biopsy specimens.[13] Bisphosphonates (pamidronate and zoledronic acid) play an important role by preventing bone resorption at sites of bone remodeling. In one study, zoledronic acid was associated with a significantly lower incidence of skeletal-related events among patients with NSCLC with bone metastasis.[50] Denosumab, another drug in a novel class of bone-targeting agents, is designed to inhibit receptor activator of nuclear factor kappa-B ligand. Compared with zoledronic acid, denosumab prolonged overall survival of patients with NSCLC with bone metastases.[51]

Brain Metastases

Lung cancer is the most common cause of brain metastases.[52] Metastases to the brain are usually symptomatic, and more than two-thirds of patients with brain metastases have some neurologic symptoms during the course of their illness.[53] The clinical manifestations of brain metastases are variable depending on the location of the lesion and the degree of associated edema. Headache is a common presenting symptom and occurs more often with multiple metastases. Focal or generalized seizures have occurred in approximately 10% of patients by the time of presentation.[53] Other symptoms of brain metastases include nausea and vomiting, focal weakness, confusion, ataxia, or visual disturbance. The signs and symptoms of brain metastases are often subtle; therefore, brain metastases should be suspected in all patients with lung cancer in whom neurologic symptoms develop. Magnetic resonance imaging (MRI) is currently the criterion standard for the diagnosis of brain metastases.

Corticosteroids can rapidly decrease the symptoms associated with brain metastases by decreasing peritumoral edema.[54] Patients with seizures should be treated with antiepileptic medication. Subsequent treatment should be used according to size, number, and location of lesions as well as the extracranial disease status and performance status of the patient. Treatment modalities for brain metastases include whole-brain radiotherapy, stereotactic radiosurgery, and surgical resection. Stereotactic radiosurgery should be considered before whole-brain radiotherapy for patients with one to three brain metastases.[55]

Leptomeningeal carcinomatosis is not rare in NSCLC[56–58] and continues to be a devastating end-stage complication of the disease. Further improvements in systemic treatment may lead to prolonged survival for more patients with stage IV disease; therefore, when all existing therapies have failed in these patients, leptomeningeal carcinomatosis may be more likely to develop. The most common ways for malignant cells to gain access to the subarachnoid space are by direct extension from preexisting tumors or by hematogenous dissemination. A high index of suspicion is required to make an early diagnosis of leptomeningeal carcinomatosis as there is a variety of neurologic manifestations. Headache, changes in mental status, cranial nerve palsies, back or radicular pain, incontinence, lower motor neuron weakness, and sensory abnormalities are typical symptoms.[59] The most informative diagnostic tool in the evaluation of leptomeningeal carcinomatosis is lumbar puncture. The opening pressure should be measured and cerebrospinal fluid sent for cytologic examination, cell count, and measurement of protein and glucose.[60] Positive findings on cerebrospinal fluid cytology examination are found on initial lumbar puncture in 50% of patients with leptomeningeal carcinomatosis and in approximately 85% of patients who have three high-volume lumbar punctures.[61,62] Therefore, patients with clinical symptoms and signs suggestive of leptomeningeal carcinomatosis should have repeated lumbar puncture if the first cytology evaluation yields negative results.

Leptomeningeal carcinomatosis is a particularly difficult challenge in the treatment of cancer. Intrathecal chemotherapy has been the mainstay of treatment, even though the extent of its benefit has not been proven in randomized clinical trials.[63] A ventriculoperitoneal shunt is also an effective palliative tool to decrease intracranial pressure.[58] Given the dismal treatment outcome and prognosis of patients with leptomeningeal carcinomatosis, new therapeutic agents or strategies are urgently needed.[64]

Spinal Cord Metastases or Spinal Compression

Spinal cord metastases or compression can be classified anatomically as intramedullary, leptomeningeal, and extradural. Extradural compression includes several mechanisms, such as continued growth of bone metastases into epidural space, blockage of neural foramina by a paraspinal mass, and destruction of vertebral bone. At the time of presentation, 90% of patients have local or radicular pain, and up to 50% of patients may have paralysis, sensory loss, and sphincter dysfunction.[65,66] If the clinical suspicion of spinal cord compression is high, immediate high-dose dexamethasone should be administered before compression is confirmed radiographically.[67] Radiotherapy is the mainstay of treatment for spinal cord metastases and should be started immediately after MRI confirmation of spinal cord compression. For patients with lung cancer who have symptomatic epidural spinal cord compression and good performance status, a neurosurgical consultation is recommended and, if appropriate, surgery should be performed immediately, followed by radiotherapy.[13]

Liver and Adrenal Gland Metastases

Liver involvement occurs frequently with lung cancer. Patients may have upper quadrant or epigastric discomfort as a result of large metastases. Most liver metastases are asymptomatic, and some patients experience vague symptoms such as fatigue, weight loss, and nausea. Liver dysfunction occurs only in the presence of extensive metastases.

The type of cancer most often associated with adrenal metastases is lung cancer, followed by gastric cancer.[68] Adrenal metastases are usually detected on CT scans, and bilateral metastases appear in approximately half of patients with lung cancer.[68,69] In most cases, these lesions are asymptomatic, although large metastatic masses may cause pain. Adrenal insufficiency is rare even in bilateral metastases because functional adrenal cortical loss occurs only when more than 90% of the adrenal gland has been destroyed.[68] However, adrenal insufficiency should be suspected in patients who present with appropriate clinical symptoms and bilateral adrenal metastases. Anecdotal reports have suggested that long-term survival can occur after resection of isolated adrenal metastasis from NSCLC,[70,71] but this has not been confirmed by randomized clinical trials and the chance of selection bias should be considered.

Other Metastatic Sites

Lung cancer metastases may occur at other sites, such as skin, soft tissue, pancreas, intraabdominal lymph nodes, bowel, ovaries, and thyroid. Management of these metastatic sites is primarily based on the patient's symptoms.

PARANEOPLASTIC SYNDROMES

Paraneoplastic symptoms are not uncommon in lung and other cancers, and can sometimes be the first clinical manifestation of the disease. Paraneoplastic symptoms are generally referred to as effects from the cancer that are not directly caused by invasion into vital organs, obstruction, or space-occupying effects from the primary cancer or remote metastasis.[72] Lung cancers have long been associated with paraneoplastic effects, which encompass a large spectrum of anatomic phenomena. They include a variety of endocrine, neurologic, dermatologic, and other body function disturbances that are indirect results of the cancer and not a result of the direct presence of cancer cells. Paraneoplastic phenomena are not specific to lung cancer, although the frequency of involvement is variable among tumor types. For instance, hypertrophic pulmonary osteoarthropathy and clubbing occur more often with lung and thoracic cancers than with other primary cancers. In addition, certain lung cancer subtypes may be more related to paraneoplastic phenomena than others, in particular SCLC, carcinoid tumors, and other neuroendocrine cancers. Paraneoplastic syndromes may be classified in several ways (Table 20.2) and in

some cases reflect common or similar pathogenic mechanisms as well as organ of involvement.

Dermatologic or Musculoskeletal Disorders

Hypertrophic Pulmonary Osteoarthropathy and Digital Clubbing

Digital clubbing, which manifests early with the loss of angle between nail and nail fold, has long been acknowledged as a possible sign of lung cancer. In a review published in 2009, authors reported that digital clubbing was found in up to 10% of patients with lung cancer and in patients with tumors metastatic to the lung.[73] Digital clubbing is associated with hypertrophic pulmonary osteoarthropathy, a condition characterized by periosteal and subperiosteal new bone formation along the shaft of long bones and the phalanges.[72] Clinically, patients often report symmetrical, painful arthropathy of the wrists, ankles, knees, and elbows. Simple radiographic examination of the long bones may show typical periosteal new bone formation, and a bone scan usually confirms bilateral diffuse uptake by the long bones. Symptoms of hypertrophic pulmonary osteoarthropathy may respond completely to surgical resection; however, for patients who are not surgical candidates, symptomatic treatment includes specific systemic treatment of the cancer in addition to bisphosphonates; analgesics, including opiates and nonsteroidal antiinflammatory agents; and, occasionally, palliative radiation therapy.[73]

Rare Skin Disorders

Tripe palm is a rare paraneoplastic syndrome associated with lung cancer, presenting with symptoms of thickened velvety palms and pronounced dermatoglyphics.[74] It can occasionally occur with acanthosis nigricans, another paraneoplastic skin condition that manifests as gray-brown hyperpigmented skin plaques. Another rare paraneoplastic syndrome linked to lung cancer is erythema gyratum repens, which is usually associated with substantial disease burden and is a cutaneous eruption with a unique wood-grain pattern morphology.[75]

Dermatomyositis

Dermatomyositis is an inflammatory myopathy associated with skin changes.[72] A typical sign of dermatomyositis is a heliotrope rash (blue-purple discoloration named after the heliotrope plant) of the upper eyelids and an erythematous rash on the face, neck, and anterior chest (V sign) or back and shoulders (shawl sign), knees, elbows, and malleoli.[76] The rash can be pruritic and may worsen after sun exposure. Another characteristic is Gottron papules, a raised violaceous rash or papules at the knuckles, prominent in metacarpophalangeal and interphalangeal joints. This chronic rash can become scaly with a shiny appearance. Dilated fingernail base capillary loops with irregular, thickened, and distorted cuticles can also be seen, and the fingers may appear like so-called mechanic hands, with cracked, horizontal lines that look dirty. Associated proximal muscle weakness can range from mild to severe and may develop before or at the time of the skin changes.

Polymyositis

Polymyositis is another paraneoplastic syndrome associated with lung cancer and presents clinically as a subacute myopathy that evolves over weeks to months, along with weakness of the proximal muscles.[77] Dermatomyositis and polymyositis can develop in different subtypes of lung cancer.[77] It is important to note that these specific paraneoplastic phenomena may be the initial symptoms of lung cancer or may develop during the course of disease progression. Anticancer therapy may help to reduce the

TABLE 20.2 Classification of Different Paraneoplastic Syndromes of Lung Cancer

Classification	Paraneoplastic Phenomena
Dermatologic or musculoskeletal	Hypertrophic pulmonary osteoarthropathy Digital clubbing Dermatomyositis/polymyositis
Endocrine or metabolic	Syndrome of inappropriate antidiuretic hormone secretion (SIADH) Hypercalcemia Cushing syndrome Carcinoid syndrome
Neurologic	Lambert-Eaton myasthenic syndrome Cerebellar ataxia Sensory neuropathy Limbic encephalitis Encephalomyelitis Autonomic neuropathy Retinopathy Opsomyoclonus
Hematologic	Anemia Leukocytosis Thrombocytosis Eosinophilia
Constitutional	Anorexia Weight loss Asthenia

symptoms of polymyositis and dermatomyositis; otherwise, corticosteroids are the standard treatment, with immunomodulators offered as an additional therapeutic option.[73]

Endocrine and Metabolic Phenomena

Most endocrine paraneoplastic syndromes result from tumor secretion of peptides or hormones that result in metabolic or homeostatic derangements. Well-known endocrine syndromes associated with lung cancer include syndrome of inappropriate antidiuretic hormone secretion (SIADH), Cushing syndrome, and carcinoid syndrome, as well as metabolic sequelae such as hypercalcemia. Other hormones known to be secreted by lung cancers include interleukin-1α, tumor necrosis factor, human chorionic gonadotropin, transforming growth factor-β, atrial natriuretic peptide, and others.[78] The paraneoplastic endocrine phenomena are typically discovered during initial evaluation of the patient or after diagnosis of lung cancer. These endocrine syndromes may not always correlate with stage or prognosis of the cancer. Anticancer treatments may improve the clinical condition.

Syndrome of Inappropriate Antidiuretic Hormone Secretion

Hyponatremia is a condition associated with many lung diseases, including lung cancer.[78] A study from the 1950s recognized SIADH as a cause of hyponatremia.[79] SIADH is more common in SCLC, affecting 10% to 45% of patients, compared with approximately 1% of patients with other types of cancer.[79] SIADH can cause anorexia, cognition change, confusion, lethargy, and seizures, because antidiuretic hormone secretion leads to persistent renal tubule overexpression of aquaporins and subsequent water resorption.[79] The duration of development and severity of the hyponatremia will influence the clinical symptoms. Life-threatening complications can occur when sodium levels fall to 120 mmol/L or lower, at which point organ failure can occur. The hallmarks of SIADH are euvolemic hyponatremia, plasma hypoosmolality, abnormally high urinary osmolality, and abnormally high urinary sodium concentration in the absence of confounders, such as volume depletion, adrenal insufficiency or hypothyroidism, and medication effects.

The diagnosis of SIADH requires exclusion of other causes, specifically volume depletion, which can confound the diagnostic algorithm and interpretation of laboratory results. The mainstay of SIADH treatment is therapy for the lung cancer, and hyponatremia may resolve within weeks from initiation of chemotherapy for SCLC. In the interval of time before response, the hyponatremia can be managed with fluid restriction, with or without demeclocycline or a vasopressin receptor antagonist (e.g., conivaptan or tolvaptan).[79] Acute severe hyponatremia may be carefully treated with hypertonic saline infusion, but the correction should be gradual so as to avoid overcorrection, thereby minimizing the risk of osmotic demyelination (central pontine demyelination).

Cushing Syndrome

Cushing syndrome has long been recognized as a paraneoplastic phenomenon in cancer, including lung cancer. Between 5% and 10% of Cushing syndrome cases are thought to be paraneoplastic in etiology, and most of these are a result of ectopic adrenocorticotropic hormone (ACTH) secretion rather than corticotropin-releasing hormone. Many cases of Cushing syndrome are related to lung cancer, especially those of neuroendocrine lineage such as SCLCs and carcinoid tumors, which are the lung cancer subtypes most likely to produce ectopic ACTH.[72,80] The symptoms of ectopic ACTH secretion in lung cancer can vary, and patients may not have all the typical features of Cushing syndrome, given the natural history of lung cancers, especially considering the aggressiveness of SCLC. In SCLC-related Cushing syndrome, there

may be aberrant processing of proopiomelanocortin, a precursor of pro-ACTH and ACTH.[81] The precursor levels are elevated more than the ACTH level and correlate with cortisol levels. Conversely, it is thought that bronchial carcinoid tumors process proopiomelanocortin normally and produce more ACTH, reminiscent of pituitary gland overproduction of ACTH.[82] Common symptoms include moon facies and proximal myopathy, as well as hypokalemia and hyperglycemia. Classic features of Cushing syndrome are more likely to occur in bronchial carcinoid tumors.

The diagnosis of Cushing syndrome is confirmed by an elevated cortisol level in a 24-hour urine sample, and an elevated serum ACTH. Failure of suppression by high-dose dexamethasone helps distinguish ectopic paraneoplastic ACTH secretion from pituitary ACTH oversecretion.[72] Imaging studies, including MRI of the pituitary, may be helpful in the differential diagnosis. Treatment should be directed at the cause of the syndrome. When surgical resection of the tumor (i.e., carcinoid) is possible, the syndrome may be resolved. In unresectable lung cancers, medical management includes the use of metyrapone, ketoconazole, somatostatin analogs, aminogluthetimide, tomidate, and mifepristone.[72,80] If medical management fails, bilateral adrenalectomy may be considered. Cushing syndrome often presents in patients with metastatic disease and portends a poor prognosis.[83]

Carcinoid Syndrome

Carcinoid syndrome, recognized by symptoms of flushing and diarrhea, is the result of secretion of serotonin and other vasoactive substances released into the circulatory system from neuroendocrine tumors. Carcinoid syndrome is mainly associated with metastatic tumors in the midgut, whereas hindgut (distal colorectal) and foregut (gastroduodenal, bronchial) carcinoid tumors are rarely a cause. Nonetheless, approximately 1% to 5% of bronchial neuroendocrine tumors may secrete ectopic serotonin and produce the syndrome.[79,84] Typical carcinoid syndrome symptoms include flushing of the chest, secretory diarrhea, bronchoconstriction, and, if the syndrome is chronic, it may lead to cardiac valvular fibrosis. Acute episodes may cause cardiovascular collapse and shock. The diagnosis of carcinoid syndrome requires evidence of an abnormal 5-hydroxy-indoleacetic acid level in a 24-hour urine collection, as this is the main metabolite of serotonin (although it may not be of as much value in bronchial carcinoids). In some cases, elevation of the serum chromogranin A levels may also have diagnostic utility, although with low specificity.[85] In terms of imaging, many neuroendocrine tumors express somatostatin receptors, so nuclear octreotide scintigraphy may be considered in addition to conventional imaging.[86] In the future, novel PET isotopes may prove useful for the localization of these tumors. Carcinoid crises, indicated by hypotension, arrhythmias, and bronchospasm, may be precipitated by surgery, anesthesia, biopsy, and drugs such as adrenergic agents or chemotherapy.[79] Acute cases may require early stabilization with octreotide treatment, and, for patients with carcinoid heart disease and severe valvular dysfunction, cardiac surgery may be necessary to improve quality of life and provide survival benefit.

Hypercalcemia

Hypercalcemia often occurs in lung cancer and is usually a result of humoral hypercalcemia of malignancy (HHM) or osteolytic bone metastases.[78,87,88] HHM is most commonly associated with squamous cell carcinoma and is caused by the production and secretion of parathyroid hormone (PTH)-related peptide by tumor cells.[80] Its discovery was the culmination of careful research, and most cases of hypercalcemia in lung cancer are now recognized as the result of HHM. The degree of hypercalcemia and the rapidity of biochemical changes influence the presentation. The symptoms of hypercalcemia include cognitive changes, fatigue, polyuria, and abdominal symptoms in conjunction with dehydration. Laboratory tests show hypercalcemia and hypophosphatemia, and electrocardiogram changes may include a prolonged PR or QRS interval, a short QT interval, bradycardia, or heart block. HHM is associated with large tumor burden, male gender, advanced disease, elevated creatinine levels, and poor prognosis.[89] Greater degrees of HHM are associated with the presence of bone metastases, and severe hypercalcemia can lead to coma and death. Diagnosis requires exclusion of other causes, such as metastatic bone involvement, and may be verified by a normal PTH level, low serum phosphorus level, and elevated PTH-related protein level. Management of hypercalcemia involves addressing the calcium levels and associated complications, especially dehydration. Therapeutic strategies include correcting the fluid balance, increasing renal excretion of calcium, and, when possible, reducing bone resorption concurrently with anticancer treatments. Substantial hypercalcemia should be promptly treated; fluid restoration with isotonic saline is beneficial in the renal clearance of calcium, which may be further enhanced by a loop diuretic once adequate hydration has been achieved. Overaggressive rehydration should be avoided because patients with lung cancer may also have coexisting cardiac disease. Bisphosphonates, and particularly other novel agents such as denosumab, are indicated to inhibit calcium release and osteoclast function. Other agents that are effective in treating hypercalcemia include mithramycin, plicamycin, and calcitonin; gallium nitrate treatment has also been used.[79,80]

Blood Disorders

Anemia

Anemia is often found in patients presenting with lung cancer, and the disorder contributes to symptoms of fatigue and dyspnea. It can be considered a form of anemia of chronic disease if the ferritin levels are either normal or elevated. Other, less common hematologic disorders such as microangiopathic hemolytic anemia, characterized by Coombs-negative, hemolytic anemia with schistocytes and thrombocytopenia, have been reported.[90]

Leukocytosis

Mild leukocytosis is relatively common in lung cancer; however, extreme elevations are rare.[91] Autonomous production of cytokines (granulocyte colony-stimulating factor and granulocyte macrophage colony-stimulating factor) has been noted in some patients with lung cancer, and leukocytosis appears to have a negative prognostic effect.[92] Conversely, hypereosinophilia is not often found in patients with lung cancer, potentially because of tumor overexpression of granulocyte macrophage colony-stimulating factor leading to a leukemoid reaction.[93]

Thrombocytosis

Reactive thrombocytosis is relatively common in cancers, including lung cancer.[94] The prevalence of thrombocytosis in lung cancer is variable, and it is thought to be an independent prognostic factor of survival in patients with primary lung cancer, including operable NSCLC.[95,96]

Hypercoagulation States

The relationship between cancer and coagulopathy was suggested by Trousseau nearly 150 years ago, and it is now definitively known that patients with lung cancer are at a higher risk of thromboembolic events compared with people who have other types of cancer or who do not have cancer. Several hypercoagulative

disorders have been associated with lung cancer, and they vary in severity. These disorders may either be present before the diagnosis of lung cancer or may occur during the course of treatment for the disease. The classic Trousseau syndrome (migratory superficial thrombophlebitis and occasionally arterial emboli) has been noted in patients with lung cancer.[97] Multiple aspects in lung cancer are associated with a higher risk of thrombosis because of patient-related, cancer-related, and treatment-related factors that combined can contribute to the risk of developing a thrombotic event.[98] Tissue factor overexpression is considered by some to be a major contributor to cancer-related thrombosis.[99]

Deep Venous Thrombosis and Thromboembolism

The authors of a large study published in 2008 reported that venous thromboembolism (VTE) developed in approximately 3% of patients with lung cancer within 2 years, and that the incidence of VTE was associated with a higher risk of death within 2 years after the diagnosis of NSCLC or SCLC.[100] Conventional anticoagulation may not be as effective for patients with lung cancer because VTE is more likely to recur in these patients compared with patients without cancer.[101] In a 2011 Cochrane review of randomized clinical trials comparing low-molecular-weight heparin, unfractionated heparin, and fondaparinux (a selective inhibitor of factor Xa) in patients with cancer and objectively confirmed VTE, low-molecular-weight heparin was potentially superior to unfractionated heparin in the initial treatment of VTE in patients with cancer.[102] A paucity of data are available on the ideal duration of anticoagulation therapy for this paraneoplastic cancer syndrome. A systematic review published in 2011 concluded that metastatic malignancy, adenocarcinoma, or lung cancer confers a higher risk of VTE recurrence than localized malignancy or some other cancers.[103] The development of VTE during lung cancer treatment is also not uncommon, and clinicians should be aware of the increased risk and introduce effective preventive measures when indicated.[104] Early data also suggest a possible link between KRAS gene mutations and an increased risk of VTE in NSCLC.[105]

Disseminated Intravascular Coagulopathy

Lung cancer may also be accompanied by disseminated intravascular coagulation, with bone marrow involvement and reduced platelet counts.[106] In addition, idiopathic thrombocytopenic purpura-like syndrome has been reported in patients with NSCLC.[107,108]

Thrombotic Microangiopathy

Thrombotic thrombocytopenic purpura, a disseminated form of thrombotic microangiopathy, has been found in patients with lung cancer.[109] Immunohistochemical (IHC) staining of lung tumor cells from patients with thrombotic thrombocytopenic purpura has demonstrated endothelial proliferative factors such as vascular endothelial growth factor and osteopontin.[110]

Paraneoplastic Neurologic Syndromes

Paraneoplastic neurologic syndromes (PNSs) are rare, affecting approximately 0.01% of patients with cancer overall, but they are more frequently found in patients with SCLC (3–5%).[111] In some cases, PNS may result from immune crossreactivity between cancer cells and antigens of the nervous system. Antibodies to neuronal surface antigens and intracellular antigens have been reported, and T cells are implicated.[112–114] Because the tumor cells do not directly produce the syndrome, treatment of the primary cancer may not always abolish the syndrome and additional immunosuppressive therapy is often required. PNS may often be identified before the cancer is diagnosed, and thus evaluation by CT and

PET imaging may be necessary. Repeated diagnostic evaluations for cancer may be needed when initial cancer screening does not identify an obvious tumor. The symptoms of PNS depend on the type of neuronal cells affected, ranging from the central nervous system to the peripheral nerves, as well as involvement of neuromuscular junctions.

Central Nervous System

Limbic Encephalitis. As a result of limbic system involvement, manifestations of limbic encephalitis include subacute seizures, memory loss, confusion, and psychiatric symptoms. SCLC is most often associated with limbic encephalitis, but NSCLC has also been linked with the syndrome.[111,115] A number of neuronal antibodies have been reported in limbic encephalitis, including voltage-gated potassium channel antibodies, GABAb, and others.[116,117]

Subacute Cerebellar Degeneration. Subacute cerebellar degeneration presents with rapidly developing cerebellar symptoms such as ataxia, nystagmus, and dysarthria. The prognosis for patients with subacute cerebellar degeneration is often poor, because the syndrome is associated with severe disability and impairment.[111] Selective loss of Purkinje fibers is causative, and cerebellar atrophy should be excluded. Associated antibodies in SCLC include anti-Hu (also called anti-neuronal nuclear antibody, type 1 or ANNA-1), anti-Ri, and anti-P/Q voltage-gated calcium channels (VGCCs).[111,118–120]

Encephalomyelitis. Encephalomyelitis is characterized by simultaneous dysfunction at various levels of the central nervous system such as the hippocampus, spinal cord, and dorsal root ganglia of myenteric plexus.[111] This condition is mostly found in patients with SCLC. The antibodies implicated include anti-Hu and anti-CV2.[121]

Peripheral Nervous System

Sensory Neuropathy. Sensory neuropathy from damage to the cells of the dorsal root ganglia manifests as subacute onset of asymmetrical numbness, pain, and involvement of the arms and lower limbs as well as proprioceptive loss.[79,111] Loss of deep tendon reflexes and panmodality sensory loss will be noted on physical examination. The diagnosis is supported by electrophysiologic demonstration of involvement of the sensory fibers. The commonly implicated antibodies in sensory neuronopathy include anti-Hu and anti-CV2, and SCLC is most often associated with this condition.[122]

Autonomic Neuropathy. Autonomic neuropathy may be subacute over weeks and involves the sympathetic, parasympathetic, and enteric systems, resulting in orthostatic hypotension, gastrointestinal tract dysfunction, sicca, bladder and bowel dysfunction, altered pupillary reflexes, loss of sinus arrhythmia, and weight loss.[72] Anti-Hu, anti-CV2, anti-nAchR, and anti-amphiphysin antibodies may be involved.

Neuromuscular Group of Peripheral Nervous System

Lambert-Eaton Myasthenic Syndrome. Lambert-Eaton myasthenic syndrome (LEMS) occurs with proximal muscle weakness, especially at the hip, with progression in cranio-caudal direction. Patients may also have an associated loss of deep tendon reflexes and autonomic dysfunction. The muscle weakness is thought to be caused by damage to VGCCs present on the presynaptic nerve terminal.[123] These same VGCCs are expressed by SCLC, and LEMS may affect up to 3% of patients with SCLC.[79] It is interesting to note that in SCLC LEMS may

precede the clinical or radiographic diagnosis of the cancer. Electromyography is helpful and shows low-voltage muscle action potential amplitude and decremental response with low-rate stimulation, but incremental response to high-rate stimulation.[72] LEMS should respond to treatment of the underlying lung cancer, and resistant LEMS may respond to plasma exchange, gamma globulin, and immunosuppression with azathioprine and corticosteroids.[124]

Less Common Peripheral Nervous Systems

Opsoclonus–Myoclonus. Opsoclonus–myoclonus is associated with anti-Ri antibodies in SCLC. Clinical features of the syndrome include myoclonus, involuntary eye movements, and truncal ataxia. Cerebrospinal fluid examination shows increased protein and mild pleocytosis. Partial or complete resolution may occur with treatment of the underlying SCLC.[79,124,125]

Cancer-Associated Retinopathy. Cancer-associated retinopathy in SCLC is thought to be caused by damage to the retinal photoreceptors, resulting in scotomas, photosensitivity, and reduced retinal arteriole caliber.[79,124,125] Leaks from retinal vessels can be seen with angiography. Spectral-domain optical coherence tomography has also been reported to be useful in the diagnosis of cancer-associated retinopathy. Progression to blindness is common and is caused by an autoantibody to the 23 kDa photoreceptor protein, recoverin. The condition may improve with corticosteroids and anticancer therapy.[126]

CLINICAL AND MOLECULAR PROGNOSTICATION OF LUNG CANCER

Lung cancer is the most common cause of cancer death in both men and women, accounting for 27% of cancer-related mortality every year.[127] At present, tumor staging is the most important prognostic factor for survival.[25] Unfortunately, patients with early-stage NSCLC are at substantial risk for recurrence and death, even after potentially curative surgical resection, with 5-year survival rates ranging from 30% to 60%. Recurrence and death will occur in as many as 40% of patients with stage I, 66% with stage II, and 75% with stage IIIA disease.[128,129] Given that some patients die of lung cancer whereas others survive without disease recurrence after surgery for an identically staged lung cancer, more factors must be considered to explain the variability of survival within each staging group. Although the TNM staging system has been the standard for determining outcome for patients with NSCLC, the stage classification may be imprecise for an individual patient. Therefore, efforts have been made to identify other prognostic factors for patients with lung cancer, including several molecular factors (Table 20.3).

Prognostic markers are patient or tumor-related factors that may provide information on the likely outcome for untreated patients; predictive markers influence and predict the outcome of a specific treatment in terms of either response or survival benefit.

Clinical Factors

Age

Many studies have shown that chemotherapy is feasible and safe in the older population of patients with NSCLC. Age on its own is not a negative predictive factor and treatment should not be withheld solely on the basis of a patient's age.[130,131] Functional impairment or comorbidity, rather than chronologic age, affects treatment tolerance and effectiveness in patients with NSCLC.[132] Many retrospective analyses have demonstrated similar efficacy outcomes between older and younger patients.[133–135] In a prospective study that enrolled

TABLE 20.3 Clinical and Molecular Prognostic Factors of Lung Cancer

Clinical Factors	Molecular Factors
Age	Nucleotide excision repair system
Performance status	ERCC1
Smoking status	RRM1
Gender	Oncogenes/tumor suppressor genes
Histology	KRAS
Findings on PET	P53
	Protein kinases
	EGFR
	ALK
	FGFR1
	Tumor cell proliferation
	Ki67
	Gene expression arrays
	Epigenetics
	Proteomic analysis
	MicroRNAs

ALK, anaplastic lymphoma kinase; *EGFR,* epidermal growth factor receptor; *ERCC1,* excision repair cross-complementation group 1; *FGFR1,* fibroblast growth factor receptor 1; *KRAS,* Kirsten rat sarcoma; *PET,* positron emission tomography; *RRM1,* ribonucleotide reductase messenger 1.

451 older patients with NSCLC (median age, 77 years), combination therapy of carboplatin plus paclitaxel was compared with either vinorelbine or gemcitabine monotherapy.[136] The median survival was 10.3 months for the combination compared with 6.2 months for single-agent chemotherapy, which was comparable with the level reported based on an unselected NSCLC population. However, it should also be noted that toxicity is greater among older patients, leading to high morbidity and mortality rates.[137,138] Additionally, published data are highly likely to be affected by selection bias in favor of good prognosis, since only the fittest older patients would have been enrolled in these trials.

Performance Status

When the IASLC International Staging Committee proposed a revised tumor staging system based on details in a very large database, performance status was found to be an important prognostic factor in NSCLC.[139–141] An independent comprehensive analysis of a separate population of approximately 27,000 patients demonstrated that good performance status is an independent predictor of prolonged survival.[142]

Smoking Status

In addition to being the major risk factor in the development of lung cancer, smoking status is known to affect the clinical outcome of patients with the disease. In a retrospective analysis of patients with NSCLC, the median overall survival was 30.0 months for never-smokers and 10.0 months for ever-smokers ($p < 0.001$).

Although smoking status was associated with histology and performance status, a never-smoking status was demonstrated to be a favorable prognostic factor.[142,143]

Gender

Lung cancer in women has a different intrinsic biologic behavior and natural history compared with men.[144] The 5-year survival rate for women with lung cancer is 15.6% compared with 12.4% for men. Women have longer survival after surgical resection of early-stage lung cancer.[145–147] However, the prognostic implication of gender should be considered along with smoking status and histology, because female patients are more likely to

be never-smokers and to have histology of adenocarcinoma.[144,148] Although it seemed there was a sex-related difference in survival in prospectively enrolled Chinese patients with NSCLC, the difference disappeared in the subgroup analysis of never-smokers with adenocarcinoma.[149] (Gender and lung cancer is addressed fully in Chapter 5.)

Histology

The identification of specific histologic type has become important in the treatment of patients with NSCLC, particularly when studies showed greater efficacy of pemetrexed for patients with a nonsquamous cell carcinoma type than for patients with squamous cell carcinoma.[150] Targetable oncogenes, such as the epidermal growth factor receptor (*EGFR*) mutation or the anaplastic lymphoma kinase (ALK) translocation, are more commonly found in adenocarcinomas.[151,152] Unlike the predictive role of histologic type, the prognostic relevance has not been fully evaluated, although several studies recently showed the favorable prognostic feature of squamous cell carcinoma.[140,141]

PET Imaging

Recent advances in FDG-PET have enabled not only a better diagnosis and staging of lung cancer but also the prediction of its malignancy grade and prognosis.[153,154] (Further explanation about the prognostic role of PET is described in Chapter 22).

Molecular Factors

Nucleotide Excision Repair System

Excision Repair Cross-Complementation Group 1. Excision repair cross-complementation group 1 (ERCC1) is the primary DNA repair mechanism that removes platinum-DNA adducts, which are the basis for platinum cytotoxicity. In a study by Simon et al.[155] the authors initially reported that high ERCC1 expression, which was measured by real-time quantitative polymerase chain reaction (qRT-PCR), is an independent predictor of longer survival for patients with surgically resected NSCLC. The International Adjuvant Lung Cancer Trial evaluated ERCC1 expression using IHC in 761 tumors from a randomized trial of adjuvant cisplatin-based chemotherapy in completely resected NSCLC.[156] Adjuvant chemotherapy significantly prolonged survival among patients with ERCC1-negative tumors ($p = 0.002$) but not among patients with ERCC1-positive tumors ($p = 0.40$). Among patients with NSCLC who did not receive adjuvant chemotherapy, patients with ERCC1-positive tumors survived longer than patients with ERCC1-negative tumors. Since then, many studies have evaluated the predictive and prognostic roles of ERCC1 in early- or advanced-stage NSCLC.[157–163] Most recently, however, the level of expression of ERCC1 protein was determined by IHC in a validation set of samples obtained from 494 patients in two independent phase III trials (the National Cancer Institute of Canada Clinical Trials Group JBR.10 and the Cancer and Leukemia Group B 9633 trial from the Lung Adjuvant Cisplatin Evaluation Biology project). This study was unable to validate the predictive effect of IHC staining for the ERCC1 protein, and none of the 16 antibodies could distinguish the four ERCC1 protein isoforms.[164]

Ribonucleotide Reductase Messenger 1. Ribonucleotide reductase messenger 1 (RRM1) is a component of ribonucleotide reductase and the molecular target of gemcitabine. Although an initial prospective trial showed an inverse correlation between RRM1 expression and disease response rates in patients treated with gemcitabine-based chemotherapy, a subsequent trial failed to demonstrate RRM1 as a predictive factor for gemcitabine-based chemotherapy.[165,166] Data about its prognostic implication are rare.

Oncogenes and Tumor Suppressor Genes

KRAS. *KRAS* is a member of the RAS family of oncogenes and encodes a protein that binds guanine nucleotides. *KRAS* mutations occur frequently in NSCLC, found in 15% to 30% of NSCLC among Western patients, although the rate is lower among Asian patients.[167–173] Most of these mutations are found in adenocarcinomas and are associated with a history of smoking. The mutation in *KRAS* results in constitutive activation and continuous transmission of growth signals to the nucleus. A meta-analysis identified *KRAS* mutations as a negative prognostic factor.[174] In addition, among patients with completely resected or advanced NSCLC, the median survival of patients with *KRAS* mutation was shorter than that for patients with *KRAS* wild-type or *EGFR* mutation.[169,173] However, in a later study, which included 1543 patients who had been enrolled in four randomized trials of adjuvant chemotherapy for completely resected NSCLC, the authors reported that *KRAS* mutation had no prognostic role in patients with completely resected NSCLC.[175]

Unlike in colorectal cancer, where *KRAS* mutation has been demonstrated as a predictive factor for poor response to an EGFR-targeting agent such as cetuximab, the predictive role of *KRAS* mutation in NSCLC has been questionable.[176,177] Although many studies have demonstrated poorer clinical outcomes after therapy with EGFR-tyrosine kinase inhibitors (TKIs) among patients with *KRAS* mutation compared with patients with *KRAS* wild-type, this result was refuted by findings that *KRAS* mutation status had no effect on clinical outcomes with EGFR-TKIs in patients with EGFR wild-type.[168,169,173,178–180]

P53. The *p53* tumor suppressor gene is the most commonly mutated gene in all human malignancies, and alterations in the *p53* gene are the most frequently found genetic mutations in human cancer. Inactivation of p53 results in diminished efficiency of DNA repair, derangements of cell cycle regulation, and overall increased genomic instability. Prognostic significance of p53 has been investigated extensively in NSCLC. A prospective study demonstrated that p53 mutations were independently predictive of decreased survival for patients with stage I tumors but not for patients with stage II or III tumors.[181] The relationship between p53 mutational status and adverse survival outcomes has been supported by the results of several other studies in which NSCLC samples of all tumor stages were analyzed.[182–186] Meta-analyses generally have indicated that *p53* gene mutations or p53 protein over-expression were associated with decreased overall survival of patients with NSCLC.[187,188]

Protein Kinases

EGFR. The EGFR pathway is a regulator of cellular proliferation, angiogenesis, apoptosis, and migration. The mutations of genes in the EGFR signaling pathway are thought to be important for the pathogenesis of lung adenocarcinoma.[189] *EGFR* mutations in lung cancer are associated with never-smoking status, female gender, East Asian ethnicity, and histology of adenocarcinoma.[190,191] Typically, *EGFR* mutations are mutually exclusive with *KRAS* mutations or ALK rearrangements.[173,180,192,193] In 2004, EGFR mutation was described to be predictive for response to EGFR-TKIs in NSCLC.[194] Since then, many prospective trials have also demonstrated that *EGFR* mutations act as strong predictors for the efficacy of EGFR-TKIs.[152,195–199] The Iressa Pan Asia Study showed that the response rate to gefitinib was 71.2% in the EGFR mutation-positive subgroup, compared with 1.1% in the mutation-negative subgroup.[152] Other prospective studies have also demonstrated that *EGFR* mutation is a powerful predictive factor for clinical outcomes in patients treated with erlotinib or afatinib. Higher objective response rates and longer progression-free survival have been reported for EGFR-TKIs compared with cytotoxic

chemotherapy for EGFR-positive tumors.[197–199] Based on these data, *EGFR* mutation testing is strongly recommended for advanced NSCLC. The prognostic role of *EGFR* mutation, however, is still controversial, particularly in surgically resected early-stage NSCLC. Although initial studies showed that *EGFR* mutation correlated with worse survival in NSCLC, other studies have shown no significant association.[191,200,201] The clinical observation that patients with *EGFR* mutation survive longer may be because EGFR mutation is more frequently associated with other good prognostic factors.

Anaplastic Lymphoma Kinase. In 2007, Soda et al.[202] identified the echinoderm microtubule-associated protein like 4 (EML4)-ALK fusion gene as a driving oncogene in a subset of NSCLC. ALK-rearranged lung cancer is a unique NSCLC subset that is characterized by ALK gene inversion or translocation. Several selective ALK inhibitors have demonstrated their effectiveness in patients with NSCLC harboring ALK rearrangement.[203–206] Although the subset of patients with ALK-rearranged lung cancer mostly benefit from ALK inhibitors, the prognosis of patients with ALK-rearranged tumors who were not treated with ALK inhibitors was comparable to patients with tumors lacking ALK rearrangement.[207,208]

Fibroblast Growth Factor Receptor 1. Fibroblast growth factor receptor (FGFR) belongs to the super-family of receptor tyrosine kinases and is encoded by four genes (*FGFR1*, *FGFR2*, *FGFR3*, and *FGFR4*). *FGFR1* has been identified as one of the emerging molecular targets for the treatment of lung cancer.[209] *FGFR1* amplification is detected in about 15% of squamous cell lung carcinomas, and it is regarded as a druggable target.[210–212] However, the data about its prognostic relevance are contradictory, and further research is warranted.[210–212]

Tumor Cell Proliferation

Ki-67. Ki-67, a nonhistone protein, is a DNA-binding nuclear protein expressed throughout the cell cycle in proliferating cells, but not in quiescent (G0) cells. Although its exact function remains unclear, Ki-67 has been used as a proliferative marker in malignant tumors.[213] The prognostic relevance of Ki-67 has been extensively investigated in NSCLC. A recent meta-analysis, which included 28 studies conducted between 2000 and 2012, indicated that the expression of Ki-67 seems to have prognostic influence in NSCLC, with a high labeling index pointing toward poor prognosis.[214] However, it is difficult to reach consensus on the prognostic value of Ki-67 expression because various cut-off levels and methods have been used across studies.[214]

Gene Expression Arrays

Molecular profiling of tumors has led to the identification of gene expression patterns that are associated with specific phenotypes and prognosis. The development of genomic techniques, particularly DNA microarray and qRT-PCR, provides an opportunity to discover groups of genes whose coordinated expression could have greater power than individual genes to predict disease outcome. Despite the diversity in the approaches used, three main steps are needed in the model of genomic prognostication.[215] First, the expression levels of several hundred to tens of thousands of genes are quantified by microarray or qRT-PCR, and the data are then processed. Second, expression data are combined and grouped by clustering and risk score generation to produce a gene signature that correlates with a clinical outcome. Third, the signature is validated in datasets of independent cohorts.

It is well accepted that alterations in the expression levels of certain genes are strongly associated with carcinogenesis. These changes in gene expression are represented by the quantitative changes in mRNA levels. In 1995, Schena et al.[216] demonstrated a gene expression profiling technique—adapted from Southern blotting that used strands of complementary DNA spotted onto a piece of glass to examine multiple mRNA expression levels at once—known as a microarray. Since then, this technology was quickly developed and many investigators found differences in gene expression profiles between lung cancer and normal lung tissue.[217,218] Bhattacharjee et al.[217] examined 186 snap-frozen lung tumors using 12,600 unique transcript-containing oligonucleotide microarrays and classified the group of lung adenocarcinomas into four distinct subgroups according to the genetic profiles. The median survival rates among the four subgroups were significantly different. Beer et al.[219] examined 86 resected lung adenocarcinomas using 6800 transcript-containing oligonucleotide microarrays. They defined a risk index based on the top 50 genes to identify low-risk and high-risk stage I lung adenocarcinomas, which differed significantly with respect to survival, showing that gene-expression profiles based on microarray analysis can be used to predict survival in early-stage lung adenocarcinoma. The first report of a qRT-PCR–based molecular signature with prognostic implications was published in 2007.[220] In this study, investigators identified 16 genes that correlated with survival among patients with NSCLC by analyzing microarray data and risk scores, and then, five genes (*DUSP6*, *MMD*, *STAT1*, *ERBB3*, and *LCK*) were selected for qRT-PCR and decision-tree analysis. The five-gene signature was demonstrated as an independent predictor of survival.[220]

Epigenetics

Epigenetic modifications are now known to significantly contribute to lung cancer carcinogenesis. For example, the aberrant promoter methylation of the tumor suppressor gene p16 leads to gene silencing, which is an early event in carcinogenesis.[221,222] Epigenetic changes are being tested as a noninvasive biomarker for the prognosis of lung cancer. Brock et al.[223] evaluated the prognostic value of methylation patterns for seven genes (*p16*, *MGMT*, *DAPK*, *RASSF1A*, *CDH13*, *ASC*, and *APC*) in resected stage I NSCLC, and they found that pairs of gene combinations of *p16*, *CDH13*, *APC*, and *RASSF1A* were a risk factor for recurrence.[223]

Proteomic Analysis

Proteomic approaches involve the comprehensive investigation of proteins using two-dimensional gel electrophoresis and mass spectrometry. Through the development of high-throughput platforms, proteomics allowed for the simultaneous measurement of multiple protein products and/or protein modifications.[224] These processes are useful in detecting the dysregulation in malignancy as well as protein function. Moreover, proteomics has some advantage over genomics because protein biomarkers can be a more accurate signature of a disease state, as proteins are the actual functional players. Proteomics was extensively used to define the prognosis of patients with lung cancer. The expression level of many proteins such as phosphoglycerate kinase 1 (PGK1), annexin A3 (ANXA3), S100A11, and cytokeratins (CKs) has been reported to be associated with prognosis in lung cancer.[225–228]

MicroRNA

MicroRNAs (miRNAs) are small noncoding RNAs approximately 22 nucleotides long that play crucial roles in lung carcinogenesis through posttranscriptional regulation of tumor suppressor genes and oncogenes. There is evidence to support that miRNAs are dysregulated during tumor initiation and progression. Currently, there are more than 1200 human miRNAs, and many studies have demonstrated major differences in miRNA expression between lung tumors and noninvolved adjacent lung tissue.[229] Many studies have investigated the role of miRNAs in lung cancer as well as their role as diagnostic, prognostic, and therapeutic targets.[230]

The association between miRNA expression signatures and prediction of prognosis has also been evaluated in several studies. The high level of miR-708 in NSCLC was found to be associated with a reduced overall survival for never-smokers with lung adenocarcinomas.[231] Lu et al.[232] found that miRNA expression patterns between lung adenocarcinoma and squamous cell carcinoma significantly differed in 171 miRNAs, including Let-7 family members and miR-205. They also found two miRNA signatures that significantly differentiate the survival rates of these lung cancers. However, the role of miRNAs in the clinical setting remains unresolved, warranting large, prospective studies that demonstrate reproducibility.

CONCLUSION

Early recognition of initial lung cancer symptoms and specific clinical syndromes is very important for all physicians and for primary care physicians in particular. Increased awareness of alarming symptoms such as cough, hemoptysis, dyspnea, and weight loss may be a key factor in earlier detection of lung cancer, resulting in better outcomes. Diagnosis of lung cancer by its clinical presentation only is, however, not sufficient for detecting all lung cancers at an early stage. Screening of asymptomatic individuals at highest risk for lung cancer with use of low-dose CT has been shown to be efficient not only for diagnosing lung cancer at an early stage but also for substantially reducing lung cancer–specific mortality. Awareness of several clinical and molecular prognostic factors of lung cancer may hopefully become more important and relevant to the physician's clinical evaluation and may optimize personalized care of patients with lung cancer in daily practice.

KEY REFERENCES

5. Ost DE, Yeung SC, Tanoue LT, Gould MK. Clinical and organizational factors in the initial evaluation of patients with lung cancer: diagnosis and management of lung cancer, 3rd ed: American College of Chest Physicians evidence-based clinical practice guidelines. *Chest*. 2013;143(suppl 5):e121S–e141S.
9. Mayor S. Cough-awareness campaign increases lung cancer diagnoses. *Lancet Oncol*. 2014;15(1).
13. Simoff MJ, Brian L, Slade MG, et al. Symptom management in patients with lung cancer: diagnosis and management of lung cancer, 3rd ed: American College of Chest Physicians evidence-based clinical practice guidelines. *Chest*. 2013;143(suppl 5):e455S–e497S.
35. Ford DW, Koch KA, Ray DE, Selecky PA. Palliative and end-of-life care in lung cancer: diagnosis and management of lung cancer, 3rd ed: American College of Chest Physicians evidence-based clinical practice guidelines. *Chest*. 2013;143(suppl 5):e498S–e512S.
53. Patchell RA. The management of brain metastases. *Cancer Treat Rev*. 2003;29(6):533–540.
72. Pelosof LC, Gerber DE. Paraneoplastic syndromes: an approach to diagnosis and treatment. *Mayo Clin Proc*. 2010;85(9):838–854.
100. Chew HK, Davies AM, Wun T, Harvey D, Zhou H, White RH. The incidence of venous thromboembolism among patients with primary lung cancer. *J Thromb Haemost*. 2008;6(4):601–608.
113. Darnell RB, Posner JB. Paraneoplastic syndromes involving the nervous system. *N Engl J Med*. 2003;349(16):1543–1554.
140. Sculier JP, Chansky K, Crowley JJ, et al. The impact of additional prognostic factors on survival and their relationship with the anatomical extent of disease expressed by the 6th Edition of the TNM Classification of Malignant Tumors and the proposals for the 7th Edition. *J Thorac Oncol*. 2008;3(5):457–466.
141. Chansky K, Sculier JP, Crowley JJ, Giroux D, Van Meerbeeck J, Goldstraw P. The International Association for the Study of Lung Cancer Staging Project: prognostic factors and pathologic TNM stage in surgically managed non-small cell lung cancer. *J Thorac Oncol*. 2009;4(7):792–801.
180. Jackman DM, Miller VA, Cioffredi L-A, Yeap BY, Jänne PA, Riely GJ, et al. Impact of epidermal growth factor receptor and KRAS mutations on clinical outcomes in previously untreated nonsmall cell lung cancer patients: results of an online tumor registry of clinical trials. *Clin Cancer Res*. 2009;15(16):5267–5273.

193. Rodig SJ, Mino-Kenudson M, Dacic S, et al. Unique clinicopathologic features characterize ALK-rearranged lung adenocarcinoma in the western population. *Clin Cancer Res.* 2009;15(16):5216–5223.

220. Chen HY, Yu SL, Chen CH, et al. A five-gene signature and clinical outcome in non–small-cell lung cancer. *N Engl J Med.* 2007;356(1):11–20.

225. Chen G, Gharib TG, Wang H, et al. Protein profiles associated with survival in lung adenocarcinoma. *Proc Natl Acad Sci USA.* 2003;100(23):13537–13542.

230. Zhang WC, Liu J, Xu X, Wang G. The role of microRNAs in lung cancer progression. *Med Oncol.* 2013;30(3):675.

See Expertconsult.com for full list of references.

21 Conventional Imaging of Lung Cancer

Patricia M. de Groot, Brett W. Carter, and Reginald F. Munden

SUMMARY OF KEY POINTS

- Low-dose multidetector computed tomography (CT) screening of active and former heavy smokers has been shown to decrease lung cancer mortality.
- The malignant potential of solid pulmonary nodules depends on their size, with larger nodules more likely to represent tumor. Nevertheless, solid nodules have a low overall malignancy rate (7%).
- Ground-glass nodules and part-solid nodules have a higher chance of malignancy than completely solid nodules, up to 63% in the case of mixed density solid and ground-glass lesions. The differential diagnosis for ground-glass lesions that persist after 3 months includes focal fibrosis, atypical adenomatous hyperplasia, and indolent adenocarcinoma.
- Chest CT with intravenous contrast is recommended for all patients with suspected or known lung cancer to assess primary tumor characteristics, nodal disease, and intrathoracic or extrathoracic metastases.
- Accurate staging of lung cancer is critical to inform management decisions and therapy. The seventh edition of tumor, node, and metastasis (TNM) staging from the International Association for the Study of Lung Cancer/American Thoracic Society is currently in use; proposed revisions for the eighth edition have been published.
- Magnetic resonance imaging (MRI) is useful in evaluating several factors that determine potential resectability of lung tumors including pericardial or myocardial invasion, brachial plexus involvement in the setting of superior sulcus tumors, and invasion of regional vasculature or the spinal cord in central tumors.
- MRI is also showing promise in detection of metastatic lymph nodes, displaying better sensitivity and accuracy compared with ^{18}F-2-deoxy-D-glucose-positron emission tomography–CT in some studies.
- Chest CT with contrast is useful in assessing lung cancer response to radiation or chemotherapy, surgical resection, and emergent conditions that may be associated with malignancy.

Primary lung cancer is the leading cause of cancer mortality worldwide and constitutes a major public health challenge. In the United States, lung cancer is as deadly as the next three causes of cancer deaths combined (prostate, colorectal, and pancreatic cancer in men; breast, colorectal, and pancreatic cancer in women).[1] In 2014, the incidence of lung cancer is estimated to be 224,210 cases, with lung cancer responsible for 86,930 deaths in men and 72,330 deaths in women in the United States.[1] In 2013 in the European Union, primary lung cancer caused approximately 187,000 deaths in men and 82,640 deaths in women, the latter constituting a 7% increase from 2009.[2] Nevertheless, the lung cancer epidemic is considered to have peaked in the developed world, and more than half of new lung cancer cases now occur in developing countries.[3,4] In countries such as China, where widespread tobacco smoking has become a more recent event, lung cancer incidence and mortality rates are increasing.[4]

Primary carcinoma of pulmonary origin includes several distinct histologic types and may be divided into small cell lung cancer (SCLC) and nonsmall cell lung cancer (NSCLC). SCLC is a pulmonary neuroendocrine tumor with aggressive features. Other neuroendocrine malignancies of the lung are carcinoid and large cell neuroendocrine tumors.[5] NSCLC is more common overall than SCLC and encompasses adenocarcinoma and squamous cell carcinoma, as well as less frequently seen tumors of the lung such as large cell carcinoma, sarcomatoid carcinoma, and spindle cell sarcoma.

A shift in the prevailing lung cancer cell type occurred in the latter decades of the 20th century. In the 1950s, cases of squamous cell carcinoma outnumbered cases of adenocarcinoma, the second most common type of lung cancer, by a ratio of 17:1. Since that time, polycyclic aromatic hydrocarbons, a known carcinogen specifically associated with squamous cell carcinoma of the lung, have been reduced in manufactured cigarettes, with a relative decline in the incidence of squamous cell carcinoma.[6] However, the incidence of primary lung adenocarcinoma has increased during the same period. These cancers have been linked to tobacco-specific nitrosamines, which are still present in cigarettes in substantial quantities.[7–9] The use of cigarette filters, although reducing the risk of squamous cell carcinoma, has had no effect on the risk of adenocarcinoma.[10]

RADIOLOGIC PRESENTATION OF LUNG CANCER

Diagnostic imaging plays an important role in the diagnosis, workup, and staging of primary lung cancer. Conventional chest radiographs and computed tomography (CT) of the chest both have a role in identifying and evaluating abnormalities in the thorax. Chest CT is an essential tool in tumor staging and in determining clinical and surgical management.

On imaging, primary lung cancers vary in their appearance from a solitary pulmonary nodule to amorphous consolidation. They may also have varying densities, ranging from ground-glass attenuation (defined as slightly increased lung density through which vessels can be seen), to mixed ground-glass and solid density lesions, to solid tumors. A lung cancer may be cavitary at presentation or may cavitate during the course of treatment. The early, common, and uncommon imaging features of lung cancer are discussed in this chapter.

SOLITARY PULMONARY NODULE CHARACTERIZATION

Many lung cancers, particularly at the early stages, present as a solitary pulmonary nodule (up to 3 cm) or mass (greater than 3 cm), but only a small fraction of pulmonary nodules are actually cancerous.[11] Several features seen on imaging may help to differentiate malignant from benign nodules, the most important of which are size, density, and enhancement. Other important characteristics include border contour, shape, patterns of calcification, presence of macroscopic fat, and cavitation (Fig. 21.1). Location and multiplicity of nodules should also be noted.

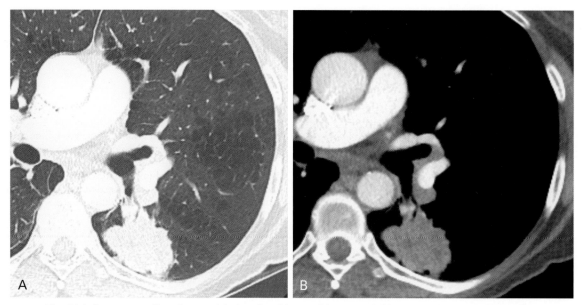

Fig. 21.1. Squamous cell carcinoma of the lung in a 71-year-old woman. Axial computed tomography image with contrast material in (A) lung windows and (B) soft-tissue windows shows a sizeable, irregular, spiculated, heterogeneously enhancing mass in the left lower lobe in a patient with severe smoking-related emphysema. The large size, irregular borders, and enhancement are all characteristics associated with malignancy.

Size

The larger a nodule is at presentation, the higher the likelihood that it is malignant. For a solid, discrete pulmonary nodule, the risk of cancer is categorized according to size. A solid nodule up to 5 mm has a 1% risk of being cancer. Nodules between 6 mm and 10 mm have a 24% chance of malignancy, which increases to 33% for nodules 11 mm to 20 mm. Solid lesions greater than 20 mm in diameter have an 80% chance of malignant histology.[12] A lesion greater than 30 mm has a 93% to 99% rate of malignancy.[13,14]

Changes in nodule size are also an important prognostic consideration. Nodules that decrease in size over time are most likely infectious or inflammatory in etiology. Conversely, nodules that enlarge while under observation are considered malignant until proven otherwise. Consequently, established algorithms for managing pulmonary nodules are promulgated by the Fleischner Society. For follow-up of solid nodules, slight variations may exist, depending on the risk stratification of the individual. In a high-risk person such as a smoker, nodules up to 4 mm should have a single follow-up 12 months after presentation. Solid nodules greater than 4 mm and up to 6 mm should be reassessed by CT at 6 months to 12 months after presentation and then at 18 months to 24 months if unchanged. For nodules greater than 6 mm to 8 mm, the initial follow-up is at 3 months to 6 months, followed by reassessment at 9 months to 12 months and again at 24 months, if unchanged. Nodules greater than 8 mm may be followed-up with CT at 3 months, 9 months, and 24 months; alternatively, dynamic contrast-enhanced CT, positron emission tomography (PET), and/or biopsy could be performed.[15] Solid nodules identified on presentation should be followed up for a minimum of 2 years to establish stability and benignity. Interval nodule growth should prompt further workup, including biopsy.[16]

Density

Solid nodules have a low overall malignancy rate of 7%.[11] Subsolid nodules have a greater chance of being malignant than solid nodules and may represent primary adenocarcinomas of the lung.

Ground-Glass Opacity

Pure ground-glass lesions, those lesions with homogeneous transparent density through which underlying architectural features are seen, have an 18% chance of being malignant.[11] Very small ground-glass nodules, up to 5 mm, may reflect atypical adenomatous hyperplasia, which is premalignant and does not require CT follow-up, according to the Fleischner Society recommendations for subsolid nodules.[17] For lesions greater than 5 mm, the differential diagnosis includes focal fibrosis, atypical adenomatous hyperplasia, and indolent primary adenocarcinoma.[18] Neoplasms with pure ground-glass attenuation usually correspond with adenocarcinoma in situ, the type A lesion in the Noguchi classification scheme of pulmonary adenocarcinomas, although rarely, they may be of mixed subtype. Heterogeneous ground-glass lesions or lesions with internal alveolar collapse are compatible with Noguchi type B lesions.[19] Ground-glass adenocarcinomas have doubling times on the order of 384 days to 567 days.[19]

The presence of solid components mixed with ground-glass attenuation denotes a mixed-density, part solid nodule (PSN). These part solid and part ground-glass nodules have the highest malignancy rate (63%).[11] The larger size of the solid features is associated with worse prognosis;[17] these lesions correspond to Noguchi types B and C (Fig. 21.2). The development of solid density within a pure ground-glass opacity (GGO) under surveillance is an indication of transformation to a more aggressive lesion. An increase in diameter in an observed GGO is also a sign of progression (Fig. 21.3).[19] Papillary, tubular, acinar, and other subtypes of lung adenocarcinoma on imaging cannot be reliably distinguished; rather, the diagnosis is histologic.[20]

Initial follow-up for both pure GGOs and PSNs is performed 3 months after presentation to distinguish a potentially infectious or inflammatory lesion, which would be expected to decrease or resolve in this period.[17] Single GGOs greater than 5 mm in diameter that persist after 3 months without change should be reassessed annually for a minimum of 3 years, unless or until they show progression. Solitary PSNs are managed according to the size of the solid component. If the solid portion is less than 5

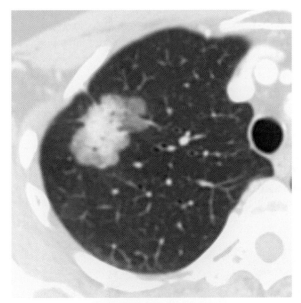

Fig. 21.2. Nonsmall cell lung cancer in a nonsmoking 63-year-old woman. Axial computed tomography image with contrast material in lung windows shows a large multilobulated right upper lobe lesion having both solid and ground-glass attenuation. The large solid component is suspicious for a more aggressive lesion. Examination of the biopsy specimen indicated invasive adenocarcinoma.

mm, follow-up for the nodule may be similar to that for a GGO, for a minimum of 3 years. Lesions with larger solid components persistent after 3 months should be reassessed by biopsy and/or resected.[17]

The presence of several GGOs and/or mixed-density lesions makes resection of all lesions impossible for some individuals. Multiple GGOs 5 mm or less should have a follow-up CT at 2 years and again at 4 years after presentation, in the absence of interval changes. Pure GGOs greater than 5 mm without a dominant lesion should undergo annual surveillance similar to that for a single GGO. Careful follow-up of these GGOs should be done in order to identify candidate tumors for limited resection based on progression or aggressive transformation. When a dominant lesion or lesions with part solid components are present in the setting of other nodules, biopsy and/or lung-sparing surgical resection is advised.[17]

Enhancement

Neoplastic pulmonary nodules have been shown to have increased vascularity compared with benign nodules, suggesting that nodule enhancement can be used as a distinguishing characteristic in evaluating indeterminate solid lesions.[21] The assessment process requires noncontrast CT images through the pulmonary nodule, which is then imaged at specific time points up to 4 minutes after administering intravenous contrast medium.[22] Hounsfield unit (HU) attenuation measurements are taken with a region of interest for every time point and the differential enhancement is calculated. A difference of 15 HU or less is strongly suggestive of benignity. With a 15-HU threshold, investigators have found 98% sensitivity but 58% specificity for malignancy.[21,22] Another study using a threshold of 30 HU with multidetector CT demonstrated 99% sensitivity for malignancy, with 54% specificity, a positive predictive value of 71%, and a negative predictive value of 87%.[22,23] Nevertheless, because of time constraints, need for technical expertise, availability of other noninvasive assessment methods such as PET–CT, and radiation dose to the patient, nodule enhancement studies are not frequently performed in the

nonacademic clinical setting. More recently, dual-energy CT, which has the capability of creating a virtual noncontrast image, has been investigated as a potential method of measuring nodule enhancement without multiple acquisitions, thus minimizing the radiation dose.[22]

Borders

A nodule with an irregular or shaggy border can raise suspicion for malignancy; however, infectious and inflammatory nodules may have a similar appearance. The degree of suspicion may rest on the overall constellation of radiographic findings, the individual's symptoms and demographic characteristics, and persistence over time. Cancers may be multilobulated, although smooth and well-circumscribed nodules may be malignant 21% of the time.[22,24] Spiculation in the periphery of a nodule correlates pathologically with a desmoplastic reaction of the nodule or tumor infiltration into the surrounding lung parenchyma and is present much more frequently in malignant nodules.[20,25] Many lung cancers are ill defined, hindering detection on radiographs.[26,27]

Shape

Although most lung cancers manifest as a nodule or mass, the overall shape of carcinomas varies. Some adenocarcinomas, particularly the mucin-producing subtype, can present as ill-defined parenchymal consolidation caused by mucin filling the alveoli; this is radiographically indistinguishable from pneumonia but will persist despite antibiotic treatment (Fig. 21.4). An uncommon manifestation of early lung cancer is a focally thickened or impacted bronchus, sometimes with peripheral inflammatory changes.[28,29]

Calcification

Calcifications within a nodule can be evaluated according to their pattern. Benign calcifications are central, diffuse, laminar, or so-called popcorn in shape.[13,28] Eccentric calcification is associated with malignancy. Nonetheless, preexisting calcifications in the lungs such as granulomas may become engulfed by a tumor, and carcinoid tumors can have punctate calcifications, making the presence of calcification less reliable in determination of benign disease.[28]

Adipose Content

Macroscopic fat within a pulmonary nodule can be identified visually and is measurable with a region of interest; HU measurement less than 1 is compatible with adipose tissue. The presence of macroscopic fat is an indication of benignity and favors the diagnosis of hamartoma, a smooth muscle neoplasm having no malignant potential. However, low attenuation in a nodule without the presence of actual fat can suggest necrosis or the presence of mucin.

Cavitation

Up to 22% of primary lung cancers demonstrate cavitation on CT imaging.[30] Squamous cell carcinomas of the lung are the most likely to exhibit this feature; however, primary lung adenocarcinomas will also cavitate. One type of cavitation occurs when tumors outgrow their blood supply and undergo central necrosis. Some adenocarcinomas exhibit a phenomenon of pseudocavitation caused by bronchial or alveolar expansion within the tumor (Fig. 21.5).[20] It is also possible for a lung cancer to arise in the wall of a preexisting cystic space.[31]

Nevertheless, infectious processes of the lung, including mycobacterial, fungal, and bacterial pneumonias, can also cavitate, as can nodules related to vasculitis. Some early studies demonstrated that cavity wall thickness measured on radiographs could be a discriminating feature in distinguishing nonmalignant from malignant disease; however, results of other studies using CT have suggested that measuring wall thickness is not as useful.[30] Both inner cavity wall irregularity and notching, or focal lobulation of the outer cavity wall, have both been shown to occur more frequently in malignant than in benign cavitary lesions.[22,32]

Multiplicity

The implication of more than one lesion also depends on size and density. Multiple small, solid nodules that are smaller than 6 mm are most likely to be postinfectious/postinflammatory and are considered low risk for malignancy.[16,33] Conversely, numerous ground-glass nodules and/or PSNs are highly suggestive of multifocal synchronous primary adenocarcinomas.[34] The presence of two synchronous primary lung carcinomas of different histologic types is also possible but uncommon.[29]

Location

Lung cancers may be located in the peripheral or central aspect of the lungs. Statistically, more malignancies are found in the upper lobes, especially the right upper lobe.[35]

IMAGING WITH CHEST RADIOGRAPHS

The chest radiograph is by far the most commonly performed radiographic study, with almost 80.5 million chest radiographs

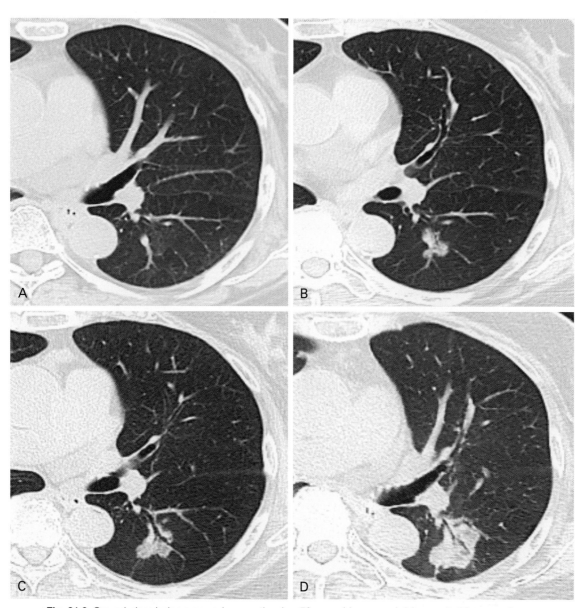

Fig. 21.3. Ground-glass lesion progressing over time in a 73-year-old woman. Axial computed tomography images in lung windows over an 8-year period. (A) Baseline image shows a nearly imperceptible ground-glass opacity in the superior segment of the left lower lobe; (B) after approximately 3 years, a small lobulated ground-glass opacity is visible in this region; (C) after another 3 years, the lesion continues to enlarge and demonstrates an air bronchogram; and (D) at the last time period, 8 years after the original presentation, the tumor has progressed in both size and density and is compatible with a primary lung adenocarcinoma. It was not resected because of multifocal adenocarcinomas in this patient.

performed in 2010 in short-term-stay US hospitals alone, not including associated facilities, specialty hospitals, and independent doctors' offices.[36] Radiographs are inexpensive and widely available, and the radiation dose is negligible (0.1 rem). Chest radiography is the first-line imaging modality for individuals with symptoms referable to the chest, such as cough, shortness of breath, hemoptysis, and chest pain. Chest radiographs are also obtained as baseline examinations before procedures, including surgery. The chest radiograph, therefore, provides an early opportunity to detect both symptomatic and asymptomatic lung cancers.

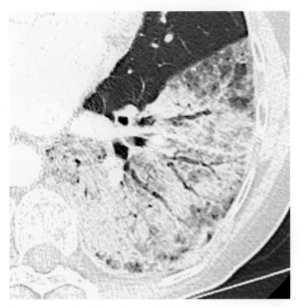

Fig. 21.4. Nonsmall cell lung cancer in a 71-year-old woman. This heterogeneous consolidation filling and expanding the left lower lobe on axial computed tomography in lung windows is proven by examination of a biopsy specimen to be a well-differentiated mucinous adenocarcinoma with bronchoalveolar features.

The error rate for the detection of lung cancer by chest radiography is generally accepted to be 20% to 50%, which is likely the result of a combination of factors.[27,28] Even with an adequate search pattern and search duration, limitations in human sight, technical aspects of the radiograph, and tumor characteristics can make identification of an early lung cancer challenging.[28]

Technical Factors

The radiograph itself may be of limited quality for a variety of technical reasons, including overpenetration or underpenetration of the chest by the photon beam or positioning variances such as rotation or lordosis. Objects external to the patient may cause artifacts. Although metal objects such as jewelry and clothing fasteners are easy to identify, nonmetal items such as buttons, hair, or clothing decorations may be confounding. Parts of the lung may be excluded from the field of view by faulty technique. Lastly, the ability of the patient to achieve full lung inspiration on the radiograph affects the conspicuity of lesions.[37] Visualization of nodules is enhanced by using higher peak kilovoltage (140 kVp), which accentuates contrast.[28]

Blind Spots on Radiography

Chest radiographs can have blind spots, many of them due to overlapping anatomic structures such as skeletal bones. Specific regions such as the hila, where the pulmonary arteries and veins and the airways converge, may also be difficult to evaluate (Fig. 21.6). Superimposed acute processes may mask findings of malignancy. Not infrequently, pneumonia can be the first indication of a central obstructing or partially obstructing lesion. Recurrent consolidations in the same location are highly suspicious (Fig. 21.7).[13] Consequently, radiographic follow-up to document resolution of pneumonia is advised. Chronic lung disease such as pulmonary fibrosis may also hinder identification of a focal abnormality. It is worth noting that preexisting chronic lung disease is a risk factor for lung cancer.

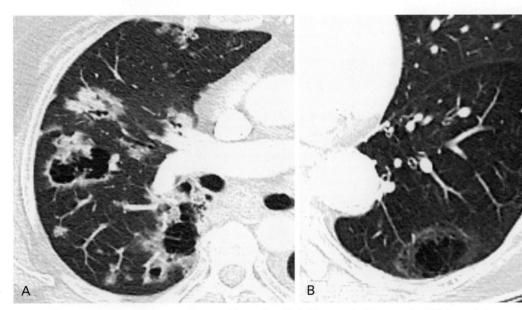

Fig. 21.5. Adenocarcinomas with central lucencies. (A) Axial computed tomography (CT) image in lung windows demonstrates multifocal lung opacities, some with pseudocavitation, in this 75-year-old man with primary lung adenocarcinoma having both mucinous and nonmucinous components, and (B) axial CT image in lung windows shows adenocarcinoma developing in the periphery of a preexisting cluster of emphysematous spaces in a 71-year-old woman.

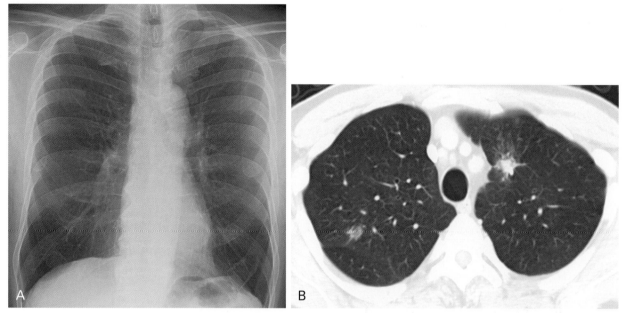

Fig. 21.6. Nonsmall cell lung cancer in an 85-year-old man. (A) Posteroanterior chest radiograph shows hyperinflated lungs compatible with chronic obstructive pulmonary disease. A small opacity is seen partially overlying the right posterior sixth rib. Hazy opacity also appears along the left paratracheal region just above the aortic arch. This example demonstrates the difficulty of visualizing subsolid lung lesions, the blind spots associated with the mediastinum and overlapping bone structures, and satisfaction of search limitations. (B) Axial computed tomography image in lung windows demonstrates bilateral lung tumors, which were proven by examination of a biopsy specimen to be synchronous adenocarcinomas.

Characteristics of Lung Cancers Missed on Radiography

Retrospective studies of lung cancers not prospectively identified on chest radiography have demonstrated several common characteristics. In general, missed lung cancers were located in the upper lobes, although one study showed no difference in the location of missed and detected lung cancers.[26,27] Another characteristic was small nodule size, on average 16 mm to 19 mm.[26,27,38] An analysis of size differences in detection rate indicated that nodules 10 mm or smaller were missed 71% of the time. Nodules 10 mm to 30 mm in size were not detected 28% of the time. However, nodules 30 mm to 40 mm were missed at a rate of 12%, and nodules greater than 40 mm were identified 100% of the time. Centrally located nodules that were missed had a larger circumference than overlooked peripheral nodules.[27] Overlying anatomic structures contributed to difficulty in detecting lung cancers.[26,27] Many of the missed cancers had ill-defined borders and relatively low levels of density.[26,27] A high pretest probability of lung cancer has been shown to promote detection rates, and in two studies, underdiagnosis of lung cancers in women appeared to be related to lower clinical suspicion.[26,37]

Use of Special Radiographic Views

Disagreement exists over the importance of lateral projection in making a diagnosis of lung cancer. The authors of several studies have discovered a few cancers that could be visualized only on the lateral radiograph; although this represents a small number of cases, there is support for continued acquisition of the lateral chest radiograph in conjunction with the posteroanterior view (Fig. 21.8).[26] Oblique radiographs may also be helpful in determining whether an abnormality seen on standard views is external to the patient.

New Technology in Radiography

Technical advances in chest radiography have been made possible by digital radiographic technology.

Computer-Aided Detection

Computer-aided detection of pulmonary nodules on chest radiographs has been subject to the limitation of a high false-positive rate, but it does provide a so-called second reader effect by supporting the reading radiologist.[39] It has been shown that double reads improve interpretation accuracy;[28] however, in the current health-care system, practical reasons preclude having two trained radiologists read the same film. The use of computer-aided detection software systems has been shown to significantly enhance the accuracy and sensitivity of even experienced radiologists in detecting lung cancers on radiographs.[39,40] In one study, the computer-aided detection program was able to identify 40.4% of subtle or very subtle cancers.[40]

Dual-Energy Subtraction Radiography

Dual-energy subtraction technology uses two exposures of the frontal view of the chest obtained milliseconds apart at two different energy levels, or kVp. A postprocessing algorithm uses these exposures to virtually subtract the osseous structures from the radiograph, producing a soft tissue, thus providing a predominant image with greater conspicuity of lesions that are surrounded by air in the lungs, and fewer blind spots from overlapping skeletal structures (Fig. 21.9). Nevertheless, persistent limitations exist, including suboptimal evaluation of the retrocardiac space, the periphery of the lungs, and the retrosternal space.

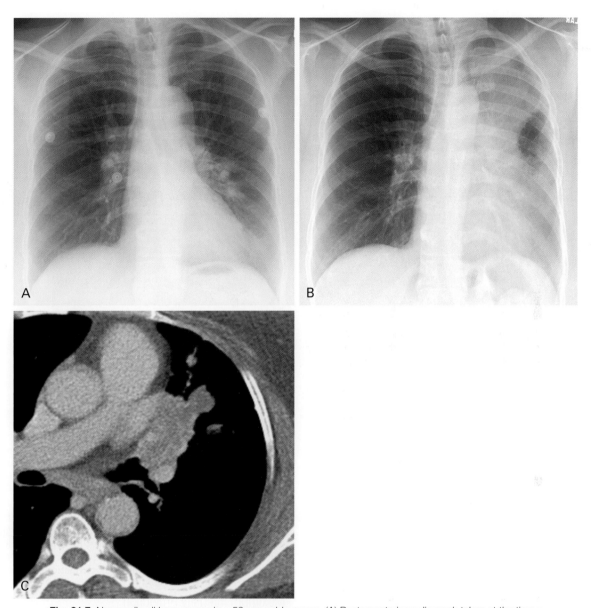

Fig. 21.7. Nonsmall cell lung cancer in a 59-year-old woman. (A) Posteroanterior radiograph taken at the time of original presentation to an emergency center for symptoms of cough. A lingular pneumonia was reported. The patient was treated but lost to follow-up. (B) A repeat radiograph was not obtained until 10 months later, when the entire left upper lobe was consolidated. (C) Chest computed tomography (CT) image was obtained several days later, and axial CT image in soft-tissue windows demonstrates an obstructing tumor in the lingula, which was determined by examination of a biopsy specimen to be squamous cell carcinoma.

Early phantom studies showed improved detection of thoracic abnormalities with dual-energy subtraction technology,[41,42] and observer studies have shown increased accuracy of lung nodule identification by both trained radiologists and residents.[43] Although dual-energy subtraction technology has improved the detectability of all lung cancers, it is particularly helpful in identifying PSNs, which are the most likely to be malignant.[44] Dual-energy subtraction technology can be used concurrently with computer-aided detection, but this combination has not yet been rigorously investigated.

IMAGING WITH CT

The discovery of a nodule or persistence of a lung opacity on radiography can be an indication for CT evaluation.[45] In a subset of the population of smokers and former smokers, screening for lung cancer with low-dose multidetector CT has been shown by the National Lung Cancer Screening Trial to decrease lung cancer mortality.[46] In addition, lung nodules may be found incidentally during CT imaging for other reasons, such as motor vehicle trauma or pulmonary embolism evaluation in the emergency department.

Chest CT is much more sensitive than radiography for detecting lung nodules and more useful for characterizing abnormalities. CT allows for more accurate description of size and density of a lesion and can identify satellite lesions below the resolution of radiography. CT permits a more detailed inspection of the pleura, the mediastinum, the thoracic lymph node basins, and extrathoracic regions, including the liver and adrenal glands, both common sites of metastases from lung cancer.

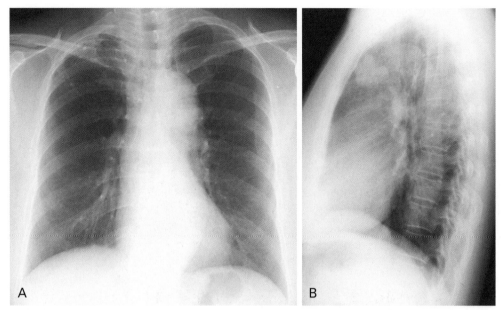

Fig. 21.8. Adenocarcinoma in a 69-year-old woman. (A) Posteroanterior radiograph of the chest has slightly increased density in the region of the aortic arch and aorticopulmonary window. (B) The lesion is much easier to visualize on the lateral projection, in which a multilobulated tumor is seen anteriorly in the retrosternal space.

Blind Spots on CT

Several factors influence the recognition and diagnosis of lung cancer on CT. Small endobronchial lesions may be very subtle and difficult to see, necessitating meticulous examination of the airways.[28,47] Small pulmonary nodules are missed on CT up to 47% of the time, usually because of central and/or peribronchovascular location (Fig. 21.10).[47] Adjacent airspace disease, including pneumonia or atelectasis, can obscure findings of malignancy.[47] However, the Golden S sign denoting a central obstructing tumor with peripheral lobar collapse (classically, the right upper lobe) is highly suggestive of malignancy.[13] On contrast-enhanced CT scans, differential enhancement of atelectasis compared with tumor or infection can help identify underlying lung lesions.[47] The presence of intravenous contrast material also facilitates recognition of lymphadenopathy, particularly in the hilar regions, and of pleural involvement.[47,48] The presence of other major findings on chest imaging can distract the reader and may hinder identification of a small malignancy.[47,49]

Characteristics of Lung Cancers Missed on CT

The characteristics of lung cancers not detected on CT have been reviewed in several studies. The diameters of cancerous lesions missed on chest CT examinations are smaller than lesions missed on radiographs; the mean diameter in one study was 12 mm and in another was 9.8 mm for detection errors and 15.9 mm for interpretation errors.[49,50] A large proportion of the missed tumors were subtle GGOs correlating mostly with well-differentiated lung adenocarcinomas.[50,51] Central endobronchial lesions were most commonly missed in one study.[49] Location in the lower lobes and in the perihilar regions contributed to detection failure, as did preexisting lung disease.[49,50] A number of cancers were not prospectively identified in nonsmoking women.[52] An acknowledged limitation in these studies is the thick 10-mm collimation and image reconstruction CT technique common to most of the examinations reviewed.[49,50] A 5-mm collimation and image reconstruction algorithm is much more common on modern CT scanners, and even thinner collimation is standard in many academic centers.

New Technology in CT

Computer-Aided Detection

Computer-aided detection programs have also been developed to identify pulmonary nodules on CT (Fig. 21.11). Studies using computer-aided detection as a second reader have shown improved sensitivity in nodule detection.[53,54] False-positive results obtained using the software application are usually caused by vessels en face, vascular branch points, and/or artifacts.[22] Although use of computer-aided detection to identify ground-glass nodules is more complicated than for solid nodules, some studies have shown that computer-aided detection also improves detection of ground-glass and mixed-attenuation nodules.[54,55]

Maximum Intensity Projection

Maximum intensity projection images can facilitate the identification of small solid pulmonary nodules.[22] The improvement in reader sensitivity is similar to that of computer-aided detection.[23]

USE OF CT IN STAGING OF LUNG CANCERS

The revised version of the TNM staging system for NSCLC is discussed in detail in Chapter 25. Adopted in 2009 after the evaluation of 67,725 cases of NSCLC, this edition of the TNM staging system categorizes TNM features into groups that best align with prognosis and treatment of the disease.[56] This edition has also been recommended for staging of SCLC and bronchopulmonary carcinoid tumors.[57,58] Chest CT is routine for baseline staging of lung cancer and for surgical planning, if the disease is potentially resectable. The study should include the adrenal glands in their entirety. As a result, much of the liver will also be within the field of view, although the entire liver is not typically imaged. Use of intravenous contrast material is preferred if not contraindicated by the patient's allergy profile or by declining renal function.[59] Multidetector CT acquires continuous volume datasets, which can then be used to create multiplanar reformatted images for additional information.[13] Axial reconstructions are most optimal at 5 mm or less.

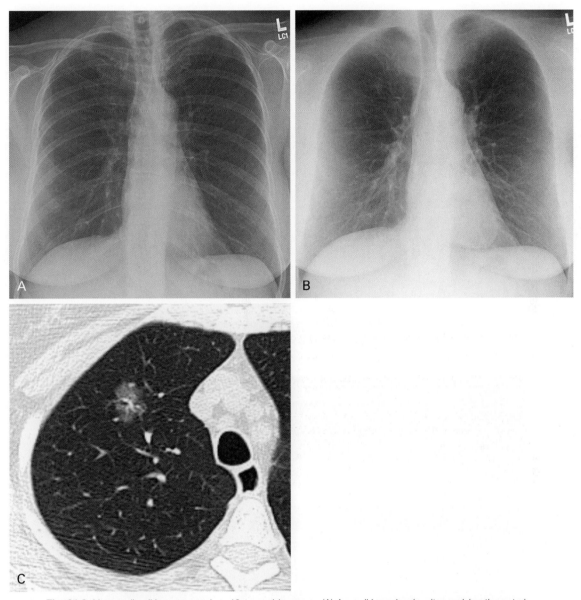

Fig. 21.9. Nonsmall cell lung cancer in a 43-year-old woman. (A) A small irregular density overlying the anterior right second rib is difficult to visualize on posteroanterior chest radiograph; (B) the dual-energy subtraction soft-tissue window projection accentuates the opacity and facilitates detection; and (C) chest computed tomography (CT) image with contrast material was obtained and axial CT image in lung windows demonstrates a focal ground-glass lesion compatible with an adenocarcinoma.

Tumor (T) Descriptors

Evaluation of lung tumors is first based on the size of the lesion, which correlates with prognosis. Smaller lesions have better outcomes: the 5-year survival for T1a lung carcinoma is 77%. By contrast, T4 lung cancer is associated with a 15% 5-year survival rate.

Accordingly, lesions up to 3 cm are T1, lesions up to 2 cm are T1a, and lesions greater than 2 cm up to 3 cm are T1b. The T2 category is divided into two parts: T2a lesions are greater than 3 cm to 5 cm, and T2b masses are 5 cm to 7 cm in size. T3 lesions are greater than 7 cm in diameter or located less than 2 cm from the carina. T4 tumors involve the carina directly.[56,60]

Attendant factors upstage the T descriptor, including invasion of adjacent structures and collapse of the surrounding lung (Fig. 21.12).

Direct Invasion of the Pleura

Tumors that abut a pleural surface, including the fissures, for a contact distance of greater than 3 cm, are considered suspicious for possible pleural invasion. Other findings that suggest invasion include eradication of the extrapleural fat plane, an obtuse angle between the tumor and pleural surface, and a tumor–pleura contact that exceeds the tumor height.[61] Nevertheless, pleural invasion is not conclusively identified by imaging in most instances, excluding frank invasion of the chest wall; the pathologic evaluation of the resected specimen is definitive. Bone destruction and/or tumor tissue extending between the ribs is consistent with chest wall invasion, considered T3, which necessitates an en bloc resection of chest wall with the tumor.[13]

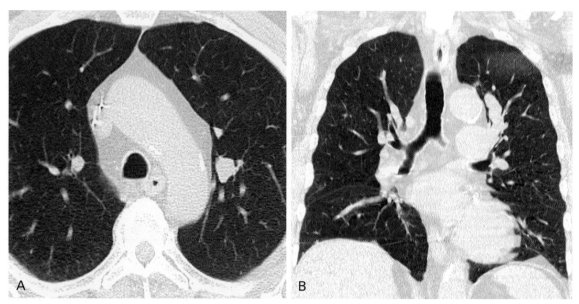

Fig. 21.10. Nonsmall cell lung cancer in a 76-year-old man. (A) Axial computed tomography (CT) image in lung windows and (B) coronal CT reformatted image in lung windows demonstrate asymmetry of the central bronchovascular structures, with an expanded tubular opacity in the left upper lobe. This is a potential blind spot on CT examinations.

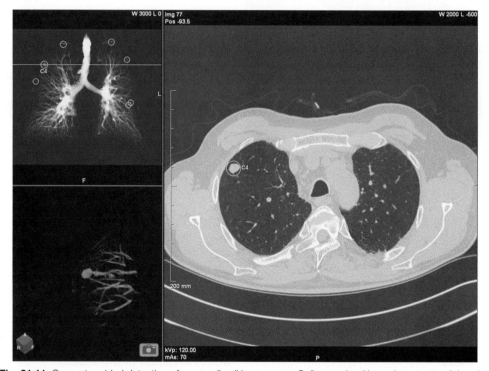

Fig. 21.11. Computer-aided detection of nonsmall cell lung cancer. Software algorithms detect potential nodular opacities on computed tomography images. Although some of the identified abnormalities are seen to be false-positive results, such as bronchovascular branch points when evaluated by the radiologist, the computer-aided detection software can also recognize lung cancers, as in this case.

Direct Invasion of the Mediastinum

Stranding of the mediastinal fat subjacent to the tumor, contact length greater than 3 cm along the mediastinal margin, and contact with the aorta of greater than 90° are suspicious for possible invasion of the mediastinum. Obliteration of the fat plane between the tumor and mediastinal structures is suspicious and also raises the possibility of mural invasion involving systemic and pulmonary vascular structures. Nevertheless, prediction of subtle mediastinal invasion with conventional imaging is low.[13,62] Frank invasion of the heart or trachea can be seen and represents T4 disease.

Satellite Nodules

The presence of small lung nodules in addition to the dominant lesion also upstages the tumor. Satellite nodules within the

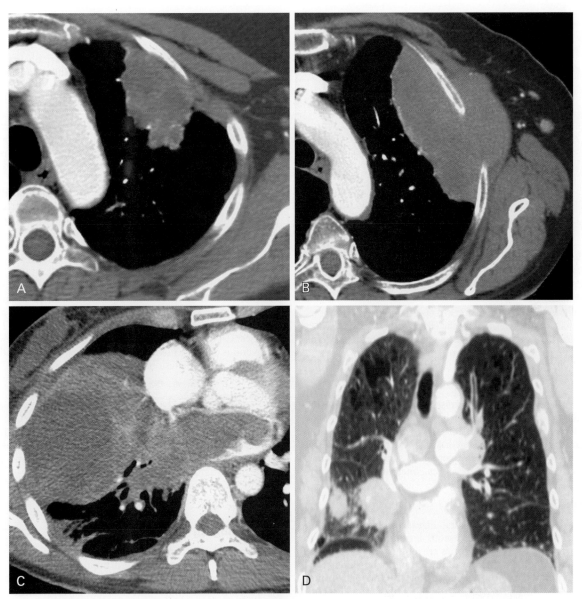

Fig. 21.12. Several findings will upstage nonsmall cell lung cancer. Axial computed tomography (CT) images in soft-tissue windows show (A) pleural invasion; (B) frank chest wall invasion through the intercostal space; and (C) cardiac invasion. Satellite nodules in the same lobe as the primary tumor are considered T3 disease, as seen on (D) coronal reformatted CT image in lung windows.

same lung lobe as the primary malignancy constitute T3 disease. Nodules ipsilateral to the tumor but in a different lung lobe represent T4 disease. If the nodules are in the contralateral lung, they are considered metastatic, M1a.[56]

Postobstructive Collapse or Pneumonitis

Lobar collapse around a central obstructing lesion constitutes T2 disease.

Lymph Node (N) Descriptors

Involvement of lymph nodes by tumor also has an effect on prognosis. Nodal basins commonly affected by lung cancer include the supraclavicular chains, the compartments of the mediastinum, and the hilar regions. Nodal disease occasionally but infrequently can be seen in the internal mammary chains, the parietal spaces, or the axillary and retropectoral spaces.

Lymph nodes that measure 1 cm or more in short-axis diameter on CT are considered to be suspicious for nodal metastatic disease despite relatively low sensitivity and specificity.[13] However, not all metastatic lymph nodes meet the size criteria for enlargement and not all enlarged nodes are metastatic. An analysis of resected nodes measuring 2 cm to 3 cm found that 37% had no metastatic involvement.[63] When nodal disease is not identified on standard CT, ^{18}F-2-deoxy-D-glucose (FDG)-PET or PET–CT can be useful for identifying small malignant nodes as well as for guiding biopsies. Lymph node sampling is performed to confirm the presence of nodal disease based on suspicious CT or PET–CT findings.[64]

Absence of nodal metastatic disease is considered N0. The presence of hilar or intrapulmonary lymphadenopathy ipsilateral to the tumor constitutes N1 disease. Metastatic adenopathy in the ipsilateral mediastinum and/or subcarinal region qualifies as N2 disease. The spread of metastases to the contralateral mediastinum, the contralateral hilum, or the supraclavicular or scalene

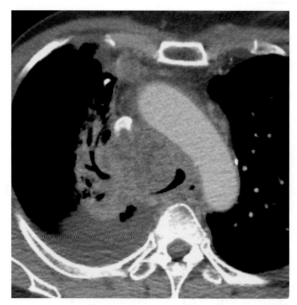

Fig. 21.13. Nonsmall cell lung cancer in a 68-year-old woman. Axial computed tomography with contrast material in soft-tissue windows demonstrates bulky metastatic disease causing severe compression of the trachea above the carina and the esophagus. Early invasion of the superior vena cava appears, although the vessel remains patent.

nodes of either side denotes N3 disease and raises the stage to IIIB, which is considered unresectable.[56,65]

When extensive bulky nodal disease is present, compression and/or frank invasion of the mediastinal vascular structures is possible, with danger of superior vena cava syndrome. Tracheal and/or esophageal compromise is also a concern (Fig. 21.13).

Metastasis (M) Descriptors

Metastatic disease includes pleural disease, contralateral pulmonary parenchymal nodules, osseous lesions, and deposits in extrathoracic organs. Two categories are designated. M1a disease comprises intrathoracic metastases, including malignant pleural disease and pulmonary nodules contralateral to the index tumor (Fig. 21.14). Pericardial and myocardial metastases are also considered to be in the M1a category. M1b disease incorporates extrathoracic metastatic lesions (Fig. 21.15).[56,66] The distribution is based on outcome data showing that survival was significantly worse among patients with metastases outside the thorax than among patients with metastatic disease confined to the lung and pleura.[66]

A pleural effusion is seen in up to 33% of individuals who present with NSCLC. Etiologies include sympathetic and parapneumonic processes in addition to neoplasm, and so definitive characterization is required. Malignant pleural effusion can be a difficult diagnosis unless pleural nodularity is clearly evident on CT, as thoracentesis is positive in 65% of cases. Nevertheless, a second thoracentesis may identify up to 30% more individuals with malignant effusion, and repeat thoracentesis is advised as the next step in the investigation. If the diagnosis remains in doubt, thoracoscopy is used, with accurate diagnosis of pleural involvement in more than 95% of patients.[67]

When clinical examination is normal, the risk of discovering extrathoracic metastases on imaging is low. However, metastatic disease is found on imaging workup in more than 50% of patients with an abnormal clinical examination.[13] The relative frequencies of metastatic deposits in extrathoracic organs from NSCLC have been reported as 3% for adrenal gland, 5% for liver, 7% for bone, and 10% for brain.[13,68]

Adrenal Gland Imaging

CT imaging through the adrenal glands is recommended for staging of lung cancer and is almost invariably included as part of the dedicated chest CT.[13] The finding of an adrenal nodule should be evaluated, but statistically, benign adrenal adenomas are present in at least 10% of the general population. Characteristics of benign adrenal nodules include smaller size (<2 cm), low attenuation (<10 HU) on noncontrast studies, sharper definition, and lack of enhancement. Conversely, malignant nodules are often larger, have heterogeneous attenuation, and are often diffuse rather than focal. In indeterminate cases, in-phase and out-of-phase MRI can identify the presence of microscopic fat consistent with benign adenoma. PET–CT may also be helpful, as adenomas generally have little or only background FDG activity. Fine-needle aspiration biopsy can resolve additional questions.[13]

Liver Imaging

Lung cancer metastases to the liver are usually seen in the context of other metastatic disease to regional nodes and so rarely alter management.[13] Liver metastases were found in 3% of asymptomatic individuals with NSCLC in one meta-analysis.[69] The staging chest CT includes most of the liver in the field of view. Use of intravenous contrast medium improves identification and characterization of hepatic lesions.

Bone Imaging

Asymptomatic bone metastases are uncommon.[13] CT is more sensitive than radiography for the detection of small osseous lesions without pathologic fracture. Ill-defined lucencies within bone on CT images raise concern about metastatic deposits. Nuclear scintigraphy with technetium-99m or PET–CT can be used for evaluation, and some lesions may exhibit FDG activity before becoming radiographically evident.

Brain Imaging

Brain metastases from lung cancer are often not clinically apparent.[13] Therefore dedicated brain imaging with contrast-enhanced head CT or brain MRI is recommended, not just for symptomatic individuals but also for asymptomatic individuals with advanced local disease who are being considered for aggressive treatment. Occult brain metastases are more likely to occur with larger primary tumors. Squamous cell carcinomas are less likely to metastasize to the brain than are adenocarcinomas or SCLC.[13]

IMAGE-GUIDED BIOPSY

Transthoracic needle biopsy for tumor cell–type analysis and for confirmation of metastatic disease is most often guided by CT (Fig. 21.16), although a superficial lesion such as in the chest wall could be accessed using ultrasound guidance.[13] CT-guided biopsy has a reported accuracy rate of 80% to 95% in positive tumor identification. By contrast, transbronchial biopsy has good results with central endobronchial lesions, but its accuracy rate is less than 80% for peripheral tumors.[13] Surgical open-lung biopsy or video-assisted thoracoscopic surgery can be useful to obtain larger tissue samples but has increased associated morbidity.[9,70]

Currently, a core-needle biopsy is recommended to provide sufficient tissue for biomarker analysis performed once the cell type has been established. In cases of necrotic or cavitary lesions, the sample should be taken from the wall of the tumor rather than the acellular center.[13]

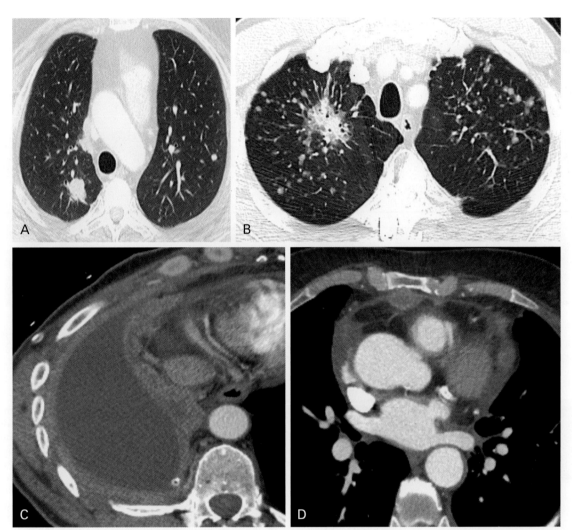

Fig. 21.14. Metastatic disease in the M1a category is limited to the thorax. (A) Axial computed tomography (CT) image in lung windows demonstrates a dominant right upper lobe tumor and a satellite nodule in the left upper lobe, compatible with metastasis in a 54-year-old man; (B) axial CT image in lung windows for another 61-year-old male never-smoker shows innumerable bilateral miliary metastases, associated in this case with a papillary adenocarcinoma; (C) axial CT image with contrast material in soft-tissue windows shows pleural nodularity and cytology-proven malignant effusion in this 63-year-old man with metastatic adenocarcinoma; and (D) axial CT image with contrast material in soft-tissue windows demonstrates several pericardial metastases in a 64-year-old woman with nonsmall cell lung cancer.

CT IMAGING OF RESPONSE TO THERAPY

Lung cancers may be treated with chemotherapy, radiation, or surgery or a combination of these modalities. Chest CT plays a crucial role in evaluating response to therapy and in assessing treatment complications.

Chemotherapy

Neoadjuvant chemotherapy may be administered in an effort to diminish tumor size before planned resection. Systemic chemotherapy is also the standard of care in cases of metastatic disease. Imaging with chest CT at regular intervals is useful to assess the efficacy of a chemotherapy regimen and to avoid unnecessary toxicity if the chemotherapy is ineffective.

Drug toxicity related to chemotherapy can manifest in the lungs as almost any pattern of interstitial pneumonia, including nonspecific interstitial pneumonia, usual interstitial pneumonia, organizing pneumonia, eosinophilia with pulmonary infiltrates, lymphocytic interstitial pneumonia, and desquamative interstitial pneumonia.[71] Drug toxicity typically occurs during treatment with a chemotherapy agent, and cessation of the offending agent usually results in improvement. Patients receiving multidrug therapy are at an increased risk of drug toxicity.[71] In some cases of pulmonary fibrosis, the damage cannot be reversed.[71]

CT findings suggesting possible drug toxicity include intralobular and interlobular septal thickening, nodular opacities, mosaic lung attenuation, diffuse alveolar opacities, migratory opacities, bronchovascular opacities, and honeycombing.[71]

Radiotherapy

Radiotherapy may be used as definitive treatment with curative intent for stage I or II lung cancer, particularly for individuals with comorbidities such as severe emphysema and cardiovascular disease that may make surgery inadvisable. In later-stage but resectable cancers, radiotherapy may be used as adjuvant therapy in conjunction with surgery for improved local control of disease; it can also be used for palliation.[72]

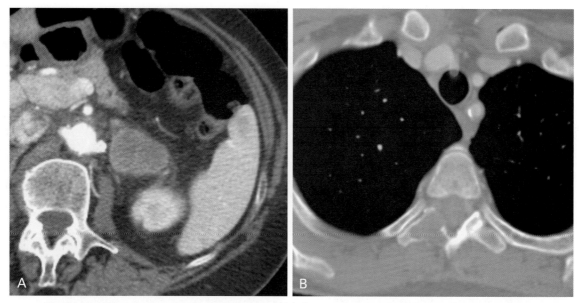

Fig. 21.15. Metastatic disease in the M1b descriptor includes metastases to the extrathoracic organs. (A) Axial computed tomography (CT) image with contrast material in soft-tissue windows shows a large, heterogeneously enhancing left adrenal mass, proven by examination of a biopsy specimen to be metastatic adenocarcinoma. (B) Axial CT image in bone windows demonstrates a lytic metastasis in the right T4 transverse process.

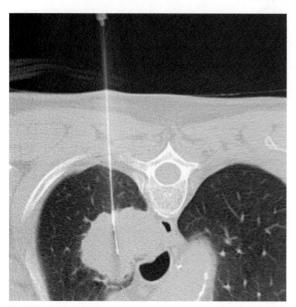

Fig. 21.16. Axial image from computed tomography–guided biopsy in lung windows with a patient in prone position shows the biopsy needle in the center of the large irregular right lung mass having histology consistent with undifferentiated small cell lung cancer.

Conventional opposed parallel beam radiotherapy has been largely supplanted in the past several years by three-dimensional (3-D) conformal radiotherapy and stereotactic ablative radiotherapy, which use multiple beams to minimize the radiation dose to normal structures while delivering a high dose to the tumor tissue.[72] Chest CT is used to ascertain response of the treated lesion, to monitor other potential effects of the radiation, and to exclude any recurrence within the radiation field or the appearance of metastatic disease outside of it.

Decreased size of the irradiated tumor is often observed soon after treatment, without any ancillary findings.[72] Radiation-induced changes in the surrounding lung parenchyma are categorized as early phase radiation pneumonitis, corresponding with the acute exudative and proliferative phases of alveolar damage and occurring 1 month to 6 months after completion of treatment, and late-phase radiation fibrosis with collagen deposition taking place from 6 months to 24 months after treatment cessation.[72–74] These changes are often progressive along a continuum, although radiation pneumonitis can spontaneously resolve. Although several factors influence radiation damage, including preexisting patient conditions, the degree of severity of the lung injury directly correlates with the radiation dose, particularly the percentage volume that receives greater than 20 Gy.[72,74] Clinically significant, symptomatic pulmonary toxicity (grade 2 and above) from radiation develops in up to 37% of patients receiving 3-D conformational radiotherapy and 4% of patients receiving stereotactic ablative radiotherapy, requiring steroid and other treatment. Some chemotherapy drugs, including bleomycin, doxorubicin, and busulfan, can increase radiation effects.[72]

The appearance of radiation-induced lung injury on CT has conventionally been described as having four patterns. Two of these, homogeneous slight ground-glass attenuation involving the radiation field and patchy consolidation within but not conforming to the radiation port, correspond with radiation pneumonitis. Discrete but nonuniform consolidation is the third pattern. Solid consolidation of the entire irradiated portion of the lung with volume loss, architectural distortion, and traction bronchiectasis represents the fourth pattern, radiation fibrosis.[73,75] Pleural effusion is also considered a treatment effect.[72]

With the newer radiation techniques, the resulting patterns of lung injury have somewhat different morphology and distribution. Focal ground glass or consolidation representing radiation pneumonitis is typically seen only in the area directly adjacent to the treated tumor, although discrete opacities can be seen in other parts of the radiation field.[72] Radiation fibrosis after 3-D conformational radiotherapy or stereotactic ablative radiotherapy can have a modified conventional pattern, similar to but less extensive than traditional radiation fibrosis. Focal fibrosis and traction bronchiectasis confined to the area around the tumor is classified as mass-like. A 1-cm wide linear

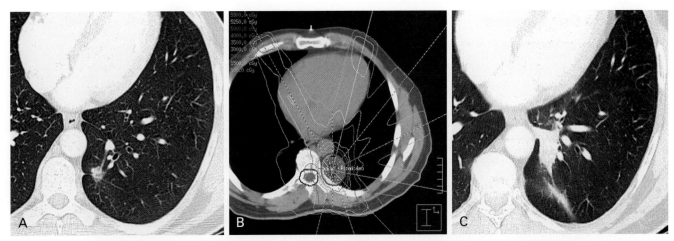

Fig. 21.17. Sequela of stereotactic ablative radiation, scar-like pattern of fibrosis. (A) Axial computed tomography (CT) image in lung windows shows a small heterogeneous left lower lobe tumor with pleural tethering compatible with a primary adenocarcinoma; (B) the beams from different directions used to treat the lesion as well as the diminishing radiation dose at specific distances from the target are documented in the radiation treatment-planning CT study; and (C) axial CT image in lung windows shows a small focal opacity in the left lower lobe with volume loss and minimal band-like scarring.

or plate-like opacity causing volume loss and replacing the original tumor is considered the scar-like pattern of fibrosis (Fig. 21.17).[72]

CT findings that should prompt suspicion of disease recurrence in the radiation field include development of a mass or cavitation within radiation fibrosis, new occlusion of dilated bronchi within the fibrosis, and/or late appearance or enlargement of an ipsilateral pleural effusion.[76] A recurrent tumor usually occurs within 2 years after completion of treatment.[72]

Surgical Resection

After surgical resection of lung tumors with lobectomy or pneumonectomy, periodic CT studies are used to exclude recurrent disease at the surgical site as well as to monitor for late metastatic disease. After surgical resection, patients are followed-up with contrast-enhanced chest CT every 3 months to 4 months for the first 2 years. In the absence of any concerning finding at the end of 2 years, these patients may have annual follow-up with noncontrast CT.

IMAGING OF EMERGENT CONDITIONS IN LUNG CANCER

In some circumstances, lung cancer can cause severe secondary abnormalities that require emergent identification and treatment.

Pulmonary Embolism

Malignancy is a known risk factor for coagulopathy, and the development of deep venous thrombosis and pulmonary thromboembolic disease is an important potential complication. Clinically unsuspected pulmonary emboli are seen in up to 4% of asymptomatic individuals with cancer on multidetector CT; the prevalence is higher with some types of malignancies, including melanoma and gynecologic tumors, among individuals with progressive disease and also among patients receiving chemotherapy.[77,78] Pulmonary emboli can manifest as pruning of pulmonary arteries distal to the clot (Westermark sign) or as a wedge-shaped infarct (Hampton hump sign) on chest radiography; however, radiographs are most often normal in the setting of pulmonary embolism. Use of contrast-enhanced

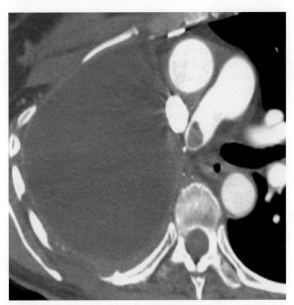

Fig. 21.18. Stump thrombus after right pneumonectomy. Axial computed tomography image with contrast material in soft-tissue windows shows a small dense opacity in the ligated right pulmonary artery, outlined by intravenous contrast material in the pulmonary arterial tree. The pneumonectomy space has an expected appearance, as it is entirely filled with fluid.

multidetector CT with thin 1.25-mm reconstructions is helpful for detection, localization, and assessment of clot burden. Emboli in the pulmonary arteries are outlined by intravenous contrast material, which is white on CT; they appear as low-density masses with often elongated shapes within the opacified vessels. The presence or absence of right ventricular strain should also be evaluated.[77]

Acute pulmonary embolism is different from stump thrombus, in which turbulent flow produces a small clot within a ligated pulmonary artery after pneumonectomy (Fig. 21.18); stump thrombosis is a recognized complication in 12% of pneumonectomy cases. Although systemic anticoagulation is not required in all cases, subsets of patients may require treatment.[79]

Superior Vena Cava Syndrome

Occlusion of the superior vena cava is associated with primary lung cancer in 50% to 80% of cases. Tumor tissue and/or metastatic lymphadenopathy can compromise the patency of the superior vena cava via extrinsic compression or vascular invasion.[77] Collateral circulation may develop if the process is sufficiently gradual, but acute obstruction may also occur. Superior vena cava syndrome is a clinical diagnosis, and associated imaging findings include widening of the mediastinum on radiographs and mediastinal soft tissue on CT, interruption of contrast material within the superior vena cava on contrast-enhanced CT, and opacification of collateral vascularity (Fig. 21.19).[77]

Central Airway Obstruction

Primary lung cancer is also the most common cause of endobronchial obstruction. The severity of clinical symptoms is related to the location of the lesion; "lesions in the upper airways can be acutely life-threatening if the airway is blocked."[77] Narrowing of the airway lumen can be extrinsic or it can result from a lesion of the bronchial wall. Stenting may be used to preserve patency if surgical resection is precluded. Radiation is also used to debulk tumors and improve air flow.[77]

IMAGING WITH MRI

Multidetector CT and FDG-PET–CT are routinely used to initially stage lung cancer, evaluate treatment response, and detect residual or recurrent disease. The role of MRI has historically been limited to evaluating superior sulcus tumors and identifying involvement of the mediastinum, chest wall, and spinal cord, but technologic advances have expanded the techniques available to radiologists and improved the image quality of MRI.[80] The applications of MRI have been extended to include the identification and characterization of pulmonary nodules, differentiation of lung cancer from other pulmonary processes, and detection of lymph node involvement and distant metastases as part of lung cancer staging.[81]

Identification of Pulmonary Nodules

Although multidetector CT is considered the standard criterion for identifying pulmonary nodules, several studies have been performed to assess the efficacy of nodule detection by MRI. In general, detection rates of 46% to 96% have been reported using a wide variety of MRI sequences on 1.5-T and 3-T systems.[82–86] The efficacy of MRI in detecting pulmonary nodules is most dependent on the size of the nodule and the specific imaging sequences used. For instance, Schroeder et al.[85] found sensitivities of 73%, 86.3%, 95.7%, and 100% for nodules measuring less than 3 mm, 3 mm to 5 mm, 6 mm to 10 mm, and greater than 10 mm, respectively, on T2-weighted half-Fourier acquisition single-shot turbo spin-echo sequences. Biederer et al.[83] demonstrated a sensitivity of 88% for 4-mm nodules on 3-D and two-dimensional gradient-echo sequences, as well as sensitivity, specificity, and positive and negative predictive values close to 100% for nodules greater than 5 mm on all MRI sequences other than T2-weighted half-Fourier acquisition single-shot turbo spin-echo.[83]

In general, the nodule detection rate is higher with spin-echo sequences than gradient-echo sequences.[82–86] Bruegel et al.[87] found sensitivities of 72%, 69%, and 63.4% for nodule detection on triggered short-tau inversion recovery, fast spin-echo, and short-tau inversion recovery sequences, respectively. This group reported that the sensitivities of sequences such as half-Fourier acquisition single-shot turbo spin-echo, inversion recovery half-Fourier acquisition single-shot turbo spin-echo, and precontrast and postcontrast volumetric interpolated 3-D gradient echo

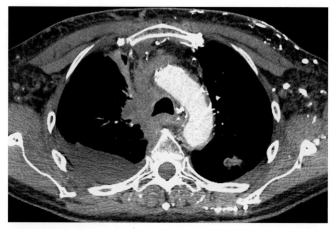

Fig. 21.19. Superior vena cava obstruction. Axial computed tomography image with contrast material in soft-tissue windows demonstrates amorphous soft-tissue density in the region of the left brachiocephalic vein and superior vena cava. Numerous opacified collateral vessels appear in the left chest wall and in the mediastinum, which provide blood return to the right atrium; intravenous contrast material has reached the systemic arterial circulation as evidenced by the opacified aortic arch.

were less than other fast spin-echo sequences.[87] Both et al.[88] demonstrated sensitivities of 85% and 90% for nodules measuring greater than 4 mm on T2-weighted half-Fourier fast spin-echo and T1-weighted gradient-echo sequences, respectively.[88] Short-tau inversion recovery sequences alone have demonstrated sensitivities greater than 90% in detecting nodules measuring 3 mm and larger.[89] The efficacy of diffusion-weighted imaging in detecting pulmonary nodules has been reported. Koyama et al.[90] demonstrated a lower detection rate for diffusion-weighted imaging (85%) compared with short-tau inversion recovery (100%), and limited ability to detect small nodules and nonsolid adenocarcinomas on diffusion-weighted imaging.

Characterization of Pulmonary Nodules

The characterization of pulmonary nodules with conventional imaging is widely used but has limitations. For example, multidetector CT provides morphologic information only, and differentiating between benign and malignant nodules is limited to classic appearances of calcium or fat within the nodule. Dynamic contrast-enhanced CT has demonstrated high sensitivity but limited specificity in differentiating between nodules secondary to overlapping enhancement patterns in active granulomatous processes, hypervascular benign nodules, and malignant nodules.[91,92] Lastly, the effectiveness of PET and PET–CT is limited by false-positive results due to infection and inflammation and false-negative results in the setting of some adenocarcinomas and carcinoids.[93]

MRI also has limitations, but investigations show promise in improving characterization of nodules. On T1-weighted and T2-weighted spin-echo images, many pulmonary nodules, lung cancers, and metastases demonstrate low or intermediate signal intensity.[94–98] Short-tau inversion recovery sequences are better than T1-weighted and T2-weighted sequences at differentiating between benign and malignant nodules; however, their sensitivity, specificity, and accuracy are 83.3%, 60.6%, and 74.5%, respectively.[82] Koyama et al.[82] evaluated the efficacy of noncontrast multidetector CT and 1.5-T MRI in detecting pulmonary nodules and differentiating between benign and malignant nodules in 161 individuals. The sensitivity of nodule detection was higher for multidetector CT (97%) than short-tau inversion recovery turbo spin-echo sequences (82.5%), but the malignant nodule detection rates were similar (100% for multidetector CT and 96.1% for MRI). Several studies evaluating the efficacy of diffusion-weighted imaging in characterizing pulmonary nodules have yielded mixed results. In general, malignant lesions demonstrate high signal intensity on diffusion-weighted imaging and low apparent diffusion coefficient due to increased cellularity, high tissue disorganization, and increased extracellular space tortuosity. Although diffusion-weighted imaging may be more beneficial than traditional T1-weighted and T2-weighted sequences, false-positive results due to infectious and inflammatory lesions and false-negative results in the setting of some low-grade adenocarcinomas and metastases limit its effectiveness.[99]

Ultrafast dynamic contrast-enhanced sequences have been used in dynamic perfusion MRI studies to differentiate between benign and malignant nodules. Malignant nodules typically demonstrate homogeneous enhancement on T1-weighted images after the administration of intravenous contrast material. Factors such as tumor angiogenesis, tumor necrosis, scarring, presence or absence of fibrosis, and tumor interstitial spaces result in some variability.[94–98,100] Information regarding enhancement patterns or blood supply obtained from dynamic contrast-enhanced MRI may be beneficial in distinguishing between benign and malignant nodules. Various dynamic MRI techniques have been used for this purpose, with reported sensitivities of 94% to 100%, specificities of 70% to 96%, and accuracies greater than 88%.[94–97,100]

Ohno et al.[98] demonstrated higher specificity and accuracy for MRI in differentiating between benign and malignant nodules compared with multidetector CT and FDG-PET. Specifically, the accuracies of dynamic contrast-enhanced MRI, dynamic contrast-enhanced multidetector CT, and PET–CT were 88.1%, 83.2%, and 83.7%, respectively. Currently, no imaging methodology is without limitations, and MRI remains an important tool in the armamentarium.

USE OF MRI IN STAGING OF LUNG CANCER

T Descriptors

MRI is superior to CT in differentiating lung cancers from other pulmonary processes such as atelectasis or consolidation. For instance, although many tumors demonstrate high signal intensity on T2-weighted imaging (Fig. 21.20), postobstructive atelectasis and pneumonitis typically demonstrate greater signal intensity than do malignancies.[101] On diffusion-weighted imaging, lung cancers demonstrate higher signal intensity than postobstructive atelectasis.[102] MRI is better than CT in evaluating the heart, pericardium, and great vessels and can be used to assess invasion of the cardiac chambers (Fig. 21.21), myocardium, or superior vena cava.[103]

One of the most important uses of MRI in the staging of lung cancer is the determination of mediastinal and/or chest wall invasion. Malignancies that invade only the mediastinal fat may be surgically resected, whereas malignancies that invade mediastinal structures are generally considered unresectable. The Radiologic Diagnostic Oncology Group first reported that MRI was significantly more accurate than CT in identifying invasion of the mediastinum.[80] In one study, Ohno et al.[103] evaluated 50 individuals with NSCLC and suspected mediastinal and/or hilar invasion with contrast-enhanced CT, cardiac-gated MRI, and noncardiac-gated and cardiac-gated MR angiography. Compared with contrast-enhanced CT and T1-weighted imaging, the reported sensitivity of 78% to 90%, specificity of 73% to 87%, and accuracy of 75% to 88% for MR angiography in identifying invasion of the mediastinum and hilum were greater.

The reported sensitivity and specificity for detection of chest wall invasion by CT are highly variable, with values of 38% to 87% and 40% to 90%, respectively.[104] Findings on MRI suggestive of chest wall invasion include infiltration or disruption of the normal extrapleural fat plane on T1-weighted sequences or hyperintensity of the parietal pleura on T2-weighted

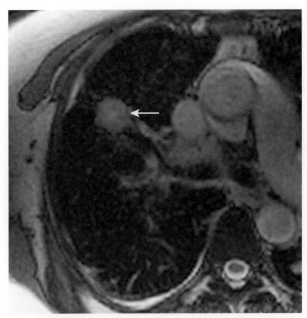

Fig. 21.20. Nonsmall cell lung cancer in a 49-year-old woman. Axial T2-weighted magnetic resonance imaging (MRI) demonstrates a hyperintense nodule *(arrow)* with irregular margins in the right lung. Examination of a biopsy specimen indicated squamous cell carcinoma. Many primary and secondary malignancies of the lung demonstrate high signal intensity on T2-weighted MRI.

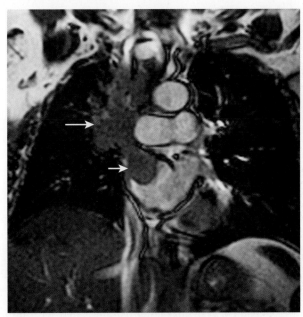

Fig. 21.21. Invasion of the cardiac chambers by a small cell lung cancer in a 57-year-old woman. Coronal balanced steady-state free precession magnetic resonance imaging (MRI) shows the primary tumor *(long arrow)* in the medial right upper lobe extending through the right superior pulmonary vein into the left atrium *(short arrow)*. MRI is superior to computed tomography in evaluating for involvement of the heart, pericardium, and great vessels.

sequences.[105,106] Short-tau inversion recovery sequences may demonstrate high signal intensity within the chest wall structures whose signal is otherwise suppressed by this technique (Fig. 21.22).[105] The administration of intravenous contrast material may assist in making the diagnosis.[105] Techniques such as cine MRI during breathing may be used to identify

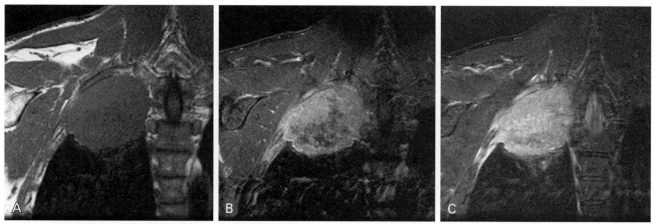

Fig. 21.22. Superior sulcus tumor invading the chest wall in a 61-year-old man. (A) Coronal T1-weighted noncontrast; (B) T1-weighted postcontrast; and (C) short-tau inversion recovery magnetic resonance images demonstrate a large mass in the right upper lobe. Note the region of tumor enhancement and short-tau inversion recovery hyperintensity extending through the intercostal space into the chest wall, consistent with invasion.

chest wall invasion, as fixation of the tumor to the chest wall suggests involvement, but free movement of the tumor along the parietal pleura suggests absence of invasion.[107] One study using both dynamic cine MRI and CT demonstrated sensitivity, specificity, and accuracy of 100%, 70%, and 76%, respectively, for cine MRI, and 80%, 65%, and 68%, respectively, for CT.[107]

N Descriptors

The MRI sequences recommended for optimal detection of metastatic lymph nodes include cardiac-triggered and/or respiratory-triggered conventional or black-blood short-tau inversion recovery turbo spin-echo sequences.[81,108] Metastatic lymph nodes typically demonstrate high signal intensity on short-tau inversion recovery sequences, whereas normal lymph nodes show low signal intensity. Estimates of the sensitivity, specificity, and accuracy of short-tau inversion recovery turbo spin-echo imaging have been reported as 83.7% to 100%, 86% to 93.1%, and 86% to 92.2%, respectively.[81,108] Compared with CT, the sensitivity and accuracy of short-tau inversion recovery are much higher.[81] Another study demonstrated that the sensitivity and accuracy of MRI using short-tau inversion recovery sequences were much better than those of PET–CT, at 90.1% and 92.2%, compared with 76.7% and 83.5%, respectively.[108] Yi et al.[109] demonstrated no significant differences between whole-body MRI and PET–CT in determining nodal involvement and also reported that specific findings such as high signal intensity and eccentric cortical thickening or obliterated fatty hilum on T2-weighted black-blood turbo spin-echo sequences were reliable indicators of malignancy (Fig. 21.23). Nomori et al.[110] demonstrated that diffusion-weighted imaging was more accurate than PET in establishing nodal disease. However, the intrinsic low spatial resolution of diffusion-weighted imaging limits detection of small lymph nodes and localization of abnormal lymph nodes.

M Descriptors

FDG-PET–CT is the imaging modality of choice for detecting metastatic disease, and the addition of FDG-PET to conventional staging examinations has resulted in greater detection

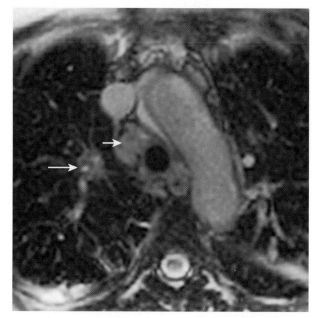

Fig. 21.23. Pathologic lymphadenopathy in a 51-year-old man with nonsmall cell lung cancer. Axial T2-weighted magnetic resonance image demonstrates an irregular nodule *(long arrow)* in the right lung that represents the patient's primary lung cancer. Note the enlarged and slightly hyperintense right paratracheal lymph node *(short arrow)*. Examination of a biopsy specimen of the lymph node indicated malignant involvement. Studies have demonstrated that specific findings such as high signal intensity and eccentric cortical thickening or obliterated fatty hilum on T2-weighted black-blood turbo spin-echo sequences are reliable indicators of malignancy.

of extrathoracic metastases.[111] One study demonstrated similar accuracy between PET–CT (88.2%) and whole-body MRI (87.7%) for detecting metastatic disease,[112] and another demonstrated no significant differences between the diagnostic value of PET–CT and MRI in the preoperative staging assessment of NSCLC.[113]

PET and PET–CT are best at demonstrating osseous and soft-tissue metastases, whereas MRI is best at identifying brain, liver, and adrenal metastases secondary to superior soft-tissue contrast.[101] The sensitivity of PET and PET–CT in detecting brain metastases is limited by hypermetabolism of the brain parenchyma. Therefore CT and/or MRI are recommended for detection of brain metastases (Fig. 21.24). Hepatic metastases typically manifest as enhancing lesions on T1-weighted

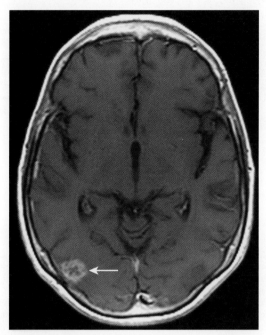

Fig. 21.24. Brain metastases in a 64-year-old man with nonsmall cell lung cancer. Axial contrast-enhanced T1-weighted magnetic resonance imaging (MRI) demonstrates a peripherally enhancing lesion *(arrow)* in the right posterior temporal/parietal lobe. Examination of a biopsy specimen indicated metastatic disease from the patient's lung cancer. Because the sensitivity of positron emission tomography (PET) and PET/computed tomography (CT) in detecting brain metastases is limited by hypermetabolism of the brain parenchyma, CT and/or MRI is preferred for identifying brain metastases.

images after the administration of intravenous contrast material.[101] Chemical-shift MRI techniques may be used to identify adrenal adenomas with a sensitivity of 100% and specificity of 81% and distinguish between adenomas and metastatic disease.[101] The loss of signal on T1-weighted out-of-phase imaging from an adrenal lesion is consistent with an adrenal adenoma (Fig. 21.25), whereas a persistent high signal is suggestive of metastasis (Fig. 21.26).

MRI OF RESPONSE TO THERAPY

Specific sequences such as dynamic contrast-enhanced and diffusion-weighted imaging with apparent diffusion coefficient have been used to assess the ability of MRI to detect response among patients treated with chemoradiation therapy. Chang et al.[114] suggested that dynamic contrast-enhanced MRI had the potential to predict early response in patients treated with bevacizumab, gemcitabine, and cisplatin. Yabuuchi et al.[115] reported a significant correlation between early changes in apparent diffusion coefficient and reduction in tumor size, as well as greater median progression-free survival and median overall survival in patients whose tumors demonstrated increases in apparent diffusion coefficient. Results from another study suggest that early changes in apparent diffusion coefficient values may be used to monitor early response of lung cancer to chemoradiation therapy.[116]

CONCLUSION

Conventional radiographic imaging studies play a crucial role in the detection and staging of lung cancer. Chest radiographs may provide the earliest opportunity to identify an unsuspected lung cancer. CT is essential for the characterization of abnormalities and determines preliminary staging for a tumor once a tissue diagnosis is established. MRI of localized regions in the chest can provide information, particularly regarding soft-tissue and neurovascular invasion. These imaging modalities work in concert with PET–CT and with surgical biopsy to guide management and treatment planning.

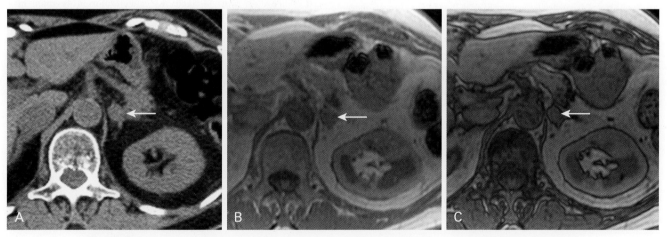

Fig. 21.25. Left adrenal adenoma in a 54-year-old woman with nonsmall cell lung cancer. (A) Noncontrast axial computed tomography (CT) image demonstrates a well-circumscribed nodule in the left adrenal gland *(white arrow)* that did not meet the CT criteria for an adenoma. Axial T1-weighted (B) in-phase and (C) out-of-phase magnetic resonance images of the same patient show loss of signal *(white arrow)* on the out-of-phase imaging, indicating the presence of microscopic fat and highly suggestive of an adenoma.

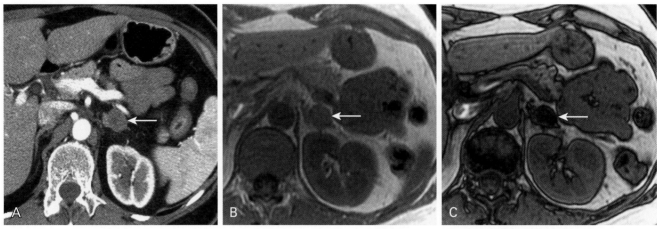

Fig. 21.26. Left adrenal metastasis in a 49-year-old woman with nonsmall cell lung cancer. (A) Noncontrast axial computed tomography (CT) image demonstrates a well-circumscribed nodule in the left adrenal gland (*white arrow*) that did not meet the CT criteria for an adenoma. Axial T1-weighted (B) in-phase and (C) out-of-phase magnetic resonance images of the same patient show persistent high signal in the nodule. Examination of the specimen after CT-guided biopsy confirmed metastasis from the patient's nonsmall cell lung cancer.

KEY REFERENCES

11. Henschke CI, Wisnivesky JP, Yankelevitz DF, Miettinen OS. Small stage I cancers of the lung: genuineness and curability. *Lung Cancer.* 2003;39(3):327–330.
13. Hollings N, Shaw P. Diagnostic imaging of lung cancer. *Eur Respir J.* 2002;19(4):722–742.
15. MacMahon H, Austin JH, Gamsu G, et al. Guidelines for management of small pulmonary nodules detected on CT scans: a statement from the Fleischner Society. *Radiology.* 2005;237(2):395–400.
17. Naidich DP, Bankier AA, MacMahon H, et al. Recommendations for the management of subsolid pulmonary nodules detected at CT: a statement from the Fleischner Society. *Radiology.* 2013;266(1):304–317.
22. Brandman S, Ko JP. Pulmonary nodule detection, characterization, and management with multidetector computed tomography. *J Thorac Imaging.* 2011;26(2):90–105.
45. American College of Radiology. *ACR Appropriateness Criteria (Reviewed 2012).* http://www.acr.org/Quality-Safety/Appropriateness-Criteria.
46. National Lung Screening Trial Research Team, Aberle DR, Adams AM, et al. Reduced lung-cancer mortality with low-dose computed tomographic screening. *N Engl J Med.* 2011;365(5):395–409.
56. Goldstraw P, Crowley J, Chansky K, et al. The IASLC Lung Cancer Staging Project: proposals for the revision of the TNM stage groupings in the forthcoming (seventh) edition of the TNM classification of malignant tumours. *J Thorac Oncol.* 2007;2(8):706–714.
57. Shepherd FA, Crowley J, Van Houtte P, et al. The International Association for the Study of Lung Cancer lung cancer staging project: proposals regarding the clinical staging of small cell lung cancer in the forthcoming (seventh) edition of the tumor, node, metastasis classification for lung cancer. *J Thorac Oncol.* 2007;2(12):1067–1077.
65. Rusch VW, Crowley J, Giroux DJ, et al. The IASLC Lung Cancer Staging Project: proposals for the revision of the N descriptors in the forthcoming seventh edition of the TNM classification for lung cancer. *J Thorac Oncol.* 2007;2(7):603–612.
66. Postmus PE, Brambilla E, Chansky K, et al. The IASLC Lung Cancer Staging Project: proposals for revision of the M descriptors in the forthcoming (seventh) edition of the TNM classification of lung cancer. *J Thorac Oncol.* 2007;2(8):686–693.
76. Choi YW, Munden RF, Erasmus JJ, et al. Effects of radiation therapy on the lung: radiologic appearances and differential diagnosis. *Radiographics.* 2004;24(4):985–997.
77. Katabathina VS, Restrepo CS, Betancourt Cuellar SL, Riascos RF, Menias CO. Imaging of oncologic emergencies: what every radiologist should know. *Radiographics.* 2013;33(6):1533–1553.
99. Koyama H, Ohno Y, Seki S, et al. Magnetic resonance imaging for lung cancer. *J Thorac Imaging.* 2013;28(3):138–150.
108. Ohno Y, Koyama H, Nogami M, et al. STIR turbo SE MR imaging vs. coregistered FDG-PET/CT: quantitative and qualitative assessment of N-stage in non-small-cell lung cancer patients. *J Magn Reson Imaging.* 2007;26(4):1071–1080.
110. Nomori H, Mori T, Ikeda K, et al. Diffusion-weighted magnetic resonance imaging can be used in place of positron emission tomography for N staging of non-small-cell lung cancer with fewer false-positive results. *J Thorac Cardiovasc Surg.* 2008;135(4):816–822.

See Expertconsult.com for full list of references.

22 Positron Emission Tomography Imaging of Lung Cancer

Jeremy J. Erasmus, Feng-Ming (Spring) Kong, and Homer A. Macapinlac

SUMMARY OF KEY POINTS

- ^{18}F-2-deoxy-D-glucose (FDG)-positron emission tomography–computed tomography (PET–CT) is routinely used clinically for diagnosis, staging, and radiation treatment planning and may have a role in prognosis and monitoring of treatment response.

- FDG-PET–CT is not optimal in determination of T descriptors (additional small lung nodules, locoregional invasion, etc.) as respiratory motion and or low-radiation-dose imaging degrade image quality.

- FDG-PET–CT has superior accuracy compared with CT in detecting hilar (N1), mediastinal (N2, N3), and extrathoracic (N3) nodal metastasis.

- FDG-PET–CT has superior accuracy compared with CT in detecting M1b and M1c (extrathoracic) metastasis.

- FDG-PET–CT detection of occult metastasis (M1b/M1c) increases as T and N descriptors increase and impact on management is greater in patients with more advanced disease.

- FDG uptake threshold such as standardized uptake value (SUV) is unreliable in differentiating inflammatory from metastatic disease.

- FDG-PET prognostic information is not dependable and may be confounded by limitations of SUV reproducibility.

- FDG-PET–CT metabolic tumor volume and total lesion glycolysis (which take into account tumor size and uptake of FDG) may be important prognostic factors.

- FDG-PET–CT may allow an early and sensitive assessment of antitumor effect after therapy.

- FDG-PET–CT improves accuracy of target delineation in radiation treatment planning.

- A PET–CT-defined tumor target is usually smaller than that defined by CT, and incorporation of PET–CT into radiotherapy planning can allow radiation-dose escalation without increasing side effects.

- FDG is the only Medicare-approved PET–CT tracer for evaluation of cancer.

- Novel PET radiotracers that interrogate different metabolic pathways beyond glycolysis, receptors, and targets are being evaluated in staging, response evaluation, and targeted therapy assessment.

PET using the radiopharmaceutical FDG, a D-glucose analog labeled with fluorine-18, complements conventional radiographic imaging for the evaluation of patients with nonsmall cell lung cancer (NSCLC). FDG-PET has an important role in the staging of NSCLC according to the tumor, node, and metastasis (TNM) system and is routinely used to improve the detection of nodal and extrathoracic metastases. FDG-PET is also currently used to improve the planning of radiation

therapy and is being evaluated for the assessment of prognosis and therapeutic response. By potentially allowing for an earlier and more sensitive assessment of the effect of antitumor therapy, FDG-PET may be predictive of the outcome of treatment and the survival of patients after treatment. This chapter will discuss the use of FDG-PET for the staging of disease, the planning of radiation therapy, and the assessment of outcome and prognosis, with an emphasis on the appropriate clinical use of FDG-PET for the treatment of patients who have NSCLC. In addition, the use of novel radiotracers that interrogate different metabolic pathways, receptors, and targets to overcome the potential limitations of FDG-PET in staging, as well as early response evaluation and monitoring of response to targeted therapies, will be reviewed.

STAGING OF LUNG CANCER

Size, Location, and Locoregional Invasion (T Descriptor)

FDG-PET is used together with CT because the integration of metabolic activity with the high-spatial resolution of CT is important for the evaluation of tumors in terms of size, location, and the degree of locoregional invasion (T descriptor) as well as for the determination of the anatomic location of regions of focally increased FDG uptake.[1,2] It is important to be aware that the relatively poor spatial resolution of PET limits its utility for the evaluation of the primary tumor. However, the CT component of integrated PET–CT also has shortcomings in terms of its ability to accurately demonstrate T descriptors such as the presence of additional small lung nodules and locoregional invasion as it is often performed during respiration and with a low-radiation-dose imaging protocol, both of which can compromise image quality. Nevertheless, FDG-PET improves the detection of nodal and distant metastases and frequently alters the treatment of patients.[3–8] Accordingly, this review of TNM staging will focus on the important role of PET imaging for the detection of nodal and distant metastases at the time of initial staging according to the seventh edition of the American Joint Committee on Cancer TNM staging system and will reference the proposals for the forthcoming eighth edition when applicable.[9–15]

Regional Lymph Nodes (N Descriptor)

The presence and location of nodal metastasis (N descriptor) are important when determining the treatment of and prognosis for patients with NSCLC and, because these descriptors adequately predict prognosis, they will be maintained in the forthcoming eighth staging system.[10,13,14] Lymph node maps, in which the node stations are numbered according to anatomic structures, are commonly used in an attempt to ensure uniformity when designating the clinical and pathologic extent of nodal metastases.[16,17] There is no universally accepted nodal map and the International Association for the Study of Lung Cancer has proposed a new lymph node map that reconciles the differences among the currently used maps.[18] However, while a precise and universally accepted nomenclature to describe lymph node involvement is essential for selecting appropriate

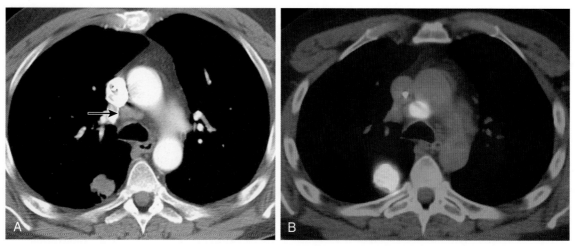

Fig. 22.1. A 49-year-old man with NSCLC who was being evaluated for surgical resection. (A) Axial contrast-enhanced CT showing a 2.5-cm nodule in the upper lobe of the right lung and a small node (short-axis diameter, 1 cm) in the ipsilateral mediastinum *(arrow)*. (B) Axial PET–CT scan showing increased FDG uptake in the nodule and in the right lower paratracheal lymph node. A biopsy was positive for nodal metastatic disease, and the patient underwent neoadjuvant chemotherapy followed by concurrent chemoradiation.

therapy and assessing the outcomes of treatment, a major shortcoming of clinical staging is the use of nodal size to detect metastatic disease. Toloza et al.,[19] in a meta-analysis of 20 studies (3438 patients) that was performed to evaluate the use of CT for staging of the mediastinum, found that the use of a short-axis diameter of more than 1 cm as the threshold for the detection of nodal metastasis was associated with a pooled sensitivity of 57% and a pooled specificity of 82%.

FDG-PET is more accurate than CT for staging of the mediastinum in terms of nodal involvement, and FDG-PET is being increasingly integrated into both surgical and radiation oncology treatment strategies for patients with NSCLC (Fig. 22.1).[3,4,6,20] Birim et al.,[4] in a meta-analysis of 17 studies (833 patients) in which PET was compared with CT for nodal metastasis detection in patients with NSCLC, reported that the overall sensitivity and specificity of FDG-PET for detecting mediastinal lymph node metastases were 83% (range, 66–100%) and 92% (range, 81–100%), respectively, whereas those of CT were 59% (range, 20–81%) and 78% (range, 44–100%), respectively. In addition, improvement in the accuracy of nodal metastasis detection has been reported in association with the use of integrated PET–CT as compared with the use of CT ($p = 0.004$) and PET ($p = 0.625$) separately.[1] However, in a recent study of 159 patients with NSCLC, the use of PET–CT for mediastinal N determination was associated with low sensitivity and accuracy.[21] Based on the evaluation of 1001 nodal stations (723 mediastinal, 148 hilar, and 130 intrapulmonary), the sensitivity, specificity, and accuracy of PET–CT for the detection of mediastinal nodal metastasis were 45.2%, 94.5%, and 84.9%, respectively. The sensitivity of PET–CT for the detection of malignant involvement was 32.4% (12 of 37) for nodes measuring less than 10 mm and 85.3% (29 of 34) for nodes measuring 10 mm or more. Although infrequently addressed, the timing of PET–CT imaging may affect N determination. Ideally, PET imaging for the evaluation of nodal metastasis in patients being evaluated for surgical resection should be performed in close temporal relationship to the anticipated date of resection. In this regard, there may be a meaningful association between the sensitivity of PET–CT and the time from imaging to resection.[22] Booth et al.[22] reported that the sensitivity and accuracy of PET–CT for N2 nodal detection were 64% and 94%, respectively, when performed less than 9 weeks before pathologic sampling,

compared with 0% and 81%, respectively, when performed 9 weeks or more before pathologic sampling.

Despite the superior accuracy of FDG-PET–CT over CT in terms of N determination, a limitation is the overlap in the appearance of malignant and benign lymph nodes as microscopic nodal metastases normally are not FDG-avid, whereas inflammatory lymph nodes can be FDG-avid. The use of an FDG uptake threshold such as the maximum standardized uptake value (SUV_{max}) to differentiate inflammatory from metastatic nodal disease has limited utility for clinical N determination as numerous factors, including the time to imaging after FDG administration and the type of scanner and image reconstruction algorithm used, can affect the thresholds selected. We are not aware of any prospective multicenter trial that has validated an FDG uptake threshold, and visual interpretation currently tends to be more accurate than SUV quantification.[23] When mediastinal lymph nodes are FDG-avid as determined on the basis of visual analysis or SUV, the number of false-positive results due to infectious or inflammatory etiologies is too high to allow for a confident diagnosis of nodal metastasis (Fig. 22.2).[21,24] In this regard, because the positive predictive value of FDG-PET is not optimal for diagnosing nodal metastasis, invasive sampling should be performed to confirm pathologically involved nodes (pN) disease when the PET and CT findings are indicative of nodal metastasis or when the CT and PET findings are incongruent.[24,25] In addition, even if PET–CT is negative for mediastinal nodal metastasis, the need for histologic confirmation persists because of the low sensitivity and accuracy of PET–CT for intrathoracic nodal staging.[21,24] However, it is important to emphasize that the precise role of FDG-PET with regard to invasive nodal evaluation is unclear. Although not universally accepted, the American College of Chest Physicians evidence-based practice guidelines recommend that invasive confirmation of the mediastinal nodes is not needed in patients with a peripheral clinical stage I NSCLC if PET of the mediastinum is negative.[25,26] Furthermore, a meta-analysis of 10 studies (1122 patients) indicated that occult nodal metastasis is not infrequent in patients with clinical stage T1-2N0 NSCLC but that PET and CT provide a favorable negative predictive value for the detection of mediastinal metastasis (0.94 for T1 disease and 0.89 for T2 disease), suggesting a low yield from invasive clinical staging for this subgroup of patients.[27]

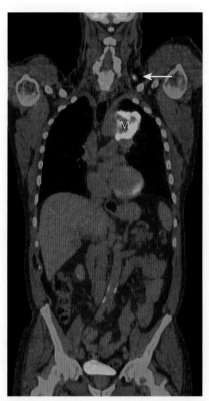

Fig. 22.2. A 62-year-old man with a NSCLC in the upper lobe of the left lung who was being evaluated for surgical resection. This coronal PET–CT shows increased FDG uptake in the mass in the upper lobe of the left lung *(M)* and a small node (short-axis diameter, 1 cm) in the left supraclavicular region *(arrow)*. A biopsy revealed findings consistent with reactive lymphoid hyperplasia (abundant lymphoid tissue, germinal center fragments, increased large cells, tingible body macrophages) and absence of metastatic carcinoma. The patient underwent left upper lobectomy.

In an attempt to determine the need for invasive sampling after PET and CT imaging, de Langen et al.[28] performed a meta-analysis to evaluate the association between the size of mediastinal nodes and the probability of malignancy. The authors reported a 5% posttest probability for N2 disease in patients with a negative result on FDG-PET imaging in whom the mediastinal nodes measured 10 mm to 15 mm on CT and suggested that these patients should be treated with thoracotomy. In comparison, they reported a 21% posttest probability for N2 disease in patients with a negative result on FDG-PET imaging in whom the lymph nodes measured more than 16 mm on CT and suggested that these patients should have mediastinoscopy prior to thoracotomy. For patients with a positive result on FDG-PET, the posttest probability of malignancy was 62% when the nodes measured 10 mm to 15 mm on CT and 90% when the nodes measured more than 16 mm. Although the authors did not suggest any management strategies regarding histologic confirmation of nodal metastasis when the result on FDG-PET is positive, N2 and N3 disease should be histologically confirmed in patients who are potentially eligible for resection or adjuvant therapy.

The expanded role of nonsurgical management for patients with early-stage NSCLC and the definitive use of FDG-PET–CT to detect mediastinal nodal metastasis in high-risk patients or patients with advanced disease who are being evaluated for nonsurgical management underscore the importance of accurate nodal evaluation. In this regard, there have been attempts to improve the detection of mediastinal nodal metastasis when using FDG-PET–CT in the staging algorithm. The SUV_{max} of

the primary tumor has been used to predict the likelihood of microscopic nodal metastatic disease and to improve the accuracy of N staging.[29–31] Trister et al.[31] reported that a high SUV for the primary tumor was an independent predictor of occult mediastinal nodal metastasis in patients with clinical stage I and II NSCLC and recommended invasive staging of the mediastinum when the SUV is more than 6. In addition, in a study of 265 patients with NSCLC, Miyasaka et al.[29] reported that the SUV_{max} of the primary tumor was a significant predictor of pathologic nodal involvement, with pN1-2 disease being detected in 25 (41%) of 61 in whom the SUV_{max} was more than 10, compared with only 26 (12.7%) of 204 patients in whom it was less than 10 ($p < 0.0001$). The detection of nodal metastasis also may be improved by the use of point spread function (PSF) reconstruction along with PET–CT scanners. PSF reconstruction recently became commercially available, and, as a result of improved image contrast and reduced image noise, may be more sensitive for the detection of small-volume nodal metastases. Lasnon et al.[32] reported that PSF PET had higher sensitivity (97%), negative predictive value (92%), and negative likelihood ratio (0.04) than did conventional iterative reconstruction ordered subset expectation maximization PET (78%, 57%, 0.31, respectively) for nodal evaluation in patients with NSCLC. While improved sensitivity increases the likelihood of false-positive results, the authors concluded, on the basis of the significant improvements in sensitivity ($p = 0.01$), negative predictive value ($p = 0.04$), and low negative likelihood ratio that were observed in association with PSF reconstruction, that preoperative invasive nodal staging may be omitted in cases in which the result of PSF FDG-PET–CT is negative. A potential further advance in nodal assessment is the use of an artificial neural network (ANN). Toney and Vesselle[33] recently reported that an ANN overcame the subjectivity associated with the interpretation of PET, outperformed an expert FDG-PET–CT reader in terms of accuracy, and differentiated malignant and benign inflammatory lymph nodes with overlapping appearances on PET–CT. The ANN used four FDG-PET–CT-derived input parameters (primary tumor SUV_{max}; tumor size; node size; and FDG uptake at the N1, N2, and N3 stations) and correctly predicted the N descriptor in 99.2% of cases, compared with 72.4% for the expert reader.

Distant Metastasis

Distant metastases (M descriptor) are common in patients with NSCLC at the time of presentation and are currently subclassified into M1a metastases (additional nodules in the contralateral lung, malignant pleural effusion, pleural nodule[s], pericardial nodule[s]) and M1b (extrathoracic) metastases.[11,12] The forthcoming eighth edition proposals for the M descriptor maintain the M1a descriptor but the M1b will now be assigned to cases with a single extrathoracic metastasis, and M1c to those with multiple extrathoracic metastases in one or more organs.[13,15]

Although FDG-PET–CT can be useful in the evaluation of the intrathoracic and extrathoracic metastases, the role of FDG-PET in detecting M disease is not clearly defined. For instance, patients with early clinical stage (T1 N0) NSCLC have a low incidence of occult metastasis; thus extensive evaluation for metastasis in these patients may not be warranted.[34] Viney et al.[35] performed a randomized controlled trial to determine the appropriate role of FDG-PET in the clinical treatment of patients who have early stage NSCLC. In that study, 183 patients with early-stage lung cancer (>90% of who had T1 2N0 involvement) were assigned to conventional workup (92 patients) or to conventional workup and PET (91 patients). Compared with conventional staging, PET confirmed staging in 61 patients, staged the tumors as benign in two patients, and upstaged the tumors in 22 patients, including 11 patients with N2 nodal metastatic disease and two patients with pleural metastasis. Distant metastases were rarely detected with PET (2 of 91 patients; <5%). Overall, the results of PET could have resulted in a change in treatment for 26% of the patients, with the avoidance of thoracotomy in 11 of 91 patients and with 13 of 91 potentially receiving neoadjuvant chemotherapy or chemoradiation therapy. However, because the general policy of the participating surgeons was to operate on patients with apparently completely resectable stage IIIA disease without any further evaluation, PET resulted in further investigation or other management changes in only 12 patients (14%).

In patients with more advanced disease, whole-body FDG-PET–CT has a greater impact on the accuracy of staging as well as on management. The American College of Surgeons Oncology Group reported that PET had a sensitivity, specificity, positive predictive value, and negative predictive value of 83%, 90%, 36%, and 99%, respectively, for M1 disease.[6] Whole-body PET imaging stages intrathoracic and extrathoracic disease in a single study and detects occult extrathoracic metastases in up to 24% of patients who are selected for curative resection (Fig. 22.3).[5,6,36] The incidence of detection of occult metastases has been reported to increase as the T and N descriptors increase (from 7.5% in early-stage disease to 24% in advanced disease).[36] In two studies with a relatively high proportion of patients with more advanced lung cancers that were considered to be resectable on the basis of standard clinical staging, PET imaging prevented nontherapeutic surgery in one of five patients.[5,6] A more recent prospective study, similar to the PLUS multicenter randomized trial conducted by van Tinteren et al.[5] but evaluating PET–CT rather than dedicated PET, demonstrated that 52 (63%) of 83 patients in the PET–CT group underwent surgery, with 13 (25%) of 52 thoracotomies being futile. By contrast, in the conventional staging group, 73 (80%) of 91 patients underwent thoracotomy, with 38 (52%) of 73 thoracotomies being futile.[5,37,38]

The widespread use of FDG-PET has changed the imaging algorithm that is used to detect metastases to specific organ sites, particularly the osseous skeleton, the adrenal glands, and extrathoracic lymph nodes. In this regard, FDG-PET–CT is particularly effective for detecting bone metastasis. A meta-analysis of 17 studies demonstrated that the pooled sensitivity and specificity for the detection of bone metastasis were 92% and 98%, respectively, for FDG-PET–CT, compared with 86% and 88%, respectively, for bone scintigraphy.[39] As a result, FDG-PET–CT has to a large extent replaced 99mTc-methylene-diphosphonate (MDP) bone scintigraphy for the evaluation of possible bone metastasis in patients with NSCLC (Fig. 22.4).[39–41] Specifically, 99mTc-MDP bone scintigraphy now has no additional utility for patients with NSCLC if FDG-PET is performed as part of the staging algorithm. In fact, discordant findings of skeletal metastasis between 99mTc-MDP scintigraphy and FDG-PET–CT have been reported to occur in 20% of patients with NSCLC.[42] This discordance is in large part due to the ability of FDG-PET to detect early bone metastasis and the failure of 99mTc-MDP scintigraphy to detect early neoplastic infiltration of bone marrow. FDG-PET–CT is also useful for detecting adrenal metastasis and for distinguishing benign from malignant adrenal masses that are detected with CT.[43] A meta-analysis of 21 studies (1391 lesions), including five studies that specifically focused on patients with lung cancer, demonstrated that FDG-PET had a combined sensitivity and specificity of 94% and 82%, respectively, for the detection of adrenal metastasis in patients with lung cancer.[43] Similar to the assessment of bone metastasis, FDG-PET has changed the imaging algorithm used to evaluate an indeterminate adrenal mass detected with CT and is now often used as the definitive imaging modality rather than magnetic resonance imaging (MRI), particularly when the adrenal mass is small (Fig. 22.5). In fact, adrenal masses

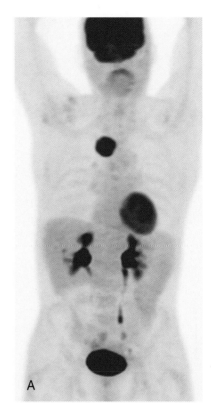

A

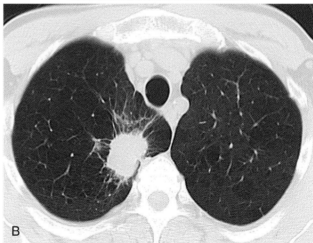

B

Fig. 22.3. A 53-year-old man with NSCLC who was being evaluated for surgical resection. (A) Axial contrast-enhanced CT showing a spiculated mass in the upper lobe of the right lung. Note the diffuse emphysematous lung disease. (B) Whole-body maximum intensity projection PET showing increased uptake of FDG in the mass. Note the absence of nodal and distant metastasis. Whole-body PET stages intrathoracic and extrathoracic disease in a single study.

can be characterized with use of FDG-PET, and subsequent imaging is usually unnecessary.[43] If an adrenal mass in a patient with potentially resectable NSCLC has normal FDG uptake on PET, curative resection should be considered without further evaluation. If an adrenal mass has increased FDG uptake, biopsy should be performed to confirm metastatic disease. FDG-PET–CT has limitations in the evaluation of liver and brain metastases. Specifically, because of the high background uptake of FDG by normal brain tissue, the ability to detect brain metastasis is not optimal.[44] MRI is the current standard of care for patients with NSCLC who are undergoing evaluation of possible brain

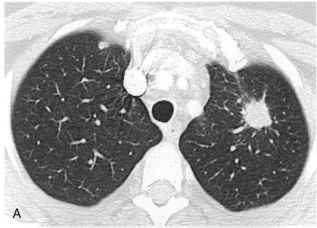

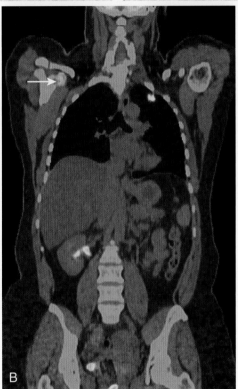

Fig. 22.4. A 46-year-old woman with NSCLC in the upper lobe of the left lung who presented with shoulder pain. (A) Axial contrast-enhanced CT showing a spiculated nodule in the upper lobe of the left lung. (B) Coronal PET–CT showing increased uptake of FDG in the nodule in the upper lobe of the left lung and in the coracoid process of the scapula (arrow), which was suspicious for metastasis. Biopsy confirmed metastatic disease, and the patient was treated palliatively.

metastases, and FDG-PET–CT lacks the sensitivity and specificity to replace this diagnostic test.[45] Similarly, FDG-PET–CT has a limited role in the detection of hepatic metastases. Although FDG-PET–CT has a high specificity for the detection of occult hepatic metastases, it has a low sensitivity, and, accordingly, FDG-PET is not routinely used for this purpose.

Whole-body FDG-PET imaging improves the accuracy of staging in patients with NSCLC. However, focal increased uptake of FDG in extrathoracic lesions that are unrelated to the primary NSCLC can mimic distant metastasis. Accordingly, all extrathoracic FDG-avid lesions that potentially would alter patient management should be further imaged or biopsied to

confirm the diagnosis of distant metastasis. The rationale for this management approach is supported by the results of a prospective study that was performed to assess the incidence and diagnosis of a single site of extrapulmonary accumulation of FDG in patients with newly diagnosed NSCLC.[46] Of the 350 patients in the study group, 72 had solitary FDG-avid lesions. Sixty-nine of these patients underwent biopsy of the lesion; of these, 37 (54%) had a solitary metastasis, whereas 32 (46%) had a lesion that was unrelated to the NSCLC, such as a benign tumor or inflammatory lesion (26 patients) or a clinically unsuspected second malignancy or recurrence of a previously diagnosed carcinoma (6 patients).

PROGNOSIS

The widespread use of CT and the increase in lung cancer screening programs have resulted in the detection of small lung cancers, typically adenocarcinomas, with indolent to aggressive malignant behavior. A recent multicenter study involving 610 patients with clinical stage IA lung cancer validated the ability of FDG-PET–CT together with high-resolution CT to predict the malignant behavior and prognosis of early adenocarcinomas of the lung (Fig. 22.6).[47] The diameter of the primary tumor was 20 mm or less in 354 patients and more than 20 mm in 256 patients. The mean duration of follow-up after surgery was 41.8 months, and the rate of disease recurrence was 9.5% (58 patients). A significant difference in recurrence-free survival was identified between tumors with an SUV_{max} of 2.9 or less and those with an SUV_{max} of more than 2.9 (5-year recurrence-free survival ratio, 95% compared with 72%; $p < 0.001$). In addition, SUV_{max} was a significant prognostic factor for cancer-specific survival ($p < 0.001$). Furthermore, when combined with a high-resolution CT ground-glass opacity ratio {(1 – [maximum dimension of solid component of tumor on lung windows/maximum dimension of tumor on lung windows]) × 100}, the data were especially useful for predicting the malignant grade of tumors and patient prognosis. The prediction of the biologic behavior of small adenocarcinomas is important for the selection of the appropriate surgical option. In this regard, the frequency of lymphatic, vessel, or pleural invasion was only 2% among tumors with an SUV of 2.9 or less and a ground-glass opacity ratio of 25% or more, and the 1% incidence of nodal metastasis or recurrence in this group suggests that sublobar resection, rather than lobectomy, could be considered as definitive management.[47] The use of SUV to identify patients with clinical stage IA lung cancers that are appropriate for limited resection was also supported by a report involving 183 patients with clinical stage IA NSCLC who were evaluated with PET–CT and underwent resection.[45] The 5-year recurrence rate was 0% for patients with a corrected SUV (the ratio of the tumor SUV_{max} to the liver SUV_{mean}) of less than 1.0, compared with 22.9% for those with a corrected SUV of 1.0 or more, and the 5-year cancer-specific survival rates for these groups were 100% and 88.7%, respectively.[48]

The level of increased FDG uptake in the primary tumor at the time of diagnosis also has been used to predict prognosis, and this level may be prefaced on the correlation of the SUV_{max} of the primary tumor with tumor differentiation, necrosis, pathologic type, size, and epidermal growth factor receptor (EGFR) protein expression.[47,49–51] Bille et al.[49] evaluated the prognostic significance of SUV_{max} of the primary tumor in a study of 404 patients with NSCLC who underwent potentially curative resection after PET–CT. SUV_{max} of the primary tumor was significantly associated with survival ($p = 0.00016$). The median survival, 2-year survival, and 5-year survival rates were 26.4%, 88.4%, and 72.1%, respectively, for the 209 patients with an SUV_{max} of less than 8.6, compared with 19.6%, 71%, and 47.8%, respectively, for the 195 patients with an SUV_{max} of 8.6 or more. Because a high tumor SUV_{max} potentially could

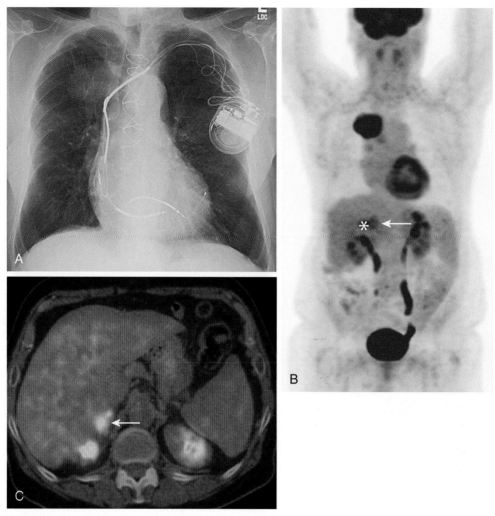

Fig. 22.5. A 70-year-old woman with NSCLC of the upper lobe of the right lung and an adrenal mass. (A) Posteroanterior radiograph of the chest, showing a mass in the upper lobe of the right lung. Note the presence of an implantable cardioverter defibrillator. (B) Whole-body PET maximum intensity projection image showing increased FDG uptake in the mass in the right lung and the right adrenal mass *(arrow)*. *Asterisk* indicates normal renal excretion of FDG in a calyx. (C) Axial PET–CT showing increased uptake of FDG in the right adrenal mass *(arrow)*, which was suspicious for metastasis. A biopsy confirmed metastatic disease.

allow more appropriate use of neoadjuvant and adjuvant therapy, a subgroup analysis of patients with stage I disease (for whom international guidelines do not recommend adjuvant treatment) was performed; this analysis showed that the SUV did not independently predict survival.[49] However, patients with stage II, III, or IV disease who had received adjuvant chemotherapy had better survival if the SUV_{max} was below 8.7, and the authors postulated that these patients would benefit most from targeted adjuvant therapy.[49] These findings are consistent with the current consensus that adjuvant chemotherapy after complete resection can result in a significant and clinically meaningful survival advantage for patients with stage II to IIIA NSCLC although not for patients with stage 1B disease.[52,53] However, Cerfolio et al.,[54] in a retrospective study of 315 patients who underwent complete resection of NSCLC, found that patients with stage IB and stage II disease who had SUV values that were greater than the median value for their respective stages had lower disease-free survival rates at 4 years. The differences in disease-free survival between patients with stage IB disease (92% for the low SUV group, compared with 51% for the high SUV group) and stage II disease (64% for the low SUV group, compared with 47% for the high SUV group) were

significant ($p = 0.005$ and 0.044, respectively). When the results were stratified according to stage, the actual 4-year survival rates for the low and high SUV groups were 80% and 66%, respectively, for patients with stage IB disease; 64% and 32%, respectively, for those with stage II disease; and 64% and 16%, respectively, for those with stage IIIA disease.

Performance status and stage are firmly established as prognostic factors for patients with NSCLC, and small studies have indicated that FGD-PET may also be useful for determining the prognosis for patients with early and advanced NSCLC.[47,49,51,55-59] However, a prospective National Cancer Institute–funded American College of Radiology Imaging Network/Radiation Therapy Oncology Group cooperative group trial evaluating posttreatment FDG-PET at approximately 14 weeks after radiotherapy in patients with stage III NSCLC demonstrated limited utility for predicting the prognosis.[60] Two hundred and twenty-six patients had pretreatment FDG-PET, and 173 patients had posttreatment FDG-PET. Pretreatment SUV_{peak} and SUV_{max} values were not associated with survival, although a posttreatment SUV_{peak} value of more than 7 was significantly associated with survival ($p < 0.001$). Overall survival (OS) based on the study's prespecified posttreatment

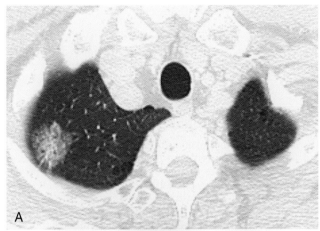

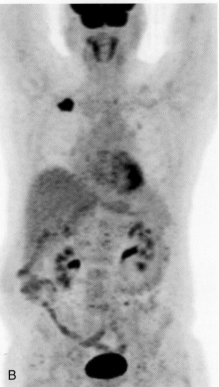

Fig. 22.6. A 72-year-old man with stage I (T1b N0 M0) adenocarcinoma of the lung. (A) Axial contrast-enhanced CT showing a 2.5-cm nodule in the upper lobe of the right lung with ground-glass opacity and solid attenuation. (B) Whole-body maximum intensity projection FDG-PET image showing focal increased FDG uptake (SUV_{max} = 12.3) in the right upper lobe nodule. Note the absence of nodal and distant metastases. Fifteen months following lobectomy of the upper lobe of the right lung, the patient developed a metastatic lesion in the left lung. Primary stage I malignancies that have a high SUV tend to have a higher rate of recurrence. *SUV*, standardized uptake value.

SUV_{peak} cutoff value of 3.5 was not significantly different in patients with an SUV_{peak} less than 3.5 compared with those with an SUV_{peak} greater than 3.5 ($p = 0.29$). The authors concluded that the use of a simple posttreatment SUV cutoff value of 3.5 after chemoradiotherapy is not useful for the clinical management of patients. The authors postulated that because patients with a high SUV (>7) after chemoradiotherapy have poor outcomes, this subpopulation could be considered for early additional treatment.[60]

FDG-PET studies are often limited by small size, their retrospective nature, and variations in treatment protocols, particularly for patients with advanced-stage NSCLC. These factors, in part, may account for the contradictory reports in the literature regarding the applicability of prognostic information provided by FDG-PET for patients with NSCLC. Hoang et al.[56] performed a retrospective review of 214 patients with advanced-stage NSCLC who underwent FDG-PET at the time of the initial diagnosis. Univariate and multivariate analysis provided no evidence that the survival times were significantly different for patient subgroups that were defined according to SUV_{max}; the median survival time was 16 months for the 106 patients in whom the primary tumor had an SUV_{max} of less than 11.1, compared with 12 months for the 108 patients in whom it had an SUV_{max} of 11.1 or more. In addition, improved outcomes may be confounded by PET-induced stage migration and selection bias.[61,62] In a retrospective analysis involving 12,395 patients with NSCLC in the pre-PET and PET periods, there was a 5.4% decrease in the number of patients with stage III disease and an 8.4% increase in the number of patients with stage IV disease in the PET period, corresponding with an increase in PET use from 6.3% to 20.1%.[58] The use of PET predicted better survival for patients with stage III and stage IV disease. These data support the notion that stage migration is at least partially responsible for an apparent improvement in the survival of these patients.

A limitation of the studies in which the level of increased FDG uptake (as indicated by SUV) is related to survival is that the threshold SUV used for analysis ranges widely and reproducibility may not be robust. To improve reproducibility of SUV between scanners, some investigators have proposed that a ratio of tumor SUV_{max} to either liver or blood SUV_{max} be used rather than an absolute SUV_{max}.[63] The use of a ratio potentially overcomes the issue of the appropriate threshold SUV_{max} to use for the purpose of predicting survival. Additionally, the ratio potentially can eliminate the effects on SUV related to the use of different data-acquisition and reconstruction-processing protocols at different institutions.[64] Westerterp et al.[64] reported differences in SUV quantitation of as much as 30% among three different institutions. Furthermore, variables such as the time between the administration of FDG and image acquisition, blood glucose level, and respiratory motion during image acquisition can affect SUV. The European Association of Nuclear Medicine has published procedural guidelines to provide a minimum standard for the acquisition and interpretation of PET and PET–CT in order to decrease the variability of SUV and to allow comparison of multicenter trials.[65] A standardized PET protocol has been instituted in The Netherlands and serves as a model for wider application.[66] The standardization includes (1) patient preparation, (2) matching of scan parameters such as scan time per bed position and image acquisition mode (two-dimensional or three-dimensional), (3) matching of image resolution by prescribing reconstruction settings, (4) matching of data-analysis procedures by defining volume-of-interest methods and SUV calculations, and (5) a quality-control procedure for verification of scanner calibration and the use of a National Electrical Manufacturers Association image-quality phantom for the verification of activity concentration recoveries. In a recent multi-institutional trial, a National Electrical Manufacturers Association body phantom was used to determine a correction coefficient for each scanner that was then used to standardize the SUV data.[47] In addition, protocol-optimized images and compliance with European Association of Nuclear Medicine guidelines have been reported to allow for a reliable pretherapy and posttherapy evaluation when using different-generation PET systems.[67]

While the quantitative analysis of PET for the determination of prognosis may be confounded by the limitations of SUV reproducibility, other proposed techniques, including dual-phase PET and assessment of metabolic tumor burden, may improve the ability to determine prognosis.[68–71] Houseni et al.[68] reported that the change in SUV_{max} between early and delayed PET imaging during a single study was a strong independent predictor of prognosis for patients with adenocarcinoma of the lung. The median survival time was 15 months for patients in whom SUV_{max} increased by more than 25% between the two time points, compared with 39 months for those in whom SUV_{max} increased by less than 25%. In addition, FDG-PET–CT-assessed parameters reflecting metabolic tumor burden, such as metabolic tumor volume (MTV) and total lesion glycolysis (TLG), which take into account the size of the tumor as well as the uptake of FDG, are currently being investigated as prognostic factors.[69,70,72] Im et al.,[72] in a recent meta-analysis of 13 studies (1581 patients) performed to evaluate the prognostic value of MTV and TLG, reported that lung cancer patients with high MTV had a worse prognosis with a hazard ratio (HR) of 2.71 (95% confidence interval [CI], 1.82–4.02, $p < 0.00001$) for adverse events and an HR of 2.31 (95% CI, 1.54–3.47, $p < 0.00001$) for death.[72] Similarly, patients with high TLG had a worse prognosis with an HR of 2.35 (95% CI, 1.91–2.89, $p < 0.00001$) for adverse events and an HR of 2.43 (95% CI, 1.89–3.11, $p < 0.00001$) for death. Importantly, the prognostic value of MTV and TLG remained significant in a subgroup analysis according to TNM stage. Measurements of whole-body metabolic tumor burden with MTV and TLG have also been reported to be better prognostic indicators than SUV_{max} and SUV_{mean} in patients with NSCLC who are being assessed for surgical resection as well as for those with advanced disease who are receiving chemotherapy.[69–71] In a retrospective study of 106 patients (including 19 with stage I–II and 87 with stage III–IV lung adenocarcinoma), the MTV and TLG of each malignant lesion were measured prior to treatment and were summated to give whole-body MTV and whole-body TLG values for each patient.[71] Univariate survival analysis of patients with stage III–IV disease identified high whole MTV values (≥90) and high whole TLG values (≥600) as being significant predictors of poor progression-free survival (PFS; $p < 0.001$) and poor prognosis ($p < 0.001$). Multivariate survival analysis identified high whole MTV values and high whole TLG values as being independent predictors of poor PFS ($p < 0.001$) and prognostic predictors of poor OS ($p < 0.001$). However, in a survival analysis of patients with stage I–II disease, MTV and TLG were not independent prognostic predictors.[71] Similarly, in a retrospective study of 50 patients who underwent stereotactic body radiation therapy (SBRT) for stage I NSCLC, MTV and TLG were not correlated with OS.[73] However, the role of volume-based parameters of FDG-PET–CT in patients with stage I NSCLC after SBRT is unclear and requires further evaluation. Another recent study of 88 patients with stage I NSCLC (including 68 patients with T1 N0 M0 disease and 20 with T2a N0 M0 disease) who had FDG-PET–CT and then SBRT indicated that MTV and TLG were significantly associated with disease-free survival.[74]

Because of the inherent limitations of data obtained from retrospective studies with small numbers of patients, the role of FDG-PET in the treatment of NSCLC remains unclear. Cerfolio et al.[54] posed several questions regarding the appropriate use of FDG-PET for patients with NSCLC that are worthy of consideration: (1) Should patients with an early clinical-stage NSCLC and a primary tumor with a high SUV undergo more extensive imaging prior to resection to detect occult metastases? (2) Would a patient with an early-stage lung cancer who has a high SUV benefit more from adjuvant therapy than one with a low SUV, and would such a patient also benefit from neoadjuvant therapy? (3) Should the SUV be considered together with the clinical stage when determining therapy? and (4) Should patients with a high SUV have more intensive postoperative surveillance? While the definitive answers to these questions require multi-institutional prospective randomized trials, the evolving experience with FDG-PET indicates that FDG-PET will have an expanded role in the treatment of NSCLC.

THERAPEUTIC RESPONSE

The use of anatomic imaging to assess response according to World Health Organization criteria and Response Evaluation Criteria in Solid Tumors (RECIST 1.1) has limitations that may be overcome by FDG-PET imaging.[75,76] FDG-PET allows for an early and sensitive assessment of antitumor effect after therapy in patients with NSCLC.[54,77–81] Lee et al.[78] evaluated the role of FDG-PET–CT in predicting the early response to therapy in a study of 31 patients with stage IIIB–IV NSCLC who received standard chemotherapy or molecular-targeted therapy. A metabolic response after one cycle of systemic therapy had a significant correlation with best overall response ($p < 0.01$). Moon et al.,[82] in a recent study of patients with advanced NSCLC, reported that FDG-PET can potentially be useful to identify a subgroup of patients who would benefit from maintenance treatment after the completion of first-line chemotherapy. In terms of the response to cytostatic treatment regimens, FDG-PET–CT has been reported to predict the histopathologic response in patients undergoing neoadjuvant EGFR inhibition therapy with erlotinib.[83–85] Similar to the assessment of prognosis, the quantitative analysis of FDG-PET for the determination of therapeutic response is affected by many factors. Wahl et al.[86,87] have accordingly proposed criteria for the systematic and structured assessment of response to therapy. These guidelines (PET Response Criteria in Solid Tumors [PERCIST 1.0]) are being increasingly used in clinical trials and in structured clinical reporting and improve the quantitative analysis of FDG-PET in the determination of therapeutic response.

FDG-PET–CT is also being used to monitor the response of tumors to radiotherapy.[88–92] The SUV of the primary tumor and regional nodes after completion of radiotherapy has been reported to predict poor treatment response and tumor control.[91] A return of the tumor SUV to normal after treatment appears to be an accurate marker for complete response and a sensitive indicator of good prognosis.[88] The detection of residual and recurrent disease with FDG-PET–CT has been reported to have a sensitivity of 100%, a specificity of 92%, a positive predictive value of 92%, a negative predictive value of 100%, and a diagnostic accuracy of 96%.[91] The value of FDG-PET–CT in monitoring the response to treatment was highlighted in a review published in the *New England Journal of Medicine*.[93]

Studies on the use of FDG-PET–CT to evaluate the response to anticancer therapies have suggested that early metabolic changes after therapy are strongly predictive of clinical outcome in many disease states. The literature has been focused on FDG-PET–CT imaging that is performed at approximately 3 months after the completion of radiation therapy. In a prospective National Cancer Institute–funded American College of Radiology Imaging Network/Radiation Therapy Oncology Group cooperative group trial evaluating the correlation between FDG-PET–CT findings approximately 3 months after the completion of conventional concurrent platinum-based chemoradiotherapy in patients with stage III NSCLC, pretreatment SUV_{peak} and SUV_{max} were not associated with survival.[60] Posttreatment SUV_{peak} was associated with survival in a continuous variable model (HR, 1.087; 95% CI, 1.014–1.166; $p = 0.020$). However, when analyzed as

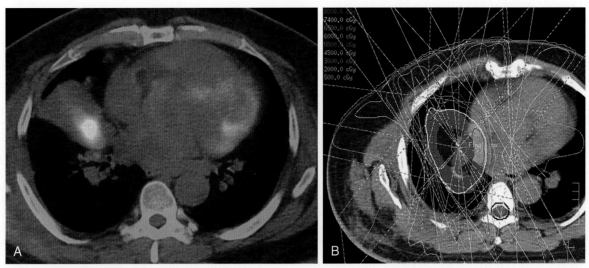

Fig. 22.7. A 53-year-old man with NSCLC and poor respiratory function was being treated with definitive intensity-modulated radiation therapy (IMRT) and concurrent chemotherapy. (A) Axial PET–CT scan, performed prior to treatment, showing complete obstructive atelectasis with consolidation of the middle lobe and focal increased uptake of FDG in the primary malignancy. (B) Computed dosimetric reconstruction used for IMRT with the highest radiation dose of 74 Gy *(white color line)* surrounding the location of the treated malignancy.

a prespecified binary value with a posttreatment SUV_{max} at a cutoff of 3.5 or greater, there was no association with survival and the authors concluded that while higher posttreatment tumor SUV is associated with worse survival, no clear prognostic threshold cutoff value is applicable for routine clinical use. While evaluation of posttreatment images is complicated by the presence of variable hypermetabolic inflammatory posttreatment changes, a limited number of studies have demonstrated that early FDG-PET–CT (performed 1 month to 2 months after treatment) is prognostic of survival and is more predictive than the CT response, stage, or pretreatment performance status.[92,94]

Recent investigators have shown an increased interest in performing FDG-PET–CT early during the course of treatment. Imaging that has been performed during the course of chemoradiation has shown markedly fewer inflammatory changes, suggesting that FDG-PET–CT during treatment may allow for an evaluation of the response to therapy. Most importantly, the ability to assess the response to therapy during the course of treatment would permit a change in therapy for patients who are not responding optimally. Researchers from The Netherlands reported a large intraindividual heterogeneity in the evolution of FDG uptake during the early course of radiation therapy.[95] The investigators reported a nonsignificant increase during the first week of radiation therapy ($p = 0.05$) and a small but significant decrease during the 2nd week ($p = 0.02$). Investigators from the University of Michigan demonstrated a greater and more significant reduction of peak FDG activity at 40 Gy to 50 Gy at 4 weeks to 5 weeks during the course of fractionated radiation therapy.[96] The regions of peak tumor FDG activity during radiation therapy correlated with those seen at 3 months after radiation therapy ($R^2 = 0.7$; $p < 0.001$). In 2008, abstracts presented by investigators from Stanford University at the meeting of the Radiological Society of North America and by investigators from Princess Margaret Hospital at the meeting of the American Society of Thoracic Radiation Oncology demonstrated a heterogeneous reduction of FDG uptake at about 4 weeks during radiation therapy. The Stanford group also reported a correlation between FDG uptake during radiation therapy and PFS. Indeed, the role of PET–CT in therapeutic monitoring is expanding rapidly because

of its ability to provide earlier and more robust identification of nonresponders or poor responders as compared with CT. Therefore PET–CT potentially can provide important benefits to individual patients by allowing early changes to alternative, more efficacious treatment or by avoiding the unnecessary toxicity related to ineffective therapy. In this regard, Choi et al.[97] reported that FDG-PET can be useful for personalizing therapeutic options for patients with advanced NSCLC who are receiving radiotherapy or chemoradiotherapy by identifying those with a high risk of residual cancer who could receive salvage therapy soon after the completion of standard therapy. In addition, RTOG 1106 is an ongoing randomized phase II trial that will perform PET–CT scan during RT with doses of around 40 Gy to 46 Gy to predict treatment response. In the experimental arm, PET–CT will be used to define the target for the boost phase of radiation therapy to raise the daily dose to the reduced target volume for the remainder of the treatment without increasing the doses to normal organs.

FDG-PET–CT FOR RADIATION TREATMENT PLANNING AND ADAPTIVE PLANNING

FDG is the only Medicare-approved PET–CT tracer for the evaluation of cancer, and FDG-PET–CT is the most widely available procedure used in daily oncology practice. FDG-PET–CT is being increasingly used for patients with NSCLC, including for diagnosis, staging, radiation treatment planning, and monitoring of the treatment response.[93,98–102] FDG-PET–CT plays an important role in target delineation during the planning of radiation treatment for patients with NSCLC[103–108] and has been shown to improve the accuracy of target definition (Fig. 22.7).[89,104,109,110] FDG-PET–CT helps differentiate the primary tumor from collapsed lung and/or adjacent normal tissue, such as large vessels, and defines the extent of disease in the chest wall. PET reduces interobserver variability compared with CT alone.[111] Integrated PET–CT further improves the consistency of target delineation.[95] A prospective clinical trial involving the use of PET–CT-based planning demonstrated isolated nodal failures in only one of 44 patients.[112] The tumor target that is defined on the basis of PET–CT is usually smaller than that defined on the basis of CT; therefore the incorporation of PET–CT into radiotherapy planning has the potential to allow radiation-dose escalation without increasing side effects.[112,113] Tumor volume can be generated reliably with use of either a rigorous visual method or source-to-background ratio-based autodelineation.[95,114] The latter method also has shown good correlation with pathologic findings. MTV after chemotherapy or radiation therapy is not well defined. Investigators who are involved in the RTOG 1106 study are testing whether increasing the radiation dose on the basis of FDG-PET during treatment will lead to higher cure rates.

Novel Tracers

PET is one of the most important advances in biomedical science and is now incorporated into medical practice, particularly for the detection of disease, the planning of treatment, the monitoring of the response to treatment, and the detection of recurrence in patients with cancer. PET radionuclides are produced and incorporated into various compounds for measuring specific molecular processes in living patients. Multiple new PET tracers have been designed to interrogate various pathways beyond glycolysis, such as FDG-PET, which is accepted clinically as a marker of general cellular metabolism but has known limitations in discriminating viable cancer from active inflammation and has lower uptake in certain tumors such as prostate and breast cancer. These new tracers are being developed for the evaluation of various cellular processes, some of which may include amino acid transport, protein synthesis, fatty acid metabolism, receptors, and proliferation.

The clinical imaging of proliferation of both normal and cancerous tissue is important for evaluating tissue function and characteristics as it has the potential to improve our ability to monitor the response to therapy and to predict the outcome of treatment. More traditional imaging methods for assessing tumor size and growth (e.g., CT, MR, and sometimes ultrasound) may be limited because of the delay associated with cell death and may not manifest early. The ability of PET to assess metabolic activity noninvasively, quantitatively, and reproducibly makes it ideal for the assessment of tumor response and prognosis. Tumor growth relies on an increasing population of cells because of cell division. In contrast with normal cells, tumors grow out of control as they fail to respond to the normal homeostatic mechanisms that maintain the appropriate number of cells in the process of cell renewal. Originally, the technique for assessing the proliferation rate or DNA synthesis as a means of monitoring the response to therapy was based on the use of radiolabeled DNA precursors or nucleosides, which are incorporated into the DNA of cells during the S phase of the cell cycle. Because thymidine (TdR) is not incorporated into RNA, it was chosen early on as the best tracer for measuring cell proliferation, and the use of ^{3}H-TdR and autoradiography allowed for the analysis of the kinetics of proliferation. These studies documented the variability of proliferative rates among tumors, and this was not unexpected since nonproliferating cells are common as well as high tumor cell death rates. Subsequently, C-11-labeled TdR was developed, which can be labeled at both the methyl and the two-ring position to noninvasively assess tumor proliferation in patients. However, kinetic analysis is required as the metabolites in the blood and CO_2 are present and need to be accounted for in the uptake analysis. Clinical studies have been performed to assess various tumors, including lung cancer. However, because of the short (20-minute) physical half-life of C-11 TdR, this procedure was limited to academic or research centers with direct proximal access to a cyclotron facility to perform these studies. More importantly, the biologic half-life of C-11 TdR was limited

because of its rapid in vivo degradation once injected intravenously in humans.

^{18}F-labeled 3′-deoxy-3′-fluorothymidine (^{18}F-FLT) was then developed partly because of its more favorable half-life as a tracer for imaging proliferation. Unlabeled FLT has been known for many years as an antiviral agent, particularly for human immunodeficiency virus therapy. In the simplified model of FLT retention (which is quite similar to FDG retention), FLT is taken up from the circulation by tumors and is transported into the cell, where it is trapped by phosphorylation by cytosolic thymidine kinase 1 (TK1). TK1 has been shown to have increased activity when cells are going through the S phase; thus FLT retention reflects proliferative activity. In vitro studies have shown a strong correlation between FLT uptake in growing cells and the S phase fraction. Tehrani et al.[115] reported that correlative PET studies of C-11 TdR and FLT showed comparable uptake patterns but that FLT had greater in vivo stability, resulting in improved imaging characteristics.

Shields et al.,[116] in a pilot study involving a patient with NSCLC, reported that PET demonstrated increased uptake of FLT in the primary lung tumor as well as in the liver and bone marrow, thereby limiting the usefulness of this tracer for identifying metastases in these sites. High liver uptake is seen only in humans (not in canines) as a result of increased glucuronidation of FLT in the human liver. FLT demonstrates minimal brain uptake, making it a better tracer than FDG (high background brain activity) for assessing brain tumor metabolism. FLT also demonstrates uptake in the gastrointestinal tract, which, like the bone marrow, has a substantial number of proliferating cells. Renal excretion with bladder accumulation was also noted.

When serial imaging is performed to assess prognosis and to evaluate the response to therapy, the reproducibility and repeatability of the PET technique is essential. de Langen et al.[117] evaluated the reproducibility of FLT PET measurements for nine patients with NSCLC and six patients with head and neck cancer. The patients were scanned twice within 7 days prior to receiving therapy. The maximum pixel value within the tumor (SUV_{max}) and a threshold-defined volume of 41% of the maximum pixel value with correction for local background (SUV41%) were used to quantify FLT uptake. SUV41% and SUV_{max} showed excellent reproducibility, and the authors concluded that when monitoring response using serial measurements of FLT, changes of more than 15% in SUV41%, and 20% to 25% in SUV_{max}, are likely due to the biologic effects of therapy rather than variability in measurements.[117] One of the strengths of PET is the ability to quantify the metabolic process being studied. Aside from the commonly used semiquantitative SUV measurements, measurements of metabolic active volumes may be a better index of viable (FDG) or proliferating (FLT) tumor. Frings et al.,[112] in a study of 20 patients with NSCLC, evaluated the repeatability of metabolic volume measurements with the use of both FDG (11 patients) and FLT (9 patients) on the basis of four semiautomated three-dimensional volume-of-interest methodologies. The study set the ranges by which significant differences in measured volumes of interest could be considered change and represented more than measurement variation.[118] The most precise quantification of PET studies has been done with proof of concept that FLT PET imaging provides a valid and independent measure of DNA synthetic rate. One such study was performed in 17 patients with 18 tumors using multiple kinetic models, which involved blood sampling with metabolite analysis.[119] This study concluded that compartmental analysis of FLT PET images can yield robust estimates of FLT uptake, which correlated with in vitro measures of tumor proliferation.

Most clinical studies of FLT PET have involved patients with lung cancer. Yamamoto et al.,[120] in a prospective study of 18 patients with newly diagnosed NSCLC, compared FDG and FLT PET findings with immunohistochemical correlation using Ki-67 as an index of proliferation. The sensitivity was 72% for FLT and 89% for FDG. False-negative FLT PET findings were reported for four of five patients with bronchioloalveolar carcinoma, which is similar to the known low FDG uptake in these slow-growing tumors. The mean FLT SUV was significantly lower than the mean FDG SUV, and a significant correlation was observed between the FLT SUV and the Ki-67 index. Although FLT uptake correlated significantly with proliferative activity, the correlation was not better than that for FDG uptake ($p < 0.0001$). Similar findings were reported in a larger study of 68 patients with NSCLC, in which FLT SUV$_{max}$ was significantly correlated with Ki-67 and CD105-MVD (microvessel density; $r = 0.550$ and $r = 0.633$, $p = 0.001$ and $p = 0.001$, respectively).[121] There was also some correlation with CD31-MVD (microvessel density) and CD34-MVD, both of which are markers of angiogenesis ($r = 0.228$ and $r = 0.235$, $p = 0.062$ and $p = 0.054$, respectively). These findings indicate a complex situation in which FLT uptake in patients with lung cancer is influenced by multiple factors, including angiogenesis. In another prospective study, involving 25 patients with suspected lung cancer, static and dynamic ^{18}F-FLT PET images were acquired prior to surgical resection and were compared with the expression of Ki-67 and TK1 as determined with immunohistochemical staining.[122] The analysis revealed that static FLT SUV$_{max}$ uptake from 60 minutes to 90 minutes correlated with the overall ($p = 0.57$, $p = 0.006$) and maximal ($p = 0.69$, $p < 0.001$) immunohistochemical expressions of Ki-67 and TK1 but not with TK1 enzymatic activity ($p = 0.34$, $p = 0.146$). Correlation between TK1 activity and TK1 protein expression was limited to immunohistochemical scoring for maximal expression. No significant correlations between TK1 enzyme activity and K (FLT) were observed. The study suggested that FLT uptake and retention within cells may be complicated by a variety of still undetermined factors in addition to TK1 enzymatic activity.

Prospective clinical studies have demonstrated that FLT uptake in lung cancers is consistently lower than FDG uptake, with lower sensitivity, higher specificity, and higher positive predictive value. In the study by Yamamoto et al.,[123] 36 of 54 patients with pulmonary nodules had lung cancer. On the basis of visual analysis, the sensitivity of FLT for the detection of lung cancer was 83%, the specificity was 83%, and the accuracy was 83%. The corresponding values for FDG were 97%, 50%, and 81%, respectively. On the basis of semiquantitative analysis, the sensitivity of FLT was 86%, the specificity was 72%, and the accuracy was 81%. The corresponding values for FDG were 89%, 67%, and 81%. The same group then studied 34 patients with NSCLC to compare FLT with FDG preoperatively.[124] For the detection of primary tumor, the sensitivity was 67% for FLT, compared with 94% for FDG ($p = 0.005$). The sensitivity, specificity, positive predictive value, negative predictive value, and accuracy of lymph node staging on a per-patient basis were 57%, 93%, 67%, 89%, and 85%, respectively, for FLT PET and 57%, 78%, 36%, 91%, and 74%, respectively, for FDG ($p > 0.1$ for all comparisons). Two of the three distant metastases were detected with FLT and FDG-PET.

Multiple studies have been performed to assess the utility of FLT PET for evaluating the response to treatment. Early response changes in ^{18}F-FLT uptake have been observed after the start of chemotherapy and radiation therapy in a pilot study of five patients with locally advanced lung cancer, with imaging performed on days 2, 8, 15, or 29 after therapy.[125] This study

provided proof of concept of the potential to monitor the changes in both tumor and normal tissues during therapy. It also provided background for the further development of response-adapted radiotherapy.

Kahraman et al.[120] compared FDG and FLT PET in a study of 30 patients with stage IV NSCLC who were being treated with erlotinib. Volumetric parameters were used to compare TLG for FDG and tumor lesion proliferation for FLT at baseline, 1 week, and 6 weeks after erlotinib therapy. A lower cutoff value of 20% or 30% reduction in FLT uptake was used to define metabolic response. Patients with lower early and late residual TLG and tumor lesion proliferation had a significantly prolonged PFS. Zander et al.[126] reported the results of a phase II trial in which 34 patients with untreated stage IV NSCLC were evaluated with both FDG and FLT PET during erlotinib therapy. Changes in FDG and FLT uptake after 1 week and 6 weeks of erlotinib treatment were compared with nonprogression as measured with CT after 6 weeks of treatment, PFS, and OS. Changes in FDG uptake after 1 week of therapy predicted nonprogression after 6 weeks of therapy, with an area under the receiver operating characteristic curve of 0.75 ($p = 0.02$). Patients with an early metabolic FDG response (cutoff value, 30% reduction in peak SUV) had significantly longer PFS and OS. Early FLT response also predicted significantly longer PFS (HR, 0.31; 95% CI, 0.10–0.95; $p = 0.04$) but did not predict OS or nonprogression after 6 weeks of therapy. The authors concluded that early FDG-PET response predicts OS, PFS, and nonprogression at 6 weeks. This prospective trial illustrates the continued value of FDG-PET for predicting therapeutic benefit even without knowledge of EGFR mutation status. Early FLT response was not predictive for identifying patients with EGFR mutations with response to therapy or with stable disease. It will be interesting to see if the advantage of FDG-PET over FLT PET imaging will be maintained in a larger cohort of patients.

Overall, FLT PET imaging technique as a noninvasive, quantitative method for measuring tumor proliferation has demonstrated a strong correlation with tumor proliferation indices, particularly Ki-67 scores, as was reviewed in a meta-analysis study.[127] Studies comparing FLT and FDG in terms of the early response to treatment and the prediction of outcome after therapy have yielded mixed results, with FDG overall demonstrating better correlation with the prediction of early response and prognosis. Finally, the natural biodistribution of FLT with high background activity in the bone marrow and liver may ultimately limit its overall clinical utility as it will fail to identify metastatic disease in these areas, which are common sites of lung cancer spread (Fig. 22.8).

Angiogenesis is the formation of new blood vessels, a process that involves the migration, growth, and differentiation of endothelial cells lining the inside wall of blood vessels. Angiogenesis inhibitors that can stop or slow the growth and spread of tumors have been developed. Bevacizumab is a Food and Drug Administration (FDA)-approved monoclonal antibody that recognizes and binds to vascular endothelial growth factor, which then is unable to activate the vascular EGFR. Bevacizumab has been approved for the management of various solid tumors, including NSCLC, in combination with other drugs.[128] The FDA has approved other drugs with antiangiogenic activity, including sorafenib, sunitinib, pazopanib, and everolimus, for cancer therapy. Several new PET angiogenesis imaging agents recently have been developed to target the αvβ3 integrin, which is expressed on activated endothelial cells during angiogenesis. The αvβ3 integrin has a pocket in which the peptide arginine–glycine–aspartic acid (RGD) can bind with high affinity. RGD is then cyclized and labeled with ^{18}F for imaging with PET. These imaging agents are intended to improve patient selection

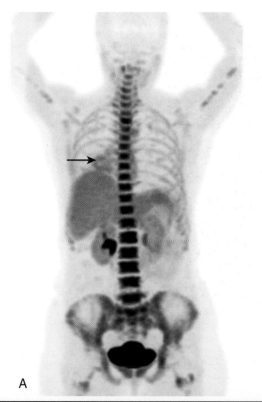

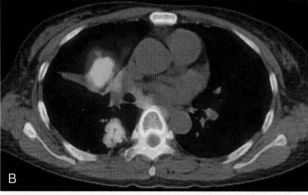

Fig. 22.8. ^{18}F-labeled 3′-deoxy-3′-fluorothymidine (^{18}F-FLT) PET–CT scanning was performed for a patient with metastatic NSCLC of the lower and middle lobes of the right lung. (A) Whole-body maximum intensity projection image showing uptake in the malignancy in the lower lobe *(arrow)*. Note the high background activity in the bone marrow and liver and the low background activity in the brain. (B) Axial FLT PET–CT scan showing FLT uptake in the tumor in the lower and middle lobes, indicating proliferating tumor at both sites. Note the intense FLT uptake in the thoracic vertebrae and sternal body, which may limit detection of osseous metastases in these sites.

and subsequent monitoring of the response to therapy because not all patients respond to these targeted therapies.[129] The first PET tracer for which clinical data are available is ^{18}F-galacto-RGD, which has been shown to have very favorable imaging characteristics, with high metabolic stability and high radiochemical yield.[130] The first pilot study involved nine patients (including 5 patients with melanoma, 1 with chondrosarcoma, 1 with soft-tissue sarcoma, 1 with renal cell cancer, and 1 with pigmented villonodular synovitis).[131] There was good uptake in tumors, with the SUV ranging from 1.2 to 10.0. There was also notable uptake in the spleen and intestines, with fast excretion

via the kidneys and minimal uptake in the other organs. Subsequent expansion of the clinical study to 19 patients with similar types of tumors (melanoma and sarcoma) again demonstrated the favorable biodistribution in humans, with higher uptake in tumors with high contrast.[132] However, the clinical acceptance of this tracer has been hampered by the complex labeling procedure for its production. More recently, ^{18}F-fluciclatide (formerly known as ^{18}F-AH111585) has been developed with a high yield and a less complex radiosynthesis procedure.[133] The initial study, which involved eight healthy volunteers, demonstrated a favorable biodistribution with a predominance of renal excretion, with high background activity noted in the liver and gastrointestinal tract.[134] The dosimetry and safety profile were comparable with those of other common clinical PET tracers. The phase I study, involving seven patients with breast cancer, demonstrated good tumor uptake, with no adverse side effects noted. The metabolic stability of the tracer was demonstrated by means of chromatographic assessment of blood samples. The tumor uptake pattern was notable for a predominant peripheral distribution along the tumor rim. One patient with liver metastases had low uptake because of the high background activity in the liver, but other sites of metastases, including bone, pleura, and nodes, showed high uptake of the PET tracer. ^{18}F-fluciclatide was further evaluated in a multicenter proof-of-concept trial that included patients with NSCLC.[135] The uptake pattern and biodistribution showed minimal activity in the lungs, mediastinum, bone marrow, and brain, and thus this could be a suitable agent for potentially identifying the primary nodal involvement and distant metastases. Most recently, ^{18}F-fluciclatide was used to assess the response of human glioblastoma xenografts to treatment with the antiangiogenic agent sunitinib.[136] ^{18}F-fluciclatide detected changes in tumor uptake after acute antiangiogenic therapy markedly earlier than any significant volumetric changes were observable (Fig. 22.9). These results suggest that this imaging agent may provide clinically important information for guiding patient care and monitoring the response to antiangiogenic therapy. These data are exciting as there are very few data on response monitoring with the use of αvβ3 PET imaging. The Stanford group recently described the pharmacokinetic and dosimetry data for imaging αvβ3 integrin levels using ^{18}F-FPPRGD2.[137] The authors demonstrated that the biodistribution of ^{18}F-FPPRGD2 is favorable and that its primary application is likely to be PET for the evaluation of patients with brain, breast, or lung cancer.

Overall, imaging of angiogenesis with PET tracers shows great potential as angiogenesis is a hallmark of cancer and several FDA-approved targeted agents are available. The biodistribution of these tracers is favorable to lung cancer imaging as there is minimal background activity in the lungs and mediastinal nodes, as well as in the brain and bone marrow (common sites of distant metastases). However, the high uptake in the liver may deter detection of small-volume metastatic disease in this site. The early data are encouraging for the potential use of these agents for patient selection, tumor staging, and monitoring of response to antiangiogenic therapy.

Numerous in vivo and in vitro studies have shown that the oxygen tension within solid tumors influences the ability of the cells to respond to radiation therapy. Hypoxia in malignant tumors can affect the outcome of anticancer treatments. Oxygen is believed to act as a potent radiosensitizer, and hypoxic tumors are relatively resistant to radiotherapy because of their lack of oxygen. In addition, hypoxia triggers several processes such as angiogenesis and enhanced glycolysis that may lead to more aggressive clinical behavior and broad therapeutic resistance. However, proven noninvasive methods to determine the degree of hypoxia within these tumors are not currently available.

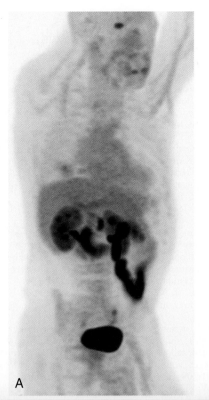

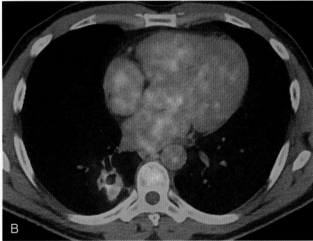

Fig. 22.9. A patient with adenocarcinoma in the lower lobe of the right lung after chemotherapy. (A) Whole-body ^{18}F-fluciclatide maximum intensity projection image showing uptake in the right lower lobe of the right lung. Note the lack of cerebral and cerebellar brain activity; the focus of uptake in the pituitary correlates with a known pituitary adenoma. Note also the high background activity in the bowel, moderate uptake in the liver, and low activity in the marrow. The primary excretion of the tracer is via the kidneys, which is seen as uptake also in the urinary collecting system and the bladder. (B) ^{18}F-fluciclatide PET–CT scan showing uptake in the cavitary adenocarcinoma in the lower lobe of the right lung.

Considerable efforts have been put forth to develop methods and imaging techniques for measuring oxygen and hypoxia in tissues. PET–CT has been used for several years as a noninvasive imaging technique to study tumor hypoxia, with several radiotracers in development. Radiolabeled 2-nitroimidazole compounds offer a minimally invasive (requiring only an

intravenous catheter), less technically demanding technique compared with the Eppendorf electrode method (the current criterion standard). In addition, because all sites of disease can be imaged, the sampling bias inherent in electrode methods is not present in association with 2-nitroimidazole PET–CT. ^{18}F-fluoromisonidazole (FMISO) was proposed as a tracer for determining tumor hypoxia in vivo with PET in 1984. Several experimental and clinical studies have indicated that FMISO uptake in tissues is correlated with tissue oxygen tension. Therefore FMISO PET–CT allows noninvasive differentiation between hypoxic and normoxic tumors. FMISO has been shown to selectively bind to hypoxic cells both in vitro and in vivo, and it has been used quantitatively to assess tumor hypoxia in different tissues in patients with cancer involving the lung, brain, head, and neck.[138–140] As hypoxia is one of the most important prognostic factors in cancer of the head and neck and NSCLC, Eschmann et al.[99] examined whether FMISO uptake could predict tumor recurrence after radiation therapy in a study involving 40 patients (including 26 patients with cancer of the head and neck and 14 patients with NSCLC). At 4 hours after injection, tumor-to-mediastinum (or tumor-to-muscle) ratios were used to quantify uptake and the kinetics of FMISO uptake were described with time-activity curves to stratify patients into defined groups. These results showed that a tumor-to-muscle cutoff of 1.6 in patients with cancer of the head and neck or a tumor-to-mediastinum ratio cutoff of 2 in patients with NSCLC could differentiate patients who subsequently had recurrence of disease from those who did not. Only three (27%) of 11 patients with ratios less than these cutoff values had recurrent disease. FMISO PET demonstrated the ability to image and quantify hypoxia. Tumor cells exhibiting hypoxia were more resistant to radiation therapy than adequately oxygenated tumor cells. The researchers found that high uptake of FMISO correlated with greater risk of tumor recurrence. They also found that a high ratio of uptake of FMISO by tumor tissue compared with uptake by muscle tissue correlated with a higher rate of tumor recurrence. Gagel et al.,[101] in a study involving a population of patients with NSCLC, reported that FMISO PET allowed for the qualitative and quantitative definition of hypoxic subareas that may correspond with the sites of local recurrences. The degree of FMISO uptake may predict response to radiotherapy and freedom from disease as well as OS. An ongoing trial (RTOG 1106/ACRIN6697) is testing the value of FMISO for predicting the response of stage III NSCLC to concurrent chemoradiation.

CONCLUSION

FDG-PET is routinely used to improve the detection of nodal and extrathoracic metastases in patients with NSCLC who are being assessed for curative resection. FDG-PET imaging has the potential to allow more appropriate selection of patients for surgical resection and neoadjuvant and adjuvant therapy and allows improved planning for radiation therapy. In a limited number of studies, FDG-PET has been useful for the evaluation of prognosis and treatment response. In addition, novel PET radiotracers may assist therapeutic decisions and overcome the potential limitations of FDG-PET in the staging of tumors, the prediction of prognosis, and the assessment of therapy. However, it is currently unclear how to appropriately incorporate FDG-PET and the novel tracers into clinical decisions regarding therapy and prognosis. Although prospective multi-institutional trials and standardization of PET imaging protocols are required for the true utility to be determined, the evolving experience with PET imaging indicates a greater role in the treatment of NSCLC.

KEY REFERENCES

5. van Tinteren H, Hoekstra OS, Smit EF, et al. Effectiveness of positron emission tomography in the preoperative assessment of patients with suspected non-small-cell lung cancer: the PLUS multicentre randomised trial. *Lancet.* 2002;359:1388–1393.

6. Reed CE, Harpole DH, Posther KE, et al. Results of the American College of Surgeons Oncology Group Z0050 trial: the utility of positron emission tomography in staging potentially operable non-small cell lung cancer. *J Thorac Cardiovasc Surg.* 2003;126:1943–1951.

35. Viney RC, Boyer MJ, King MT, et al. Randomized controlled trial of the role of positron emission tomography in the management of stage I and II non-small-cell lung cancer. *J Clin Oncol.* 2004;22:2357–2362.

36. MacManus MP, Hicks RJ, Matthews JP, et al. High rate of detection of unsuspected distant metastases by PET in apparent stage III non-small-cell lung cancer: implications for radical radiation therapy. *Int J Radiat Oncol Biol Phys.* 2001;50:287–293.

37. Fischer B, Lassen U, Mortensen J, et al. Preoperative staging of lung cancer with combined PET-CT. *N Engl J Med.* 2009;361:32–39.

46. Lardinois D, Weder W, Roudas M, et al. Etiology of solitary extrapulmonary positron emission tomography and computed tomography findings in patients with lung cancer. *J Clin Oncol.* 2005;23:6846–6853.

47. Uehara H, Tsutani Y, Okumura S, et al. Prognostic role of positron emission tomography and high-resolution computed tomography in clinical stage IA lung adenocarcinoma. *Ann Thorac Surg.* 2013;96:1958–1965.

54. Cerfolio RJ, Bryant AS, Ohja B, Bartolucci AA. The maximum standardized uptake values on positron emission tomography of a non-small cell lung cancer predict stage, recurrence, and survival. *J Thorac Cardiovasc Surg.* 2005;130:151–159.

56. Hoang JK, Hoagland LF, Coleman RE, Coan AD, Herndon 2nd JE, Patz Jr EF. Prognostic value of fluorine-18 fluorodeoxyglucose positron emission tomography imaging in patients with advanced-stage non-small-cell lung carcinoma. *J Clin Oncol.* 2008;26:1459–1464.

59. Paesmans M, Berghmans T, Dusart M, et al. Primary tumor standardized uptake value measured on fluorodeoxyglucose positron emission tomography is of prognostic value for survival in non-small cell lung cancer: update of a systematic review and meta-analysis by the European Lung Cancer Working Party for the International Association for the study of lung cancer staging project. *J Thorac Oncol.* 2010;5:612–619.

60. Machtay M, Duan F, Siegel BA, et al. Prediction of survival by [18F] fluorodeoxyglucose positron emission tomography in patients with locally advanced non-small-cell lung cancer undergoing definitive chemoradiation therapy: results of the ACRIN 6668/RTOG 0235 trial. *J Clin Oncol.* 2013;31:3823–3830.

65. Boellaard R, Delgado-Bolton R, Oyen WJ, et al. FDG PET/CT: EANM procedure guidelines for tumour imaging: version 2.0. *Eur J Nucl Med Mol Imaging.* 2015;42:328–354.

67. Lasnon C, Desmonts C, Quak E, et al. Harmonizing SUVs in multicentre trials when using different generation PET systems: prospective validation in non-small cell lung cancer patients. *Eur J Nucl Med Mol Imaging.* 2013;40:985–996.

72. Im HJ, Pak K, Cheon GJ, et al. Prognostic value of volumetric parameters of 18F-FDG PET in non-small-cell lung cancer: a meta-analysis. *Eur J Nucl Med Mol Imaging.* 2015;42:241–251.

78. Lee DH, Kim SK, Lee HY, et al. Early prediction of response to first-line therapy using integrated 18F-FDG PET/CT for patients with advanced/metastatic non-small cell lung cancer. *J Thorac Oncol.* 2009;4:816–821.

86. Wahl RL, Jacene H, Kasamon Y, Lodge MA. From RECIST to PERCIST: evolving considerations for PET response criteria in solid tumors. *J Nucl Med.* 2009;50(suppl 1):122S–150S.

94. Mac Manus MP, Hicks RJ, Matthews JP, Wirth A, Rischin D, Ball DL. Metabolic (FDG-PET) response after radical radiotherapy/chemoradiotherapy for non-small cell lung cancer correlates with patterns of failure. *Lung Cancer.* 2005;49:95–108.

104. MacManus M, Nestle U, Rosenzweig KE, et al. Use of PET and PET/CT for radiation therapy planning: IAEA expert report 2006-2007. *Radiother Oncol.* 2009;91:85–94.

109. Nestle U, Kremp S, Grosu AL. Practical integration of [18F]-FDG-PET and PET-CT in the planning of radiotherapy for non-small cell lung cancer (NSCLC): the technical basis, ICRU-target volumes, problems, perspectives. *Radiother Oncol.* 2006;81:209–225.

121. Yang W, Zhang Y, Fu Z, Sun X, Mu D, Yu J. Imaging proliferation of 18F-FLT PET/CT correlated with the expression of microvessel density of tumour tissue in non-small-cell lung cancer. *Eur J Nucl Med Mol Imaging.* 2012;39:1289–1296.

136. Battle MR, Goggi JL, Allen L, Barnett J, Morrison MS. Monitoring tumor response to antiangiogenic sunitinib therapy with 18F-fluciclatide, an 18F-labeled alphaVbeta3-integrin and alphaV beta5-integrin imaging agent. *J Nucl Med.* 2011;52:424–430.

140. Lin Z, Mechalakos J, Nehmeh S, et al. The influence of changes in tumor hypoxia on dose-painting treatment plans based on 18F-FMISO positron emission tomography. *Int J Radiat Oncol Biol Phys.* 2008;70:1219–1228.

See Expertconsult.com for full list of references.

23 Diagnostic Workup for Suspected Lung Cancer Confined to the Chest

Nicholas Pastis, Martina Bonifazi, Stefano Gasparini, and Gerard A. Silvestri

SUMMARY OF KEY POINTS

- In the context of disease confined to the chest, mediastinal staging is crucial for determining the best curative treatment strategy, especially for nonsmall cell lung cancer (NSCLC).
- Urgent referral for chest imaging is recommended for patients who present with hemoptysis or any of several symptoms or signs that are unexplained or persistent.
- Chest radiograph is the main radiographic investigation in the primary care setting in the diagnostic workup for suspected lung cancer.
- Features suggestive of intrathoracic invasion are important clues that help to distinguish between benign and malignant nodules.
- ^{18}F-2-deoxy-D-glucose-positron emission tomography is an essential tool for the diagnosis and staging of disease in patients with radiographic and clinical findings consistent with lung cancer.
- Indeterminate nodules or negative mediastinal findings require additional procedures to obtain a tissue diagnosis.
- The method for definitive diagnosis and staging of lung cancer depends on the suspected cell subtype (small cell lung cancer or NSCLC), the size and location of the primary tumor, the presence or absence of radiographic findings suggestive of mediastinal involvement, and the overall clinical status of the patient.
- Flexible bronchoscopy should be offered to every patient with central lesions on computed tomography for whom nodal staging does not influence treatment.
- Transbronchial needle aspiration is increasingly being supplanted by endobronchial ultrasound fine-needle aspiration.
- Endoscopic ultrasound may be used to increase the number of mediastinal node stations amenable to nonsurgical sampling.
- Staging the mediastinum is of paramount importance in the diagnostic workup for suspected lung cancer confined to the chest, as it dictates treatment options and prognosis.

Lung cancer remains the leading cause of cancer-related death worldwide, with a 5-year survival rate of approximately 15%, as more than two-thirds of patients present with locally advanced or metastatic disease for which curative treatment is no longer feasible.[1,2] Hence, the prevention and early detection of lung cancer are crucial to achieving a substantial reduction in mortality. An early diagnosis could be obtained by systematic screening of high-risk individuals or by prompt referral of symptomatic patients. Patients with lung cancer present a diagnostic challenge in that they often present with myriad symptoms and signs that are common and nonspecific (e.g., weight loss and fatigue) or that are directly related to the primary lesion, to intrathoracic spread, to paraneoplastic syndromes, or to distant metastasis.[3] Because of this ambiguity in presentation, risk factors need to be identified in patients with a higher likelihood of having lung cancer. Smoking is the leading risk factor, but lung cancer does not develop in all long-term heavy smokers and cancer is developing in an increasing proportion of patients with no history of tobacco smoking.[4] In fact, older age, previous diagnoses of other cancers, family history of lung cancer, and exposure to occupational carcinogens seem to increase long-term risk independent of smoking.[5]

The initial evaluation should focus on careful physical examination and history taking to identify patients with suspected lung cancer who should have additional studies, such as a serum chemistry profile, a complete blood count, a calcium level, and testing of liver function, as well as noninvasive imaging studies such as radiographs, computed tomography (CT), and positron emission tomography (PET). According to the third edition of the American College of Chest Physicians (ACCP) evidence-based clinical practice guidelines on the diagnosis and management of lung cancer (2013),[6] the goal of the initial evaluation of patients with suspected lung cancer is to assess key issues related to the patient's overall health, the probability of cancer, and the probability of metastatic disease, as these factors have an impact on every other step of the diagnosis, staging, and treatment process. To optimize the management of lung cancer, the most appropriate biopsy target must be identified and any comorbidities that might limit treatment options should be addressed. The first step should be to identify whether the disease is still confined to the chest, as this factor has an impact on the need for and location of biopsies as well as on the prognosis. In this context, mediastinal staging becomes crucial for determining the best curative treatment strategy, especially for nonsmall cell lung cancer (NSCLC).[7]

If surgery is being considered, the final component of the initial evaluation should be a physiologic assessment of pulmonary function. To stratify the patient's operative risk, testing of lung function—specifically, measurements of forced expiratory volume in 1 second and carbon monoxide diffusion in the lung—is a helpful predictor of morbidity and mortality in those undergoing lung resection.[8]

This chapter focuses on the diagnostic workup for suspected lung cancer that is confined to the chest and provides an extensive description of potential clinical and radiographic features as well as a practical approach to establishing the final diagnosis and staging.

CLINICAL FEATURES

Symptoms related to the primary tumor include cough, breathlessness, hemoptysis, and chest discomfort. A persistent cough and dyspnea, likely due to an endobronchial mass or postobstructive pneumonia, are the most common symptoms. These symptoms occur in up to 75% and 60% of patients, respectively, and may be associated with wheezing and stridor. Intermittent, aching chest discomfort is noted by approximately 50% of patients at the time of diagnosis. Hemoptysis is rarely severe and usually only consists of blood streaking of the sputum.[8,9] Forty percent of patients present with symptoms and signs related to intrathoracic spread involving the nerves, chest wall, pleura, vascular system, and/or viscera as a result of either direct extension or lymphatic spread. Recurrent laryngeal nerve palsy is more common in left-sided tumors and usually causes hoarseness. Phrenic nerve paralysis leads to an elevated hemidiaphragm and presents as breathlessness in patients who already have compromised respiratory function. A Pancoast tumor involves either the right or left apex in the superior sulcus near the brachial plexus and commonly infiltrates the eighth cervical and first and second thoracic nerve roots, causing pain, cutaneous temperature change, and muscle wasting along the relevant nerve root. It may present with Horner syndrome as a result of involvement of the sympathetic chain and stellate ganglion, causing unilateral enophthalmos, ptosis, miosis, and ipsilateral anhidrosis. Chest wall invasion can cause painful soft-tissue masses or rib destruction. Pleural effusion may be related to direct extension of the primary tumor, to implantation of tumor metastasis, or to mediastinal lymphatic obstruction and is typically heralded by dyspnea or chest pain.[8,9]

Superior vena cava syndrome is the result of direct obstruction of the superior vena cava by the primary tumor or by enlarged right paratracheal metastatic lymph nodes, causing face or arm swelling; dyspnea; venous distention in the neck, upper chest, and arms; headache; upper limb edema; dizziness; drowsiness; blurring of vision; cough; and dysphagia. Lung cancer accounts for 46% to 75% of all cases of superior vena cava obstruction, and the most common histologic subtype is small cell lung cancer (SCLC).[8,9]

Paraneoplastic syndromes represent a group of clinical disorders that are associated with malignant lesions but are not directly related to the physical effects of primary or metastatic tumors. Paraneoplastic syndromes occur in at least 10% of patients with lung cancer, especially SCLC, irrespective of the extension and size of the primary tumor, and may be the first manifestation of the disease. They include a myriad of endocrine, neurologic, skeletal, renal, metabolic, hematologic, cutaneous, and collagen vascular syndromes, which are likely due to the production of bioactive substances either by the tumor or in response to the tumor (e.g., polypeptide hormones, hormone-like peptides, antibodies or immune complexes, prostaglandins, or cytokines; Table 23.1). Hypercalcemia, the syndrome of inappropriate antidiuretic hormone secretion, Cushing syndrome, digital clubbing, hypertrophic osteoarthropathy, hematologic abnormalities, and hypercoagulable disorders are the most common syndromes observed.[8,9] Nonspecific symptoms include weakness and weight loss.

Delays in achieving a final diagnosis after the initial onset of symptoms can occur at several steps. First, the patient may notice a new symptom or a change in the usual respiratory symptoms, but some months may pass before he or she sees a physician.[10] Additional time may then be required for the physician to obtain imaging studies of the chest, for the patient to be referred to a specialist, or for the specialist to establish a final diagnosis.[11] Hamilton et al.[12] evaluated the positive predictive values of symptoms and physical signs and identified so-called red flags that were independently associated with lung cancer in multivariable analyses; these red flags included hemoptysis, anorexia, weight loss, fatigue, dyspnea, persistent cough, chest pain, and digital clubbing.

According to the National Institute for Health and Clinical Excellence (NICE) clinical guideline on the diagnosis and treatment of lung cancer, an urgent referral for chest imaging is recommended for patients who present with hemoptysis or any of several symptoms or signs (including cough, chest and/or shoulder pain, dyspnea, weight loss, hoarseness, finger clubbing, features suggestive of metastasis from a lung cancer, and cervical and/or supraclavicular lymphadenopathy) that are unexplained or persistent (lasting for more than 3 weeks). Smokers and ex-smokers who are older than 40 years of age and have persistent hemoptysis, signs of superior vena cava obstruction, and stridor should be offered an urgent referral to a member of the lung cancer multidisciplinary team, usually the chest physician, while awaiting the results of chest imaging.[13]

HISTORY

History taking should focus on major baseline risk factors, including smoking, occupational exposure (mainly to asbestos),[14] family history of lung cancer, previous diagnosis of other malignancy, preexisting nonmalignant lung diseases (e.g., chronic obstructive pulmonary disease, idiopathic pulmonary fibrosis,

TABLE 23.1 Paraneoplastic Syndromes

Syndrome	Type of Lung Cancer	Causative Agents
Acromegaly	Carcinoid tumors; small cell	Growth hormone-releasing hormone; growth hormone
Carcinoid syndrome	Carcinoid tumors; large cell Small cell	Serotonin
Ectopic adrenocorticotropic hormone (ACTH) syndrome	Small cell Carcinoid tumors	ACTH corticotropin-releasing hormone
Encephalomyelitis/subacute sensory neuropathy	Small cell	Anti-Hu antibody and Hu-D antigen
Granulocytosis	Nonsmall cell	Colony-stimulating factor (CSF); granulocyte–CSF Granulocyte-macrophage CSF Interleukin (IL)-6
Hypercalcemia	Nonsmall cell (usually squamous cell)	Parathyroid hormone-related peptide; parathormone
Hyponatremia	Small cell Nonsmall cell	Arginine vasopressin Atrial natriuretic peptide
Lambert–Eaton syndrome	Small cell	Anti-P/Q channel antibody and P/Q-type calcium channel (antigen)
Retinopathy	Small cell	Antirecoverin antibody and specific antigen specific to photoreceptor cells (recoverin)
Thrombocytosis	Nonsmall cell Small cell	IL-6
Thromboembolism	Nonsmall cell Small cell	Procoagulants Inflammatory cytokines Tumor interaction with host cells

tuberculosis, and previous pneumonia), and socioeconomic deprivation.[8] Finally, residence in or travel to an area with endemic fungal pathogens could suggest a benign infectious disease in the correct clinical context.

IMAGING FEATURES AND DIAGNOSTIC ACCURACY

Radiography plays a crucial role in the diagnostic workup for suspected lung cancer.[15] The main investigation in the primary care setting is the chest radiograph. The radiographic appearance of lung cancer at the time of the initial presentation may vary. Lung cancer occurs more often on the right side rather than on the left side and in the upper lobes rather than in the lower lobes, with a predominance in central locations.[8] Up to 40% of the radiographic findings associated with lung cancer are related to central tumors causing airway obstruction with secondary atelectasis and lung parenchyma consolidation. However, although a radiograph of the chest may lead to the identification of a suspected lung mass, it lacks sufficient resolution to differentiate benign from malignant disease, and, if a previous radiograph is not available to demonstrate stability over 2 years, the patient will need additional evaluation.[7] A negative result does not exclude lung cancer, especially if there is a high pretest probability. Stapley et al.[16] retrospectively reviewed the medical records of 247 patients with lung cancer to assess radiographic findings in the primary care setting and reported that more than 10% of patients had had negative radiographic findings in the 3 months before diagnosis. Moreover, negative findings on chest radiographs may occur with any cancer symptom other than hoarseness.[16] Therefore the standard imaging study for patients with suspected lung cancer is conventional contrast-enhanced CT of the chest, as it provides anatomic details such as the location, shape, margins, and attenuation characteristics of the primary lesion; the proximity of the lesion to surrounding structures; the extent of invasion of the chest wall; and the presence or absence of suspected mediastinal lymph node involvement.[17] Other advantages of CT are its widespread availability and its relatively low cost in comparison with more advanced imaging modalities, such as PET–CT (PET combined with CT) or magnetic resonance imaging (MRI).

In the case of a solitary lesion without any apparent evidence of lymph node involvement, atelectasis, or postobstructive pneumonia, specific morphologic characteristics may help to differentiate benign disease from malignant disease (Table 23.2). For this purpose, CT images should be thin slice, with contiguous 1-mm slices made through nodules. Lesions that are larger than 3 cm and that are located in the upper lobe are more likely to be malignant. Spiculated, lobulated, and ragged margins as well as notches and concavity in the margins are highly predictive of

lung cancer, whereas smooth borders usually suggest a benign lesion. However, as many as one-third of lesions with smooth borders are malignant. A ground-glass attenuation surrounding a nodule may signify hemorrhagic infarction and is known as the so-called CT halo sign. This finding has been associated with aspergillosis, Kaposi sarcoma, granulomatosis with polyangiitis, and metastatic angiosarcoma. Adenocarcinoma in situ (previously known as bronchioalveolar carcinoma) also can produce a halo as a result of its lepidic growth. Tentacle or polygonal margins occur in association with fibrosis, alveolar infiltration, and collapsed alveoli.[17] Regarding calcifications, laminated or concentric calcifications with a dense central core, diffuse and solid calcifications, or popcorn calcifications suggest a benign lesion. Although there is no specific pattern associated with malignancy, punctate and eccentric calcifications may be associated with lung cancer. Cavitation can occur in association with malignant nodules (most commonly squamous cell carcinoma) as well as benign diseases, including abscesses, infectious granulomas, vasculitides, early Langerhans cell histiocytosis, and pulmonary infarction. A cavity wall thickness of less than 5 mm is suggestive of a benign etiology, whereas irregular walls and a wall thickness of more than 15 mm are usually (although not always) associated with malignant lesions.[17]

Lung nodules can be classified as solid or subsolid. Subsolid nodules can be part solid and part ground glass or can be pure ground-glass nodules (GGNs), defined as focal increased lung attenuation through which normal parenchymal structures such as airways, vessels, and interlobular septa are still visible. GGNs are frequently multiple, and the approach to these nodules is beyond the scope of this chapter. According to the International Association for the Study of Lung Cancer, the American Thoracic Society, and the European Respiratory Society, the presence of solid components in the GGN is associated with more invasive pathologic features, as subsolid nodules frequently represent the histologic spectrum of adenocarcinomas, including atypical adenomatous hyperplasia, adenocarcinomas in situ, minimally invasive adenocarcinomas, and lepidic-predominant adenocarcinomas. However, because of their slow growth rate and low metabolic activity, the differential diagnosis between benign and malignant subsolid lesions remains quite problematic. In fact, another relevant factor to take into account, which requires the availability of previous CT images, is the growth rate. Malignant nodules have a volume-doubling time of 20 days to 400 days, although the majority of cancers double in volume within 100 days. A doubling time of more than 400 days is usually associated with benign disease, whereas a doubling time of less than 20 days indicates very rapid growth and strongly suggests infectious processes.

TABLE 23.2 Morphologic Features on Computed Tomography Suggestive of Malignant or Benign Disease[17]

Morphologic Characteristics	Malignant Disease	Benign Disease
Size	>3 cm	≤3 cm
Margins	Spiculated, lobulated, ragged, notches and concavity, halo (adenocarcinoma in situ, Kaposi sarcoma, angiosarcoma), rarely smooth (up to a third of cases)	Smooth, halo (aspergillosis, granulomatosis with polyangiitis), polygonal, rarely spiculated (lipoid pneumonia, focal atelectasis, tuberculoma, and progressive massive fibrosis)
Calcifications/attenuations	Punctate, eccentric	Laminated and concentric, dense central core, diffuse and solid, popcorn (hamartoma)
Cavitations	Irregular and thicker walls (>15 mm)	Cavity wall thickness <5 mm (abscesses, infectious granulomas, vasculitides, early Langerhans cell histiocytosis, pulmonary infarction)
Ground glass[3]	Subsolid GGNs (atypical adenomatous hyperplasia, adenocarcinomas in situ, minimally invasive adenocarcinomas and lepidic-predominant adenocarcinomas)	Pure GGNs
Growth rate	Doubling time, 20 to 400 days	Doubling time, <20 days (infectious process) or >400 days

GGN, Ground-glass nodule.

The presence of features suggestive of intrathoracic invasion is an important clue that helps to distinguish between benign and malignant nodules. Although numerous criteria have been used to define lymph node involvement, the most widely used criterion is a short-axis diameter of more than 1 cm on a transverse CT image. In a systematic review of the medical literature relating to the accuracy of CT staging of the mediastinum, the median sensitivity and specificity of CT for identifying mediastinal lymph node metastasis were 55% and 81%, respectively.[7] Although these studies were statistically heterogeneous, the findings are similar to the results of meta-analyses addressing the accuracy of CT for staging of the mediastinum in NSCLC, which have demonstrated very low sensitivity, ranging from 51% to 64%.[18,19] In fact, as many as 20% of patients who have T1 N0 M0 disease diagnosed on the basis of CT imaging are still found to have positive lymph node involvement on the basis of surgical lymph node sampling. Moreover, although pooled specificity values (range, 76% to 84%) are higher overall than the sensitivity values, a consistent rate of lymph nodes that are defined as malignant on the basis of CT is actually benign.[20]

The increasing availability of ^{18}F-2-deoxy-D-glucose (^{18}FDG)-PET in clinical practice has allowed the technique to become an essential tool for the diagnosis and staging of disease in patients with radiographic and clinical findings consistent with lung cancer. ^{18}FDG-PET is very accurate for differentiating benign from malignant lesions with nodules as small as 1 cm and may also detect clinically unexpected distant metastasis. Increased cellular uptake, defined as a standardized uptake value of more than 2.5, is a common property of both neoplastic and inflamed tissues. However, the sensitivity for lesions smaller than 1 cm is quiet low, likely due to lower metabolic activity, well-differentiated low-grade malignancies not being detected, and a high false-positive rate from inflammation. For mediastinal staging, PET has been shown to have both higher sensitivity and specificity than CT. A meta-analysis of data on PET demonstrated pooled estimates of 74% (95% confidence interval [CI], 69% to 79%) and 85% (95% CI, 82% to 88%) for sensitivity and specificity, respectively.[21] However, in the context of a cancer that is still confined to the chest and thus is potentially curable, the rate of false-positive findings, which may result in missed opportunities for surgical resection, is too high. Moreover, some studies have shown a direct correlation between the accuracy of PET and increasing lymph node size on CT, where the sensitivity is higher (but specificity is lower) when nodes are enlarged.[21]

Newer-generation integrated PET–CT imagers have combined the advantages of both modalities, allowing correlation between CT (which demonstrates anatomic details) and ^{18}FDG-PET (which identifies aspects of tumor function and metabolism). For differentiating between malignant and benign lung nodules, PET–CT is associated with a significantly higher specificity than CT or PET alone because of the ability to discard false-positive uptake on PETs on the basis of the morphologic findings on CT.

Lastly, dynamic MRI is an emerging diagnostic tool for the differential diagnosis and staging of lung cancer. One advantage of this tool is that it does not involve the use of ionizing radiation. Available data suggest that MRI is at least as accurate as CT in evaluating the mediastinum,[22,23] and because MRI can detect differences in intensity between normal tissues and tumor, it may be superior in the ability to detect tumor invasion into the mediastinum, chest wall, diaphragm, or vertebral bodies.[22,24–27] In fact, MRI excels in the delineation of superior sulcus tumors, including tumors that involve the neural foramina, spinal canal, and brachial plexus.[28] ACCP and NICE guidelines currently state that MRI should not routinely be performed to assess the stage of the primary tumor, but that MRI is useful for patients with superior sulcus tumors.[7,13]

Overall, the available data indicate that when the findings of noninvasive imaging (combined PET–CT, PET or CT alone, and MRI) suggest malignancy, it represents an excellent guide to determine the proper technique to achieve the final diagnosis and staging. However, especially in the context of a suspected lung cancer that is confined to the chest and a high baseline suspicion of disease, indeterminate nodules or negative mediastinal findings require additional procedures to obtain a tissue diagnosis.

DIAGNOSTIC APPROACH FOR ESTABLISHING A DEFINITIVE DIAGNOSIS AND STAGING

As previously stated, the method for definitive diagnosis and staging of lung cancer depends on the suspected cell subtype (SCLC or NSCLC), the size and location of the primary tumor, the presence or absence of radiographic findings suggestive of mediastinal involvement, and the overall clinical status of the patient.[21]

The ACCP guidelines recommend that, for patients in whom SCLC is suspected on the basis of radiographic and clinical findings, the diagnosis should be confirmed with whatever method is easiest (sputum cytology, thoracentesis, bronchoscopy, or transthoracic fine-needle aspiration).[21] For patients in whom NSCLC is suspected, the method of achieving a diagnosis is usually dictated by the presumptive stage of the disease, as the main goal is to maximize the yield of the selected procedure by establishing both diagnosis and staging with one test and avoiding unnecessary invasive tests.[7] The NICE guidelines also recommend choosing investigations that give the most information about diagnosis and staging with the least risk to the patient.[13] After distant metastases have been ruled out, lung cancer presentation can be separated into four categories with respect to intrathoracic radiographic characteristics: (1) extensive mediastinal infiltration by tumor, (2) enlarged discrete N2 or N3 nodes, (3) central tumor or a tumor with enlarged N1 nodes but a normal mediastinum, and (4) peripheral small tumor with normal-sized lymph nodes.[7] For patients who have extensive infiltration of the mediastinum, defined as a mass that infiltrates and encircles the vessels and airways such that mediastinal lymph nodes are no longer visible, the diagnosis of lung cancer should be established with the least-invasive and safest method. In cases in which mediastinal involvement (stage III) is suspected, sampling the mediastinum rather than the primary tumor offers the advantage of diagnosis and staging in one procedure.

In patients with discrete mediastinal lymph node enlargement on CT or PET, mediastinal involvement must be confirmed, and, for that purpose, endoscopic techniques such as endobronchial ultrasound (EBUS) or endoscopic ultrasound (EUS)-guided sampling are preferred as a first step over surgical staging, as they are less invasive and less costly than mediastinoscopy. However, in cases in which the results of EBUS or EUS are negative, mediastinoscopy is recommended. The absence of findings suggestive of mediastinal involvement on both CT and PET images has a high negative predictive value, except in the case of a centrally located tumor or N1 lymph node enlargement. These factors make the chance of N2 or N3 involvement relatively high (20% to 25%) and the use of a technique such as EBUS, EUS, or combined EBUS and EUS-guided needle aspiration is suggested to confirm the staging. Conversely, in the presence of peripheral lung nodules, the chance of mediastinal involvement is quite low.[7]

Different techniques are available to achieve the diagnosis of the primary tumor, and the choice among them is largely guided by the size and location of the lesion. Sputum cytology is particularly useful for the evaluation of patients who have a centrally located tumor and patients who have hemoptysis. However, if sputum cytology is negative for carcinoma, additional testing is recommended.

For patients with suspected lung cancer who have a pleural effusion, thoracentesis is recommended to diagnose the cause of the effusion. If cytologic examination of pleural fluid is negative, image-guided pleural biopsy or medical or surgical thoracoscopy is recommended. However, if CT of the chest shows pleural thickening or pleural nodules and/or masses, image-guided needle biopsy may be considered as a first approach.[21]

Endoscopic Techniques for Diagnosis and Staging

Over the past decade, endoscopic techniques (bronchoscopy and esophageal endoscopy) have emerged as procedures of choice for the diagnosis and staging of lung cancer. With the addition of real-time ultrasound guidance, endoscopic procedures have demonstrated accuracy for mediastinal staging, with pooled sensitivities comparing favorably with that of the traditional criterion standard, mediastinoscopy.[7] In addition, endoscopic techniques are associated with lower morbidity and mortality and are more cost effective than mediastinoscopy.[29,30]

Flexible Bronchoscopy

Flexible bronchoscopy should be offered to every patient with central lesions on CT for whom nodal staging does not influence treatment. In addition, patients with suspected lung cancer may have symptoms due to endobronchial involvement that require airway inspection with bronchoscopy for tissue sampling in order to make a diagnosis or to guide further interventions. Endobronchial biopsies provide the highest sensitivity (74%), followed by brushings (61%), and washings (47%).[31] A combination of these methods provides a diagnosis in 88% of cases.[26] Endobronchial needle aspiration may provide deeper penetration with less hemorrhage, and the use of this method in addition to forceps biopsies and brushings may improve sensitivity to 95%.[32,33]

The sensitivity of bronchoscopy for peripheral nodules is lower than for central lesions. Transbronchial needle aspiration (TBNA) and transbronchial biopsy have provided the highest sensitivity, followed by transbronchial brushings and lavage or washing.[34,35] However, the overall diagnostic accuracy largely depends on the size of the suspected primary tumor, as it has been reported to be 34% for lesions smaller than 2 cm.[21] Therefore for patients with suspected peripheral lung nodules with an indeterminate likelihood of malignancy, for whom a tissue diagnosis is required before surgical resection, appropriate techniques of sampling include fluoroscopic guidance, radial EBUS, electromagnetic navigation bronchoscopy, and transthoracic needle aspiration (TTNA). When the lesion is moderately to highly suspicious for lung cancer, an upfront surgical excision performed via thoracoscopy is the most definitive method for establishing a diagnosis.[21]

EBUS Fine-Needle Aspiration

Although still associated with high diagnostic yield in expert hands, TBNA is increasingly being supplanted by EBUS fine-needle aspiration. At best, TBNA can be used for selective mediastinal staging, as only subcarinal and right paratracheal lymph nodes are reliably sampled by most bronchoscopists.[36] Because of its limitations, TBNA has a low pooled sensitivity of 39% (95% CI, 17% to 61%), as reported by Holty et al.[37] in a meta-analysis of 13 studies.[7] The use of real-time ultrasound to directly visualize the target during EBUS fine-needle aspiration has solved major deficiencies associated with traditional TBNA.[38] EBUS–TBNA is a versatile and accurate tool for the simultaneous diagnosis and staging of mediastinal and hilar lymph nodes or masses. Its range includes the highest mediastinal lymph nodes (station 1), upper paratracheal lymph nodes (stations 2R and 2L), lower paratracheal lymph nodes (stations 4R and 4L), subcarinal lymph nodes (station 7), hilar lymph nodes (station 10), and interlobar lymph nodes (station 11). From a technical standpoint, para-aortic lymph nodes (station 6) and aortopulmonary window

or subaortic lymph nodes (station 5) typically require a surgical approach, whereas paraesophageal lymph nodes (station 8) and pulmonary ligament lymph nodes (station 9) are usually best accessed with use of EUS fine-needle aspiration (Fig. 23.1).

Because of its safety and accuracy, the uses of EBUS have been expanded to include preoperative mediastinal staging and tissue acquisition for the purposes of molecular analysis and immunohistochemical staining.[39–41] Complications such as severe bleeding and infection are almost negligible, and the rate of pneumothorax is 0.07% to 0.2%.[42–45]

Clearly, EBUS–TBNA is superior to CT and PET for mediastinal staging.[46] Two meta-analyses of studies evaluating the use of EBUS–TBNA for mediastinal staging, by Adams et al.[36] (disease prevalence, 46%) and Gu et al.[42] (disease prevalence, 68%), showed pooled sensitivities of 88% (95% CI, 79% to 94%) and 93% (95% CI, 91% to 94%), respectively.

In addition, in a large systematic review of related studies by the ACCP in which 2756 patients met the criteria for mediastinal staging, the median sensitivity was 89% (range, 46% to 97%), the median negative predictive value was 91%,[7,36,42] and the overall specificity and positive predictive value were both 100%.[1,12,17]

The sensitivity of EBUS–TBNA is higher for enlarged and/or PET-positive lymph nodes (94%; 95% CI, 93% to 96%) than for normal-sized and PET-negative lymph nodes (76%; 95% CI, 65% to 85%).[42] Without rapid on-site evaluation, at least three aspirations per node should be obtained. The use of rapid on-site evaluation can further reduce the number of aspirations without reducing the accuracy of the method.[34,47,48] Unlike the traditional TBNA, needle size (i.e., 22 gauge vs. 21 gauge) does not substantially change the sensitivity of EBUS–TBNA.[48,49]

EUS Needle Aspiration

Primarily because of its superior ability to sample the posterior mediastinum through the esophageal wall, EUS may be used to increase the number of mediastinal node stations amenable to nonsurgical sampling.[50] Like EBUS, EUS is performed with use of real-time ultrasound. EUS needle aspiration can be used to sample inferior pulmonary ligament, paraesophageal, subcarinal, left paratracheal, and aortopulmonary window node stations (stations 9, 8, 7, 4L, and 5). Anterolateral paratracheal locations (stations 2R, 2L, and 4R) are commonly involved in patients with lung cancer but are not sampled reliably with this technique.[50,51] No major complications have been reported in association with this technique, and minor complications such as transient fever, sore throat, cough, nausea, and vomiting are rare (prevalence, 0.8%).[52]

A systematic review in the 2013 ACCP guidelines and a meta-analysis by Micames et al.[52] demonstrated that the overall sensitivities of EUS needle aspiration for mediastinal staging were 89% and 83%, respectively.[7] The sensitivities of the method were higher for enlarged lymph nodes (50% to 66%) than for normal-sized lymph nodes (87% to 92%). The overall false-negative rate was 14%.[7,52]

In a pooled analysis of data from 2433 patients with evaluable lung cancer, EUS was shown to have a sensitivity and specificity of 89% and 100%, respectively.[53–76] For patients with lung cancer without adenopathy on CT, EUS has been shown to sample nodes as small as 3 mm in diameter, which is useful given the high incidence of metastasis in normal-sized lymph nodes in patients with lung cancer.[77] The findings of surgical studies indicate that it may be possible to predict the location of mediastinal lymph node metastases at certain levels based on the location of the tumor. This relationship may influence the use of EUS for some patients without adenopathy on CT images of the chest. Lymphatic pathways favor spread to aortopulmonary window nodes from left upper lobe tumors and to subcarinal nodes from left and right lower lobe lesions.[78] EUS has been studied for the evaluation of

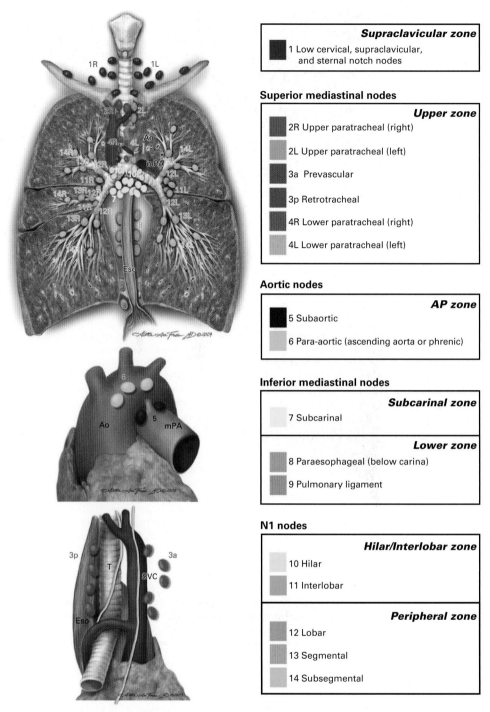

Supraclavicular zone
1 Low cervical, supraclavicular, and sternal notch nodes

Superior mediastinal nodes

Upper zone
2R Upper paratracheal (right)
2L Upper paratracheal (left)
3a Prevascular
3p Retrotracheal
4R Lower paratracheal (right)
4L Lower paratracheal (left)

Aortic nodes

AP zone
5 Subaortic
6 Para-aortic (ascending aorta or phrenic)

Inferior mediastinal nodes

Subcarinal zone
7 Subcarinal

Lower zone
8 Paraesophageal (below carina)
9 Pulmonary ligament

N1 nodes

Hilar/Interlobar zone
10 Hilar
11 Interlobar

Peripheral zone
12 Lobar
13 Segmental
14 Subsegmental

Fig. 23.1. International Association for the Study of Lung Cancer map of regional lymph nodes for the determination of N descriptor during tumor, node, and metastasis (TNM) staging of lung cancer. *Ao,* Aorta; *AP,* aortopulmonary, *Eso,* esophagus; *SVC,* superior vena cava, *T,* trachea. *(Reprinted with permission from International Association for the Study of Lung Cancer. Staging Manual in Thoracic Oncology. Orange Park, FL: Editorial Rx Press; 2009.)*

patients with known lung cancer without enlarged mediastinal lymph nodes on CT and has detected mediastinal involvement (stage III or IV disease) in up to 42% of cases.[53]

Unlike other methods of mediastinal staging, EUS has the capability to stage lung cancer from locations outside the mediastinum. The left lobe of the liver, a substantial part of the right lobe of the liver, and the left (but not the right) adrenal gland can be identified and sampled in 97% of patients.[79] In addition, left pleural effusions can be visualized and sampled during EUS.

Combined EBUS and EUS Needle Aspiration

When combined, EUS and EBUS have shown superior yield to that than when the techniques are used alone. A pooled analysis of data from seven studies (811 patients) showed a sensitivity and specificity of 91% and 100%, respectively.[7,55,59,60,80–83] When used in tandem, these procedures are complementary by providing near-complete access to the mediastinum for staging and are particularly useful for evaluation of a radiographically normal mediastinum.[55,60] In a randomized controlled trial of patients with (suspected) NSCLC, staging with EUS and mediastinoscopy was compared with mediastinoscopy alone and was shown to have greater sensitivity for detecting mediastinal node metastases and also led to fewer unnecessary thoracotomies.[80]

The combined use of EBUS and EUS provides the opportunity to reach nearly all mediastinal lymph nodes except for para-aortic and prevascular nodes.[81,84] The procedure may be performed either with the sequential use of two dedicated echo-endoscopes or with an EBUS scope placed first in the airway and then in the esophagus.[85] In a 2013 meta-analysis, Zhang et al.[86] found that combined EBUS and EUS needle aspiration had a pooled sensitivity of 86% and had greater sensitivity than either EBUS–TBNA alone (75%) or EUS needle aspiration alone (69%) for staging the mediastinum of patients with lung cancer. Wallace et al.[74] reported that combined EBUS and EUS needle aspiration can decrease the requirement for further surgical procedures by approximately 30%. In a systematic review of seven studies (811 patients), combined EBUS and EUS needle aspiration had an overall sensitivity and negative predictive value of 91% and 96%, respectively, which were slightly higher than those of each technique alone.[7]

TTNA and Core Biopsy

TTNA and core samples are commonly obtained from pulmonary nodules or masses via CT guidance but may be obtained with ultrasound guidance in select cases in which the tumor abuts the pleural surface. The sensitivity and specificity of CT-guided TTNA are 90% and 97%, respectively.[31]

It should be noted that in most cases, TTNA or other nonsurgical biopsy techniques for peripheral pulmonary lesions do not eliminate the need for surgery, especially in patients with a high pretest probability of cancer, unless a clear noncancerous diagnosis can be made.[87] Nonetheless, TTNA may be unavoidable for patients who are not candidates for surgery but must have tissue diagnosed before treatment, patients who are likely to have noncancerous lesions, patients who request that a diagnosis be confirmed before surgery, and patients who must have confirmation of metastatic disease.

The major risks of TTNA include a 15% rate of pneumothorax and a 1% rate of major hemorrhage.[88] Although pneumothorax may be life threatening and may lead to tension physiology without treatment, most cases do not require treatment (tube thoracostomy is necessary in 6% of biopsies).[88,89] The major risk factors for the development of pneumothorax include the presence of emphysema, a smaller lesion size, and a greater depth of needle penetration from the pleural surface to the edge of the lesion.

CONCLUSION

Staging the mediastinum is of paramount importance in the diagnostic workup for suspected lung cancer confined to the chest, as it dictates treatment options and prognosis. Despite advances in imaging modalities and the increased accuracy of PET–CT for noninvasive staging of the mediastinum, tissue sampling remains necessary to confirm mediastinal node disease. Endoscopic techniques, including EBUS, EUS, or combined EBUS, should now be considered first-line procedures for mediastinal staging because of their excellent accuracy and safety profile. These techniques are complementary to a thorough history, physical examination, and imaging modalities.

KEY REFERENCES

1. National Comprehensive Cancer Network. NCCN Clinical Practice Guidelines in Oncology: Non-Small Cell Lung Cancer; 2017. http://www.nccn.org.
2. Morgensztern D, Ng S, Gao F, et al. Trends in stage distribution for patients with non-small cell lung cancer: a National Cancer Database survey. *J Thorac Oncol*. 2010;5(1):29–33.
5. Collins LG, Haines C, Perkel R, et al. Lung cancer: diagnosis and management. *Am Fam Physician*. 2007;75(1):56–63.
6. Ost DE, Yeung SC, Tanoue LT, et al. Clinical and organizational factors in the initial evaluation of patients with lung cancer: diagnosis and management of lung cancer, 3rd ed: American College of Chest Physicians evidence-based clinical practice guidelines. *Chest*. 2013;143(suppl 5):e121S–e141S.
7. Silvestri GA, Gonzalez AV, Jantz MA, et al. Methods for staging non-small cell lung cancers; diagnosis and management of lung cancer, 3rd ed: American College of Chest Physicians evidence-based clinical practice guidelines. *Chest*. 2013;143(suppl 5):e211S–e250S.
8. Spiro SG, Gould MK, Colice GL, et al. Initial evaluation of the patient with lung cancer: symptoms, signs, laboratory tests, and paraneoplastic syndromes: ACCP evidenced-based clinical practice guidelines (2nd edition). *Chest*. 2007;132(suppl 3):149S–160S.
12. Hamilton W, Peters TJ, Round A, et al. What are the clinical features of lung cancer before the diagnosis is made? A population based case-control study. *Thorax*. 2005;60(12):1059–1065.
13. National Institute for Health and Clinical Excellence. NICE Clinical Guideline 121: The Diagnosis and Management of Lung Cancer; 2011. http://www.nice.org.uk/nicemedia/live/13465/54202/54202.pdf.
19. Gould MK, Kuschner WG, Rydzak CE, et al. Test performance of positron emission tomography and computed tomography for mediastinal staging in patients with non-small-cell lung cancer: a meta-analysis. *Ann Intern Med*. 2003;139(11):879–892.
20. Silvestri GA, Gould MK, Margolis ML, et al. Noninvasive staging of non-small cell lung cancer: ACCP evidenced-based clinical practice guidelines (2nd edition). *Chest*. 2007;132(suppl 3):178S–201S.
21. Rivera MP, Mehta AC, Wahidi MM. Establishing the diagnosis of lung cancer: diagnosis and management of lung cancer, 3rd ed: American College of Chest Physicians evidence-based clinical practice guidelines. *Chest*. 2013;143(suppl 5):e142S–e165S.
27. Shiotani S, Sugimura K, Sugihara M, et al. Diagnosis of chest wall invasion by lung cancer: useful criteria for exclusion of the possibility of chest wall invasion with MR imaging. *Radiat Med*. 2000;18(5):283–290.
28. Ravenel JG. Evidence-based imaging in lung cancer: a systematic review. *J Thorac Imaging*. 2012;27(5):315–324.
30. Steinfort DP, Liew D, Conron M, et al. Cost-benefit of minimally invasive staging of non-small cell lung cancer: a decision tree sensitivity analysis. *J Thorac Oncol*. 2010;5(10):1564–1570.
31. Rivera MP, Mehta AC. American College of Chest Physicians. Initial diagnosis of lung cancer: ACCP evidence-based clinical practice guidelines (2nd edition). *Chest*. 2007;132(3):131S–148S.
33. Govert JA, Dodd LG, Kussin PS, et al. A prospective comparison of fiberoptic transbronchial needle aspiration and bronchial biopsy for bronchoscopically visible lung carcinoma. *Cancer*. 1999;87(3):129–134.
34. Trisolini R, Cancellieri A, Tinelli C, et al. Rapid on-site evaluation of transbronchial aspirates in the diagnosis of hilar and mediastinal adenopathy: a randomized trial. *Chest*. 2011;139(2):395–401.
35. Gasparini S, Ferretti M, Secchi EB, et al. Integration of transbronchial and percutaneous approach in the diagnosis of peripheral pulmonary nodules or masses. Experience with 1,027 consecutive cases. *Chest*. 1995;108(1):131–137.
49. Yarmus LB, Akulian J, Lechtzin N, et al. Comparison of 21-gauge and 22-gauge needle in endobronchial ultrasound-guided transbronchial needle aspiration. Results of the American College of Chest Physicians Quality Improvement Registry, Education, and Evaluation Registry. *Chest*. 2013;143(4):1036–1043.
50. Silvestri GA, Hoffman BJ, Bhutani MS, et al. Endoscopic ultrasound with fine-needle aspiration in the diagnosis and staging of lung cancer. *Ann Thorac Surg*. 1996;61(5):1441–1445. discussion 1445–1446.
54. Fritscher-Ravens A, Bohuslavizki KH, Brandt L, et al. Mediastinal lymph node involvement in potentially resectable lung cancer: comparison of CT, positron emission tomography, and endoscopic ultrasonography with and without fine-needle aspiration. *Chest*. 2003;123(2):442–451.
55. Wallace MB, Pascual JM, Raimondo M, et al. Minimally invasive endoscopic staging of suspected lung cancer. *JAMA*. 2008;299(5):540–546.
68. Annema JT, Versteegh MI, Veselic M, et al. Endoscopic ultrasound-guided fine-needle aspiration in the diagnosis and staging of lung cancer and its impact on surgical staging. *J Clin Oncol*. 2005;23(33):8357–8361.

69. Annema JT, Versteegh MI, Veselič M, et al. Endoscopic ultrasound added to mediastinoscopy for preoperative staging of patients with lung cancer. *JAMA*. 2005;294(8):931–936.

79. Chang KJ, Erickson RA, Nguyen P. Endoscopic ultrasound (EUS) and EUS-guided fine-needle aspiration of the left adrenal gland. *Gastrointest Endosc*. 1996;44(5):568–572.

80. Annema JT, van Meerbeeck JP, Rintoul RC, et al. Mediastinoscopy vs endosonography for mediastinal nodal staging of lung cancer: a randomized trial. *JAMA*. 2010;304(20):2245–2252.

84. McComb BL, Wallace MB, Pascual JM, et al. Mediastinal staging of nonsmall cell lung carcinoma by endoscopic and endobronchial ultrasound-guided fine needle aspiration. *J Thorac Imaging*. 2011;26(2):147–161.

85. Tournoy KG, Keller SM, Annema JT. Mediastinal staging of lung cancer: novel concepts. *Lancet Oncol*. 2012;13(5):e221–e229.

88. Wiener RS, Schwartz LM, Woloshin S, et al. Population-based risk for complications after transthoracic needle lung biopsy of a pulmonary nodule: an analysis of discharge records. *Ann Intern Med*. 2011;155(3):137–144.

89. Ost D, Fein AM, Feinsilver SH. The solitary pulmonary nodule. *N Engl J Med*. 2003;348(25):2535–2542.

See Expertconsult.com for full list of references.

24 Preoperative and Intraoperative Invasive Staging of the Mediastinum

Gail E. Darling, Ramón Rami-Porta, and Kazuhiro Yasufuku

SUMMARY OF KEY POINTS

- Staging of the mediastinum is a key component in the evaluation of patients with lung cancer and includes both preoperative and intraoperative components.
- The International Association for the Study of Lung Cancer lymph node map provides standard definitions of each nodal station and allows precise, uniform nomenclature when staging mediastinal and pulmonary lymph nodes.
- The importance of lymph node assessment in the staging of nonsmall cell lung cancer is well recognized, but despite this, inadequate lymph node assessment is too common.
- Variation in the extent of mediastinal lymph node staging has been a source of confusion in the literature.
- Systematic sampling may be performed by endobronchial ultrasound–transbronchial needle aspiration (EBUS–TBNA) or endoscopic ultrasound (EUS) or mediastinoscopy prior to a planned resection or at the time of the planned resection.
- Minimally invasive needle techniques including EBUS–TBNA and EUS–fine-needle aspiration are now considered the tests of first choice to confirm mediastinal disease in accessible lymph node stations.

Staging of the mediastinum is a key component in the evaluation of patients with lung cancer and includes both preoperative and intraoperative components. The purpose of mediastinal staging is to distinguish those patients who may benefit from surgery from those who should have other forms of treatment. The preoperative assessment of the mediastinum includes computed tomography (CT) and positron emission tomography (PET) scans and has been addressed in Chapters 21 and 22. Invasive or operative mediastinal staging includes the techniques of mediastinoscopy, mediastinotomy, thoracoscopic staging, staging at the time of planned resection, and needle biopsy techniques such as endobronchial ultrasound (EBUS) or endoscopic ultrasound (EUS). Invasive mediastinal staging provides histologic or cytologic confirmation of the status of the mediastinal lymph nodes. It is important to differentiate mediastinal node assessment for the purpose of staging versus a possible therapeutic benefit. Whether mediastinal lymph node dissection (MLND) improves survival is controversial.

Patients who have proven metastases in mediastinal lymph nodes have a poor prognosis because of increased risk of systemic disease. Identification of N2 disease prior to resection is preferable to avoid a noncurative resection as surgery alone is inadequate, whereas patients without mediastinal node involvement are candidates for surgery.

Pathologic confirmation of nodal status by the techniques described in this chapter is important because the diagnostic accuracy of imaging tests such as CT and PET is insufficient for clinical decision making. The positive predictive value of CT ranges from 0.18 to 0.88. On average, the likelihood of an enlarged node on CT being positive for metastatic disease is only 60%. Similarly, nodes that are positive on PET are pathologically positive for metastatic disease only 75% to 85% of the time.[1] This means that 15% to 40% of the time patients may be denied curative intent therapy because of imaging tests. Abnormal imaging should be confirmed or refuted pathologically.

This chapter will address the relevant anatomy with respect to the International Association for the Study of Lung Cancer (IASLC) lymph node map (Fig. 24.1), the definitions used in discussing staging of the mediastinum, the indications for invasive staging, the techniques available for invasive staging, and the appropriate use of these techniques.

LYMPH NODE ANATOMY OF THE MEDIASTINUM AND THE IASLC LYMPH NODE MAP

The IASLC lymph node map was published in 2009 (see Fig. 24.1).[2] The map illustrates the key lymph node anatomy of the mediastinum and lung. The goal of the IASLC Staging Committee in creating this new map was to reconcile the differences between the Japanese and Mountain–Dresler lymph node maps and to provide specific anatomic definitions of the lymph node stations.[2] The key changes include the description of level 1 nodes as supraclavicular and suprasternal nodes, the division between right- and left-sided nodes defined as the left lateral border of the trachea, definition of the subcarinal nodes as level 7 (not level 7 and 10 as on the Japanese map), and the clear division of lymph node levels based on clearly identified anatomic landmarks (Table 24.1). This map provides standard definitions of each nodal station and allows precise, uniform nomenclature when staging mediastinal and pulmonary lymph nodes. Mediastinal nodes (N2 and N3) are numbered 1–9. Hilar and intrapulmonary (N1) nodes are numbered 10–14.

LYMPH NODE STATIONS AND CHOICE OF STAGING TECHNIQUE

Standard mediastinoscopy or videomediastinoscopy can access lymph node stations 1, 2R/L, 4R/L, 7, and 10R. Stations 5 and 6 can be accessed by extended mediastinoscopy, parasternal mediastinotomy (Chamberlain procedure) or anterior mediastinoscopy, and video-assisted thoracic surgery (VATS). Prevascular nodes (3a) may be accessible by parasternal mediastinotomy or anterior mediastinoscopy and VATS. VATS can access ipsilateral nodal stations as well as hilar nodes and even interlobar nodes if the fissure is explored.

Needle techniques include EBUS–transbronchial needle aspiration (EBUS–TBNA) and EUS–needle aspiration (EUS–NA).

EBUS–TBNA can access all the nodes accessed by mediastinoscopy and additionally stations 11 and 12 bilaterally. EUS–NA can access stations 8 and 9 as well as the same stations as mediastinoscopy, but not the hilar nodes.

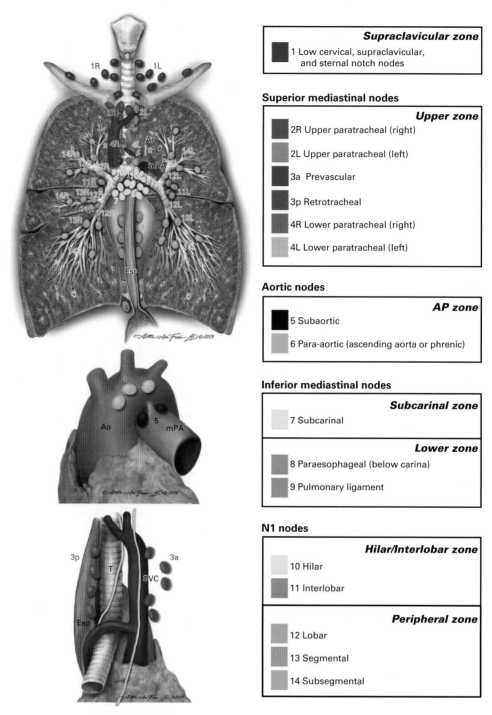

Fig. 24.1. International Association for the Study of Lung Cancer map of regional lymph nodes for the determination of N descriptor during tumor, node, and metastasis staging of lung cancer. *Ao,* Aorta; *Eso,* esophagus; *mPA,* main pulmonary artery; *SVC,* superior vena cava; *T,* trachea. *(Reprinted with permission from International Association for the Study of Lung Cancer. Staging Manual in Thoracic Oncology. Orange Park, FL: Editorial Rx Press; 2009.)*

Techniques such as video-assisted mediastinal lymphadenectomy (VAMLA) and transcervical extended mediastinal lymphadenectomy (TEMLA) have been used for staging, but are more appropriately considered as techniques for mediastinal node dissection. These techniques may have therapeutic as well as staging applications.

INDICATIONS FOR INVASIVE MEDIASTINAL STAGING

The American College of Chest Physicians (ACCP) evidence-based clinical practice guidelines,[3] the European Society of Thoracic Surgeons (ESTS) guidelines,[4] and Cancer Care Ontario (CCO) Program in Evidence-Based Care Practice Guidelines[5] are concordant in their recommendations for indications and techniques for invasive staging (Table 24.2). Invasive staging by needle techniques is recommended if available, but surgical biopsies are recommended if the needle techniques are negative because of the low negative predictive value of needle biopsy techniques.[3]

ACCP does not recommend invasive staging for patients with extensive mediastinal infiltration.[3] However, invasive staging techniques may be used for diagnostic purposes. ACCP, ESTS, and

TABLE 24.1 Anatomical Definitions for Each Lymph Node Station and Station Grouping by Nodal Zones in the Map Proposed by the International Association for the Study of Lung Cancer

Lymph Node Station	Anatomical Limits
SUPRACLAVICULAR ZONE	
1: Low cervical, supraclavicular, and sternal notch nodes	Upper border: lower margin of cricoid cartilage. Lower border: clavicles bilaterally and, in the midline, the upper border of the manubrium. 1R designates right-sided nodes, 1L left-sided nodes in this region. For lymph node station 1, the midline of the trachea serves as the border between 1R and 1L.
UPPER ZONE	
2: Upper paratracheal nodes	2R: Upper border: apex of the right lung and pleural space, and, in the midline, the upper border of the manubrium. Lower border: intersection of the caudal margin of innominate vein with the trachea. As for lymph node station 4R, 2R includes nodes extending to the left lateral border of the trachea. 2L: Upper border: apex of the lung and pleural space, and, in the midline, the upper border of the manubrium. Lower border: superior border of the aortic arch.
3 Prevascular and retrotracheal nodes	3a: Prevascular. On the right: Upper border: apex of chest. Lower border: level of carina. Anterior border: posterior aspect of sternum. Posterior border: anterior border of superior vena cava. On the left: Upper border: apex of chest. Lower border: level of carina. Anterior border: posterior aspect of sternum. Posterior border: left carotid artery. 3p: Retrotracheal. Upper border: apex of chest. Lower border: carina.
4: Lower paratracheal nodes	4R: includes right paratracheal nodes, and pretracheal nodes extending to the left lateral border of the trachea. Upper border: intersection of the caudal margin of innominate vein with the trachea. Lower border: lower border of the azygos vein. 4L: includes nodes to the left of the left lateral border of the trachea, medial to the ligamentum arteriosum. Upper border: upper margin of the aortic arch. Lower border: upper rim of the left main pulmonary artery.
AORTOPULMONARY ZONE	
5: Subaortic (aortopulmonary window)	Subaortic lymph nodes lateral to the ligamentum arteriosum. Upper border: the lower border of the aortic arch. Lower border: upper rim of the left main pulmonary artery.
6: Para-aortic nodes (ascending aorta or phrenic	Lymph nodes anterior and lateral to the ascending aorta and aortic arch. Upper border: a line tangential to the upper border of the aortic arch. Lower border: the lower border of the aortic arch.
SUBCARINAL ZONE	
7: Subcarinal nodes	Upper border: the carina of the trachea. Lower border: the upper border of the lower-lobe bronchus on the left; the lower border of the bronchus intermedius on the right.
LOWER ZONE	
8: Paraesophageal nodes (below carina)	Nodes lying adjacent to the wall of the esophagus and to the right or the left of the midline, excluding subcarinal nodes. Upper border: the upper border of the lower-lobe bronchus on the left; the lower border of the bronchus intermedius on the right. Lower border: the diaphragm.
9: Pulmonary ligament nodes	Nodes lying within the pulmonary ligament. Upper border: the inferior pulmonary vein. Lower border: the diaphragm.
HILAR/INTERLOBAR ZONE	
10: Hilar nodes	Includes nodes immediately adjacent to the mainstem bronchus and hilar vessels including the proximal portions of the pulmonary veins and the main pulmonary artery. Upper border: the lower rim of the azygos vein in the right; upper rim of the pulmonary artery on the left. Lower border: interlobar region bilaterally.
11: Interlobar nodes	Between the origin of the lobar bronchi. 11s: between the upper-lobe bronchus and bronchus intermedius on the right.[a] 11i: between the middle and lower bronchi on the right.[a]
PERIPHERAL ZONE	
12: Lobar nodes	Adjacent to the lobar bronchi.
13: Segmental nodes	Adjacent to the segmental bronchi.
14: Subsegmental nodes	Adjacent to the subsegmental bronchi.

[a]Nodal station number.

Reprinted with permission from Rusch VW, Asamura H, Watanabe H, et al. The IASLC Lung Cancer Staging Project. A proposal for a new international lymph node map in the forthcoming seventh edition of the TNM classification for lung cancer. J Thorac Oncol. 2009;4:568–577.

CCO guidelines on preoperative mediastinal lymph node staging recommend that invasive mediastinal staging is not required for peripheral stage IA tumors with no suspicion of mediastinal lymph node involvement on CT and PET scans (Fig. 24.2).[3–5]

DEFINITIONS OF MEDIASTINAL LYMPH NODE STAGING

Variation in the extent of mediastinal lymph node staging has been a source of confusion in the literature. The standard

TABLE 24.2 Indications for Invasive Mediastinal Staging

American College of Chest Physician Guidelines[2]
Absence of metastatic disease and one of the following:
   discrete mediastinal node enlargement with or without PET uptake
   PET-positive mediastinal nodes and abnormal nodes on CT
   high suspicion of N2 or N3 based on enlarged nodes on CT or PET uptake
   intermediate suspicion of N2 or N3 with a central tumor or N1 disease
European Society of Thoracic Surgeons Guidelines[3]
Any of the following:
   abnormal lymph nodes on CT
   uptake on PET scan
   central tumors
   suspected N1 disease
   low PET uptake by primary tumor
Cancer Care Ontario[4]
Any of the following:
   enlarged mediastinal nodes on CT
   uptake in mediastinal nodes on PET
   central tumors T2–T4
   suspected N1 disease

CT, Computed tomography; *PET*, positron emission tomography.

descriptions listed in Table 24.3 should be used when describing the extent of mediastinal lymph node assessment: sampling or random sampling, systematic sampling (SS), complete MLND, extended MLND, and lobe-specific systematic lymph node dissection (see Table 24.3).[6] The term systematic nodal dissection refers to a combination of mediastinal as well as hilar and intrapulmonary node dissection.[7]

Random sampling is not considered adequate for staging purposes. Certainly any suspicious or enlarged nodes should be removed as part of a lung cancer operation or when performing a staging procedure, but removal of only an enlarged or suspicious node is not sufficient. SS is the minimum assessment considered acceptable and is defined as the removal or biopsy of lymph nodes from predetermined lymph node stations based on the location of the tumor and known lymphatic drainage patterns. The specified stations represent the minimum number of stations to be assessed. MLND is a formal dissection of the lymph node bearing areas of the mediastinum including the paratracheal zone, the subcarinal space, the inferior mediastinum, and, on the left, the subaortic space and the para-aortic space. It is not simply the removal of individual lymph nodes from those regions but rather removal of all the lymph node bearing tissue within predetermined anatomic boundaries.

Extended mediastinal dissection is the formal removal of bilateral mediastinal and cervical lymph nodes. It is usually performed by VAMLA or TEMLA or by open techniques. This may be used for staging, but is more often a therapeutic technique.

Lobe-specific systematic lymph node dissection refers to the formal dissection of lymph node bearing tissues based on the anatomic location of the cancer. For example, for a left lower lobe tumor, the lymph node dissection would include the subcarinal and inferior mediastinal node dissection. Systematic node dissection refers to the combination of systematic mediastinal lymph node sampling (SS) and systematic hilar and intrapulmonary lymph node dissection.

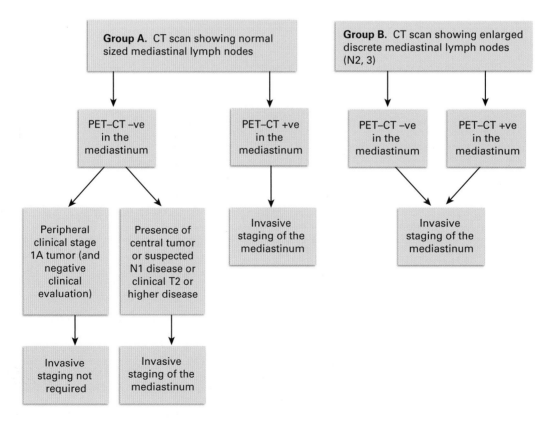

Fig. 24.2. Cancer Care Ontario (CCO) invasive mediastinal staging recommendations. *CT,* Computed tomography; *PET,* positron emission tomography

REQUIRED LYMPH NODE STATIONS FOR INVASIVE STAGING

Recommended sampling includes stations 2R/L, 4R/L, and station 7. Any nodes that are enlarged, show increased uptake on PET–CT, or are suspicious in any way should also be sampled. Guidelines from ESTS, National Institute for Health and Care Excellence (NICE), Scottish Intercollegiate Guidelines Network (SIGN), and CCO recommend that appropriate lymph node assessment include SS of at least three mediastinal lymph node stations (preferably 5), one of which should be station 7.[4,5,9]

CHOICE OF STAGING TECHNIQUE

SS may be performed by EBUS–TBNA or EUS or mediastinoscopy prior to a planned resection or at the time of the planned resection. If mediastinal nodes are suspicious for metastases, it is preferable to schedule the staging procedure in advance of the planned resection. If performed at the time of planned resection,

TABLE 24.3 Definitions of Mediastinal Lymph Node Assessment

Sampling or random sampling: sampling of lymph nodes guided by preoperative or intraoperative findings; for example, sampling of single enlarged lymph node.

Systematic sampling: sampling of predetermined lymph nodes and lymph node stations; for example, sampling of stations 2R, 4R, 7, and 10R for right-sided tumors.

Mediastinal lymph node dissection: complete removal of all mediastinal lymph node bearing tissue based on anatomic landmarks.

Extended lymph node dissection: removal of bilateral paratracheal and cervical lymph nodes by formal dissection.

Lobe-specific systematic node dissection: removal of mediastinal lymph node bearing tissue based on the location of the tumor.

Source: Lardinois D, De Leyn P, Van Schil P, et al. ESTS guidelines for intraoperative lymph node staging in non-small cell lung cancer. Eur J Cardiothorac Surg. 2006;30:787–792.

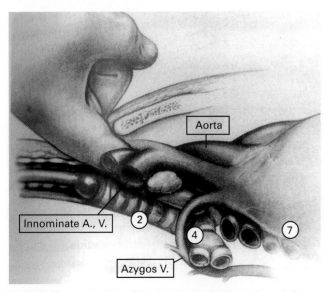

Fig. 24.3. Finger palpation of the superior mediastinum through the collar incision for mediastinoscopy. The innominate artery is palpated anteriorly. *A*, artery; *V*, vein; *2, 4, 7,* lymph node stations. *(Reprinted with permission from Pass HI, Carbone DP, Johnson DH, Minna JD, Scagliotti GV, Turrisi AT, eds.* Principles & Practice of Lung Cancer. The Official Reference Text of the IASLC. *3rd ed. Philadelphia, PA: Wolters Kluwer/Lippincott Williams and Wilkins; 2009.)*

on-site cytopathology or frozen section analysis is required as the finding of metastases in mediastinal lymph nodes is considered an indication for either nonoperative therapy or perhaps neoadjuvant therapy in selected cases. MLND is usually performed at the time of planned resection and may be performed by open thoracotomy or VATS. MLND may be performed as an alternative to SS based on surgeon preference. If no preresection invasive mediastinal staging has been done, MLND should be performed. MLND also should be performed if any N1 nodes are found to contain metastases or if at the time of resection, SS has identified N2 disease.

There has been considerable controversy over the role of SS compared with MLND. As a staging procedure, SS is adequate in patients with early stage only (clinical T1 or T2, N0 or nonhilar N1 nonsmall cell lung cancer [NSCLC] based on the ACOSOG Z0030 trial). If SS is negative for metastases in such patients, SS is adequate and further dissection by MLND does not confer a survival advantage even though 3.8% of patients in the ACOSOG Z0030 trial were identified by MLND as having occult N2 disease. However, the ACOSOG Z0030 results do not apply to patients with larger tumors (T3/T4) or hilar nodal disease. In such patients, MLND is still recommended.[10]

The importance of lymph node assessment in the staging of NSCLC is well recognized, but despite this, inadequate lymph node assessment is too common.[11,12] The consequence of inadequate staging will be reduced lung cancer survival if nodal disease goes undetected and untreated.

INVASIVE/SURGICAL STAGING TECHNIQUES

Mediastinoscopy

Definition

Mediastinoscopy is a surgical endoscopic technique that allows the exploration of the superior mediastinum along the tracheobronchial axis, from the sternal notch to the subcarinal space and along both main bronchi.[13]

Technique

Under general anesthesia and orotracheal intubation, with the patient in the supine position and the neck slightly extended, a 3-cm to 5-cm collar incision over the sternal notch is performed and carried through the subcutaneous tissue and platysma. The pretracheal muscles are separated laterally to expose the trachea. The pretracheal fascia is incised with scissors and the pretracheal plane is developed. The mediastinum is explored by finger dissection as far caudally as possible (Fig. 24.3). Finger palpation of the superior mediastinum allows the surgeon to identify anatomic landmarks, such as the innominate artery and the aortic arch, and to assess the texture of the mediastinal tissues, the consistency of the paratracheal lymph nodes, and the relation of central tumors to the mediastinal structures.

Finger palpation creates a mediastinal space into which the mediastinoscope is inserted. With the mediastinoscope in place, peritracheal dissection is completed by gently sweeping the adjacent tissues away from the airway with the dissection–suction–coagulation device (Fig. 24.4). Before taking any biopsies, the following structures should be identified: the innominate artery lying anterior to the trachea, the aortic arch lying over the trachea on the left, the azygos vein at the right tracheobronchial angle, and the pulmonary artery anterior to the carina (Fig. 24.5).

Mediastinoscopy allows biopsies of the pretracheal nodes (station 1), the right and left, superior and inferior, paratracheal nodes (stations 2R/2L and 4R/4L, respectively), the subcarinal nodes

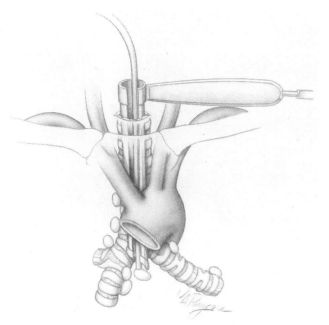

Fig. 24.4. The mediastinoscope is inserted into the superior mediastinum. *(Reprinted with permission from Shields TW, Locicero III J, Reed CE, Feins RH, eds. General Thoracic Surgery. 7th ed. Vol. 1. Philadelphia, PA: Wolters Kluwer/Lippincott Williams and Wilkins; 2009.)*

(station 7), and the right and left hilar nodes (stations 10R/10L; see Fig. 24.1, Table 24.1). For a clinically acceptable mediastinoscopy in standard clinical practice, the upper and lower paratracheal spaces and the subcarinal space should be explored and any lymph nodes identified should be subjected to biopsy. Any nodes that are enlarged on CT or show metabolic activity on PET scan should be explored and subjected to biopsy.

Nodal exploration should start on the contralateral side of the tumor to rule out N3 disease and then proceed in a systematic way to explore and perform biopsy on all accessible nodal stations. Mediastinoscopy also allows assessment of mediastinal invasion by either the primary tumor (T4) or by mediastinal nodes, which would preclude surgical resection. All biopsy sites should be controlled for bleeding before the incision is closed in two layers.[14]

Results

A review of 26 reports published between 1983 and 2011, including 9267 patients who had undergone conventional mediastinoscopy, reported a median sensitivity of 0.78 and a median negative predictive value of 0.91. An additional series of 995 patients who had undergone video-assisted mediastinoscopy and were reported in seven papers published from 2003 to 2011 showed a median sensitivity of 0.89 and a median negative predictive value of 0.92. By convention, specificity and positive predictive value of mediastinoscopy is 1, although positive results are not confirmed by other tests.[3] Videomediastinoscopy is reported to be more thorough in terms of number of nodes and nodal stations explored but there is no clear evidence of greater safety or improved staging although it has educational advantages.[15]

Complications

Reported complications include pneumothorax, wound infection, mediastinitis, esophageal perforation, tracheobronchial injury, left recurrent laryngeal nerve palsy, chyle leak, hemothorax, and bleeding from any of the vessels of the superior mediastinum,

but complications are rare and occur in about 3% of cases.[16,17] Serious bleeding complications occur in about 0.4% of cases and may be managed by packing, but may require median sternotomy.[18] Mortality related to mediastinoscopy usually is below 0.5%.[19,20]

Limitations

Mediastinoscopy does not reach the subaortic, para-aortic, prevascular, retrotracheal, and inferior mediastinal lymph nodes.

Technical Variants for Mediastinoscopic Lymphadenectomy

VAMLA and TEMLA are procedures performed from the collar incision used for mediastinoscopy;[21–23] their objective is not the taking of biopsies of the mediastinal nodes, but their systematic removal. Experience with these techniques is limited to a few centers.

VAMLA is performed with a two-blade spreadable mediastinoscope and has the objective to remove en bloc the subcarinal and the right inferior paratracheal lymph nodes, and to remove individually the left inferior paratracheal lymph nodes. The initial results from the two groups that developed VAMLA were very good, with sensitivity and negative predictive value of 1.[21,22]

TEMLA is also performed from the cervical incision, but the sternum is elevated with a sternal retractor fixed to a metal frame. The objective of TEMLA is to perform a complete mediastinal lymphadenectomy from the supraclavicular lymph nodes in the midline to the paraesophageal nodes. Most of the operation is performed in the open fashion; the mediastinoscope is used to complete the subcarinal and paraesophageal nodal dissection, and the thoracoscope to facilitate the removal of subaortic and para-aortic lymph nodes.[23] Staging results of TEMLA based on 256 patients are as follows: sensitivity, 0.94; negative predictive value, 0.97; and diagnostic accuracy, 0.98.[24] TEMLA is reported to be superior to mediastinoscopy[25] and to EBUS, EUS, or their combination both for staging and restaging lung cancer after induction therapy.[26]

Parasternal Mediastinotomy

Definition

Parasternal mediastinotomy is a procedure that allows the exploration of the anterior mediastinum through a right or left parasternal incision.[27,28]

Indicatio\ns

The ACCP and the ESTS guidelines on mediastinal staging recommend the exploration of the subaortic (station 5) and para-aortic (station 6) lymph nodes in patients with cancer of the left upper lobe when all other explored lymph nodes are negative. The natural lymphatic dissemination of left upper lobe tumors is to these two nodal stations, which cannot be reached with mediastinoscopy.[3,4] Prevascular lymph nodes (station 3a) if abnormal on CT or PET scan can be accessed by right or left parasternal mediastinotomy. Left parasternal mediastinotomy is especially valuable to explore tumors of the aortopulmonary window and to assess whether there is contact or tumor infiltration of the aortic arch.

Technique

A 4-cm to 7-cm transverse incision is performed over the second costal cartilage on the right or on the left down to the pectoralis muscle. The fibers of the pectoralis major muscle are separated in a craniocaudal fashion exposing the costal

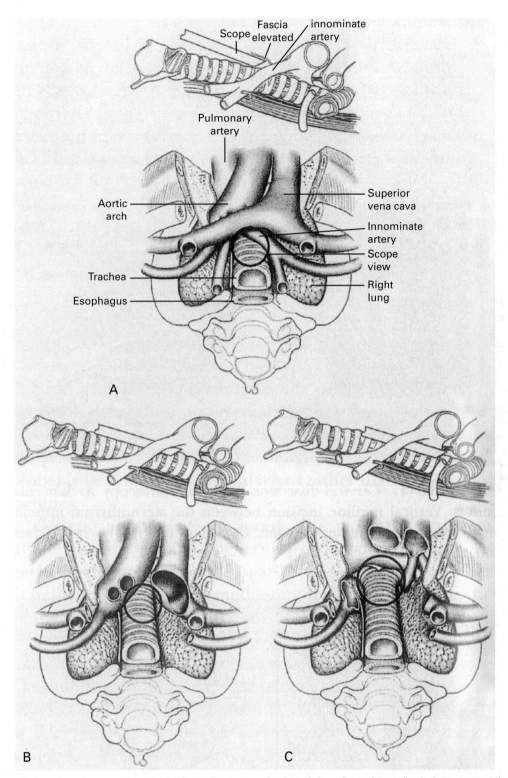

Fig. 24.5. Craniocaudal view from the surgeon's perspective and corresponding lateral view of superior mediastinal structures at three levels: (A) upper trachea, (B) mid trachea, and (C) carina. *(Reprinted with permission from Shields TW, Locicero III J, Reed CE, Feins RH, eds. General Thoracic Surgery. 7th ed. Vol. 1. Philadelphia, PA: Wolters Kluwer/Lippincott Williams and Wilkins; 2009.)*

cartilage. The cartilage is usually excised subperichondrially or, alternatively, the exploration may be carried out through the intercostal space without cartilage resection. The internal mammary vessels may be ligated or retracted. After this, the mediastinal pleura is separated laterally with finger dissection to expose the anterior mediastinum. On the left, the subaortic space and the ascending aorta can be explored, either directly or with the assistance of a mediastinoscope (anterior mediastinoscopy; Fig. 24.6). On the right, the prevascular nodes can be reached. Parasternal mediastinotomy is a versatile procedure. Besides the exploration of the anterior mediastinum, it also allows the opening of the mediastinal pleura and the

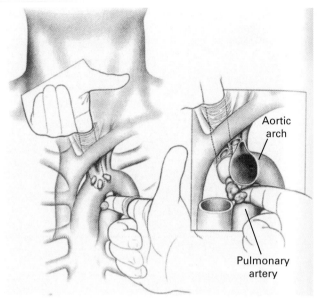

Fig. 24.6. Digital exploration of subaortic space during combined cervical and anterior mediastinotomy. *(Reprinted with permission from Shields TW, Locicero III J, Reed CE, Feins RH, eds. General Thoracic Surgery. 7th ed. Vol. 1. Philadelphia, PA: Wolters Kluwer/Lippincott Williams and Wilkins; 2009.)*

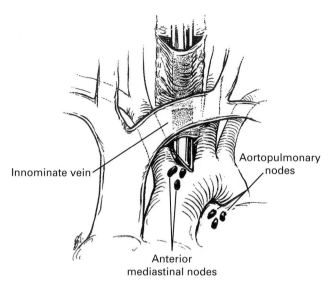

Fig. 24.7. Extended cervical mediastinoscopy. From the cervical incision used for mediastinoscopy, the mediastinoscope is advanced obliquely over the aortic arch. *(Reprinted with permission from Pearson FG, Cooper JD, Deslauriers J, et al., eds. Thoracic Surgery. Oxford, UK: Churchill Livingstone; 1995.)*

exploration of the hilum and pleural space. The pericardium can also be opened and explored to rule out direct tumor invasion or metastatic dissemination. Lung biopsies can also be performed from this incision. These additional procedures are best performed with unilateral ventilation.

For closure, the perichondrium and the muscular fibers are approximated in two layers. The subcutaneous tissue and the skin are also sutured in two layers. No pleural drainage is necessary unless the mediastinal pleura is opened during the procedure. A chest tube can be left in place till the last skin suture and then removed after the lung is kept insufflated for a few seconds to allow removal of any intrapleural air.

Results

A combined analysis of four series including a total of 238 patients, published from 1983 to 2006, showed a median sensitivity of 0.71 and a median negative predictive value of 0.91.[3] VATS is increasingly replacing these techniques for staging purposes.

Complications

Complications of parasternal mediastinotomy are rare and include injury to the phrenic nerve and to the left laryngeal recurrent nerve, mediastinitis, and pneumothorax.

Extended Cervical Mediastinoscopy

Definition

Extended cervical mediastinoscopy is an alternative technique to left parasternal mediastinotomy to explore the subaortic space from the cervical incision used for mediastinoscopy.[29]

Indications

For lung cancer staging, extended cervical mediastinoscopy has the same indications as left parasternal mediastinotomy.[3,4] In addition, it may be indicated to diagnose mediastinal tumors that are within its range of exploration.[30]

Technique

Once standard mediastinoscopy is completed and frozen section analyses reveal that there are no lymph node metastases in the superior mediastinum, a passage is created by finger dissection over the aortic arch, between the innominate artery and the left carotid artery. By finger dissection, the plane between the arteries is developed to facilitate the insertion of the mediastinoscope. The mediastinoscope is then introduced into the superior mediastinum and advanced obliquely from the cervical incision over the aortic arch, either anterior or posterior to the left innominate vein (Fig. 24.7). The pulsating aortic arch is clearly seen when the mediastinoscope is advanced. At this point the subaortic nodes are found. By rotating the tip of the scope medially, the para-aortic lymph nodes can be identified and subjected to biopsy. However, the rigid anterior chest wall limits the range of movement of the mediastinoscope in this area.[29,30] Palpation of the subaortic space is also limited from the cervical incision. If palpation is really needed to differentiate mere contact from tumor invasion, it is better to rely on parasternal mediastinotomy that allows not only direct inspection but also finger and instrumental palpation.

Results

Extended cervical mediastinoscopy is infrequently performed, but the few experiences that have been published show that the results are reproducible by different surgeons. VATS is increasingly used to assess the station 5/6 nodes. The combined analyses of 456 patients reported in five articles published between 1987 and 2012 reveal a median sensitivity of 0.71 and a median negative predictive value of 0.91.[3] An additional reported series of 82 patients with left lung carcinoma and suspected N2 disease on PET–CT or T3–T4 tumors underwent extended cervical mediastinoscopy after standard mediastinoscopy. Nodal involvement in subaortic or para-aortic lymph node stations was confirmed in 20 patients and T4 disease in 2, thereby changing the stage in 22 (27%) patients.[31]

Complications

In the largest series published to date, four (2.3%) complications occurred in 221 patients: mediastinitis, treated with antibiotics and drainage; ventricular fibrillation, treated with defibrillation;

superficial wound infection; and bleeding, treated with compression.[32] Other reported complications are pneumothorax and hoarseness, although these may happen in standard mediastinoscopy and are not specific to extended cervical mediastinoscopy.[33,34] One intraoperative death from aortic injury has been reported.[31]

Other Variants of Extended Mediastinoscopy

Retrosternal or Prevascular Mediastinoscopy. In this variant, the mediastinoscope is inserted behind the sternum, in front of the mediastinal vessels. It is rarely indicated for lung cancer staging, but is useful for the occasional patient who presents with lesions in the retrosternal region.

Mediastinoscopic Biopsy of the Scalene Lymph Nodes. From the cervical incision of mediastinoscopy, the mediastinoscope can be advanced behind the insertions of the sternocleidomastoid muscle to reach the scalene fat pad and nodes. Added to mediastinoscopy that has proved N2 disease, unsuspected N3 disease in scalene lymph nodes is found in 15% of patients, and in 68% of those with mediastinal N3 disease at mediastinoscopy.[35]

Mediastino-thoracoscopy: In cases of concomitant mediastinal and pleural lesions, the mediastinal pleura can be opened during mediastinoscopy to reach the pleural space. On the right this is best done between the trachea and the superior vena cava. On the left, the route over the aortic arch used for extended cervical mediastinoscopy can be used to reach and open the mediastinal pleura. Pleural effusion, pleural nodules, or peripheral lung nodules are the main indications of mediastino-thoracoscopy.[36–38]

Mediastinal Lymph Node Dissection

Definition

MLND is a formal dissection of all lymph node bearing tissues within anatomic boundaries and is usually performed at the time of planned resection and therefore only accesses the ipsilateral lymph nodes.

Indications

MLND is indicated when no invasive staging has been performed prior to resection. MLND is performed if at the time of resection SS identifies N1 or N2 disease, or after neoadjuvant therapy.

Technique

The right paratracheal dissection extends from the level of the right innominate artery to the right tracheobronchial angle, from the lateral border of the superior vena cava to the right anterolateral border of the trachea anterior to the right vagus nerve, to the ascending aorta. The mediastinal pleura overlying the superior vena cava posterior to the phrenic nerve is opened and the fatty tissue is dissected off the posterolateral aspect of the superior vena cava. The dissection is performed over the anterior aspect of the trachea to the ascending aorta and then posterolaterally to the vagus nerve. At the lower extent the right tracheobronchial angle and azygos vein are skeletonized. For the subcarinal dissection the mediastinal pleura is opened just at the lower edge of the right main bronchus; then the lymph node bearing tissue is dissected off the carina, the pericardium, and the left main bronchus. The inferior mediastinal dissection extends from the subcarinal space down to the diaphragm, exposing the esophagus and pericardium and taking the inferior pulmonary ligament tissues. On the left the para-aortic dissection removes all the lymph node bearing tissue between the phrenic and vagus nerves baring the aortic arch. The subaortic dissection removes

all the lymph node bearing tissue from the ligamentum arteriosum to the left upper lobe pulmonary artery, from the inferior aspect of the aortic arch to the superior aspect of the left main pulmonary artery. The left recurrent nerve is carefully dissected and preserved.

Complications

Complications of MLND based on the ACOSOG Z0030 trial include recurrent laryngeal nerve injury (0.9%), chylothorax (1.7%), and bleeding (1.1%). In the ACOSOG Z0030 trial, there were no significant differences in complication rates between MLND and SS.[39]

Thoracoscopy and VATS

Definition

Thoracoscopy is the inspection of the chest cavity for diagnostic, staging, or therapeutic purposes.

Indications

Classic thoracoscopy was limited to the assessment of lung cancer with an accompanying pleural effusion and to the taking of small biopsies; however, video thoracoscopy and VATS, performed with the assistance of several ports, allow the surgeon to perform resections of ipsilateral and contralateral additional peripheral nodules to confirm or rule out T3, T4, or M1a disease; to explore the ipsilateral mediastinum from the apex of the pleural cavity to the diaphragmatic dome; to assess the hilar and interlobar lymph nodes; to explore the inferior mediastinal nodes (station 8, paraesophageal nodes, and station 9, pulmonary ligament nodes); and even to open and assess the pericardial cavity to confirm T3, T4, or M1a disease. Thoracoscopy can replace left parasternal mediastinotomy and extended cervical mediastinoscopy to explore the subaortic and para-aortic lymph nodes. Performed immediately before lung resection, thoracoscopy or VATS may help assess tumor extent and disclose unsuspected involvement that may change the therapeutic strategy.[40,41]

Technique

Conventional thoracoscopy or video thoracoscopy for the assessment of pleural effusion or the taking of small pleural, lung, or mediastinal biopsies may be performed under local anesthesia and sedation. The operative thoracoscope has a working channel and, therefore, only one intercostal incision for the insertion of a single port is needed. Alternatively a 7mm semirigid pleuroscope with a 2.8 mm biopsy channel may be used through a 8 mm port. After drainage of the pleural fluid and taking of samples for cytopathologic examination, the parietal and the visceral pleurae are inspected for any abnormalities. Biopsies are taken from all abnormalities with a biopsy forceps. If frozen section examination reveals pleural dissemination, talc pleurodesis may be performed if the lung retains its capacity to reexpand. Lung and mediastinal biopsies can also be taken.

VATS is performed under general anesthesia with lung isolation. Multiple ports are usually required: one for the video thoracoscope and one or more for instruments. VATS offers flexibility for more advanced procedures such as the resection of additional pulmonary nodules, the assessment of hilar or intrapulmonary nodes, the extensive sampling of mediastinal nodes or MLND, and pericardioscopy. The mediastinal pleura may be opened to access paratracheal, hilar, subcarinal, and paraesophageal lymph nodes or even perform MLND. The interlobar nodes may be evaluated by opening the fissure. It is easy to perform a biopsy on pulmonary ligament lymph nodes, or they can be removed by opening the pulmonary ligament from the diaphragm to the inferior pulmonary vein.

Results

For mediastinal nodal staging, the median sensitivity and negative predictive value in 246 patients from four series published between 2002 and 2007 were 0.95 and 0.96, respectively.[3] In a series of 1306 patients with resectable tumors by standard clinical staging, video thoracoscopy, performed immediately before resection, revealed that 4.4% had unresectable tumors.[42] The most common cause of unresectability was pleural dissemination (2.5%) followed by mediastinal infiltration (1.7%). Global tumor staging was significantly better for video thoracoscopy (73.3%) than for CT (48.7%). Video thoracoscopy correctly matched the T stage with the final pathology report in 96.2% of cases. It also reduced the exploratory thoracotomy rate from 11.6%, before the introduction of routine exploratory video thoracoscopy, to 2.5%, after the implementation of its routine use.[40] In another series of 1381 patients with resectable tumors by standard staging, exploratory video thoracoscopy was possible in 1277, and in 141 cases (10.2%), tumors were considered unresectable by video thoracoscopy because of mediastinal invasion in 81 patients, pleural dissemination in 38, both in 6, and infiltration of the adjacent fissure in patients who could not tolerate pneumonectomy in 16. Exploratory thoracotomy was performed in 43 (3.1%) patients.[41] The same group performed transpleural video pericardioscopy in 91 patients with suspicion of pericardial involvement. Video pericardioscopic findings revealed that 61 patients had resectable tumors, whereas 30 had different degrees of invasion that precluded complete resection: pulmonary artery in 17, pulmonary artery and superior pulmonary vein in 6, pulmonary artery and superior vena cava in 2, and left atrium and pulmonary veins in 5.[41]

Complications

Complications are rare, occurring in about 5% of cases, and include air leak, subcutaneous emphysema, chest pain, bleeding, wound infection, and empyema.

Inferior Mediastinoscopy and Subxiphoid Pericardioscopy

Definition

Inferior mediastinoscopy refers to the inspection of the inferior mediastinum through a subxiphoid approach, whereas subxiphoid pericardioscopy is used to inspect the pericardial cavity. These are uncommon procedures.

Indications

Inferior mediastinoscopy is indicated to diagnose mediastinal lesions located between the anterior pericardium and the sternum or at the cardiophrenic angles that fall out of reach of cervical mediastinoscopy.[43,44] Subxiphoid pericardioscopy is especially indicated in patients with lung cancer and pericardial effusion that has not been diagnosed by pericardiocentesis and cytopathologic examination of the pericardial fluid.[45,46]

Technique

Both operations are performed under general anesthesia and orotracheal intubation. With the patient in the supine decubitus position, a 5-cm vertical incision is made over the xiphoid. The xiphoid is generally excised. For inferior mediastinoscopy, the mediastinoscope is inserted between the anterior pericardium and the sternum. The anterior surface of the pericardium can be explored and the

exploration can be continued to both cardiophrenic angles. Biopsy of lymph nodes or masses is performed with biopsy forceps as for cervical mediastinoscopy. If the mediastinal pleura is not opened, drainage is not necessary. The incision is closed in three layers: midline of the rectus abdominis muscles, subcutaneous tissue, and skin.

The same approach is used for subxiphoid pericardioscopy. Once the xiphoid is excised, the pericardium is grasped and incised. A sample of fluid is taken for cytopathologic examination. After drainage of the pericardial fluid, the mediastinoscope is inserted into the pericardial cavity and the internal surface of the parietal pericardium, the surface of the heart, and the intrapericardial segments of the great vessels are explored. In case of malignancy, pericardiodesis can be performed. A portion of the pericardium also can be excised to create a pericardial window that will drain the pericardial fluid into the subcutaneous tissue. A soft drain is inserted into the pericardium and the incision is closed in three layers as for inferior mediastinoscopy.

Results

Both techniques provide cytohistologic proof of tumor extent, thus increasing the certainty of the staging process. Although they are rarely indicated, they should be kept in mind when the target lesions are beyond the reach of more standard techniques.

Complications

Complications are rare and include wound infection, bleeding, and intraoperative arrhythmias, especially in pericardioscopy.

Endobronchial Ultrasound and Endoscopic Ultrasound

Definitions

EBUS-guided TBNA (EBUS–TBNA) and EUS-guided fine-needle aspiration (EUS–FNA) are minimally invasive endoscopic techniques, which are alternatives to mediastinoscopy and may replace the routine use of mediastinoscopy for invasive staging of NSCLC.

Mediastinal lymph nodes are subjected to biopsy by needle puncture under real-time ultrasound guidance under local or general anesthesia.[47,48]

EUS allows ultrasonographic imaging of structures adjacent to the gastrointestinal tract, which is useful for lymph nodes in the posterior mediastinum and upper retroperitoneum. However, the reach of EUS–FNA does not correspond completely to the reach of mediastinoscopy. EBUS–TBNA can access the same nodes as mediastinoscopy, but also extends to the hilar and interlobar lymph nodes (N1 nodes).[49] The combination of EBUS and EUS allows sampling of most mediastinal lymph nodes as well as N1 nodes (Fig. 24.8). Sonographic features of lymph nodes considered suspicious for malignancy include lymph nodes larger than 1 cm in short axis, round shape, distinct margins, heterogeneous echogenicity, evidence of necrosis, and loss of central hilar structures.[50] Lymph node assessment should be performed in a systematic manner beginning with the N3 nodes followed by N2 and then N1 nodes to avoid contamination and upstaging. Nodes are described and numbered according to the IASLC map.

Technique

Anesthesia. EBUS–TBNA and EUS–FNA can be performed on an outpatient basis using topical anesthesia and conscious sedation. For EBUS–TBNA, the bronchoscope is usually

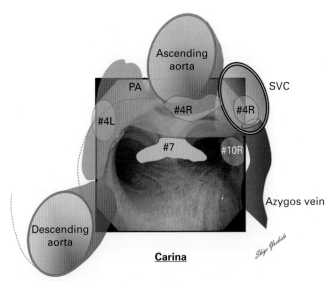

Fig. 24.8. Relevant anatomy for endobronchial ultrasound. *PA,* pulmonary artery; *SVC,* superior vena cava. *(Image courtesy Shige Yoshida.)*

inserted orally, because the size of the ultrasound probe on the tip limits nasal insertion. General anesthesia may be used instead and minimizes the cough reflex for EBUS. An endotracheal tube (size 8 or larger) may be used but causes the bronchoscope to lie in the central position within the airway, thus creating difficulty in bringing the ultrasound probe in contact with the wall of the airway. A laryngeal mask airway is a good alternative.

EBUS–TBNA. A standard flexible bronchoscopy is first performed, then the Convex Probe-EBUS (CP-EBUS) scope is passed through the vocal cords by visualizing the anterior angle of the glottis and advanced into the airway until the desired lymph node station is reached. The balloon is inflated with normal saline to achieve a maximum contact with the airway wall, then the tip of the CP-EBUS is flexed and gently pressed against the airway. Specific lymph node stations are identified using ultrasonically visible vascular landmarks (see Fig. 24.8). The Doppler mode is used to confirm and identify surrounding vessels as well as the blood flow within lymph nodes. The bronchoscopic image of the airway is simultaneously visualized to localize the insertion point of the needle. The TBNA needle is advanced through the working channel of the bronchoscope until the sheath can be visualized on the endoscopic image. The tip of the bronchoscope is then flexed up and the lymph node is visualized again on the ultrasonographic image. The needle is passed through the airway into the lymph node avoiding the cartilage. Once the needle is confirmed to be inside the lymph node, the internal stylet is used to clear out the internal lumen, which may become clogged with bronchial epithelium. The internal stylet is then removed and negative pressure is applied with a syringe. For hypervascular nodes, samples may be taken without suction to avoid bloody samples. The needle is moved back and forth inside the lymph node to obtain samples. The needle is then retracted inside the outer sheath and the entire needle is removed from the bronchoscope. The internal stylet is used to push out samples. If on-site cytopathology is available, the initial sample is placed on a slide glass, and smears are made for rapid on-site cytologic evaluation. The rest of the specimen is placed in a 50-mL conical tube filled with normal saline for cell-block preparation. Otherwise the sample is placed in standard cytology preservation solution.

The overall risk of EUS–FNA is approximately 0.5% and may include perforation of the esophagus or posterior pharynx, infection, and hemorrhage.

Complications related to EBUS–TBNA are similar to those of bronchoscopy and conventional TBNA and include pneumothorax, pneumomediastinum, hemomediastinum, mediastinitis, bacteremia, and pericarditis. To date, there are no major complications reported in the literature.

EUS–FNA. The radial EUS scope or radial miniprobe may be inserted first to identify lymph nodes of interest. Next the linear EUS scope is advanced into the stomach and then slowly withdrawn while making circular movements. Anatomic landmarks such as the inferior vena cava, right and left atrium, azygos vein, main pulmonary artery, and aorta are identified. Lymph nodes are described and numbered according to the IASLC map. Biopsy is then performed on lymph nodes using a 22-gauge needle under real-time ultrasound guidance with monitoring of the needle during insertion and aspiration. Similar to EBUS–TBNA, suction may be applied and multiple passes are made in the lymph node.

Results: EBUS–TBNA

Multiple studies have demonstrated high sensitivity, specificity, and diagnostic accuracy of EBUS–TBNA for mediastinal lymph node staging. Prospective studies of EBUS–TBNA for mediastinal staging report sensitivity of 0.94, specificity of 1, positive predictive value of 1, and diagnostic accuracy of 0.96 for mediastinal lymph node staging. The negative predictive value varies from 0.11 to 0.89 depending on the prevalence of malignancy.[51,52] Furthermore, multiple prospective series and meta-analyses have demonstrated the safety, efficacy, and high diagnostic yield of EBUS–TBNA.[53-55]

Comparison of EBUS–TBNA and mediastinoscopy in 153 potentially resectable patients with lung cancer demonstrated that in 91% of patients, there was excellent agreement between the two techniques regarding the staging of the mediastinum, and test characteristics were similar. The specificity and positive predictive value of both tests were 1. The sensitivity, negative predictive value, and diagnostic accuracy for mediastinal lymph node staging for EBUS–TBNA and mediastinoscopy were 0.81, 0.91, and 0.93, and 0.79, 0.90, and 0.93, respectively.[56]

Results: EUS–FNA

EUS–FNA offers a minimally invasive method of examining the posterior and inferior mediastinum in patients with lung cancer with a sensitivity of 0.74–0.92.[42,57-59] Unlike other invasive staging modalities such as EBUS–TBNA and mediastinoscopy, the sensitivity of EUS–FNA seems to be affected by variables such as size of the nodes, size of the tumor, and nodal station. EUS–FNA is reported to have a low negative predictive value of 0.73 and is not a very reliable test in ruling out lymph node spread. Most investigators agree that negative results of EUS–FNA should be verified by other invasive staging modalities, especially in the presence of suggestive imaging.

Comparing EUS–FNA with mediastinoscopy in a prospective study of 60 patients, the sensitivity of EUS–FNA for station 4R was 0.67, versus 0.33 for mediastinoscopy. At station 4L, EUS–FNA was also more sensitive than mediastinoscopy (0.80 vs. 0.33). The sensitivity of EUS–FNA at the subcarinal station (station 7) was 1, versus only 0.70 for mediastinoscopy. In this report the results of the yield for mediastinoscopy are much lower than previously reported; however, for lymph node stations out of the reach of mediastinoscopy, EUS–FNA is appropriate.[58]

Results: Combined EBUS and EUS

By combining EBUS–TBNA and EUS–FNA, the majority of the mediastinum as well as the hilar lymph nodes can be sampled. Using the combined approach for invasive staging, even using a single EBUS–TBNA scope for both procedures, sensitivity of 0.91 to 1 and negative predictive value of 0.91 to 0.95 have been reported.[60–62] To date, the combined EBUS–EUS approach has been shown to be more sensitive than using EBUS or EUS independently, with a significantly better negative predictive value.

A multicenter randomized controlled trial in 241 patients with resectable NSCLC compared surgical staging alone with a combined EBUS–EUS approach followed by surgical staging if no metastases were found by endosonography.[63] Of the 123 patients who started with endosonography,[64] patients underwent mediastinoscopy, with nodal metastases identified in only 4 patients. The sensitivity of the combined approach was 0.94 and negative predictive value was 0.93. In the mediastinoscopy-alone group, the sensitivity was 0.80 and the negative predictive value was 0.86, which was statistically no different from the combined approach. Despite the lack of difference in negative predictive value, the study demonstrated that the number of unnecessary thoracotomies was reduced by half in the combined-approach group. Based on this study, a new strategy for invasive staging was suggested, which begins with combined EBUS–EUS followed by mediastinoscopy if the lymph node metastasis is not demonstrated.

MEDIASTINAL RESTAGING

Stage IIIA NSCLC represents a heterogeneous group of patients with metastatic disease to N2 lymph nodes as well as T3N1 disease. The management of patients with N2 stage IIIa disease varies widely from resectable tumors with occult microscopic nodal metastases to unresectable bulky multistation nodal disease. The treatment for patients with N2 disease varies depending on the extent of N2 lymph node involvement. Neoadjuvant therapy (chemotherapy ± radiotherapy) followed by surgery for known stage IIIA (N2) disease as a routine therapeutic option is not generally recommended except as a part of a clinical trial.[65] Initial invasive mediastinal staging to confirm N2 disease is mandatory for patients treated with induction chemoradiotherapy as part of a clinical trial. The purpose of restaging is to evaluate whether there is residual involvement of the mediastinal lymph nodes after induction therapy, which would change subsequent treatment for these patients.

Restaging of the mediastinum after induction therapy has been reported by noninvasive imaging modalities (CT and PET scan). CT scan alone is a poor restaging test with false-negative (FN) and false-positive (FP) rates of approximately 40%.[66] PET scan appears to perform better than CT scan alone, although radiation therapy can cause ^{18}F-2-deoxy-D-glucose uptake due to inflammation after induction treatment. The FN and FP rates of PET scan for restaging are 25% and 33%, respectively, based on a systematic review.[66]

Invasive restaging can be performed by remediastinoscopy, VATS, and minimally invasive endoscopic NA modalities such as EBUS–TBNA and EUS–FNA, but there are a very limited number of studies looking at the role of invasive restaging. Remediastinoscopy can be performed safely in experienced hands, but only a few institutions actually perform the procedure because it can be extremely difficult due to fibrotic changes after the initial mediastinoscopy and induction therapy. Based on a systematic review, the results of remediastinoscopy are consistently worse than the initial mediastinoscopy with a pooled sensitivity of 63% and FN rate of 22%.[66] By contrast, EBUS and EUS can be performed with ease with slightly better results with a pooled sensitivity of 84% and FN rate of 14%.[64,67–69] Two studies looked at the role of first-time cervical mediastinoscopy after induction therapy for restaging after initial invasive staging with EBUS and/or EUS.[70,71] This strategy has results similar to initial staging with mediastinoscopy with an excellent sensitivity of 89% and FN rate of 9%.

Minimally invasive needle techniques including EBUS–TBNA and EUS–FNA are now considered the tests of first choice to confirm mediastinal disease in accessible lymph node stations. Thus an ideal algorithm for invasive staging of patients with N2 stage IIIa disease would be to perform initial invasive staging by ultrasound-guided needle-based techniques followed by restaging with needle-based techniques and reserve mediastinoscopy for EBUS/EUS negative cases.

CONCLUSION

Invasive staging of the mediastinum is an essential component of the evaluation of patients with NSCLC. Pathologic confirmation of imaging abnormalities is important because of the frequency of FP imaging tests. Patients at increased risk of mediastinal lymph node metastases such as those with central, larger, or higher T stage tumors or those with evidence of N1 disease should also have invasive mediastinal staging. Needle biopsy techniques offer less invasive options with equivalent results to open techniques for invasive staging. VATS provides access to the entire ipsilateral hemithorax, which increases its utility over some of the older techniques. Regardless of the technique used, it is important to perform a systematic approach by either SS or MLND.

KEY REFERENCES

3. Silvestri GA, Gonzalez AV, Jantz MA, et al. Methods for staging non-small cell lung cancer: diagnosis and management of lung cancer, ed 3, American College of Chest Physicians evidence-based clinical practice guidelines. *Chest.* 2013;143(Suppl 5):e211S–e250S.

5. Darling G, Dickie J, Malthaner R. Kennedy E, Tey R. *Invasive Mediastinal Staging of Non-Small Cell Lung Cancer.* http://www.cancer-care.on.ca/toolbox/qualityguidelines/clin-program/surgery-ebs/; 2013.

8. Scottish Intercollegiate Guidelines Network. *Management of Patients With Lung Cancer. A National Clinical Guideline.* Edinburgh: Scotland; 2005.

9. National Collaborating Centre for Acute Care. *The Diagnosis and Treatment of Lung Cancer.* London, UK: National Institute for Health and Clinical Excellence; 2005.

10. Darling GE, Allen MS, Decker PA, et al. Randomized trial of mediastinal lymph node sampling versus complete lymphadenectomy during pulmonary resection in the patient with N0 or N1 (less than hilar) non-small cell carcinoma: results of the ACOSOG Z0030 Trial. *J Thorac Cardiovasc Surg.* 2011;141:662–670.

39. Allen MS, Darling GE, Pechet TT, et al. Morbidity and mortality of major pulmonary resections in patients with early-stage lung cancer: initial results of the randomized, prospective ACOSOG Z0030 trial. *Ann Thorac Surg.* 2006;81:1013–1019.

42. Annema JT, Versteegh MI, Veselic M, et al. Endoscopic ultrasound-guided fine needle aspiration in the diagnosis and staging of lung cancer and its impact on surgical staging. *J Clin Oncol.* 2005;23:8357–8361.

50. Fujiwara T, Yasufuku K, Nakajima T, et al. The utility of sonographic features during endobronchial ultrasound-guided transbronchial needle aspiration for lymph node staging in patients with lung cancer: a standard endobronchial ultrasound image classification system. *Chest.* 2010;138:641–647.

51. Yasufuku K, Chiyo M, Koh E, et al. Endobronchial ultrasound guided transbronchial needle aspiration for staging of lung cancer. *Lung Cancer.* 2005;50:347–354.

56. Yasufuku K, Pierre A, Darling G, et al. A prospective controlled trial of endobronchial ultrasound-guided transbronchial needle aspiration compared with mediastinoscopy for mediastinal lymph node staging of lung cancer. *J Thorac Cardiovasc Surg.* 2011;142:1393–1400.

60. Wallace MB, Pascual JM, Raimnondo M, et al. Minimally invasive endoscopic staging of suspected lung cancer. *JAMA.* 2008;299:540–546.

63. Annema JT, Van Meerbeeck JP, Rintoul RC, et al. Mediastinoscopy vs endosonography for mediastinal nodal staging of lung cancer: a randomized trial. *JAMA.* 2010;304:2245–2252.

See Expertconsult.com for full list of references.

25 The Eighth Edition of the Tumor, Node, and Metastasis Classification of Lung Cancer

Ramón Rami-Porta, Peter Goldstraw, and Harvey I. Pass

SUMMARY OF KEY POINTS

- Size counts: From less than or equal to 1-cm to less than or equal to 5-cm tumor size, every centimeter has prognostic impact and separates into different T categories, and tumors greater than 5 cm but less than 7 cm are now T3; and those greater than 7 cm are now T4.
- Distance to carina does not count: Tumors with endobronchial location less than 2 cm from the carina have similar outcomes to those greater than 2 cm from the carina.
- N status remains largely the same.
- An oligometastasis is now classified as M1b.
- Descriptors for same lobe as well as other lobe intrapulmonary nodules as metastases or synchronous primary lesions are delineated.
- Part-solid adenocarcinoma size will be defined by the size of the solid component on computed tomography and of the invasive component on microscopic examination.

The tumor, node, and metastasis (TNM) classification of malignant tumors is promulgated by the Union for International Cancer Control and the American Joint Committee on Cancer.[1] The TNM classification undergoes periodical revisions based on the reports from the National TNM Committees and on the annual assessment of original articles.[2,3] For the latest two editions of the TNM classification of lung cancer (7th edition of 2009 and 8th edition of 2016), the revisions were based on two international databases collected by the International Association for the Study of Lung Cancer (IASLC).[4,5] These databases were stored, managed, and analyzed by Cancer Research And Biostatistics, a not-for-profit data center based in Seattle, WA, USA, in collaboration with the members of the IASLC Staging and Prognostic Factors Committee. This chapter presents the process of revision leading to the eighth edition of the TNM classification of lung cancer, the innovations introduced, and their clinical implications. The eighth edition of the TNM classification of malignant tumors will be enacted on January 1, 2017.

THE INTERNATIONAL ASSOCIATION FOR THE STUDY OF LUNG CANCER DATABASE FOR THE EIGHTH EDITION

For the second consecutive time, the IASLC registered data from around 100,000 patients with lung cancer. For this revision, the period of diagnosis was from 1999 to 2010. Data originated in 35 different databases in 16 countries of 5 continents. Their geographical origin and number of patients are as follows: Europe, 46,560; Asia, 41,705; North America, 4660; Australia, 1593; and South America, 190, for a total of 94,708 patients. After exclusions, 77,156 patients met the requirements

for analysis: 70,967 with nonsmall cell lung cancer (NSCLC) and 6189 with SCLC. Table 25.1 shows the type of databases contributing to the IASLC Staging Project and the nature of the data.[5] Most data were retrospective, that is, contributors around the world already were registering data on patients with lung cancer and submitted their databases to the IASLC. These databases contained the minimum information regarding TNM descriptors, but some of them lacked the necessary detail needed for deeper analyses. By contrast, data registered through the electronic data capture online system are smaller in numbers but richer in detail and were useful, for example, to analyze the descriptors of the M component because they contained the information on number and location of metastases. Table 25.2 shows the type of treatment undergone by the registered patients with SCLC and NSCLC.[5] The proportion of patients treated with tumor resection either alone or in combination with chemotherapy and/or radiotherapy is higher in this database than in the one used for the seventh edition. This is due to the fact that databases of clinical trials, usually collected for advanced disease, were not submitted. However, surgical registries have complete information on the descriptors of the anatomic extent of the disease and are readily available for analysis. Despite this lack of patients with advanced lung cancer, all findings potentially leading to recommendations for changes were validated in the populations of patients with clinically and pathologically staged tumors, except those of the M component that were exclusively based on clinically staged tumors.

INNOVATIONS IN THE T, N, AND M DESCRIPTORS

T Descriptors

The T component of the classification is complex to analyze because it has many descriptors: tumor size, endobronchial location, atelectasis/pneumonitis, and invasion of various anatomic structures surrounding the lung. For their analyses, the prognostic impact of each descriptor was analyzed individually in five different populations of patients: three with pathologically staged tumors (pT1–4 N0 M0 completely resected [R0]; pT1–4 any N M0 R0; and pT1–4 any N M0 any R, i.e., including resections with microscopic [R1] and macroscopic [R2] evidence of residual tumor) and two with clinically staged tumors (cT1–4 N0 M0 and cT1–4 any N M0). Additional univariate and multivariate analyses were performed after adjustment by histopathologic type, geographical region of origin, age, and sex. These analyses generated multiple survival curves that were closely analyzed to see if the different descriptors were properly assigned to their T category.[6] The results of these analyses can be summarized as follows:

- The 3-cm landmark still separates T1 from T2 tumors.
- Tumor size, analyzed at 1-cm intervals, has more prognostic impact than previously shown in past editions of the TNM classification. From less than or equal to 1-cm to less than or equal to 5-cm tumor size, every centimeter counts and separates different T categories.

- The prognosis of tumors greater than 5 cm to less than or equal to 7 cm was similar to that of T3 tumors.
- The prognosis of tumors greater than 7 cm was similar to that of T4 tumors.
- The prognosis of tumors with endobronchial location less than 2 cm from the carina (a T3 descriptor in the 7th edition) was found to be similar to that of their T2 counterparts (endobronchial location >2 cm from the carina).
- The prognosis of tumors with total atelectasis/pneumonitis (a T3 descriptor in the 7th edition) was found to have a T2 prognosis, similar to that of tumors with partial atelectasis/pneumonitis.

TABLE 25.1 Data Sources and Type of Data of the IASLC Database Used for the Eighth Edition of the TNM Classification of Lung Cancer[5]

Type of Database	Retrospective	Prospective (EDC)	Total
Consortium	41,548	2089	43,637
Registry	26,122		26,122
Surgical series	5373	592	5965
Institutional series		1185	1185
Institutional registries	208		208
Unknown		39	39
Total	73,251	3905	77,156

EDC, electronic data capture; *IASLC,* International Association for the Study of Lung Cancer; *TNM,* tumor, node, and metastasis.

TABLE 25.2 Treatment Modalities for Submitted Patients With Small and Nonsmall Cell Lung Cancer in the IASLC Database Used for the Eighth Edition of the TNM Classification of Lung Cancer[5]

Treatment Modality	%
Surgery alone	57.7
Chemotherapy and surgery	21.1
Radiotherapy and surgery	1.5
Trimodality	4.4
Chemotherapy alone	9.3
Chemotherapy and radiotherapy	4.7
Radiotherapy alone	1.5

IASLC, International Association for the Study of Lung Cancer; *TNM,* tumor, node, and metastasis.

- The prognosis of tumors with invasion of the diaphragm (a T3 descriptor in the 7th edition) was found to be similar to that of T4 tumors.
- The invasion of the mediastinal pleura was rarely used as a unique descriptor.

Based on the aforementioned findings, the recommendations for changes in the T categories are as follows:

- Subdivide T1 into three new subcategories: T1a (≤1 cm), T1b (>1 cm but ≤2 cm), and T1c (>2 cm but ≤3 cm).
- Subdivide T2 into two new subcategories: T2a (>3 cm but ≤4 cm) and T2b (>4 cm but ≤5 cm).
- Reclassify tumors greater than 5 cm but less than or equal to 7 cm as T3.
- Reclassify tumors greater than 7 cm as T4.
- Reclassify tumors with endobronchial location less than or equal to 2 cm from the carina, but without involvement of the carina, as T2.
- Reclassify tumors with total atelectasis/pneumonitis as T2.
- Reclassify tumors with invasion of the diaphragm as T4.
- Delete the invasion of the mediastinal pleura as a descriptor.

When survival is analyzed according to these new T descriptors, survival curves separate well and do not cross over. All survival differences are significant and there is a clear difference between T3 and T4 that was not seen in the seventh edition (Fig. 25.1).

Visceral pleural invasion, defined as the invasion of its elastic layer, is well assigned to the T2 category (Fig. 25.2).[7] There are survival differences between PL1 and PL2, but these are only identifiable at pathologic staging, so they cannot be used to modify the present T2 descriptor based on the extent of visceral pleural invasion. However, they are useful to refine postoperative prognosis in those patients with resected tumors in which visceral pleural invasion is identified. Because visceral pleura involvement impacts prognosis, the use of elastic stains is emphasized again in the eighth edition of the TNM classification of lung cancer, if it is not evident on hematoxylin and eosin stains.

N Descriptors

The N descriptors were analyzed in the population of patients with clinically and pathologically staged tumors. In both

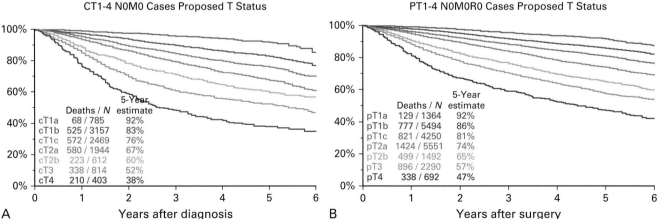

Fig. 25.1. Survival according to the clinical (A) and pathologic (B) T descriptors of the eighth edition of the tumor, node, and metastasis (TNM) classification of lung cancer. *(Reprinted with permission from Rami-Porta R, Bolejack V, Crowley J, et al. The IASLC Lung Cancer Staging Project: proposals for the revisions of the T descriptors in the forthcoming 8th edition of the TNM classification for lung cancer. J Thorac Oncol. 2015;10:990–1003.)*

populations, the present N descriptors (N0, N1, N2, and N3) separate tumors with statistically significant prognosis (Fig. 25.3). Therefore, there is no need to suggest any modification in the N component.[8]

Exploratory analyses on the quantification of nodal disease also were performed. Survival was analyzed according to the number of nodal stations involved in the population of patients with pathologically staged tumors and adequate information on the nodal stations explored. There are five groups of tumors according to the number of nodal stations involved:

- N1a: single-station N1
- N1b: multiple-station N1
- N2a1: single-station N2 without N1 disease (skip metastasis)
- N2a2: single-station N2 with N1 disease
- N2b: multiple-station N2.

Fig. 25.4 shows the survival of patients with pathologically staged tumors and nodal disease classified according to the number of nodal stations involved. All survival differences are statistically significant except those between N1b (multiple-station N1) and N2a1 (single-station N2 without N1). When these analyses are performed in the clinical staging setting, these differences cannot be replicated. This is the reason why this suggested subclassification cannot be used to modify the N descriptors, because, in principle, clinical and pathologic descriptors must be identical. However, this subclassification is clinically relevant as it may be used to refine postoperative prognosis for those patients with resected lung cancers harboring nodal disease.[8]

The IASLC regional lymph node map proposed in 2009 was the result of a multidisciplinary and international consensus (Fig. 25.5). No map or anatomic scheme is perfect, and this map is not perfect either. One advantage of this map over the others previously proposed is that this one has clear definitions for each nodal station that can be recognized by radiologists, endoscopists, and thoracic surgeons performing mediastinoscopy and systematic nodal dissection at the time of lung resection (Table 25.3). The IASLC Staging and Prognostic Factors Committee recommends the use of this map for nodal labeling and the prospective collection of data to examine its potential limitations and suggest modifications in the future.[9]

M Descriptors

The electronically captured data, that is, data registered prospectively online, were used for the revision of the M descriptors because they had adequate detail for the planned analyses. Patients with resected metastases were excluded from these analyses. Regarding the M1a descriptors, those defined in the seventh edition (metastasis within the pleural space: contralateral separate

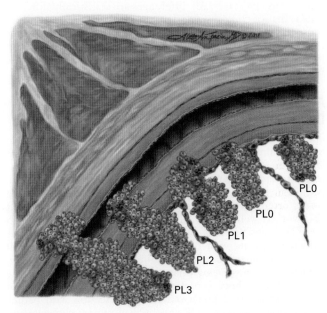

Fig. 25.2. Visceral pleura invasion. *PL0*, tumor within the subpleural lung parenchyma or invading superficially into the pleural connective tissue; *PL1,* tumor invades beyond the elastic layer; *PL2,* tumor invades the pleural surface; *PL3,* tumor invades any component of the parietal pleura. *(Copyright 2008 Aletta Ann Frazier, MD.) (Reprinted with permission from Travis WD, Brambilla E, Rami-Porta R, et al. Visceral pleural invasion: pathologic criteria and use of elastic stains. Proposal for the 7th edition of the TNM classification for lung cancer. J Thorac Oncol. 2008;3:1384–1390.)*

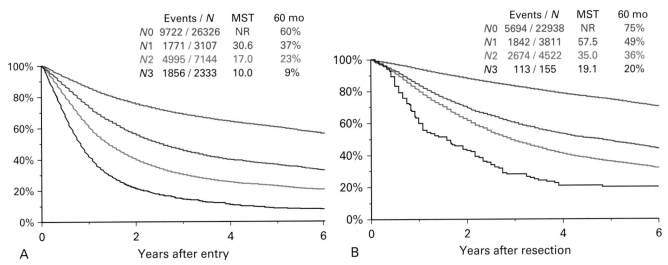

	Events / N	MST	60 mo
N0	9722 / 26326	NR	60%
N1	1771 / 3107	30.6	37%
N2	4995 / 7144	17.0	23%
N3	1856 / 2333	10.0	9%

	Events / N	MST	60 mo
N0	5694 / 22938	NR	75%
N1	1842 / 3811	57.5	49%
N2	2674 / 4522	35.0	36%
N3	113 / 155	19.1	20%

A — Years after entry

B — Years after resection

Fig. 25.3. Survival according to clinical (A) and pathologic (B) N categories. *(Reprinted with permission from Asamura H, Chansky K, Crowley J, et al. The IASLC Lung Cancer Staging Project: proposals for the revisions of the N descriptors in the forthcoming 8th edition of the TNM classification for lung cancer. J Thorac Oncol. 2015;10:1675–1684.)*

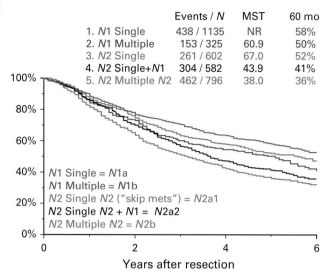

Location and Number of POS Stations N1-N2 any R

	Events / N	MST	60 mo
1. N1 Single	438 / 1135	NR	58%
2. N1 Multiple	153 / 325	60.9	50%
3. N2 Single	261 / 602	67.0	52%
4. N2 Single+N1	304 / 582	43.9	41%
5. N2 Multiple N2	462 / 796	38.0	36%

N1 Single = N1a
N1 Multiple = N1b
N2 Single N2 ("skip mets") = N2a1
N2 Single N2 + N1 = N2a2
N2 Multiple N2 = N2b

Fig. 25.4. Survival according to nodal involvement classified by the number of nodal stations involved at pathologic staging. *(Reprinted with permission from Asamura H, Chansky K, Crowley J, et al. The IASLC Lung Cancer Staging Project: proposals for the revisions of the N descriptors in the forthcoming 8th edition of the TNM classification for lung cancer. J Thorac Oncol. 2015;10:1675–1684.)*

tumor nodules, pleural and pericardial nodules, and malignant pleural and pericardial effusions) could be validated with the database of the eighth edition. Fig. 25.6A shows how similar the survival curves for all these descriptors are. Therefore, there is no need to modify them. For extrathoracic metastases (M1b), it was found that patients with single extrathoracic metastasis had similar survival to that of those with M1a tumors, but significantly worse than those with multiple extrathoracic metastases. The survival of those with multiple extrathoracic metastases in one organ and that of those with multiple extrathoracic metastases in several organs was similar. These analyses showed that the number of extrathoracic metastases had more prognostic impact than their location (Fig. 25.6B). According to these results, the recommendations for changes were the following:

- Keep the M1a descriptors as they are
- Redefine M1b to code tumors with a single extrathoracic metastasis
- Create a new category, M1c, to code tumors with multiple extrathoracic metastases either in one or in several organs.

M1a and M1b tumors have similar prognoses, but it makes sense to code them differently as they represent different anatomic forms of metastatic disease and have a different diagnostic and therapeutic approach.[10]

Stage Grouping

Table 25.4 shows the definitions of the T, N, and M descriptors for the eighth edition of the TNM classification of lung cancer. For the stage grouping, several models were discussed. Table 25.5 shows the model eventually chosen because it is the one that best separates tumors with different prognoses. Stage IA is divided into stages IA1, IA2, and IA3 to accommodate the new T1a, T1b, and T1b tumors with no nodal involvement and no metastasis. Stages IB and IIA will now group T2a and T2b tumors with no spread beyond the lung, respectively. All N1M0 tumors will be grouped in stage IIB,

together with T3 N0 M0, except for T3–T4 N1 M0 tumors that are grouped in stage IIIA. Similarly, all N2M0 tumors are stage IIIA, except for T3–T4 N2 M0 tumors that are in stage IIIB, together with all N3M0 tumors, except for T3–T4 N3 M0 for which a new stage IIIC was created. Finally, stage IV is divided into stage IVA to group M1a and M1b tumors, and stage IVB to include M1c tumors.[11] Fig. 25.7 shows the survival of patients according to clinical and pathologic stages, respectively. The expected worsening in survival is observed as tumor stage increases. All differences are statistically different except that of clinical stages IIIC and IVA. However, it makes sense to separate these tumors into two different stages as they represent different types of anatomic spread of the tumor: locoregional for those in stage IIIC and metastatic for those in stage IVA.

Applicability to SCLC and Bronchopulmonary Carcinoids

The applicability of the TNM classification to SCLC and to bronchopulmonary carcinoids was explored in the revisions leading to the seventh edition. The TNM classification was found to discriminate more prognostic groups at clinical and pathologic staging than the dichotomous classification "limited versus extensive disease" traditionally used for SCLC.[12,13] It also worked well for bronchopulmonary carcinoids, although the TNM classification was analyzed exclusively in the population of patients with resected tumors. The higher survival rates for all categories and stages, including metastatic disease, reflected the more benign nature of this neoplasm.[14] For the eighth edition, there were 4848 patients with clinically staged SCLC tumors; 582 underwent tumor resection with pathologic classification; and 428 patients had tumors clinically and pathologically staged. The analyses performed in these populations showed that the TNM classification works for SCLC, although the different natural history of this disease is clearly reflected in the lower survival rates for most categories and stages. However, it is important to realize that prognosis for early stages (IA1 to IA3) is not so different from that of NSCLC in the same stages.[15]

CLASSIFICATION OF TUMORS THAT DO NOT FIT IN THE DESCRIPTORS

Situations that are not included in the TNM descriptors are difficult to classify. These situations are uncommon, and there are no recommendations based on data. The alternative has been to agree to classify them in a certain way so that everybody classifies them similarly. Table 25.6 shows most of these situations and their recommended classification.[16]

NEW SPECIFIC RULES FOR LUNG CANCER

Measurement of Tumor Size in Part-Solid Nonmucinous Adenocarcinomas

The new classification of adenocarcinoma proposed by the IASLC, the American Thoracic Society, and the European Respiratory Society defined adenocarcinoma in situ, minimally invasive adenocarcinoma, and invasive adenocarcinomas of different cell types.[17] This new classification has been accepted by the World Health Organization and has been included in the latest edition of its book on the pathology of thoracic cancers.[18] These tumors may present as part-solid lesions on computed tomography (CT), with solid and ground-glass components. In general, the solid component on CT corresponds to the invasive part of the tumor at microscopic examination, and the ground-glass component corresponds to the lepidic part, which is the noninvasive

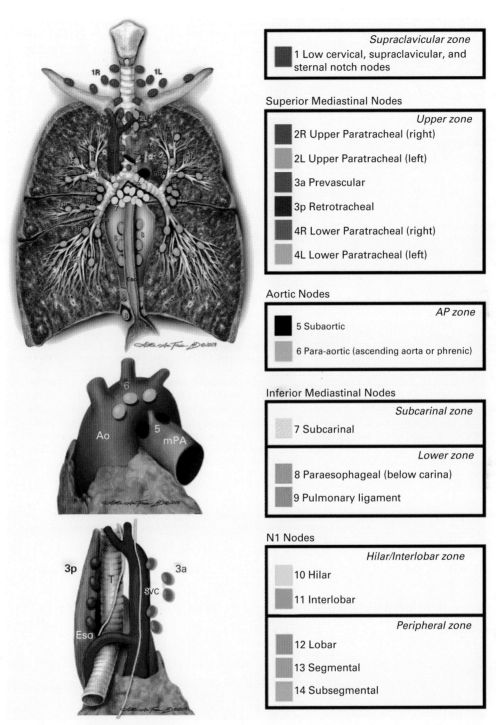

Supraclavicular zone
1 Low cervical, supraclavicular, and sternal notch nodes

Superior Mediastinal Nodes

Upper zone
2R Upper Paratracheal (right)
2L Upper Paratracheal (left)
3a Prevascular
3p Retrotracheal
4R Lower Paratracheal (right)
4L Lower Paratracheal (left)

Aortic Nodes

AP zone
5 Subaortic
6 Para-aortic (ascending aorta or phrenic)

Inferior Mediastinal Nodes

Subcarinal zone
7 Subcarinal

Lower zone
8 Paraesophageal (below carina)
9 Pulmonary ligament

N1 Nodes

Hilar/Interlobar zone
10 Hilar
11 Interlobar

Peripheral zone
12 Lobar
13 Segmental
14 Subsegmental

Fig. 25.5. International Association for the Study of Lung Cancer lymph node map. Copyright © 2009 Aletta Ann Frazier, MD. *Ao*, aorta; *Eso*, esophagus; *mPA*, main pulmonary artery; *SVC*, superior vena cava; *T*, thorax. *(Reprinted with permission from Rusch VW, Asamura H, Watanabe H, Giroux DJ, Rami-Porta R, Goldstraw P. The IASLC Lung Cancer Staging Project. A proposal for a new international lymph node map in the forthcoming seventh edition of the TNM classification for lung cancer. J Thorac Oncol. 2009;4:568–577.)*

portion of the tumor. There is a growing body of evidence indicating that prognosis is led by the size of the solid component of the tumor.[19–21] Therefore for these part-solid adenocarcinomas, size will be defined by the size of the solid component on CT and of the invasive component on microscopic examination. However, it is recommended to register both the size of the solid/invasive component and the size of the whole tumor in radiology/pathology reports.[22]

Measurement of Tumor Size After Induction Therapy

There are no rules for the measurement of tumor size after induction therapy when there has been some tumor response. A practical way to do it is to multiply the percent of viable tumor cells by the size of the total mass. This is applicable to a single focus or multiple foci of viable tumor.[22]

TABLE 25.3 Limits of the Nodal Stations of the IASLC Lymph Node Map[9]

Lymph Node Station No. (#)	Anatomic Limits
SUPRACLAVICULAR ZONE	
#1: Low cervical, supraclavicular, and sternal notch nodes	• Upper border: lower margin of cricoid cartilage. • Lower border: clavicles bilaterally and, in the midline, the upper border of the manubrium. 1R designates right-sided nodes, 1L left-sided nodes in this region. • For lymph node station 1, the midline of the trachea serves as the border between 1R and 1L.
UPPER ZONE	
#2: Upper paratracheal nodes	• 2R: Upper border: apex of the right lung and pleural space, and, in the midline, the upper border of the manubrium. • Lower border: intersection of caudal margin of the innominate vein with the trachea. • Similar to lymph node station 4R, 2R includes nodes extending to the left lateral border of the trachea. • 2L: Upper border: apex of the lung and pleural space, and, in the midline, the upper border of the manubrium. • Lower border: superior border of the aortic arch.
#3 Prevascular and retrotracheal nodes	• 3a: Prevascular • On the right: upper border: apex of chest. Lower border: level of carina. Anterior border: posterior aspect of sternum. Posterior border: anterior border of the superior vena cava. • On the left: upper border: apex of chest. Lower border: level of carina. Anterior border: posterior aspect of sternum. Posterior border: left carotid artery. • 3p: Retrotracheal • Upper border: apex of chest. Lower border: carina.
#4: Lower paratracheal nodes	• 4R: includes right paratracheal nodes, and pretracheal nodes extending to the left lateral border of the trachea. • Upper border: intersection of caudal margin of the innominate vein with the trachea. • Lower border: lower border of the azygos vein. • 4L: includes nodes to the left of the left lateral border of the trachea, medial to the ligamentum arteriosum. • Upper border: upper margin of the aortic arch. • Lower border: upper rim of the left main pulmonary artery.
AORTOPULMONARY ZONE	
#5: Subaortic (aortopulmonary window)	• Subaortic lymph nodes lateral to the ligamentum arteriosum. • Upper border: the lower border of the aortic arch. • Lower border: upper rim of the left main pulmonary artery.
#6: Para-aortic nodes (ascending aorta or phrenic)	• Lymph nodes anterior and lateral to the ascending aorta and aortic arch. • Upper border: a line tangential to the upper border of the aortic arch. • Lower border: the lower border of the aortic arch.
SUBCARINAL ZONE	
#7: Subcarinal nodes	• Upper border: the carina of the trachea. • Lower border: the upper border of the lower lobe bronchus on the left; the lower border of the bronchus intermedius on the right.
LOWER ZONE	
#8: Paraesophageal nodes (below carina)	• Nodes lying adjacent to the wall of the esophagus and to the right or the left of the midline, excluding subcarinal nodes. • Upper border: the upper border of the lower lobe bronchus on the left; the lower border of the bronchus intermedius on the right. • Lower border: the diaphragm.
#9: Pulmonary ligament nodes	• Nodes lying within the pulmonary ligament. • Upper border: the inferior pulmonary vein. • Lower border: the diaphragm.
HILAR/INTERLOBAR ZONE	
#10: Hilar nodes	• Includes nodes immediately adjacent to the main stem bronchus and hilar vessels including the proximal portions of the pulmonary veins and the main pulmonary artery. • Upper border: the lower rim of the azygos vein in the right; upper rim of the pulmonary artery on the left. • Lower border: interlobar region bilaterally.

#11: Interlobar nodes	• Between the origin of the lobar bronchi.
	• Optional notations for subcategories of station:
	  • #11s: between the upper lobe bronchus and bronchus intermedius on the right.
	  • #11i: between the middle and lower bronchi on the right.

PERIPHERAL ZONE	
#12: Lobar nodes	• Adjacent to the lobar bronchi
#13: Segmental nodes	• Adjacent to the segmental bronchi
#14: Subsegmental nodes	• Adjacent to the subsegmental bronchi

IASLC, International Association for the Study of Lung Cancer.

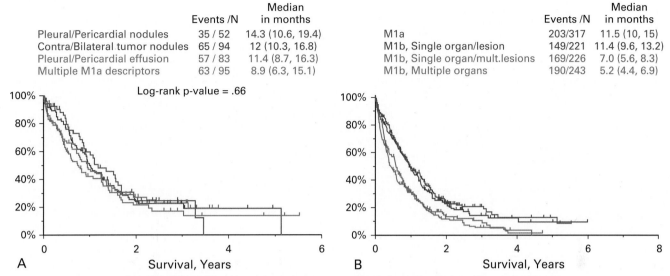

Fig. 25.6. Survival according to (A) M1a and (B) M1b descriptors and the multiplicity of extrathoracic metastases. *EDC,* electronic data capture. *(Reprinted with permission from Eberhardt WE, Mitchell A, Crowley J, et al. The IASLC Lung Cancer Staging Project: proposals for the revision of the M descriptors in the forthcoming eighth edition of the TNM classification of lung cancer.* J Thorac Oncol. *2015;10:1515–1522.)*

TABLE 25.4 Categories, Subcategories, and Descriptors of the Eighth Edition of the TNM Classification of Lung Cancer[11]

T: PRIMARY TUMOR

Category	Subcategory	Descriptors
TX		Primary tumor cannot be assessed, or tumor proven by the presence of malignant cells in sputum or bronchial washings but not visualized by imaging or bronchoscopy.
T0		No evidence of primary tumor.
Tis		Carcinoma in situ: Tis(AIS): adenocarcinoma Tis(SCIS): squamous cell carcinoma
T1		Tumor 3 cm or less in greatest dimension, surrounded by lung or visceral pleura, without bronchoscopic evidence of invasion more proximal than the lobar bronchus (i.e., not in the main bronchus).[a]
	T1mi	Minimally invasive adenocarcinoma.
	T1a	Tumor 1 cm or less in greatest dimension.[a]
	T1b	Tumor more than 1 cm but not more than 2 cm in greatest dimension.[a]
	T1c	Tumor more than 2 cm but not more than 3 cm in greatest dimension.[a]
T2		Tumor more than 3 cm but not more than 5 cm; or tumor with *any* of the following features:[b] • involves main bronchus regardless of distance to the carina, but without involving the carina • invades visceral pleura • associated with atelectasis or obstructive pneumonitis that extends to the hilar region, either involving part of the lung or the entire lung.
	T2a	Tumor more than 3 cm but not more than 4 cm in greatest dimension.
	T2b	Tumor more than 4 cm but not more than 5 cm in greatest dimension.
T3		Tumor more than 5 cm but not more than 7 cm in greatest dimension or one that directly invades any of the following: parietal pleura (PL3), chest wall (including superior sulcus tumors), phrenic nerve, parietal pericardium; or associated separate tumor nodule(s) in the same lobe as the primary tumor.
T4		Tumors more than 7 cm or one that invades any of the following: diaphragm, mediastinum, heart, great vessels, trachea, recurrent laryngeal nerve, esophagus, vertebral body, carina; or separate tumor nodule(s) in a different ipsilateral lobe to that of the primary tumor.

N: REGIONAL LYMPH NODES

NX		Regional lymph nodes cannot be assessed.
N0		No regional lymph node metastasis.
N1		Metastasis in ipsilateral peribronchial and/or ipsilateral hilar lymph nodes and intrapulmonary nodes, including involvement by direct extension.
N2		Metastasis in ipsilateral mediastinal and/or subcarinal lymph node(s).
N3		Metastasis in contralateral mediastinal, contralateral hilar, ipsilateral or contralateral scalene, or supraclavicular lymph node(s).

Continued

TABLE 25.4 Categories, Subcategories, and Descriptors of the Eighth Edition of the TNM Classification of Lung Cancer[11]—cont'd

M: DISTANT METASTASIS

M0		No distant metastasis
M1		Distant metastasis
	M1a	Separate tumor nodule(s) in a contralateral lobe; tumor with pleural nodules or malignant pleural or pericardial effusion.[c]
	M1b	Single extrathoracic metastasis in a single organ and involvement of a single distant (nonregional) node.
	M1c	Multiple extrathoracic metastases in one or several organs.

[a]The uncommon superficial spreading tumor of any size with its invasive component limited to the bronchial wall, which may extend proximal to the main bronchus, is also classified as T1a.

[b]T2 tumors with these features are classified T2a if 4 cm or less or if size cannot be determined, and T2b if greater than 4 cm but not larger than 5 cm.

[c]Most pleural (pericardial) effusions with lung cancer are due to tumor. In a few patients, however, multiple microscopic examinations of pleural (pericardial) fluid are negative for tumor, and the fluid is nonbloody and is not an exudate. Where these elements and clinical judgment dictate that the effusion is not related to the tumor, the effusion should be excluded as a staging descriptor.

TNM, tumor, node, and metastasis.

TABLE 25.5 Stage Grouping of the Eighth Edition of the TNM Classification of Lung Cancer[11]

Stage	T	N	M
Occult carcinoma	TX	N0	M0
0	Tis	N0	M0
IA1	T1mi	N0	M0
	T1a	N0	M0
IA2	T1b	N0	M0
IA3	T1c	N0	M0
IB	T2a	N0	M0
IIA	T2b	N0	M0
IIB	T1a, b, c	N1	M0
	T2a, b	N1	M0
	T3	N0	M0
IIIA	T1a, b, c	N2	M0
	T2a, b	N2	M0
	T3	N1	M0
	T4	N0	M0
	T4	N1	M0
IIIB	T1a, b, c	N3	M0
	T2a, b	N3	M0
	T3	N2	M0
	T4	N2	M0
IIIC	T3	N3	M0
	T4	N3	M0
IVA	Any T	Any N	M1a
	Any T	Any N	M1b
IVB	Any T	Any N	M1c

TNM, tumor, node, and metastasis.

Classification of Lung Cancers With Multiple Lesions

The rules for classifying lung cancers with multiple lesions are ambiguous and prone to multiple interpretations. An ad hoc subcommittee was created within the IASLC Staging and Prognostic Factors Committee to study this problem and to reach a consensus on a homogeneous way to classify these tumors. The subcommittee established four disease patterns to define the different presentations of lung cancer with multiple lesions and recommended the following rules for their classification.[23]

- *Synchronous and metachronous primary lung cancers*: These should be classified separately with a TNM for each tumor. This classification is applied regardless of the tumor location (different lungs, different ipsilateral lobes or same lobe) to grossly identified tumors and to those identified on microscopic examination. Table 25.7 shows the clinical and pathologic criteria for distinguishing second primary tumors from related tumors.[24]
- *Separate tumor nodules of the same histopathologic type (intrapulmonary metastases)*: The classification of these tumors depends

on the lobar location of the separate tumor nodules. If the separate tumor nodule(s) is/are in the same lobe of the primary tumor, they are classified as T3; if they are in a different ipsilateral lobe, they are classified as T4; and finally, if they are in the contralateral lung, they are classified as M1a. However, if there were extrathoracic metastases, the tumor would be classified as M1b or M1c depending on the number of metastases. This classification applies to separate tumor nodes identified clinically or grossly and also to those identified microscopically on pathologic examination. Table 25.8 shows the clinical and pathologic criteria for categorizing a separate tumor nodule (intrapulmonary metastasis).[23,25]

- *Multifocal pulmonary adenocarcinomas with ground-glass/lepidic features*: These tumors should be classified by the highest T with the number (#) or (m) for multiple in parentheses, and N and M categories applying to all of the multiple tumors collectively. The largest dimension of the tumor is that of the solid component by CT or of the invasive component on microscopic examination. This classification applies regardless of the location of the tumors—same lobe, same lung, or contralateral lung—and to grossly recognizable tumors as well as those identified on pathologic examination. Table 25.9 presents the clinical and pathologic criteria for characterizing these tumors.[26]
- *Diffuse pneumonic-type lung adenocarcinoma*: If there is one focus of disease, the general TNM classification for lung cancer is applied, with the T category defined by tumor size. In cases of multiple sites, the T and the M categories are defined by the location of the involved areas: T3 if they are in one lobe, including miliary involvement; T4 if other ipsilateral lobes are involved; and M1a if there is involvement of the contralateral lung. In this case, the T category is defined by the T category of the largest tumor. T4 also is applied when size is difficult to determine, but there is evidence of invasion into another ipsilateral lobe. The N category should apply to all pulmonary sites, and the appropriate M category is chosen depending on the anatomic location of the metastases. As for the other disease patterns described, this classification applies to grossly identified tumors and to those discovered on pathologic examination. Table 25.10 shows the clinical and pathologic criteria for characterizing these tumors.[26]

Table 25.11 summarizes the basic radiographic and pathologic features, the recommended TNM classification, and the conceptual view of the four patterns of lung cancer with multiple lesions.[23]

IMPLICATIONS FOR CLINICAL PRACTICE

One of the most important findings that prompted revisions in the eighth edition of the TNM classification of lung cancer is

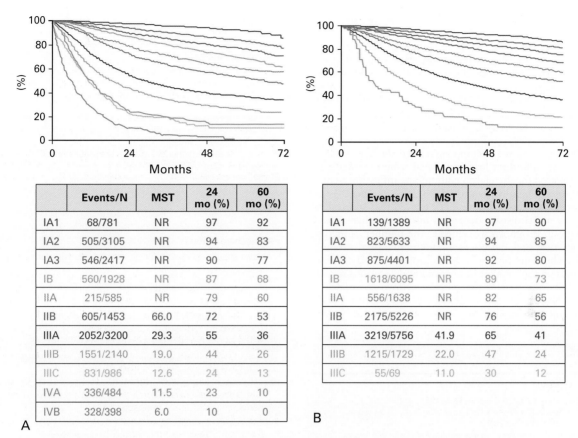

	Events/N	MST	24 mo (%)	60 mo (%)
IA1	68/781	NR	97	92
IA2	505/3105	NR	94	83
IA3	546/2417	NR	90	77
IB	560/1928	NR	87	68
IIA	215/585	NR	79	60
IIB	605/1453	66.0	72	53
IIIA	2052/3200	29.3	55	36
IIIB	1551/2140	19.0	44	26
IIIC	831/986	12.6	24	13
IVA	336/484	11.5	23	10
IVB	328/398	6.0	10	0

A

	Events/N	MST	24 mo (%)	60 mo (%)
IA1	139/1389	NR	97	90
IA2	823/5633	NR	94	85
IA3	875/4401	NR	92	80
IB	1618/6095	NR	89	73
IIA	556/1638	NR	82	65
IIB	2175/5226	NR	76	56
IIIA	3219/5756	41.9	65	41
IIIB	1215/1729	22.0	47	24
IIIC	55/69	11.0	30	12

B

Fig. 25.7. Survival by (A) clinical and (B) pathologic stages. *MST,* Median survival time; *NR,* not reached. *(Reprinted with permission from Goldstraw P, Chansky K, Crowley J, et al. The IASLC Lung Cancer Staging Project: proposals for the revision of the stage grouping in the forthcoming (8th) edition of the TNM classification of lung cancer. J Thorac Oncol. 2016;11:39–51.)*

TABLE 25.6   Guide to Uniform Classification When the Rules Do Not Fit[16]

Description of the Tumor	Classification
Direct invasion of an adjacent lobe, across the fissure or directly if the fissure is incomplete, unless other criteria assign a higher T classification	T2a
Invasion of phrenic nerve	T3
Paralysis of the recurrent laryngeal nerve, superior vena caval obstruction, compression of the trachea or esophagus related to direct extension of the primary tumor	T4
Paralysis of the recurrent laryngeal nerve, superior vena caval obstruction, compression of the trachea or esophagus related to lymph node involvement	N2
Involvement of great vessels: aorta, superior vena cava, inferior vena cava, main pulmonary artery (pulmonary trunk), intrapericardial portions of the right and left pulmonary arteries, intrapericardial portions of the superior and inferior right and left pulmonary veins	T4
Pancoast tumors with evidence of invasion of the vertebral body or spinal canal, encasement of the subclavian vessels, or unequivocal involvement of the superior branches of the brachial plexus (C8 or above)	T4
Pancoast tumors without the above criteria for T4 classification	T3
Direct extension to visceral pericardium	T4
Invasion into hilar fat, unless other criteria assign a higher T	T2a
Invasion into mediastinal fat	T4
Discontinuous tumor nodules in the ipsilateral parietal or visceral pleura	M1a
Discontinuous tumor nodules outside the parietal pleura in the chest wall or in the diaphragm	M1b or M1c

the increased relevance of tumor size as a prognostic factor. Now the smallest coded invasive tumor is that of 1 cm or less in greatest dimension. Nearly 60% of tumors identified in screening programs have this dimension, and they will now be clearly differentiated from others by the new T1a category.[27] These small tumors will be the base ground for further research on growth rate, tumor density, intensity of standardized uptake value, type of resection, and investigation of alternative therapies such as stereotactic body radiation therapy or radiofrequency ablation, molecular profile, and genetic signatures. The presence of tumor size as a descriptor in all T categories will be useful to better

stratify tumors in future clinical trials and will improve our capacity to prognosticate. This means that determining the greatest dimension of the tumor will be more clinically relevant than it was in the previous editions of the TNM classification and, therefore, a greater responsibility for the managing physician.

The fact that the recently described adenocarcinoma in situ (AIS), Tis(AIS), and minimally invasive adenocarcinoma, T1mi,[17] have been included in the classification and have specific categories will increase awareness of them and facilitate the prospective collection of data.[22] In addition, attention will have to be paid when determining the size of the solid component of part-solid tumors, as the size of the solid component (not the size of the whole tumor) leads prognosis.[22]

Visceral pleura invasion has been confirmed as an important prognostic factor. Even its two categories (PL1 and PL2) have prognostic impact. Therefore, the recommendation for pathologists is to use elastic stain when the invasion of the visceral pleura cannot be determined adequately with hematoxylin and eosin stains. Failure to use elastic stains may underestimate visceral pleura invasion in about 20% of patients thought to have stage IA tumors.[28]

The descriptors of the N component have not been modified, but there is an important learning drawn from the analyses of the database used for the eighth edition: quantification of nodal disease matters. This already was evident from the analyses performed for the seventh edition. They proved that survival rate according to nodal disease depended on the number of nodal zones involved. Prognosis worsened as the number of involved nodal zones increased, but it was also found that single-zone N2 disease had the same prognosis as multiple-zone N1 disease.[29] The analyses on the number of involved nodal stations revealed similar results: the greater the number of involved nodal stations, the worse the prognosis. They also showed other results that have practical implications: there are survival differences

TABLE 25.7 Clinical Criteria for Separate Versus Related Pulmonary Tumors[24]

CLINICAL CRITERIA[a]

Tumors may be considered separate primary tumors if:
  They are clearly of a different histologic type (e.g., squamous carcinoma and adenocarcinoma).
Tumors may be considered to be arising from a single tumor source if:
  Matching breakpoints are identified by comparative genomic hybridization.
Relative arguments that favor separate tumors:
  • Different radiographic appearance or metabolic uptake.
  • Different pattern of biomarkers (driver gene mutations).
  • Different rates of growth (if previous imaging is available).
  • Absence of nodal or systemic metastases.
Relative arguments that favor a single tumor source:
  • The same radiographic appearance.
  • Similar growth patterns (if previous imaging is available).
  • Significant nodal or systemic metastases.
  • The same biomarker pattern (and same histotype).

PATHOLOGIC CRITERIA (I.E., AFTER RESECTION)[b]

Tumors may be considered separate primary tumors if:
  • They are clearly of a different histologic type (e.g., squamous carcinoma and adenocarcinoma).
  • They are clearly different by a comprehensive histologic assessment.
  • They are squamous carcinomas that have arisen from carcinoma in situ.
Tumors may be considered to be arising from a single tumor source if:
  • Exactly matching breakpoints are identified by comparative genomic hybridization.
Relative arguments that favor separate tumors (to be considered together with clinical factors):
  • Different pattern of biomarkers.
  • Absence of nodal or systemic metastases.
Relative arguments that favor a single tumor source (to be considered together with clinical factors):
  • Matching appearance on comprehensive histologic assessment.
  • The same biomarker pattern.
  • Significant nodal or systemic metastases.

[a]Note that a comprehensive histologic assessment is not included in clinical staging, as it requires that the entire specimen be resected.
[b]Pathologic information should be supplemented with any clinical information that is available.

TABLE 25.8 Criteria to Categorize a Lesion as a Separate Tumor Nodule (Intrapulmonary Metastasis)[23,25]

CLINICAL CRITERIA

Tumors should be considered to have a separate tumor nodule(s) if:
  • There is a solid lung cancer and a separate tumor nodule(s) with a similar solid appearance and with (presumed) matching histologic appearance.
  • This applies whether or not a biopsy has been performed on the lesions, provided that there is strong suspicion that the lesions are histologically identical.
  • This applies whether or not there are sites of extrathoracic metastases.
AND provided that:
  • The lesions are NOT judged to be synchronous primary lung cancers.
  • The lesions are NOT multifocal GG/L lung cancer (multiple nodules with GG/L features) or pneumonic-type of lung cancer.

PATHOLOGIC CRITERIA

Tumors should be considered to have a separate tumor nodule(s) (intrapulmonary metastasis) if:
  • There is a separate tumor nodule(s) of cancer in the lung with a similar histologic appearance to a primary lung cancer.
AND provided that:
  • The lesions are NOT judged to be synchronous primary lung cancers.
  • The lesions are NOT multiple foci of LPA, MIA, and AIS.

A radiographically solid appearance and the specific histologic subtype of solid adenocarcinoma denote different things.
AIS, adenocarcinoma in situ; *GG/L,* ground glass/lepidic; *LPA,* lepidic predominant adenocarcinoma; *MIA,* minimally invasive adenocarcinoma.

TABLE 25.9 Criteria Identifying Multifocal Ground-Glass/Lepidic Lung Adenocarcinoma[26]

CLINICAL CRITERIA

Tumors should be considered multifocal GG/L lung adenocarcinoma if:
  • There are multiple subsolid nodules (either pure ground glass or part-solid), with at least one suspected (or proven) to be cancer.
  • This applies whether or not a biopsy has been performed of the nodules.
  • This applies if the other nodules are found on biopsy to be AIS, MIA, or LPA.
  • This applies if a nodule has become >50% solid but is judged to have arisen from a GGN, provided there are other subsolid nodules.
  • GGN lesions <5 mm or lesions suspected to be AAH are not counted for the TNM classification.

PATHOLOGIC CRITERIA

Tumors should be considered multifocal GG/L lung adenocarcinoma if:
  • There are multiple foci of LPA, MIA, or AIS.
  • This applies whether a detailed histologic assessment (i.e., proportion of subtypes) shows a matching or different appearance.
  • This applies if one lesion(s) is LPA, MIA, or AIS and there are other subsolid nodules for which a biopsy has not been performed.
  • This applies whether the nodule(s) are identified preoperatively or only on pathologic examination.
  • Foci of AAH are not counted for the TNM classification.

A radiographically solid appearance and the specific histologic subtype of solid adenocarcinoma denote different things.
AAH, atypical adenomatous hyperplasia; *AIS,* adenocarcinoma in situ; *GG/L,* ground glass/lepidic; *GGN,* ground-glass nodule; *LPA,* lepidic predominant adenocarcinoma; *MIA,* minimally invasive adenocarcinoma; *TNM,* tumor, node, and metastasis.

between patients whose tumors are classified as single-station N2 without N1 disease and those with single-station N2 with N1 disease. The former has better survival than the latter and similar survival to those with multiple-station N1 disease.[8] All these findings are derived from pathologic staging and could not be reliably replicated at clinical staging, which precluded its use to subclassify the present N descriptors. However, they have clinical relevance. First, they will help the managing physician to refine postoperative prognosis of those patients whose tumors have been removed and who are found to have nodal disease. Second, the fact that single-station N2 without N1 disease has the same prognosis as multiple-station N1 disease will raise the question of whether upfront surgery could be indicated for these patients. The problem is that determining whether a tumor has single-station N2 disease without N1 at clinical staging is difficult with the staging methods currently used. One study that tried to determine single-zone N2 disease with systematic CT, positron emission tomography, and selective mediastinoscopy failed in doing so in 19% of the patients who were eventually found to have multiple-zone N2 disease.[30] Third, it seems obvious that if we want to offer upfront tumor resection to patients with single-station N2 disease, we have to preoperatively stage their tumors beyond CT, positron emission tomography, and standard mediastinoscopy. Only with a properly performed transcervical mediastinal lymphadenectomy can single-station or single-zone N2 disease be reliably identified. This may be an argument in favor of video-assisted mediastinoscopic lymphadenectomy and transcervical extended mediastinal lymphadenectomy, which have the objective to remove the mediastinal lymph nodes and the surrounding fatty tissue. Their sensitivity and negative predictive values are 1 or close to 1.[31–35]

Although it would have been very desirable, the fact is that the regional and pulmonary lymph node map proposed by the IASLC has not been universally used.[8,9] This may account for the important differences found when survival according to the N categories is studied by geographic region.[8] The IASLC lymph node map is the first map developed from an international and multidisciplinary consensus. It is our responsibility to use it properly to classify nodal disease in a homogeneous way. This will improve our understanding of the implications of nodal disease in the different anatomic areas.

The M component has undergone an important change in the eighth edition of the TNM classification. Subdividing extrathoracic metastases according to their number (M1b for single extrathoracic metastasis and M1c for multiple extrathoracic metastases in one or in several organs) identifies a group of metastases (M1b) that can be the base for further and deeper research on metastatic disease. Oligometastatic disease and oligoprogression are not uniformly defined because they may comprise tumors with one to five metastatic deposits. There can also be circulating cancer cells and micrometastases that are different forms of metastatic dissemination.[36] Therefore, an immediate implication for clinical practice is that the number and location of metastasis must be registered to determine the M1 category. Pathologic confirmation is desirable, as well as the registration of the largest dimension of the metastasis or the largest dimension of the largest metastases if there are several. The organ location is also important because there might be prognostic differences, although these could not be proved in the analyses leading to the eighth edition of the TNM classification.[10] The new M1b category represents the least extensive disease of extrathoracic dissemination and may constitute the basic component of oligometastatic

TABLE 25.10 Criteria Identifying the Pneumonic Type of Adenocarcinoma[26]

CLINICAL CRITERIA

Tumors should be considered pneumonic-type of adenocarcinoma if:
- The cancer manifests in a regional distribution, similar to a pneumonic infiltrate or consolidation.
- This applies whether there is one confluent area or multiple regions of disease. The region(s) may be confined to one lobe, in multiple lobes, or bilaterally, but should involve a regional pattern of distribution.
- The involved areas may appear to be ground glass, solid consolidation, or a combination thereof.
- This can be applied when there is compelling suspicion of malignancy whether or not a biopsy has been performed of the area(s).
- This should not be applied to discrete nodules (i.e., GG/L nodules).
- This should not be applied to tumors causing bronchial obstruction with resultant obstructive pneumonia or atelectasis.

PATHOLOGIC CRITERIA

Tumors should be considered pneumonic type of adenocarcinoma if:
- There is diffuse distribution of adenocarcinoma throughout a region(s) of the lung, as opposed to a single well-demarcated mass or multiple discrete well-demarcated nodules.
- This typically involves an invasive mucinous adenocarcinoma, although a mixed mucinous and nonmucinous pattern may occur.
- The tumor may show a heterogeneous mixture of acinar, papillary, and micropapillary growth patterns, although it is usually lepidic predominant.

A radiographically solid appearance and the specific histologic subtype of solid adenocarcinoma denote different things.
GG/L, ground glass/lepidic.

TABLE 25.11 Schematic Summary of Patterns of Disease and TNM Classification of Patients With Lung Cancer With Multiple Pulmonary Sites of Involvement[23]

	Second Primary Lung Cancer	Separate Tumor Nodule (Intrapulmonary Metastasis)	Multifocal GG/L Nodules	Pneumonic Type of Adenocarcinoma
Imaging features	Two or more distinct masses with imaging characteristic of lung cancer (e.g., spiculated)	Typical lung cancer (e.g., solid, spiculated) with separate solid nodule	Multiple ground-glass or part-solid nodules	Patchy areas of ground glass and consolidation
Pathologic features	Different histotype or different morphology by comprehensive histologic assessment	Distinct masses with the same morphologic features by comprehensive histologic assessment	Adenocarcinomas with prominent lepidic component (typically varying degrees of AIS, MIA, LPA)	Same histologic features throughout (most often invasive mucinous adenocarcinoma)
TNM classification	Separate cTNM and pTNM for each cancer	Location of separate nodule relative to primary site determines if T3, T4, or M1a; single N and M	T based on highest T lesion with (#/m) indicating multiplicity; single N and M	T based on size or T3 if in single lobe, T4 or M1a if in different ipsilateral or contralateral lobes; single N and M
Conceptual view	Unrelated tumors	Single tumor, with intrapulmonary metastasis	Separate tumors, albeit with similarities	Single tumor, diffuse pulmonary involvement

AIS, adenocarcinoma in situ; *c*, clinical; *GG/L*, ground glass/lepidic; *LPA*, lepidic-predominant adenocarcinoma; *MIA*, minimally invasive adenocarcinoma; *p*, pathologic; *TNM*, tumor, node, and metastasis.

disease. This difference is important because, in contradistinction with polymetastatic disease, where palliation is the main therapeutic objective, the aim of therapy in oligometastatic disease and oligoprogression is radical (that is, the elimination of all known disease) with whatever means are available or are suitable to the size and location of the metastases: surgical resection, standard radiotherapy, stereotactic radiotherapy, radiofrequency ablation, microwave ablation, chemotherapy, or targeted therapy, either alone or in combination.

Finally, the new stage grouping will surely raise questions about the indication for therapy for those tumors that have changed stage by virtue of reclassification. Although therapeutic indications are stage based, the taxonomic changes introduced in the eighth edition of the TNM classification do not necessarily imply an automatic change of therapy.[11] Therapy should be based on properly designed clinical trials. The clinical judgment of the multidisciplinary team will decide the best therapy for the individual patient and tumor after assessment of the best available evidence.[37–39]

In conclusion, the eighth edition of the TNM classification of lung cancer improves our understanding of the anatomic extent of the tumor, enhances our capacity to indicate prognosis at clinical and pathologic staging, and increases the possibilities of research by facilitating tumor stratification in future clinical trials.

KEY REFERENCES

4. Goldstraw P, Crowley JJ. The International Association for the Study of Lung Cancer international staging project on lung cancer. *J Thorac Oncol.* 2006;1:281–286.

5. Rami-Porta R, Bolejack V, Giroux DJ, et al. The IASLC Lung Cancer Staging Project: the new database to inform the eighth edition of the TNM classification of lung cancer. *J Thorac Oncol.* 2014;9:1618–1624.

6. Rami-Porta R, Bolejack V, Crowley J, et al. The IASLC Lung Cancer Staging Project: proposals for the revisions of the T descriptors in the forthcoming 8th edition of the TNM classification for lung cancer. *J Thorac Oncol.* 2015;10:990–1003.

8. Asamura H, Chansky K, Crowley J, et al. The IASLC Lung Cancer Staging Project: proposals for the revisions of the N descriptors in the forthcoming 8th edition of the TNM classification for lung cancer. *J Thorac Oncol.* 2015;10:1675–1684.

10. Eberhardt WE, Mitchell A, Crowley J, et al. The IASLC Lung Cancer Staging Project: proposals for the revision of the M descriptors in the forthcoming eighth edition of the TNM classification of lung cancer. *J Thorac Oncol.* 2015;10:1515–1522.

11. Goldstraw P, Chansky K, Crowley J, et al. The IASLC Lung Cancer Staging Project: proposals for the revision of the stage grouping in the forthcoming (8th) edition of the TNM classification of lung cancer. *J Thorac Oncol.* 2016;11:39–51.

14. Travis WD, Giroux DJ, Chansky K, et al. The IASLC Lung Cancer Staging Project: proposals for the inclusion of bronchopulmonary carcinoid tumors in the forthcoming (seventh) edition of the TNM classification for lung cancer. *J Thorac Oncol.* 2008;3:1213–1223.

15. Nicholson AG, Chansky K, Crowley J, et al. The IASLC Lung Cancer Staging Project: proposals for the revision of the clinical and pathologic staging of small cell lung cancer in the forthcoming eighth edition of the TNM classification for lung cancer. *J Thorac Oncol.* 2016;11:300–311.

22. Travis WD, Asamura H, Bankier A, et al. The IASLC Lung Cancer Staging Project: proposals for coding T categories for subsolid nodules and assessment of tumor size in part-solid tumors in the forthcoming eighth edition of the TNM classification of lung cancer. *J Thorac Oncol.* 2016;11(8):1204–1223.

25. Detterbeck FC, Bolejack V, Arenberg DA, et al. The IASLC Lung Cancer Staging Project: background data and proposals for the classification of lung cancer with separate tumor nodules in the forthcoming eighth edition of the TNM classification for lung cancer. *J Thorac Oncol.* 2016;11:681–692.

26. Detterbeck FC, Marom EM, Arenberg DA, et al. The IASLC Lung Cancer Staging Project: background data and proposals for the application of TNM staging rules to lung cancer presenting as multiple nodules with ground glass or lepidic features or a pneumonic-type of involvement in the forthcoming eighth edition of the TNM classification. *J Thorac Oncol.* 2016;11:666–680.

See Expertconsult.com for full list of references.

26 | Preoperative Functional Evaluation of the Surgical Candidate

Alessandro Brunelli and Pieter E. Postmus

SUMMARY OF KEY POINTS

- Predicted postoperative forced expiratory volume in 1 second (ppoFEV$_1$) has been shown to be inaccurate in predicting actual postoperative FEV$_1$ in patients with chronic obstructive pulmonary disease (COPD). It should not be used alone to select patients for surgery.
- FEV$_1$ and carbon monoxide lung diffusion capacity (DLCO) and their derivate ppoFEV$_1$ and predicted postoperative DLCO (ppoDLCO) should be measured and calculated in all candidates for lung resection by estimating the number of functioning segments to be removed during an operation.
- ppoDLCO has been shown to be a reliable predictor of pulmonary morbidity and mortality in both patients with and patients without COPD.
- Low-technology exercise tests (i.e., Shuttle Walk Test and Stair-Climbing Test) may be used to screen patients before surgery. However, poor performance at these tests (i.e., <25 shuttles or 400 m at Shuttle Walk Test or <22 m at Stair-Climbing Test) indicates functional limitation. These patients should be referred to cardiopulmonary exercise test (CPET).
- CPET assesses the global fitness of the patient expressed as the rate of maximum oxygen (VO$_{2peak}$) consumption and several other direct and derivate measures, which can be used to identify the limiting factor in the oxygen transport system.
- A VO$_{2peak}$ less than 10 mL/kg/min or over 35% of the predicted value indicates high risk for anatomic lung resection.
- Cardiac risk stratification should be performed in all candidates for lung resection. The use of a risk score, such as thoracic Revised Cardiac Risk Index (ThRCRI), is a simple and reliable means to refer patients to noninvasive cardiac evaluation (i.e., ThRCRI >1.5).
- Appropriately aggressive cardiac interventions should be instituted before surgery only for patients who would need such interventions irrespective of the planned surgery. However, prophylactic coronary revascularization before surgery in patients who otherwise do not need such a procedure does not appear to reduce perioperative risk.
- Minimally invasive thoracic surgery (video-assisted thoracoscopic surgery) has been shown to be associated with reduced risk of morbidity and mortality, particularly in high-risk patients.

For stage I and II nonsmall cell lung cancer, resection is the best validated treatment option with the aim of cure. In order for this aim to be achieved, not only should the tumor be resectable, but also the patient should be operable (i.e., fit enough to undergo the resection as well as to have satisfactory postoperative quality of life). Deciding on resectability typically is a team effort and depends on staging based on adequate imaging of the tumor and its potentially metastatic sites, both locoregional and systemic. Operability is based first on the risk of immediate perioperative and postoperative complications and second on the risk of long-term disability after resection of parts of the affected lung (or lungs). Consequently, the decision to proceed with curative-intent surgery should take into account both aspects of operability. This decision is becoming increasingly critical as alternative strategies for resection are gaining ground and outcomes are promising, particularly for patients with smaller (stage 1A) tumors, despite the fact that many patients who are judged to be inoperable receive stereotactic radiotherapy and are not selected for inclusion in phase II studies.[1]

Many patients with lung cancer have been smokers and have comorbidities resulting from damage to sensitive organs and organ systems. Damage to lung tissue resulting in COPD with reduced pulmonary function and atherosclerotic cardiovascular disease are the most common findings in these patients. The presence of such comorbidities makes it critical to evaluate the possibly increased risks of both long-term disability and possible perioperative complications. Preoperative physiologic assessment aims to quantify the magnitude of this risk.

Furthermore, lung cancer is a disease of elderly people and logically many of these patients may have comorbid conditions such as diabetes or renal disease.

EVALUATION OF COMORBIDITY

Comorbid conditions are best evaluated with use of the Charlson Comorbidity Index (Table 26.1),[2] which has been shown to be an independent predictor of surgical mortality as well as long-term survival. A subset of 1844 patients with lung cancer who had had surgical resection in Norway from 1993 to the end of 2005 was evaluated according to the Charlson Comorbidity Index, and potential factors influencing 30-day mortality were analyzed. The overall mortality rate within 30 days postoperatively was 4.4%. Male gender (odds ratio, 1.76), older age (odds ratio, 3.38 for an age between 70 and 79 years), right-sided tumors (odds ratio, 1.73), and extensive procedures (odds ratio, 4.54 for pneumonectomy) were identified as risk factors for postoperative mortality in multivariate analysis. The Charlson Comorbidity Index was identified as an independent risk factor for postoperative mortality ($p = 0.017$).[2]

TABLE 26.1 Charlson Comorbidity Index Scoring

Score	Condition
1	Coronary artery disease
	Congestive heart failure
	Chronic pulmonary disease
	Peptic ulcer disease
	Peripheral vascular disease
	Mild liver disease
	Cerebrovascular disease
	Connective tissues disease
	Diabetes
	Dementia
2	Hemiplegia
	Moderate-to-severe renal disease
	Diabetes with end-organ damage
	Any prior tumor (within 5 y of diagnosis)
	Leukemia
	Lymphoma
3	Moderate-to-severe liver disease
6	Metastatic solid tumor
	AIDS (not only HIV positive)

AIDS, acquired immune deficiency syndrome; *HIV,* human immunodeficiency virus.

In a study of 433 consecutive patients (340 men and 93 women) who underwent curative resection for the treatment of nonsmall cell lung cancer, the Charlson Comorbidity Index was used to estimate the risk of mortality. The overall 5-year survival rate was 52% among patients with a Charlson Comorbidity Index of 0, 48% among those with an index of 1 or 2, and 28% among those with an index of 3 or more. Multivariate analysis showed that age; a Charlson comorbidity grade of 1 or 2; a Charlson comorbidity grade of 3 or more; bilobectomy; pneumonectomy; and pathologic stages IB, IIB, IIIA, IIIB, and IV were associated with impaired survival.[4]

Combining the score with physiologic parameters should therefore help in deciding whether a patient may be a candidate for surgery.

ESTIMATION OF CARDIAC RISK

The risk of major cardiac events, defined as the occurrence of ventricular fibrillation, pulmonary edema, complete heart block, cardiac arrest, or cardiac death, during admission has been reported to be approximately 3% after major anatomic lung resection.[5,6] Typical candidates for pulmonary surgery for the management of lung cancer usually have both pulmonary and cardiac diseases as a result of cigarette smoking and are potentially at increased risk for perioperative cardiovascular complications. Unfortunately, the available literature specific to cardiac risk in patients undergoing surgery for the management of lung cancer is minimal, and most of what can currently be recommended must be extrapolated from literature on intraabdominal surgery and suprainguinal vascular surgery, both of which, like lung resection, are regarded as high-risk procedures from a cardiac standpoint.[5,7]

A recent study using Surveillance, Epidemiology, and End Results Medicare data on patients undergoing resection for the management of lung cancer within 1 year after coronary stenting showed that patients who had been treated with stenting had higher rates of major cardiovascular events and mortality (9.3% and 7.7%, respectively) in comparison with those who had not (4.9% and 4.6%, respectively; $p < 0.0001$ for both comparisons).[8]

Two organizations have produced guidelines on the evaluation and treatment of cardiac risk factors in candidates for lung resection: (1) the European Respiratory Society/European Society of Thoracic Surgeons (ERS/ESTS) joint task force and (2) the American College of Chest Physicians (ACCP).[9,10]

In general, a detailed evaluation for coronary heart disease is not recommended for patients who have an acceptable exercise tolerance or a Revised Cardiac Risk Index (RCRI) of less than 2.5.[7,11,12]

The RCRI, as originally described by Lee et al.,[5] is a four-class cardiac risk score with six factors, including a history of coronary artery disease, cerebrovascular accident, insulin-dependent diabetes, congestive heart failure, a serum creatinine level of greater than 2 mg/dL, and high-risk surgery. All factors are equally weighted, and one point is assigned for the presence of each factor.[5]

Although the RCRI was cited as the preferred cardiac risk score in the recently published American College of Cardiology/American Heart Association (ACC/AHA) and European Society of Cardiology/European Society of Anaesthesiology guidelines as well as by the joint ERS/ESTS task force on fitness for radical treatment of patients with lung cancer,[7,9,13] this score originally was developed from a generic surgical population that included only a small group of thoracic patients. Brunelli et al.[6] recently recalibrated the RCRI in a study involving a large population of candidates for major anatomic lung resection to obtain a more specific tool for our setting. In that study, only four of the original six factors were found to be reliably associated with major cardiac morbidity and these four factors were assigned different weights (history of coronary artery disease, 1.5 points; cerebrovascular disease, 1.5 points; serum creatinine level of greater than 2 mg/dL, 1 point; and pneumonectomy, 1.5 points). The resulting aggregate score, ranging from 0 to 5.5 points and named the ThRCRI, was found to be more accurate than the traditional score in this population (c index, 0.72 compared with 0.62; $p = 0.004$). The risk of major cardiac events was 23% for patients with an aggregate score of more than 2.5 (class D), compared with 1.5% for those with a score of 0 (class A).

The ThRCRI was subsequently validated in a number of studies.[6,15] Most recently, the score was tested and validated in a large population of patients who were included in the Society of Thoracic Surgeons (STS) database.[16] Major cardiovascular complications were reported in 4.3% of more than 26,000 patients who underwent pulmonary anatomic resection. The average ThRCRI score for patients without major cardiovascular complications was half of that for patients with complications (0.6 compared with 1.1; $p < 0.0001$). Incremental differences in the risk of major cardiovascular complications were noted among the score categories (grade A, 2.9%; grade B, 5.8%; grade C, 11.9%; grade D, 11.1%; $p < 0.0001$). On the basis of this recent evidence, the ACCP guidelines included this parameter in their updated cardiac algorithm.

According to the ACC/AHA guidelines,[7] noninvasive cardiac evaluation is recommended for patients with limited capacity for exercise, those with a ThRCRI of more than 1.5, and those with a known or newly suspected cardiac condition to identify the relatively small proportion of patients who need intensified intervention to control heart failure or arrhythmias or to treat underlying myocardial ischemia.

Appropriately aggressive cardiac interventions should be instituted before surgery only for patients who would need such interventions irrespective of the planned surgery. However, prophylactic coronary revascularization before surgery in patients who otherwise do not need such a procedure does not appear to reduce perioperative risk.[17] McFalls et al.[17] recently demonstrated that, in a population of patients undergoing major elective vascular surgery who had concomitant stenosis of more than 70% in one or more coronary vessels, prophylactic percutaneous coronary intervention or coronary artery bypass grafting did not change the risk of 30-day mortality, postoperative myocardial ischemia, or long-term survival.

Recent data from the Perioperative Ischemic Evaluation study group indicated that although commonly used regimens of perioperative beta-blockers reduced the risk of cardiovascular death and nonfatal myocardial ischemia (hazard ratio, 0.84), they actually increased the risk of stroke (hazard ratio, 2.17) and overall mortality (hazard ratio, 1.33), perhaps by interfering with stress responses in critically ill patients.[18] Therefore, the new institution of a beta-blocker therapy is not recommended for patients with ischemic heart disease who are not already taking them.

Finally, CPET has been shown to be a useful tool for detecting both overt and occult exercise-induced myocardial ischemia with a diagnostic accuracy similar to single-photon emission computed tomographic myocardial perfusion testing and superior to standard electrocardiographic stress testing.[19–21] For this reason, CPET can be proposed as a noninvasive test for detecting and quantifying myocardial perfusion defects in patients who are at increased risk for coronary artery disease.

PREDICTED POSTOPERATIVE FORCED EXPIRATORY VOLUME IN 1 SECOND

ppoFEV$_1$, which is estimated on the basis of the number of functioning, nonobstructed segments to be removed during an operation, traditionally has been used to stratify respiratory risk in candidates for lung resection. The following equations can be applied to estimate the residual lung function.

For candidates for pneumonectomy, the perfusion method is used with the following formula:

$$ppoFEV_1 = preoperative\ FEV_1 \times$$
$$(1 - fraction\ of\ total\ perfusion\ for\ the\ resected\ lung)$$

A quantitative radionuclide perfusion scan is performed to measure the fraction of total perfusion for the resected lung. For candidates for lobectomy, the anatomic method is used with the following formula:

$$ppoFEV_1 = preoperative\ FEV_1 \times (1 - a/b)$$

The number of functional or unobstructed lung segments to be removed is represented by a, and the total number of functional segments is represented by b.[22]

The findings of bronchoscopy and computerized tomographic scanning should be used to assess and estimate the patency of the bronchus and segmental structure.

Many studies have investigated the role of ppoFEV$_1$ in predicting postoperative complications and in selecting patients for surgery. Olsen et al.[23] were the first to suggest a safety threshold value of 0.8 L as the lower limit for surgical resection. However, Pate et al.[24] found that patients with a mean ppoFEV$_1$ of as low as 0.7 L tolerated thoracotomy for the resection of lung cancer. The main limitation of those early studies is that they used an absolute value of ppoFEV$_1$. This method might prevent older patients, patients of small stature, and female patients, all of whom might tolerate a lower absolute FEV$_1$, from having a potentially curative resection for the management of lung cancer.

Markos et al.[25] were the first to propose using a percentage of the predicted value as the cutoff value. They found that half of the patients with a ppoFEV$_1$ of less than 40% of the predicted value died in the perioperative period. Other authors confirmed that perioperative risk increases substantially when the ppoFEV$_1$ is less than 40% of the predicted normal value.[26-32] The predictive role of ppoFEV$_1$ recently was challenged in investigations that showed an acceptable mortality rate among patients with prohibitive FEV$_1$ or ppoFEV$_1$ values who underwent lung resection.[33,34]

Alam et al.[35] demonstrated that the odds ratio for the development of postoperative respiratory complications increased as the ppoFEV$_1$ and ppoDLCO decreased (with a 10% increase in the

risk of complications for every 5% decrease in predicted postoperative lung function). Brunelli et al.[33] showed that ppoFEV$_1$ was not associated with an increased risk of complications in those with FEV$_1$ less than 70%.

These findings may be partly explained by the so-called lobar volume reduction effect, which can reduce functional loss in patients with airflow limitations. In candidates for lobectomy with lung cancer and moderate-to-severe COPD, resection of the most affected parenchyma may determine an actual improvement in the elastic recoil, a reduction of the airflow resistance, and an improvement in pulmonary mechanics and ventilation–perfusion matching, similar to what happens in typical candidates for lung volume reduction surgery with end-stage heterogeneous emphysema.

In this regard, many studies already have shown the minimal loss or even improvement of pulmonary function after lobectomy in patients with obstruction, calling into question the traditional operability criteria that are primarily based on pulmonary parameters.[36–43]

Brunelli et al.[42] recently found that patients with COPD had significantly lower losses of FEV$_1$ and DLCO compared with patients without COPD at 3 months after lobectomy for the management of lung cancer (8% compared with 16% and 3% compared with 12%, respectively). In that series, 27% of patients with COPD actually had improvement in FEV$_1$ and 34% had improvement in DLCO at 3 months after the operation.

This lobar volume reduction effect takes place very early after lung resection. In fact, 17% of patients with airflow limitation who undergo pulmonary lobectomy actually may have improvement in FEV$_1$ at the time of discharge as compared with preoperative measurement.[44]

The early lobar volume reduction effect was confirmed by Varela et al.[45] who showed that the percentage loss of FEV$_1$ on the first postoperative day after lobectomy was lower in patients with a higher degree of COPD. These findings indicate that ppoFEV$_1$ may not work properly in patients with obstructive disease and cannot be used alone to select patients for surgery, especially those with limited pulmonary function.

Although many studies have shown that ppoFEV$_1$ is fairly accurate for predicting the definitive residual FEV$_1$ at 3 months to 6 months after surgery, Varela et al.[46] recently demonstrated that it substantially overestimates the actual FEV$_1$ in the first postoperative days, when most complications occur. On the first postoperative day, the actual FEV$_1$ was measured to be about 30% lower than predicted.[46] This finding may have serious clinical implications whenever ppoFEV$_1$ is used for patient selection and risk stratification before surgery.

CARBON MONOXIDE LUNG DIFFUSION CAPACITY

In 1988, Ferguson et al.[47] reported that DLCO was a predictor of adverse outcomes after pulmonary resection; in that study, patients with a DLCO of less than 60% had mortality rates as high as 20% and pulmonary complication rates as high as 40%. These findings were subsequently confirmed by other authors.[25,26]

In addition to being a good predictor of immediate postoperative complications, DLCO is probably the objective parameter that is most closely associated with postoperative quality of life.[48]

ppoDLCO, calculated in the same manner as ppoFEV$_1$, was first shown to be a reliable predictor of pulmonary complications and mortality in 1995.[49] In that series, patients with a ppoDLCO of less than 40% had a mortality rate as high as 23%. Those results were subsequently confirmed by Santini et al.[50] who found an inverse linear correlation between pulmonary complications and ppoDLCO. Patients with a ppoDLCO of less than 30% may have a risk of pulmonary complications of greater than 80%. Recent studies have shown that FEV$_1$ and DLCO are poorly correlated and that more than 40% of patients with a normal

FEV_1 (an FEV_1 of more than 80%) may have a DLCO of less than 80% and that 7% of patients with FEV_1 >80% may have a ppoDLCO of 40%.[51] Other studies have demonstrated that a reduced ppoDLCO is a reliable predictor of cardiopulmonary morbidity and mortality not only in patients with reduced FEV_1 but also in those with normal respiratory function.[51,52] In a recent large study involving approximately 8000 patients from the STS General Thoracic Surgery Database who were treated with lung resection, the percentage of predicted DLCO was strongly associated with the occurrence of pulmonary complications.[53] This association was independent from the COPD status.

On the basis of this evidence, recent functional guidelines have recommended the measurement of DLCO in all candidates for lung resection, regardless of the preoperative FEV_1 value.[9,10]

Many patients undergoing major lung resection for the management of cancer receive preoperative chemotherapy. Recent reports have suggested that chemotherapy can be associated with a 10% to 20% reduction in DLCO despite stable or improved spirometric values.[54–57] These changes are associated with drug-induced structural lung damage and have been associated with an increase in postoperative respiratory complications.[55,56,58,59] Therefore reassessment of pulmonary status and DLCO after induction therapy and prior to resection is recommended to ensure that the operative risk has not increased as a result of newly impaired DLCO.[9,10]

VIDEO-ASSISTED THORACOSCOPIC SURGERY

Several reports have shown reduced rates of morbidity among patients who are treated with minimally invasive video-assisted thoracoscopic surgery (VATS) lobectomy.[60–63] This finding is likely explained by the minimal impact of this operation on the chest wall mechanics. This effect is particularly evident in patients with compromised pulmonary function. Berry et al.[64] reported that, in patients with an FEV_1 of less than 60% or a DLCO of less than 60% who underwent pulmonary lobectomy with use of either thoracotomy or VATS, thoracotomy was a strong predictor of complications on multivariable analysis (odds ratio, 3.46; $p = 0.0007$).[64] FEV_1 and DLCO remained predictors of complications in patients undergoing thoracotomy but not thoracoscopy.

Similarly, in a large population of patients in the STS database who underwent lobectomy, multivariable regression analysis showed that thoracotomy (odds ratio, 1.25; $p < 0.001$), decreasing FEV_1% predicted (odds ratio, 1.01 per unit; $p < 0.001$), and DLCO% predicted (odds ratio, 1.01 per unit; $p < 0.001$) independently predicted pulmonary complications.[65] Among patients with an FEV_1 of less than 60%, the rate of pulmonary complications was markedly increased among those who underwent thoracotomy as compared with those who underwent VATS ($p = 0.023$).[65] No significant difference was noted among patients with an FEV_1 of more than 60% of the predicted value. More recently, Burt et al. (Burt BM, Kosinski AS, Shrager JB, Onaitis MW, Weigel T. Thoracoscopic lobectomy is associated with acceptable morbidity and mortality in patients with predicted postoperative forced expiratory volume in 1 second or diffusing capacity for carbon monoxide less than 40% of normal. J Thorac Cardiovasc Surg. 2014 Jul;148(1):19–28) have shown that patients operated on through VATS and with prohibitive ppoFEV$_1$ or ppoDLCO below 40% of predicted value have a far lower risk of mortality compared with case-matched counterparts operated on through thoracotomy. For patients with ppoFEV$_1$% less than 40%, mortality was 4.8% in the open group versus 0.7% in the VATS group ($p = 0.003$). Similar results were seen for ppoDLCO% less than 40% (5.2% open, 2.0% VATS, $p = 0.003$).[65a]

Other studies have shown better preservation of pulmonary function compared with preoperative values in patients undergoing VATS lobectomy than in those undergoing thoracotomy.[66,67]

At this time, the evidence is still too limited to justify a change in the current functional guidelines. However, it appears likely that with the increasing number of patients who are treated with the VATS approach, we will be able to verify whether traditional pulmonary thresholds of operability (mostly derived from series of patients undergoing thoracotomy) should be updated.

EXERCISE TESTING

Exercise testing is increasingly used in the preoperative workup of candidates for lung resection. These tests can be used to assess the entire oxygen-transport system and to detect possible deficits that may predispose to postoperative complications.[68]

In fact, exercise increases the utilization of oxygen peripherally and requires the entire interlocking lung–heart–vascular oxygen transport system to react.[68] In the lung, exercise determines an increase in ventilation, VO_2, carbon dioxide excretion, and blood flow, similar to those experienced after lung resection. Therefore the potential exists to evaluate much of the cardiopulmonary system with just one test.

Several tests can be used in clinical practice. These tests can be classified as low-technology tests, involving a limited use of resources and personnel, and high-technology tests, such as the cardiopulmonary test, involving direct measurement of the expired gases during incremental exercise on a bicycle or treadmill.

Low-Technology Tests

The most frequently used low-technology tests in our specialty are the 6-Minute Walking Test, Shuttle Walk Test, and Stair-Climbing Test.

6-Minute Walking Test

Conflicting reports have been published regarding the 6-Minute to 12-Minute Walking Test for the evaluation of candidates for lung resection. Some investigators have not found this type of exercise to be predictive of complications,[25,69] whereas others have found it to be predictive of mortality in patients with high respiratory risk (an FEV_1 of less than 1.6 L). Pierce et al.[26] found that the 6-Minute Walking Test was predictive of respiratory failure but not of mortality or other complications. The test is not a maximal exercise test and may not be stressful enough in all patients to reveal deficits of the oxygen-transport system. Because of these inconsistent findings, the recent ERS/ESTS joint task force on fitness for radical therapy did not recommend its use for preoperative risk-stratification before lung resection.[9]

Shuttle Walk Test

The Shuttle Walk Test is certainly more reproducible than the 6-Minute Walk Test. In one study, regression analysis indicated that 25 shuttles on the Shuttle Walk Test indicate a VO_{2peak} of 10 mL/kg/min.[70]

However, more recent studies have challenged this conclusion, showing that the distance walked on the Shuttle Walk Test did not differ between patients with and without complications and that the test appeared to underestimate exercise capacity at the lower range compared with peak oxygen consumption.[71] Benzo and Sciurba[72] recently showed that VO measured during the Shuttle Walk Test is highly correlated with the level (or minute) of the test. A cutoff of 25 shuttles walked had a positive predictive value of 90% for predicting a VO_{2peak} of more than 15 mL/kg/min. The recent ACCP functional guidelines recommend use of the Shuttle Walk Test or the Stair-Climbing Test as low-technology exercise tests for patients with lung cancer who are being considered for surgery if either the $ppoFEV_1$ or ppoDLCO is less than 60% of the predicted value and both are above 30% of the predicted value.[10]

Stair-Climbing Test

The Stair-Climbing Test has several advantages in that it is familiar to patients; is economic, requires little in terms of resources, personnel, and equipment; and is rapid and non-invasive. However, it is very stressful for patients in that they are pushed to reach a visible objective represented by the next landing.

The Stair-Climbing Test has been used for decades.[73] Van Nostrand et al.,[74] in what we believe to have been the first published retrospective report in which the Stair-Climbing Test was included in the preoperative evaluation, found that patients who were unable to climb two flights of stairs had a 50% rate of mortality after pneumonectomy.

In a report on 54 patients who performed the Stair-Climbing Test before lung resection, Olsen et al.[75] found that the ability to climb three flights of stairs most clearly separated patients who had a longer hospital stay, postoperative intubation, and a greater frequency of complications. Holden et al.,[28] in a series of high-risk patients with an FEV_1 of less than 1.6 L, found that those who had fatal complications after lung resection had climbed fewer steps than those who had few or no complications (42 compared with 71; $p < 0.05$). Climbing more than 44 steps was predictive of a successful surgical outcome.

In 2001, Girish et al.,[76] in a prospective evaluation of 83 patients undergoing thoracotomy or upper abdominal laparotomy surgery, found that patients with complications climbed significantly fewer flights of stairs than those without complications (2.1 compared with 4.4; $p = 0.00002$). The inability to climb two flights of stairs was associated with a positive predictive value of 80%; conversely, the ability to climb more than five flights of stairs was associated with a negative predictive value of 95%.

In a series on 160 patients, Brunelli et al.[77] found that only 6.5% of patients who climbed more than 14 m in altitude had complications. However, 29% of patients who climbed between 12 m and 14 m and 50% of those who climbed less than 12 m had complications. This progressive increase in the rate of cardiopulmonary morbidity with the reduction in the altitude climbed preoperatively indirectly demonstrates that stair climbing is a stressful test that is capable of revealing severe deficits in maximum aerobic capacity. In the same study, Brunelli et al.[77] observed only four complications and no mortality in a high-risk group of 17 patients with a $ppoFEV_1$ of less than 35% and/or a ppoDLCO of less 35% who were judged to be operable on the basis of the satisfactory performance on the Stair-Climbing Test.

These findings were subsequently confirmed in a larger series of 640 major anatomic resections,[78] in which the height climbed during the preoperative Stair-Climbing Test discriminated between patients with and without complications. In particular, compared with patients who were able to climb more than 22 m, those who did not reach 12 m had a 2.5-fold higher rate of cardiopulmonary complications, a 3-fold higher rate of cardiac complications, and a 13-fold higher mortality rate (13% compared with only 1%). In the 73 patients with prohibitive pulmonary function (a $ppoFEV_1$ <40% or a ppoDLCO <40%, or both), all of those who climbed more than 22 m survived the operation, whereas 2 of the 10 who climbed less than 12 m died.

Brunelli et al.[79] showed a direct correlation between the height climbed and the VO_2 measured during the Stair-Climbing Test with a portable gas analyzer. Ninety-eight percent of patients who climbed more than 22 m had a VO_{2peak} of more than 15 mL/kg/min. The cutoff value of 22 m had a positive predictive value of 86% for predicting a VO_{2peak} of more than 15 mL/kg/min.

On the basis of these findings, the ERS/ESTS guidelines on fitness for radical therapy recommended the Stair-Climbing Test as an alternative screening test in cases in which formal CPET is not readily available.[9] However, in cases of reduced performance (i.e., height of <22 m), patients should be referred for CPETs for a better evaluation of aerobic reserve. Furthermore, the recent ACCP functional guidelines recommended the use of this test as a first-line test for patients with either a $ppoFEV_1$ or a ppoDLCO of between 60% and 30% predicted.[10] For patients climbing less than 22 m, however, a formal CPET is recommended to exactly detect the deficit in the oxygen-transport system.

Cardiopulmonary Exercise Test

The CPET is the criterion standard for the preoperative evaluation of candidates for lung resection. It is performed in a controlled environment with continuous monitoring of various cardiologic and pulmonary parameters, it is standardized and easily reproducible in different settings, and, in addition to VO_{2peak}, which certainly remains the most important parameter associated with exercise capacity, it provides several other direct and derived measures that can be used, in cases of limited aerobic reserve, to precisely identify possible deficits in the oxygen-transport system.[80,81]

Responses such as the VT, VE/VCO_2 slope, VE/VCO_2 at peak exercise, oscillatory ventilation, oxygen uptake on kinetics, rate of recovery of VO_2, and oxygen uptake efficiency slope have been used with greater frequency to classify functional limitations and to stratify risk in patients with heart disease. Many of these responses are expressions of ventilatory efficiency and reflect the various underlying pathophysiologic factors leading to inefficient breathing associated with heart failure or pulmonary disease.

Findings from the CPET have important clinical implications as it allows for the institution of specific treatments to optimize perioperative management (such as optimization of COPD treatment, management of ischemic heart disease, rehabilitation) to improve the overall status of the cardiopulmonary system and reduce surgical risk.

The ERS/ESTS functional guidelines emphasized the role of high-technology exercise testing. Ideally, all patients with an FEV_1 or DLCO (or both) of less than 80% of the predicted value and those with a history of cardiac disease should perform this test.[9]

The recent ACCP functional guidelines also emphasize this methodology.[10] A CPET is recommended for patients with lung cancer and candidates for lung resection with either a $ppoFEV_1$ or a ppoDLCO of less than 30% predicted, an altitude of less than 22 m reached on the Stair-Climbing Test, or a positive high-risk cardiac evaluation. This recommendation is based on several studies that showed the importance of VO_{2peak} in predicting cardiopulmonary complications and mortality in our specialty. The importance of maximum rate of oxygen consumption (VO_{2max}) in our specialty was first suggested by Eugene et al.[82] in 1982.

In that small study of 19 patients, the authors found that a VO_{2max} of less than 1000 mL was associated with a 75% mortality, whereas FEV_1 and forced vital capacity (FVC) had no predictive value in terms of postoperative complications. Subsequently, other small studies in the 1980s and early 1990s confirmed these findings.[83–85]

In 1995, Bolliger et al.[86] demonstrated that VO_{2max} had a better discriminatory ability when expressed as percentage of predicted value rather than as an absolute value. The authors found that the probability of complications was only 10% in patients with a VO_{2max} of greater than 75% of the predicted value, whereas it was as high as 90% in those with VO_{2max} below 40% of the predicted value.

The same group subsequently confirmed the importance of this parameter in a different group of patients.[87] They were able to develop a model predicting the risk of cardiopulmonary complications on the basis of the extent of resection and preoperative VO_{2max}. For instance, in a patient undergoing pneumonectomy with a VO_{2peak} of 50%, the risk of morbidity may be as high as 86%. In that series, the authors found that the morbidity rate was as high as 86% for patients with VO_{2peak} of lower than 60% of the predicted value, compared with only 12% for those with VO_{2peak} of greater than 90%.

In a large series involving more than 400 patients from the Cancer and Leukemia Group B national multicenter database, Loewen et al.[88] showed that patients with complications had a significantly lower VO_{2max} compared with patients without complications and confirmed the findings of the aforementioned studies.

Brunelli et al.,[89] in a recent study of more than 200 patients undergoing major anatomic lung resections with complete CPET evaluation before surgery, confirmed the safety threshold of 20 mL/kg/min (with a 0% rate of mortality and a 7% rate of cardiopulmonary morbidity) but found that values of VO_{2peak} below 12 mL/kg/min increased the risk of mortality. In such patients, the cardiopulmonary morbidity and mortality rates may be as high as 33% and 13%, respectively. Interestingly, in that large series, 43% of all patients had a preoperative VO_{2peak} below 15 mL/kg/min (with only 14% of patients having a VO_{2peak} of greater than 20 mL/kg/min), reflecting the case mix of patients who undergo modern thoracic surgery. These patients are generally elderly and unfit, with underlying cardiopulmonary comorbidities, and we should be ready to accept such levels of VO_{2peak} in our practices.

A recent meta-analysis confirmed the importance and the ability of VO_{2peak} to predict cardiopulmonary complications or mortality after pulmonary resection.[90] The authors of most studies generally agreed that a VO_{2max} value below 10 mL/kg/min to 15 mL/kg/min should be regarded as a high-risk threshold for lung resection and that values above 20 mL/kg/min are safe for any kind of resection, including pneumonectomy.

Similar to ppoFEV₁ and ppoDLCO a segmental estimation of VO_{2max} was suggested by Bolliger et al.,[27] who found that a value of $ppoVO_{2max}$ of less than 10 mL/kg/min (or 35% of the predicted value) was the only parameter that retrospectively identified all three patients who died in a subgroup of 25 patients at increased risk for postresectional complications.

In addition to VO_{2max}, CPET can provide several other direct and indirect measures, which can help to refine the preoperative risk stratification. Several authors have reported on such derived parameters (i.e., efficiency slope, oxygen pulse, VE/VCO₂ slope), which proved to be predictive of cardiac and pulmonary complications.[80,91,92]

ALGORITHMS

For practical reasons, published evidence on operability and functional assessment is often summarized in algorithms or flowcharts. Algorithms should be used as guides to standardize the preoperative clinical practice by minimizing variations and inappropriate exclusions. However, this schematic representation cannot capture the entire spectrum of patients, and exceptions may occur. Patients should always be evaluated individually.

The two most recent functional algorithms are those proposed by the ERS/ESTS joint task force on fitness for radical therapy and the ACCP lung cancer guidelines.[9,10] Both algorithms emphasize the importance of a preliminary cardiologic evaluation.

Patients with low cardiologic risk or with an optimized cardiologic treatment may proceed with the rest of the functional workup. Both algorithms recommend measurement of FEV₁ and DLCO in all patients. These two parameters must be expressed as percentages of predicted values.

In the ERS/ESTS flowchart (Fig. 26.1), patients without active cardiac problems and low cardiac risk and with both FEV₁ and DLCO greater than 80% of predicted values can be safely treated with the planned resection, including pneumonectomy. All other patients with an FEV₁ and/or DLCO below 80% of the predicted value should undergo an exercise test. Ideally, a formal CPET with VO_{2peak} measurement should be performed. However, in many settings, this test is not readily available because of logistic or organizational reasons. In these circumstances, a low-technology exercise test, preferably the Stair-Climbing Test, can be used as a screening test. Patients showing optimal performance on these tests (more than 22 m on the Stair-Climbing Test or more than 400 m on the Shuttle Walk Test) can proceed to surgery, whereas all other patients (those with <22 m on the Stair-Climbing Test or <400 m on the Shuttle Walk Test) should undergo a formal CPET to better define aerobic capacity.

In patients with borderline VO_{2peak} (between 10 mL/kg/min and 20 mL/kg/min or between 35% and 75% of predicted values), split lung function should be taken into consideration with estimation of ppoFEV₁ and ppoDLCO. Patients with borderline ergometric parameters and both ppoFEV₁ and ppoDLCO greater than 30% of the predicted value can proceed with the planned surgery. In all the others, $ppoVO_{2peak}$ should be estimated in a similar fashion as ppoFEV₁. If $ppoVO_{2peak}$ is lower than 10 mL/kg/min or 35% of the predicted value, the patient should be advised to choose alternative treatments as lobectomy or pneumonectomy is not recommended.

In the ACCP flowchart (Fig. 26.2), patients who are deemed to be at low cardiologic risk and who have ppoFEV₁ and ppoDLCO values that are both greater than 60% of predicted values are regarded as low risk for surgery (with a risk of mortality <1%). Patients with either a ppoFEV₁ or a ppoDLCO between 30% and 60% should perform a low-technology exercise test as a screening test. If the performance on the low-technology exercise test is satisfactory, the patient is regarded as being at moderate risk (morbidity and mortality rates may vary according to the values of split lung function, exercise tolerance, and extent of resection). A CPET is indicated only in cases in which the ppoFEV₁ or ppoDLCO values are lower than 30% or when the performance on the Stair-Climbing Test or Shuttle Walk Test is not satisfactory (i.e., an altitude of <22 m on the Stair-Climbing Test or a distance of <400 m on the Shuttle Walk Test). As in the European algorithm, VO_{2peak} values lower than 10 mL/kg/min or 35% of the predicted value indicate a high risk for major anatomic resection through thoracotomy; in such patients the risk of mortality may be higher than 10%, and considerable risk of severe cardiopulmonary morbidity and residual functional loss is expected. Conversely, VO_{2peak} values of greater than 20 mL/kg/min or 75% of predicted value indicate low risk.

SMOKING CESSATION

Although many patients with lung cancer stop smoking years before a tumor becomes symptomatic, a considerable number of patients are still current smokers at the time of diagnosis. Literature on whether stopping smoking preoperatively

26

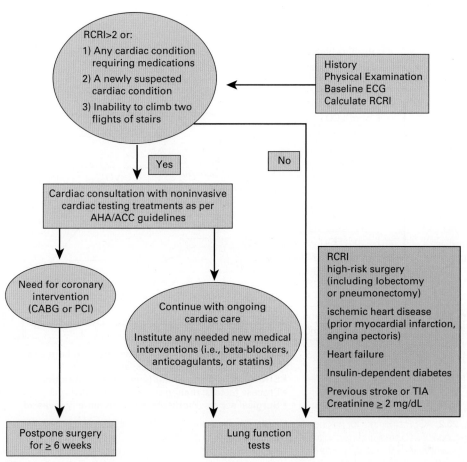

Fig. 26.1. ERS/ESTS algorithm for preoperative functional evaluation. *AHA/ACC*, American Heart Association/American College of Cardiology; *CABG*, coronary artery bypass grafting; *ECG*, electrocardiogram; *ERS/ESTS*, European Respiratory Society/European Society of Thoracic Surgeons; *PCI*, percutaneous coronary intervention; *RCRI*, Revised Cardiac Risk Index; *TIA*, transient ischemic attack. *(Reproduced from Brunelli A, Charloux A, Bolliger CT, et al. ERS/ESTS clinical guidelines on fitness for radical therapy in lung cancer patients (surgery and chemo-radiotherapy). Eur Respir J. 2009;34:17–41.)*

improves outcome is far from robust, and the systematic review by Schmidt-Hansen et al.[93] did not lead to any firm conclusions. Retrospective studies have demonstrated a reduced number of pulmonary complications as well as a reduced rate of perioperative mortality for nonsmokers as compared with current and former smokers, with longer abstinence associated with a favorable trend.[94,95] The effect of smoking cessation might extend beyond the perioperative period as the quality of life in quitters is much better than in persistent smokers.[96] In a population of patients with lung cancer with a clear difference in histologic findings between first and second primary tumors, there was a trend for a much higher risk of developing a second primary tumor among those who continue to smoke.[97] Overall, physicians should encourage their patients to quit smoking prior to the operation and should emphasize that the earlier they quit, the better, as the effects of smoking cessation are immediate and long-lasting.

PULMONARY REHABILITATION

In general, there is growing evidence that preoperative conditioning is advantageous; however, these standard programs generally last 6 weeks to 12 weeks. Because it is necessary for patients with malignant disease to undergo surgery without delay, effective short-term preoperative pulmonary rehabilitation programs should be adopted. Data to support the routine use of pulmonary rehabilitation are not robust.[98] Patients in poor condition who are expected to have the highest risk of perioperative problems seem to benefit most from a short (4-week) training program.[98] This may as well have consequences for the patients who are preoperatively treated with chemotherapy and have a considerable risk of weight loss as well as deconditioning.

CONCLUSION

Patients with lung cancer often have several problems related to the harmful effects of smoking. It is therefore necessary to evaluate these patients in a timely and effective way to find out if there is a possibility for those staged with resectable disease. These evaluations should clarify the potential cardiopulmonary risks during and after the operation. For patients who are found to be operable, measures should be taken to prevent perioperative and postoperative complications as much as possible. Smoking cessation and rehabilitation are part of this risk reduction.

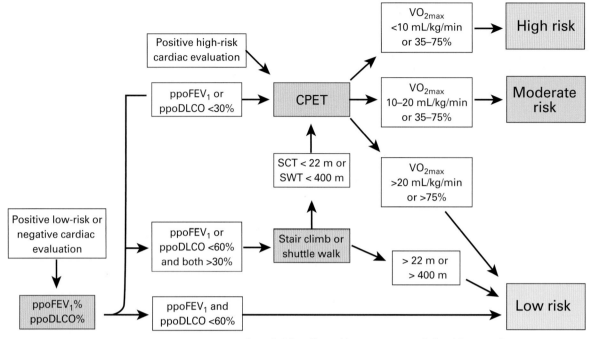

Fig. 26.2. ACCP algorithm for preoperative functional evaluation. *ACCP,* American College of Chest Physicians; *ppoDLCO,* predicted postoperative carbon monoxide lung diffusion capacity; *ppoFEV₁,* predicted postoperative forced expiratory volume in 1 second; *CPET,* cardiopulmonary exercise test; *SCT,* Stair-Climbing Test; *SWT,* Shuttle Walk Test. *(Reproduced with permission from Brunelli A, Kim AW, Berger KI, Addrizzo-Harris DJ. Physiologic evaluation of the patient with lung cancer being considered for resectional surgery: diagnosis and management of lung cancer, 3rd ed: American College of Chest Physicians evidence-based clinical practice guidelines. Chest. 2013;143(5 Suppl):e166S–190S.)*

KEY REFERENCES

6. Brunelli A, Varela G, Salati M, et al. Recalibration of the revised cardiac risk index in lung resection candidates. *Ann Thorac Surg.* 2010;90(1):199–203.
7. Fleisher LA, Beckman JA, Brown KA, et al. ACC/AHA 2007 guidelines on perioperative cardiovascular evaluation and care for noncardiac surgery: a report of the American College of Cardiology/American Heart Association Task Force on Practice Guidelines (Writing Committee to Revise the 2002 Guidelines on Perioperative Cardiovascular Evaluation for Noncardiac Surgery) developed in collaboration with the American Society of Echocardiography, American Society of Nuclear Cardiology, Heart Rhythm Society, Society of Cardiovascular Anesthesiologists, Society for Cardiovascular Angiography and Interventions, Society for Vascular Medicine and Biology, and Society for Vascular Surgery. *J Am Coll Cardiol.* 2007;8(50):e159–e241.
9. Brunelli A, Charloux A, Bolliger CT, et al. ERS/ESTS clinical guidelines on fitness for radical therapy in lung cancer patients (surgery and chemo-radiotherapy). *Eur Respir J.* 2009;34:17–41.
10. Brunelli A, Kim AW, Berger KI, Addrizzo-Harris DJ. Physiologic evaluation of the patient with lung cancer being considered for resectional surgery: diagnosis and management of lung cancer, 3rd ed: American College of Chest Physicians evidence-based clinical practice guidelines. *Chest.* 2013;143(suppl 5):e166S–e190S.
13. Poldermans D, Bax JJ, Boersma E, et al. Guidelines for pre-operative cardiac risk assessment and perioperative cardiac management in non-cardiac surgery: the task force for preoperative cardiac risk assessment and perioperative cardiac management in non-cardiac surgery of the European Society of Cardiology (ESC) and endorsed by the European Society of Anaesthesiology (ESA). *Eur Heart J.* 2009;30:2769–2812.
17. McFalls EO, Ward HB, Moritz TE, et al. Coronary-artery revascularization before elective major vascular surgery. *N Engl J Med.* 2004;351(27):2795–2804.
19. Pinkstaff S, Peberdy MA, Kontos MC, Fabiato A, Finucane S, Arena R. Usefulness of decrease in oxygen uptake efficiency slope to identify myocardial perfusion defects in men undergoing myocardial ischemic evaluation. *Am J Cardiol.* 2010;106(11):1534–1539.
43. Sekine Y, Iwata T, Chiyo M, et al. Minimal alteration of pulmonary function after lobectomy in lung cancer patients with chronic obstructive pulmonary disease. *Ann Thorac Surg.* 2003;76(2):356–361.
47. Ferguson MK, Little L, Rizzo L, et al. Diffusing capacity predicts morbidity and mortality after pulmonary resection. *J Thorac Cardiovasc Surg.* 1988;96(6):894–900.
51. Brunelli A, Refai MA, Salati M, Sabbatini A, Morgan-Hughes NJ, Rocco G. Carbon monoxide lung diffusion capacity improves risk stratification in patients without airflow limitation: evidence for systematic measurement before lung resection. *Eur J Cardiothorac Surg.* 2006;29(4):567–570.
52. Ferguson MK, Vigneswaran WT. Diffusing capacity predicts morbidity after lung resection in patients without obstructive lung disease. *Ann Thorac Surg.* 2008;85(4):1158–1164.
60. Paul S, Altorki NK, Sheng S, et al. Thoracoscopic lobectomy is associated with lower morbidity than open lobectomy: a propensity-matched analysis from the STS database. *J Thorac Cardiovasc Surg.* 2010;139(2):366–378.
64. Berry MF, Villamizar-Ortiz NR, Tong BC, et al. Pulmonary function tests do not predict pulmonary complications after thoracoscopic lobectomy. *Ann Thorac Surg.* 2010;89(4):1044–1051.

86. Bolliger CT, Jordan P, Solèr M, et al. Exercise capacity as a predictor of postoperative complications in lung resection candidates. *Am J Respir Crit Care Med*. 1995;151:1472–1480.

89. Brunelli A, Belardinelli R, Refai M, et al. Peak oxygen consumption during cardiopulmonary exercise test improves risk stratification in candidates to major lung resection. *Chest*. 2009;135:1260–1267.

92. Brunelli A, Belardinelli R, Pompili C, et al. Minute ventilation-to-carbon dioxide output (VE/VCO$_2$) slope is the strongest predictor of respiratory complications and death after pulmonary resection. *Ann Thorac Surg*. 2012;93(6):1802–1806.

See Expertconsult.com for full list of references.

27 Results of Video-Assisted Techniques for Resection of Lung Cancer

Frank C. Detterbeck, Alberto Antonicelli, and Morihito Okada

SUMMARY OF KEY POINTS

- Many meta-analyses, outcomes and matched cohort studies demonstrate equal long-term outcomes for video-assisted thoracoscopic surgery (VATS) and open lobectomy.
- Matched comparisons generally demonstrate equal long-term survival for VATS versus open lobectomy for lung cancer, suggesting that the improved survival seen in unmatched studies is due to confounding factors.
- Many meta-analyses, outcomes, and matched cohort studies demonstrate similar operative mortality for VATS and open lobectomy.
- Pain, hospital length of stay, and complications are lower after VATS than after open lobectomy.
- There is no difference in the incidence of N2 nodal upstaging; the effect on N1 upstaging is unclear.
- The ability to deliver adjuvant chemotherapy may be better after VATS lobectomy.
- VATS lobectomy is associated with a learning curve of about 50 cases.

Over 100 years ago, Jacobaeus[1] first reported the diagnosis and treatment of pleural effusions using a thoracoscope. Since then, the application of thoracoscopy to pulmonary resection has advanced as a useful adjunct for surgeons, perhaps most prominently for wedge resection or pleural procedures. From the late 1980s to the 1990s, surgeons began using VATS for lobectomies to treat patients with early stage nonsmall cell lung cancer (NSCLC). In 1992, VATS simultaneously stapled lobectomy without rib spreading was reported by Lewis et al.[2] and with individual vessel and bronchial ligation was reported by Roviaro et al.[3] During the following year, the outcomes of VATS lobectomy were published by Walker et al.,[4] Coosemans et al.,[5] Kirby et al.,[6] and Hazelrigg et al.[7] The surgical approach has become far less invasive as the instrumentation has gradually improved over the past two decades and VATS has evolved into a basic and vital thoracic surgical technique.

However, the penetration of VATS anatomic resections (lobectomy and segmentectomy) has been slow to occur, and currently about 30% of anatomic resections in the United States are performed using VATS.[8–11] These VATS lobectomies in the United States are performed primarily by dedicated thoracic surgeons.[12] As reported in the database of the Society of Thoracic Surgeons (STS), which represents predominantly dedicated thoracic surgeons in the United States, the proportion of lobectomies done via VATS has increased from 19% in 2005 to 44% in 2009 and is currently 66%.[13] A similar increase from 20% to 54% from 2007 to 2011 has been reported in Denmark, which has a highly centralized health-care system.[14] Robust data about the overall proportion of lobectomies that are performed using VATS in Europe or Asia are not available, but estimates put this well below the penetration currently seen in the United States.[15]

DEFINITIONS

Video-assisted thoracoscopic surgery (VATS) is used for wedge resection, segmentectomy, lobectomy, pneumonectomy, sleeve lobectomy, lobectomy with chest wall resection, and extrapleural pneumonectomy.[16] The approaches vary substantially: reports on VATS lobectomy alone describe the use of one to six incisions from 4 cm to 10 cm in length, with and without rib spreading.[1,17,18] In general, however, VATS lobectomy is interpreted to mean an anatomic lobectomy with ligation of individual bronchi and vessels and lymph node dissection or sampling using a minimal number of ports without a retractor or rib spreading.

A clear definition of VATS lobectomy is needed. The Cancer and Leukemia Group B established a definition of VATS lobectomy for a prospective, multi-institutional trial, and this definition has been widely adopted.[19] A VATS lobectomy is defined as involving no rib spreading; maximum incisions of 8 cm; dissection of individual veins, arteries, and airways for the lobe in question; and node sampling or dissection identical to open thoracotomy.[19] This definition was endorsed by most of the 55 experts participating in the 20th Anniversary of VATS Lobectomy Conference: The Consensus Meeting, organized by the Scientific Secretariat and the International Scientific Committee of the International VATS Lobectomy Consensus Group.[20] However, several participants thought that a small retractor should be acceptable in specific circumstances, for example, when performing complex procedures such as bronchoplasty or when delivering a large specimen.

Some surgeons have suggested that VATS should include only procedures done exclusively with visualization on a monitor. This criterion should be abandoned for several reasons. The most important issues for patients with malignant diseases are the incisional trauma, achievement of curative surgery, and subsequent oncologic outcomes. Occasional viewing through a 4-cm, non–rib-spreading incision does not change the nature of the procedure. A hybrid VATS approach using both a monitor and direct vision without rib spreading or a robotic approach can provide a three-dimensional understanding of anatomy as well as magnified proximity visualization and would surely clinically facilitate complex procedures such as sleeve lobectomy or segmentectomy.[21–23]

Technical aspects of how to accomplish a VATS lobectomy are beyond the scope of this chapter and are the subject of surgical atlases. Styles vary in how surgeons perform different steps of the operation. The essential feature, however, is a hilar dissection and individual division of the vessels and bronchus of the lobe. Most often, these structures are divided using an endostapler, but ligation, division between clips, or sealing with energy devices is also feasible for smaller vessels.

Patient Selection

Patient selection ultimately depends on the surgeon's judgment about the ability to accomplish an oncologically appropriate resection of a given patient's tumor. However, some general guidance can be obtained from the opinions of experts at the

TABLE 27.1 Video-Assisted Thoracoscopic Surgery (VATS) Lobectomy Recommendations Derived From Consensus Statement of the International VATS Lobectomy Consensus Group[18]

INDICATIONS FOR VATS LOBECTOMY	
≤7 cm (T1, T2a, and T2b)	Recommended
N0 or N1 status	Recommended
Patients with previous thoracic surgery or pleurisy	Highly recommended
CONTRAINDICATIONS FOR VATS LOBECTOMY	
Chest wall involvement including rib(s)	Contraindicated
Central tumor invading hilar structure(s)	Contraindicated
FEV_1 <30%	Contraindicated
DLCO <30%	Contraindicated
PREOPERATIVE INVESTIGATIONS	
PET/CT and sampling of positive mediastinal lymph nodes	Highly recommended
Sampling of positive lymph nodes by EBUS/EUS	Recommended
VATS assessment at the time of surgery	Highly recommended
Total ipsilateral lymph node dissection in all patients	Recommended
INDICATIONS FOR CONVERSION TO OPEN THORACOTOMY	
Major bleeding	Highly recommended
Significant chest wall involvement	Recommended
Vascular sleeve	Highly recommended
Bronchial sleeve	Highly recommended
Bronchovascular sleeve	Highly recommended
TRAINING	
Number of cases to overcome steep learning curve: 50	Highly recommended
Resident case volume of a training center: >50/y	Recommended
Minimum case volume to maintain VATS skills: >20/y	Recommended
Proctoring should be necessary in all new VATS surgeons	Highly recommended
FUTURE DIRECTIONS	
Establishment of multi-institutional database	Recommended
Increased exposure of VATS lobectomy to trainees	Highly recommended
Establishment of standardized VATS lobectomy workshops	Highly recommended

Data taken from Yan T, Cao C, D'Amico TA, et al. Video-assisted thoracoscopic surgery lobectomy at 20 years: a consensus statement. *Eur J Cardiothorac Surg.* 2014;45(4):633–639.

CT, computed tomography; *DLCO,* diffusing capacity of the lungs for carbon monoxide; *EBUS,* endobronchial ultrasound; *EUS,* endoscopic ultrasound; *FEV_1,* forced expiratory volume in 1 second; *PET,* positron emission tomography.

recent Consensus Meeting (Table 27.1). Most of these experts consider VATS to be appropriate for stage I and II tumors unless there is substantial hilar involvement or the need for chest wall, bronchial, or vascular sleeve resection.

OUTCOMES: COMPARISON OF VATS AND OPEN LOBECTOMY

The scope of what can be successfully performed thoracoscopically includes pneumonectomy,[24,25] segmentectomy,[23,26] sleeve lobectomy,[21,27] and lobectomy with chest wall resection.[28] However, the literature is too limited for most of these procedures to define outcomes, and the results are confounded by patient selection, making assessment of the impact of the VATS approach per se difficult at best.

By contrast, the literature on VATS lobectomy for cancer is so abundant that we have chosen to focus our review on meta-analyses and large outcomes studies. Only a few randomized controlled trials were conducted; these were early in the VATS

experience and were small, underpowered studies. As the procedure matured and experience grew, increasing amounts of nonrandomized data showed that VATS lobectomy for cancer was safe, with outcomes similar to or better than those of open lobectomy. In the United States, the decision was made that a randomized controlled trial of VATS compared with open lobectomy would require a design to prove equivalence, which would necessitate too many patients and would not be worth the expense.[9] Hence, the strongest data come from large outcomes and propensity-matched studies and not randomized controlled trials.

To provide an evidence base for this chapter, a comprehensive literature search was carried out for studies comparing VATS with open lobectomy or segmentectomy for lung cancer. We included reports that involved a meta-analysis, a randomized controlled trial, a propensity-matched or otherwise case-matched study, or an outcomes study using a large multi-institutional database. We did not include reports of individual, single-institution comparative series without case matching. Two systematic reviews were not included because a quality assessment judged them to be poor, and they included studies that were otherwise already captured.[29,30] One meta-analysis was excluded because it focused only on three propensity-matched studies, which were already included individually.[31] Another was excluded because it used an erroneous code for VATS lobectomy.[32]

Short-Term Outcomes

The results of many studies have demonstrated that VATS lobectomy is a safe procedure (Table 27.2). These studies, including meta-analyses, propensity-matched series, case-matched series, and randomized controlled trials, demonstrate that the conversion rate from VATS to open procedure is about 5% to 10%. Most of these conversions resulted from oncologic or technical factors; bleeding was the reason for conversion in only a few studies. Furthermore, conversion from VATS to an open procedure is not associated with increased perioperative mortality or complications when compared with planned open thoracotomy.[30]

The studies included in this review (Table 27.2) almost universally show no significant difference in perioperative mortality between VATS and open lobectomy (Fig. 27.1).[9,10,14,33–54] Closer examination shows that, in fact, the trend to lower perioperative mortality rates with VATS is consistent. This lower mortality rate is true even among special populations of patients (e.g., older, frail, high pulmonary risk) in case-matched series. The length of hospital stay has been significantly lower for VATS resection in most studies (Fig. 27.2). The difference is approximately 1 day to 3 days, on average. Comparison between studies is difficult, however, because the average length of stay varies markedly, most likely reflecting differences in regional standards and the structure of the health-care system.

The overall rate of complications is also significantly lower in VATS resection in most studies (Table 27.2, Fig. 27.3).[10,33–35,37,39–47,50–54] Comparison of complications among studies is difficult because of the varying definitions of a complication and the degree of severity of complications that were counted. Certain specific relevant complications have been reported in some studies (Table 27.3).[10,34–45,50,52–55] A fairly consistent trend toward lower rates of pneumonia, prolonged air leak, arrhythmia, and need for postoperative mechanical ventilation has been demonstrated, with the difference being significant in less than half of the studies.

Some of the studies have included VATS resections performed with rib spreading. Comparisons of VATS resection done with and without rib spreading show lower rates of complications when rib spreading is avoided.[34,36] Specifically, avoidance of rib spreading is associated with significantly less pain,

TABLE 27.2 Short-Term Outcomes of VATS Compared With Open Procedures

First Author	Year	N (Total)	Inclusion Criteria, Comments	Conversion Rate %	Operative Mortality %			Complications (Overall) %			Hospital Stay (Days, Median)		
					VATS	Open	p	VATS	Open	p	VATS	Open	p
META-ANALYSES													
Cheng[34]	2007	3589	About 20% rib spr	6	1.2	1.7	NS	13	20	0.0002	Lower	—	0.007
Chen[66]	2013	3457	Stage I	—	—	—	—	20	29	<0.0001	Lower	—	<0.01
Yan[35]	2009	2641	20% Rib spr	8	0.4	0.7	NS	—	—	—	12	12	—
Cai[68]	2013	1564	Stage I	—	—	—	—	Lower		0.013	—	—	—
PROPENSITY-MATCHED SERIES													
Paul[76]	2013	41,039	NIS	—	1.6	2.3	NS	41	45	<0.001	5	7	<0.001
Yang[11]	2016	18,780	NCDB	—	1.5	1.8	NS	—	—	—	5	6	<0.01
Falcoz[15]	2016	5442	ESTS DB	—	1.0	1.9	0.02	29	32	<0.04	6	8	0.0003
Cao[77]	2013	3634		—	1.3	1.8	NS	25	35	0.0001	Lower	—	<0.00001
Cao[78]	2013	2916	Chinese DB	8	0.8	1.1	—	—	—	—	—	—	—
Paul[76]	2010	2562	STS	—	0.9	1	NS	26	35	<0.0001	4	6	<0.0001
Scott[79]	2010	752	Stage cI	—	0	1.6	NS	27	48	NS	5	7	<0.001
Flores[55]	2009	741	Stage cIa	18	0.3	0.3	NS	24	30	0.05	5	7	<0.001
Villamizar[80]	2009	568	Prospective DB	5	3	5	0.02	31	49	—	4	5	<0.0001
Lee[47]	2013	416	Cornell U	2	1	3	NS	15	18	—	4	5	0.02
Ilonen[56]	2011	232	Stage cI	14	2.6	3.4	NS	16	27	<0.03	8	11	0.001
Jeon[81]	2013	182	COPD, Stage cI	11	0	3.3	NS	22	33	NS	6	9	0.04
Scott[79]	2010	136	Stage cI	7	1.4	1.6	NS	34	39	NS	4	7	<0.0001
Yang[11]	2016	60	Preop chemo		3	7	NS	40	57	NS	4	5	0.007
CASE-MATCHED SERIES													
Cattaneo[39]	2008	164	Elderly	1	0	3.6	NS	28	45	0.04	5	6	0.001
Jones[33]	2008	78	Converted	11	0	2	NS	50	48	NS	8	8	NS
Demmy[40]	1999	38	Old, frail	14	16	5	—	32	32	—	5	12	0.02
OUTCOMES STUDIES (ADJUSTED DATA)[a]													
Ceppa[44]	2012	12,970	STS	—	—	—	—	Lower		0.001	—	—	—
Ceppa[44]	2012	—	Hi pulm risk	—	—	—	—	Lower		0.02	—	—	—
Farjah[9]	2009	12,958	SEER Medicare	—	Lower	—	NS	—	—	—	4	8	<0.001
Park[73]	2012	6292	NIS	—	—	—	NS	Lower		0.004	Lower	—	0.001
Swanson[74]	2012	3961	Premiere DB	—	—	—	—	Lower		0.02	6	8	<0.0001
Licht[58]	2013	1513	Stage cI. DLCR	—	1.1[b]	2.9[b]	0.02[b]	—	—	—	—	—	—
RANDOMIZED CONTROLLED TRIALS													
Craig[51]	2001	110	—	—	0	0	NS	3	8	—	(9)[c]	(8)[c]	(NS)[c]
Kirby[52]	1995	55	Stage cI	10	—	—	—	24	53	<0.05	7	8	NS

[a]Reported data are that adjusted for multiple predictive factors (multivariate analysis).
[b]Unadjusted data.
[c]Study protocol demanded a minimum 7-day hospitalization.

COPD, chronic obstructive pulmonary disease; *DB,* database; *DLCR,* Danish Lung Cancer Registry; *ESTS DB,* European Society of Thoracic Surgery Database; *Hi pulm risk,* high pulmonary risk; *NCDB,* National Cancer Database (US); *NIS,* National Inpatient Sample (a representative large sample of US hospital admissions); *NS,* not significant; *NS (italics);* not significant, but a trend (i.e., $p \leq 0.1$ but > 0.05); *preop chemo,* preoperative chemotherapy; *rib spr,* rib spreading; *SEER,* Surveillance, Epidemiology and End-Result database; *STS,* Society of Thoracic Surgeons Database; *U,* university; *VATS,* video-assisted thoracoscopic surgery.

shorter hospital stay, lower perioperative complications, and lower mortality rates.[34,56]

Postoperative pain is significantly less after VATS lobectomy than following open thoracotomy. In a 2007 meta-analysis of the available data, the pain level, analgesic dose, and frequency and duration of analgesic use over the first postoperative week were significantly lower after VATS lobectomy than after open lobectomy ($p = 0.008$ to 0.0001).[34] Pain, measured with a visual analog scale, was less with VATS throughout the first month, but by postoperative month 3, there was no difference (Fig. 27.4).[34]

Limited data show that VATS significantly improves the proportion of patients who are functioning independently and without limitations. The time to full mobility is significantly reduced, and patients are quicker to regain arm mobility.[57] Overall quality of life appears to be better for patients who have received VATS compared with those who received open lobectomy.[58] Pulmonary function tests at 1 year are better after VATS lobectomy.[34]

Lastly, older and frail patients seem to be better able to tolerate a VATS lobectomy.[47–49]

Long-Term Outcomes

Many series have reported long-term outcomes associated with VATS compared with open resection for lung cancer (Table 27.4).[9,14,33–36,38,41,43,48,55,59–63] In large meta-analyses, the 5-year survival is reported to be better following VATS resection, with most studies indicating a significant difference. However, this comparison is potentially confounded if patients with smaller, earlier stage tumors are more likely to be selected for a VATS resection. Some authors have tried to address this by focusing only on stage I NSCLC and have shown either better or equal survival after VATS resection (Fig. 27.5).[34,59,61] Others have addressed this by propensity matching or other ways of case matching. These comparisons have shown no difference in long-term outcomes, either for all matched patients

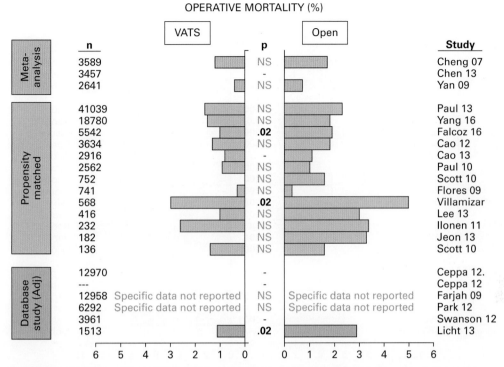

Fig. 27.1. Operative mortality for VATS versus open lobectomy. Graphic representation of the percent operative mortality for VATS versus open lobectomy in meta-analyses, propensity-matched comparisons, and outcome studies reporting adjusted results. In most studies this represents 30-day mortality. *Adj,* results adjusted for other factors (e.g., age, stage, comorbidities, health-care structural characteristics); *NS,* not significant; *VATS,* video-assisted thoracoscopic surgery.

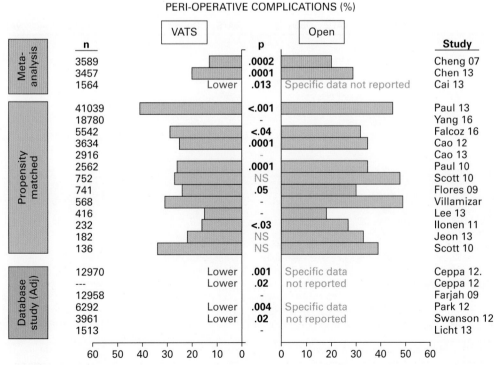

Fig. 27.2. Perioperative complications for VATS versus open lobectomy. Graphic representation of the percent perioperative complications for VATS versus open lobectomy in meta-analyses, propensity-matched comparisons, and outcome studies reporting adjusted results. *Adj.,* results adjusted for other factors (e.g., age, stage, comorbidities, health-care structural characteristics); *NS,* not significant; *VATS,* video-assisted thoracoscopic surgery.

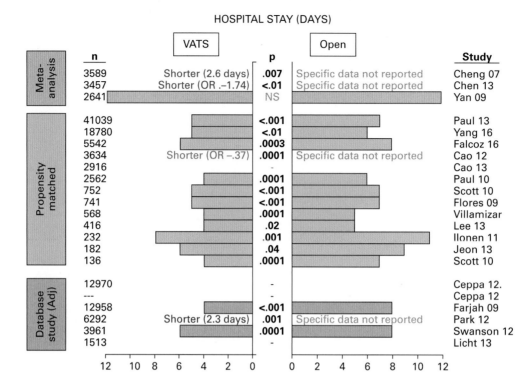

Fig. 27.3. Hospital length of stay for VATS versus open lobectomy. Graphic representation of hospital length of stay in days for VATS versus open lobectomy in meta-analyses, propensity-matched comparisons, and outcome studies reporting adjusted results. *Adj,* results adjusted for other factors (e.g., age, stage, comorbidities, health-care structural characteristics); *NS,* not significant; *OR,* odds ratio; *VATS,* video-assisted thoracoscopic surgery.

TABLE 27.3 Short-Term Outcomes of VATS Compared With Open Procedures: Specific Complications

First Author	Year	N (Total)	Inclusion Criteria, Comments	% Pneumonia			% Prolonged Air Leak			% Arrhythmia			% Mechanical Ventilation		
				VATS	Open	p	VATS	Open	p	VATS	Open	p	VATS	Open	p
META-ANALYSES															
Cheng[34]	2007	3589	~20% Rib Spr	Lower		NS	Higher[a]		NS	Same	Same	NS	Lower		NS
Chen[66]	2013	3457	Stage I	2	5	0.03	5	7	NS	10	12	NS	—	—	—
Yan (all)[35]	2009	2641	20% Rib Spr	2	10	*NS*	5	6	NS	10	10	NS	—	—	—
Cai[68]	2013	1564	Stage I	Lower	—	NS	Lower	—	NS	Lower	—	0.05	—	—	—
Yan (no Rib Spr)[35]	2009	925	No Rib Spr	0.5	2	*NS*	2	2	NS	4	4	NS	—	—	—
PROPENSITY-MATCHED SERIES															
Paul[76]	2013	41,039	NIS	7	8	NS	—	—	—	14	18	<0.001	5	6	*NS*
Falcoz[15]	2016	5442	ESTS	6	6	NS	10	9	NS	5	5	NS	0.7	1.4	<0.008
Cao[77]	2013	3634		3	5	0.008	8	10	0.02	7	12	<0.00001	—	—	—
Paul[76]	2010	2562	STS	3	4	*NS*	8	9	NS	7	12	0.0004	0.5	0.6	NS
Scott[79]	2010	752	Stage cl	—	—	—	2	7	NS	9	13	NS	0	4	—
Flores[55]	2009	741	Stage cla	—	—	—	4	4	NS	10	11	NS	—	—	—
Villamizar[80]	2009	568	Prospective DB	5	10	0.05	13	19	0.05	13	21	0.01	—	—	—
Lee[47]	2013	416	Cornell U	1	3	—	6	6	—	6	6	NS	1	3	—
Ilonen[56]	2011	232	Stage cl	4	3	—	4	10	—	1	3	—	0	1	—
Jeon[81]	2013	182	COPD, Stage cl	1	11	0.01	11	15	NS	8	9	NS	—	—	—
Yang[11]	2015	60	Preop chemo	7	13	NS	10	20	NS	23	23	NS	0	3	NS
OUTCOMES STUDIES (ADJUSTED DATA)[b]															
Ceppa[44]	2012	12,970	STS	3[c]	5[c]	<0.001	—	—	—	—	—	—	0.4[c]	0.8[c]	0.002
Swanson[74]	2012	3961	Premiere DB	Same	Same	NS	Lower	—	*NS*	Lower[c]	—		—	—	—
RANDOMIZED CONTROLLED TRIALS															
Craig[51]	2001	110	—	0	6	—	—	—	—	0	2	—	2	0	—
Kirby[52]	1995	55	Stage cl	—	—	—	12	27	NS	—	—	—	—	—	—

[a]Patients discharged early with chest tube in place counted as air leak until postoperative visit.
[b]Reported data are that adjusted for multiple predictive factors (multivariate analysis).
[c]Unadjusted data.
COPD, chronic obstructive pulmonary disease; *DB,* database; *ESTS,* European Society of Thoracic Surgery Database; *NIS,* National Inpatient Sample (a representative large sample of US hospital admissions); *NS,* not significant; *NS (in italics),* not significant, but a trend (i.e., $p \leq 0.1$ but > 0.05); *preop chemo,* preoperative chemotherapy; *Rib Spr,* rib spreading; *STS,* Society of Thoracic Surgeons Database; *U,* university; *VATS,* video-assisted thoracoscopic surgery.

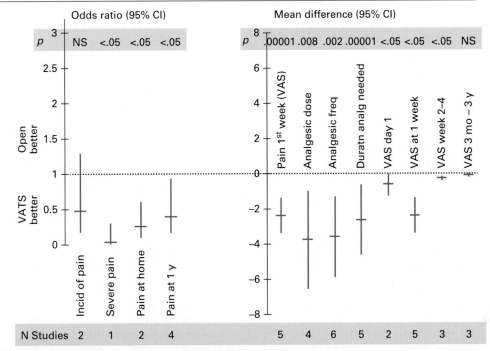

Fig. 27.4. Pain after VATS versus open lobectomy. Graphic summary of a meta-analysis of pain after VATS versus open lobectomy. *CI,* confidence interval; *Incid,* incidence; *NS,* not significant; *VAS,* visual analog scale; *VATS,* video-assisted thoracoscopic surgery. *(Data taken from Cheng D, Downey RJ, Kernstine K, et al. Video-assisted thoracic surgery in lung cancer resection: a meta-analysis and systematic review of controlled trials.* Innovations (Phila). *2007;2(6):261–292.)*

TABLE 27.4 Long-Term Outcomes of VATS Compared With Open Procedures

| First Author | Year | Inclusion Criteria, Comments | N (Total) | % 5 Year Survival | | | | | | % Recurrence | | | | | |
| | | | | All | | | Stage I | | | Local | | | Systemic | | |
				VATS	Open	p	VATS	Open	p	VATS	Open	p	VATS	Open	p
META-ANALYSES															
Zhang[41]	2013		5389	Better	—	<0.01	—	—	—	3	5	0.03	8	13	0.0001
Taioli[67]	2013		4767	Better		0.001	—	—	—	—	—	—	—	—	—
Cheng[34]	2007	~20% Rib Spr	3589	Better	—	0.03	—	—	NS	13	19	*NS*	—	—	—
Chen[66]	2013	Stage I	3457	Better	—	0.00001	Better	—	0.01	—	—	—	—	—	—
Yan (all)[35]	2009		2641	Better	—	0.04	—	—	—	4	8	NS	6	11	0.03
Cai[68]	2013	Stage I	1979	Better	—	<0.001	Better	—	<0.001	Higher	—	0.001	Same	Same	NS
Li[42]	2012	Stage I	1362	88	80	<0.0001	88	80	<0.0001	5	8	*NS*	7	11	0.02
Yan[35]	2009	No Rib Spr	925	—	—	NS	—	—	—	0.5	0.6	NS	1.1	1.5	*NS*
PROPENSITY-MATCHED SERIES															
Yang[11]	2016	NCDB	18,780	(87)[a]	(86)[a]	<0.04	—	—	—	—	—	—	—	—	—
Cao[77]	2013	Chinese DB	2916	62	60	NS	—	—	NS	—	—	—	—	—	—
Su[48]	2014	Stage cl	752	72	66	NS	—	—	—	Same	Same	NS	Same	Same	NS
Flores[55]	2009	Stage cla	741	79	75	NS	—	—	—	—	—	—	—	—	—
Berry[28]	2014	Duke U	560	55	48	NS	61	55	NS	—	—	—	—	—	—
Lee[47]	2013	Cornell U	416	76	77	NS	79	84	NS	4	5	—	6	10	—
Yang[11]	2015	Preop chemo	60	50	50	NS	—	—	—	—	—	—	—	—	—
CASE-MATCHED SERIES															
Jones[33]	2008	Converted	78	66	44	NS	—	—	—	—	—	—	—	—	—
Demmy[40]	1999	Old, frail	38	—	—	—	—	—	—	0	0	NS	—	—	—
OUTCOMES STUDIES (ADJUSTED DATA)[b]															
Farjah[9]	2009	SEER MC	12,958	Same	Same	NS	—	—	—	—	—	—	—	—	—
Licht[58]	2013	cl. DLCR	1513	Same	Same	NS	—	—	—	—	—	—	—	—	—
RANDOMIZED CONTROLLED TRIALS															
Sugi[50]	2000	Stage cla	100	90	85	NS	—	—	—	6	6	NS	4	13	NS

[a]2-year data.
[b]Reported data are that adjusted for multiple predictive factors (multivariate analysis).
DB, database; *DLCR,* Danish Lung Cancer Registry; *NCDB,* National Cancer Database (US); *NS,* not significant; *NS (in italics),* not significant, but a trend (i.e., $p \leq 0.1$ but > 0.05); *Rib Spr,* rib spreading; *SEER MC,* Surveillance, Epidemiology and End-Result-Medicare database; *U,* university; *VATS,* video-assisted thoracoscopic surgery.

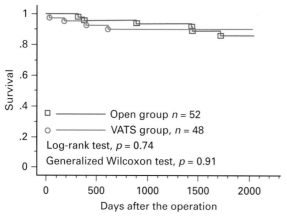

Fig. 27.5. Overall survival of VATS versus open lobectomy. Overall survival in a randomized study of VATS versus open lobectomy for patients with clinical stage Ia lung cancer. *VATS,* video-assisted thoracoscopic surgery. *(Reproduced with permission from Sugi K, Kaneda Y, Esato K. Video-assisted thoracoscopic lobectomy achieves a satisfactory long-term prognosis in patients with clinical stage IA lung cancer.* World J Surg. *2000;24(1):27–31.)*

or for patients within a subset of stage I disease (Table 27.4). Outcomes studies have typically shown a long-term survival benefit for unadjusted results but no significant difference when the results are adjusted for prognostic factors.[14,50,64] It should be noted that these adjustments include structural and treatment factors such as center volume, center type, stage, staging tests, node dissection, and adjuvant therapy; however, patient-related and tumor-related factors (i.e., comorbidities, stage, histology) are usually not available in these databases. In large series (>500 patients) that include stage-specific outcomes after VATS, long-term survival rates for VATS have been similar stage-for-stage to the average rates for resected NSCLC in general.[65,66]

Many authors have examined the rate of either local or systemic recurrence. These studies have shown a fairly consistent trend to lower recurrences of both types in patients who have VATS resection, with about one-third of these demonstrating that the difference was significant (Table 27.4). However, these analyses have the disadvantage of not being matched or randomized. Nevertheless, consistent results are seen in randomized controlled trials, propensity-matched studies, and larger outcomes studies.[43,62,63] It has been suggested that better oncologic outcomes after VATS resection may be because VATS causes fewer inflammatory mediators in the early postoperative period,[53] but this suggestion remains speculative.

In summary, the data in aggregate demonstrate that survival after VATS resection is essentially the same as after open resection. Suggestions of possibly better outcomes are likely related to confounding factors because such differences generally disappear when propensity matching or adjustment for structural or treatment variables are made.

Specific Issues

Node Dissection/Staging N1 and N2

Data from a large number of unmatched, nonrandomized comparisons have shown no difference in mediastinal node staging between VATS and open lobectomy, specifically no difference in the number of nodes or the number of node stations sampled in a meta-analysis (14 studies, $p = 0.63$).[31] This issue has also been addressed in two randomized and several prospective trials, which showed no difference.[54,63,67,68] A propensity-matched study of the

National Cancer Database (NCDB) found that significantly more nodes were examined during VATS versus open resections (10.3 vs. 9.7, $p < 0.01$).[69] A systematic review and meta-analysis specifically addressing node staging found no difference between VATS and open procedures.[41] Although a difference in staging has been reported in some retrospective studies, the investigators of these studies have stated that the difference resulted from intentional omission of sampling of some node stations on clinical grounds, not because of technical limitations of the approach.[41,44]

In 2012, Boffa et al.[13] examined nodal upstaging in 11,531 patients with clinical stage I primary lung cancers who had lobectomy or segmentectomy from 2001 to 2010 in the STS database (7137 open procedures and 4394 VATS). There was no difference between VATS and thoracotomy in the rate of upstaging to N2 involvement, but there was a significantly lower rate of N1 upstaging in the VATS group. This difference was interpreted as suggesting that less attention is paid to assessing N1 nodes during VATS resection. A follow-up study was carried out by Licht et al.[14] using the Danish National Lung Cancer Registry. Although the number of dissected node stations was the same, VATS resulted in lowering of both N2 and N1 nodal upstaging (3.8% vs. 11.5%, $p < 0.001$ and 8.1% vs. 13.1%, $p < 0.001$, respectively) than did open lobectomy for clinical stage I NSCLC.[13] However, multivariate analysis showed no difference in survival, suggesting that nodal upstaging either did not matter or reflected confounding by unknown selection or recording factors.

Two recent studies, both using a propensity-matched analysis of T1,2N0M0 patients in the NCDB, came to conflicting conclusions.[69,11] One study found no difference in N1 or N2 upstaging (7.7 vs. 8.1 [N1] and 3.8 vs. 4.1 [N2], $p = 0.53$ in 9380 matched pairs of VATS/robotic vs. open patients, respectively),[69a] whereas the other found lower N1 and a trend to lower N2 upstaging (6.9 vs. 8.0, $p = 0.046$ [N1] and 3.2 vs. 3.9, $p = 0.098$ [N2] in 4437 matched pairs of VATS vs. open patients, respectively).[69] The reason for the discrepancy is unclear. There were only slight differences in factors included in the propensity matching and the years included (2010–2012[11] and 2010–2011[69]). There was no difference whatsoever in nodal upstaging between VATS and robotic procedures in the study that included robotic resections,[11] which has also been confirmed by others.[70] Other unmatched retrospective studies have suggested a lower rate of N1 and N2 upstaging via VATS or similar rates of N2 upstaging.[62,71,72]

It may be that the rate of nodal upstaging is a reflection of other factors and not actually the approach used. Boffa et al.[13] found that there was no difference in N1 upstaging by VATS versus open approaches when the analysis was restricted to sites that performed one or the other approach in most (≥80%) of their resections (8.7% vs. 8.7% in 989 VATS cases vs. 3668 open cases).[13] Medbery et al.[69] found no difference in N1 or N2 upstaging when the analysis was restricted to academic/teaching centers (10.5 vs. 12.2 VATS vs. open, $p = 0.084$ in 2008 matched pairs), although they did find an overall lower rate of N upstaging by VATS in an analysis restricted to cases that had seven or more nodes examined (12.1 vs. 14.0 VATS vs. open, $p = 0.031$ in 2825 matched pairs).[69] Finally, although the propensity-matched studies attempted to account for tumor characteristics such as T stage and size, none of the studies could account for factors such as whether the tumor was central versus peripheral, or mostly solid versus ground glass (characteristics that are known to affect the incidence of nodal involvement).

Taken together, the data suggest that there is little, if any, inherent difference in the ability to carry out intraoperative staging between VATS and open resections. There are some data suggesting the possibility of a lower rate of N1 node assessment with VATS, but the validity and impact of a rate difference, if any, are unclear.

Ability to Tolerate Adjuvant Chemotherapy

The ability of patients to receive adjuvant chemotherapy is improved following VATS lobectomy, as assessed in several studies.[67,73-77] Retrospective studies without adjustment for other patient characteristics have all shown a better ability to administer adjuvant chemotherapy after VATS resection. For example, in one study, the ability to deliver more than 75% of the planned dose was higher with VATS (89% vs. 71%).[67] Furthermore, chemotherapy toxicity appears to be reduced after a VATS resection.[67] However, in a registry study in which adjustments were made for comorbidities and other factors, VATS resection was not associated with better delivery of adjuvant chemotherapy (only age, comorbidities, and the N1 or N2 node status were associated with better delivery).[74]

A few authors have reported long-term outcomes for VATS compared with open resections in patients who were given adjuvant chemotherapy. Some findings have suggested that survival is better in the VATS group.[67,74] However, in a multivariate analysis of this issue in the Danish National Lung Cancer Registry, it appears that survival was statistically associated with comorbidity, pathology, and compliance but not with the surgical approach.[74]

Learning Curve

Without question, VATS lobectomy is associated with a learning curve, as are all surgical procedures. The experts at the VATS Consensus Meeting estimated that, in general, most surgeons become reasonably proficient and comfortable with the procedure after approximately 50 cases. This learning curve is consistent with the findings of several investigations that have also indicated 50 cases as a number that achieves a reasonable comfort level.[78-80] Furthermore, the results of studies suggest that training of thoracic surgical residents in VATS lobectomy can be accomplished safely.[79] According to a study by Boffa et al.,[64] most thoracic surgical trainees in the United States, especially those with a predominant focus on thoracic surgery, thought that their training had prepared them to perform VATS lobectomy.

Robotic Versus VATS Lobectomy

The rate of robotic lobectomy is still quite low, although the number of robotic lobectomies has increased significantly (10.4% of lobectomies in 2012 in the NCDB were performed using robotics).[11] Available matched or adjusted comparative studies suggest there is no major difference in outcomes of VATS versus robotic lobectomy.[11] Specifically, no difference was observed in 30-day mortality, length of stay, or nodal upstaging in propensity-matched comparisons (295 and 1938 matched pairs),[82] or in comparisons adjusted for patient and hospital characteristics.[83] Some studies have found no difference in total major or minor complications,[82,83] but Paul et al.[83] found a significantly higher rate of iatrogenic complications (accidental laceration or bleeding) that persisted after adjustment for patient and hospital characteristics (odds ratio, 2.64 [1.58–4.43]). The cost of robotic lobectomy appears to be higher than for VATS (by about $4500), even without accounting for the capital cost of the robot itself.[82,83]

DISCUSSION

VATS lobectomy was first described in the early 1990s, and an abundance of literature has been published on the subject. The data reviewed in this chapter demonstrate that VATS lobectomy is safe, is associated with lower rates of complications and mortality than open lobectomy, and results in equivalent long-term outcomes. Thus VATS lobectomy is well established and should be considered the standard of care from a patient perspective. Indeed, the 2013 lung cancer guidelines of the American College of Chest Physicians recommend a minimally invasive resection as the preferred method for resection of early stage NSCLC in experienced centers (evidence level, grade 2C).[84]

Some of the advantages of VATS are seen only transiently; for example, pain is nearly resolved at 3 months with either a VATS or open approach. However, other advantages, such as lower operative mortality rates, have long-term implications. Whether other potential advantages, such as long-term survival or the ability to deliver adjuvant chemotherapy, are attributable to the VATS approach or to patient selection is, as yet, unclear.

The appropriate place for VATS lobectomy from a societal perspective is more difficult to define. Many factors besides patient experience and outcomes play a role. The availability of equipment and expertise are important factors, as is the balance between material and personnel costs (e.g., How does an extra day in the hospital compare with an extra staple cartridge used in the surgical suite?). The structure of the health-care system and cultural norms of the society have a considerable influence on these factors, which will balance differently in specific settings.

Resistance to change may be one of the major factors inhibiting wider adoption, despite the data supporting the technique. Time is needed to fully assess a new technique, but surely 20 years and thousands of studies have provided sufficient assessment. The learning curve is inarguable, but certainly it can be overcome, as many centers have demonstrated. Reviewing the data and investing in learning a new technique are needed for greater adoption of VATS.

CONCLUSION

VATS lobectomy is well established and supported by a large body of literature. The evidence has been summarized in several meta-analyses, large-scale outcomes studies, many propensity-matched studies, and small randomized controlled trials. The propensity-matched studies and adjusted outcomes data generally demonstrate that short-term mortality and long-term survival rates are equivalent between VATS and open lobectomy. However, simple comparisons and meta-analyses demonstrate that VATS resections are associated with less morbidity, fewer complications, lower mortality rates, and decreased length of stay compared with thoracotomy. Therefore we conclude that lobectomy should be performed by VATS whenever possible.

KEY REFERENCES

11. Yang CF, Sun Z, Speicher PJ, et al. Use and outcomes of minimally invasive lobectomy for stage I non-small cell lung cancer in the National Cancer Database. *Ann Thorac Surg*. 2016;101(3):1037–1042.

15. Falcoz PE, Puyraveau M, Thomas PA, et al. Video-assisted thoracoscopic surgery versus open lobectomy for primary non-small-cell lung cancer: a propensity-matched analysis of outcome from the European Society of Thoracic Surgeon database. *Eur J Cardiothorac Surg*. 2016;49(2):602–609.

32. Gopaldas RR, Bakaeen FG, Dao TK, Walsh GL, Swisher SG, Chu D. Video-assisted thoracoscopic versus open thoracotomy lobectomy in a cohort of 13,619 patients. *Ann Thorac Surg*. 2010;89(5):1563–1570.

49. Port JL, Mirza FM, Lee PC, Paul S, Stiles BM, Altorki NK. Lobectomy in octogenarians with non-small cell lung cancer: ramifications of increasing life expectancy and the benefits of minimally invasive surgery. *Ann Thorac Surg*. 2011;92(6):1951–1957.

69. Medbery RL, Gillespie TW, Liu Y, et al. Nodal upstaging is more common with thoracotomy than with VATS during lobectomy for early-stage lung cancer: an analysis from the National Cancer Data Base. *J Thorac Oncol*. 2016;11(2):222–233.

71. Higuchi M, Yaginuma H, Yonechi A, et al. Long-term outcomes after video-assisted thoracic surgery (VATS) lobectomy versus lobectomy via open thoracotomy for clinical stage IA non-small cell lung cancer. *J Cardiothorac Surg*. 2014;9:88.

73. Park HS, Detterbeck FC, Boffa DJ, Kim AW. Impact of hospital volume of thoracoscopic lobectomy on primary lung cancer outcomes. *Ann Thorac Surg*. 2012;93(2):372–379.

74. Swanson SJ, Meyers BF, Gunnarsson CL, et al. Video-assisted thoracoscopic lobectomy is less costly and morbid than open lobectomy: a retrospective multiinstitutional database analysis. *Ann Thorac Surg*. 2012;93(4):1027–1032.

75. Teh E, Abah U, Church D, et al. What is the extent of the advantage of video-assisted thoracoscopic surgical resection over thoracotomy in terms of delivery of adjuvant chemotherapy following non-small-cell lung cancer resection? *Interact Cardiovasc Thorac Surg*. 2014;19(4):656–660.

76. Paul S, Altorki NK, Sheng S, et al. Thoracoscopic lobectomy is associated with lower morbidity than open lobectomy: a propensity-matched analysis from the STS database. *J Thorac Cardiovasc Surg*. 2010;139(2):366–378.

83. Paul S, Jalbert J, Isaacs AJ, Altorki NK, Isom OW, Sedrakyan A. Comparative effectiveness of robotic-assisted vs thoracoscopic lobectomy. *Chest*. 2014;146(6):1505–1512.

See Expertconsult.com for full list of references.

28 Robotic Surgery: Techniques and Results for Resection of Lung Cancer

Ayesha Bryant, Benjamin Wei, Giulia Veronesi, and Robert Cerfolio

SUMMARY OF KEY POINTS

- Robotic surgery can be used for completely portal (no utility incision) or robotic-assisted (uses utility incision) techniques.
- Appropriate patient and port positioning are critical for a successful performance of robotic lobectomy.
- Perioperative morbidity and mortality for robotic lobectomy are comparable to that for video-assisted thoracoscopic surgical (VATS) lobectomy.
- Robotic lobectomy may have advantages in terms of surgeon ergonomics, mediastinal lymph node dissection, and intraoperative blood loss over VATS lobectomy.
- Robotic lobectomy can be done safely and is being increasingly used for anatomic pulmonary resections.

DEFINITIONS

A general thoracic operation is defined as any operative procedure for lesions or structures in the thorax, including but not limited to lesions or pathology in the mediastinum, pulmonary parenchyma, chest wall muscles or skeletal structures, diaphragm, or esophagus.

A robotic system is defined as any machine or mechanical device that uses a computer to translate human movements into the movement of robotic instruments. The robotic instruments or tools, not the surgeon's hands, interact with the patient's tissue.

A robotic thoracic operation is defined as a general thoracic operation that is minimally invasive (i.e., no rib spreading) and in which the surgeon's and assistant's views of the operative field are via a monitor rather than through an incision. Moreover, the procedure utilizes a robotic system for all or mostly all of the crucial aspects of the operation. For pulmonary resection, crucial surgical aspects include dissection and ligation of the pulmonary arteries and veins, dissection and removal of the mediastinal and hilar lymph nodes, and bagging of the specimen. For mediastinal operations, dissection and removal of the mediastinal lesion are robotically performed. For esophageal operations, dissection of the esophagus and/or the esophageal lesion, resection and/or bagging of the specimen, removal of the thoracic lymph nodes, and possibly anastomosis of the esophagus to the stomach or other chosen conduit are crucial tasks completed with the robotic system.

We have suggested a nomenclature that differentiates completely portal robotic operations (CPRs) from operations in which a utility incision is used, which are referred to as robotic-assisted operation or robotic-assisted thoracic surgery. Such a nomenclature specifies the number of robotic arms implemented and is defined as follows.

A CPR is defined as an operation that uses ports only (incisions that are only as large as the size of the trocars placed in them). In this case the air in the pleural space or chest cavity does not communicate with the ambient air in the operating room, carbon dioxide is used to insufflate the chest, and the only port incision that is larger than the trocars that go through them is one through which a specimen contained in a protective bag is removed.

A robotic-assisted operation is defined as a procedure in which a utility incision is used (defined as either an incision in the chest that may or may not have trocars or robotic arms placed through it or an incision that allows communication between the ambient air in the operating room and the pleural space), which does not involve spreading of the ribs, and in which carbon dioxide insufflation is used selectively (only as needed).

The number of robotic arms used during the operation is included in the nomenclature and is separated by a hyphen after the type of operation is specified. The abbreviation for the type of operation also includes a one-letter initial to indicate the specific procedure. For example, a CPR lobectomy using four arms is a CPRL-4, and a CPR segmentectomy using three arms is a CPRS-3 (Table 28.1).

HISTORY OF SURGICAL ROBOTICS

Industrial robots are mechanical arms that, working alone or in cooperation, perform precise, complex, repetitive tasks, and manipulations under computer control. Robot arms are increasingly flexible in terms of the objects they can work on and the tasks they perform, including capabilities that require visual and other sensing systems linked to powerful computers with artificial intelligence software.

Surgical robots also consist of mechanical arms that attach to surgical instruments. However, although computers filter and scale the movements and manipulations carried out by these arms, surgeons always directly control the arms. Robotic surgical systems have been in development since the 1980s.[1] Intuitive Surgical Inc. and Computer Motion Inc. emerged as the two main companies producing robotic systems for minimally invasive surgery in the first decade of the 21st century.[2] Intuitive Surgical's robot arms are controlled manually by the surgeon; Computer Motion's system employed voice control too. Both companies obtained limited approval from the US Food and Drug Administration (FDA) for their systems. The two companies merged in 2003. Several other companies in Europe and the United States are developing robotic surgical systems: most are intended for minimally invasive surgery, but others are being developed to perform open surgery or remote surgery.

The da Vinci Surgical System (Intuitive Surgical Inc., Sunnyvale, CA, USA) is currently the only FDA-approved robotic system for lung surgery.[2] The surgeon sits at a console some distance from the patient, who is positioned on an operating table in close proximity to the robotic unit with its three or four robotic arms.[3–9] The robotic arms incorporate remote center technology, in which a fixed point in space is defined, and the surgical arms move around it to minimize stress on the thoracic wall during manipulations. The system's small

TABLE 28.1 Operative Characteristics for the Proposed Nomenclature System for General Thoracic Robotic Operations

	Completely Portal Robotic	Robotic Assisted
Suggested abbreviations	CPR	RA
Designation includes the number of robotic arms used	Yes (e.g., CPRL-4, completely portal robotic lobectomy using 4 arms)	Yes (e.g., RAL-4, robotic-assisted lobectomy using 4 arms)
Rib spreading	No	No
Access or utility incision made	No	Yes
Carbon dioxide insufflation used	Yes	Sometimes
Communication between pleural space air and ambient air in operating room	No	Yes
Trocars placed though all incisions	Yes	No
Incisions bigger than size of trocars used	No	Yes
Site of specimen removal	Usually over the anterior aspect of the tenth rib	Usually over the anterior aspect of the fourth rib

proprietary EndoWrist instruments, which are attached to the arms, are capable of performing a wide range of high-precision movements. The surgeon's hand movements with the so-called master instruments at the console control the EndoWrist instruments. These master instruments sense the surgeon's hand movements and translate them electronically into scaled-down micromovements to manipulate the small surgical instruments. Hand tremor is filtered out by a 6-Hz motion filter. The surgeon observes the operating field through console binoculars. The image comes from a maneuverable high-definition stereoscopic camera (endoscope) attached to one of the robot arms. The console screen can also display digital input from electrocardiography, computed tomography, and other imaging modalities. The Firefly Fluorescence Imaging (Intuitive Surgical, Inc) involves a camera head with laser-based illuminator to visualize vascular and lymph node flow in three dimensions after injection of fluorescent dye.

The console also has foot pedals that allow the surgeon to engage and disengage different instrument arms, reposition the master controls on the console without moving the instruments themselves, and activate electric cautery. A second optional console allows tandem surgery and training.

ROBOTIC LOBECTOMY: TECHNICAL ASPECTS

The number of robotic pulmonary resections continues to increase. The team learning curve for robotic surgery is steep; however, the learning curve for the typical thoracic surgeon may be less than that for VATS lobectomy, especially for lymph node dissection. This difference may be one reason why the popularity of robotic resection is increasing among surgeons. A review of the guidelines and pathways to team building and credentialing for robotic pulmonary resections follows.

Operating Room Configuration

As with any operation, planning each stage of the operation is crucial to ensure success. The robot adds anxiety to inexperienced robotic surgeons and anesthesiologists. Thus planning the room layout before the operation is essential and includes positioning the bedside cart, robot, nurses' table, monitors, and patient relative to the anesthesia equipment. The robot is driven in over the patient's head during lobectomy; thus precise planning and communication of the position of two monitors and the distance between the operating surgeon at the console and the scrub nurse and surgical assistant(s) at the patient's bedside are needed (Fig. 28.1).

Console

The surgeon's console should be positioned in such a way that good communication with the surgical team at the bedside can be established. The da Vinci Surgical System console contains a

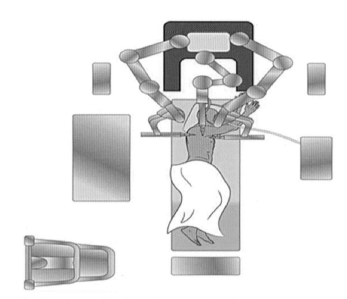

Fig. 28.1. A potential universal room setup for all robotic operations, regardless of specialty.

microphone that amplifies the voice of the surgeon to the rest of the team. The presence of a second console permits easy exchange of control between surgeon, medical student, resident, or fellow for training purposes; this second console, if used, should be located fairly close to the primary console.

Robot/Bed

The approach of the robot to the patient's side should be clear of any obstacles. The robot is driven over the patient's head on a 15-degree angle to open up robotic arm 3 over the head and shoulder (Fig. 28.2). In addition, monitors are positioned so that the bedside assistants and scrub nurse have a clear view.

Depending on the size of the room and the arrangement of immobile structures within it, the patient's bed may need to be turned such that the patient's head is located well away from the ventilator and anesthesia console. A long extension for the endotracheal tubing should be used if necessary.

When the robot is set up, robotic arm 3 should be placed on the robot side opposite the side of the lobectomy (e.g., if performing a right lobectomy, robot arm 3 should be located on the robot's left when facing the robot).

Surgical Team

The surgical bedside assistant should be in position at the patient's ventral side (i.e., in front of the patient's abdomen

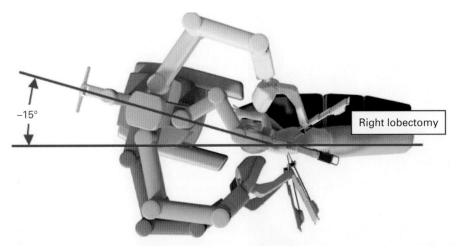

Fig. 28.2. The optimal angle for driving the robot over the patient's head to maximize the use of robotic arm 3 and prevent external collisions.

and chest), with a monitor on the opposite side. The scrub nurse should be in position with the instrument stand near or over the patient's feet, as in conventional thoracotomy or VATS.

Patient Positioning

The patient is placed in the supine position, general anesthesia is induced, and the patient is intubated with a left-sided double-lumen endotracheal tube. Proper placement of the double-lumen tube is assisted greatly by the use of a flexible pediatric bronchoscope and is crucial to a smooth operation because access to the patient's head and endotracheal tube will be limited by their positioning and the presence of the robot after docking.

After the double-lumen tube is secured, the patient is placed in the lateral decubitus position with the operative side up. An axillary roll is placed. We do not use an arm board; rather, we place the patient's back at the edge of the table, leaving space in front of the face to fold the arms and expose the axilla for port placement (Fig. 28.2). We have used this positioning for more than 17 years for our thoracotomies because when a four-arm robotic approach is used, robotic arm 3 can move on a plane that is below the bed and avoid conflicts with that arm and the operative bed itself. Padding should be used around the arms and head to prevent nerve damage during the surgery. We use large foam pads to protect the patient's head and arms. This easy, quick, and cost-effective technique requires no special equipment and is reproducible.

Port Placement/Docking

The ports are inserted in the seventh intercostal space over the top of the eighth rib for upper/middle lobectomy and in the eighth intercostal space over the top of the ninth rib for lower lobectomy (Fig. 28.3).

The ports are marked as follows: robotic arm 3, a 5-mm port is located 1 cm to 2 cm lateral from the spinous process of the vertebral body; robotic arm 2, an 8-mm port is located 10 cm medial to robotic arm 3; the camera port (we prefer a 12-mm camera) is located 9 cm medial to robotic arm 2; and robotic arm 1 (a 12-mm port) is placed directly above the diaphragm anteriorly. The assistant port (12 mm) is placed as low as possible in the chest, triangulated exactly halfway between the most anterior robotic port (which is robotic arm 1 in the right chest and robotic arm 2 in the left chest) and the camera port, and as

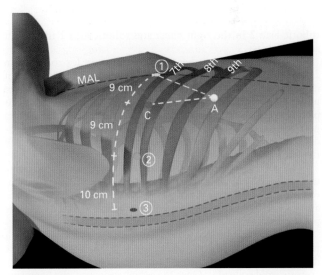

Fig. 28.3. (Right side). The optimal port placement for a completely portal robotic lobectomy using all four arms. The four ports are placed over the same rib: over the top of the ninth rib for lower lobectomy and over the top of the eighth rib for upper lobectomy. The 12-mm access port *(A)* is placed halfway between the camera port *(C)* and robotic arm 1 *(1)* for upper and lower lobes and between the camera and robotic arm 2 *(2)* for middle lobectomy. The port is placed as low as possible staying just above the diaphragm as carbon dioxide is insufflated to help push the diaphragm down. *3*, robotic arm 3; *MAL*, midaxillary line.

low as possible to remain just above the diaphragm, which is being pushed downward by the insufflating humidified carbon dioxide gas.

Sequence of Port Placement

A 5-mm port is placed first in the camera port position, and carbon dioxide insufflation is initiated at a pressure of 10 mmHg. We use humidified warm carbon dioxide. An intercostal nerve block with 0.25% bupivacaine with epinephrine (Marcaine) is then performed from ribs 3 to 8 by injecting a wheel of bupivacaine subpleurally under direct vision. Then the 5-mm thoracoscope is used to help assist the placement of all other ports, which are placed under direct vision. The camera port is placed first, robotic arm 3 is placed second, and

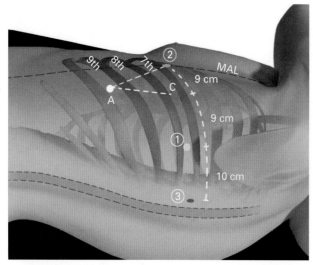

Fig. 28.4. (Left side). As in Fig. 28.3, but showing left side.

robotic arm 2 in the right chest and robotic arm 1 in the left are placed last.

The 5-mm camera is then moved to the port for robotic arm 2, and the two most anterior ports (robotic arm 1 in the right chest and robotic arm 2 in the left) and the access port are placed under direct vision using a seeking needle. Our techniques completely avoid all of the diaphragmatic fibers. The 5-mm camera port is then replaced by a 12-mm camera port. We use a zero-degree scope for the entire procedure to help prevent torquing of the intercostal nerve.

The port placement for left-sided lobectomy is a mirror image to that previously described (Fig. 28.4). The difference is that robotic arm 3 is next to robotic arm 1, rather than next to robotic arm 2. The numbering is different; however, the locations of the ports are the same.

The robot is moved at a 15-degree angle toward the patient's face off the long axis of the bed (Fig. 28.2). The robotic arms are docked to the ports, maximizing the amount of space between the arms to avoid collisions. Once the system is docked, the operating table cannot be moved.

The instruments used to start the surgery are an 8-mm Cadiere forceps in the left robotic arm, an 8-mm bipolar curved thoracic dissector in the right robotic arm, and a 5-mm thoracic grasper in robotic arm 3.

For their initial placement, robotic instruments should be inserted under direct vision during thoracic surgery. Once instruments are safely positioned, they can be quickly and safely inserted or changed for other instruments by properly using the memory feature of the robot, which automatically inserts any new instrument to a position that is exactly 1 cm proximal to the latest position. However, when this memory feature is used, the surgeon must ensure that no vital structures have moved into the path of the newly placed instrument. The most common structure to move is the lung.

The insertion of robotic instruments deserves special attention, as does the passing of vascular staplers around fragile structures such as the pulmonary artery and vein. Carefully orchestrated movements and clear communication are needed between the surgeon and the surgical bedside assistant, a resident, fellow, physician assistant, or nurse practitioner who acts as the surgeon's link to the patient. We have developed our own communication system between the bedside assistant and the surgeon to prevent iatrogenic injuries. This communication system uses the anvil of the stapler as the hour hand of a clock so that the degree of articulation can be quantified and communicated.

Mediastinal Lymph Node Dissection

The pleural surface is inspected before initiating node dissection and lobectomy to confirm that there are no metastatic lesions. We perform mediastinal lymph node dissection before lobectomy not only to evaluate the lymph nodes but also to access arterial and venous branches and the bronchus.

Right Side

The inferior pulmonary ligament is divided to gain access to station 9 lymph nodes, which are removed along with station 8 lymph nodes. Robotic arm 3 is used to retract the lower lobe medially and anteriorly to remove lymph nodes from station 7. Care is taken to control the two feeding arteries that make the subcarinal lymph node bloody. Robotic arm 3 is used to retract the upper lobe inferiorly, whereas robotic arms 1 and 2 are used to dissect lymph nodes at stations 2R and 4R, clearing the space between the superior vena cava anteriorly, the esophagus posteriorly, and the azygos vein inferiorly. Avoiding dissection too far superiorly can prevent injury to the right recurrent laryngeal nerve that wraps around the subclavian artery.

Left Side

The inferior pulmonary ligament is divided to facilitate removal of lymph nodes at station 9. The nodes in station 8 are then removed. Station 7 is accessed in the space between the inferior pulmonary vein and lower lobe bronchus, lateral to the esophagus. The lower lobe is retracted medially/anteriorly with robotic arm 3 during this process. Absence of the lower lobe facilitates dissection of lymph nodes at station 7 from the left. Because of enhanced magnification and 360-degree vision, the robot has a distinct advantage compared with VATS for the dissection of station 7 lymph nodes from the left chest. Lastly, robotic arm 3 is used to wrap around the left upper lobe and press the lobe inferiorly to allow dissection of stations 5 and 6 lymph nodes. Care should be taken while working in the aortopulmonary window to avoid injury to the left recurrent laryngeal nerve. Station 2L cannot typically be accessed during left-sided mediastinal lymph node dissection because of the presence of the aortic arch, but the 4L node is commonly removed.

General Concepts

In general, for a right-handed surgeon, a blunt instrument such as a Cadiere forceps is placed in robotic arm 2, which is always the left hand, and the right hand, which controls robotic arm 1, uses a thoracic dissector.

The stapler may be placed through one of three ports: the access port, robotic arm 1, or robotic arm 2. The current design of commercially available white or gray vascular staplers requires a 12-mm port; the green-loaded stapler commonly used for the bronchus requires a 15-mm port. We prefer to remove the trocar and leave it docked to the robotic arm and then place the stapler through the skin incision. We prefer to place a vessel loop under a vessel to be stapled to help elevate it while the stapler is passed beneath it.

We commonly use a prerolled sponge to absorb blood from the operative field or facilitate blunt dissection to improve visibility.

Removal of lymph nodes from surrounding structures should be done before stapling them in the interests of both ensuring an oncologically sound operation and facilitating isolation and division of structures.

Adhesions, if substantial, may be lysed via the assistant port using VATS techniques until safe placement of all the robotic instruments is permitted.

The order in which the structures are isolated and divided during lobectomy varies somewhat, depending on patient anatomy.

TABLE 28.2 Outcomes for Robotic Surgery

Author (y), Type of Study	No. of Patients; Indication	Type of Operation[a]	Average No. of Lymph Nodes Removed	Size of Access Port (cm)	No. of Ports	Rate of Major Morbidity (%)	Operative Mortality Rate (%)	Rate of Conversion to Open Procedure (%)	Operative Time (min) (Range)	Length of Stay (Mean Days) (Range)	Overall Survival Rate (%)
Kent et al. (2014),[12] Review of national database	430; all-comers	Lobectomy and segmentectomy	NR	NR	NR	44 (any)	0.2	NR	NR	4	NR
Wilson et al. (2014),[13] Multicenter	302; clinical stage I primary lung cancer	Lobectomy (257) Segmentectomy (45)	20.9	NR	NR	NR	0	NR	NR	3.4	2 y: 87.6
Cerfolio et al. (2011),[11] Single center	168; primary lung cancer	Lobectomy (106) Segmentectomy (16) Wedge resection (26)	8	>1.5	4	5	0	11.9	132	2 (1–7)	NR
Dylewski et al. (2011),[10] Single center	200; 125 primary lung cancer cases and 75 other cases	Lobectomy (160) Bilobectomy (1) Segmentectomy (35) Pneumonectomy (1)	5	2–4	3	26 (overall)	1.5	1.5	175 (82–370)	3 (1–44)	NR
Veronesi et al. (2011),[14] Single center	91; primary lung cancer	Lobectomy	5	3	4	4–11	0	10	239 (85–411)	5	2 y: 88
Gharagozloo et al. (2009),[6] Single center	100; pathologic stages I–IIIA primary lung cancer	Lobectomy	NR	2–3	3–4	21 (overall)	3	1	216 ± 27	4 (3–42)	32 mo: 99
Park (2012),[15] Multicenter	325; primary lung cancer	Lobectomy (324) Bilobectomy (1)	5	<8	3–4	4	0.3	8.3	206 (110–383)	5 (2–28)	5 y: 80 Stage IA: 91 Stage IB: 88 Stage II: 49

[a]In the studies by Cerfolio et al. and Dylewski et al., some patients had a procedure other than a robotic one.
NR, not recorded.

OUTCOMES

The outcomes after robotic surgery for lung cancer have been reported in several series[6,10–15] (Table 28.2).

Short-Term Results

Two studies showed that short operative times (132 min and 175 min, respectively) are possible as the experience of each surgeon grows.[11,12] Despite decreasing operative times, these two series also demonstrated extremely low operative mortality rates and outstanding mediastinal lymph node removal, and both used a completely portal technique that eliminated an access incision except at the end of the operation for extraction of the bagged specimen.

An updated series of 282 patients undergoing robotic lobectomy demonstrated an average blood loss of 20 mL, 0.5% rate of intraoperative/postoperative transfusion, 107-minute mean operative time, and median 2-day hospital length of stay with low rates of perioperative major morbidity (9.6%) and mortality (0.25% 30-day and 0.5% 90-day mortality).[16] Operative times have been shown to decrease with surgeon experience.[17]

Similarly, as detailed in Chapter 27, surgeons who used a VATS access incision also have reported outstanding results with a low 30-day mortality rate. The hospital length of stay for robotic surgery has been comparable to that for VATS lobectomy, ranging from a mean of 2 days to 5 days.

One study comparing results from 120 robotic lobectomies with those from VATS cases in the Society of Thoracic Surgeons database from 2009 to 2010 demonstrated lower postoperative blood transfusion rates (0.9% vs. 7.8%, $p = 0.002$), fewer air leaks greater than 5 days (5.2% vs. 10.8%, $p = 0.05$), decreased chest tube duration (3.2 days vs. 4.8 days, $p < 0.001$), and decreased length of stay (4.7 days vs. 7.3 days, $p < 0.001$) compared with open lobectomy, and trending in favor of robotic lobectomy over VATS.[18] Studies of the rate of nodal upstaging with robotic lobectomy versus VATS are conflicting, with some showing an advantage, whereas others have not.[19,20]

Long-Term Results

The success of oncologic procedures is measured by the 5-year survival rate. Because robotic anatomic pulmonary resection is relatively new, few studies have reported an actuarial 5-year survival rate. One study with a median follow-up of 27 months demonstrated 5-year survival of 91% for stage IA patients, 88% for stage IB patients, and 49% for stage II patients and a 43% 3-year survival for patients with stage IIIA disease.[20] A theoretical advantage of minimally invasive procedures is that they produce a lower level of inflammatory response and thus may improve 5-year survival. Further studies are needed and are ongoing.

CONCLUSION

The future of minimally invasive surgery will involve robotics. The use of robotic technology for the performance of anatomic lung resection is increasing.[13] Although there is currently only one robotic system for thoracic surgery, other prototypes are being explored. To maintain safe and effective robotic surgery, surgeons must continue to design evidence-based pathways to the credentialing of robotic surgical teams. Despite the small number of studies reported in the literature from several single centers and a handful of surgeons, the results show good intraoperative results with anatomic pulmonary resection and promising long-term survival rates. Further studies on the true cost to society (not solely to the hospital or patient) and the actual 5-year to 10-year survival rates for people with cancer treated robotically are needed. In addition, literature that evaluates the reproducibility of this type of robotic surgery across centers and its feasibility in impoverished or Third-World countries is also needed.

KEY REFERENCES

5. Park BJ, Flores RM, Rusch VW. Robotic assistance for video-assisted thoracic surgical lobectomy: technique and initial results. *J Thorac Cardiovasc Surg*. 2006;131(1):54–59.
7. Veronesi G, Galetta D, Maisonneuve, et al. Four-arm robotic lobectomy for the treatment of early-stage lung cancer. *J Thorac Cardiovasc Surg*. 2010;140(1):19–25.
11. Cerfolio RJ, Bryant AS, Skylizard L, Minnich DJ. Initial consecutive experience of completely portal robotic pulmonary resection with 4 arms. *J Thorac Cardiovasc Surg*. 2011;142(4):740–746.
12. Kent M, Want T, Whyte R, Curran T, Flores R, Gangadharan S. Open, video-assisted thoracic surgery, and robotic lobectomy: review of a national database. *Ann Thorac Surg*. 2014;97:236–244.
13. Wilson JL, Louie BE, Cerfolio RJ, et al. The prevalence of nodal upstaging during robotic lung resection in early stage non-small cell lung cancer. *Ann Thorac Surg*. 2014;97:1901–1906.
16. Nasir BS, Bryant AS, Minnich DJ, Wei B, Cerfolio RJ. Performing robotic lobectomy and segmentectomy: cost, profitability, and outcomes. *Ann Thorac Surg*. 2014;98(1):203–208.
17. Melfi FM, Davini F, Romano G, et al. Robotic lobectomy for lung cancer: evolution in technique and technology. *Eur J Cardiothorac Surg*. 2014;46:626–630.
18. Adams RD, Bolton WD, Stephenson JE, et al. Initial multicenter community robotic lobectomy experience: comparisons to a national database. *Ann Thorac Surg*. 2014;97:1893–1898.
19. Lee BE, Shapiro M, Rutledge JR, Korst RJ. Nodal upstaging in robotic and video assisted thoracic surgery lobectomy for clinical N0 lung cancer. *Ann Thorac Surg*. 2015;100:229–233.
20. Park BJ, Melfi F, Mussi A, et al. Robotic lobectomy for non-small cell lung cancer (NSCLC): long-term oncologic results. *J Thorac Cardiovasc Surg*. 201;143:383–389.

See Expertconsult.com for full list of references.

29 Extent of Surgical Resection for Stage I and II Lung Cancer

Hisao Asamura and Dominique Grunenwald

SUMMARY OF KEY POINTS

- With the realization that many more lung cancers are being detected, which may not only be indolent but also smaller than 2 cm, thoracic surgeons are considering sublobar resections in their practice.
- There are conflicting data from meta-analyses and large databases regarding the efficacy of segmentectomy or wedge resection compared with lobectomy.
- Despite promising data from propensity-matched trials of lobectomy compared with sublobar resection, the results of the Japanese and American randomized trials for management of the less than 2-cm nodule should define the proper resection for this population.

Present-day surgery for lung cancer with curative intent consists of resecting (removing) the proper extent of the lung parenchyma bearing the cancer lesion, along with the local–regional lymph nodes, which may contain cancer metastasis.[1] For resecting the lung parenchyma, the following surgical procedures may be performed, depending on the extent of the disease: pneumonectomy (removal of the entire lung on either side), bilobectomy (removal of two adjacent lobes), lobectomy (removal of a single lobe), segmentectomy (segmental resection, removal of a single segment or adjacent segments), and wedge or partial resection (removal of wedge-shaped parenchyma regardless of the bronchovascular anatomy). When the proximal portion of the bronchus is involved by the direct extension of the tumor or by lymph node metastasis at the hilum and the resected end of the bronchus with lobectomy or pneumonectomy cannot be tumor-free, a sleeve resection, which entails resection of the proximal portion of the bronchus and reconstruction, might be considered in conjunction with lobectomy (sleeve lobectomy) or pneumonectomy (sleeve pneumonectomy) to ensure a safe surgical margin. Sleeve resection enables tumor-free resection without sacrificing the noninvolved lung parenchyma.

With respect to the pulmonary hilum, these procedures can be divided into anatomic resection (pneumonectomy, bilobectomy, lobectomy, and segmentectomy) and nonanatomic resection (wedge resection). In anatomic resection, the extent of the pulmonary parenchyma for resection is determined by the extent of perfusion of the pulmonary vessels as well as by the extent of aeration of the bronchi, which are divided at the hilum. In nonanatomic resection, the extent of the parenchymal resection is determined solely by the location of the target lesion. Although segmentectomy and wedge resection are both referred to as sublobar resection, the technical characteristics of these two procedures are quite different (Fig. 29.1).

In this chapter, we discuss the proper selection of the mode of parenchymal lung resection, with particular focus on stage I and II lung cancer, from both oncologic and technical viewpoints. We also present an overview of the evolution of lung cancer surgery since the 1930s, when the only option available for surgical resection for lung cancer was pneumonectomy.

OVERVIEW OF THE EVOLUTION OF LUNG CANCER SURGERY

Historically, lung cancer surgery has evolved so as to minimize the extent of parenchymal resection (Fig. 29.2). Surgeons have been trying to achieve an optimal balance between radical surgery and surgery that preserves postoperative lung function. Kummel[2] presented the earliest report, published in 1911, of a pneumonectomy of the right side; the patient was a 40-year-old man who died on the sixth postoperative day. After a series of early postoperative deaths after pneumonectomy in the 1920s, Evarts Graham Churchill[3] in St. Louis, Missouri, reported the first successful pneumonectomy, using a tourniquet technique, on a 48-year-old male doctor with lung cancer in 1932. After this landmark operation, reports of successful pneumonectomies for lung cancer were presented by Rienhoff and Broyles,[4] Alexander,[5] Archibald,[6] Sauerbruch,[7] and Overholt.[8] In 1940, Overholt[9] reviewed 110 pneumonectomies, including his own 15 cases, for benign and malignant lung diseases and found a mortality rate of 65% for procedures performed for malignant disease. He noted that the operability of primary lung cancer was 25%. In the 1940s, pneumonectomy was established as the standard mode of pulmonary resection for lung cancer. Allison[10] performed pneumonectomy with intrapericardial ligation of the pulmonary vessels, and more importantly, adding local–regional lymph node dissection to pneumonectomy was proposed as radical surgery for lung cancer. Cahan and coworkers[11] called this procedure radical pneumonectomy, which indicated the combination of parenchymal resection and lymph node dissection.

In the 1950s and 1960s, lobectomy gradually replaced pneumonectomy. In 1950, Churchill et al.[12] reported that the 5-year survival rate with lobectomy (19%) was better than that with pneumonectomy (12%). Belcher[13] reported a 5-year survival rate after lobectomy of 61%, which was outstanding at that time. In 1960, Cahan[14] again defined radical lobectomy as an operation in which one or two lobes of an entire lung are excised in a block dissection, along with certain regional hilar and mediastinal lymphatics (Fig. 29.3). The extent of lymph node dissection was also defined according to the primary site of the lung cancer. Cahan analyzed the outcomes of 48 radical lobectomies for primary and metastatic lung cancers and concluded that survival for 5 or more years could be attributed in large part to radical lobectomy associated with more extensive lymphatic dissection. In the 1970s and 1980s, lobectomy was considered the standard mode of resection for primary lung cancer and pneumonectomy was no longer the standard approach.

Although lobectomy came to be considered the standard of care for primary lung cancer, lesser resections—segmentectomy and wedge resection—for peripheral lung cancer have always been reserved for patients who are not able to tolerate more extensive procedures such as lobectomy or pneumonectomy. Churchill and Belsey[15] originally introduced segmental resection in 1939 as segmental pneumonectomy for the treatment of benign lung diseases. This technique was later advocated for use in patients who had operable lung cancer and limited pulmonary reserve. In 1972, Le Roux[16] reported on 17 patients with peripheral tumors who had undergone segmental resection. In 1973, Jensik et al.[17]

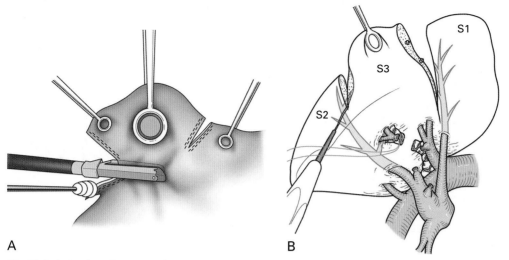

Fig. 29.1. Anatomic and nonanatomic sublobar resections. (A) A segmentectomy (segmental resection) with the division of bronchovascular structures at the hilum (anatomic) S1-S3 represent individual segments. *S1,* Apical segment of the right upper lobe; *S2,* posterior segment of the right upper lobe; *S3,* anterior segment of the right upper lobe. (B) A wedge resection. No anatomic division of bronchovascular structures. *(Courtesy Hisao Asamura, MD.)*

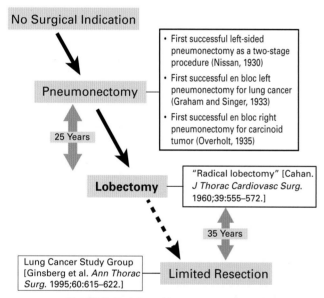

Fig. 29.2. Evolution of lung cancer surgery.

suggested that anatomic pulmonary segmentectomy could be effectively applied to small primary lung cancers when the surgical margins were sufficient.

The results of some subsequent nonrandomized studies showed that excellent outcomes could be achieved with segmental resection for patients with early cancers. These reports stimulated a debate about the optimal resection technique for early-stage non-small cell lung cancer (NSCLC), which the Lung Cancer Study Group addressed in a prospective, randomized trial conducted with 247 patients with stage IA NSCLC.[18] The investigators examined postoperative prognosis and pulmonary function after limited pulmonary resection, including anatomic segmentectomy and non-anatomic wide wedge resection, or lobectomy. They found a 75% increase in the recurrence rate ($p = 0.02$) and a 30% increase in the overall death rate ($p = 0.08$) for limited resection. With regard to pulmonary function, the investigators judged the follow-up and reporting to be somewhat unreliable because study funding was terminated early. The authors concluded that limited resection did not confer improved perioperative morbidity, mortality, or late postoperative pulmonary function. Because of the higher rates of

death and local–regional recurrence associated with limited resection, lobectomy still must be considered the surgical procedure of choice for patients with peripheral T1 N0 NSCLC. Because this landmark trial is the only randomized trial in which limited resection was directly compared with lobectomy, the results are still considered valid.

In 2006 and 2011, Allen et al.[19] and Darling et al.[20] published results from a prospective, randomized trial—the American College of Surgery Oncology Group Z0030 study—designed to evaluate the prognostic significance of lymph node dissection in lung cancer. In this trial, systematic sampling was compared with lymph node dissection for N0 or nonhilar N1, T1, or T2 NSCLC (stage I and II). In short, the results of this study did not support a prognostic advantage of lymph node dissection over sampling. The authors concluded that if systematic and thorough presection sampling of the mediastinal and hilar lymph nodes is negative, mediastinal lymph node dissection does not improve survival for patients with early-stage NSCLC; the authors added that these results cannot be generalized to patients who have radiographic staging or higher-stage tumors.

On the basis of the results of these two important prospective studies, it is widely accepted that the present-day standard of care should be at least lobectomy with lymph node sampling or dissection for stage I and II lung cancer.

RESULTS OF SURGICAL RESECTION FOR STAGE I AND II LUNG CANCER

The outcome of surgery for stage I and II lung cancer has been best demonstrated in publications in 2006 and 2007 by the International Association for the Study of Lung Cancer (IASLC), with results based on the largest and latest global database.[21,22] In 1998, for the preparation of the forthcoming seventh edition of the *TNM Classification of Malignant Tumours* (published in 2009),[23] the IASLC established its Lung Cancer Staging Project. Data were contributed from 46 sources in more than 19 countries. Adequate data were available for 67,725 cases of NSCLC and 8088 cases of small cell lung cancer (SCLC) treated with all modalities of care between 1990 and 2000. In these studies, the survival rates for clinical (c) and pathologic (p) stage I and II NSCLC were given according to the seventh edition of the tumor, node, and metastasis (TNM) system. The 5-year survival rates were 50% for cIA, 43% for cIB, 36% for cIIA, and 25% for cIIB lung cancer. The corresponding 5-year survival rates for

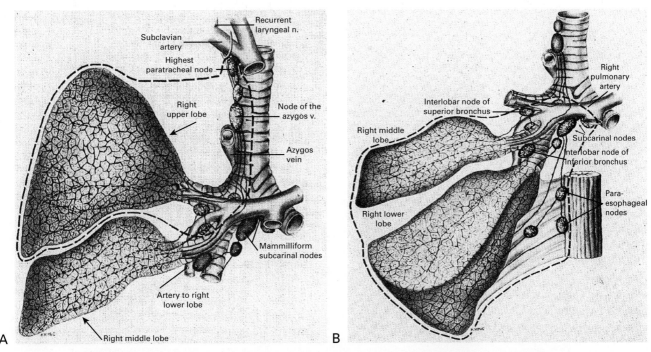

Fig. 29.3. Radical lobectomy. (A) The extents of parenchymal resection (lobe) and (B) lymph node dissection are both determined by the location of the primary tumor. A, Right upper and middle lobe. B, Right middle and lower lobe. *(Reprinted with permission from Cahan WG. Radical lobectomy.* J Thorac Cardiovasc Surg. *1960;39:555–572.)*

pathologic stage lung cancer were 73% for pIA, 58% for pIB, 48% for pIIA, and 36% for pIIB. Current consensus is that postoperative adjuvant chemotherapy improves survival for patients with lung cancer of stage II or higher, as indicated by the results of a series of large-scale clinical trials in the late 1990s and early 2000s.[24–26] Although the IASLC database contained 349 cases of resected SCLC with pathologic TNM staging available, the survival data were given only for clinical stages. With regard to c-stage I and II, the 5-year survival rates were 38% for cIA, 21% for cIB, 38% for cIIA (only 8 patients), and 18% for cIIB.[27]

Detailed survival data for patients with resected lung cancer were reported in a series of Japanese lung cancer registry studies. A retrospective registry study has been performed three times for patients who had resections in 1994, 1999, and 2004.[28–30] The latest report was based on 11,663 patients with all histologic types who had resections in 2004 and for whom survival data were provided according to tumor classification with use of the seventh edition of the TNM classification.[30] Among these 11,663 patients, 243 (2.1%) had tumors with small cell histology. The 5-year survival rates for c-stage lung cancer were 82% for cIA, 66.1% for cIB, 54.5% for cIIA, and 46.4% for cIIB. The 5-year survival rates for p-stage lung cancer were 86.8% for pIA, 73.9% for pIB, 61.6% for pIIA, and 49.8% for pIIB.

A new classification of adenocarcinoma of the lung, which included earlier forms of adenocarcinoma, was published in 2011 to provide uniform terminology and diagnostic criteria.[31] In short, new concepts were introduced, such as adenocarcinoma in situ (AIS) and minimally invasive adenocarcinoma (MIA), for small solitary adenocarcinomas with either pure lepidic growth or predominant lepidic growth smaller than 5 mm to define patients who, if they were to undergo complete resection, would be expected to have 100% or near-100% disease-specific survival, respectively. By contrast, adenocarcinomas are also classified according to their predominant pattern, with comprehensive histologic subtyping as lepidic, acinar, papillary, or solid. Earlier forms such as AIS and MIA were recognized only after the advent of high-resolution computed tomography and the dissemination of computed tomography screening programs. In

the Japanese Registry Study,[30] these early-stage lung cancers had been included with stage IA cancers, and the proportion of these cancers may be associated with a difference in survival, especially for stage IA disease. The surgical significance of these classifications has also been analyzed.[32] In studies published in 2011 and 2013, the prognosis of 545 radiographically determined noninvasive adenocarcinomas of the lung that showed ground-glass opacity (GGO) was described; a consolidation-to-tumor ratio of 0.25 or less in cT1a was used as a radiographic criterion of noninvasive cancer, and the lesion was resected using lobectomy.[33,34] The 5-year survival rates for noninvasive and invasive adenocarcinomas were 96.7% and 88.9%, respectively. This surgical outcome indicates the realistic possibility of lesser resections, such as segmentectomy and wedge resection, for early lung cancers.

POSSIBILITY OF SUBLOBAR, LIMITED RESECTION FOR STAGE I AND II LUNG CANCER

Technical and Pathologic Considerations

When we think of sublobar resection, especially segmental resection, as a possible radical resection for lung cancer, in which no tumor tissue must be left behind, we must consider several factors. In sublobar resection, the lung parenchyma must be transected and divided for the procedure to be complete, whereas in lobectomy, the fissure is divided to remove the entire lobe. Sublobar resection has some technical limitations associated with tumor size, location, histologic type, and node involvement. In particular, tumor size and location are closely related to the safe surgical margin in a radical resection.

Tumor size and local recurrence after sublobar resection have been studied extensively. Bando et al.[35] studied 74 patients who had sublobar resections and found that the local–regional recurrence rate was 2% for tumors less than 2 cm and 33% for tumors larger than 2 cm. Fernando et al.[36] and Okada et al.[37] also found that tumor size less than 2 cm was an independent, favorable predictor of a smaller chance of recurrence and better survival after sublobar resection. If we consider the distance between the tumor and the surgical margin of the lung parenchyma, it is easy to understand why larger tumors have a greater chance of local recurrence (Fig. 29.4A). Another important factor is the location of the tumor in relation to the pleural surface and the hilum. A fundamental, geometric understanding of a lung segment is that the segment is fan-shaped, with the base on the pleural surface and the apex at the pulmonary hilum. Therefore, the distance between the tumor and the resection line is inevitably smaller for a tumor that is close to the hilum, even if the tumor is small (Fig. 29.4B). In general, even for a tumor diameter of 2 cm or less, segmentectomy or wedge resection should be performed only if the tumor is located in the outer third of the lung parenchyma. Other unfavorable factors for limited resection are an aggressive histology, such as SCLC, and lymph node involvement. These conditions indicate a higher likelihood of tumor spread in the lobe that contains the segment.

Oncologic Considerations

Limited, sublobar resection should be considered for lung cancer in the following three situations:

- T1 N0 M0 lung cancer in individuals with limited cardiopulmonary reserve, regardless of the type of lesion;

- early lung cancer with a predominantly GGO appearance (pathologic AIS or MIA);
- small but invasive lung cancers located in the periphery of the lung.

As noted earlier, considerable interest in sublobar resection arose in the 1970s and 1980s when the feasibility of limited resection for patients with a compromised cardiopulmonary reserve was demonstrated. At that time, the 5-year survival and recurrence rates for sublobar resection were considered inferior to the rates for lobectomy, and sublobar resection was restricted to patients with impaired cardiac function or substantial comorbidities that precluded conventional lobectomy. In fact, in 1994, Warren and Faber[38] demonstrated decreased survival and increased recurrence among 173 patients with stage I NSCLC who had sublobar resection or lobectomy. However, the results of single-institution retrospective investigations published between 1997 and 2004, in which the equivalency of sublobar resection to lobectomy for patients with limited cardiopulmonary reserve was evaluated, contradict earlier results and demonstrate that stage I disease portends a survival advantage regardless of the extent of surgical resection or the histologic subtype. Campione et al.[39] found no significant difference in survival between lobectomy and anatomic segmentectomy in a series of 121 patients with stage IA lung cancer. Other studies demonstrated similar

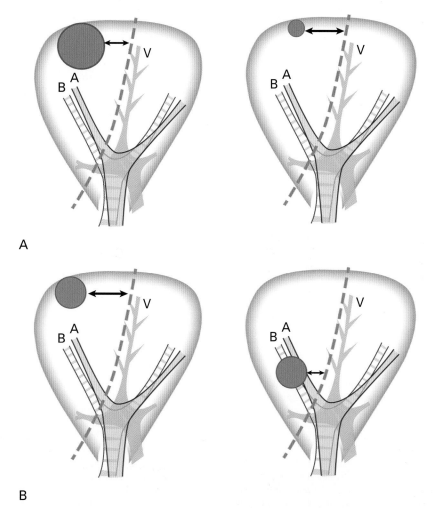

Fig. 29.4. Relationship between the tumor and the surgical margin. (A) For larger tumors, the distance between the tumor and the surgical margin becomes inevitably smaller. (B) When the tumor is located close to the pulmonary hilum, the distance between the tumor and the surgical margin also becomes smaller, despite the tumor size. *A,* Pulmonary artery; *B,* bronchus; *V,* pulmonary vein. *(Courtesy Hisao Asamura, MD.)*

results for segmentectomy and lobectomy.[40–50] The surgical indication of limited resection for patients with stage IA lung cancer with limited cardiopulmonary reserve is the reasonable treatment of choice.

As discussed previously, AIS (formerly bronchioloalveolar carcinoma) and MIA are novel concepts that indicate the noninvasive or minimally invasive nature of adenocarcinoma with the unique radiographic presentation of GGO. In a variety of retrospective Japanese studies, the use of limited resection for patients with nonsolid (pure) or part-solid (mixed) GGO tumors has been assessed. In each of these studies, patients with an AIS or an MIA had prolonged survival and lower recurrence after resection compared with patients with other subtypes of NSCLC. The use of sublobar resection for these early tumors was based on a clinical–pathologic study of the correlation between the degree of invasive growth (stromal invasion) and the prognosis. Sakurai et al.[51] classified 380 resected adenocarcinomas of 2 cm or less in diameter according to the degree of invasive growth (structural deformity and its location in the adenocarcinoma) and showed that 100% survival could be achieved for patients with AIS or MIA, despite the mode of pulmonary resection. On the basis of these clinical–pathologic observations, it would be reasonable to consider sublobar resection for AIS and MIA with GGO according to the location and size of the tumor.

The indication for sublobar resection must be considered from not only an oncologic but also an anatomic perspective. In the case of a tumor that is located deep inside the lung parenchyma, sublobar resection cannot ensure a safe surgical margin because the surgical margin is close to the hilar structures. As noted previously, the shortest distance between a tumor and the resected margin falls in the area close to the hilum. The tumor diameter also affects the distance to the surgical margin. Therefore as with segmentectomy or wedge resection, sublobar resection should be used only when the tumor is located in the outer third of the lung parenchyma and, preferably, is 2 cm or less in diameter. For tumors that are located in the inner two-thirds of the lung parenchyma or that are larger than 2 cm in diameter, lobectomy should still be selected, regardless of the tumor pathology.

However, for a histologically invasive lung cancer that is a small (≤2 cm, T1a), solitary nodule located in the periphery of the lung, the feasibility of limited, sublobar resection must be assessed from the perspective of the present day. Such an assessment would entail revision of the Lung Cancer Study Group study performed in the late 1980s.[18] Indeed, the present-day routine workup for patients with resectable lung cancer is different from the workup done in the 1980s. To investigate sublobar resection for early lung cancer, a few prospective studies are ongoing. As summarized by Iwata,[52] the role of sublobar resection has been explored in large databases such as Surveillance, Epidemiology, and End Results Program and the National Cancer Database (NCDB). Veluswamy et al.'s[53] analysis of 2008 adenocarcinomas and 1139 squamous cell carcinomas all less than 2 cm in patients older than 65 revealed that wedge was always inferior to other resections independent of histology; however, for adenocarcinoma, overall survival and lung cancer–specific survival of segmentectomy were equivalent to lobectomy, but not for squamous cell carcinoma. By contrast, Khullar et al.'s[54] and Speicher's et al.'s[55] analyses of clinical stage I patients in the NCDB revealed that overall survival was inferior for sublobar resections compared with lobectomy. These analyses, however, were limited in that only 290 of 987 propensity-matched patients in the NCDB could be analyzed for survival because survival was not available past 2006. Meta-analyses investigating the role of sublobar resections also failed to have consensus. In Cao et al.'s analysis of 54 studies,[56] intentional use of sublobar resections resulted in similar overall survival to lobes while this was not seen in cases where a sublobar resection was performed for compromised patients. The disease-free survival

always favored lobectomies. Bao et al.'s[57] survival analysis of 22 studies found equivalent overall survival between segmentectomy and lobectomy only for tumors smaller than 2 cm. Finally, in an analysis of 4564 lobectomies and 2287 sublobar resections, Taioli et al.[58] concluded that the high degree of heterogeneity of study design for these analyses might preclude useful conclusions using conventional meta-analyses to study these resections. Five propensity-matched studies with 69 to 312 matched sublobar and lobectomy patients with 3-year to 10-year overall survival data have been published.[59–63] Common matching parameters have included age, sex, and tumor size, and all studies found no differences in disease-free survival or overall survival comparing segmentectomy with lobectomy. Kodama et al.'s[63] study is notable in that it summarized 10-year intermediate end points from surgery revealing that freedom from local–regional recurrence for segmentectomy and lobectomy was 95.3% and 97%, respectively, and no differences in overall survival were recorded for 10-year survival (segmentectomy, 83.2%; lobectomy, 88%). With regard to the use of video-assisted thoracoscopic surgery (VATS) segmentectomy, two studies have revealed equal overall survival and disease-free survival for VATS segmentectomy compared with VATS lobectomy,[62,64] whereas Ghaly et al.[65] have reported no difference in disease-free survival or overall survival for 91 VATS segmentectomies compared with 102 open chest segmentectomies.

Randomized clinical trials with peripheral lung cancers no more than 2 cm in diameter as the target lesions are being conducted in the United States by the Cancer and Leukemia Group B (CALGB 140503; ClinicalTrials.gov identifier: NCT00499330)[38] and in Japan by the Japan Clinical Oncology Group and the West Japan Oncology Group (JCOG0802/WJOG4607L).[66] For the CALGB trial, the primary end point is disease-free survival and the secondary end points are overall survival, rate of local–regional and systemic recurrence, and pulmonary function; the estimated enrollment is 1258. For the Japanese trial, the end points are overall survival (primary) and postoperative pulmonary function (secondary), and the targeted accrual is 1100 patients (Fig. 29.5). If the prognosis for patients who have segmentectomy is not significantly inferior to that for patients who have lobectomy and if the postoperative pulmonary function is significantly better for patients who have segmentectomy, we can definitively conclude that the standard surgical modality for these early tumors should be segmentectomy.

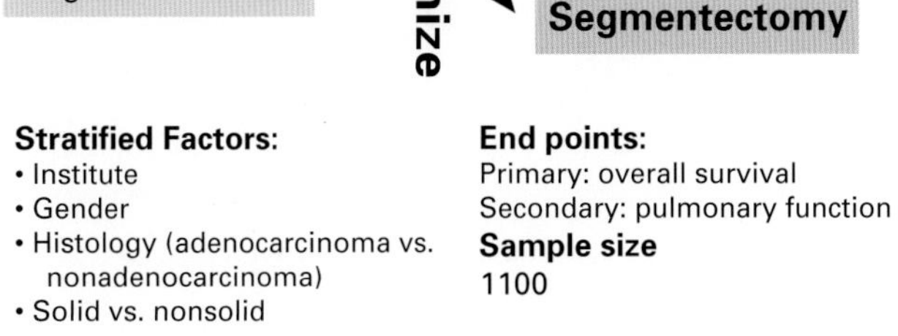

JCOG0802/WJOG4607L

Fig. 29.5. The design of JCOG0802/WJOG4607L, an ongoing phase III randomized trial comparing segmentectomy and lobectomy for small lung cancers (part-solid ground-glass opacities or solid tumors) that are 2 cm or less in diameter.

CONCLUSION

The present-day standard of care for lung cancer resection is still at least lobectomy with hilar and mediastinal lymph node sampling or dissection. It is reasonable to perform sublobar resection, such as segmentectomy and wedge resection, for patients with limited cardiopulmonary reserve. The use of sublobar resection may be justified for most early lung cancers with minimal or no invasive features located in the outer region of the lung parenchyma. The feasibility of sublobar resection for lung cancer with overt invasive features is under investigation, with particular focus on tumors 2 cm or less in diameter. The results of several ongoing trials are awaited. Lobectomy should be recognized as the standard mode of resection for appropriate patients.

KEY REFERENCES

18. Ginsberg RJ, Rubinstein LV. Randomized trial of lobectomy versus limited resection for T1 N0 non-small cell lung cancer. Lung Cancer Study Group. *Ann Thorac Surg*. 1995;60:615–622.
20. Darling GE, Allen MS, Decker PA, et al. Randomized trial of mediastinal lymph node sampling versus complete lymphadenectomy during pulmonary resection in the patient with N0 or N1 (less than hilar) non-small cell carcinoma: results of the American College of Surgery Oncology Group Z0030 Trial. *J Thorac Cardiovasc Surg*. 2011;141:662–670.
22. Goldstraw P, Crowley J, Chansky K, et al. International Association for the Study of Lung Cancer International Staging Committee; Participating Institutions. The IASLC Lung Cancer Staging Project: proposals for the revision of the TNM stage groupings in the forthcoming (seventh) edition of the TNM classification of malignant tumours. *J Thorac Oncol*. 2007;2:706–714.
29. Asamura H, Goya T, Koshiishi Y, et al. Japanese Joint Committee of Lung Cancer Registry. A Japanese Lung Cancer Registry study: prognosis of 13,010 resected lung cancers. *J Thorac Oncol*. 2008;3:46–52.
31. Travis WD, Brambilla E, Noguchi M, et al. International Association for the Study of Lung Cancer/American Thoracic Society/European Respiratory Society international multidisciplinary classification of lung adenocarcinoma. *J Thorac Oncol*. 2011;6:244–285.
34. Asamura H, Hishida T, Suzuki K, et al. Japan Clinical Oncology Group Lung Cancer Surgical Study Group radiographically determined noninvasive adenocarcinoma of the lung: survival outcomes of Japan Clinical Oncology Group 0201. *J Thorac Cardiovasc Surg*. 2013;146:24–30.
37. Okada M, Nishio W, Sakamoto T, et al. Effect of tumor size on prognosis in patients with non-small cell lung cancer. The role of segmentectomy as a type of lesser resection. *J Thorac Cardiovasc Surg*. 2005;129:87–93.
48. Okada M, Koike T, Higashiyama M, Yamato Y, Kodama K, Tsubota M. Radical sublobar resection for small-sized non-small cell lung cancer: a multicenter study. *J Thorac Cardiovasc Surg*. 2006;132:769–775.
49. El-Sherif A, Gooding WE, Santos R, et al. Outcomes of sublobar resection versus lobectomy for stage I non-small cell lung cancer: a 13-year analysis. *Ann Thorac Surg*. 2006;82:408–416.
59. Altorki NK, Kamel MK, Narula N, et al. Anatomical segmentectomy and wedge resections are associated with comparable outcomes for small cT1N0 non-small cell lung cancer. *J Thorac Oncol*. 2016;11(11):1984–1992.
60. Tsutani Y, Miyata Y, Nakayama H, et al. Oncologic outcomes of segmentectomy compared with lobectomy for clinical stage IA lung adenocarcinoma: propensity score-matched analysis in a multicenter study. *J Thorac Cardiovasc Surg*. 2013;146:358–364.
61. Landreneau RJ, Normolle DP, Christie NA, et al. Recurrence and survival outcomes after anatomic segmentectomy versus lobectomy for clinical stage I non-small-cell lung cancer: a propensity-matched analysis. *J Clin Oncol*. 2014;32:2449–2455.
62. Hwang Y, Kang CH, Kim HS, Jeon JH, Park IK, Kim YT. Comparison of thoracoscopic segmentectomy and thoracoscopic lobectomy on the patients with non-small cell lung cancer: a propensity score matching study. *Eur J Cardiothorac Surg*. 2015;48:273–278.

See Expertconsult.com for full list of references.

30 Extended Resections for Lung Cancer: Chest Wall and Pancoast Tumors

Valerie W. Rusch and Paul E. Van Schil

SUMMARY OF KEY POINTS

Chest Wall:

- Invasion of parietal pleura and chest wall indicates T3; involvement of vertebral body indicates T4 chest wall tumor.
- Extensive resection required.
- Long-term survival possible postresection if:
  - No distant metastases
  - No mediastinal lymph node involvement
  - Complete (R0) resection.
- Systematic lymph node dissection should be performed as part of resection.
- Choice of prosthesis for chest wall reconstruction determined by size and location of chest wall defect.

Pancoast:

- Superior pulmonary sulcus: uppermost extent of costovertebral gutter.
- Challenging to treat due to involvement of adjacent vital structures, including brachial plexus, subclavian vessels, and spine.
- By definition, stage IIB or higher; mediastinal staging via endobronchial ultrasound or mediastinoscopy recommended.
- Induction chemoradiotherapy followed by surgical resection is the standard of care.
- Operative approaches:
  - Posterior (Paulson) approach
  - Modified posterolateral periscapular (Masaoka) approach
  - Anterior (Dartevelle/Spaggiari) transmanubrial approach.

CHEST WALL TUMORS

General Principles

Invasion of the parietal pleura or chest wall by a primary lung cancer is a relatively rare occurrence, reported in 5% to 8% of all cases of lung cancer.[1] Invasion of the parietal pleura and the chest wall suggests a T3 tumor, and involvement of the vertebral bodies suggests a T4 tumor. Tumors infiltrating the second or first rib and surrounding structures usually are considered to be superior sulcus or Pancoast tumors when neurologic symptoms are present.[1] Pancoast tumors are described in detail in the latter part of this chapter.

Extensive resection is required to remove tumors invading the chest wall. Although such tumors once were considered to have a dismal prognosis, many series have shown that long-term survival may be possible when the patient has no distant metastases, no involvement of mediastinal nodes, and evidence of complete (R0) resection as demonstrated by histologically negative margins in the ribs as well as in the muscles and soft tissues of the chest wall. In addition, a thorough lymph node evaluation by means of either systematic node dissection or at least a lobe-specific node dissection related to the location of the primary tumor is required. A minimum of six lymph node stations must be removed, of which three must be located in the mediastinum and must include the subcarinal station.[7] According to the definition of complete resection as proposed by Rami-Porta et al.[2] there must be no extracapsular extension and the highest mediastinal lymph node must be negative. Complete (R0) resection can be challenging in cases of posterior tumors located near the costovertebral angle or involving vertebral bodies, and analysis of frozen sections is not feasible for tumors with osseous margins.

Staging

The goal of surgical treatment in cases of T3 and T4 lung cancers is to obtain an R0 resection. Surgical treatment may be part of a multimodality approach that includes induction chemotherapy or chemoradiation therapy to reduce the tumor volume and to optimize resection margins. A thorough preoperative evaluation is necessary. Functional operability depends on a detailed cardio-pulmonary assessment as outlined by a working group of the ERS together with the ESTS.[3] T3 and T4 tumors require at least a lobectomy, but no specific criteria have been developed to determine whether a patient will tolerate a planned chest wall resection. Nevertheless, as it is clear that a chest wall resection may induce additional respiratory compromise, clinical judgment by an experienced thoracic surgeon and discussion of each individual case by a multidisciplinary tumor board are necessary when this procedure is anticipated. Published series report that mediastinal nodal involvement is a poor prognostic factor and that extensive surgery is not warranted when mediastinal lymph node metastases are present.[4,5]

Computed tomography (CT) of the chest with use of intravenous contrast medium is the preferred method for defining the extent of the primary tumor and evaluating the involvement of hilar and mediastinal lymph nodes (Fig. 30.1). Findings on CT images that are used to identify osseous or soft-tissue chest wall invasion include obliteration of the extrapleural fat plane, the length of tumor contact with the pleural surface, the angle of the tumor with the pleura, and clear evidence of chest wall invasion.[6] A combination of several criteria increases sensitivity.[4] For para-vertebral and superior sulcus tumors, magnetic resonance imaging (MRI) of the chest is required to determine neural or vertebral involvement. Respiratory dynamic MRI has been shown to have a sensitivity of 100% and a specificity of 83% for determining chest wall invasion but has not been widely adopted.[7] Ultrasonography of the chest wall also may be helpful but does not show superior sulcus tumors.[8] Positron emission tomography (PET), preferably, integrated PET–CT, should be performed for every patient to evaluate local–regional extension and possible distant spread precluding surgical intervention.

The pathologic status of the mediastinal nodes should be confirmed before a large chest wall resection is planned.[9] Endobronchial ultrasound and endoscopic ultrasound with transbronchial or transesophageal biopsy are currently the procedures of choice. In selected cases, these procedures are supplemented with mediastinoscopy to reduce the false-negative rate as much as possible.

Surgical Resection

Depending on the location of the primary tumor and its extension into the chest wall, the incision is carefully chosen and may be centered on the anterior, lateral, or posterior chest wall. The thoracic cavity is entered away from the primary tumor, as every attempt should be made to obtain an en bloc resection with complete removal of the primary tumor together with the invaded chest wall to avoid any spillage of tumor cells in the pleural cavity.[10] Video-assisted thoracoscopic surgery may be helpful for initial evaluation.[11]

The precise margins to be obtained around the primary tumor have not been exactly determined, but most authors have agreed that at least 1 cm is required.[4] Once the pleural space has been entered, chest wall involvement is evaluated and a determination is made as to whether an extrapleural resection or a full-thickness chest wall resection is required. Stoelben and Ludwig[1] described four categories of chest wall involvement for determining the subsequent resection (Table 30.1). When the tumor easily detaches from the chest wall in the extrapleural plane by finger dissection, this usually indicates only inflammatory adhesions that do not require chest wall resection. Frozen section analysis of

suspicious areas of the parietal pleura may clarify this. When the tumor is densely adherent or frankly invades the chest wall, rib resection is indicated. For anterior tumors, resection of part or all of the sternum may be needed. For posterior tumors, resection of transverse processes or vertebral bodies may be needed, and a spine surgeon (either an orthopedic surgeon or a neurosurgeon) should work collaboratively with the thoracic surgeon.[12] However, resection of these vertebral structures is infrequently seen outside the classic Pancoast (superior sulcus) position. To reduce trauma to the uninvolved extrathoracic muscles, rib resection can be performed from inside the chest with use of the technique described by Cerfolio et al.[13]

Lobectomy or bilobectomy is the procedure of choice for pulmonary resection. A pneumonectomy is necessary in some cases, but it is a high-risk procedure when combined with extensive chest wall resection and should be performed only in centers with extensive experience.[14]

Multiple techniques are available for reconstruction of the chest wall. No reconstruction is required for defects of 3 cm or less that are covered by the scapula. However, when the defect is located at the tip of the scapula, chest wall reconstruction is required to prevent entrapment of the scapula, which is a highly symptomatic complication that is associated with poor cosmetic results.[4] Polypropylene and polyglactin meshes, polytetrafluoroethylene patches, and the so-called Marlex mesh with methylmethacrylate (MMM) sandwich technique are options for the reconstruction of large defects.[15] Close cooperation with a plastic surgeon is required in situations in which soft-tissue reconstruction is needed to cover a chest wall prosthesis. Polytetrafluoroethylene is frequently used as the standard material. However, for large anterior or anterolateral defects, the MMM sandwich technique provides greater immediate chest wall stability (Figs. 30.2A and 30.2B) with the lowest risk of postoperative respiratory insufficiency.[16] A new moldable system composed of titanium with connecting bars and rib clips is useful for obtaining a rigid basis when reconstructing the chest wall.[17,18] This system is particularly useful for large defects associated with skin ulceration and infection, for which the MMM sandwich technique is contraindicated (Fig. 30.3A–B). Synthetic material should be covered by viable muscle or musculocutaneous flaps to reduce the risk of infection.

Results and Long-Term Survival

At experienced centers, the mortality and morbidity rates associated with these procedures have decreased. The mean postoperative mortality rate is about 6%, with the majority of deaths being caused by pulmonary complications and respiratory failure.[4] This finding underlines the importance of careful preoperative cardiorespiratory evaluation and discussion within a multidisciplinary team before the decision is made to proceed with an extensive resection. In addition to standard complications after thoracotomy, specific complications related to the chest wall resection include infection necessitating removal of the prosthetic material, herniation of the scapula, paradoxical respiration (flail chest), and, in cases involving dissection close to the spinal cord, paraplegia and leakage of cerebrospinal fluid.

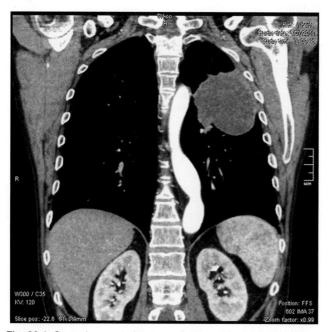

Fig. 30.1. Coronal computed tomography image demonstrating large tumor invading the chest wall in a 58-year-old patient.

TABLE 30.1 Intraoperative Categories of Chest Wall Involvement and Subsequent Resection[a]

Intraoperative Findings	T Status[b]	Procedure
Lung and tumor not fixed to chest wall	Not T3	Standard resection
Inflammatory adhesions between tumor and parietal pleura or previous inflammatory pleuritic	Not T3	Extrapleural resection
Tumor has penetrated visceral pleura to the parietal pleura	T3	Extrapleural lobectomy probably possible
Tumor has infiltrated soft-tissue or osseous chest wall	T3 or T4	Lung and chest wall resection

[a]Adapted from Stoelben E, Ludwig C. Chest wall resection for lung cancer: indications and techniques. *Eur J Cardiothorac Surg.* 2009;35(3):450–456.
[b]Related to chest wall.

In selected cases, induction chemotherapy or chemoradiation therapy may be helpful for decreasing the tumor volume and limiting the subsequent chest wall resection, but such therapy has not been standard treatment except for Pancoast tumors. Adjuvant chemotherapy or radiotherapy also remains controversial, and no specific guidelines exist for patients who have chest wall resection. Radiotherapy may be indicated for patients with close or positive surgical margins, but no randomized evidence is available to support its routine use.

In most large series, the 5-year overall survival rate has been approximately 30% to 40%. Long-term survival depends on lymph node involvement and the completeness of resection. In 1999, in a large series of 334 chest wall resections, Downey et al.[19] showed that the 5-year survival rate was 32% for patients with apparently complete (R0) resections but only 4% for those with incomplete (R1 and R2) resections. These findings were confirmed in later studies.[4] In a large series of 531 patients with pT3 lung cancer, a relatively uniform prognosis was found for the different subgroups of T3 involvement.[20] For the 407 patients with chest wall involvement, the 5-year survival rate was 43%. In a comparative study involving the seventh edition of the tumor, node, metastasis classification system, the prognosis for 140 patients with T3 chest wall invasion was not significantly different from that for 28 patients with tumors measuring more than 7 cm in size without chest wall invasion.[21] In a multivariate analysis of 107 patients who had chest wall resection for the management of lung cancer invading the chest wall, the completeness of resection, tumor size, node status, depth of invasion, and completeness of adjuvant chemotherapy were independent prognostic factors.[22] In that series, the overall 5-year survival rate was 26%.

With regard to the extent of pulmonary resection, a recent series showed that pneumonectomy combined with chest wall resection is feasible for highly selected patients.[14] In that series of 34 patients, the mortality rate was 2.9%, the morbidity rate was 38%, and the overall 5-year survival rate was 47%. For patients with N0, N1, and N2 disease, the 5-year survival rates were 60%, 56%, and 17%, respectively. After complete (R0) resection, the rate of local recurrence is very low.[10] N2 involvement can be considered to be a marker for systemic disease, and most patients with N2 involvement will die of distant metastases.[1]

Quality of life after chest wall resection is important to consider, but published data are sparse. In a retrospective series of 51 patients who were treated with chest wall resection, quality of life was only moderately impaired.[23] Subjective parameters, including dyspnea, correlated well with quality of life, whereas objective measurements of pulmonary function did not.

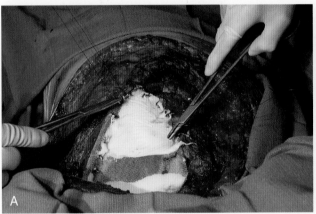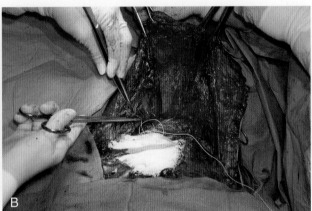

Fig. 30.2. Intraoperative photographs made during reconstruction of a large anterior chest wall and sternal defect with use of a so-called MMM sandwich (Marlex mesh with methylmethacrylate) prosthesis (viewed from the foot of the operating room table). The prosthesis is secured to the remaining half of the sternum medially and to the ribs inferiorly and laterally. (A) The polypropylene mesh has been infiltrated with methylmethacrylate, with an area left open for tissue ingrowth, and (B) prior to closure of the incision, absorbable sutures are used to tack the overlying muscle flaps to the prosthesis to prevent the formation of a seroma.

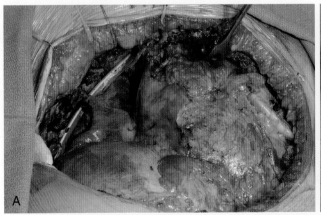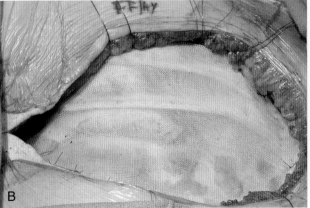

Fig. 30.3. (A) Intraoperative photograph made during sternal and chest wall reconstruction at the site of a large anterior defect following resection for the management of osteoradionecrosis, and (B) titanium rods provide chest wall stability and are covered with a polypropylene mesh in preparation for myocutaneous flap soft-tissue coverage.

TABLE 30.2 Studies Reporting Results of Induction Chemoradiotherapy Plus Surgical Resection for Patients With Pancoast Tumors

Author (y)	No. of Patients	Induction Therapy	Rate of Complete Resection (R0) (%)	5-Year Overall Survival Rate (%)
Marra et al.[63] (2007)	31	Cisplatin + etoposide + 45 Gy	94	46
de Perrot[84] (2008)	44	Cisplatin + etoposide + 45 Gy	89	59
Pourel et al.[62] (2008)	107	Cisplatin + etoposide + 45 Gy	90	40
Kunitoh et al. (JCOG 9806)[67] (2008)	76	Mitomycin, vinblastine, and cisplatin + 45 Gy (split course)	89	56

PANCOAST TUMORS

Historical Background

Nonsmall cell lung cancer (NSCLC) of the superior sulcus, commonly termed Pancoast tumors, is challenging to treat because of its involvement of adjacent vital structures, including the brachial plexus, subclavian vessels, and spine. Originally described by a radiologist, Henry Pancoast, in 1932,[24] Pancoast tumors were thought to be uniformly fatal until the 1950s, when, on the basis of anecdotal experience, induction radiotherapy and resection were found to be curative.[25,26] During the next 40 years, this approach remained the standard of care, with advances limited to the development of novel surgical techniques for T4 tumors involving the subclavian vessels and spine.[27–29] However, complete resection was usually achieved in only 60% of patients, and the overall 5-year survival rate remained at about 30%, indicating a need for novel therapy.[30] During the 1990s, concurrent cisplatin-based chemotherapy and radiotherapy followed by resection was shown to be safe and effective for the management of some stage III NSCLC.[31] The findings of small studies suggested that this treatment might be appropriate for Pancoast tumors,[32] which led to a large North American trial, the results of which established the use of induction chemoradiation therapy followed by resection as the standard of care. Other studies subsequently corroborated the results of the North American trial (see Table 30.2).

Anatomic Definition

The original definition of a Pancoast tumor was a carcinoma of uncertain origin, arising in the extreme apex of the chest, that was associated with shoulder and arm pain, atrophy of the hand muscles, and Horner syndrome. Anatomically, the pulmonary sulcus is synonymous with the costovertebral gutter, which extends from the first rib to the diaphragm. The term superior pulmonary sulcus is used to describe the uppermost extent of this recess.[33,34] Unbeknown to Pancoast, the most accurate description of this type of tumor was reported in 1932 by Tobias, who recognized it as a peripheral lung cancer.[35]

This original definition has been expanded to include tumors that do not involve the brachial plexus or stellate ganglion. Tumors involving the chest wall at the level of the second rib or below do not meet the criteria for classification as Pancoast tumors. Chest wall involvement may be limited to invasion of the parietal pleura in the superior sulcus but typically extends to involve the upper ribs, vertebral bodies, subclavian vessels, nerve roots of the brachial plexus, or stellate ganglion.

The thoracic inlet can be divided into three compartments on the basis of the insertions of the anterior and middle scalene muscles on the first rib and the posterior scalene muscle on the second rib. The anterior compartment, located anterior to the anterior scalene muscle, contains the subclavian and internal jugular veins and the sternocleidomastoid and omohyoid muscles. The middle compartment, located between the anterior and middle scalene muscles, includes the subclavian artery, the trunks of the brachial plexus, and the phrenic nerve. The posterior compartment contains the nerve roots of the brachial plexus, the stellate ganglion, and the vertebral column.

Originally, Pancoast tumors were considered to be located only posteriorly. However, they also may be located anteriorly, with predominantly vascular involvement rather than neurologic or vertebral involvement. Surgeons should be adept at both anterior and posterior approaches, as a combined procedure may be necessary to obtain a complete resection.

Pretreatment Evaluation

The presence of a Pancoast syndrome is not always associated with NSCLC. Other diseases, including lymphoma, tuberculosis, and primary chest wall tumors, may be associated with an apical mass and chest wall involvement. Transthoracic needle biopsy should be performed to establish a diagnosis before treatment.

Pancoast tumors are, by definition, classified as stage IIB or higher and require an extent-of-disease evaluation before treatment is initiated, including contrast-enhanced CT of the chest and upper abdomen, whole-body PET, and MRI of the brain (Fig. 30.4A–B). Because Pancoast tumors with mediastinal node metastases (N2 or N3 disease) have a poor prognosis, mediastinal staging via either endobronchial ultrasound or mediastinoscopy should be considered.

MRI with use of intravenous contrast medium is the modality of choice for evaluating structures of the thoracic inlet, including the brachial plexus, subclavian vessels, spine, and neural foramina and is crucial for preoperative planning.[36] The extent of nerve root involvement must be assessed. Resection of the T1 nerve root usually does not cause motor function deficit, but resection of the C8 nerve root or lower trunk of the brachial plexus leads to loss of hand and arm function. A careful neurologic examination is informative and supplements MRI findings.[37] Pain extending along the ulnar aspect of the forearm and hand is consistent with T1 involvement. Weakness of the intrinsic muscles of the hand indicates involvement of the C8 nerve root or lower trunk of the brachial plexus. Resection of a Pancoast tumor should be planned jointly with a spine neurosurgeon to allow optimal patient selection and the best chance of complete resection.

Patients must be evaluated to determine whether they can tolerate combined-modality therapy. Performance status, renal function, and neurologic function must be adequate in order for the patient to receive platinum-based chemotherapy. Pulmonary function tests and, when necessary, cardiac stress tests are done to evaluate the ability of the patient to tolerate pulmonary resection.

Multimodality Treatment

The management of NSCLC of the superior sulcus during the past 70 years can be classified into four eras. Pancoast first described these tumors as "a peculiar neoplastic entity found in the upper portion of the pulmonary sulcus of the thorax . . . evidently epithelial in its histopathology, but its exact origin is uncertain."[24] During the ensuing 20 years, these tumors became

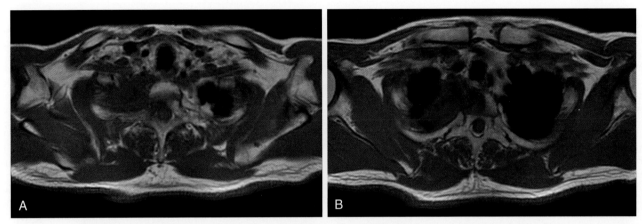

Fig. 30.4. Preoperative magnetic resonance imaging showing a T4 Pancoast tumor that has invaded the thoracic spine. After induction chemoradiation therapy, complete (R0) resection was achieved by means of combined posterior resection of the involved area of the spine and posterolateral thoracotomy to complete the lobectomy and chest wall resection. (A) The tumor has filled the superior sulcus but has not invaded the brachial plexus or subclavian vessels, and (B) the tumor has invaded and destroyed part of the vertebral body.

TABLE 30.3 Historical Experience With Induction Therapy (Primarily Radiotherapy) and Surgery for Superior Sulcus NSCLCs (Pancoast Tumors)[a]

Author (y)	No. of Patients	Preoperative Treatment	Rate of Complete Resection (R0) (%)	2-y Survival (%)	5-y Survival (%)
Paulson et al.[33] (1975)	61	Radiotherapy	NS	34	26
Miller et al.[76] (1978)	26	Radiotherapy	NS	NS	32
Attar et al.[77] (1979)	73	Radiotherapy	48	23 (3 y)	NS
Stanford et al.[78] (1980)	16	Radiotherapy	NS	NS	49
Anderson et al.[79] (1986)	28	Radiotherapy	50	NS	34
Devine et al.[80] (1986)	40	Radiotherapy	70	NS	10
Shahian et al.[81] (1987)	18	Radiotherapy	50	64	56
Wright et al.[82] (1987)	21	Radiotherapy	NS	55	27
Sartori et al.[40] (1992)	42	Radiotherapy	NS	38	25
Dartevelle et al.[27] (1993)	29	None (postoperative radiotherapy)	NS	50	31
Ginsberg et al.[48] (1994)	124	Radiotherapy	56	45	26
Maggi et al.[41] (1994)	60	Radiotherapy	60	NS	17.4
Martinez-Monge et al.[32] (1994)	18	Chemoradiation therapy	76	NS	56 (4 y)
Muscolino et al.[83] (1997)	15	Radiotherapy	73	NS	26.6
Rusch et al.[30] (2000)	225	Radiotherapy	64 (T3), 39 (T4)	NS	46 (T3), 13 (T4)

[a]Adapted from Rusch et al. Factors determining outcome after surgical resection of T3 and T4 lung cancers of the superior sulcus. *J Thorac Cardiovasc Surg.* 2000;119(6):1147–1153.

NS, not stated.

recognized as NSCLC but were considered inoperable and incurable. In 1956, Chardack and MacCallum[25] reported the case of a patient in whom a poorly differentiated squamous cell carcinoma was managed with en bloc resection of the right upper lobe, involved chest wall, and nerve roots, followed by adjuvant radiotherapy (65.28 Gy over 54 days). The patient was alive and disease-free 5 years later. In 1956, Shaw[38] reported on a patient with the typical Pancoast syndrome who was referred for palliative radiotherapy. After treatment with 3000 cGy of radiation, the pain resolved and the tumor decreased in size, so Shaw performed a radical resection similar to that described by Chardack and MacCallum. The complete resection and long-term survival that were achieved in that case prompted Shaw et al.[26] to test this treatment strategy in additional patients. In 1961, they reported excellent local control and longer-than-anticipated survival in a study of 18 patients who were treated with 3000 to 3500 cGy of radiation over 2 weeks, followed by complete en bloc resection of the involved lobe, chest wall, and nerve roots 1 month later.

After that report, induction radiation (3000 cGy in 10 fractions over 2 weeks) and en bloc resection via an extended posterolateral thoracotomy became the standard of care for superior sulcus NSCLC. For 30 years (the second era in the management of Pancoast tumors), the basic therapeutic strategy for these

tumors remained unchanged. The findings of multiple series (Table 30.3) confirmed the original results reported by Shaw and Paulson but also identified adverse prognostic factors, including the presence of mediastinal node metastases (N2 disease), involvement of the spine or subclavian vessels (T4 disease), and incomplete (R1 or R2) surgical resection.[33,37,39–47] The largest published series, which included 225 patients who were treated at Memorial Sloan-Kettering Cancer Center between 1974 and 1988, confirmed the importance of these prognostic factors.[30,48] Although the operative mortality rate was low (4%), R0 resection was achieved for only 64% of T3 N0 tumors and 39% of T4 N0 tumors and local–regional recurrence was common.[30] The survival rate after lobectomy was better than that after limited pulmonary resection, and the addition of intraoperative brachytherapy to resection did not appear to improve the survival rate.[48] The overall 5-year survival rate was 46% for T3 N0 tumors, 13% for T4 N0 tumors, and 0% for N2 disease.[30] These results emphasized the need for new treatment strategies to improve both local control and overall survival.

During the late 1980s and the 1990s (the third era in the management of Pancoast tumors), several thoracic surgery groups developed novel approaches for the resection of tumors involving the spine and subclavian vessels. Dartevelle et al.[27] developed an anterior transcervical approach for the management of tumors involving the subclavian vessels and reported a 5-year survival rate of 31%. This experience led to widespread acceptance of the anterior approach involving resection of the subclavian artery and graft reconstruction for the management of T4 tumors. Modifications of this approach included the development of a transmanubrial osteomuscular sparing approach that avoids clavicular resection or disarticulation, the addition of a posterior or anterolateral thoracotomy to facilitate exposure of the lung and spine, and the use of a hemiclamshell thoracotomy (anterior thoracotomy and partial median sternotomy).[49–52] For superior sulcus carcinomas involving the spine, groups from Memorial Sloan-Kettering Cancer Center, from MD Anderson Cancer Center, and from institutions in France developed techniques for multilevel vertebrectomy and spine reconstruction that were designed to be performed in conjunction with pulmonary resection. Such techniques were facilitated by improvements in the materials available for spine stabilization.[28,29,53–55] The development of techniques allowing for complete resection of these technically challenging groups of T4 tumors was an important advance in the surgical management of Pancoast tumors. However, the overall 5-year survival rate remained approximately 30%.

During this same time period, several studies were performed to evaluate the results of treatment with radiation only. The results of these studies are difficult to interpret because they were retrospective, they included small numbers of patients, the tumors were only clinically staged, and the treatment techniques were highly variable.[56–58] The 5-year survival rate ranged from 0% to 40%, depending on tumor stage, total radiation dose, and other prognostic factors such as weight loss. The results in terms of local control and survival appeared to be inferior to those reported after surgical treatment, but this difference reflects in part the patient population and the variable treatment techniques. The brain was a common site of disease progression.[58]

The success of combined-modality therapy for stage IIIa (N2) NSCLC during the 1980s and 1990s led directly to the development of a large multicenter North American phase II trial (SWOG 9416, INT 0160),[59] representing the fourth era in the management of Pancoast tumors. Induction chemoradiation therapy followed by resection is a logical treatment strategy for a group of tumors that present a formidable challenge in terms of local control. The induction regimen used in this trial had been tested in previous trials and was known to be feasible and effective in the multi-institutional setting.

This phase II study enrolled 111 eligible patients with mediastinoscopy-negative, clinical T3–4 N0–1 tumors of the superior sulcus.[59] Induction therapy consisted of two cycles of etoposide and cisplatin with 45 Gy of concurrent radiation. Patients with stable disease or tumor regression had thoracotomy and anatomic pulmonary resection followed by two additional cycles of postoperative chemotherapy. Of the 111 patients who were enrolled, 83 (75%) ultimately had thoracotomy. Induction therapy was well tolerated and had a significant ability to sterilize the primary tumor. One-third of the patients had a complete pathologic response and another one-third had minimal residual microscopic disease in the resected specimen. R0 resection was obtained for 91% of T3 tumors and 87% of T4 tumors.

Three additional observations from this study are important. First, the rate of postoperative complications was not significantly greater after induction chemoradiation therapy than with historical experience with radiation therapy. Second, CT imaging after induction therapy overstaged the disease in a significant proportion of patients; specifically, 55% of patients who had stable disease on CT had either a complete pathologic response or only residual microscopic disease. Lastly, as has been the experience with NSCLC in general, only a small proportion of patients (42%) were able to successfully complete the course of postoperative chemotherapy.

The final results of this trial were reported in 2007.[60] The 5-year survival rate was 44% for all patients and 54% for those who had a complete resection. The pathologic response, but not the tumor stage, predicted the overall survival rate. Relative to previous experience with induction radiotherapy, the pattern of relapse changed predominantly to one of distant failure rather than local recurrence.[44] The excellent results in this trial with respect to the response to induction treatment, the rate of operative mortality, the rates of R0 resection and local control, and the overall rate of long-term survival effectively established the treatment regimen as a new standard of care for both T3 and T4 tumors. Additional single-institution studies and a multicenter phase II trial from Japan demonstrated similar results.[32,61–67]

Accrual to the North American Pancoast tumor trial was completed within the planned time frame but required the efforts of 76 surgeons from all North American cooperative groups to enroll 111 eligible patients. This difficulty in accrual indicates that it may not be possible to complete future randomized phase III trials that include resection within an acceptable length of time for this uncommon NSCLC subset. This trial highlights several issues that could be studied in future trials. First, induction therapy regimens involving the use of more contemporary chemotherapy drug combinations may lead to even better outcomes, but these regimens would need to be no more toxic when combined with radiotherapy and surgery. The induction regimen theoretically also could be intensified by increasing the dose of radiation. Krasna et al.[68,69] reported on 23 patients who were treated with a median radiation dose of 59.4 Gy in combination with platinum-based chemotherapy before surgical resection. The pathologic complete response rate to induction therapy was 46%, and the overall 5-year survival rate was 49%, results that were not clearly superior to those of the INT 0160 trial. Second, this trial emphasized the difficulty of delivering cisplatin-based therapy postoperatively to this group of patients. Lastly, the high risk of brain metastases in this trial was similar to that reported in other combined-modality trials for patients with locally advanced NSCLC.

Technical Approaches to Resection

Posterior (Paulson) Approach

The patient is placed in the lateral decubitus position and rotated slightly anteriorly, and the chest is entered via a posterolateral thoracotomy. The pleural cavity is examined to determine resectability, and then the incision is carried superiorly, midway between the scapula and the spinous processes, to the seventh cervical vertebra, dividing the trapezius and rhomboid muscles. Exposure is obtained by placing the upper blade of the rib-spreading retractor under the scapula and the lower blade on the chest wall or by elevating the scapula with an internal mammary retractor (Fig. 30.5). The scalene muscles are detached from the first and second ribs.

The chest wall resection is then performed. The anterior border of the resection specimen is divided, allowing for a 4-cm margin from the tumor. After anterior division of the first rib, dissection is carried posteriorly in the subperiosteal plane to the T1 transverse process. The erector spinae muscle is retracted away from the thoracic spine, exposing the costovertebral angle. Although the ribs can be disarticulated from the transverse processes of the vertebral bodies, resection of the transverse processes along with the heads of the involved ribs is the best way to achieve a complete (R0) resection. This part of the operation is best performed by a spine surgeon or neurosurgeon. To prevent leakage of cerebrospinal fluid, the intercostal nerves are ligated with vascular clips. The posterior resection is carried to the first rib, and the T1 nerve root is ligated and divided if it is encased in tumor. Resection of the T1 nerve root can result in some weakness of the intrinsic muscles of the hand, although the hand

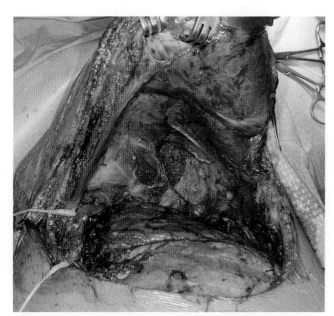

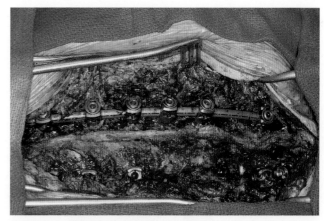

Fig. 30.6. Intraoperative photograph showing a rod-and-screw system, similar to the type used for the correction of scoliosis, that was inserted for spine stabilization after the resection of a T4 Pancoast tumor involving several vertebral bodies.

Fig. 30.5. Intraoperative photograph made during exposure for the resection of a Pancoast tumor. The incision (performed with use of the hook approach as described by Masaoka et al.)[79] follows the contours of the scapula, which is then elevated away from the chest wall with an internal artery retractor. The entire chest wall, including the first and second ribs, is well exposed. The erector spinae muscle has been mobilized and retracted posteriorly with use of so-called fish hooks, exposing the costovertebral junction in preparation for en bloc resection of the involved rib heads and transverse processes.

usually remains functional. Resection of the C8 nerve root and/or lower trunk of the brachial plexus results in permanent paralysis of the intrinsic muscles of the hand. If frozen-section analysis demonstrates no residual viable tumor involving the nerve roots, the nerve roots can be spared.

After the chest wall resection, the specimen is allowed to drop into the chest cavity and the lobectomy and mediastinal lymph node dissection are performed. Chest wall reconstruction is unnecessary if the chest wall defect is small and is limited to the upper three ribs. If a defect is present at the scapular tip, chest wall reconstruction is performed with use of a 2-mm-thick Gore-Tex patch (W.L. Gore and Associates, Flagstaff, AZ, USA). The thoracotomy incision is then closed.

Resection of Vertebral Body and Epidural Tumors

Tumors involving the vertebral body and posterior elements of the spine and extensive epidural tumors are resected via a posterior approach with use of posterior cervicothoracic spinal fixation (performed by a spine neurosurgeon) followed by anterior resection and reconstruction. The patient is placed in the prone position, and a midline incision is performed. Resection of the involved area of the spine is accomplished with a high-speed drill. A multilevel rhizotomy of the involved nerve roots is performed, and the chest wall is disarticulated from the vertebral bodies. Posterior segmental fixation is performed with a single screw-and-rod system similar to the type used for the correction of pediatric scoliosis (Fig. 30.6). Through a posterolateral thoracotomy, the chest wall resection and reconstruction and the lobectomy are then completed.

Anterior Approaches

Masaoka et al.[70] were the first to describe the use of an anterior approach for the resection of tumors involving the structures of

the thoracic inlet. With this technique, the patient is placed in the supine position and a partial median sternotomy is extended into the anterior fourth intercostal space as well as to a transverse incision at the base of the neck (a so-called trap door incision). The neck strap muscles are divided, the anterior chest wall is retracted, and the pleural cavity is opened to expose the vascular and nerve structures of the thoracic inlet. The scalene muscles are divided, and the lung and chest wall resections are performed.

Subsequently, Masaoka et al.[71] described a modification of the posterior approach for Pancoast tumors (the so-called hook approach) because resection of the transverse processes and the heads of the ribs was difficult through the anterior approach. A long curved periscapular skin incision, extending from the level of the seventh cervical vertebra around to the midclavicular line and ending anteriorly above the nipple, is performed. Tilting the operating table and moving the arm affords complete exposure of the entire thoracic inlet and allows resection and reconstruction of the subclavian vessels (Fig. 30.7A).

Dartevelle et al.[27] was the first to describe a transclavicular approach to the thoracic inlet. The patient is placed in the supine position with the neck hyperextended and the head turned away from the involved side. An incision is made along the anterior border of the sternocleidomastoid muscle and is extended horizontally, below and parallel to the clavicle at the level of the second intercostal space, to the deltopectoral groove (Fig. 30.7B).[27,72] Next, the pectoralis major muscle is dissected away from the clavicle, and a myocutaneous flap is folded back, exposing the thoracic inlet. The scalene fat pad and the medial half of the clavicle are excised. The distal parts of the internal, external, and anterior jugular veins are divided to expose the subclavian and innominate veins. If the subclavian vein is involved, it is resected.

The anterior scalene muscle is divided, the phrenic nerve is preserved, and the subclavian artery is mobilized. If the subclavian artery is involved, it is resected and reconstructed, usually with a polytetrafluoroethylene vascular graft.

The middle scalene muscle is divided above its insertion on the first rib. The C8 and T1 nerve roots are identified and are dissected up to the confluence of the lower trunk of the brachial plexus. The ipsilateral prevertebral muscles are resected along with the paravertebral sympathetic chain and stellate ganglion and the T1 nerve root.

The chest wall resection is then performed. The first rib is divided at the costochondral junction anteriorly. The second rib is divided at its midpoint, the dissection is carried along the superior border of the third rib to the costovertebral angle, and the ribs are disarticulated from the transverse processes.

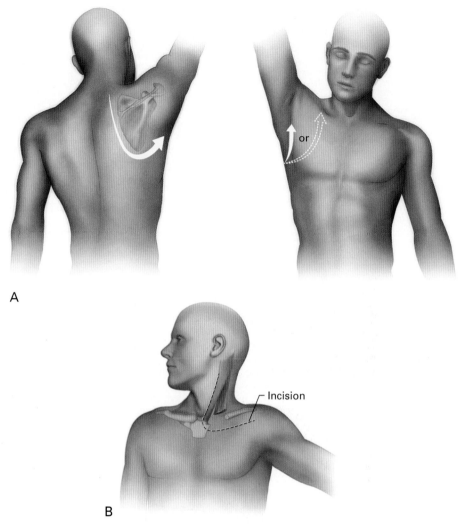

Fig. 30.7. (A) Illustration depicting the trans-scapular (hook) approach for the resection of a Pancoast tumor. The anterior part of the incision can be brought into the midaxillary line rather than the midclavicular line. This incision provides the exposure shown in Fig. 30.5. (B) Illustration depicting the transclavicular approach as described by Dartevelle et al.[26] for the resection of a Pancoast tumor involving the subclavian vessels.

Through this cavity, an upper lobectomy is performed and the cervical incision is closed. If exposure is inadequate, the anterior incision is closed and the resection is completed via a posterolateral thoracotomy.

The transclavicular approach, which includes resection of the medial half of the clavicle, has been the subject of concern because of its functional and aesthetic consequences. Grunenwald and Spaggiari[49] described a transmanubrial osteomuscular sparing approach that avoids division or disarticulation of the clavicle. An L-shaped cervicotomy is performed as described by Dartevelle et al.[27] The manubrium is exposed and divided via an L-shaped incision, with the sternoclavicular articulation being left intact. The first costal cartilage is resected, permitting mobilization of an osteomuscular flap that is progressively elevated.[73] Additional refinements of this approach were reported by Spaggiari and Pastorino[50] and Klima et al.[74] Pancoast tumors invading the anterior structures of the thoracic inlet can now be completely resected because of the development of approaches that allow exposure to critical neurovascular structures. These approaches have been summarized by Macchiarini.[75]

CONCLUSION

Resection of a lung cancer tumor invading the chest wall is a major procedure that should be performed by experienced surgeons, preferably at high-volume centers. Multidisciplinary care is necessary to determine the optimal diagnostic and therapeutic strategy for each individual patient. Good long-term results can be achieved after R0 resection in the absence of mediastinal lymph node involvement. Prospective studies are required to determine the precise role of induction and adjuvant therapy, especially for larger tumors and in cases of R1 resection.

Superior sulcus NSCLCs pose a therapeutic challenge because of their proximity to numerous vital structures. During the past 40 years, the development of effective combined-modality therapy and of novel surgical approaches has dramatically improved the rates of local control and overall survival for patients with these tumors. Future studies are needed to address the continuing problems of systemic relapse after surgery, especially in the brain.

KEY REFERENCES

5. McCaughan BC, Martini N, Bains MS, McCormack PM. Chest wall invasion in carcinoma of the lung. Therapeutic and prognostic implications. *J Thorac Cardiovasc Surg*. 1985;89(6):836–841.
16. Weyant MJ, Bains MS, Venkatraman E, et al. Results of chest wall resection and reconstruction with and without rigid prosthesis. *Ann Thorac Surg*. 2006;81(1):279–285.
26. Shaw RR, Paulson DL, Kee JL. Treatment of the superior sulcus tumor by irradiation followed by resection. *Ann Surg*. 1961;154(1):29–40.
27. Dartevelle PG, Chapelier AR, Macchiarini P, et al. Anterior transcervical-thoracic approach for radical resection of lung tumors invading the thoracic inlet. *J Thorac Cardiovasc Surg*. 1993;105(6):1025–1034.
28. Bilsky MH, Vitaz TW, Boland PJ, Bains MS, Rajaraman V, Rusch VW. Surgical treatment of superior sulcus tumors with spinal and brachial plexus involvement. *J Neurosurg*. 2002;97(suppl 3):301–309.
30. Rusch VW, Parekh KR, Leon L, et al. Factors determining outcome after surgical resection of T3 and T4 lung cancers of the superior sulcus. *J Thorac Cardiovasc Surg*. 2000;119(6):1147–1153.
50. Spaggiari L, Pastorino U. Transmanubrial approach with anterolateral thoracotomy for apical chest tumor. *Ann Thorac Surg*. 1999;68(2):590–593.
60. Rusch VW, Giroux DJ, Kraut MJ, et al. Induction chemoradiation and surgical resection for superior sulcus nonsmall cell lung carcinomas: long-term results of Southwest Oncology Group Trial 9416 (Intergroup Trial 0160). *J Clin Oncol*. 2007;25(3):313–318.
67. Kunitoh H, Kato H, Tsuboi M, et al. Phase II trial of preoperative chemoradiotherapy followed by surgical resection in patients with superior sulcus nonsmall cell lung cancers: report of Japan Clinical Oncology Group Trial 9806. *J Clin Oncol*. 2008;26(4):644–649.
72. Macchiarini P, Dartevelle P, Chapelier A, et al. Technique for resecting primary and metastatic nonbronchogenic tumors of the thoracic outlet. *Ann Thorac Surg*. 1993;55(3):611–618.

See Expertconsult.com for full list of references.

Extended Resections for Lung Cancer: Bronchovascular Sleeve Resections

Shun-ichi Watanabe

SUMMARY OF KEY POINTS

- Bronchovascular sleeve resection is an essential technique for general thoracic surgeons to preserve as much as possible the patient's lung function and quality of life after pulmonary resection.
- Previous reports suggested that the incidence rates of bronchopleural fistula and surgical mortality after sleeve lobectomy and sleeve pneumonectomy were 3% and 2.5%, and 5.5% and 20.9%, respectively.
- In the tissue-healing process of the anastomotic site after bronchial sleeve resection, previous reports suggested that the blood flow in the bronchial arteries proximal to the anastomosis comes from the aorta, but the blood flow distal to the anastomosis comes from the pulmonary artery.
- There are controversies in techniques of bronchial sleeve resections regarding suturing methods, suturing layers, types of anastomosis, types of sleeve resection, and the necessity of wrapping the anastomosis.
- There are controversies in techniques of pulmonary artery angioplasty regarding types of resection, types of reconstruction, order of reconstruction in a double sleeve resection, and the necessity of anticoagulant therapy.

Bronchoplastic and angioplastic procedures are essential techniques in general thoracic surgery. When performing lung cancer operations, thoracic surgeons sometimes encounter situations that require these techniques; therefore thoracic surgeons should know how to perform these procedures. This chapter describes the history of, and strategy and techniques for, bronchoplastic and angioplastic surgical procedures.

HISTORY AND SURGICAL OUTCOMES OF BRONCHOVASCULAR SLEEVE RESECTION

Bronchial Sleeve Resection

The first bronchoplastic surgical procedure was described by Bigger in 1932.[1] The patient was a 14-year-old boy with a tumor in the left main bronchus, and the tumor was removed with an incision in the bronchus. Postoperative examination of the pathologic specimen indicated that the resected tumor was malignant. Therefore a week after the surgical procedure, a left pneumonectomy was done. However, the patient died of infectious pericarditis after these repeated thoracotomy procedures. The first bronchial sleeve resection was performed by Thomas in 1947.[2] The patient was a young man who was awaiting a commission in the Royal Air Force. An adenoma on the right upper lobe bronchus was detected at clinical examination, and the tumor was found to be occluding the right main bronchus. A sleeve resection and an end-to-end anastomosis of the right main bronchus were performed. The patient

was able to serve as an Air Force pilot in active flying duties after this lung-preserving operation.

In 1959, Johnston and Jones[3] described the first successful sleeve lobectomy for primary lung cancer, a procedure that had been performed by Allison in 1952. In 1955, Paulson and Shaw[4] named this procedure a "bronchoplastic surgery." In the 1970s and 1980s, Jensik et al.,[5] Bennett and Smith,[6] and Faber et al.[7] reported on case series of patients who had sleeve lobectomies. The first report of a carinal resection was made by Mathey et al.[8] in 1966, and in 1978, Grillo[9] reported success with 38 cases.

The results of bronchoplastic procedures have been reported in several studies (Table 31.1).[10–20] In most of these reports, 5-year survival rates were 40% to 50% and mortality rates were relatively low, ranging from 0% to 7.5%. Tedder et al.[10] reviewed the results of 1915 bronchoplastic procedures for primary lung cancer that were performed over 12 years, starting in 1979. According to that report, the incidence rates of bronchopleural fistula, bronchovascular fistula, and surgical mortality after sleeve lobectomy and sleeve pneumonectomy procedures were 3% and 10.1%, 2.5% and 2.9%, and 5.5% and 20.9%, respectively.

Pulmonary Artery Angioplasty

Gundersen[21] published the first report of a pulmonary artery sleeve resection in 1967. That report described two cases of successful pulmonary artery sleeve resection and end-to-end anastomosis. After the publication of these results, many successful cases were reported.[22,23] More recently, an increasing number of studies have described the results of concurrent bronchoplasty and pulmonary artery angioplasty procedures (Table 31.2).[13,16,17,24–27] For example, Rendina et al.[17] reported on 40 cases of concurrent procedures. The 5-year survival rate was 38.6%, which was equivalent to the 5-year survival rate of 38.7% recorded for 80 cases of only bronchoplastic surgical procedures.[17]

HEALING OF THE ANASTOMOTIC SITE AFTER BRONCHIAL SLEEVE RESECTION

Ishihara et al.[28] detailed the results obtained in animal models regarding the tissue-healing process of the anastomotic site after bronchial sleeve resection. He injected silicone rubber of different colors into the bronchial artery and pulmonary artery after a sleeve lobectomy. The results confirmed that the blood flow in the bronchial arteries proximal to the anastomosis came from the aorta, but the blood flow distal to the anastomosis came from the pulmonary artery (Fig. 31.1). Inui et al.[29] evaluated bronchial blood flow by laser Doppler velocimetry in dogs. Their results suggested that the bronchial mucosal blood flow was reduced when the peribronchial tissue was detached, and blood flow was restored by dressing the anastomosis with the greater omentum.[29]

According to some reports, systemic administration of small doses of steroids after the bronchoplastic procedure prevented an inflammatory reaction and edema in the tissue around the anastomotic site.[30,31] Consequently, this treatment was believed to improve blood flow and promote healing of the anastomosis. However, Inui et al.[29] suggested that treatment with steroids did

TABLE 31.1 Results for the Bronchial Sleeve Resection: Previous Reports With More Than 100 Cases

Reference	No. of Patients	Mortality (%)	5-Year Survival Rate (%)
Tedder et al. (1992)[10]	1915	7.5	40
Van Schil et al. (1996)[11]	145	4.8	46
Rea et al. (1997)[12]	217	6.2	49
Icard et al. (1999)[13]	110	2.8	39
Kutlu et al. (1999)[14]	100	2.0	49
Tronc et al. (2000)[15]	184	1.6	52
Okada et al. (2000)[16]	151	0	48
Rendina et al. (2000)[17]	145	3.0	38
Deslauriers et al. (2004)[18]	300	2.7	54
Ludwig et al. (2005)[19]	116	4.3	43
Yildizeli et al. (2007)[20]	218	4.1	43

TABLE 31.2 Results for Concurrent Bronchoplastic and Angioplastic Procedures

Reference	No. of Patients	Mortality (%)	5-Year Survival Rate (%)
Icard et al. (1999)[13]	16	NA	39
Rendina et al. (2000)[17]	40	0	39
Okada et al. (2000)[16]	21	0	48
Fadel et al. (2002)[24]	11	0.7	52
Chunwei et al. (2003)[25]	21	NA	33
Lausberg et al. (2005)[26]	67	1.5	43
Nagayasu et al. (2006)[27]	29	17.2	24

NA, not available.

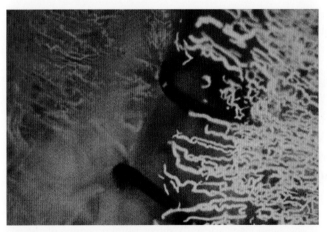

Fig. 31.1. Stereomicroscopic view of the bronchial circulation at the anastomosis site. The bronchial arteries were perfused with different colors of silicone rubber. Bronchial arteries proximal to the anastomosis are filled with orange silicone rubber, which was injected into the aorta. Bronchial arteries distal to the anastomosis are filled with yellow silicone rubber, which was injected into the pulmonary artery. *(Reprinted with permission from Ishihara T, Nemoto E, Kikuchi K, Kato R, Kobayashi K. Does pleural bronchial wrapping improve wound healing in right sleeve lobectomy?* J Thorac Cardiovasc Surg. *1985;89(5):665–672.)*

not improve blood flow at the anastomotic site in animal models as evaluated by laser Doppler velocimetry. Rendina et al.[30] reported that treatment with steroids in the clinical setting substantially decreased the incidence of postoperative morbidity and shortened the postoperative intensive care unit and hospital stays. The patients in that study received postoperative aerosol steroid inhalation three times per day and intravenous injections of 10 mg methylprednisolone twice a day.

SURGICAL TECHNIQUES AND CONTROVERSIES REGARDING BRONCHIAL SLEEVE RESECTIONS

Suturing Method: Interrupted or Continuous?

The first question for the optimal selection of a suturing method is whether an interrupted or continuous suture should be used. It is generally thought that a continuous suture allows less blood flow at the anastomotic site than an interrupted suture. Reduced blood flow could lead to anastomotic dehiscence or stenosis; therefore the interrupted suture has been adopted in many institutions. However, Kutlu and Goldstraw[14] and Aigner et al.[32] reported good results with a continuous suture technique. Bayram et al.[33] found no pathologic differences in the healing process between dogs treated with interrupted and continuous sutures.

The greatest concern about a continuous suture technique is that if part of an anastomosis develops dehiscence, the defect might propagate over the whole anastomosis. This possibility may explain why many thoracic surgeons are reluctant to adopt the continuous suture technique. Hamad et al.[34] reported a new bronchial anastomosis technique, which uses three running sutures. They showed that this technique could be performed easily and quickly with few knots, and it minimized the risk of a whole anastomosis dehiscence, even after difficult sleeve resections.

The advantage of a continuous suture is that it is technically easier than an interrupted suture, particularly for a mini-thoracotomy procedure. The innovation of absorbable monofilament sutures made continuous suture techniques easy and safe. Nevertheless, the advantage of the interrupted suture is that it maintains good blood flow at the anastomosis. Furthermore, if a partial dehiscence occurs, the whole anastomosis would not be compromised. The disadvantage of the interrupted suture is that tying several posterior sutures with knots on the outside of the anastomosis is technically difficult. However, current advances have made it possible to place several posterior suture knots on the inside of an anastomosis, which should be more convenient and technically easier to perform. When absorbable monofilament sutures are used in this procedure, airway complications can be avoided because the knots are readily absorbed, provoke little tissue reaction, and create minimal bronchial obstruction.

Suturing Layers: Through-and-Through or Submucosal Suture?

Two methods are used for suturing the cartilaginous portion of the bronchus. One method is to place the suture outside the mucosal layer, for the so-called submucosal suture; the other method is to pierce through the whole wall of the bronchus, for the so-called through-and-through suture. Paulson and Shaw[4] demonstrated the effectiveness of the submucosal suture using interrupted fine cotton or cable-wire sutures. Rendina et al.[35] also recommended using the submucosal suture with the aid of magnifying loupes. However, no evidence has supported the usefulness of the submucosal suture; thus in many institutions, the whole-wall suture has been performed with use of an absorbable monofilament thread. This method is preferred for two reasons. First, the submucosal suture is technically more difficult than the whole-wall suture. Second, the monofilament absorbable suture is unlikely to develop anastomotic complications from infection associated with the thread. This type of infection may occur with either a submucosal suture or a through-and-through suture and may result in collection of sputum and anastomotic stenosis.

Type of Anastomosis: Telescope or End-To-End?

Two methods are used for creating a bronchial anastomosis: the telescope and the end-to-end methods. The telescope anastomosis is currently used when a large-caliber mismatch is present

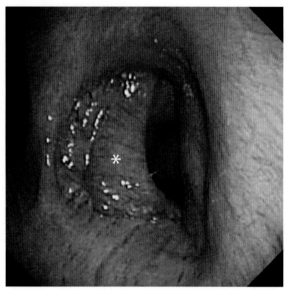

Fig. 31.2. Endoscopic view of a bronchial anastomosis after a wedge sleeve resection of the right upper lobe. The wedge sleeve resection caused a deformation to develop in the airway mucosa *(asterisk)*, which may cause sputum retention at the anastomotic site.

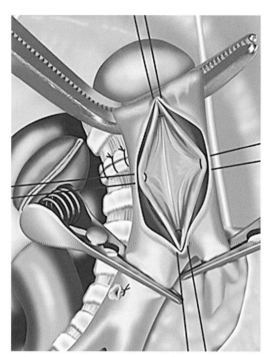

Fig. 31.3. Illustration of a patch reconstruction after a tangential resection of the pulmonary artery. The advantage of the patch reconstruction is that the suture line of the pulmonary artery does not touch the bronchial anastomosis; this is advantageous particularly after a left upper bronchovascular sleeve resection.

between the bronchial ends.[36] This method does not require a tissue wrapping for the anastomosis, and many good results have been reported to date, particularly in lung transplantation procedures. However, some transplant surgeons have reported disadvantages of the telescope anastomosis. The primary disadvantage is that the retrograde collateral blood flow from the pulmonary artery of the residual lung may be insufficient at the overlapping edges of the distal bronchus; therefore this method may lead to necrosis and stenosis at the anastomosis. The mortality rate for patients with stenosis after a telescope anastomosis is reportedly 2% to 3%.[37] Aigner et al.[32] reported that the incidence of anastomotic complications associated with the telescope technique was 30% in the early 1990s. Converting to the end-to-end bronchial anastomosis markedly reduced the complication rate to less than 4%.[32] Rabinov et al.[38] suggested that the "reverse telescope" anastomosis technique greatly reduced the incidence of anastomotic stenosis.

Type of Sleeve Resection: Wedge or Conventional?

When the tumor invades a very small area of the central bronchial wall or when it is considered to be a low-grade malignant tumor that requires only a small surgical margin, a wedge sleeve resection can be performed instead of a conventional sleeve resection. The wedge resection maintains the blood flow of the bronchial anastomosis because a small area of the bronchial wall remains connected. However, this procedure may cause a deformed airway to develop, which may result in sputum retention at the anastomotic site (Fig. 31.2). Moreover, tension at the anastomosis may become excessive. In such cases, it is recommended to convert to the conventional sleeve resection. Rendina et al.[35] suggested that a sleeve resection is always preferable to a wedge sleeve resection because the latter procedure caused a number of complications as a result of excessive tension.

Bronchial Anastomosis: Wrap or No Wrap?

Several tissues may be used as an autologous material for wrapping the bronchial anastomosis, including the pericardial fat pad, the intercostal muscle, and the parietal pleura, among others. Wrapping the bronchial anastomosis may cover the small

dehiscence site and prevent the formation of a bronchopleural fistula. This procedure also prevents erosion at the surface of the pulmonary artery adjacent to the anastomosis, thereby preventing the development of a bronchovascular fistula. No clear evidence indicates that wrapping the bronchial anastomosis promotes angiogenesis around the anastomosis.[28,29]

SURGICAL TECHNIQUES AND CONTROVERSIES REGARDING PULMONARY ARTERY ANGIOPLASTY

Pulmonary Artery Resections and Reconstructions: Tangential Resection or Sleeve Resection?

Tangential Resection

The tangential resection is performed when the tumor invades part of the pulmonary artery. A direct running suture of the resected pulmonary artery wall may cause stenosis and thromboembolism in the pulmonary artery; therefore direct running suture should be applied only when the tumor invades a small area of the pulmonary artery. Cerfolio and Bryant[39] suggested that when a direct suture is estimated to reduce the pulmonary artery diameter by 20% to 30%, a sleeve resection of the pulmonary artery should be performed instead of a direct suture in order to prevent stenosis and occlusion of the pulmonary artery. When the resected area of the pulmonary artery is too large for a direct suture but not large enough for a sleeve resection (i.e., <50% of the arterial wall), a patch reconstruction should be applied. The advantage of a patch reconstruction compared with a sleeve resection of the pulmonary artery is that the suture line of the pulmonary artery does not touch the bronchial anastomosis; this is advantageous, particularly after a left upper bronchovascular sleeve resection (Fig. 31.3).

Autologous pericardium is the preferred material for a pulmonary artery patch because of its many advantages. The autologous pericardial patch can be taken readily from the pericardial sac, anterior to the phrenic nerve. The autologous pericardial patch shrinks substantially immediately after excision. Thus care must be taken to obtain a piece of the pericardium that appears much wider than the size of the pulmonary artery defect. The patch is sutured to the pulmonary artery with continuous 5-0 or 6-0 non-absorbable monofilament sutures.[17,39] The edge of the autologous pericardium also tends to recoil during suturing. Therefore several sutures should be placed around the edge of the recoiled pericardial patch prior to the running suture in order to ensure that the pericardium remains flat and to make suturing easy (Fig. 31.3). Bovine pericardium is stiffer than autologous pericardium, so using bovine pericardium can eliminate the recoiling problem, but bovine pericardium is expensive.

Sleeve Resection

Compared with a direct suture, a sleeve resection of the pulmonary artery is associated with a lower incidence of stenosis and, consequently, a lower frequency of thromboembolism. An end-to-end anastomosis is typically performed with a 5-0 or 6-0 monofilament nonabsorbable suture. A sleeve resection of the pulmonary artery is usually performed along with a sleeve resection of the bronchus; therefore tension at the pulmonary artery anastomosis is minimal. However, when a bronchial sleeve resection is not required, a pulmonary artery sleeve resection should be performed with a conduit interposition reconstruction. A synthetic or autologous graft is used as the material for the conduit, and a 2-cm section should be sufficient for the length of the conduit. Rendina et al.[40] reported that the autologous conduit could be prepared from a section of the pericardium. A conduit is constructed by wrapping the pericardium around a 28-F chest tube and then suturing the sides longitudinally with a 6-0 monofilament nonabsorbable suture. Cerezo et al.[41] described a new method for reconstruction of an autologous pulmonary artery conduit; they used a pulmonary vein graft collected from the resected lung.

Which Should Be Reconstructed First in a Double Sleeve Resection: The Bronchial or Vascular Anastomosis?

Much controversy has focused on the order of reconstruction in a double sleeve resection. Rendina et al.[40] suggested that the vascular reconstruction should be performed before the bronchial anastomosis because it reduces the time that the pulmonary artery must be clamped. However, other authors have noted that it is preferable to perform the bronchial anastomosis before the vascular anastomosis.[42] Two reasons are cited for the latter preference. First, once the pulmonary artery is reconstructed, it is difficult to perform the bronchial anastomosis because it requires retracting the pulmonary artery, which may cause a thromboembolism or dehiscence at the pulmonary artery anastomosis. Second, inflation of the lung after a bronchial anastomosis allows the surgeon to check the tension and detect kinking at the pulmonary artery anastomosis.

Postoperative Anticoagulant Therapy: Necessary or Unnecessary?

Controversy persists regarding the use of postoperative anticoagulant therapy. Rendina et al.[35] administered a dose of heparin (3000 U, single venous injection) before the anastomosis and a subcutaneous injection of heparin (15,000 U/day) for 7 days to 10 days after surgical procedures. Cerfolio and Bryant[39] suggested that only a small dose of heparin (1500 U, single venous injection) should be used before the anastomosis to avoid the risk of postoperative bleeding. At the National Cancer Center Hospital in Tokyo, we do not administer heparin either during or after surgical procedures, and we have not found any cases of thromboembolism of the pulmonary artery.

CONCLUSION

Bronchovascular sleeve resection is an indispensable surgical technique for thoracic surgeons. This technique is performed to preserve the patient's lung function and quality of life after the operation; thus special care must be taken to avoid postoperative morbidity and mortality. Thoracic surgeons can optimize outcomes by understanding the essential techniques and controversies involved in this procedure.

KEY REFERENCES

1. Bigger IA. Diagnosis and treatment of primary carcinoma of lung. *South Surg.* 1935;4:401–415.
3. Johnston JB, Jones PH. The treatment of bronchial carcinoma by lobectomy and sleeve resection of the main bronchus. *Thorax.* 1959;14(1):48–54.
4. Paulson DL, Shaw RR. Bronchial anastomosis and bronchoplastic procedures in the interest of preservation of lung tissue. *J Thorac Surg.* 1955;29(3):238–259.
6. Bennett WF, Smith RA. A twenty-year analysis of the results of sleeve resection for primary bronchogenic carcinoma. *J Thorac Cardiovasc Surg.* 1978;76(6):840–845.
9. Grillo HC. Tracheal tumors: surgical management. *Ann Thorac Surg.* 1978;26(2):112–125.
10. Tedder M, Anstadt MP, Tedder SD, Lowe JE. Current morbidity, mortality, and survival after bronchoplastic procedures for malignancy. *Ann Thorac Surg.* 1992;54(2):387–391.
21. Gundersen AE. Segmental resection of the pulmonary artery during left upper lobectomy. *J Thorac Cardiovasc Surg.* 1967;54(4):582–585.
22. Venuta F, Ciccone AM, Anile M, et al. Reconstruction of the pulmonary artery for lung cancer: long-term results. *J Thorac Cardiovasc Surg.* 2009;138(5):1185–1191.
28. Ishihara T, Nemoto E, Kikuchi K, Kato R, Kobayashi K. Does pleural wrapping improve wound healing in right sleeve lobectomy? *J Thorac Cardiovasc Surg.* 1985;89(5):665–672.
29. Inui K, Wada H, Yokomise H, et al. Evaluation of a bronchial anastomosis by laser Doppler velocimetry. *J Thorac Cardiovasc Surg.* 1990;99(4):614–619.
30. Rendina EA, Venuta F, Ricci C. Effects of low-dose steroids on bronchial healing after sleeve resection. A clinical study. *J Thorac Cardiovasc Surg.* 1992;104(4):888–891.
39. Cerfolio RJ, Bryant AS. Surgical techniques and results for partial or circumferential sleeve resection of the pulmonary artery for patients with non-small cell lung cancer. *Ann Thorac Surg.* 2007;83(6):1971–1976.
40. Rendina EA, Venuta F, de Giacomo T, Rossi M, Coloni GF. Parenchymal sparing operations for bronchogenic carcinoma. *Surg Clin North Am.* 2002;82(3):589–609.

See Expertconsult.com for full list of references.

32 Multiple Nodules: Management of Synchronous and Metachronous Lung Cancers

Jessica S. Donington

SUMMARY OF KEY POINTS

- Multiple primary lung cancers (MPLCs) are increasing in incidence as imaging accuracies improve and resections are better tolerated.
- Differentiating MPLCs from intrathoracic metastatic disease is challenging and based primarily on clinical judgment.
- Molecular analysis for tumor clonality has the potential to increase accuracy of differentiation between MPLCs and intrathoracic metastatic disease.
- Complete resection is the treatment of choice for MPLCs, but preservation of pulmonary parenchyma is essential and therefore the use of sublobar resections is common.
- Survival rates following complete resection of synchronous MPLCs are reported as between 35% and 75% with prognosis being decreased in those with N1 and N2 involvement.
- Metachronous MPLCs are almost always diagnosed at an early stage in asymptomatic patients as part of surveillance imaging. Survival following resection is typically 40% and determined by the stage of the second cancer.
- Stereotactic body radiotherapy is an attractive treatment alternative for early stage MPLC because of its ability to preserve pulmonary parenchyma.

The concept of MPLCs was introduced by Beyreunther in 1924,[1] but remained a rarity for many decades. From 1960 to 1990 only sporadic case series were reported,[2–6] but it was not until the integration of computed tomography (CT) scanning into lung cancer care that the true magnitude was appreciated. Today, rapid improvements in imaging accuracy, decreased mortality associated with lung cancer resections, increased use of CT scans for routine postoperative surveillance, and integration of mutational analysis for resected cancers are all contributing to a growing cohort of MPLC. Whether presenting as synchronous or metachronous tumors, one of the greatest challenges is differentiating MPLCs from intrathoracic metastatic disease. The first step in that distinction is appropriately recognizing the frequency of MPLCs in the modern era. Rates of less than 5% of all nonsmall cell lung cancers (NSCLCs) from older series are now believed to greatly underestimate the true incidence of MPLCs.[7] High-resolution CT scans also allow for the detection of ground-glass opacities, which are not evident on standard chest x-ray or early generation CT scans. These precancerous lesions and early stage adenocarcinomas have a lepidic growth pattern with a predilection for indolence and multiplicity. Risk factors and prognosis for multifocal adenocarcinomas are different from traditional MPLCs reported in older series. The management and treatment decisions for MPLCs follow the same general principles used for other early stage NSCLCs with special consideration for the preservation of pulmonary parenchyma and vigilant post-treatment surveillance.

DIFFERENTIATING MPLCs FROM METASTATIC DISEASE

Patients with multiple nodules at the time of NSCLC diagnosis or a new pulmonary nodule following successful treatment of an early stage NSCLC pose a significant clinical challenge due to the lack of clear criteria that differentiate intrapulmonary metastasis from MPLC. The most widely referenced definition is from 1975, from Martini and Melamed.[8] It is applied most appropriately to metachronous tumors, or to those that have already been resected or found at autopsy, and relies heavily on cell type (i.e., adenocarcinoma or squamous cell carcinoma). Further factors used to refine the criteria include origin in an area of carcinoma in situ, lack of carcinoma in common lymphatics, and lack of extrathoracic metastasis (Table 32.1).[9] This definition is becoming outdated in an era when mutational and molecular analysis can differentiate tumors on a genetic basis.

Some investigators have suggested that individual adenocarcinomas can be distinguished based on differences in the proportion of histologic subtypes (i.e., lepidic, papillary, acinar, micropapillary).[10,11] By contrast, other investigators report that mutational and molecular analysis of somatic changes in tumor DNA can better discriminate between MPLC and metastatic disease. Mutational analysis of the epidermal growth factor receptor and K-ras mutations can be used to differentiate between metastatic and second primary adenocarcinomas of the lung.[11–13] The utility of this approach is limited by the facts that this type of analysis is only relevant to adenocarcinomas, not all adenocarcinomas harbor these mutations, and expression can be heterogeneous throughout the tumor. Cytogenetic profiles can be used to evaluate the clonal relationship between tumors.[14,15] Genomic DNA copy number alterations are key events in tumor development and array comparative genomic hybridization can distinguish between clonal tumors (metastasis) and MPLCs.[12,16] Investigators from the Massachusetts General Hospital reported on 68 patients with multiple resected adenocarcinomas whose tumors were classified as MPLC or metastasis by a comprehensive histologic profiling, including profiling using SNaPshot multiplex polymerase chain reaction. In their study, the 3-year survival rate was significantly improved in patients classified as MPLC by molecular profiling, but not by histologic profiling, indicating improved accuracy with molecular analysis.[17] Although this molecular profiling appears to be more precise than histologic profiling, it is time consuming, expensive, and requires large amounts of genomic DNA. Molecular analysis may not currently be reasonable for use on a case-by-case basis, but it is helping to redefine the frequency and clinical characteristics associated with MPLCs.

Clinical judgment remains critically important in these cases, with biopsy typically having only a small and supplemental role.[18] Patients are generally placed into management categories based on the appearance, location of nodules, and the presence of nodal or extra thoracic metastatic disease. Biopsies are often difficult and typically not helpful in differentiating metastasis and second primaries without molecular analysis because the majority of MPLCs are of the same histology.

TABLE 32.1 Criteria From Martini and Melamed[8] for Multiple Primary Lung Cancers

Metachronous	**DIFFERENT HISTOLOGY**	
	Same histology if	Prolonged interval between tumors (typically >2 years)
		Development from separate area of carcinoma in situ
		Different lobes with:
		• no shared lymph node basins
		• no extrathoracic metastasis
Synchronous	**DIFFERENT HISTOLOGY**	
	Same histology if	Development from separate area of carcinoma in situ
		Different lobes with:
		• no cancer in shared lymph node basins
		• no extrathoracic metastasis

MPLCs in the Lung Cancer Staging System

The previous editions of the tumor, node, and metastasis (TNM) classification for lung cancer have been somewhat vague with respect to the classification of lung cancer with multiple pulmonary sites of involvement, which has resulted in marked variability in how these tumors are classified.[19,20] The creation of homogeneous groups is a goal of cancer staging, but this task is challenging when lung cancer occurs in different pulmonary sites, and the individual cancers exhibit distinct patterns of biologic behavior, recurrence, and survival. In previous lung cancer staging systems, there has been a lack of clarity regarding these distinct patterns of disease as well as ambiguity about how to best apply stage classification.

Definitions have evolved over time for multiple intrathoracic sites of lung cancer in the TNM system. Prior to 1993, all separate tumor nodules were classified as M1. They were then defined as T4 if in a different lobe. In 1997, separate tumor nodules were classified as T4 if in the same lobe and M1 if in a different lobe (ipsilateral or contralateral). In 2010, separate nodules were reclassified as T3 for a same lobe, as T4 if in a different ipsilateral lobe, and as M1 if in a contralateral lobe.[19,20] However, none of these definitions addressed the concept of variability in appearance and behavior of these additional sites of disease. Furthermore, the seventh edition contained only an elusive mention of ground-glass or lepidic lesions (GG/L) and predated the classification of adenocarcinoma histologic subtypes.[21,22]

In the eighth edition of TNM classification, four distinct disease patterns were identified for lung cancers with multiple sites of pulmonary involvement and clear instructions were provided on how to apply the TNM classifications to each pattern of disease.[23] The four disease patterns include: (1) synchronous primary lung cancers, (2) multiple GG/L nodules, (3) solid primary lung cancer with one or more separate solid tumor nodule(s) of the same histologic type, and (4) pneumonic type of lung cancer, a diffuse form that is radiologically similar to pneumonia. The radiographic and pathologic features of each of these four disease categories are outlined in Table 32.2. Second primary lung cancers and GG/L are each recognized as variants of MPLCs. In patients with second primary cancers, each tumor is staged with a unique TNM. GG/L cases are also viewed as independent tumors, but are more interrelated with a strong predilection for multiplicity and lack of lymphatic involvement and are therefore recommended to be staged with the T based on the highest T lesion and "#/m" indicating multiplicity and a single N and M designation. Solid tumors with separate solid nodules and pneumonic lung cancer are not variants of MPLC, but are rather variants of advanced intrathoracic spread of a single tumor and are therefore staged as T3 if spread is limited to a single lobe, T4 if spread is to a single lung, and M1 if bilateral.[24]

Synchronous Primary Lung Cancers

The improved resolution of CT imaging has led to increased rates of NSCLC patients presenting with multiple nodules at initial diagnosis. The definitions for synchronous MPLC remain ambiguous, even though treatment algorithms and prognosis are dramatically different from those for patients with multiple nodules from the same tumor. Prognosis for these patients is not as good as those who present with a single primary tumor, but far better than those with widely metastatic disease. Most feel that classifying all of these as intrathoracic metastatic disease greatly "over stages" a significant number of patients with synchronous primary early stage tumors, and denying local therapy may miss the potential for cure. The lack of uniformity for precise identification and definitions for synchronous primary NSCLC has resulted in a paucity of large series of homogeneously treated patients.

Patient Evaluation

Recent trials support an aggressive approach to the treatment of patients with more than one nodule suspicious for early stage NSCLC with the understanding that these may represent MPLC, but a thorough preoperative assessment is essential to rule out metastatic disease and assure the patient has adequate cardiopulmonary reserve to tolerate local therapy for both cancers. Preoperative assessment includes routine pulmonary function tests because these patients may require multiple resections, CT scan of the chest, and whole-body positron emission tomography (PET). Additional tests considered essential include brain imaging by magnetic resonance imaging (MRI) or CT and pathologic mediastinal staging, even in cases of CT-negative and PET-negative mediastinal nodes.[18] Every attempt should be made to exclude the possibility that this may represent intrathoracic metastatic disease prior to local intervention.

Surgical Resection and Outcome

Once two nodules are deemed to be synchronous early stage MPLCs, careful planning is needed to adequately treat each while preserving pulmonary parenchyma. The vast majority of large series of synchronous MPLCs involve patients who undergo resection of both cancers.[18] Five-year survival for resected patients ranges from 16% to 76% but is improved in more recent series and in those with a predominance of multifocal adenocarcinoma, which has a more indolent behavior (Table 32.3).[10,25–34] A 2013 meta-analysis specifically looked at prognostic factors and outcomes of resections for synchronous MPLCs.[35] The authors specifically attempted to exclude carcinoid tumors and pure adenocarcinoma in situ from the analysis, because of their indolent nature. Tumors were considered synchronous if they occurred within 2 years of initial resection. Four hundred and sixty-seven patients were analyzed from six different studies conducted from 1983 to 2011,[10,25,30,36–38] which coincides with the integration of CT scanning into NSCLC care. The majority of patients (67%) had the same histology in both tumors. Between 16% and 78% of patients were treated with at least one sublobar resection, and half of the tumors were unilateral. Two tumors were seen in most patients, but 11% had three or more. Median overall survival was 52 months, far more in line with survival for early stage than metastatic NSCLC. Risk factors for poor outcome included male gender, increasing age, nodal involvement, and unilateral tumors, with N2 involvement being the strongest predictor of poor outcome. Those patients with favorable status with regard to these four prognostic factors

TABLE 32.2 Schematic Summary of Patterns of Disease and TNM Classification of Patients With Lung Cancer With Multiple Pulmonary Sites of Involvement

Eighth Edition Staging Category	Multiple Primary Lung Cancer		Single Lung Cancer With Intrathoracic Spread	
	Second Primary Lung Cancer	Multifocal GG/L Nodules	Separate Tumor Nodule	Pneumonic Type of Lung Cancer
Imaging Features	≥2 distinct masses with imaging characteristic of lung cancer (e.g., spiculated)	Multiple ground-glass or part-solid nodules	Typical lung cancer (e.g., solid, spiculated) with separate solid nodule	Patchy areas of ground glass and consolidation
Pathologic Features	Different histotype or different morphology by comprehensive histologic assessment	Adenocarcinomas with prominent lepidic component (typically varying degrees of AIS, MIA, and LPA)	Distinct masses with the same morphology by comprehensive histologic assessment	Same histology throughout (most often invasive mucinous adenocarcinoma)
Staging	Separate cTNM and pTNM for each cancer	T based on highest T lesion with "#/m" indicating multiplicity; single N and M	Location of separate nodule relative to primary site determines if T3, T4, or M1a; single N and M	T based on size if in single lobe, T4 or M1a if in different ipsilateral or contralateral lobe; single N and M

AIS, adenocarcinoma in situ; *GG/L,* ground glass/lepidic; *LPA,* lepidic predominant adenocarcinoma; *MIA,* minimally invasive adenocarcinoma; *TNM,* tumor, node, and metastasis.

(gender, age, lymph nodes, and laterality) had a 5-year survival of 82% in a pooled survival estimate from the six trials compared with only 43% for those with any poor prognostic risk factors.[35] Factors such as lung function, tumor size, and adjuvant therapies were not included in the analysis.

A consistent finding throughout the literature is that approximately one-third of synchronous MPLCs are detected incidentally at the time of resection.[2,10,35,39–41] Frozen section is typically not informative in these circumstances because histology is typically the same. An R0 resection is recommended, and this typically requires a sublobar resection for one or both of the lesions. If an R0 resection is not possible, a diagnostic biopsy is recommended to help direct further care.[18] Hilar and mediastinal lymph node evaluation is essential for these patients. As with other early stage NSCLC patients, there is a risk of a false-negative result on preoperative evaluation and N2 involvement is strongly associated with poor prognosis.

Metachronous Primary Lung Cancers

Incidence

Similar to synchronous MPLCs, the definition for metachronous tumors remains somewhat ambiguous. Increases in the incidence of metachronous MPLC in recent literature can be attributed to (1) more patients presenting with early stage NSCLC, (2) more patients surviving treatment for early stage NSCLC, and (3) increased use of CT scans as part of routine postoperative surveillance. Series of resected NSCLC patients prior to the year 2000 typically reported rates of 0.5% to 3.2% in resected patients.[42–45] Large series from 2001 and 2002 reported rates of 4.1% and 4.6%, and a 2013 report of 1294 patients from the Memorial Sloan Kettering Cancer Center (MSKCC) found 7% incidence of second primary lung cancers.[39,46,47] Although this was substantially higher than that reported by previous series, it is important to note that this is lower than the rate of recurrence within the same population (20%). In the MSKCC series, the rate of tumor recurrence following resection begins to decrease after 4 years, whereas the rate of a second primary NSCLC increased steadily over time, going from a rate of 3/100 person-years in the first 2 postoperative years to 6/100 person-years 5 years from resection. Most series report an average interval of 30 months to 50 months between initial and subsequent tumors (Table 32.4).[40,46,48–50]

The majority of second primary NSCLCs (93%) in the MSKCC series were detected by scheduled surveillance CT scan.

The augmented rate of MPLCs in this series is attributed to the increased use of routine postoperative surveillance scans. Patients received on average 1.9 CT scans in year 1 and 1.5 scans in year 2, which decreased to 0.8 scans/year through year 7. A 2010 analysis of the Surveillance, Epidemiology, and End Results (SEER) database found only 1.5% incidence of second primary NSCLC, but only 25% of resected early stage NSCLC patients in SEER receive any postoperative surveillance by CT.[51] Differences in the incidence of MPLC in the SEER and MSKCC are likely related to the decreased use of postoperative CT surveillance in the SEER population.

Similar to synchronous tumors, approximately two-thirds of metachronous MPLCs are of the same histology,[2,3,25,40,41,45,52] but that histology is changing over time. Squamous cell carcinomas were once the most common, but adenocarcinoma is reported more frequently in modern series.[47] This shift in histology may impact prognosis, as multifocal adenocarcinomas are thought to have a more indolent course, predilection toward multiplicity, and excellent survival following resection.[9]

Evaluation

Patients suspected of having a metachronous MPLC require careful evaluation to rule out the possibility of recurrent disease. Whole-body PET and brain MRI are considered essential, but the role for invasive mediastinal staging is less clear. The use of mediastinoscopy and the extent of systematic mediastinal lymph node evaluation used for the initial NSCLC may limit the ability to perform invasive mediastinal staging for the subsequent cancer. Endobronchial ultrasound with biopsy is an attractive alternative in a patient who has previously undergone mediastinoscopy, but accuracy is decreased in this setting.

Surgical Resection and Outcome

Almost all cases (75% to 90%) of metachronous MPLCs are detected at an early stage, and treatment therefore centers on local strategies with the grand majority undergoing surgery. Sublobar reactions are common, being used in approximately 40%, and this appears unchanged between older and more recent series. Survival following resection is approximately 40% at 5 years, somewhat disappointing for early stage NSCLC, but much better than would be expected for metastatic disease (Table 32.4).[25,40,46,48–50] Stage of the second tumor is the most consistent predictor of survival. Survival rates are improved in patients undergoing resection of metachronous multifocal GG/Ls.[9]

TABLE 32.3 Series Reporting Outcomes for Resected Synchronous MPLCs Since the Integration of CT Scanning in NSCLC Care

Author(s)	Years	N	Multiple Adenocarcinoma (%)	Bilateral (%)	5-y Survival (%)	Poor Prognostic Factors
Riquet et al.[25]	1983–2005	118	57.6	7	23.4	Location in different lobe
Okada et al.[40]	1985–1996	28	21	25	70	Stage III or IV
Trousse et al.[26]	1985–2006	125	52	27	34	Low FEV$_1$
						Sublobar resection
						Pneumonectomy
						Male
						pN1-2 symptoms
Vansteenkiste et al.[27]	1990–1994	35	14	20	33	pN1-2
Chang et al.[28]	1990–2006	92	87	12	35	pN1-2
De Leyn et al.[33]	1990–2007	36	12	100	38	N/R
Bae et al.[49]	1990–2008	19	36	37	51	Histologic discordance
						Primary tumor stage
Rostad et al.[32]	1993–2000	94	52	4	28	Adenocarcinoma
						Male
						Older age
						Pneumonectomy
Finley et al.[10]	1995–2006	175	76	45	64 (3 y)	>Stage IA
						Male gender
Mun and Kohno[31]	1995–2008	19	84	100	76	N/R
Fabian et al.[30]	1996–2009	67	31	66	53	Higher clinical stage
						Incomplete preoperative staging
Shah et al.[29]	1997–2010	47	N/R	100	35 (3 y)	None identified
Zhang et al.[34]	2010–2014	285	88	33	78	Male gender
						Symptoms
						LN involvement

CT, computed tomography; *FEV$_1$,* forced expiratory volume in 1 second; *LN,* lymph node; *MPLC,* multiple primary lung cancer; *N/R,* not reported; *NSCLC,* nonsmall cell lung cancer.

TABLE 32.4 Series Reporting Outcomes Following Resection for Metachronous MPLCs Since the Integration of CT Scanning Into NSCLC Care

Author(s)	Years	N	Multiple Adenocarcinoma (%)	Median DFI (mo)	5-y Survival (%)[a]	Poor Prognostic Factors
Riquet et al.[25]	1983–2005	116	44	N/R	32	Age
						pN2
Okada et al.[40]	1985–1996	29	17	49	33	Stage 2 tumor
Aziz et al.[46]	1985–1999	41	N/R	46	44	Short DFI
						Histologic concordance
Battafarano et al.[48]	1988–2002	69	29	29	33.4	Stage 2 tumor
Carretta et al.[50]	1988–2005	23	96	52	70	Stage 2 tumor
Bae et al.[49]	1990–2008	23	52	31	77	Discordant histology
						Stage 2 tumor

[a]From second tumor resection.
CT, computed tomography; *DFI,* disease-free interval; *MPLC,* multiple primary lung cancer; *N/R,* not reported; *NSCLC,* nonsmall cell lung cancer.

Metachronous Tumors Following Pneumonectomy

Development of subsequent lung cancer in the remaining lung after a pneumonectomy poses a unique treatment problem, and surgery is often considered contraindicated. There are a limited number of small series documenting feasibility of resection of second primary lung cancer following pneumonectomy,[53–56] but overall information on this select group of patients is limited. The largest series from the Mayo Clinic reports on 14 patients over a 20-year period.[57] Similar to other series of metachronous MPLC, the overwhelming majority of subsequent tumors were found in asymptomatic patients on routine surveillance CT scans and all were stage I. The 1-year, 3-year, and 5-year survival rates after resection for metachronous MPLC were 86%, 71%, and 50%, respectively. Wedge resection was the preferred mode of resection, with improved short- and long-term outcomes compared with more extensive procedures.[57]

Stereotactic Body Radiotherapy

Stereotactic body radiotherapy (SBRT) is an emerging option for patients with MPLC. SBRT for synchronous MPLC has been investigated in multiple small, single-institution retrospective series. Many patients in these series are treated with resection of one focus and SBRT of the other, but several report SBRT for both foci (Table 32.5).[58–61] The largest series to date is from the Netherlands, where 62 patients with synchronous NSCLCs were treated.[62] Fifty-six had SBRT to both lesions and six underwent resection for one tumor and SBRT for the other. There were no grade 4 or 5 adverse events; primary tumor control was 84% at 2 years, and 2-year overall survival was 56%. An exploratory analysis between unilateral and bilateral tumors noted no differences in toxicity, but a significant decrease in local and regional control for unilateral MPLCs.

SBRT is particularly attractive in this setting of metachronous MPLC because these are almost always diagnosed at an early stage and there is an increased need to preserve pulmonary parenchyma. Multiple small series studies on SBRT for metachronous MPLC reported excellent local control and 2-year overall survival rates similar to those of surgery (Table 32.6).[59,62,63] In a retrospective series of 48 metachronous MPLCs treated at Washington University, the 2-year overall survival rate was

TABLE 32.5 Series Reporting Results for SBRT for Synchronous MPLC

Author(s)	Years	N	Treatment	Dose	Duration of Follow-Up (mo)	Adverse Events ≥ Grade 3 (%)	Local Control (%)	Overall Survival (%)
Sinha and McGarry[61]	2001–2005	8	N/R	48–66 Gy in 3–4 fx	21	0	93 (1.5 y)	100 (1.5 y)
Creach et al.[59]	2004–2009	15	3 surgery + SBRT 12 SBRT × 2	40–54 Gy in 3–5 fx	24	0	94	27.5 (2 y)
Griffioen et al.[58]	2003–2012	62	56 surgery + SBRT 6 SBRT × 2	54–60 Gy in 3–8 fx	44	4.8	84 (2 y)	56 (2 y)
Shintani et al.[60]	2007–2012	18	3 surgery + SBRT 15 SBRT × 2	48–60 Gy in 4–10 fx	34	11	78 (3 y)	69 (3 y)

fx, fractions; *MPLC*, multiple primary lung cancer; *SBRT*, stereotactic body radiotherapy.

TABLE 32.6 Series Reporting Results for SBRT for Metachronous MPLC

Author(s)	Years	N	Median Interval (mo)	Treatment	Dose	Duration of Follow-Up (mo)	Adverse Events ≥ Grade 3 (%)	Local Control (%)	Overall Survival (%)
Griffioen et al.[62]	2003–2013	107	48	98 surgery + SBRT 9 CRT + SBRT	54–60 Gy in 3–8 fx	46	3.7	89 (3 y)	60 (3 y)
Creach et al.[59]	2004–2009	48	N/R	46 surgery + SBRT 2 SBRT × 2	40–54 Gy in 3–5 fx	24	0	92	68 (2 y)
Hayes et al.[63]	2007–2014	17	115	17 surgery + SBRT	48–60 Gy in 3–8 fx	18		93 (2 y)	88 (2 y)

CRT, conformal radiotherapy; *fx*, fractions; *MPLC*, multiple primary lung cancer; *SBRT*, stereotactic body radiotherapy.

TABLE 32.7 Series Reporting on SBRT for Metachronous Second Primary Lung Cancer Arising After Pneumonectomy

Author(s)	Years	N	Pathologic Confirmation	Dose	Duration of Follow-Up (mo)	Adverse Events ≥ Grade 3% (%)	Local Control (%)	Overall Survival (%)
Testolin et al.[64]	2015	12	0%	25–48 Gy in 1–4 fx	28	0	64 (2 y)	80 (2 y)
Simpson et al.[65]	2014	2	50%	48 Gy in 4 fx, 50 Gy in 5 fx	12–16	50	100	50
Thompson et al.[66]	2004–2013	13	21%	48 Gy in 4 fx	24	15	100	61 (2 y)
Haasbeek et al.[67]	2003–2008	15	20%	54–60 Gy in 3–8 fx	16.5	13	100 (2 y)	91% (2 y)

fx, fractions; *SBRT*, stereotactic body radiotherapy.

68%; in comparison 15 synchronous MPLCs treated over the same period had a 2-year survival of only 27.5%.[59] The largest reported series of SBRT for metachronous MPLC is from the Netherlands, with 107 patients treated between 2003 and 2013.[62] The majority had an anatomic resection for their initial NSCLC, and median interval between tumors was 48 months. At 2 years, local control was 89% and overall survival 60%, which were very similar to early survival results for single primary NSCLC.

A growing body of evidence suggests that SBRT is also a safe and effective treatment option in selected patients with metachronous MPLC following pneumonectomy (Table 32.7).[64–67] Testolin et al.[64] reported a series of 12 patients treated for MPLC after pneumonectomy for NSCLC. All patients completed the planned treatment with 2-year disease-free survival and overall survival rates of 36.1% and 80%. Haasbeek et al.[67] reported on SBRT in 15 postpneumonectomy patients, with a disease-free survival and overall survival of 91% and 80.8%. Pathologic confirmation of disease is challenging in this population due to fear of pneumothorax with single lung and is therefore frequently deferred.

EVIDENCE-BASED PRACTICE GUIDELINES

Both the American College of Chest Physicians and the European Society for Medical Oncology address MPLCs in their most recent evidence-based guidelines. In the European Society for Medical Oncology guidelines for treatment of metastatic NSCLC, it is recommended that solitary oligometastatic disease to the contralateral lung in most cases should be considered as a second primary tumor and treated if possible with surgery or definitive radiation.[68]

The most recent lung cancer guidelines from the American College of Chest Physicians address MPLCs under the "Special Treatment Issues" heading. The guideline details the importance of a multidisciplinary approach to the evaluation and management of patients with two intrathoracic foci of NSCLC.[18] The guidelines also recommend that diagnosis of MPLC can be based on the judgment of a multidisciplinary team and that clinical expertise best defines care with biopsy providing only supplemental information. The guidelines go on to recommend invasive mediastinal staging and extrathoracic imaging with whole-body PET and brain MRI for those patients being considered for curative resection. The final recommendation is that tumors found incidentally in a different lobe at the time of surgery should be resected if the patient has adequate pulmonary reserve and there is no evidence for mediastinal node involvement.[18]

Upcoming guidelines from the American Society for Radiation Oncology for the use of SBRT in NSCLC also address MPLCs. Similar to other society recommendations, they encourage a multidisciplinary approach and thorough pretreatment staging to help differentiate MPLC from intrathoracic metastasis. SBRT is recommended as a curative treatment option for patients with synchronous and metachronous MPLCs with equivalent rates of local control, toxicity, and overall survival compared with single NSCLCs treated with SBRT.

CONCLUSION

Patients with lesions suspicious for MPLCs pose a challenge to the thoracic oncologic community. The discrimination between multiple independent primaries and intrathoracic metastatic disease is currently based on nonspecific criteria including location, size, timing, CT appearance, and evidence for nodal or metastatic disease. We are moving into an era where that determination can be made far more precisely based on molecular analysis of tumor clonal relationships and DNA alternations. As imaging technologies improve, resection becomes less invasive, and CT screening and surveillance become more widely integrated, the incidence of MPLCs should continue to rise. Thus an increased understanding of the biology of MPLC is required to help identify these patients for cancer prevention strategies and to better define treatment algorithms and prognosis. Clinicians require increased guidance as to which tumors can be treated by conservative local measures (observation, sublobar resection, SBRT) and which are responsible for the poor 5-year survival rates reported through the literature.

KEY REFERENCES

8. Martini N, Melamed MR. Multiple primary lung cancers. *J Thorac Cardiovasc Surg.* 1975;70:606–612.
11. Zhang Y, Hu H, Wang R, et al. Synchronous non-small cell lung cancers: diagnostic yield can be improved by histologic and genetic methods. *Ann Surg Oncol.* 2014;21:4369–4374.
12. Arai J, Tsuchiya T, Oikawa M, et al. Clinical and molecular analysis of synchronous double lung cancers. *Lung Cancer.* 2012;77:281–287.
13. Girard N, Deshpande C, Azzoli CG, et al. Use of epidermal growth factor receptor/Kirsten rat sarcoma 2 viral oncogene homolog mutation testing to define clonal relationships among multiple lung adenocarcinomas: comparison with clinical guidelines. *Chest.* 2010;137:46–52.
17. Mino-Kenudson M, Myamoto A, Dias-Santagata D, et al. The role of molecular profiling to differentiate multiple primary adenocarcinomas from intrapulmonary metastases from a lung primary. *J Clin Oncol.* 2013;31(suppl). [abstr 7555].
18. Kozower BD, Larner JM, Detterbeck FC, Jones DR. Special treatment issues in non-small cell lung cancer: Diagnosis and management of lung cancer, 3rd ed: American College of Chest Physicians evidence-based clinical practice guidelines. *Chest.* 2013;143:e369S–e399S.
23. Detterbeck FC, Bolejack V, Arenberg DA, et al. The IASLC Lung Cancer Staging Project: background data and proposals for the classification of lung cancer with separate tumor nodules in the forthcoming eighth edition of the TNM classification for lung cancer. *J Thorac Oncol.* 2016;11:681–692.
24. Detterbeck FC, Nicholson AG, Franklin WA, et al. The IASLC Lung Cancer Staging Project: summary of proposals for revisions of the classification of lung cancers with multiple pulmonary sites of involvement in the forthcoming eighth edition of the TNM classification. *J Thorac Oncol.* 2016;11:639–650.
34. Zhang Z, Gao S, Mao Y, et al. Surgical outcomes of synchronous multiple primary non-small cell lung cancers. *Sci Rep.* 2016;6:23252.
35. Tanvetyanon T, Finley DJ, Fabian T, et al. Prognostic factors for survival after complete resections of synchronous lung cancers in multiple lobes: pooled analysis based on individual patient data. *Ann Oncol.* 2013;24:889–894.
49. Bae MK, Byun CS, Lee CY, et al. Clinical outcomes and prognostic factors for surgically resected second primary lung cancer. *Thorac Cardiovasc Surg.* 2012;60:525–532.
52. van Bodegom PC, Wagenaar SS, Corrin B, Baak JP, Berkel J, Vanderschueren RG. Second primary lung cancer: importance of long term follow up. *Thorax.* 1989;44:788–793.
54. Spaggiari L, Grunenwald D, Girard P, et al. Cancer resection on the residual lung after pneumonectomy for bronchogenic carcinoma. *Ann Thorac Surg.* 1996;62:1598–1602.
61. Sinha B, McGarry RC. Stereotactic body radiotherapy for bilateral primary lung cancers: the Indiana University experience. *Int J Radiat Oncol Biol Phys.* 2006;66:1120–1124.
62. Griffioen GH, Lagerwaard FJ, Haasbeek CJ, Slotman BJ, Senan S. A brief report on outcomes of stereotactic ablative radiotherapy for a second primary lung cancer: evidence in support of routine CT surveillance. *J Thorac Oncol.* 2014;9:1222–1225.
63. Hayes JT, David EA, Qi L, Chen AM, Daly ME. Risk of pneumonitis after stereotactic body radiation therapy in patients with previous anatomic lung resection. *Clin Lung Cancer.* 2015;16:379–384.
66. Thompson R, Giuliani M, Yap ML, et al. Stereotactic body radiotherapy in patients with previous pneumonectomy: safety and efficacy. *J Thorac Oncol.* 2014;9:843–847.

See Expertconsult.com for full list of references.

Surgical Management of Patients Considered Marginally Resectable

Hiran C. Fernando and Paul De Leyn

SUMMARY OF KEY POINTS

- Up to 25% of patients with stage I nonsmall cell lung cancer are considered medically inoperable or high risk for surgery.
- Therapies such as stereotactic body radiation therapy or ablation offer a less invasive alternative to surgery for marginally resectable patients.
- Guidelines have been developed to determine fitness for lung cancer surgery (see text).
- Guidelines to determine optimal therapy (e.g., surgery vs. stereotactic body radiation therapy/ablation) are not well established.
- The American College of Chest Physicians has determined that patients with a forced expiratory volume in 1 second or percentage of lung diffusion capacity for carbon monoxide less than 40% are at an increased risk for resection.
- The American College of Surgeons Oncology Group has defined criteria for patients considered to be high-risk for lobectomy but who are still candidates for sublobar resection or nonoperative therapy.
- Resection is still feasible in such patients defined as high risk.
- Sublobar resection can be undertaken with low mortality by experienced surgeons.
- Sublobar resection does not result in significant declines in pulmonary function in high-risk patients.
- Evaluation in a multidisciplinary setting that includes an experienced thoracic surgeon is recommended when determining therapy for marginally resectable patients.

The standard treatment of stage I nonsmall cell lung cancer (NSCLC) is lobectomy with systematic node dissection. Unfortunately, up to 25% of patients with stage I NSCLC are considered to be medically inoperable or are at high risk for surgery.[1] The increasing use of computed tomography (CT) screening often results in the detection of small tumors. This increase in the number of people with small tumors raises the following question: "What is the appropriate extent of pulmonary resection, particularly in older patients or in patients who, for other reasons, have marginally resectable disease?" The role of sublobar resection is further challenged by the introduction of new techniques associated with low rates of mortality and morbidity, such as stereotactic ablative radiotherapy (SABR) and radiofrequency ablation (RFA).

WHICH PATIENTS ARE CONSIDERED MARGINALLY RESECTABLE?

Respiratory failure and pulmonary complications represent the most substantial risks following lung resection, and preprocedure risk assessment is based primarily on pulmonary function. Algorithms for differentiating risk levels for patients who are candidates for lung resection have been published.[2] These guidelines provide general cutoffs for additional assessment and suggest threshold values to differentiate low-risk patients from high-risk patients. Cardiac evaluation and lung function testing—including lung diffusion capacity for carbon monoxide (DLCO)—are recommended for every patient who is to have pulmonary resection. Most centers use predictive postoperative forced expiratory volume in 1 second (FEV_1) and DLCO. If both values are higher than 30%, resection may still be feasible. According to the American College of Chest Physicians guidelines on the physiologic evaluation of patients for pulmonary resection,[3] patients with an estimated postoperative FEV_1 or DLCO of less than 40% are considered to be at increased risk for postoperative complications. The American College of Surgeons Oncology Group (ACOSOG) has initiated two studies in high-risk patients who have had sublobar resection and patients who are medically inoperable and are treated with RFA.[4,5] Although the same physiologic criteria were used for both studies (Table 33.1), an important factor was that a credentialed surgeon evaluated patients and deemed each patient to be either a poor candidate for lobectomy but a candidate for a more limited resection or a potential candidate for RFA because the patient was medically inoperable. Criteria that define marginally resectable as contrasted with unresectable are not standardized, and clinical evaluation by an experienced surgeon is essential. Ideally, the cases of all patients who are considered to have marginally resectable disease should be reviewed at a multidisciplinary meeting with an experienced thoracic surgeon participating in the discussion. In some cases of heterogeneous emphysema, pulmonary function may even improve after resection when the tumor is in the most emphysematous zone. This improvement is demonstrated by the results of lung volume–reduction surgery, and patients with this type of disease should not be denied the benefits of a curative lung resection.

It is difficult to know how many patients with stage I NSCLC are considered marginally resectable; however, we can get an estimate from some large database studies, such as those using data from the Surveillance, Epidemiology, and End Results (SEER) database. In one study involving 14,555 patients with stage I and II lung cancer, approximately 30% of patients aged 75 years or older were not offered surgery, compared with 8% of patients younger than 65 years.[6] It is unclear how many of these patients were not surgical candidates, and how many, if evaluated by an experienced surgeon, would have been offered sublobar resection. In another analysis of data from the SEER database, 10,761 patients with stage IA NSCLC had resection, with sublobar resection performed in 2234 (20.7%) of these patients.[7]

ROLE OF SUBLOBAR RESECTION IN THE TREATMENT OF NONSMALL CELL LUNG CANCER

The use of segmentectomy for treatment of lung cancer was initially described in 1973, when Jensik et al.[8] reported on patients who had segmental resection for lung cancer, thereby questioning the standard of lobectomy at that time. The only prospective

TABLE 33.1 Major and Minor Eligibility Criteria in the American College of Surgeons Oncology Group Z4032 Trial[a]

Major Criteria	Minor Criteria
FEV_1 ≤50%	FEV_1, 51% to 60%
DLCO ≤50%	DLCO, 51% to 60%
	Age ≥75 years
	Pulmonary hypertension (defined as pulmonary artery systolic pressure >40 mmHg)
	Poor left ventricular function (defined as an ejection fraction ≤40%)
	Resting or exercise arterial pO_2 ≤55 mmHg or SpO_2 ≤88%
	pCO_2 >45mmHg
	Modified Medical Research Council Dyspnea Scale score ≥3

[a]Eligible patients had to meet one major criterion or two minor criteria.[4]
DLCO, lung diffusion capacity for carbon monoxide; FEV_1, forced expiratory volume in 1 second; pCO_2, partial pressure of carbon dioxide; pO_2, partial pressure of oxygen; SpO_2, peripheral capillary oxygen saturation.

study comparing sublobar resection with lobar resection for the treatment of NSCLC is the Lung Cancer Study Group (LCSG) trial.[9] In this study, 122 patients were randomly assigned to limited resection (segmentectomy [67%] or wedge resection) and 125 patients to lobectomy. A threefold increase in local recurrence was associated with lobectomy, as was a trend suggesting a survival benefit ($p = 0.088$). Since the early 2000s, a large body of literature consisting of single-institution studies has demonstrated equivalent rates of regional recurrence and survival for segmentectomy and lobectomy for small (≤2 cm) node-negative tumors.[10–15] In an effort to increase the level of evidence to support limited resection for these small tumors, two prospective randomized studies are ongoing: one in the United States and Canada, with an expected enrollment of 1258 patients over 5 years (CALGB 140503; ClinicalTrials.gov identifier: NCT00499330); and the other in Japan, with an accrual of 1100 patients over 3 years (JCOG0802/WJOG4607L). Inclusion criteria in both trials are peripheral small (≤2.0 cm) NSCLC, excluding noninvasive lung cancer on CT (pure ground-glass opacity [GGO]). Until the data in these ongoing randomized trials are mature, it is recommended that, for standard-risk patients with operable disease, anatomic segmentectomy should be reserved for pure GGO lesions or partly solid lesions (<25%) smaller than 2 cm, located in the peripheral third of the lung. These pure GGO lesions are known to be noninvasive and are associated with no spread to the nodes. When segmentectomy is performed, the tumor should be situated in the central aspect of a typical pulmonary segment and the T1a N0 M0 status should be confirmed by examination of an intraoperative frozen section of N1 and N2 nodes. In addition, the surgeon should always resect all intersegmental lymph nodes to ensure they are tumor free. Otherwise, the procedure should be converted to a lobectomy. In patients considered marginally resectable, sublobar resection can be performed more liberally. To decrease rates of local recurrence, this procedure is combined with intraoperative brachytherapy at some centers.[16]

Sublobar resection can be performed by anatomic segmentectomy or wedge resection. In the case of wedge resection, the intersegmental and interlobar lymph nodes are usually not removed, and the margin between the staple line and the tumor is more likely to be smaller, especially in central lesions. In the LCSG trial, segmentectomy was associated with a decreased risk of recurrence in the involved lobe compared with wedge resection.[9] The superiority of segmentectomy over wedge resection for non-GGO lesions has been demonstrated in multiple studies. In one study of SEER data for patients with stage IA NSCLC, the survival associated with segmentectomy was compared with the survival associated with wedge resection. After adjusting for propensity scores, overall and lung cancer-specific survival rates were significantly better after segmentectomy (hazard ratio, 0.80 [95% confidence interval, 0.69–0.93] and hazard ratio, 0.72 [95% confidence interval, 0.59–0.88], respectively).[17]

IMPACT OF SUBLOBAR RESECTION ON LUNG FUNCTION AND MORBIDITY

In the LCSG trial, pulmonary function tests were measured preoperatively and at 6-month intervals.[9] At 6 months, the changes from baseline for FEV_1, forced vital capacity, and maximum voluntary ventilation were significantly better in patients who had sublobar resection than in patients who had lobar resection. At 12 months to 18 months, only the FEV_1 was significantly better for patients who had sublobar resection compared with lobectomy. DLCO was not routinely measured in the LCSG trial. Keenan et al.[18] analyzed pulmonary function tests from 147 patients who underwent lobectomy and 54 patients who underwent segmentectomy. One year after lobectomy, there were significant decreases from the preoperative values for forced vital capacity, FEV_1, maximal voluntary ventilation, and DLCO capacity in patients who received lobectomy. However, the lung volume did not change substantially after segmentectomy. The only significant change after segmentectomy was in DLCO. The preoperative pulmonary function in patients who underwent segmentectomy was significantly reduced compared with that in patients who underwent lobectomy (FEV_1, 75.1% vs. 55.3%; $p < 0.001$). A 2009 study demonstrated that a substantial decline in postoperative function after lung resection is less likely among patients with low FEV_1.[19] In this study, investigators compared the outcomes for patients older than 75 years with stage I NSCLC who received segmentectomy (78 patients) or lobectomy (106 patients). The 30-day operative mortality rate was 1.3% for segmentectomy and 4.7% for lobectomy. Patients who received segmentectomy had fewer major complications (11.5% vs. 25.5%; $p = 0.02$). The 5-year overall and disease-free survival rates were equivalent.

The role of brachytherapy in marginally resectable (≤3 cm) stage I NSCLC treated by sublobar resection was evaluated in a multicenter randomized trial (Z4032). In a preliminary report from this trial, multivariable regression analysis showed no significant impact of brachytherapy, video-assisted thoracoscopic surgery (VATS), or thoracotomy on 3-month FEV_1, DLCO, or dyspnea score.[20] A 10% change in FEV_1 or DLCO was regarded as clinically meaningful. The FEV_1 decreased by 10% in 22% of patients who received sublobar resection of the lower lobe compared with 9% of patients who received sublobar resection of the upper lobe ($p = 0.04$; odds ratio, 2.79). An updated analysis of this study was recently reported.[21] Pulmonary function tests were obtained at baseline, 3 months, 12 months, and 24 months after therapy. This updated analysis only included 69 patients who had measurement at all four time points. The median change from baseline for FEV_1% was +2%, +1%, and +1% at 3 months, 12 months, and 24 months, respectively. The median change from baseline for DLCO% was –1%, –2%, and –2% at the same time points, respectively. A decline of 10% or more was seen after lower lobe resections at 3 months, but was not seen at 12 months or 24 months. A decline of 10% or more in DLCO was seen after thoracotomy at 3 months but not at 12 months or 24 months.

This trial also demonstrated that sublobar resection was associated with a 30-day and 90-day mortality of 1.4% and 2.7%, respectively.[22] Grade 3 or higher complications occurred in 27.9% of patients. Segmental resections were more likely to be associated with grade 3 or higher adverse events (41.5%) compared with wedge resections (29.7%). DLCO less than the median of 46% was also associated with a greater risk of grade 3 or higher toxicity.

A recent study evaluated the ACOSOG criteria in 490 stage I lung cancer patients undergoing resection at their institution.[23]

Patients were divided into high risk and low risk based on the inclusion criteria from Z4032, with 180/490 patients defined as high risk. No differences in postoperative mortality were seen between high-risk and standard-risk patients, however, length of stay was longer in the high-risk groups. Major (15.6% vs. 6.7%) and minor (48.3% vs. 22.3%) morbidity were also significantly increased in the high-risk groups. Three-year survival was 59% for high-risk and 76% for standard-risk patients. This study not only supports the classification used in the ACOSOG studies, but also underscores the continued role of surgery for these patients with no differences in mortality and acceptable 3-year survival.

VIDEO-ASSISTED THORACOSCOPIC SURGERY

Segmentectomy can also be routinely performed with minimally invasive surgical techniques.[24] In one single-institution series, 225 segmental resections were performed for stage I NSCLC patients (104 VATS and 121 open procedures).[25] There were no deaths among the patients who had VATS; however, two patients (1.6%) who had an open procedure died. Compared with open segmentectomy, VATS segmentectomy was associated with a shorter hospital stay (5 days vs. 7 days) and a lower rate of pulmonary complications (15.4% vs. 29.8%). The operative time, estimated blood loss, mortality rate, recurrence rate, or survival rate did not differ between the two groups. In a later series published by the same group, data on 785 patients who had segmentectomy or lobectomy were reviewed.[26] Among patients with stage IA NSCLC, there were no differences in time to recurrence and overall recurrence between the two procedures.

SUBLOBAR RESECTION VERSUS OTHER LOCAL THERAPIES

Although surgical resection remains the standard of care for early stage lung cancer, new techniques, including sublobar resection, SABR, and RFA, are now available for local therapy for high-risk patients with stage I NSCLC. These techniques are associated with lower procedure-related morbidity and mortality rates but increased rates of locoregional recurrence compared with lobectomy. One advantage of surgical resection is that lymph nodes can be removed and evaluated to confirm histology. Surgical and anesthetic techniques continue to improve, requiring updates to current guidelines. The identification of patients who are at high risk for lobectomy remains a complex clinical decision, and therefore the cases of such patients should be discussed by a multidisciplinary team.[27]

In many retrospective studies, selection bias has been demonstrated. An example of this bias was seen in a study by Crabtree et al.,[28] in which data for 462 patients who received surgery were compared with 76 patients who received SABR. Patients had a clinical stage IA/B NSCLC that was determined by the results of CT and positron emission tomography. In an unmatched comparison, the overall 5-year survival was 55% for patients who received surgery and the 3-year survival was 32% for patients who received SABR. After final pathologic examination, disease was upstaged in 35% of the patients who had surgery, with 13.8% of patients found to have N1 disease and 3.5% to have N2 disease. In the remaining 17.7% of patients, the T stage was upstaged from T1 to T2–T4. The analysis showed that patients who had surgery were younger, had lower comorbidity scores, and had better pulmonary function compared with the patients who received SABR. When a propensity analysis was used, the rates of local recurrence and disease-specific survival were similar for both groups of patients. The investigators matched 57 high-risk surgical patients to 57 patients who received SABR and found that the operative mortality rate for the high-risk surgical group was 7.0%, with no treatment-related deaths associated with SABR. In the matched comparison of this subgroup, there were no differences between surgery and SABR in terms of freedom from local recurrence (88% vs. 90%), disease-free survival (77% vs. 86%), and overall survival (54% vs. 38%) at 3 years.

In another study, the risk factors from three cooperative group trials involved RFA or SABR for patients who were medically inoperable and sublobar resection for patients who were deemed marginally operable.[29] The lowest values for DLCO were found among patients who received RFA. On initial evaluation, the 30-day rate of grade 3 or higher adverse events was higher for patients who had sublobar resection than for patients who received SABR. Nevertheless, in a propensity-matched comparison, there was no difference in grade 3 or higher adverse events at 30 days. These findings support the need for randomized trials to better compare these therapies.

Optimization of Oncologic Outcomes With Sublobar Resection

Because a better margin is more likely to be achieved when segmentectomy is performed, oncologic outcomes are likely to be improved by the preferential use of segmentectomy instead of wedge resection and by paying close attention to ensure an adequate surgical margin is achieved. Ideally, lymph node dissection or sampling should be done, and, as stated earlier, intersegmental lymph nodes are more likely to be removed with a segmental resection. In the Z4032 study, segmentectomy was associated with higher lymph node counts and, not surprisingly, higher rates of node upstaging.[30]

More recent data have supported the superior results with segmentectomy compared with wedge resection in the LCSG trial.[9] An analysis of data from the SEER database also demonstrated superior results for patients treated with segmental resection compared with wedge resection, even in tumors that were 2 cm or smaller.[17]

A strict definition for an adequate margin in sublobar resections remains unresolved, but a margin distance of 1 cm or more than the maximum tumor diameter is generally recommended.[31] To prevent local relapse, some institutions have used adjuvant intraoperative brachytherapy in conjunction with sublobar resection. Initial results from retrospective studies have suggested that this technique is effective in reducing rates of local recurrence.[16,32,33] Subsequently, the results of a prospective randomized study were reported.[4] There was no decrease in local recurrence rates associated with brachytherapy among patients with stage I NSCLC (≤3 cm in maximum diameter), which may have been a result of participating surgeons paying closer attention to margins. Only 6.6% of patients had positive results on cytologic examination of a sample taken from the staple line following resection, and it was in this group that the strongest trend favoring the use of brachytherapy was demonstrated. Three-year survival following resection was 70.8% in this group of patients with marginally resectable disease.

CONCLUSION

Sublobar resection should be considered the standard of care for patients with NSCLC who are deemed marginally resectable. Oncologic outcomes are improved with wide surgical margins, which are easier to achieve when segmental resection is performed. In addition, lymph node dissection or sampling should be done if resection is planned. Removal of lymph nodes will likely lead to a higher incidence of node upstaging, but will also help in identifying patients who are appropriate candidates for adjuvant chemotherapy. This added information would not be possible with alternative therapies such as SABR or RFA. Despite initial enthusiasm, adjuvant brachytherapy does not appear to offer oncologic advantages when applied routinely; however, brachytherapy may be useful for patients in whom the surgical margin will likely be close, and perhaps for patients with larger tumors, for whom sublobar resection is thought to be the best therapeutic option.

KEY REFERENCES

2. Brunelli A, Charloux A, Bolliger CT, et al. ERS/ESTS clinical guidelines on fitness for radical therapy in lung cancer patients (surgery and chemoradiotherapy). *Eur Respir J*. 2009;34:17–41.
3. Colice GL, Shafazand S, Griffin JP, et al. Physiological evaluation of the patient with lung cancer being considered for resectional surgery: ACCP evidence-based clinical practice guidelines (2nd edition. *Chest*. 2007;132(suppl 3):161s–177s.
4. Fernando HC, Landreneau RJ, Mandrekar SJ, et al. The impact of adjuvant brachytherapy with sublobar resection on local recurrence rates after sublobar resection: results from the ACOSOG Z4032 (Alliance), a phase III randomized trial for high-risk operable non-small cell lung cancer. *J Clin Oncol*. 2014;32:2456–2462.
5. Dupuy DE, Fernando HC, Hillman S, et al. Radiofrequency ablation of stage IA non-small cell lung cancer in medically inoperable patients: results from the American College of Surgeons Oncology Group Z4033 (Alliance) trial. *Cancer*. 2015;121:3491–3498.
9. Ginsberg RJ, Rubinstein LV. Randomized trial of lobectomy versus limited resection for T1 N0 non-small cell lung cancer. *Ann Thorac Surg*. 1995;60:615–623.
21. Kent MS, Mandrekar SJ, Landreneau R, et al. Impact of sublobar resection on pulmonary function: long-term results from American College of Surgeons Oncology Group Z4032 (Alliance). *Ann Thorac Surg*. 2016;102:230–238.

22. Fernando HC, Landreneau RJ, Mandrekar SJ, et al. Thirty- and ninety-day outcomes after sublobar resection with and without brachytherapy for non-small cell lung cancer: results from a multicenter phase III study. *J Thorac Cardiovasc Surg*. 2011;142:1143–1151.
23. Sancheti MS, Melvan JN, Medbery RL, et al. Outcomes after surgery in high-risk patients with early stage lung cancer. *Ann Thorac Surg*. 2016;101:1043–1051.
27. Donington J, Ferguson M, Mazzone P, et al. American College of Chest Physicians and Society of Thoracic Surgeons Consensus Statement for evaluation and management for high-risk patients with stage I non-small cell lung cancer. *Chest*. 2012;142:1620–1635.
29. Crabtree T, Puri V, Timmerman R, et al. Treatment of stage I lung cancer in high-risk and inoperable patients: comparison of prospective clinical trials using stereotactic body radiotherapy (RTOG 0236), sublobar resection (ACOSOG Z4032), and radiofrequency ablation (ACOSOG Z4033). *J Thorac Cardiovasc Surg*. 2013;145:692–699.

See Expertconsult.com for full list of references.

34   Technical Requirements for Lung Cancer Radiotherapy

Fiona Hegi, Todd Atwood, Paul Keall, and Billy W. Loo, Jr.

SUMMARY OF KEY POINTS

- Radiotherapy plays a central role in the treatment of lung cancer for patients in both the palliative and curative settings.
- Major advances in the technologic aspects of both radiotherapy and medical imaging have dramatically increased the accuracy and precision of treatment, resulting in less toxic and more curative treatment.
- In the developed world, the minimum standard for curative intent radiotherapy is linear accelerator-based three-dimensional (3-D) conformal radiotherapy with computed tomography (CT)-based computerized planning. Other technologies, such as cobalt teletherapy with two-dimensional (2-D) planning, may still be appropriate in low-resource settings.
- New approaches to radiotherapy treatment integrate information from multiple imaging sources, together with information about respiratory motion, and utilize sophisticated computerized approaches to planning to accurately model conformal dose distribution in the patient.
- Increased precision of treatment has permitted safe dose escalation for both early stage lung cancer and pulmonary metastases through stereotactic approaches, as well as making curative treatment easier to safely deliver for locally advanced lung cancer patients.
- Ongoing technologic developments in particle therapy and image guidance systems may further benefit lung cancer patients by increasing the precision of treatment and reducing the low-dose wash seen in current intensity-modulated planning approaches.
- The rapid evolution of radiotherapy technology means that ongoing education is required to maintain an up-to-date understanding of the imaging, planning, and delivery processes of modern radiotherapy in order to optimize the use of technology for lung cancer patients.

Radiotherapy plays a key role in the treatment of lung cancer potentially at any stage of the disease. Because lung cancer is predominantly in advanced stages at the time of diagnosis,[1] perhaps the largest overall clinical impact of radiotherapy has been in palliation of symptomatic sites. Even so, radiotherapy can be used with curative intent for a larger proportion of patients than can any other treatment modality. Major advances in the technologic aspects of both radiotherapy and medical imaging since the mid-1990s have dramatically increased the accuracy and precision of tumor targeting and treatment delivery, translating into less toxic and more curative treatment for both more advanced and earlier stage disease than has historically been treated with

radiotherapy treatment.[2] By contrast, radiotherapy generally requires a substantial technologic infrastructure, and lack of this infrastructure has been a barrier to access for patients in much of the world. It is estimated that in low-income to middle-income countries where over one-half of the global burden of cancer arises, only 25% of patients who would benefit from radiotherapy have access to it, and more than 20 countries have no access to radiotherapy at all.[3,4]

Sophistication of radiotherapy technology ranges from relatively simple to highly complex. Radiotherapy that is purely palliative in intent can result in substantial symptom relief, such as reduction of pain, airway or vascular obstruction, and hemoptysis, using relatively low doses of radiation that are tolerable even when delivered to relatively large volumes of the body.[5] In this application, highly accurate tumor localization and precise dose sculpting are less critical than simply having access to expeditious treatment with radiotherapy, and basic equipment is generally adequate. Conversely, obtaining the highest chance of local tumor control and cure with radiotherapy requires the most accurate possible determination of the tumor extent and spatial distribution and the delivery of highly dose-intensive radiation to all macroscopic tumor deposits without exceeding the tolerances of critical and sometimes sensitive normal organs.

The latter requires exquisite shaping of the radiation dose in space while ensuring highly accurate delivery to cover the entire tumor while minimizing any unnecessary radiation dose to the surrounding normal tissues. The technologies enabling such advanced radiotherapy continue to evolve rapidly and include multimodality imaging, such as x-ray CT, positron emission tomography (PET), and magnetic resonance imaging (MRI); technologies to characterize and manage tumor and organ motion, such as four-dimensional (4-D) imaging and multiple approaches to control, mitigate, or compensate for respiratory motion; advanced linear accelerator technologies, including multidirectional-shaped or intensity-modulated beams; computerized radiation planning and optimization; and particle beams with more favorable physical and/or biologic properties than conventional high-energy x-rays.

Multiple professional societies and expert panels have published guidelines on the management of lung cancer, with several providing recommendations specifically on radiotherapy techniques (see following list). In the developed world, the minimum technical standard for curative-intent lung cancer radiotherapy is considered to be linear accelerator-based 3-D conformal radiotherapy with CT-based computerized planning. This chapter will primarily focus on this technology as the base as well as on more advanced technologies. Nevertheless, we recognize that, for decades, curative radiotherapy has been accomplished with more basic technologies that may still be the best available in more-limited-resource settings. In such settings, an expert panel of the International Atomic Energy Agency has identified the baseline level of technology as cobalt megavoltage therapy with 2-D planning.[6]

In this chapter, we summarize the technologies of lung cancer radiotherapy and their use, technical requirements and quality assurance, and challenges and future directions.

Annotated List of Resources From Expert Organizations on the Treatment of Lung Cancer, Including Clinical and Technical Aspects of Radiotherapy

National Comprehensive Cancer Network (NCCN) Clinical Practice Guidelines in Oncology: Nonsmall cell lung cancer (NSCLC) [http://www.nccn.org]

Guidelines that serve as a statement of evidence and consensus of the authors regarding their views of currently accepted approaches to the treatment of NSCLC.

NCCN Clinical Practice Guidelines in Oncology: Small cell lung cancer (SCLC) [http://www.nccn.org]

Guidelines that serve as a statement of evidence and consensus of the authors regarding their views of currently accepted approaches to treatment of SCLC.

American College of Chest Physicians (ACCP) Evidence-Based Clinical Practice Guidelines: Treatment of stage I and II NSCLC [Howington et al. *Chest.* 2013(5 Suppl):e278S–313S]

Collection of recommendations that address the diagnosis and management of stages I and II NSCLC.

ACCP Evidence-Based Clinical Practice Guidelines: Treatment of stage III NSCLC [Ramnath et al. *Chest.* 2013;143(5 Suppl):e314S–340S]

Collection of recommendations that address the diagnosis and management of stage III NSCLC.

ACCP Evidence-Based Clinical Practice Guidelines: Treatment of SCLC [Jett et al. *Chest.* 2013;143(5 Suppl):e400S–419S]

Collection of recommendations that address the diagnosis and management of SCLC.

ACR Appropriateness Criteria: Radiation therapy for SCLC [Kong et al. *Am J Clin Oncol.* 2013;36(2):206–213]

Report focused on developing acceptable medical practice guidelines for SCLC used by the Agency for Healthcare Research and Quality (AHRQ), as designed by the Institutes of Medicine (IOM).

ACR Appropriateness Criteria: Nonsurgical treatment for NSCLC: poor performance status or palliative intent [Rosenzweig et al. *J Am Coll Radiol.* 2013;10(9):654–664]

Report focused on developing acceptable medical practice guidelines for NSCLC used by AHRQ, as designed by the IOM.

European Society for Medical Oncology (ESMO) Clinical Practice Guidelines: early-stage and locally advanced NSCLC [Vansteenkiste et al. *Ann Oncol.* 2013;24 (Suppl 6):vi89–vi98]

European guidance document on the diagnosis, staging, and management of early and locally advanced NSCLC.

ESMO Clinical Practice Guidelines: SCLC [Früh et al. *Ann Oncol.* 2013;24 (Suppl 6):vi99–vi105]

European guidance document on the diagnosis, staging, and management of SCLC.

American Association of Physicists in Medicine (AAPM) Task Group (TG) 179: Quality assurance for image-guided radiation therapy (IGRT) utilizing computed tomography (CT)-based technologies [Bissonnette et al. *Med Phys.* 2012;39(4):1946–1963]

Report that provides consensus recommendations for quality-assurance protocols that ensure patient safety and patient treatment fidelity for CT-based IGRT systems, allowing for the widespread management of geometric variations in patient setup and internal organ motion.

ACR and ASTRO Practice Guideline: Intensity-modulated radiation therapy (IMRT) [Hartford et al. *Am J Clin Oncol.* 2012;35(6):612–617]

Guidance document designed to serve as an educational tool to assist practitioners in providing appropriate radiation oncology care for patients, with a focus on IMRT.

American Society for Radiation Oncology (ASTRO) Evidence-Based Clinical Practice Guideline: Palliative thoracic radiotherapy in lung cancer [Rodrigues et al. *Pract Radiat Oncol.* 2011;1(2):60–71]

Guidance document that provides information on the use of external beam radiotherapy, endobronchial brachytherapy, and concurrent chemotherapy in the setting of palliative thoracic treatment of lung cancer, based on available evidence complemented by expert opinion.

ASTRO and ACR Practice Guidelines: IGRT [Potters et al. *Int J Radiat Oncol Biol Phys.* 2011;76(2):319–325]

Guidance document designed to serve as an educational tool to assist practitioners in providing appropriate radiation oncology care for patients, with a focus on IGRT.

ACR and ASTRO Practice Guideline: 3-D external-beam radiation planning and conformal therapy (2011) [http://www.acr.org/guidelines]

Guidance document designed to serve as an educational tool to assist practitioners in providing appropriate radiation oncology care for patients, with a focus on 3-D conformal radiation therapy.

AAPM TG 101: Stereotactic ablative radiation therapy (SABR) [Benedict et al. *Med Phys.* 2010;37(8):4078–4101]

Report that outlines the best practice guidelines for SABR.

ASTRO and American College of Radiology (ACR) Practice Guideline: Performance of SABR [Potters et al. *Int J Radiat Oncol Biol Phys.* 2010;76(2):326–332]

Guidance document designed to serve as an educational tool to assist practitioners in providing appropriate radiation oncology care for patients with a focus on SABR.

ACR Appropriateness Criteria: Nonsurgical treatment for NSCLC: good performance status/definitive intent [Gewanter et al. *Curr Probl Cancer.* 2010;34(3):228–249]

Report focused on developing acceptable medical practice guidelines for NSCLC used by the AHRQ, as designed by the IOM.

ACR Appropriateness Criteria: Induction and adjuvant therapy for stage N2 non-small cell lung cancer [Gopal et al. *Int J Radiat Oncol Biol Phys.* 2010;78(4):969–974]

Report focused on developing acceptable medical practice guidelines for NSCLC adjuvant therapy used by the AHRQ, as designed by the IOM.

ACR Technical Standard: Performance of radiation oncology physics for external-beam therapy (2010) [http://www.acr.org/guidelines]

Technical guidance document that is designed to serve as an educational tool to assist practitioners in providing appropriate radiation oncology care for patients by outlining the role of radiation physics for external beam therapy.

AAPM TG 142: Quality assurance of medical accelerators [Klein et al. *Med Phys.* 2009;36(9):4197–4212]

Report that provides a comprehensive overview of the necessary quality assurance for a successful radiation oncology program.

ACR Technical Standard: Medical physics performance monitoring of IGRT (2009) [http://www.acr.org/guidelines]

Technical guidance document designed to serve as an educational tool to assist practitioners in providing appropriate radiation oncology care for patients, with a focus on monitoring IGRT.

ACR Practice Guideline: Radiation oncology (2009) [http://www.acr.org/guidelines]

Guidance document designed to serve as an educational tool to assist practitioners in providing overall appropriate radiation oncology care for patients.

AAPM TG 104: Role of in-room kilovoltage x-ray imaging for patient setup and target localization (2009) [https://www.aapm.org/pubs/reports/]

Report that includes a review of image-guided processes in the clinical setting and strategies for effective modification of these processes based on clinical data.

AAPM TG 75: Management of imaging dose during IGRT [Murphy et al. *Med Phys.* 2007;34(10):4041–4063]

Report that compiles an overview of image-guided techniques and their associated radiation dose levels, identifies ways to reduce the total imaging dose without sacrificing essential imaging information, and recommends optimization strategies.

AAPM TG 76: Management of respiratory motion in radiation oncology [Keall et al. *Med Phys.* 2006;33(10):3874–3900]

Continued

Annotated List of Resources From Expert Organizations on the Treatment of Lung Cancer, Including Clinical and Technical Aspects of Radiotherapy—cont'd

Report that describes the magnitude of respiratory motion, discusses radiotherapy-specific problems caused by respiratory motion, explains techniques that explicitly manage respiratory motion, and gives recommendations and guidelines for these devices and their use with conformal and IMRT.

AAPM TG 65: Tissue inhomogeneity corrections for megavoltage photon beams (2004) [https://www.aapm.org/pubs/reports/]

Report that provides physical and mathematical insight into the inhomogeneity problem, including the capabilities and limitations of the particular methods available, in order to help guide oncologists and physicists to deliver the correct radiation dose.

AAPM IMRT Subcommittee: Guidance document on delivery, treatment planning, and clinical implementation of IMRT [Ezzell et al. *Med Phys.* 2003;30(8):2089–2115]

Report that provides the framework and guidance to allow clinical radiation oncology physicists to make judicious decisions in implementing a safe and efficient IMRT program in their clinics.

AAPM TG 58: Clinical use of electronic portal imaging [Herman et al. *Med Phys.* 2001;28(5):712-737]

Report that provides materials to help medical physicists and colleagues succeed in the clinical implementation of electronic

portal imaging devices for various radiation oncology procedures.

AAPM TG 53: Quality assurance for clinical radiotherapy treatment planning [Fraass et al. *Med Phys.* 1998;25(10):1773–1829]

Report that provides the framework and guidance to allow radiation oncology physicists to design comprehensive and practical treatment planning quality-assurance programs for their clinics.

AAPM TG 6: Managing the use of fluoroscopy in medical institutions (1998) [https://www.aapm.org/pubs/reports/]

Report designed to provide practicing medical physicists with information regarding managing fluoroscopic dose and resource materials that may be used in an education program for nonradiologists who use fluoroscopy.

AAPM TG 28: Radiotherapy portal imaging quality (1987) [https://www.aapm.org/pubs/reports/]

Report that describes the trade-offs in portal imaging quality and dose as they apply to successful treatments in radiation oncology.

International Agency for Research on Cancer Lung Cancer Consortium (IARC) [http://ilcco.iarc.fr/]

The IARC group shares comparable data from ongoing lung cancer case–control and cohort studies.

RADIOTHERAPY EQUIPMENT

Imaging and Simulation Systems

Imaging and simulation systems for radiotherapy have evolved rapidly since their introduction in the early 1950s. Dedicated radiotherapy simulators initially consisted of diagnostic x-ray tubes simply mounted to replicate radiotherapy treatment geometries. Over time, simulator improvements were iteratively introduced to provide more information for 2-D, and eventually 3-D and 4-D, target localization and treatment planning. In the developed world, a combination of 3-D simulation systems, such as x-ray CT, PET, and MRI, has become the standard of care for modern lung cancer staging and radiotherapy. As simulation and imaging systems have become more sophisticated, high-quality diagnostic and functional information has become readily available, leading to more accurate lung tumor localization, treatment planning, and treatment delivery.[7]

2-D Simulation

Conventional 2-D simulators consist of a diagnostic x-ray tube that is able to image in both static and fluoroscopic modes, while reproducing the radiation properties and geometric movements of the radiotherapy treatment unit. Although the information from a conventional simulator is inherently 2-D, acquiring images at orthogonal angles can produce simplified 3-D information. It is possible to design treatment fields that encompass the target volume and spare normal tissues using 2-D simulation, but the process is typically limited to simplified or palliative lung cancer cases where more complex imaging techniques are not necessary or not available. The major disadvantage of conventional simulation is the lack of true 3-D information. This technique does not provide enough information for lung cancer treatments requiring complex beam geometries and sophisticated dose distributions.

Computed Tomography

CT simulators have become the standard of care for radiotherapy in the developed world. CT imaging data provide a complete 3-D view of the patient's anatomy, allowing for more accurate delineation of the tumor and the surrounding normal tissues. In addition, the CT data inherently include the associated tissue density information, which is a necessity for 3-D radiotherapy treatment planning.

Dedicated CT simulators are based on diagnostic CT scanners, with a few modifications. CT simulators typically include a laser alignment system as a reference for patient positioning, a 3-D imaging workstation for image visualization and manipulation, a larger bore size to accommodate patient immobilization devices, and a flat tabletop to replicate the radiotherapy treatment unit couch. CT data sets can be reconstructed in any orientation to provide coronal or sagittal slices of the anatomy, and digitally reconstructed radiographs can be created from CT data sets to resemble planar x-ray images from any angle or orientation. These characteristics allow for treatment geometries to be visualized that are possible on the treatment unit, but not possible on a conventional 2-D simulator.

Modern CT simulators are also capable of acquiring 4-D data. Four-dimensional CT simulation allows for the tumor to be evaluated at multiple time points in the respiratory cycle and for the most beneficial respiratory phase to be selected for treatment planning and delivery. The combination of these CT imaging advancements provides a simulation technique that allows for more accurate tumor localization, treatment visualization, and subsequent treatment delivery.[8]

Positron Emission Tomography

Combined PET/CT simulators are becoming increasingly common in radiation oncology departments worldwide. In the developed world, ^{18}F-2-deoxy-D-glucose (FDG)-PET–CT scans are consistently being used to provide detailed anatomic information combined with functional metabolic information for patients with lung cancer. PET–CT images have been shown to be effective for selecting patients with unresectable lung cancer for definitive radiotherapy, lung cancer staging, and delineating lung cancer target volumes.[8,9]

Combined PET–CT simulators include all of the radiotherapy-specific additions described in the previous section, with an additional PET detector ring integrated into the simulator housing. Although PET images alone are able to provide the same useful metabolic information, combined PET–CT simulation systems mitigate image registration issues that arise when PET and CT images are acquired separately for tumor localization and treatment planning. Newer PET–CT simulators also include 4-D imaging capabilities. Like 4-D CT simulation, 4-D PET–CT allows for tumor metabolism to be evaluated at multiple time points in the respiratory cycle.

Magnetic Resonance Imaging

The use of MRI in radiation oncology is becoming increasingly common. MRI offers a way to combine high-quality anatomic and functional information, without the use of ionizing radiation. As a whole, MRI is capable of generating anatomic images with excellent soft-tissue contrast and functional images that demonstrate perfusion, diffusion, and chemical information.

MRI is often used in lung cancer radiotherapy when high soft-tissue contrast information is needed to delineate the tumor from surrounding tissues or when tumor respiratory motion analysis would benefit from images with a very high temporal and spatial resolution.[10] Although the inherent density in CT data is currently considered to be the standard for radiotherapy treatment planning, MRI units are increasingly being installed in radiation oncology departments to complement PET–CT simulators. In addition, many MRI vendors now offer larger bore sizes to accommodate patient immobilization devices and a flat tabletop to resemble other imaging modalities and the treatment unit. However, because MRI units are not integrated into CT simulators, proper image registration is necessary when MR images are used to delineate lung tumors.

Immobilization

Lung cancer immobilization devices are designed to reproduce the patient position from the time of simulation to the completion of radiotherapy. Ideal immobilization techniques and devices are able to comfortably secure the patient in an optimal position for simulation and therapy, while minimizing intrafraction motion, limiting beam attenuation, and not interfering with patient localization systems.

Immobilization systems for lung cancer radiotherapy commonly include polyurethane foam casts or evacuated vacuum bags/cushions placed underneath the patient's thorax, combined with a device to help position the patient's arms overhead. Additional pads and wedges are often added to make the patient more comfortable and increase the overall positioning reproducibility. With the rise of hypofractionated lung cancer regimens, additional abdominal compression techniques have also been used to further decrease the allowable respiratory tumor motion during simulation and the subsequent radiotherapy treatments.[11]

Treatment Planning Systems

Modern radiotherapy treatment planning systems are an integral part of the successful treatment of cancer with radiation. Treatment planning systems provide a set of computerized tools that allow the radiation oncologist, medical physicist, and treatment planner to create and visualize radiotherapy treatments, given the imaging data available. Early treatment planning systems relied solely on 2-D simulation techniques for tumor localization and treatment beam arrangement. In these systems, orthogonal pairs of 2-D images could be used to infer 3-D information for tumor localization, but treatment visualization was restricted to the available imaging planes, and dose distributions did not accurately reflect variations in tissue density.

As imaging systems and dose-calculation algorithms have advanced, so have treatment planning system capabilities. Current 3-D treatment planning systems are able to superimpose radiotherapy treatment beams on 3-D image sets with any geometry or orientation, allowing the use of a so-called beam's eye view technique to visualize the radiation beam in conjunction with the relevant patient anatomy. Furthermore, images from multiple imaging modalities can be rigidly registered to the treatment planning CT, and additional anatomic and functional information can be examined with respect to the treatment plan. Many treatment planning systems are now incorporating deformable image registration algorithms as well to accommodate the increased use of MR and PET imaging in radiotherapy. Current treatment planning systems are also able to integrate 4-D image data into the treatment planning process. Sophisticated treatment planning systems provide tools to analyze the extent of tumor motion throughout the respiratory cycle. This analysis allows the radiation oncologist to determine the optimal treatment phases for each individual tumor, while evaluating the dose distributions for any portion of the respiratory-gated treatment. 4-D treatment planning system functionality is especially beneficial for lung cancer radiotherapy.

Modern treatment planning systems also include advanced tools for treatment plan optimization and analysis. Treatment planners and medical physicists can easily adjust beam angles and weighting factors for conventional forward-calculated plans, whereas optimization parameters and associated weightings can easily be altered for inverse planning tasks. These treatment planning system capabilities streamline the overall treatment planning process. In addition, advanced treatment planning system analysis tools, such as dose–volume histograms, provide a more thorough investigation of the dose delivered to the radiotherapy target and the surrounding normal tissues. The combination of these advanced treatment planning system tools allows for accurate and efficient treatment planning for lung tumors and other cancers.

Target and Normal Tissue Delineation

Computerized 3-D treatment planning requires the identification of the spatial extent of both where the radiation dose needs to be deposited and what regions should be spared. The delineation of the target(s) and normal organs, also known as contouring, is generally made on 3-D images acquired during the simulation process, most often CT. At present, this process is primarily performed manually by an expert human observer, who draws the structures on cross-sectional image slices. However, computer software tools are often used to automate portions of this process with rapidly increasing sophistication.

Medical imaging technologies have advanced over time to provide increasingly exquisite detail that improves the accuracy of target and normal tissue delineation. The addition of metabolic imaging, particularly FDG-PET, provides increased sensitivity and specificity to guide the inclusion or exclusion of targets in the treatment volume. Nevertheless, it is important to understand the uncertainties in contouring and account for them in the treatment plan. The International Commission on Radiation Units and Measurements (ICRU) has developed a nomenclature for contouring that incorporates these concepts in the context of 3-D treatment planning and intensity-modulated radiation therapy (IMRT).[12,13] In brief, within this paradigm, the gross tumor volume refers to the extent of macroscopic tumor (i.e., visible on imaging or physical examination), whereas the clinical target volume refers to the regions at highest risk for microscopic tumor involvement. Uncertainties in the target definition are addressed by defining a larger volume that incorporates margins around these target volumes, and it is this planning target volume to which the radiation dose is prescribed. The margins used to form the planning volume include an internal margin to account for physiologic target motion, such as respiratory motion, and a set up margin to account for uncertainties in patient-positioning reproducibility, machine calibration, and other technical factors.

In order to optimize the treatment plan, in addition to ensuring adequate dose coverage of the targets, doses to the normal organs at risk of injury must be constrained, which requires contouring the normal organs at highest risk of injury by radiation. In the thorax, these organs generally include the lungs, esophagus, spinal cord, heart, and potentially other organs depending on the anatomic extent of the treatment volume and the dosing regimen. Atlases for standardized, consensus-based contouring for thoracic radiation therapy are useful references.[14] In addition, guidelines for normal organ dose constraints, based on a combination of clinical data, expert consensus, and constraints associated with acceptable toxicity in clinical trials are summarized in the National Comprehensive Cancer Network Guidelines for nonsmall cell lung cancer and quantitative analysis of normal tissue effects in the clinic reports.[15–19]

Dose Calculation for Lung Cancer Radiotherapy

In lung cancer radiotherapy, the transport of radiation originates in the therapy device and ends with energy deposition in the patient and beyond. There are many different types of interactions of photons and electrons, and the likelihood and characteristics of these interactions depend on the particle type, particle energy, and the material or tissue that the particles are passing through. These interactions are covered in detail in medical physics texts such as texts by Khan,[20] Johns and Cunningham,[21] and Metcalfe et al.[22] The complexity of radiation transport is exacerbated in lung cancer radiotherapy, where the density of lung tissue is approximately one-quarter of that of most other soft tissues and can range from a density very close to air in emphysematous regions to near that of soft tissue in high-density lung. Adding to this complexity are the sharp tissue density boundaries between the lung and chest wall or abdomen, lung and mediastinum, and the lung and lung tumor.

Independent of the complexity of radiation transport in lung cancer radiotherapy, a method to estimate the dose is needed for each patient's course of treatment. As imaging technology and computational power have advanced, so has the ability of dose-calculation algorithms to account for the complexity of radiation transport, resulting in algorithms in general use today having fewer and smaller errors than those of the past. Accurate radiation transport simulations of photons and electrons in lung cancer radiotherapy and the subsequent dose calculations are challenging, particularly in the following anatomic regions:

- In the lungs where the photon range and electrons set in motion by the photons will travel 3 to 10 times as far as the same particles in the rest of the soft tissue in the body due to the lower density of the lungs
- At the lung–tumor boundary lateral to the beam where there is lateral disequilibrium as more charged particles from the tumor enter the lung than vice versa resulting in a dose gradient
- At the lung–tumor boundary proximal to the beam where there is a rebuild-up of dose due to the step-up in density from the lung to the tumor
- At the tumor–lung boundary distal to the beam where there is a reduction of dose due to the step-down in density from the tumor to the lung
- Near the trachea and the main bronchi where the density inside the airways is typically 1/1000 of the density of soft tissue, and therefore there is very little attenuation of the photons and electrons
- At the chest wall and lung interface where the density changes can cause dose buildup and build-down

Knowledge of dose in the regions is important, both for the tumor where local control is related to dose and for normal tissue toxicity,[23] as pneumonitis,[16] rib fractures,[24] and other sequelae are side effects of radiation therapy. In particular, in the case of stereotactic ablative radiotherapy (SABR), in which often small treatment fields are used to treat tumors surrounded by low-density lung tissue, there is evidence that less accurate dose calculation may adversely impact treatment outcomes.[25,26]

The complexity of dose-calculation algorithms in general is higher for higher beam energies, smaller field sizes, lower density regions, and the use of IMRT or volumetric modulated radiation therapy (VMAT). Dose-calculation algorithm accuracy is also limited by the quality of the input data that are used to generate the beam models and heterogeneity corrections. Therefore both the measured beam data and the patient anatomy,[27] typically determined from CT,[28] are important parameters influencing the overall accuracy.

Dose-calculation algorithms have evolved since the 1960s to include more physics and to model the interactions of radiotherapy beams with human tissue in a more natural manner that reflects the known interaction and transport processes. The American Association of Physicists in Medicine (AAPM) Task Group 76 report on respiratory motion management recommends "that the most accurate dose calculation available be used."[29]

These algorithms can be grouped into several classes: photon transport correction methods, superposition/convolution methods, Monte Carlo methods, and finite-element methods.

Photon Transport Correction Methods

The first dose-calculation algorithms used in radiotherapy accounted for variations in tissue density by correcting for the photon transport. These algorithms, such as effective depth, effective tissue-to-air ratio, and Batho power law, account well for body surface changes and source-skin distance changes; however, in the lung, the dose relative to a homogeneous calculation assuming water only would be increased. For small fields, due to the increase in electron range, the dose to the lung actually decreases relative to a homogeneous calculation and therefore homogenous (no correction) algorithms often were used. These uses of these algorithms are declining, and if any of the following algorithms are clinically commissioned and available, they should be used.

Superposition/Convolution Methods

In superposition algorithms, the primary photon interactions from the treatment beam are determined very accurately by ray tracing. From the photon interaction sites, the dose deposited by electrons set in motion by the primary photons is computed by scaling energy deposition kernels based on the density path length between the interaction site and the deposition site. The energy deposition kernels are normally computed via Monte Carlo methods by forcing photons to interact at a point in water. The dose from the interaction of scattered photons is also computed in a similar manner. Superposition algorithms accurately account for photon transport, and account for electron transport in variable density tissue. The accuracy of superposition algorithms can be reduced at boundaries with large density differences, such as the lung–chest wall, lung–tumor, and lung–mediastinum boundaries. Given other uncertainties in lung cancer radiotherapy, such as target delineation and motion, the superposition algorithm should be sufficiently accurate for most clinical purposes.

Monte Carlo Methods

Considered the most accurate dose-calculation algorithms available, Monte Carlo methods explicitly model the transport of photons and electrons from the treatment head and into the patient using physics principles based on our understanding of the interactions of particles with matter, including quantum mechanics. Monte Carlo methods are clinically available; however, there are still many uncertainties with Monte Carlo, including the model of the specific linear accelerator used, the modeling of the patient anatomy, and the statistical uncertainty inherent in Monte Carlo calculations. A comprehensive guideline for those clinicians planning to use Monte Carlo dose-calculation methods is the AAPM Task Group 105 report.[30]

Finite-Element Methods

Another more recent class of dose-calculation algorithms uses finite-element methods to propagate radiation beams in patients. The incident particle fluence is discretized into spatial, energy, and angular distributions. This particle fluence is then propagated through the absorbing media in a grid, accounting for the attenuation and scattering of particles. This method yields results similar to those with Monte Carlo calculations.[31]

Many treatment planning systems have, at a minimum, a superposition-class algorithm as the most accurately available option. Often treatment planning systems will have more than one algorithm and use a faster algorithm; for example, the multiple iterations required for IMRT optimization. For the final dose calculation, the most accurate algorithm available should be used. The most accurate algorithm will yield the best estimate of dose to the patient that will guide the plan review process and alert the clinician to high-dose or low-dose areas of concern that need to be monitored or, in some cases, require plan modifications. The more accurate algorithm also improves the quality of data used for dose reporting and outcome analysis. A useful summary, still relevant to many algorithms in use today, is from Fogliata et al.,[32] who compared the performance of seven algorithms from four treatment planning system vendors with Monte Carlo calculations in consistent geometries. They found that as the complexity of the model of particle transport increased, so did the improved match to the Monte Carlo–calculated result, particularly with larger variations in density and higher energies.

Treatment Delivery Systems

Linear Accelerator

Most lung cancer radiotherapy in the developed world is delivered by linear accelerators (linacs). 4-Megavoltage (4-MV) linacs with onboard kilovoltage (kV) or MV planar imaging panels and CT planning are standard in most radiotherapy departments and are sufficient to deliver 3-D conformal radiotherapy for most patients with lung cancer. Developments in beam modulation by multileaf collimators have led to the implementation of increasingly sophisticated techniques in lung cancer radiotherapy, such as IMRT and VMAT, and the integration of image guidance technology, such as cone-beam CT and optical image guidance systems, has led to the development of sophisticated radiotherapy delivery systems that can deliver radiotherapy to moving targets with high precision. Modulated techniques that deliver precisely sculpted radiotherapy fields are attractive because they can reduce the exposure of normal tissue to radiation dose but are more complex to deliver due to the increased risk of geographically missing the radiotherapy target. In situations where the tumor is small and highly mobile, or during SABR where very large radiotherapy doses are delivered over

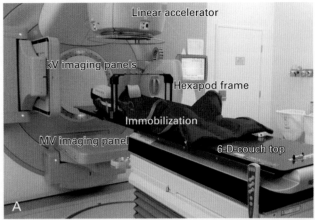
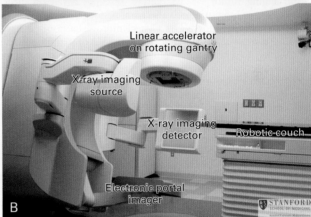
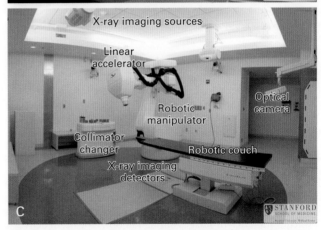

Fig. 34.1. Examples of modern image-guided linear accelerator radiation therapy systems. (A and B) The most common systems in clinical use have a C-arm configuration and may be used for conventionally fractionated radiation therapy as well as stereotactic ablative radiotherapy (with appropriate technical implementation). (C) A dedicated stereotactic radiotherapy system using a compact linear accelerator mounted on a robotic manipulator. *kV,* kilovoltage; *MV,* megavoltage. *(Image A Courtesy J. Barber, Nepean Cancer Care Centre, Penrith, Australia.)*

a short period using highly conformal radiotherapy fields, the use of more sophisticated radiotherapy delivery systems may be advantageous.

The most common linear accelerator systems have a C-arm geometry in which an open gantry rotates in a circular motion and the radiation beam is directed toward the isocenter of the gantry perpendicular to its axis of rotation (Fig. 34.1). Noncoplanar beam arrangements are possible by combining gantry rotation with rotations of the patient couch. Imaging systems may be mounted on the gantry to provide rotating views to produce cone-beam CT images or in fixed configurations in the treatment room. Descriptions of some commercially available linacs with novel configurations of linac heads with image guidance systems follow.

The CyberKnife (Accuray, Sunnyvale, CA, USA) is a dedicated stereotactic radiotherapy system and has a 6-MV linac mounted on a robotic arm.[33,34] The robotic arm permits treatment with six degrees of freedom, and the CyberKnife is equipped with a number of image guidance systems that permit tracking of mobile radiotherapy targets. Two orthogonal kV imaging systems can image bony anatomy or fiducial markers before every one to few beams, and respiratory motion can be monitored by either external optical sensors or by assessing the motion of fiducials within a lung tumor.[35,36] Markerless tracking based on direct visualization of lung tumors is also possible for selected peripherally located lung tumors. The CyberKnife uses a nonisocentric planning technique, in which a large number of planning nodes are assigned to a treatment volume, and each node can receive a modulated beamlet given in six degrees of freedom, resulting in dose distributions that are precisely sculpted to the shape of the radiotherapy target volume. With tight dose conformity and high levels of accuracy, the CyberKnife system lends itself to stereotactic radiotherapy approaches in which extremely high doses are delivered to small moving targets within the lung parenchyma.[37,38]

TomoTherapy (TomoTherapy Inc., Madison, WI, USA) machines have a linac mounted in a CT-based ring gantry, allowing the delivery of a fan-shaped radiotherapy beam as the linac head rotates around the patient. An MV CT is incorporated to allow the acquisition of MV CT images for image guidance. TomoTherapy is capable of rapidly delivering long, precisely shaped radiotherapy fields without the need for junctions between fields.[39]

Cobalt Therapy Systems

Cobalt-based radiotherapy delivery systems are in widespread use throughout the developing world.[4] These permit the delivery of MV radiotherapy beams, with less complex quality assurance and maintenance than linear accelerators.

There have been developments in cobalt technology, which allow the delivery of sophisticated radiotherapy plans in combination with image-guided radiotherapy. The ViewRay (ViewRay Inc., Oakwood Village, OH, USA) system has three Cobalt-60 heads with multileaf collimators mounted in a rotating gantry. This is combined with a split-magnet MRI system, which allows the acquisition of MR images during radiotherapy beam delivery. These images can be used to assess the accuracy of radiotherapy beam delivery to the target or to facilitate real-time adaptation of the radiotherapy treatment plan.

Hadron Therapy Systems

Proton therapy is the most common form of hadron therapy. Protons are positively charged particles that are accelerated to very high energies (70 MeV to 250 MeV) by cyclotrons or synchrotrons, then transported through a series of vacuum tubes and magnets into treatment delivery rooms where they are delivered through a snout (collimator) that shapes the proton beam.[40] The main advantage of proton beams is that the beams deposit most of their energy abruptly in a confined spatial extent, reducing the incidental irradiation of surrounding tissues for a given dose to the target. Proton-beam delivery systems have evolved from fixed gantries with a single beam to rotating gantries that can deliver multiple proton beams capable of delivering radiotherapy plans

of high precision and complexity. The size and expense of proton therapy systems have limited their widespread availability. However, a large number of proton radiotherapy facilities are under development with many lung cancer clinical trials for proton therapy ongoing at the time of publication.[41]

TREATMENT DELIVERY FOR NONSMALL CELL LUNG CANCER

The evolution of radiotherapy treatment techniques for nonsmall cell lung cancer has been largely driven by innovations in our ability to image the tumor during the planning process and increasingly accurate image verification techniques during treatment delivery. The use of 3-D CT-based planning is now commonplace in many departments, permitting the development of more refined dosimetric assessments, such as using dose–volume histograms and volumetric analyses to analyze the relationship between dosimetry and toxicity. In turn, incorporation of this knowledge has led to a search for greater conformity with the development of 3-D conformal radiotherapy and the increasing use of IMRT and VMAT.

2-D Planning Simulation

2-D planning is based on landmarks, which are palpable externally, or visible on planar simulation films. 2-D planning does not permit the assessment of doses to individual internal organs, and the ability to predict toxicity or to ensure accuracy of treatment delivery is limited in comparison with 3-D conformal radiotherapy. The process of 2-D planning follows.

- *Image acquisition:* Planar images of the lung tumor are acquired using a simulator. The degree of respiratory excursion can be assessed to some extent on the planar images, which may be used as a guide to choosing an appropriate field size.
- *Patient contour acquisition:* An external surrogate, such as a strip of lead, is used to acquire an external patient contour at the level of the tumor.
- *Planning:* The external patient contour and the size and approximate position of the tumor are mapped, and a cross-sectional representation of the patient is constructed. The isodoses of the fields that have been selected are then mapped onto this cross section, allowing calculation by hand of the monitor units required to deliver the dose.

Conformal Radiotherapy: 3-D Conformal Radiotherapy, IMRT, and VMAT

The introduction of 3-D CT-based planning was a tremendous innovation in radiotherapy planning, permitting for the first time the 3-D visualization of tumors and organs at risk. The information from CT could be used for more accurate planning of lung radiotherapy for patients, based on the electron-density information provided by CT. The relationship between doses to the lung and pulmonary toxicity began to be explored, which permitted the development of 3-D conformal radiotherapy and eventually the introduction of IMRT and VMAT. In the contemporary practice of lung radiotherapy, the planning CT may be fused with functional imaging such as PET or MRI to facilitate accurate delineation of the tumor.

Planning concepts have developed in parallel with the dissemination of CT technology. The planning concepts for 3-D conformal radiotherapy were defined in ICRU 50 and 62.[12,42] The concepts of gross tumor volume, clinical target volume, and planning target volume were defined, and adequate coverage of the planning target volume specified that the planning target volume required coverage between 95% and 107% of the prescribed dose.

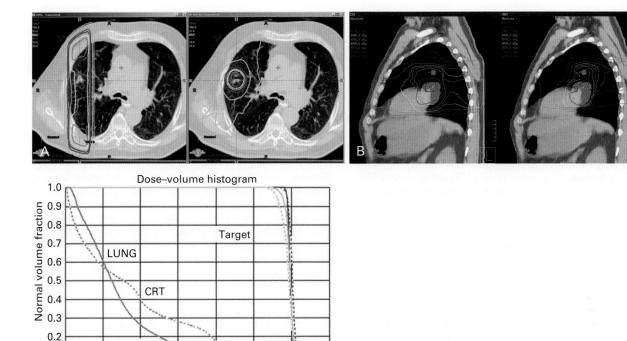

Fig. 34.2. (A) Comparison of conventional anterior–posterior postage stamp fields for medically inoperable early stage lung cancer (left) with an arc-based stereotactic ablative radiotherapy (SABR) plan (right). In the conventional plan, the highest doses are in normal tissues, preventing the use of ablative doses, whereas the conformal SABR plan minimizes normal tissue irradiation and permits ablative treatment of the tumor. *(Courtesy B.W. Loo, Stanford, CA.)* (B) Comparison of 3-D conformal radiotherapy (left) and volumetric modulated arc therapy (VMAT; right) plans for locally advanced lung cancer. Conformity of the high-dose region (95% isodose in *steel pink*) is improved with VMAT compared with 3-D conformal radiotherapy, with smaller amounts of normal lung exposed to potentially damaging radiotherapy (20-Gy isodose in *green*). *(Courtesy K. Anslow, Nepean Cancer Care Centre, Penrith, Australia.)* (C) Dose–volume histograms comparing VMAT *(solid lines)* and 3-D conformal radiotherapy *(dotted lines)* plans for locally advanced lung cancer. The volume of normal lung exposed to potentially damaging radiotherapy is reduced with VMAT, but the low-dose wash of 5 Gy covers a larger volume. Radiotherapy planning target volume coverage is equivalent with lower exposure to normal lung. *CRT,* conformal radiotherapy. *(Courtesy K. Anslow, Nepean Cancer Care Centre, Penrith, Australia.)*

In 3-D conformal radiotherapy, beams are placed and adjusted by the dosimetrist or physicist. The beam weighting and angles can be adjusted, but there is no modulation of the beam during treatment. IMRT uses multiple small beams for which fluence may be modulated during treatment delivery. In addition, the process of planning is inverse rather than forward planned, that is, the objectives of the plan that the planner wishes to achieve are specified at the beginning of the planning process, and the planning software optimizes the plan to meet these prespecified criteria. In comparison with 3-D conformal radiotherapy plans, IMRT plans may have a large number of highly modulated beams. This permits great conformity as the high-dose region can be precisely sculpted to match the shape of the planning target volume. However, the large number of beams increases the low-dose wash in IMRT plans, and IMRT plans can be much more heterogeneous than 3-D conformal radiotherapy plans with steep dose gradients. In lung cancer, the heterogeneity of IMRT plans may be exacerbated by the low electron density of pulmonary tissue. In addition, though evidence is contradictory, it is possible that the risk of pneumonitis is related to the low-dose wash in normal lung,[43] which is increased with IMRT because beams are delivered from a large number of angles. The implementation of IMRT requires care to minimize the risk of geographic miss associated with increased conformity of the high-dose regions, particularly with mobile lung tumors. Incorporating an evaluation of low-dose wash is also important to minimize the risk of toxicity. Despite these risks, the use of IMRT confers great benefits for patients receiving lung radiotherapy, permitting greater sparing of normal tissue and the ability to deliver a higher dose to the tumor; IMRT has also been safely demonstrated in several large series.[44,45]

VMAT is a later development that differs from IMRT as the modulated beam rotates continuously in one or more arcs around the patient. VMAT has been shown in a number of studies to be able to deliver highly conformal dose distributions.[46,47] However, the major advantage of VMAT is the rapid delivery time in comparison with conventional multiple-beam IMRT. VMAT treatment techniques have varying degrees of dose conformity for early stage and locally advanced lung cancer (Fig. 34.2).

The search for methods to reduce toxicity led to the recognition that there was a limited understanding of tumor and normal tissue organ motion during radiotherapy treatment. Evidence from other sites demonstrated the dangers of geographic miss of the tumor with a tightly conformal radiotherapy field. 4-D CT images the tumor over at least a full respiratory cycle and then binds images from each part of the respiratory cycle together to create a composite image of the movement of the tumor over time. The use of 4-D CT has allowed clinicians to restrict treatment of the tumor to a specific part of the respiratory cycle (gating) and to create radiotherapy target volumes that are more likely to reflect the true position range of the tumor during radiotherapy treatment.

Hadron Therapy

Charged-particle (hadron) radiotherapy can deliver superior dose distributions compared with photon radiotherapy techniques. Unlike photons, the energy loss of a charged particle is relatively small until the end of the range of the particle. The remaining energy is lost over a small distance, forming the Bragg peak. Radiotherapy planning with charged particles exploits these physical characteristics, concentrating the Bragg peaks of multiple charged-particle beams within the radiotherapy target. A number of different charged particles have been used in radiotherapy for lung cancer, but most patients have been treated with protons. Studies in patients with lung cancer treated with proton therapy have demonstrated the safety and efficacy of this technique.[47–49] As the dose to normal tissue can be reduced when compared with standard photon-based techniques, the use of charged-particle therapy may also permit safer dose escalation in patients receiving lung radiotherapy.[50]

Delivery of Conformal Radiotherapy: Image-Guided Radiotherapy

The development of radiotherapy planning technology has facilitated new treatment approaches, such as SABR in which high doses are delivered to small moving targets using highly conformal radiotherapy plans. The increasing conformity of radiotherapy plans potentially reduces the risk of toxicity to surrounding organs at risk, but demands increasingly sophisticated image guidance technology to ensure accurate delivery to the target volume.

- *Electronic portal imaging:* Electronic portal imaging panes are standard on modern linacs and may be used to take orthogonal images prior to treatment. The electronic portal imaging panels may be used for set up based on bone landmarks but are unable to provide sufficient resolution of soft-tissue anatomy to allow soft-tissue matching in general.[51]
- *Cone-beam CT:* An increasing number of linacs are equipped with either kV or MV cone-beam CT. The image quality obtained from cone-beam CT is inferior to diagnostic CT but is still sufficient to permit matching on the basis of soft-tissue anatomy.[52] Some vendors have also made 4-D cone-beam CT available,[53] permitting the assessment of tumor motion on the linac.
- *ExacTrac (Brainlab AG, Feldkirchen, Germany):* The ExacTrac system uses two kV imaging panels that take orthogonal kV images of the bony anatomy and radiotherapy target. This system may be coupled with external optical sensors that can be used to track patient motion during radiotherapy beam delivery or for respiratory motion management.[54]
- *Intrafraction imaging approaches:* A number of approaches have been developed to assess patient and tumor motion while the radiotherapy beam is being delivered.
- *CyberKnife:* During a CyberKnife treatment, more than 100 small radiotherapy beamlets deliver the dose to the target. kV images may be acquired prior to every beam or every few beams, allowing compensation for patient motion or tumor motion.[34] The motion of targets that move with respiration can be predicted by combining external optical sensor tracing of respiratory motion with direct visualization of fiducial markers or the tumor.

- *Implanted markers with radiofrequency guidance:* The Calypso System (Varia Medical Systems, Palo Alto, CA, USA) and other similar systems use markers that emit radiofrequency signals. The position of the marker can be determined by triangulation of the signals, and the radiotherapy beam delivery can be adapted to match the position of a moving tumor target.[55]

MOTION MANAGEMENT

As modern radiation therapy has enabled the delivery of increasingly conformal dose distributions, the importance of understanding and addressing uncertainties in target localization relative to the treatment plan correspondingly increases. One substantial source of uncertainty arises from the fact that targets in the thorax generally move from a number of causes, especially breathing. The magnitude of respiratory motion depends on several factors, such as anatomic location within the thorax, and conditions, such as chronic obstructive pulmonary disease, but also exhibits wide individual patient variability.[56,57] While most tumors move only a small amount, motions of up to several centimeters is possible. The primary objectives of respiratory motion management are to ensure adequate dose coverage of the tumor and to reduce incidental irradiation of normal organs. The process involves characterizing tumor and organ motion, selecting a motion management strategy, and verifying accurate implementation of that strategy by image guidance at the time of treatment. Recommendations for implementation of respiratory motion management strategies are summarized in the report of AAPM Task Group 76.[29]

The most basic approach to managing respiratory motion is to individualize the target design to cover the range of motion during free breathing for each given patient. This is appropriate for most patients as respiratory motion is limited in most. The magnitude of motion can be assessed as part of CT-based simulation by a number of techniques, including slow scanning CT, two-phase inhale/exhale CT, and respiratory-correlated (4-D) CT. Fluoroscopy may also be used as an adjunct to CT to estimate the degree of respiratory excursion. Targeting based on individual patient motion assessment avoids the over-targeting and under-targeting inherent when using a single population-derived respiratory motion target expansion for all patients.

Many more sophisticated options are available for respiratory motion management, requiring different levels of technology, procedural invasiveness, and cooperation from the patient. Some of these approaches depend on the implantation of fiducial markers in or near the tumor or other anatomic structures as surrogates for localizing the corresponding structures. A procedure must be performed to implant internal markers, generally by bronchoscopy or endoscopy or percutaneously under CT or other image guidance. These markers are most commonly used with planar x-ray images or fluoroscopy, in which case they are metallic radio-opaque markers. They may also be radiofrequency transponders whose positions can be read nearly continuously by an external electromagnetic array.

Motion management techniques may also be categorized as those that reduce respiratory motion and those that compensate for free-breathing motion. Methods for reducing respiratory motion include mechanical restriction of motion, such as by external compression of the abdomen to restrict diaphragmatic excursion or by modifications of breathing, such as breath hold or shallow breathing. By contrast, methods for free-breathing motion management include respiratory gating, in which the radiation beam is turned on only during a portion of the breathing cycle in which the target is at a prespecified location, and dynamic tumor tracking, in which the radiation beam follows the target as it moves with breathing. Fig. 34.3 shows an example of respiratory-gated radiation therapy.

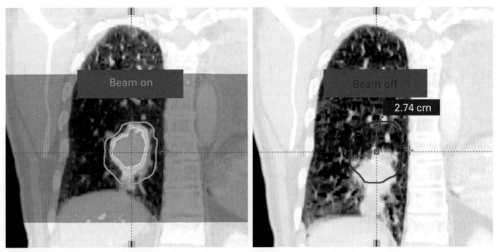

Fig. 34.3. A conceptual example of respiratory gating for a tumor with a large excursion during breathing. The beam is on only during a portion of the respiratory cycle (during exhale in this example). This permits use of smaller treatment margins and less irradiation of normal lung tissue. It is important to use image-guidance techniques to verify that this complex treatment is delivered accurately.

The lung cancer radiotherapy process

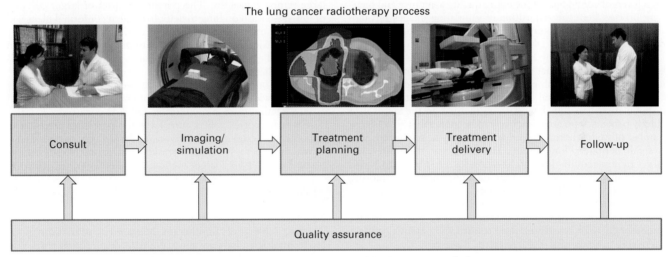

Fig. 34.4. Quality assurance underpins each step of the lung cancer radiotherapy process.

With all of these strategies, particularly the more complex ones used with the intent of reducing treatment margins, it is important to ensure that the strategies are achieving the intended result by confirming that the tumor location is as planned when the beam is being delivered. This confirmation is primarily accomplished through image guidance (previously discussed), with each motion management method having specific image guidance strategies that are most appropriate. Particularly, when external surrogates of internal anatomy (such as surface markers) are used to control the radiation beam, imaging should be used to confirm that they correspond accurately to the internal anatomy locations at all times during treatment delivery. Each motion management approach has its strengths and weaknesses, and it is most important that practitioners fully understand the uncertainties in the method of choice and how to mitigate them.

QUALITY ASSURANCE FOR LUNG CANCER RADIOTHERAPY

Cancer radiotherapy uses large doses of radiation that when misused can, and has, caused harm to patients and operators alike. Quality assurance in all aspects of the radiotherapy process is

critical to achieve the highest likelihood of treatment success and to reduce the likelihood and impact of errors (Fig. 34.4). The traditional approach to radiation therapy is being transformed into a more industrial approach using analyses to determine potential errors, or failure modes characterized as most likely, most severe, and hardest to detect, and allocate a proportionate amount of the quality-assurance budget to these failure modes.[58] The forthcoming AAPM Task Group 100 Report will detail this new approach.

In lung cancer, similar to other cancer sites, radiotherapy development and adherence to written guidelines for patient selection, patient immobilization devices, 3-D/4-D CT and/or PET imaging, target and normal tissue delineation, margin determination, planning approach, and dose–volume constraints, and treatment delivery are important.[59]

Lung cancer radiotherapy requires additional quality-assurance procedures over many other radiotherapy procedures due to the dose-calculation challenges from the low-density lung and the motion management methods previously discussed.[29] For example, if respiratory monitors are being used for breath-hold, gated, or tumor-tracking treatments, then the accuracy of these monitoring systems, in isolation and as part of an internal/external correlation model, needs to be verified. Breath-hold methods require patient training, and therefore staff training is necessary to coach and advise the patients. Due to the respiratory motion occurring during imaging and treatment, special procedures and care should be taken when implementing image-guided radiotherapy procedures. Another challenge of respiratory motion is the interplay effect,[60] a phenomenon introducing dose uncertainty when the motion of the beam and tumor are uncorrelated, which is exacerbated with IMRT procedures.

As with all radiotherapy procedures, constant vigilance by the treatment staff is important. Training and education for all staff involved with lung cancer radiotherapy, as well as periodic retraining, is recommended. A physicist should be available to solve any hardware-related problems. Staffing levels appropriate to the technology, workflow, and patient load are essential.

FUTURE DIRECTIONS IN LUNG CANCER RADIOTHERAPY

Early Stage Lung Cancer and Pulmonary Metastases

SABR is a newer technology in which high doses per fraction are given over a short period of time. The delivery of SABR demands high levels of confidence in the entire quality assurance and planning process from the acquisition of simulation images through the use of complex planning techniques, right through to beam delivery.[61]

A large and increasing body of evidence indicates that SABR is highly effective and that it may be delivered with minimal toxicity. In comparison with conventionally fractionated radiotherapy, SABR has high local control rates and has been associated in population-based analysis with an increase in the survival of elderly patients, who are more likely to be inoperable.[62,63] A large number of studies have shown that SABR may be safely delivered to small, peripheral lung tumors. However, centrally located and larger tumors require dose modification for safe treatment,[64] and ongoing investigations at the time of publication are exploring optimization of SABR for these tumors.

SABR may also be used to treat pulmonary metastases, and there is an increasing body of evidence for the role of ablative radiotherapy to increase both local control and potentially affect survival in patients with oligometastatic disease.[65]

Locally Advanced Lung Cancer

Locally advanced lung cancer remains challenging to treat, with poor local control and high rates of systemic relapse. While the results of the Radiation Therapy Oncology Group (RTOG) 0617 trial have demonstrated that radiation dose escalation to 74 Gy compared with 60 Gy with or without the addition of cetuximab to carboplatin/paclitaxel-based chemoradiation does not increase the survival in locally advanced lung cancer and may increase the patient-assessed toxicity of treatment,[66–68] the results of standard-dose chemoradiation with the high level of quality assurance maintained on that study were nevertheless favorable compared with historical outcomes in this patient population. Future directions related to dose optimization include isotoxic and individualized adaptive dose intensification, an approach that is being tested in the RTOG 1106 trial using metabolic imaging (FDG-PET) as the basis for defining the target volume for higher doses.

Considering the high rates of systemic progression in locally advanced lung cancer, the integration of systemic therapies with radiotherapy continues to be an active area of research. The optimal approach to integrating molecular diagnostics and molecularly targeted therapies and immunotherapies into the curative treatment of locally advanced lung cancer is the subject of numerous active and developing clinical trials.

Individualizing Treatment

Increasingly, thoracic oncologists are focusing on personalizing the approach to patients with lung cancer. Genetic profiling of tumors is already being used to select systemic therapies for patients with lung cancer. Recent work is examining tumor cell burden during and after treatment and may be able to provide prognostic information for patients receiving radiotherapy for lung cancer, eventually identifying patients who could benefit from dose escalation or de-escalation.

A number of investigators are also examining the role of adaptive radiotherapy based on planning using the individual patient's lung biology.[69,70] Assessments of regional lung function may facilitate avoidance of normal lung, reducing the risk of radiotherapy-induced lung toxicity, and imaging assessments during treatment may permit adaptive radiotherapy to mirror the changes seen in tumor size and shape during radiotherapy.[71]

Technical Advances in Radiotherapy Planning and Imaging

The introduction of complex planning techniques has allowed the delivery of highly conformal radiotherapy plans to increasingly large tumor volumes.[72] The potential impact of larger volumes of low-dose wash on lung toxicity from such conformal plans will need to be understood better, and clinical data are continually emerging. Meanwhile, developments in proton and heavy-ion therapy will ultimately reduce both high-dose and low-dose incidental irradiation of normal organs.

Finally, ongoing developments in image guidance will likely lead to the widespread introduction of imaging technologies, such as intrafraction motion monitoring and 4-D cone-beam CT.[53,73] These technologies will in turn facilitate increasing precision in radiotherapy planning and delivery, as the delivery of highly conformal radiotherapy plans and tracking and gating of lung tumors become possible for a larger number of radiotherapy departments.

CONCLUSION

Radiotherapy plays a crucial role in the treatment of lung cancer. The technologies of radiotherapy, bolstered by advances in imaging technologies, have advanced dramatically in recent years, creating new opportunities for improved clinical outcomes in lung cancer. The current technical baseline in developed countries is CT-planned 3-D conformal radiotherapy. Much more sophisticated and promising technologies are being adopted rapidly and being evaluated in clinical trials. By contrast, access to basic radiotherapy is sorely lacking for large populations worldwide. The future of radiotherapy for lung cancer will include both optimizing the use of advanced technologies and increasing its access globally for the treatment of this leading cause of cancer death worldwide.

KEY REFERENCES

2. McCloskey P, Balduyck B, Van Schil PE, Faivre-Finn C, O'Brien M. Radical treatment of non-small cell lung cancer during the last 5 years. *Eur J Cancer*. 2013;49(7):1555–1564.
5. Rodrigues G, Macbeth F, Burmeister B, et al. Consensus statement on palliative lung radiotherapy: third international consensus workshop on palliative radiotherapy and symptom control. *Clin Lung Cancer*. 2012;13(1):1–5.
9. Mac Manus MP, Hicks RJ. The role of positron emission tomography/computed tomography in radiation therapy planning for patients with lung cancer. *Semin Nucl Med*. 2012;42(5):308–319.
12. ICRU. *Prescribing, Recording and Reporting Photon Beam Therapy (Supplement to ICRU Report 50), ICRU Report 62*. Bethseda, MD: ICRU; 1999:62.

13. [No Authors Listed] Prescribing, recording, and reporting photon-beam intensity—modulated radiation therapy (IMRT): contents. *J ICRU*. 2010;10(1). NP.

16. Marks LB, Bentzen SM, Deasy JO, et al. Radiation dose-volume effects in the lung. *Int J Radiat Oncol Biol Phys*. 2010;76(suppl 3):S70–S76.

17. Gagliardi G, Constine LS, Moiseenko V, et al. Radiation dose-volume effects in the heart. *Int J Radiat Oncol Biol Phys*. 2010;76(suppl 3):S77–S85.

18. Kirkpatrick JP, van der Kogel AJ, Schultheiss TE. Radiation dose-volume effects in the spinal cord. *Int J Radiat Oncol Biol Phys*. 2010;76(suppl 3):S42–S49.

19. Werner-Wasik M, Yorke E, Deasy J, Nam J, Marks LB. Radiation dose-volume effects in the esophagus. *Int J Radiat Oncol Biol Phys*. 2010;76(suppl 3):S86–S93.

28. Papanikolaou N, Battista JJ, Boyer AL, et al. *Tissue Inhomogeneity Corrections for Megavoltage Photon Beams. AAPM Report No 85*. Alexandria, VA: American Association of Physicists in Medicine; 2004:1–142.

29. Keall PJ, Mageras GS, Balter JM, et al. The management of respiratory motion in radiation oncology report of AAPM Task Group 76. *Med Phys*. 2006;33(10):3874–3900.

30. Chetty IJ, Curran B, Cygler JE, et al. Report of the AAPM Task Group No. 105: issues associated with clinical implementation of Monte Carlo-based photon and electron external beam treatment planning. *Med Phys*. 2007;34(12):4818–4853.

53. Sonke JJ, Zijp L, Remeijer P, van Herk M. Respiratory correlated cone beam CT. *Med Phys*. 2005;32(4):1176–1186.

58. Kutcher GJ, Coia L, Gillin M, et al. Comprehensive QA for radiation oncology: report of AAPM Radiation Therapy Committee Task Group 40. *Med Phys*. 1994;21(4):581–618.

59. De Ruysscher D, Faivre-Finn C, Nestle U, et al. European Organisation for Research and Treatment of Cancer recommendations for planning and delivery of high-dose, high-precision radiotherapy for lung cancer. *J Clin Oncol*. 2010;28(36):5301–5310.

63. Shirvani SM, Jiang J, Chang JY, et al. Comparative effectiveness of 5 treatment strategies for early-stage non-small cell lung cancer in the elderly. *Int J Radiat Oncol Biol Phys*. 2012;84(5):1060–1070.

See Expertconsult.com for full list of references.

35 Radiobiology of Lung Cancer

Jose G. Bazan, Quynh-Thu Le, and Daniel Zips

SUMMARY OF KEY POINTS

- The hallmarks of radiobiology are the "4 Rs": *r*epair, *r*eassortment, *r*eoxygenation, *r*epopulation.
- Radiation exerts its biologic effects by causing damage to DNA.
- The linear–quadratic model provides a convenient method to compare different radiation dose and fractionation schedules.
- Radiobiologic principles have underpinned the rationale for many early clinical trials in lung cancer testing including the use of alternative fractionation schedules.
- Ultra-high doses of radiation may have other mechanisms of cell killing in addition to causing DNA damage.
- Chemotherapy is most often used to sensitize the effects of radiation and improve local control in patients with locally advanced lung cancer.
- Tumor hypoxia is a major problem in treating lung tumors; clinical trials that have tried to reverse hypoxia have shown mixed results.
- Predictive biomarkers of radiation response are the subject of continued research.

Radiobiology is central to an understanding of the principles of radiotherapy today. In the early 20th century, the use of large, single doses of radiation declined as scientists and clinicians recognized that these doses caused considerable damage to normal tissues. Radiation oncologists then began applying smaller daily doses over a period of several weeks as a way to reduce this damage yet still achieve tumor control. In the 21st century, radiation oncologists have again been using large doses of radiation, over one to several days, as advances in technology now enable them to more precisely target the tumor while minimizing the amount of normal tissue exposed. In this chapter, we explore the basic tenets of radiation biology in order to understand the rationale behind these vastly different approaches as they apply specifically to the treatment of lung cancer. We also examine ways to exploit the radiobiology of lung cancer by using various strategies, including alternative fractionation schedules, concurrent chemotherapy with radiation, and modifiers of tumor hypoxia. We conclude with a look toward the future of personalized care, by examining potential biomarkers that may be used to predict response to radiotherapy.

RADIOBIOLOGIC BASIS OF CONVENTIONALLY FRACTIONATED RADIOTHERAPY

This section provides a review of the basic principles of radiobiology, including the mechanism of action of x-rays, the linear–quadratic (LQ) model of cell survival, and the four Rs of radiobiology. Taken together, these fundamentals help explain why radiation is most commonly delivered as a fractionated course over 5 weeks to 6 weeks.

DNA: The Critical Target for the Biologic Effects of Radiation Damage

The biologic effects of radiation result principally from damage to a cell's DNA. The damage induced by radiation can be direct or indirect. Direct DNA damage occurs when the absorption of a photon by an atom releases an electron (a secondary electron) that then directly interacts with the DNA molecule. Indirect damage occurs when the secondary electron reacts with a water molecule to produce a free radical. It is the production of this free radical that leads to the DNA damage. Most of the DNA damage produced by the high-energy photons used in most medical linear accelerators is indirect damage.[1]

The types of DNA damage produced by radiation include base damage (>1000 lesions per cell per Gy), single-strand breaks (approximately 1000 per Gy), and double-strand breaks (approximately 20–40 per Gy).[1] Among these lesions, DNA double-strand breaks correlate best with cell killing, because they can lead to certain chromosomal aberrations (dicentrics, rings, anaphase bridges) that are lethal to the cell. Lethality, from the perspective of radiation biology, means the loss of reproductive integrity of tumor clonogens; that is, the tumor cells may still be physically present or intact and may still be able to undergo a few cell divisions, but they are no longer able to form a colony of cells.[1]

The Linear–Quadratic Model

Cell survival curves have a characteristic shape when plotted on a log-linear scale with radiation dose on the x-axis and the log of cell survival on the y-axis. At low doses, the curve tends to be straight (linear). As the dose increases, the curve bends over a region of several Gy; this region is often referred to as the shoulder of the survival curve. At very high doses, the curve tends to straighten out again.[1]

Many biophysical models have been proposed to mathematically capture this relationship between radiation dose and cell survival. A comprehensive review of all of these models is beyond the scope of this chapter but can be found in Hall and Giaccia[1] and Brenner et al.[2] The most commonly used model is the LQ model, which assumes that there are two components to cell killing: one that is proportional to the radiation dose and another that is proportional to the square of the dose.[1] Cell survival in this model is represented by the following exponential function:

$$S(D) = e^{-(\alpha D + \beta D^2)} \qquad \text{[Eq. 35.1]}$$

where S is the fraction of cells surviving a dose, D; e is the mathematical constant approximately equal to 2.71828; and α and β are constants that represent the linear and quadratic components of cell killing, respectively. At dose $D = \alpha/\beta$, the contributions from the linear and quadratic components of cell killing are equal.

The LQ model is convenient in that it depends on only two parameters (α and β) and it is relatively easy to manipulate mathematically. However, there is also a biologic rationale for using this model. As mentioned earlier, DNA double-strand breaks are believed to be the primary mechanism leading to cell death.

A single hit of radiation (one electron) can cause lethal injury by inducing breaks on two adjacent chromosomes (αD component). However, when two separate electrons cause the two chromosome breaks, cumulative injury can occur, and the probability of this occurrence is proportional to the square of the dose (βD^2).[1]

The Four Rs of Radiobiology

The principles underlying fractionated radiotherapy can best be understood in terms of the classical four Rs of radiobiology: *r*epair, *r*eassortment, *r*eoxygenation, and *r*epopulation.[1]

Repair

Repair refers primarily to the ability of normal tissues to recover from sublethal DNA damage. Sublethal damage repair is the operational term for the increase in cell survival that is seen when a given radiation dose is split into two fractions separated by a time interval. Sublethal damage repair is simply the repair of DNA double-strand breaks.[1] In terms of the LQ model, tissues that have a greater capacity for DNA double-strand break repair have larger values for β and, therefore, a low α/β ratio. By contrast, most tumors and acutely responding tissues have a low capacity for repair and, therefore, a high α/β ratio.

Reassortment

Experiments have demonstrated that the most radiosensitive phases of the cell cycle are the M and G_2 phases and the most radioresistant phase is the late S phase.[1] Reassortment is the principle that cells progress through the cell cycle during the interval between two doses of radiation. Cells that were not killed by the first dose of radiation were likely in a radioresistant phase of the cell cycle at that time. Between the first and second doses of radiation, these cells would have time to progress to the M or G_2 phase, and thus they would be more sensitive to the second dose of radiation.

Reoxygenation

The presence of oxygen within microseconds of radiation exposure is crucial for radiation-induced cell killing. Oxygen acts at the level of free radicals to effectively fix the radiation damage by inducing a permanent conformational change in the DNA molecule.

In the absence of oxygen (hypoxic conditions), as much as triple the amount of radiation may be needed to induce as much cell killing as would occur in the presence of oxygen.[1] Most tumors have areas of hypoxia. Hypoxia can be acute or chronic: acute hypoxia results from the temporary closing or blockage of a blood vessel, whereas chronic hypoxia results from the limited diffusion distance (70 μ) of oxygen.[1]

In the late 1960s, Van Putten and Kallman[3] performed a set of experiments to determine the proportion of hypoxic cells in a transplantable sarcoma in a mouse model. They measured the proportion of hypoxic cells in the untreated tumor at 14%. They then administered five fractions of daily radiotherapy (1.9 Gy per fraction) to the tumor on Monday through Friday. The subsequent Monday, the hypoxic fraction was nearly the same, at 18%. They repeated the experiment except that they administered four fractions of 1.9 Gy each to the tumor on Monday through Thursday, and the hypoxic fraction measured on Friday was again constant at 14%.

These experiments provided some of the first evidence that reoxygenation occurs between deliveries of fractions of radiation. If reoxygenation did not occur, the proportion of hypoxic tumor cells would be expected to increase by the end of a fractionated course of treatment. Therefore if enough time is allowed for reoxygenation to occur, the negative effects of hypoxia can be overcome.

Repopulation

Fractionation of radiation can lead to an increase in the surviving fraction of cancer cells if the interval between the two doses of radiation exceeds the length of the cell cycle time needed for the tumor cells to divide. Therefore repopulation of tumor cells as a result of fractionation can be detrimental. In addition, treatment with any cytotoxic agent (e.g., chemotherapy drug or radiation) can trigger surviving tumor cells to divide faster than their normal cell cycle time or can reduce the number of cells lost; this phenomenon is known as accelerated repopulation.[4] A high level of evidence supports this phenomenon in human tumors, including tumors of the lung and squamous cell carcinomas of the head and neck and the cervix. Because of this phenomenon, it is recommended that radiotherapy courses be completed without interruption.

Summary

The use of conventionally fractionated radiotherapy can now be understood in terms of the four Rs of radiobiology. Advantages of fractionation include reoxygenation of tumor cells to overcome hypoxia, reassortment of tumor cells into more sensitive phases of the cell cycle, and repair of sublethal damage in normal tissues to help reduce radiation toxicity. The main disadvantage of a fractionated course of radiation is that repopulation of tumor cells may occur, especially if the treatment course is prolonged beyond the expected time frame for completion.

Biologically Effective Dose (BED)

The biologically effective dose is a single dose value that can be used to compare the effectiveness of different fractionation schemes. This quantity is derived from the LQ model.[1] For a treatment schedule of n fractions each of size D, Eq. 35.1 can be rewritten as

$$S = e^{-\left(\alpha D + \beta D^2\right)} \text{ or, alternatively,}$$

$$\text{as } \frac{1ns}{\alpha} = nD\left(1 + \frac{D}{\frac{\alpha}{\beta}}\right) \qquad \text{[Eq. 35.2]}$$

The quantity $1nS$ is referred to as the biologically effective dose. When calculating the biologically effective dose for most tumors and tissues that respond acutely to radiation injury, the α/β ratio is usually set at 10 Gy; these tumors and tissues have a low capacity for repair, so the α term dominates the ratio. Late-responding tissues (e.g., the spinal cord) have a greater capacity for repair between fractions of radiation, so the β term dominates the ratio α/β; when calculating the biologically effective dose for these tissues, $\alpha/\beta = 3$ Gy is the most common convention.

As an example, a common fractionation schedule used to treat nonsmall cell lung cancer (NSCLC) is 60 Gy in 30 fractions of 2 Gy each. Assuming $\alpha/\beta = 10$ for the tumor and $\alpha/\beta = 3$ for late-responding tissue, the biologically effective dose for this schedule would be given as follows:

$$\text{BED}_{tumor} = (30 \text{ fractions})(2 \text{ Gy/fraction})$$
$$1 + \frac{2\,\text{Gy}}{10\,\text{Gy}} = 72 \text{ Gy} \qquad \text{[Eq. 35.3]}$$

$$\text{BED}_{late-responding\ tissue} = (30 \text{ fractions})(2 \text{ Gy/fractions})$$
$$1 + \frac{2\,\text{Gy}}{3\,\text{Gy}} = 100 \text{ Gy} \qquad \text{[Eq. 35.4]}$$

Alternatively, a fractionation schedule now used to treat patients who have a poor performance status or who are not candidates for concurrent chemotherapy is 60 Gy in 15 fractions of 4 Gy each. Again assuming $\alpha/\beta = 10$ for the tumor and $\alpha/\beta = 3$ for late-responding tissue, the biologically effective dose for this approach is

$$\mathrm{BED_{tumor}} = (15 \text{ fractions}) (4 \text{ Gy/fractions}) \\ 1 + \frac{4 \text{ Gy}}{10 \text{ Gy}} = 72 \text{ Gy} \qquad [\text{Eq. 35.5}]$$

$$\mathrm{BED_{late-responding\ tissue}} = (15 \text{ fractions}) (4 \text{ Gy fraction}) \\ 1 + \frac{4 \text{ Gy}}{3 \text{ Gy}} = 100 \text{ Gy} \qquad [\text{Eq. 35.6}]$$

Although the total dose was the same in both cases (60 Gy), the treatment schedule of 15 fractions of 4 Gy each has a higher tumor effective dose than the schedule of 30 fractions of 2 Gy each, but the 15-fraction schedule confers a higher risk to the late-responding tissue, such as the spinal cord if it is kept in the high-dose areas. The biologically effective dose is therefore a very useful tool that radiation oncologists often use when varying the fraction size from the standard 2 Gy/d. However, this simple concept does not take into account other factors that affect the biologically effective dose, such as repopulation, reassortment, and reoxygenation. In addition, the applicability of the LQ model for estimating the biologically effective dose at larger doses per fraction is under debate, as will be discussed.[5]

ALTERNATIVE FRACTIONATION SCHEDULES AND DOSE ESCALATION

In 1980, the Radiation Therapy Oncology Group (RTOG) conducted a prospective randomized study of various radiation dose and fractionation schedules among patients with unresectable stage III lung cancer.[6] Most of these patients were treated with conventional fractionation (CF) of 2 Gy/d to a dose of 40 Gy, 50 Gy, or 60 Gy. One group of patients received 40 Gy in a split-course fashion (20 Gy in 4 Gy/d over 5 days, 2-week rest period, 20 Gy in 4 Gy/d over 5 days). This trial showed a small benefit in local control for patients who received 50 Gy or 60 Gy compared with patients who received 40 Gy, although this benefit was no longer present after 2 years of follow-up. Nonetheless, this trial established 60 Gy given over 6 weeks as the optimal dose for stage III NSCLC.

Since that time, numerous approaches have been studied in an effort to improve the survival of individuals with locally advanced or early stage unresectable lung cancer. Alternative fractionation schedules can be used as a means of improving outcomes without worsening toxicity.

Hyperfractionated Radiation Therapy in Lung Cancer

Hyperfractionation refers to giving an increased number of fractions but smaller fraction sizes (e.g., <1.8 Gy to 2.0 Gy) to deliver a higher total dose over the same overall treatment time as with CF.[1] Hyperfractionation is most commonly performed by delivering the radiation treatments two or three times per day, as opposed to once daily with conventional fractionation. The final total dose delivered is often higher than the total dose administered on a conventional schedule. The overall goal of a hyperfractionated schedule is to achieve dose escalation and intensification while minimizing the likelihood of the late effects of radiotherapy.

Clinical Applications of Hyperfractionation

The role of hyperfractionation in treating NSCLC has been studied extensively. One of the first cooperative group trials examining this question was RTOG 81-08.[7] In this dose-finding and toxicity trial, all patients received 1.2 Gy twice daily (with 4 hours to 6 hours between fractions) to a dose of 50.4 Gy, 60 Gy, 69.6 Gy, or 74.4 Gy. No treatment-related deaths occurred, and severe toxicity (pneumonitis, esophagitis, or pulmonary fibrosis) developed in only six patients (<9%). In the long-term update, the 5-year overall survival rate was 8.3% for patients who received 69.6 Gy, which compared favorably with the rate of 5.6% seen among patients who received 60 Gy with CF in RTOG 78-11/79-17.[8]

In RTOG 83-11, 848 patients were randomly assigned to one of five arms: 60.0 Gy, 64.8 Gy, 69.6 Gy, 74.4 Gy, or 79.2 Gy.[9] The fractionation schedule for all arms was 1.2 Gy twice daily separated by 4 hours to 8 hours. No significant differences were found in early or late effects of radiotherapy across all the treatment arms. In addition, no significant differences were found in overall survival (60 Gy, 9.2 months; 64.8 Gy, 6.3 months; 69.6 Gy, 10.0 months; 74.4 Gy, 8.7 months; and 79.2 Gy, 10.5 months). In a subgroup analysis of patients with favorable characteristics as defined by Cancer and Leukemia Group B criteria (Karnofsky Performance Status 70–100 and <6% weight loss), a significant dose–response was found for median overall survival among the three arms with lowest total dose, favoring the 69.6 Gy arm: 60 Gy, 10 months; 64.8 Gy, 7.8 months; and 69.6 Gy, 13.0 months ($p = 0.02$). No significant improvements in median overall survival occurred with dose escalation beyond 69.6 Gy in this trial.

The RTOG and Eastern Cooperative Oncology Group (ECOG) conducted an intergroup trial in which they performed a direct comparison of hyperfractionation and CF in NSCLC. In RTOG 88-08/ECOG 4588,[10] patients were randomly assigned to one of three arms: CF to 60 Gy (2 Gy daily), hyperfractionation to 69.6 Gy (1.2 Gy twice daily), or induction chemotherapy followed by conventional fraction to 60 Gy. In this trial, induction chemotherapy was found to be superior to the treatments in the other two arms. In a direct comparison of patients who received hyperfractionation and patients who received CF (without chemotherapy), no significant difference in median overall survival was found (12.3 months vs. 11.4 months, respectively).

Fu et al.[11] also conducted a phase III trial comparing CF and hyperfractionation in NSCLC. In this trial, patients were randomly assigned to receive 63.9 ± 1.1 Gy CF (1.8 Gy to 2.0 Gy daily) or 69.6 ± 2.1 Gy hyperfractionation (1.2 Gy twice daily). Toxicity and overall survival did not differ significantly between the two arms. In a subset analysis of patients with stages I–IIIA disease only, 2-year overall survival and local control were significantly superior in the hyperfractionation arm (32% vs. 6% and 28% vs. 13%, respectively; $p < 0.05$ for both).

Summary

In conclusion, although there is a strong radiobiologic rationale for a hyperfractionation approach, modest dose escalation (above 60 Gy) has not led to a convincing survival advantage in the randomized setting. Nonetheless, these trials were conducted at a time when computed tomography and three-dimensional planning were not widely available, thereby leading to large radiation-treatment fields often including elective node radiation. In addition, the accuracy of staging was limited, especially because of the lack of positron emission tomography. With the technology available today and the unexpected initial results of RTOG 06-17 (to be discussed), radiation oncologists may now be able to fully exploit the expected radiobiologic advantages of hyperfractionation and other alternative fractionation regimens.

Accelerated Fractionation Schedules in Lung Cancer

Accelerated fractionation is defined as delivering the same total dose of radiation as in CF in a shorter overall treatment time by giving two or more fractions of radiation daily.[1] The rationale for using accelerated fractionation is to overcome repopulation of clonogenic tumor cells during fractionated radiotherapy, which should result in an increase in local control for a given total radiation dose. Practically speaking, pure accelerated fractionation (e.g., delivering 60 Gy in 2-Gy fractions over 3 weeks) is not possible because acute effects of radiation become limiting. As a result, accelerated fractionation schedules in the clinic must reduce the daily fraction size, introduce a predetermined rest period (split course), or reduce the final total dose. Most accelerated fractionation schedules incorporate smaller fraction sizes given multiple times daily and are therefore hybrids of accelerated fractionation and hyperfractionation.

Clinical Applications of Accelerated Fractionation

The Medical Research Council of United Kingdom compared CF with an accelerated fractionation regimen for patients with stage I–III or unresectable lung cancer.[12] Of these patients, 37% had stage I or II disease and 82% had tumors with squamous cell histology. In this trial, the accelerated fractionation regimen consisted of continuous hyperfractionated accelerated radiotherapy (CHART). CHART was delivered to a total dose of 54 Gy given in 1.5-Gy fractions three times per day (with a 6-hour interfraction interval) over 12 consecutive days (including weekends). Patients in the CF arm received 60 Gy in 30 fractions over 6 weeks. Despite the lower total dose, patients in the CHART arm had a significant reduction in the risk of death, with a hazard ratio of 0.76, which corresponded to an increase in 2-year overall survival of 9% (29% vs. 20%; $p = 0.004$).[12] Patients in this arm had a similar relative risk reduction with respect to local disease progression, with a hazard ratio of 0.77. As indicated in a subsequent report on the trial, the results for overall survival and disease progression were maintained with longer follow-up.[13] As expected, short-term toxicity was worse in the CHART arm, with severe dysphagia occurring at a rate of 19% compared with 3% in the CF arm. The rates of late toxicity were not different between the two arms.

More recently, ECOG 2597 compared CF with accelerated fractionation radiation after induction chemotherapy (two cycles of carboplatin and paclitaxel) for patients with stage III lung cancer.[14] Patients in the CF arm received a total dose of 64 Gy (2 Gy daily). Patients in the accelerated fractionation arm received hyperfractionated accelerated radiotherapy (HART) to a total dose of 57.6 Gy in three daily fractions of 1.5 Gy (fraction 1), 1.8 Gy (fraction 2), and 1.5 Gy (fraction 3) given over 12 days. This trial was terminated early because of poor accrual. The median overall survival in the HART arm was numerically superior to that in the CF arm (20.3 vs. 14.9 months), but this difference did not reach significance. Overall, acute grade 3 or higher toxicity did not differ between the two arms, although rates of esophagitis tended to be higher in the HART arm (25% vs. 18%). The results of this study are provocative, but induction chemotherapy followed by radiotherapy is no longer the standard of care for this group of patients.

In a similar study, termed CHARTWEL (CHART weekend less), investigators compared CF given as 66 Gy in 33 fractions over 6.5 weeks with the CHARTWEL regimen of 60 Gy in 1.5 Gy fractions three times per day over 2.5 weeks.[15] No difference in overall survival or local control was found for patients in either arm, but increased acute toxicity was found among patients in the CHARTWEL arm. However, in the subset of patients with more advanced cancer and among patients who received neoadjuvant chemotherapy, patients who received the CHARTWEL regimen had a significant local control advantage.[15]

Modestly Hypofractionated Radiation Schedules

Problems with the CHART and CHARTWEL regimens include inconvenience to the patient and the radiation therapy department due to the multiple visits per day. Another way to shorten the treatment duration while maintaining once-daily treatments is to increase the daily fraction size (e.g., >3 Gy/d). This still results in dose intensification. This strategy is attractive for situations in which concurrent chemotherapy and radiation would be recommended, but the patient is unfit for combined modality therapy. Although the structures in the mediastinum (heart, esophagus) may be more sensitive to larger fraction sizes of radiation, advances in radiation treatment planning and delivery now enable more accurate targeting of the tumor volume while minimizing dose to normal tissues.

In 2013, Osti et al.[16] performed a prospective, phase II study of patients with unresectable stage III or oligometastatic stage IV NSCLC who were unfit for chemotherapy. The prescription dose was 60 Gy in 20 fractions (3 Gy/fraction). The target volumes included gross disease (tumor and involved lymph nodes) with small margins (4 mm to 5 mm for clinical target volume expansion; 5 mm for planning target volume expansion) and daily image guidance with cone-beam computed tomography scans. A total of 30 patients were enrolled. This regimen resulted in low rates of grade 3 toxicity and a 2-year overall survival of 38%.

The University of Texas-Southwestern and Stanford led a phase I dose escalation study in patients with stage II–IV (oligometastatic) or recurrent NSCLC in which the patients were not amenable to surgery, concurrent chemotherapy, or stereotactic body radiation therapy.[17] The maximum tolerated dose was defined as the dose at which over one-third of patients experienced a grade 3 toxicity up to 90 days postradiation. All patients received 15 fractions of radiation therapy at one of three different dose levels: 50 Gy (3.33 Gy/fraction); 55 Gy (3.67 Gy/fraction); or 60 Gy (4 Gy/fraction). This study also required small margins with daily image guidance. A total of 55 patients were enrolled: 50 Gy ($n = 15$); 55 Gy ($n = 21$); and 60 Gy ($n = 19$). While there were three deaths (1 in the 55-Gy arm and 2 in the 60-Gy arm), the maximum tolerated dose was not reached. The regimen of 60 Gy in 15 fractions is now being compared in a randomized trial with 60 Gy in 30 fractions in this group of patients with poor performance status (NCT01459497).

Summary

Overall, the results of accelerated fractionation regimens for treating lung cancer appear promising. Although the CHART data in particular appear to correspond well with the expected radiobiologic results of an accelerated fractionation schedule, the inclusion of a large percentage of patients with early stage (stages I–II) cancer and the high percentage of patients with squamous cell histology make it hard to extrapolate the findings to current patients with locally advanced NSCLC among whom the proportion of squamous cell histology is declining. In addition, as a result of trials such as RTOG 9410,[18] the current standard of care for patients with locally advanced lung cancer is concurrent chemoradiation therapy. Modestly hypofractionated regimens may be reasonable for patients who are not candidates for chemotherapy.

A meta-analysis of individual data from 2000 patients treated in 10 trials showed a significantly improved overall survival with modified fractionation (i.e., hyperfractionation or accelerated fractionation) for patients with nonmetastatic NSCLC (p = 0.009). For patients with small cell lung cancer (SCLC), a positive trend toward improved overall survival was found. As expected, dose intensification resulted in higher rates of acute esophageal toxicity.[19]

STEREOTACTIC ABLATIVE RADIOTHERAPY

Stereotactic ablative radiotherapy (SABR), also known as stereotactic body radiotherapy, employs extreme acceleration by delivering a large radiation dose per fraction over one to five treatments. This type of therapy has long been used to treat malignant (and benign) conditions in the brain (stereotactic radiosurgery). In the 1990s, investigators began applying the principles of stereotactic radiosurgery to tumor sites outside the brain, such as the lung, the liver, and the spine. SABR has become the treatment of choice for patients with medically inoperable stage I lung cancer.

Radiobiology of Stereotactic Ablative Radiotherapy
The Linear–Quadratic Model

If we apply the LQ formalism to the fractionation schemes used in lung SABR, we can see that SABR delivers a large biologically effective dose (biologically effective dose in the equation) to the tumors. For example, one of the most commonly used schedules is 60 Gy given in three fractions of 20 Gy each. Using the assumption that α/β = 10, the BED_{10} of this regimen is BED_{10} = 60 Gy (1 + 20/10) = 180 Gy. In order to achieve this same BED_{10} using CF with 2 Gy per fraction, one would have to deliver a total dose of 150 Gy in 75 fractions. If these treatments were given once a day, it would take more than 15 weeks to complete the treatment course and efficacy would be lost because of repopulation. Simply put, one could argue that the success of SABR is due mostly to the delivery of very high doses of radiation to the tumor in a short time. By contrast, loss of treatment efficacy may result from hypoxia-related radioresistance when large doses per fraction are used.[20]

Universal Survival Curve

Whether the LQ model appropriately applies to the high doses per fraction used in SABR is a subject of debate. Some investigators have argued that because the LQ model is continuously curving downward as the dose increases, this model actually overestimates clonogenic cell killing in the SABR dose ranges. This has led to the proposal for a piecemeal function for cell survival, termed the universal survival curve.[21] This function combines the LQ model for low doses per fraction and another model, known as the multitarget model,[22] for larger doses per fraction. These authors found that the fit for the survival curve of an NSCLC cell line (H460) up to more than 15 Gy per fraction was vastly improved using the universal survival curve rather than the LQ model, especially as the dose per fraction increased above 10 Gy.[21]

Effects of SABR: New Mechanisms of Cell Killing?

As discussed earlier, the principles of classic radiobiology can be understood in terms of DNA double-strand break damage and the four Rs of radiobiology. However, this understanding has been driven in large part by experiments that used CF (1.8 Gy to 2 Gy per fraction). Despite the finding that the LQ model may overestimate cell killing in vitro (because the βD^2 component

predicts a continuously bending curve as the dose increases but experimental models are more consistent with a linear curve at these high doses), clinical studies have shown that the LQ model may actually underestimate tumor control by stereotactic radiosurgery and SABR.[23] Thus several groups have hypothesized that mechanisms other than DNA double-strand breaks may be responsible for the enhanced effects of SABR.

One hypothesis is that the vascular endothelium is a unique target of the high-dose radiation used in SABR. More specifically, the hypothesis is that large, single fractions of radiation (>8 Gy to 10 Gy) activate the acid sphingomyelinase pathway, ultimately resulting in the generation of ceramide, which stimulates endothelial cell apoptosis.[24,25] Another hypothesis is that SABR doses of at least 10 Gy induce substantial vascular damage, disrupting the intratumoral microenvironment and thereby indirectly leading to tumor cell death.[26] Another potential mechanism for the increased efficacy of SABR is that radiation creates a large amount of tumor antigens, which may augment the immune response, leading to further tumor cell death.[27]

Although these proposed mechanisms are intriguing and may well help to explain the excellent clinical results seen with SABR, some experts believe that SABR is successful because of the large biologically effective dose delivered to the tumor. A group of investigators pooled the data from nearly 2700 patients with medically inoperable stage I NSCLC who were treated with three-dimensional conformal radiotherapy or single-fraction or multifraction SABR.[5] Using both the LQ model and the universal survival curve, they calculated the biologically effective dose for each patient. They then plotted the tumor control probability as a function of the BED, and the results were consistent in that the tumor control probability increased as the biologically effective dose increased, regardless of which treatment patients received. At least for patients with stage I NSCLC, the results of this analysis indicated that different biologic mechanisms are not necessarily responsible for the success of SABR. The analysis does not, however, rule out the existence of these alternative or supplementary mechanisms.

MODIFICATION OF RADIATION RESPONSE

Chemotherapy

Conceptually, chemotherapy combined with radiotherapy has been explored to improve the therapeutic ratio. Chemotherapy may be integrated with radiotherapy in a variety of ways.[28] In induction therapy, chemotherapy is given before local therapy (radiotherapy or surgery). This approach, which reduces the local tumor burden and addresses micrometastatic disease up front, may be advantageous in that a reduced tumor size would result in smaller radiation treatment volumes, which could reduce acute and long-term toxicity. However, using induction chemotherapy followed by a course of radiotherapy extends the patient's overall treatment time. From a radiobiologic perspective, the extended treatment time could allow for accelerated repopulation in the primary tumor and thereby result in inferior outcomes.

Another approach is to give concurrent chemotherapy, that is, to deliver chemotherapy during the course of radiotherapy. With this approach, the overall treatment time is not extended because the definitive local and systemic therapies are given together. A disadvantage of this approach is that it often results in more acute toxicity, both local and systemic (myelosuppression).

Clinical Application: Radiation-Dose Escalation in the Setting of Concurrent Chemotherapy

Dose–response curves for local tumor control with radiotherapy have a sigmoidal shape:[1] as the radiation dose increases, the probability of tumor control also increases. Likewise, the risk of toxicity also increases as the radiation dose increases. The hyperfractionation studies mentioned earlier included modest dose escalations, mostly without concurrent chemotherapy. Since the mid-1990s, it has become clear that concurrent chemoradiation therapy is superior to other strategies of combining the two modalities. Of note is that the better survival achieved with concurrent chemoradiation therapy is due mainly to better local–regional tumor control and not to a lower rate of distant metastases.[29] Nonetheless, long-term survival, even with chemoradiation therapy to doses of 60 Gy to 66 Gy, remained low. Efforts have since been made to safely combine escalated radiation doses with concurrent chemotherapy as a way to improve patient outcomes.

In the early 2000s, several groups conducted prospective trials of radiation-dose escalation for patients with lung cancer; in these trials, doses in the range of 74 Gy to 78 Gy were consistently found to be safe.[30–32] Therefore the RTOG conducted a phase III randomized trial in protocol 06-17.[53a] This study had a 2 × 2 factorial design in which patients were randomly assigned to either 60 Gy or 74 Gy of radiotherapy, with or without cetuximab. All patients received concurrent chemotherapy with carboplatin and paclitaxel.

The preliminary results for the 60-Gy or 74-Gy assignment were initially presented at the 2011 meeting of the American Society for Radiation Oncology shortly after an interim analysis led to closure of the randomization to 60 Gy versus 74 Gy, and the results were published in 2015.[33] The median overall survival was higher for the 60 Gy versus 74 Gy arms: 28.7 months versus 20.3 months ($p = 0.0007$). When examining cases only in which there were no protocol violations of doses administered to normal tissues and when selecting cases in which at least 90% of the planning target volume received over 95% of the prescription dose (another measure of quality), the differences in survival remained significantly in favor of the 60-Gy arm. There were significantly higher rates of grade 3 or greater esophagitis in the 74-Gy arm. Radiation dose to the heart (V5Gy) was associated with increased mortality, and further analysis regarding this finding is yet to be completed. Local failure rates were numerically higher in the 74-Gy arm, although this result was not statistically significant (2-year local failure 39% vs. 30%, $p = 0.19$).

The clinical results of RTOG 06-17 are in conflict with our current understanding of basic radiobiology. As a result of this trial, dose escalation to 74 Gy is not recommended and the standard radiation dose in the setting of concurrent chemotherapy remains 60 Gy to 66 Gy.[53a]

Addressing Tumor Hypoxia

As mentioned earlier, tumor hypoxia may reduce the efficacy of radiotherapy. Intraoperative measurement of tumor partial pressure of oxygen (pO_2) among patients undergoing resection of early stage NSCLC demonstrated that tumor hypoxia existed to a certain degree in these tumors and correlated with higher expression of hypoxia-induced genes such as carbonic anhydrase IX (*CAIX*).[34] In addition, tumor hypoxia and elevated expression of osteopontin correlated with worse prognosis in these patients. Therefore investigators are interested in targeting hypoxia with radiotherapy in NSCLC. Two classes of drugs have been investigated to help overcome the detrimental effects of tumor hypoxia: hypoxic cell radiosensitizers and hypoxic cytotoxins.

Hypoxic Cell Radiosensitizers

In the 1960s, investigators began searching for compounds that mimic oxygen and that could therefore overcome chronic hypoxia by diffusing deep into the poorly vascularized portions of a tumor. These efforts led to the development of a class of drugs known as azoles, which have been extensively studied in the clinical setting. The results of earlier meta-analyses indicated that the

benefit of using these agents (and other modifiers of hypoxia) is most pronounced for patients with head and neck cancers and less pronounced for patients with lung cancer.[35,36]

Investigators are showing a renewed interest in the azoles, for their use in combination with single-fraction SABR.[37] A potential shortcoming of single-fraction SABR from the perspective of classic radiobiology is that this treatment does not take advantage of tumor reoxygenation. Multifraction SABR regimens could potentially be converted to single-fraction regimens in combination with a hypoxic radiosensitizer. Clinical trials with patients with NSCLC are needed to fully address this question.

Hypoxic Cytotoxins

An alternative to radiosensitizing hypoxic tumor cells is to develop a compound that selectively targets hypoxic cells. One common hypoxic cytotoxin is mitomycin C, which is a component of chemotherapy regimens used to treat squamous cell carcinomas of the anal canal. This drug has also been used as part of chemotherapy regimens for NSCLC, but it is no longer in widespread use for this indication.

Another hypoxic cytotoxin, tirapazamine, has been prospectively studied in patients with locally advanced NSCLC and limited-stage SCLC in several trials.[38–40] The results have been mixed. Two prospective nonrandomized trials examining tirapazamine added to concurrent chemoradiation therapy for patients with SCLC have showed promising results.[38,39] However, among patients with NSCLC, adding tirapazamine to standard chemoradiation therapy did not improve survival but did result in increased toxicity.[40] At this time, modifying hypoxia by adding tirapazamine or other hypoxic cytotoxins is not routinely performed for patients with lung cancer.

Future Directions

The U.S. National Cancer Institute has recognized that in order to continue improving the therapeutic index of radiotherapy, the technologic innovations that have occurred in radiation oncology must be supplemented with biologic innovations such as new radiosensitizing agents.[41] The National Cancer Institute recommends a series of steps to promote the rapid development of combined radiotherapy with targeted agents. However, appropriate preclinical models are needed to test the benefit of radiation combined with targeted therapy, especially agents targeting the tumor microenvironment or tumor hypoxia. One study has shown that the level of tumor oxygenation, as reflected by hypoxia imaging and the uptake of a hypoxic cell marker (pimonidazole), is highly dependent on the location of the xenograft tumor; the same tumor growing in the lungs showed considerably less hypoxia than it did growing subcutaneously. Moreover, the level of imaging hypoxia correlated well with tumor response to hypoxic cell cytotoxin.[42] The results of studies like this one indicate that judicious selection of a preclinical model may improve the link between preclinical research and clinical practice.

BIOMARKERS PREDICTIVE OF RADIATION RESPONSE

At a time when we are moving toward personalized health care, oncologists are highly interested in finding biomarkers to help tailor treatment strategies for a given patient. With the increasing number of gene mutations being discovered in NSCLC, medical oncologists are now able to select patients who may have a higher probability of having a response to the available targeted therapies specific to those mutations. For example, patients with NSCLC tumors that contain activating mutations in the epidermal growth factor receptor (EGFR) are known to have a better response to tyrosine kinase inhibitors, such as gefitinib and erlotinib.[43] Although it is widely recognized that SCLC is more radiosensitive than NSCLC, the underlying molecular mechanisms for this difference remain unknown. Among patients with NSCLC, response to radiation varies widely, both in vitro and in the clinical setting.[44] Traditional predictive biomarkers of radiation response have included tumor hypoxia, tumor repopulation, and intrinsic radiosensitivity.[45] However, measuring these parameters is difficult and cumbersome in the clinical setting.

The expression of ERCC1, a protein involved with DNA excision repair, has emerged as a potential biomarker of interest for predicting radiation response. In a study of two separate lung cancer cell lines, increased expression of ERCC1 was found in the more radioresistant cell line.[46] In a retrospective analysis of NSCLC patients with mediastinal lymph node involvement who all received neoadjuvant concurrent chemoradiation therapy, increased expression of ERCC1 in the tumor (as demonstrated by immunohistochemistry) was prognostic of worse overall survival; however, ERCC1 expression was not predictive of clinical or pathologic response.[47] Emerging data suggest that no reliable immunohistochemical means exists to specifically detect the unique functional ERCC1 isoform. The epitopes recognized by 16 commercially available ERCC1 antibodies were mapped and investigated for their capacity to identify the different ERCC1 isoforms.[48] Unfortunately, none of these antibodies could distinguish among the four ERCC1 protein isoforms and detect the one isoform that is critical for nucleotide excision repair. Until a better tool is developed, the role of ERCC1 as a biomarker for predicting radiation response among patients is unclear.

Similarly, expression of mutations in the tyrosine kinase domain of the EGFR has been found to correlate with increased radiation sensitivity in vitro.[49] In a retrospective analysis, patients with EGFR-mutant NSCLC had a better response to chemoradiation therapy than did patients with EGFR-wild-type tumors.[50] In addition, preclinical work demonstrated that radiation sensitivity was enhanced when tumors with wild-type EGFR were treated with erlotinib and radiation.[51] Although the preclinical data are promising, results from phase III trials examining the combination of thoracic radiotherapy and an EGFR inhibitor are lacking.

Several preclinical studies have been undertaken to address the need to find gene expression signatures that correlate with radiation response in NSCLC and other human cancer cell lines.[52-54] One such signature has been validated in cancers of the rectum, esophagus, head and neck, and breast.[54-56] However, this signature has not yet been evaluated in lung cancers. A robust and simple gene expression signature panel for the response of lung cancer to radiotherapy is still lacking.

The introduction of next-generation sequencing has added to what we know about the mutation patterns in lung cancers.[57] Circulating tumor DNA carrying tumor-specific sequence alterations can be found in the plasma or serum and may represent a new way of tracking tumor response during therapy. Advances in sequencing technologies have enabled the rapid identification of somatic genomic alterations in individual tumors, and these alterations can be used to design personalized assays to monitor circulating tumor DNA. In a study of patients with metastatic breast cancer, circulating tumor DNA levels showed a greater correlation with changes in tumor burden than did cancer antigen 15-3 or circulating tumor cells. This study also provided the earliest measure of treatment response in more than half the patients tested.[58] We envision a future biomarker for predicting response to radiation that involves a panel of specific single-nucleotide variations, deletions, and insertions derived directly from the patient's own tumor DNA and identified in his or her circulating DNA. This panel will be quantified and monitored during the course of radiotherapy, and this information will help the radiation oncologist determine the dose needed to eradicate such a tumor. Instead of a one-size-fits-all 60-Gy dose for all patients with NSCLC, some patients will need a lower dose for a tumor highly sensitive to radiation and some will need a higher dose for a less sensitive tumor.

CONCLUSION

Radiotherapy remains a critical treatment modality for patients with lung cancer. Use of the fundamental principles of radiation biology has led to the development of novel radiation treatment approaches, including alternative fractionation schedules, combined chemoradiation therapy, and SABR, and these approaches have had a substantial effect in the clinical setting. Nonetheless, unanswered questions remain that can be resolved by coordination between radiation biologists and clinicians, eventually translating these into meaningful applications for patient care: Are there truly new mechanisms of cell death at play in SABR? Is the LQ model valid at the doses used in SABR? What is the optimal radiation dose for treating locally advanced lung cancer? How can we best combine existing and emerging targeted agents and immunotherapy agents with radiation? The ultimate goal of answering these types of questions is to improve the outcomes for patients with lung cancer.

KEY REFERENCES

1. Hall EJ, Giaccia AJ. *Radiobiology for the Radiologist*. 7th ed. Philadelphia, PA: Wolters Kluwer Health/Lippincott Williams & Wilkins; 2012.
2. Brenner DJ, Hlatky LR, Hahnfeldt PJ, Huang Y, Sachs RK. The linear-quadratic model and most other common radiobiological models result in similar predictions of time-dose relationships. *Radiat Res.* 1998;150(1):83–91.
5. Brown JM, Brenner DJ, Carlson DJ. Dose escalation, not "new biology," can account for the efficacy of stereotactic body radiation therapy with non-small cell lung cancer. *Int J Radiat Oncol Biol Phys.* 2013;85(5):1159–1160.
6. Perez CA, Stanley K, Rubin P, et al. A prospective randomized study of various irradiation doses and fractionation schedules in the treatment of inoperable non-oat-cell carcinoma of the lung. Preliminary report by the Radiation Therapy Oncology Group. *Cancer.* 1980;45(11):2744–2753.
17. Westover KD, Loo Jr BW, Gerber DE, et al. Precision hypofractionated radiation therapy in poor performing patients with non-small cell lung cancer: phase 1 dose escalation trial. *Int J Radiat Oncol Biol Phys.* 2015;93(1):72–81.
18. Curran Jr WJ, Paulus R, Langer CJ, et al. Sequential vs. concurrent chemoradiation for stage III non-small cell lung cancer: randomized phase III trial RTOG 9410. *J Natl Cancer Inst.* 2011;103(19):1452–1460.
21. Park C, Papiez L, Zhang S, Story M, Timmerman RD. Universal survival curve and single fraction equivalent dose: useful tools in understanding potency of ablative radiotherapy. *Int J Radiat Oncol Biol Phys.* 2008;70(3):847–852.
24. Fuks Z, Kolesnick R. Engaging the vascular component of the tumor response. *Cancer Cell.* 2005;8(2):89–91.
26. Park HJ, Griffin RJ, Hui S, Levitt SH, Song CW. Radiation-induced vascular damage in tumors: implications of vascular damage in ablative hypofractionated radiotherapy (SBRT and SRS). *Radiat Res.* 2012;177(3):311–327.
28. Bentzen SM, Harari PM, Bernier J. Exploitable mechanisms for combining drugs with radiation: concepts, achievements and future directions. *Nat Clin Pract Oncol.* 2007;4(3):172–180.
33. Bradley JD, Paulus R, Komaki R, et al. Standard-dose versus high-dose conformal radiotherapy with concurrent and consolidation carboplatin plus paclitaxel with or without cetuximab for patients with stage IIIA or IIIB non-small-cell lung cancer (RTOG 0617): a randomised, two-by-two factorial phase 3 study. *Lancet Oncol.* 2015;16(2):187–199.
43. Lynch TJ, Bell DW, Sordella R, et al. Activating mutations in the epidermal growth factor receptor underlying responsiveness of non-small-cell lung cancer to gefitinib. *N Engl J Med.* 2004;350(21):2129–2139.
57. Cancer Genome Atlas Research Network. Comprehensive genomic characterization of squamous cell lung cancers. *Nature.* 2012;489(7417):519–525.

See Expertconsult.com for full list of references.

36 Patient Selection for Radiotherapy

Dirk De Ruysscher, Michael Mac Manus, and Feng-Ming (Spring) Kong

SUMMARY OF KEY POINTS

- Patient selection is crucial to ensure treatment selection and optimal outcome.
- The performance status, described by, for example, the Karnofsky or the Eastern Cooperative Oncology Group (ECOG) score, is the most important prognostic parameter.
- The benefit of concurrent chemotherapy and radiotherapy has only been demonstrated in patients with an ECOG score of 0–1.
- Patients with a bad performance status (ECOG 3 or even 4) with important local symptoms, for example, pain, obstruction, or superior venous cava syndrome, may still benefit from palliative radiotherapy.
- A poor pulmonary function either because of the presence of tumor or due to chronic lung disease is not a contraindication to high-dose radiotherapy.
- Comorbidities significantly impair the long-term survival of lung cancer patients, but are not necessarily a contraindication for high-dose radiotherapy; for example, patients with extensive emphysema show less pulmonary damage after stereotactic ablative radiotherapy.
- Interstitial lung disease and autoimmune disorders such as systemic lupus erythematosus and scleroderma have been associated with enhanced intrinsic radiosensitivity of normal tissues and, therefore, a higher risk of serious toxicity resulting from radiotherapy.
- Older and/or frail patients have a higher risk for important side effects, but should not necessarily be treated with palliative intent.
- Even in elderly patients with thoroughly staged stage III nonsmall cell lung cancer, 5-year survival rates of 15% to 20% are consistently reported with radiotherapy alone.
- Continued smoking during curative-intent radiotherapy reduces local tumor control and survival; smoking cessation is therefore essential.
- Adequate calorie and protein intake should be ensured.
- Physical activity should be encouraged; it also reduces fatigue.

Patient selection is of central importance in the management of lung cancer as it ensures that each patient receives the optimal treatment. However, in order to achieve this objective, clinically relevant parameters that are reproducible and quantifiable should be identified. A highly accurate prognostic model (or, even better, a predictive model) that has been validated on the basis of external data sets or, ideally, randomized studies should be the ultimate goal.[1] However, no such model is currently available. An international task force failed to identify high-quality data for selecting patients for radical radiotherapy.[2] Nevertheless, knowledge regarding these criteria is increasing and is needed in daily practice. In this review, we will discuss the most relevant patient and tumor-related factors that may influence the selection of patients for potentially curative radiotherapy.

PATIENT-RELATED FACTORS

Patient-related factors are often associated with overall survival, quality of life, and response to radiation. These factors (including, but not limited to, age, gender, race, performance status, weight loss, baseline pulmonary function, comorbidities, and smoking status) should be taken into consideration when the decision regarding high-dose radiotherapy is made.

Performance Status

Performance status, a measure of general well-being and activities of daily life, is one of the most important factors associated with outcome for patients with cancer. Various systems are used to evaluate performance status. The most generally used measures are the Karnofsky score and the Zubrod score (also known as the World Health Organization or ECOG score).[3] The Karnofsky score, named after David A. Karnofsky, ranges from 100 to 0, with 100 indicating "perfect" health and 0 indicating death. The Zubrod score, named after C. Gordon Zubrod, ranges from 0 to 5, with 0 denoting "perfect" health and 5 denoting death. Translation between the Zubrod and Karnofsky scales was validated in a large sample of patients with lung cancer.[4] A Zubrod score of 0 or 1 corresponds with a Karnofsky score of 80–100, a Zubrod score of 2 corresponds with a Karnofsky score of 60–70, and a Zubrod score of 3 or 4 corresponds with a Karnofsky score of 10–50.

In general, a poor performance status is not a contraindication to radiotherapy. However, the value of definitive radiotherapy for a patient with a poor performance status may be limited, as survival times are often shorter for these patients.[5] The benefit of radiotherapy in terms of survival time should be weighed against the risk of treatment toxicity and the time needed to complete the definitive course of treatment. Similar to chemotherapy, radiotherapy may offer notable benefit to selected patients with a poor performance status.[6,7] Radiotherapy is therefore recommended for this population.[8] The regimen of radiotherapy and its combination with other therapy should be individualized for each patient to achieve a maximum therapeutic effect.[8] Meanwhile, palliative radiotherapy often can be used to improve the quality of life for patients with poor performance status and, therefore, should be recommended for those with advanced disease in whom the tumor is causing clinical symptoms or syndromes. For example, a patient with an ECOG score of 3 or 4 as a result of superior venous cava syndrome, obstructive lung disease, or chest pain may have substantial improvement in quality of life after a short course of palliative radiotherapy. Patient selection for radiotherapy should thus be individualized on the basis of a balanced consideration of both the potential benefits and the potential side effects of such treatment.

Lung Function

Patients with lung cancer often present with poor baseline lung function because of the presence of a tumor or a chronic lung

337

condition. Although it is clear that a patient who has poor lung function caused by a local tumor would benefit from radiotherapy, the impaired baseline lung condition from noncancer reasons can often make high-dose radiotherapy challenging. Traditionally, definitive radiotherapy has been considered to be contraindicated for patients with poor lung function. For example, some Radiation Therapy Oncology Group (RTOG) studies, such as RTOG 9311, have excluded patients with a forced expiratory volume in 1 second (FEV_1) of less than 0.85 L or 0.75 L from treatment with high-dose radiation. Other studies, such as RTOG 0617 and RTOG 1106, allow such treatment only for patients with an FEV_1 of 1.3 L or more. However, baseline lung function has not consistently been shown to be a risk factor for radiation-induced lung toxicity after conventionally fractionated three-dimensional conformal radiotherapy or hypofractionated stereotactic ablative radiotherapy (SABR). Moreover, the results of pulmonary function tests often are not changed remarkably after modern conformal radiotherapy.[9,10] Modern dose-escalation studies such as that from the University of Michigan did not limit lung function for very high-dose radiation.[11] In a study of 47 patients, the incidence of lung toxicity had no significant correlation with the results of pulmonary function tests after concurrent chemotherapy and radiotherapy.[12] In a study of 438 patients, FEV_1 along with other patient-related factors seemed to be more important than dosimetric factors for predicting radiation pneumonitis.[13] In a study of 260 patients, the addition of FEV_1 and age to the mean lung dose (MLD) slightly improved the predictability of clinically important radiation-induced lung toxicity.[14] Similar to the SABR series,[10] the study showed that patients with higher baseline lung function tests had significantly more clinical lung toxicity.[14]

In summary, pulmonary function should be considered on an individual basis by balancing the improvement in lung function related to tumor shrinkage with the reduction in lung function related to radiotherapy. In the modern era, poor pulmonary function should not be considered a contraindication to definitive radiotherapy.

Comorbidities

Serious comorbidities are very common in patients with lung cancer and can severely affect outcomes. Long-term tobacco consumption is associated with chronic obstructive pulmonary disease (COPD), ischemic heart disease, cerebrovascular disease, and peripheral vascular disease. Furthermore, other tobacco-related cancers, including head and neck cancers, may be diagnosed before, after, or synchronously with lung cancer, thereby complicating the management of the lung cancer, the other cancer, or both. Luchtenborg et al.[15] studied 3152 patients with nonsmall cell lung cancer (NSCLC) who had surgical resection and reported that serious comorbidity caused a decrement in survival equivalent to a single increment in stage grouping. Comorbidities also reduce the tolerability of chemotherapy to patients with NSCLC.[16] High-dose radiotherapy is poorly tolerated by patients with limited cardiorespiratory reserve due to heart or interstitial lung disease,[17] who are at risk of severe dyspnea or even death if they have insufficient reserve to tolerate impaired organ function after treatment. Smith et al.[18] reported that for patients with NSCLC who were managed with curative-intent radiotherapy, a worse score on the Charlson Comorbidity Index correlated with inferior overall survival but not cause-specific survival. Paradoxically, the scarred lungs of patients with severe COPD may be less likely to be affected by severe radiation pneumonitis after SABR.[19] SABR should not be withheld from patients solely because of COPD.[20]

Although the risks of curative radiotherapy can be difficult to estimate for individual patients, it is usually possible to make a reasonable estimate of the consequences related to loss of a substantial proportion of residual lung or heart function. Apart from general comorbidities such as heart disease, several specific conditions may exacerbate the toxicity of radiotherapy.

Autoimmune disorders such as systemic lupus erythematosus and scleroderma have been associated with enhanced intrinsic radiosensitivity of normal tissues and, therefore, a higher risk of serious toxicity resulting from radiotherapy.[21]

Age and Frailty

Age and frailty are obviously two separate entities: the former is expressed as an objective, trivial number, and the latter is derived from the Latin word *fragilis*, which means "fragile" (i.e., weak). Frailty clearly increases with age, but a young individual can be frail as well. In most geriatric literature, frailty has been defined as either a threshold beyond which the functional reserve of a person is critically reduced and the tolerance of stress is negligible or as a progressive reduction of functional reserve due to a progressive accumulation of deficits.[22] Thus functional reserve should be measured objectively and used as a prognostic indicator of the survival of the patient and/or the tolerance of the treatment.

Many authors have shown that the older population is a very heterogeneous group in terms of physical, biologic, emotional, and cognitive functions. Nevertheless, increased age is associated with comorbidities as well as higher rates of hospitalization and chemotherapy-related toxicity,[23–25] shifting the overall risk-to-benefit ratio.[26] Older patients and patients with important comorbidities are underrepresented in clinical trials.[26,27] Because of the lack of data as well as the fear of iatrogenic complications, older patients generally receive less aggressive treatment,[28–30] which may result in suboptimal survival rates.[31] In selected patients, it has been shown that intensive, state-of-the art therapy benefits older patients.[32–37] Remarkably, the 5-year survival rate is 15% to 20% with radiotherapy alone for patients with stage III disease who are older than 75 years, have good performance status, and have thorough staging.[37] Defeatism thus is definitively not appropriate. Moreover, oncologic assessment methods specifically designed for older patients have been developed.[38–40] The clinical implementation of these methods will lead to more rational and appropriate care of older patients with cancer. These methods probably are also useful for younger, frail patients. These developments should move the field forward.

Concurrent Medication (Other Than Chemotherapy)

Many patients take medications because of comorbidities. The influence of common medications on the side effects associated with radiotherapy in patients with lung cancer is unknown. Angiotensin-converting enzyme inhibitors and statins are the groups of medications that have received the most interest as being potential protectors against radiation pneumonitis. However, at the present time, their influence on side effects has not been clarified.[41,42]

Molecular Factors

Molecular and genetic markers that could be used to select patients for a specific radiation schedule are of great interest. However, although some single-nucleotide polymorphisms have been associated with radiation pneumonitis and although C4b-binding protein alpha chain and vitronectin have been associated with toxicity,[43,44] these and other findings need to be validated in other data sets and their therapeutic role needs to be investigated in prospective trials.

A worse survival rate has been reported for patients with a high pretreatment level of C-reactive protein or interleukin-6 in addition to classic prognostic factors.[45] Again, the practical utility of these findings needs to be determined.

Smoking Status

Tobacco consumption is the primary cause of most lung cancers, and smoking during treatment can have a substantial negative effect on outcomes. In a study of 237 patients with complete smoking histories who were treated with definitive radiotherapy or chemoradiotherapy between 1991 and 2001, Fox et al.[46] reported worse survival for smokers with early-stage disease. Similarly, Rades et al.,[47] in a study of 181 patients who received radiotherapy for the treatment of NSCLC, reported that improved local–regional control was associated with a lower T stage ($p = 0.007$) and with no smoking during radiotherapy ($p = 0.029$) but not with hemoglobin levels or respiratory insufficiency. Jin et al.,[48] in a study of 576 patients, found that smoking status, when corrected for dose–volume effects, was the only factor that appeared to reduce the risk of treatment-related pneumonitis. Nguyen et al.[49] reported that smoking at the time of the initial consultation was associated with reduced local and local–regional control in patients who were treated with radiotherapy after surgery for the management of NSCLC.[49] It is therefore important to ensure that patients with lung cancer have access to smoking-cessation programs and that concerted efforts are made to help them to stop smoking before, during, and after treatment.[50,51]

Nutrition

The nutritional status of patients with lung cancer can be compromised as a direct result of cancer-induced alterations in metabolism and the side effects of radiotherapy. Koom et al.[52] reported malnutrition in more than one-third of patients with cancer in a multi-institutional study. Malnutrition can lead to weight loss and, in the most serious cases, cachexia. Nutritional status may be associated with survival and ideally should be assessed before the initiation of any treatment, including radiotherapy.[53,54] Weight loss is associated with poor survival among patients who are treated with radiation, and cachexia is characterized by involuntary weight loss, muscle wasting, decreased quality of life, and poor survival. In general, these conditions are not contraindications to radiotherapy. Nutritional assessment and weight monitoring are vital during radiotherapy for the treatment of lung cancer. Patients who maintain good nutrition are more likely to tolerate the side effects of treatment. Adequate calories and protein can help to maintain strength and prevent further catabolism. Individuals who do not consume adequate calories and protein use stored nutrients as an energy source, which leads to protein wasting and further weight loss. Patients with lung cancer need to be educated about radiation esophagitis, a common side effect that decreases oral intake and compromises nutritional status.

Fatigue and Physical Activity

Fatigue is one of the most common and distressing patient-reported symptoms associated with cancer. Rather than being a selection measure for radiotherapy, fatigue is a condition that needs to be managed in order for treatment to be successful. Physical training has been shown to be beneficial for patients with breast and colorectal cancer.[55,56] Patients with lung cancer often have a higher incidence and longer duration of cancer-related fatigue, leading to decreased lung function and increased functional impairment in daily living and dramatically reducing the tolerability of treatment, the quality of life, and the chance for prolonged survival.[57] Physical activity has been shown to reduce fatigue in patients with lung cancer and COPD,[58] and studies have indicated that exercise therapy may be an important consideration in the management of both early- and advanced-stage lung cancer.[59,60] For patients receiving concurrent radiotherapy, the value of physical training or pulmonary rehabilitation is limited, although the level of physical activity appears to be an additional prognostic factor to the level of performance. Preliminary evidence from a small pilot study suggested that physical training was associated with an improvement in 6-minute walking distance.[61] Until more evidence is available, we believe that patients who receive radiation-based therapy would behave similarly to those who have surgery or chemotherapy alone and would equally benefit from physical training. These patients should be advised to remain as active as possible and to continue to engage in regular physical activity and pulmonary training to the level of their tolerance.

Repeat Radiation

As the prognosis of patients with cancer improves, more individuals are at risk for the development of a local recurrence or a new primary tumor in organs that were previously treated with radiation. New radiation techniques, better imaging, and more knowledge of dose–volume relationships have led to the use of repeat radiation at high doses.

We are aware of only one prospective study of repeat radiotherapy for recurrent lung cancer,[62] with the rest being retrospective.[63–72] In the prospective trial, which included 23 patients with a local recurrence after external radiotherapy, the median interval between primary and repeat radiotherapy was 13 months.[62] The median first dose was 66 Gy, and the median second course was 51 Gy (range, 46 Gy to 60 Gy), delivered in 1.8 Gy to 2 Gy per fraction. No clinically severe toxicity was noted, but the 1-year and 2-year survival rates were only 59% and 21%, respectively. The results of the prospective study were in line with those of the retrospective series, which included 29–48 patients.[63–72] However, in one study, severe toxicity, including lethal bleeding, was reported in 3 of 11 patients with centrally located tumors that were treated with SABR.[70] Cumulative doses in excess of a cumulative biologically effective dose of 120 Gy to the aorta clearly should be avoided.[72]

Repeat radiotherapy can be considered for selected patients. In the future, individual radiosensitivity measurements, possibly with genetic profiles, may contribute to appropriate patient selection.

TUMOR-RELATED FACTORS

The management of lung cancer is determined largely by the extent of the disease. Patients who are selected for treatment with definitive radiotherapy must have disease that can be encompassed within a tolerable radiotherapy target volume, and they should have no distant metastasis. The great majority of patients who are treated with curative-intent radiotherapy have stage III disease, but there has been an increasing trend toward the use of SABR for the management of stage I disease in patients who are unable to tolerate surgical resection.[73] Accurate determination of stage involves a synthesis of all available sources of information, which may include the results of bronchoscopy, the operative findings at the time of thoracoscopy or thoracotomy, the results of pathologic evaluation of lymph node samples obtained by transbronchial biopsy,[74] and the findings on imaging studies, both structural and functional. Only a small proportion of patients who are treated with definitive radiotherapy or chemoradiation therapy would have had full mediastinal staging at the time of thoracotomy, and therefore imaging plays the central role both in selecting patients for curative therapy and in defining the target for treatment. Ultrasound-guided transbronchial biopsy has been assuming an increasing role in confirming the status of suspicious nodes that are detected on imaging studies,[75] ensuring both that patients with false-negative nodes are not inappropriately excluded from surgery and that equivocal nodes can be included within the radiotherapy target volume if they are true positive.

Accurate staging of patients with NSCLC involves correct allocation of T, N, and M stages according to the international staging system, the current edition of which resulted from the International Association for the Study of Lung Cancer Lung Cancer Staging Project.[76] The most accurate imaging staging modality currently available is ^{18}F-2-deoxy-D-glucose-positron emission tomography–computed tomography (^{18}FDG-PET–CT), which has rapidly supplanted CT and ^{18}FDG-PET alone when the newer modality has become available.[77] There is a large and growing body of evidence that shows that PET and PET–CT are superior to CT for the determination of mediastinal node status and for the detection of distant metastasis.[78,79] However, ^{18}FDG-PET does not provide accurate staging of the brain,[80] and therefore candidates for curative radiotherapy who are at high risk for occult brain metastasis (e.g., patients with involvement of mediastinal nodes) should have separate imaging of the brain, ideally with magnetic resonance imaging.

Three prospective studies have evaluated the use of PET and PET–CT to select patients for definitive radiotherapy. In the first study, 153 candidates for radical radiotherapy had staging with PET after being found suitable for radiotherapy on the basis of conventional imaging.[81] PET and conventional staging evaluations were discordant approximately 40% of the time, and only two-thirds of the patients actually received definitive radiotherapy because, in the remaining patients, PET showed either distant metastasis (18%) or intrathoracic disease that was too extensive for high-dose radiotherapy (12%). The predominant impact of PET was upstaging, and this effect was greatest for patients with the most advanced tumors. In the second study, a group of Polish investigators reported that only 75 of 100 patients with NSCLC remained eligible for curative radiotherapy after PET–CT.[82] In the third study, 25 of 75 candidates were found to be unsuitable for definitive radiotherapy after PET–CT was performed with the patient in the radiotherapy planning position.[83] The survival rate for patients who actually received definitive radiotherapy after PET–CT was remarkably good, with 32% of patients with stage IIIA disease being alive at 4 years. Only 4% of patients who received palliative treatment in the study survived for 4 years, suggesting that that PET-based patient selection had been appropriate.

Radiated Volume and Toxicity

The relationship between the volume of normal tissue that is radiated and the risk of serious pulmonary toxicity, including radiation pneumonitis and later radiation-induced fibrosis, is complex. It is made even more complex by the interaction of radiation-induced lung damage and serious preexisting cardiopulmonary comorbidities that may influence the capacity of the patient to endure high-dose radiation without becoming disabled or even dying as a result of toxicity. Consequently, the volume of lung and other normal tissue, such as heart tissue, that will be included in the target volume is an important factor that determines the suitability of a patient for definitive radiotherapy. If the volume of normal tissue, especially lung tissue, is too great, curative radiotherapy is simply not possible and other therapeutic approaches, such as palliation, must be preferred.

This consideration raises the question "What volume of normal tissue is too large?" This decision often was subjective in the past, but the advent of advanced radiotherapy planning systems has made it possible to precisely estimate the volume of lung tissue that will be radiated to any particular dose level. With the increase in computing power, it has become straightforward to display radiation lung volumes as dose–volume histograms, and these dosimetric parameters have been compared with clinical outcomes in large numbers of patients. The risk of pneumonitis can be estimated from a number of different but related dosimetric parameters. These parameters include the percentage of total lung volume radiated to 5 Gy (V5), 20 Gy (V20), and 30 Gy (V30) and the MLD. As these values increase, the risk of complications increases. The risk tends to increase with concurrent chemotherapy and may be decreased by smoking. The use of intensity-modulated radiotherapy may lead to an increase in the volume of lung tissue that is exposed to lower doses of radiation, and this increase should be accounted for to avoid potentially fatal complications.[84] The Quantitative Analysis of Normal Tissue Effects in the Clinic report recommended that V20 (the volume of both lungs minus the planning target volume receiving 20 Gy) should be limited to no more than 30% to 35% and that the total MLD should be limited to no more than 20 Gy to 23 Gy (with conventional fractionation) to limit the risk of radiation pneumonitis to 20% or less in patients with NSCLC who are treated with definitive radiotherapy.[85]

These dose limits cannot be relied on in all cases. For example, patients who have had previous pneumonectomy or other major lung resections will be less capable of surviving pneumonitis, and it has been suggested that a V5 of less than 60%, a V20 of less than 4% to 10%, and an MLD of less than 8 Gy are reasonable dose limits for intensity-modulated radiotherapy in the setting of mesothelioma after pneumonectomy.[86] Although these parameters are useful for conventional daily fractionation, limited data on their utility for multiple daily fractionation or accelerated schedules are available.[87] Similarly, dose constraints for SABR applied to the lung are in the process of being established.[88] Severe pneumonitis is relatively rare after SABR, but it is clear that increasing values of V20 and MLD are associated with an increased risk of pneumonitis.[89]

F-2-Deoxy-D-Glucose Uptake

In lung lesions, the association between increased glucose metabolism and malignancy is powerful. Intensely metabolically active lesions are much more likely to be malignant than lesions with little or no FDG uptake on PET. Lesions with low FDG avidity are commonly benign or are of low-grade malignancy. The results of a systematic review showed that primary malignant tumors with greater FDG uptake are generally aggressive and are associated with a worse prognosis.[90] However, it is less clear whether FDG uptake is an independent prognostic factor because FDG avidity is strongly correlated with the extent of disease and the size of the tumor. In surgically treated patients with stage I or II NSCLC, a higher standard uptake value (SUV) is associated with lower rates of disease-free survival and overall survival.[91,92] It also has been reported that a higher SUV and metabolic tumor volume are associated with worse prognosis in patients with stage I NSCLC who are treated with SABR.[93] A number of retrospective studies have indicated that a higher SUV is associated with a worse prognosis for patients who have definitive chemoradiation therapy for the management of locally advanced disease. However, a large prospective multicenter trial involving patients with locally advanced NSCLC who were managed with definitive chemoradiation therapy (ACRIN 6668/RTOG 0235) did not confirm a significant effect of the pretreatment SUV but did suggest that the posttreatment SUV was important.[94] In that study, pretreatment SUV was evaluable for 226 patients and posttreatment SUV was evaluable for 173 patients. The mean pretreatment SUV_{peak} and SUV_{max} values (10.3 and 13.1, respectively) were not associated with survival. However, the posttreatment SUV_{peak} value was associated with survival in a continuous variable model (hazard ratio, 1.087;

95% confidence interval, 1.014–1.166; $p = 0.020$). The authors concluded that a higher posttreatment SUV (SUV_{peak} or SUV_{max}) was associated with worse survival in cases of stage III NSCLC, although a clear cutoff value for routine clinical use could not be recommended.

Computed Tomography and Positron Emission Tomography Metrics

Although small tumor volume may be associated with a better prognosis, this benefit is no longer evident at 5 years, and tumor size per se should not be a factor influencing radical chemoradiation therapy.[95,96] Increasingly, researchers are aware that, in addition to the volume of tumors, which is partly reflected in the T stage, images show many other features that could be both prognostic and predictive. In addition to the primary tumor, all regional and distant metastatic deposits could be evaluated and classified on the basis of imaging studies.

PET has been used for this purpose. Beyond FDG, PET-labeled drugs such as ^{11}C-docetaxel and ^{11}C-erlotinib and other molecules that could be used together with radiotherapy are of great interest for the future.[97,98]

As CT is widely available and highly standardized, features of CT images increasingly have been investigated. For example, texture on CT images is quantified as mean gray-level intensity, entropy, and uniformity.[99] Goh et al.[100] found a relationship between the texture features of NSCLC on noncontrast-enhanced CT and tumor metabolism and stage. In the study by Win et al.,[101] univariate analysis demonstrated CT-derived heterogeneity, [18]FDG-PET–derived heterogeneity, diffusion-enhanced (dynamic contrast-enhanced)-CT–measured permeability, and stage were prognostic for survival of patients with NSCLC.[101] In the same study, multivariate analysis showed that permeability was the most important survival predictor, followed by stage and CT-derived textural heterogeneity. The same technology also could be used to characterize organs at risk in order to improve the individual therapeutic ratio.[102]

Mutation Status

Although most NSCLC tumors do not express a molecular target that can be blocked with currently available drugs, it is conceivable that this proportion will grow dramatically in the coming years. The question arises whether these molecular characteristics influence the sensitivity for radiotherapy.

Unfortunately, we are not aware of any prospective studies on this subject. Overexpression of epidermal growth factor receptor (EGFR) is associated with resistance to chemotherapy and radiotherapy.[103] EGFR modulates DNA repair via an association with the catalytic subunit of DNA protein kinase. However, although in vitro EGFR expression correlates with both cellular and tumor response to radiation, in vivo EGFR expression does not.[104] In addition, the type of EGFR inhibition turned out to be important: only the monoclonal antibody cetuximab improved local tumor control in some, but not all, tumors, whereas EGFR tyrosine kinase inhibitors were not synergistic.[105] Although several retrospective reports have indicated that patients who have a tumor with *EGFR* mutation have a better response to radiotherapy and a longer progression-free survival than patients who have a tumor with wild-type *EGFR*, it remains to be shown if the long-term survival will be increased.

The relationship between radiosensitivity and the echinoderm microtubule-associated protein-like 4-anaplastic lymphoma kinase (*EML4-ALK*) fusion gene has not been investigated in depth. Contrasting results have been reported on the radiosensitivity of tumor cells bearing an ALK fusion protein with or without crizotinib treatment.[106,107] To our knowledge, at the time of writing, no clinical data are available.

At the present time, mutational status does not affect the treatment strategy with regard to the use of radiotherapy.

CONCLUSION

Many known and unknown factors influence the decision with regard to which patients will receive high-dose radiotherapy. Among the patient-related factors, performance status remains the most important. Comorbidities are mostly important for overall survival but have not consistently been associated with cause-specific survival and toxicity. Tumor-related parameters such as size and volume, and, probably, genetic characteristics, are of prognostic value.

The knowledge regarding the selection of patients for the most appropriate therapy will surely evolve markedly in the coming years with the combination of all types of information into a clinical algorithm.

KEY REFERENCES

2. Brunelli A, Charloux A, Bolliger CT, et al. The European Respiratory Society and European Society of Thoracic Surgeons clinical guidelines for evaluating fitness for radical treatment (surgery and chemoradiotherapy) in patients with lung cancer. *Eur J Cardiothorac Surg.* 2009;36(1):181–184.

10. Guckenberger M, Klement RJ, Kestin LL, et al. Lack of a dose-effect relationship for pulmonary function changes after stereotactic body radiation therapy for early-stage non-small cell lung cancer. *Int J Radiat Oncol Biol Phys.* 2013;85(4):1074–1081.

11. Kong FM, Hayman JA, Griffith KA, et al. Final toxicity results of a radiation-dose escalation study in patients with non-small-cell lung cancer (NSCLC): predictors for radiation pneumonitis and fibrosis. *Int J Radiat Oncol Biol Phys.* 2006;65(4):1075–1086.

13. Dehing-Oberije C, De Ruysscher D, van Baardwijk A, Yu S, Rao B, Lambin P. The importance of patient characteristics for the prediction of radiation-induced lung toxicity. *Radiother Oncol.* 2009;91(3):421–426.

14. Wang J, Cao J, Yuan S, et al. Poor baseline pulmonary function may not increase the risk of radiation-induced lung toxicity. *Int J Radiat Oncol Biol Phys.* 2013;85(3):798–804.

47. Rades D, Setter C, Schild SE, Dunst J. Effect of smoking during radiotherapy, respiratory insufficiency, and hemoglobin levels on outcome in patients irradiated for non-small-cell lung cancer. *Int J Radiat Oncol Biol Phys.* 2008;71(4):1134–1142.

See Expertconsult.com for full list of references.

37 Stage I Nonsmall Cell Lung Cancer and Oligometastatic Disease

Suresh Senan, Umberto Ricardi, Matthias Guckenberger, Kenneth E. Rosenzweig, and Nisha Ohri

SUMMARY OF KEY POINTS

- Stereotactic ablative radiotherapy (SABR) is recommended in treatment guidelines as the nonoperative therapy of choice for early-stage nonsmall cell lung cancer (NSCLC).
- SABR can be adequately performed using either traditional linear accelerators equipped with suitable image-guidance technology or linear accelerators specifically adapted for SABR and using dedicated delivery systems.
- Clinical assessment, staging of disease, and multidisciplinary discussion should be based on published guidelines for early-stage NSCLC.
- Guideline-specified nodal staging should be performed before SABR, as nodal regions are not radiated.
- SABR dose constraints, which are based on the constraints used in the RTOG 0618, 0813, and 0915 SABR trials, are summarized in the current National Comprehensive Cancer Network guidelines.
- Results of SABR have been consistent, with both the high local control rates and low toxicity found in prospective clinical trials also being reported in large single-institution series and pooled multi-institutional analyses.
- A widely used working definition for so-called central lung tumors is tumors located either adjacent to the proximal bronchial tree or located 1 cm or less from the heart or mediastinum.
- Three distinct cohorts of patients with oligometastases can be identified: patients with oligometastatic disease at the time of diagnosis, patients with oligoprogressive disease after cytoreductive therapy, and patients with oligorecurrent disease after curative local–regional therapy.
- Results appear generalizable across centers when current SABR guidelines are followed.

Changes in the epidemiology of lung cancer are particularly relevant for the field of radiation oncology. Globally, lung cancer represents the leading cause of cancer death in men and is the second leading cause in women.[1] A key challenge is that older patients are the fastest growing population—nearly 25% of patients are 75 years of age or older.[2] Approximately 20% of all patients diagnosed with nonsmall cell lung cancer (NSCLC) have stage I disease, and surgery is currently the guideline-specified treatment for fit patients who are willing to accept the procedure-related risks.[3] However, a population study from the Netherlands showed that, among patients with stage I disease, resection was done in 49% of patients 75 years of age or older compared with 91% of patients who were 60 years of age or younger.[4] Similarly, in an analysis of data in the Surveillance, Epidemiology and End Results (SEER)-Medicare database for the period 1998 to

2007, the percentage of patients who had a surgical procedure decreased over time (75.2% in 1998 vs. 67.3% in 2007) and the percentage of patients who did not receive any local treatment increased (14.6% in 1998 vs. 18.3% in 2007).[5] These findings were explained by the increase in the proportion of patients 85 years of age or older (from 4.5% to 9%), as well as an increase in patients with three or more comorbidities (from 15% to 30%) during the study period. The reluctance to operate on older patients is mainly due to their frailty, as comorbidities are more common in the older population.[6] Although severe comorbidity has the greatest impact on outcomes during the first month following surgery, the increased death rate associated with impaired performance status persists with longer follow-up.[7]

The apparent reluctance of clinicians to refer older patients for conventional radiotherapy was partly due to the 30 or more once-daily treatments that were typically required, which is cumbersome for frail older patients. In the era before stereotactic ablative radiotherapy (SABR), outcomes of radiotherapy in early-stage NSCLC were poor despite treatment with doses ranging from 60 to 66 Gy. Local tumor recurrences occurred in approximately 40% of patients, with an overall survival rate at 3 years of approximately 30%.[8] Furthermore, a modest 6-month increase in median survival was reported in an analysis of 2010 SEER data when older radiotherapy techniques were applied.[9]

SABR: BACKGROUND AND DEFINITIONS

In the mid-1990s, the principles of cranial stereotactic radiotherapy (or radiosurgery) were transferred to extracranial sites by work pioneered at the Karolinska Hospital in Sweden.[10] Stereotactic body radiation therapy (SBRT) and SABR are equivalent terms for this technique in the body. This stereotactic approach was further developed by centers in Japan and Germany.[11-13] In subsequent years, encouraging results from both prospective and retrospective studies resulted in rapid adoption of SABR for early-stage NSCLC. A national survey in the United States found that 57% of all responding physicians used SABR for the treatment of lung cancer in 2010,[14] whereas a similar survey in Italy found that 41% of responding radiotherapy centers used SABR in 2009.[15] At present, SABR is recommended in treatment guidelines as the nonoperative therapy of choice for early-stage NSCLC.[3]

Guidelines for SABR have been released by several professional groups: the American Association of Physics in Medicine Task Group 101,[16] the American Society for Therapeutic Radiology and Oncology and the American College of Radiology,[17] the Canadian Association of Radiation Oncology-Stereotactic Body Radiotherapy,[18] the National Radiotherapy Implementation Group of the UK,[19] and the working group Stereotactic Radiotherapy of the Germany Society of Radiation Oncology.[20] Current definitions of SABR adhere to the following criteria: a high degree of accuracy, use of high doses of radiation, and delivery of radiation in one or a few treatment fractions to an extracranial target.

The rationale of SABR for early-stage NSCLC is that higher radiation doses are more effective for local control of the tumor, which translates into longer overall survival.[21,22] SABR differs from conventional radiotherapy in that SABR involves delivery of very high radiation doses only to the visible tumor, with planning and delivery of treatment optimized to ensure safety margins of a few millimeters. In addition, radiation doses to surrounding normal organs are often lower than with conventional techniques.[23] As a result, local tumor control rates of 90% and higher can be achieved and rates of severe toxicity are typically below 10%.

SABR for lung cancer is a multidisciplinary endeavor, involving all disciplines related to the diagnosis and treatment of the disease, but particularly specialists working on a radiotherapy team. Accuracy of delivery is achieved using an optimized workflow and appropriate quality assurance procedures, including development of written protocols, which is an essential component of the process.

SABR can be adequately performed using either traditional linear accelerators equipped with suitable image-guidance technology or linear accelerators specifically adapted for SABR and using dedicated delivery systems. The SABR procedure was initially defined by the use of frame-based patient set-up, the goal of which was stable and reproducible patient positioning. However, frame-based stereotactic patient set-up has been replaced by image guidance, which makes the term stereotactic somewhat misleading. With non–frame-based patient set-up, external stereotactic coordinates are replaced by visualization of a patient's anatomy using images acquired on-table and subsequently compared with pretreatment planning images. Soft-tissue images of the tumor itself, or of an implanted fiducial marker, can be used for setting up the target (Fig. 37.1).

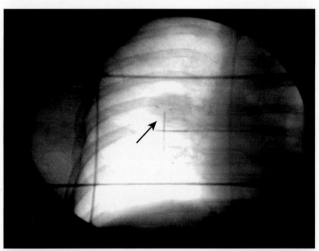

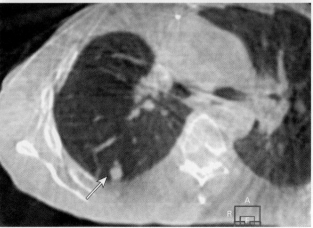

Fig. 37.1. Some techniques used for image guidance in stereotactic ablative radiotherapy for lung cancer, showing tumor visualization using a cone-beam computed tomography and implanted fiducial markers.

SABR Protocol Development, Implementation, and Quality Assurance

A dedicated SABR team should consist of radiation oncologists, medical physicists, and technicians (e.g., radiographers, radiation therapists), all of whom should have attended appropriate training courses organized by professional bodies and/or industry in accordance with the above-mentioned guidelines. Written treatment protocols that are consistent with national regulations, institution-specific equipment, and training and education of the individual radiotherapy team members should be available. SABR requires additional and more frequent physical quality assurance: verification and quality assurance of the entire SABR treatment chain is mandatory, and end-to-end tests for overall uncertainty estimation are recommended. It is paramount to verify that the radiation isocenter coincides with the mechanical isocenter, including couch rotation, room lasers, and, especially, the imaging isocenter.

CLINICAL ASSESSMENT

Clinical assessment, staging of disease, and multidisciplinary discussion should be based on published guidelines for early-stage NSCLC.[24] Unlike the toxicity found following surgery in older individuals,[25] no increased toxicity or treatment-related mortality has been noted when SABR has been extensively applied to patients between 75 and 80 years old.[26,27] The poorer overall survival rates reported in this older population after SABR are related to comorbidities, and the number of comorbidities predicts overall survival after both SABR and surgery.[7,28] SABR-related toxicity is also not increased in patients with very poor pretreatment pulmonary function,[29,30] and the available data suggest that SABR should be offered to all patients regardless of age and preexisting pulmonary comorbidities, unless their predicted survival time is short.

Diagnosis and Staging Before SABR

Diagnosis and confirmation of NSCLC based on tissue biopsy is recommended before starting any local treatment for early-stage NSCLC.[24] However, obtaining a histologic diagnosis may not be possible for peripheral lung lesions or may pose a high risk of toxicity in a patient group with considerable medical and/or pulmonary comorbidities. In the latter case, radiographic criteria of malignancy are used to establish a diagnosis. Models that predict the probability of malignancy in solitary pulmonary nodules based on both clinical and radiographic characteristics have been described and validated.[31,32] It is important to note that these criteria may not hold true in geographic regions with a high incidence of infectious and/or granulomatous lung diseases. Therefore, current guidelines state that any treatment for a possible early-stage NSCLC without a pathologic diagnosis should proceed only after assessment by an experienced multidisciplinary tumor board.[24] If the clinical and radiographic findings are inconclusive, repeated imaging to evaluate the growth pattern is an option for some patients, but careful follow-up is required because patients with malignancy are at risk for early disease progression.[33]

Guideline-specified nodal staging should be performed before SABR, as nodal regions are not radiated. Staging with ^{18}F-2-deoxy-D-glucose-positron emission tomography (FDG-PET) is essential because of its higher diagnostic accuracy for the detection of node metastases (negative predictive value, 90%)[34,35] and also because unsuspected distant metastases and second primary tumors can be excluded.[36] In the event of pathologic FDG uptake in regional lymph nodes, further evaluation by endobronchial ultrasound or endoscopic ultrasound is recommended and, if the findings are inconclusive, a mediastinoscopy may be necessary. Staging with PET–computed tomography (CT) should ideally be performed within 6 to 8 weeks before SABR is given because of the risk of disease progression in the interim.[37]

TECHNICAL OVERVIEW FOR RADIATION ONCOLOGISTS

Target Volume Definition and Treatment Planning

All imaging should be acquired in the treatment position, with standard practice dictating that planning CT images encompass the entire lung volume, and a slice thickness of 2 mm to 3 mm is used.[23] Using intravenous contrast medium may improve the delineation of centrally located primary tumors. As conventional three-dimensional (3-D) CT risk introduces artifacts and systematic errors, four-dimensional (4-D) CT, also known as respiration-correlated CT, is the recommended technique for SABR planning.[38] Although a single 4-D CT planning image provides only a snapshot of a patient's breathing pattern, several studies have demonstrated that the motion pattern and amplitude are stable over time,[39–41] making routine repeated 4-D CT imaging unnecessary. The use of FDG-PET alone is not appropriate for a reliable assessment of target motion in SABR planning.[42]

Target Volume Concept and Motion Management Strategy

Gross tumor volume is determined on the basis of CT findings in the lung and soft-tissue window. Current guidelines do not recommend the use of clinical target volume margins when SABR is delivered,[17,23] as the high radiation doses combined with rather flat dose profiles in pulmonary tissue of low electron density result in sufficient coverage of potential microscopic disease extension.[43] Integration of breathing-induced target motion into the target volume concept will ensure patient-tailored tumor targeting, with clinical implementation dependent on the chosen motion management strategy. Several different approaches are used in routine clinical practice.[44,45] Continuous radiation in free breathing is performed using the internal target volume concept, the mean target position concept, or real-time tumor tracking. Tumor tracking is possible using dedicated robotic delivery machines,[46] by dynamic multileaf tracking,[47] a gimbaled multileaf collimator,[48] or a dynamic treatment couch.[49] Noncontinuous radiation of the tumor in a reproducible position is performed using gated beam delivery in predefined phases of the breathing cycle,[50] in voluntary breath-hold,[51] or in breath-hold using the active breathing coordinator.[52]

It is important to emphasize that active motion management strategies, such as gating and tracking, require continuous intrafractional monitoring; however, continuous intrafractional monitoring is less critical for passive strategies, such as the internal target volume or mean tumor position concept. Although patient-specific motion management is strongly recommended, data from the available prospective trials did not involve the use of advanced motion management strategies. Of the individualized 4-D motion management strategies used, resulting field sizes are largest for the internal target volume concept; however, this motion management strategy is straightforward to implement and ensures adequate target coverage. Even if all uncertainties in treatment planning and delivery are minimized by currently available technologies, residual errors still remain and require minimum planning target volume (PTV) margins of about 5 mm.[53]

Dose Fractionation and Prescription

Dose prescription and reporting should comply with the International Committee on Radiation Units and Measurements Report on Prescribing, Recording, and Reporting Intensity-Modulated Photon-Beam Therapy as closely as possible, but historical practice and experiences need to be considered as well. Most prospective and retrospective studies used inhomogeneous dose distributions within the PTV, with maximum doses ranging between 105% and 150% of the prescribed dose. Inhomogeneous dose distributions offer the opportunity to deliver an extra dose to the center of the PTV, where the (potentially hypoxic) macroscopic tumor is located, without increased doses to the peripheral normal tissue.[54]

As a result of large differences in single-fraction and total doses between SABR studies, a comparison of physical doses is less meaningful. The linear quadratic model has been widely used for modeling of SABR outcomes data, but it has not been validated for very high single doses.[55] Despite uncertainty surrounding the linear quadratic model, several groups have independently demonstrated a clear dose-effect relationship for local tumor control using biologic effective doses (BEDs), with a minimum PTV dose of more than 100 Gy BED (α/β ratio, 10 Gy) required for local tumor control rates of higher than 90%.[56–58] The current recommended tumor dose for SABR of lung tumors is a minimum of 100 Gy BED, prescribed to the target volume encompassing isodose.[24] A meta-analysis demonstrated a potential detrimental effect of SABR doses exceeding more than 146 Gy BED.[59]

Total doses are typically delivered in one to eight fractions, but insurance reimbursement rules have resulted in a widespread use of five or fewer fractions in the United States. However, use of very high single-fraction doses and total doses (e.g., delivery of three fractions of 20 Gy) can damage normal tissues in or adjacent to the target volume.[60] Consequently, treatment of tumors in proximity to critical normal organs has led to the use of so-called risk-adapted fractionation schemes that deliver the required dose of 100 Gy BED in a larger number of treatment fractions with lower single-fraction doses. Fractionation appears to spare some critical normal organs while ensuring sufficiently high doses to achieve local tumor control.[61]

Fractionation appears to be especially valuable in SABR for centrally located tumors, as it allows for radiobiologic sparing of critical organs such as large bronchi, vessels, heart, and esophagus. High-quality prospective data on the safety and efficacy of SABR for centrally located lesions are limited, but a systematic review of the literature demonstrated local control rates of 85% or greater when the prescribed BED to the tumor was 100 Gy or higher. The overall treatment-related mortality was 2.7%, and when the BED to normal tissue was 210 Gy or lower (α/β ratio, 3 Gy), the rate was 1.0%.[61] Until mature prospective multicenter data become available, a recommended fractionation scheme for experienced centers is 8×7.5 Gy, with D_{max}(PTV) of 125%.

Treatment Planning

The voxel size of the dose calculation grid should be 2 mm or less, and both heterogeneity correction and use of type B algorithms improve accurate dose calculation, especially at the interface of lung tissue and soft tissue.[62] Monte Carlo dose-calculation algorithms achieve the most accurate results, but differences to collapsed cone algorithms appear small. All published prospective trials have used 3-D conformal treatment planning. Intensity-modulated radiation therapy and advanced rotational techniques such as volumetric modulated arc therapy have the potential to increase dose conformity and homogeneity and reduce treatment delivery times.[63] More data are needed on the biologic consequences of potential interplay effects between multileaf collimator motion and tumor motion. The effects of using flattening filter-free radiation, in particular, for faster delivery remain unclear.[64] Single-institution data suggest that the flattening filter-free technique is both safe and effective.[65-66] Published tolerance doses for SABR have largely not been validated, although adherence to published protocols appears reasonable at this time, as rates of severe toxicity were low as a result (Table 37.1). These dose constraints, which are based on the constraints used in the RTOG 0618, 0813, and 0915 SABR trials, are summarized in the current National Comprehensive Cancer Network guidelines.[67]

Patient Immobilization and Set-Up

Customized patient immobilization devices such as the stereotactic body frame or vacuum cushions have been used, but are not considered essential; although they may improve intrafractional patient stability, they do not negate the need for image guidance. A number of studies demonstrated that image-based verification of the target position has the single largest effect on improving the accuracy of lung SABR. Average internal shifts of 5 mm to 7 mm of the pulmonary target relative to the osseous structure are regularly found, and this shift may exceed 2 cm in individual patients.[68,69] Therefore, daily pretreatment imaging is performed with online correction of set-up errors and baseline shifts—imaging needs to demonstrate the lung tumor directly, or implanted markers as a surrogate, for the tumor position (see Fig. 37.1). Imaging during or after completion of SABR serves as a quality assurance purpose, especially in single-fraction SABR. Several technologies for image guidance are commercially available, and superiority of one method over the other has not been demonstrated. Use of volumetric imaging, as opposed to only implanted fiducial markers, has the advantage of allowing for assessment of changes in target shape and position relative to the position of organs at risk.

CLINICAL RESULTS OF SABR

The strongest evidence in support of SABR for treating early-stage NSCLC comes from population-based data.[70] In one population-based study from the Netherlands, survival rates for patients 75 years of age and older were improved after widespread access to SABR.[69] This finding was attributed to both a reduction in the proportion of untreated patients after short-course SABR became available, as well as to local control rates of up to 90% found with this modality. Of the nearly 30% of older Dutch patients who remained untreated despite the availability of SABR, the 30- and 90-day mortality rates measured from the date of diagnosis for untreated patients were 17.9% and 33.3%, respectively.[71] The 90-day mortality rate may be a result of extensive comorbidity with competing causes of death in this patient population. Therefore, overtreatment in very frail patients, even with SABR, may be avoided by carefully reassessing some less-fit patients a few weeks after diagnosis. Another population-based analysis of the National Cancer Data Base (NCDB) demonstrated improved survival in elderly (aged ≥70 years) patients with early-stage medically inoperable NSCLC receiving SABR compared with observation alone.[3,72] In an analysis of SEER data, survival rates following SABR were similar to those after lobectomy, with poorer outcomes following conventional radiotherapy or observation only.[73]

The results of SABR have been very consistent, with both the high local control rates and low toxicity found in prospective clinical trials also being reported in large single-institution series and pooled multi-institutional analyses (Table 37.2).[74–82] Data from these sources demonstrate an average 90% rate of freedom from local progression at 2 years to 3 years. The timing of

TABLE 37.1 Normal Tissue Constraints Used in Major Clinical Trials[a]

Organ at Risk	One Fraction (RTOG 0915)	Three Fractions (RTOG 0618/1021)	Four Fractions (RTOG 0915)	Five Fractions (RTOG 0813)	Eight Fractions[65]
Trachea and large bronchus	D_{max} 20.2 Gy	D_{max} 30 Gy	D_{max} 34.8 Gy 15.6 Gy < 4 cc	D_{max} 105%[b] 18 Gy < 5cc[c]	D_{max} 44 Gy
Heart	D_{max} 22 Gy 16 Gy < 15 cc	D_{max} 30 Gy	D_{max} 34 Gy 28 Gy < 15 cc	D_{max} 105%[b] 32 Gy < 15 cc	—
Esophagus	D_{max} 15.4 Gy 11.9 Gy < 5 cc	D_{max} 25.2 Gy 17.7 Gy < 5 cc	D_{max} 30 Gy 18.8 Gy < 5 cc	D_{max} 105%[b] 27.5 Gy < 5 cc[c]	D_{max} 40 Gy
Brachial plexus	D_{max} 17.5 Gy 14 Gy < 3 cc	D_{max} 24 Gy 20.4 Gy < 3 cc	D_{max} 27.2 Gy 23.6 Gy < 3 cc	D_{max} 32 Gy 30 Gy < 3 cc	D_{max} 36 Gy
Chest wall	D_{max} 30 Gy 22 Gy < 1 cc	30 Gy < 30 cc 60 Gy < 3 cc	D_{max} 27.2 Gy 32 Gy < 1 cc	30 Gy < 30 cc 60 Gy < 3 cc	—
Spinal cord	D_{max} 14 Gy 10 Gy < 0.35 cc	D_{max} 18 Gy	D_{max} 26 Gy 20.8 Gy < 0.35 cc	D_{max} 30 Gy 22.5 Gy < 0.25 cc	D_{max} 28 Gy

[a]Radiation Therapy Oncology Group (RTOG) protocols can be found on the RTOG website at www.rtog.org/ClinicalTrials/ProtocolTable.aspx.
[b]Planning target volume prescription.
[c]Volume constraint for nonadjacent wall.

TABLE 37.2 Overview of Results of Sterotactic Ablative Radiotherapy After Delivery of Radiation at More Than 106 Gy Biologic Effective Dose

Author (Year)	No. of Patients	Patients With Histopathologic Confirmation of NSCLC (%)	Overall Survival at 2–3 Years (%)	Freedom From Local Progression at 2–3 Years (%)
PROSPECTIVE PHASE II TRIALS				
Nagata et al. (2005)[71]	45	100	75	98
Baumann et al. (2009)[72]	57	67	60	92
Fakiris et al. (2009)[73]	70	100	43	88
Ricardi et al. (2010)[74]	62	65	51	88
Bral et al. (2010)[75]	40	100	52	84
Timmerman et al. (2010)[76]	54	100	38	98
All prospective studies[a]	*328*	*87.6*	*52.1*	*91.2*
LARGE RETROSPECTIVE SERIES				
Grills et al. (2010)[77]	434	64	60	94
Senthi et al. (2012)[78]	676	35	55	95
Guckenberger et al. (2013)[79]	514	85	46	80
			62[b]	93[b]
All retrospective studies[a]	*1624*	*58.8*	*53.5*	*90.0*

[a]The weighted average values are calculated for the summary of all prospective and retrospective studies.
[b]Subgroup of 164 patients treated with ≥106 Gy biologic effective dose.

disease recurrence following SABR was reported in a series of 676 patients, all of whom were treated with a BED of more than 100 Gy (Table 37.3).[61] At a median follow-up of 33 months, median overall survival was 40.7 months; actuarial 2-year rates of local, regional, and distant recurrence were 4.9%, 7.8% and 14.7%; and actuarial 5-year rates were 10.5%, 12.7%, and 19.9%, respectively.

Three randomized trials were initiated to evaluate SABR versus surgery for early-stage NSCLC. All three closed early due to poor accrual. A pooled analysis of two of the trials was reported. The rate of 3-year overall survival was 79% in the surgery group and 95% in the SABR group ($p = 0.037$). The rate of recurrence-free survival at 3 years was similar in the SABR and surgery groups (86% vs. 80%, respectively; $p = 0.54$).[83] Since there were only 58 patients in the pooled analysis, it is difficult to make conclusions on the superiority of either treatment. However, it does confirm the efficacy of SABR in the absence of patient selection bias that is inherent in phase I and II trials and the use of SABR as an alternative to surgery.

Patterns of early disease recurrence after curative SABR in early-stage NSCLC are similar to recurrences after primary surgery, where the predominant pattern of disease recurrence is also one of distant recurrence, despite staging FDG-PET.[84] This pattern suggests that occult distant metastases at the time of initial diagnosis remain a major challenge. In an analysis of nearly 1300 patients who had resection, the risk of subsequent disease recurrence ranged from 6% to 10% per person-year during the first 4 years after surgery, but decreased thereafter to 2%.[84] Conversely, the risk of second primary lung cancer ranged from 3% to 6% per person-year after surgery and did not diminish over time, a finding similar to the 6% incidence of second primary lung tumors after SABR.[61]

Toxicity

After a median follow-up of 1.6 years following SABR, the most common toxicity reported for 505 patients was pneumonitis; the rate of grade 2 or higher pneumonitis was 7%, the rate of grade 3

or higher pneumonitis was 2%, and the rate of grade 5 pneumonitis was 0.2%.[80] The median time to onset of pneumonitis was 0.4 years. The other most common toxicities included rib fracture (3%), dermatitis (2%), and myositis (1%). Serial measurements of pulmonary function parameters showed an average decrease of 3.6% in the forced expiratory volume in 1 second and of 6.8% in the diffusing capacity for carbon monoxide within 6 months and 7 to 24 months after SABR.[30] Changes in lung function correlated strongly with pretreatment pulmonary functions, with the largest decreases in function occurring in patients with the best pretreatment values, whereas pulmonary function was stable or even improved in patients with the worst pretreatment values. In addition, symptomatic radiation pneumonitis is uncommon following the treatment of peripheral lung tumors measuring 5 cm or smaller.[75,79,85]

Doses to the contralateral lung predicted for the risk of pneumonitis when larger tumors are treated using a volumetric modulated arc therapy delivery technique. Limiting volumes of the contralateral lung receiving 5 Gy to less than 26% reduces risk of acute pneumonitis,[86] and an analysis in a larger patient group indicated that both the mean dose to the contralateral lung and tumor size were strong predictors of grade 3 or higher radiation pneumonitis after treatment.[87] The findings of this study suggested that limiting the mean dose to the contralateral lung to below 3.6 Gy was optimal.

A higher incidence of severe radiation pneumonitis has been reported for patients with preexisting pulmonary fibrosis.[88] Patients with idiopathic pulmonary fibrosis have an increased risk for grade 3 or higher pneumonitis after both conventionally fractionated radiotherapy[89] and chemoradiation therapy,[90] as well as after surgical resection.[91] Although accurate estimates of the risk of high-grade radiation pneumonitis in idiopathic pulmonary fibrosis are unknown, clinicians should be aware that interstitial lung abnormalities are found on nearly 9% of CT images among individuals over 50 years of age, with definite fibrosis in 2% in a study population of patients over 50 years old.[92] A genetic polymorphism, the *MUC5B* promoter, has been found to be associated with interstitial lung disease.

The chest wall and ribs are at risk for toxicity when tumors are located in the proximity. Current guidelines recommend limiting doses to the chest wall to 30 Gy or less,[23] with approximately 3% of patients reporting severe chest wall pain and rib fractures (Fig. 37.2) after SABR using similar constraints.[93]

Less common toxicities after SABR include myositis, skin toxicity, and neuropathy.[94] Brachial plexus injury can occur following SABR for apical lung tumors, with neuropathic pain developing in the shoulder or arm, motor weakness, or sensory alteration.[95] Limiting the total dose delivered to the plexus in three or four fractions to less than 26 Gy can lower the risk of

TABLE 37.3 Stereotactic Ablative Radiotherapy for Early-Stage Nonsmall Cell Lung Cancer: Timing of Recurrences and Development of Second Primary Tumors in a Series of 676 Patients[61]

Event	Median Time to Event (Mo)
Recurrence	
Local	14.9 (95% CI, 11.4–18.4)
Regional	13.1 (95% CI, 7.9–18.3)
Distant	9.6 (95% CI, 6.8–12.4)
Second primary tumors	18 (95% CI, 12.5–23.5)

CI, Confidence interval.

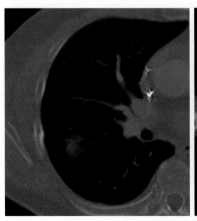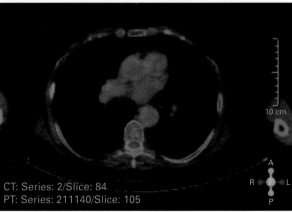

Fig. 37.2. Development of a rib fracture following treatment of a subpleural tumor.

this complication. Both tracheoesophageal fistulae and esophageal perforations have been reported following SABR to vertebral or lung SABR target in the proximity of the esophagus.[96] Careful treatment planning is necessary when performing SABR in this situation; guidelines for contouring normal organs in the thorax, as well as a summary of normal organ dose recommendations, have been published.[97]

SABR FOR CENTRAL LESIONS

A widely used working definition for so-called central lung tumors is tumors located either adjacent to the proximal bronchial tree or located 1 cm or less from the heart or mediastinum (Fig. 37.3).[66] A higher incidence of complications has been reported after SABR for central tumors;[98,99] however, in a systematic review of the literature, SABR was found to be a relatively safe and effective curative treatment, provided that appropriate fractionation schedules are used for central tumors.[61] Preliminary analysis of the RTOG 0813 trial, which is a phase I/II study designed specifically to determine the maximum tolerated dose and efficacy of SABR for centrally located tumors, showed a 7.2% rate of grade 3 or worse toxicity using a 12 Gy × 5 fraction SABR regimen. A phase II analysis will examine efficacy rates.[100] A similar single institution study was performed at Washington University in St. Louis, USA, which revealed that 11 Gy × 5 fractions was a safe effective dose. There was a single episode of fatal hemoptysis among the 42 patients treated.[101] Further progress in the use of SABR for central tumors requires ongoing prospective multi-institution trials in order to establish reliable normal organ tolerance dose constraints. However, even the use of so-called risk-adapted fractionation schemes cannot completely preclude a risk of bronchial stenosis when central lung tumors are treated,[96,102,103] but the continued use of this technique in less-fit patients is justified in light of the reported toxicity associated with surgery.[104]

FOLLOW-UP AFTER SABR

Approximately 6% of patients are diagnosed with second primary lung cancers during follow-up after SABR.[61,105] This finding supports the recommendation that patients treated with radical intent should be followed up for detection of treatable relapse, or the occurrence of a second primary lung cancer.[24] While disease progression or recurrence typically occurs within the first 2 years after treatment, current and former smokers remain at elevated risk for developing second primary lung cancers beyond 2 years.[105] A follow-up visit every 3 months to 6 months is recommended during the second and third year after SABR, with annual thoracic CT thereafter. In addition, patients with NSCLC should be offered a smoking-cessation program, as smoking cessation leads to superior treatment outcomes.

Persistent radiographic changes are common after lung SABR (Fig. 37.4), with some degree of late change being nearly universal.[106] Radiation induced lung injury surrounding the treated tumor has been found to correlate with radiation

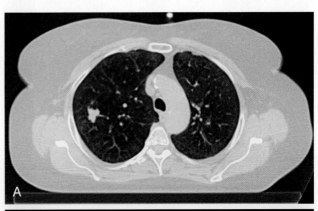

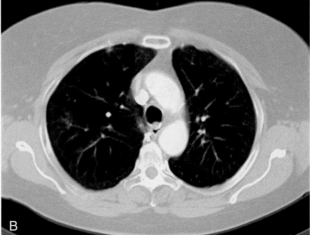

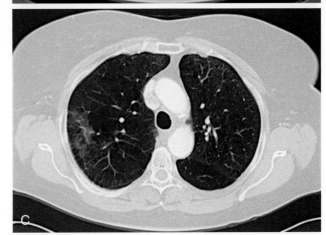

Fig. 37.4. Radiographic changes after stereotactic ablative radiotherapy (SABR). Serial computed tomography images up to 48 months after SABR showing evolution of a so-called modified conventional pattern of fibrosis. Before treatment (A), 12 months after SABR (B), and 48 months after SABR (C).

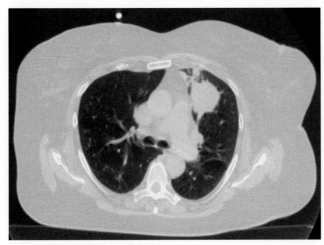

Fig. 37.3. A central tumor in the left upper lobe, adjacent to the mediastinum and pulmonary artery. The patient was treated using an eight-fraction stereotactic ablative radiotherapy scheme, to a dose of 60 Gy.

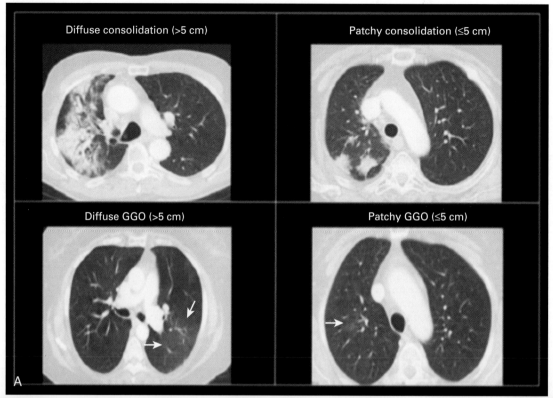

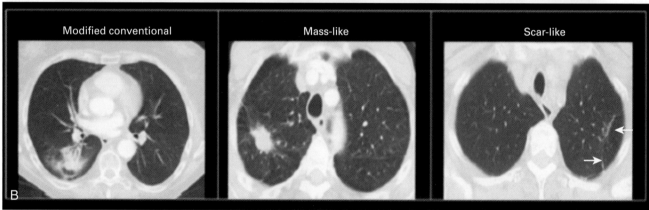

Fig. 37.5. A standardized classification system for benign changes after stereotactic ablative radiotherapy classified as (A) acute (within 6 months after treatment) or (B) late (beyond 6 months after treatment). *GGO, (Reprinted with permission from Dahele M, Palma D, Lagerwaard F, Slotman B, Senan S. Radiological changes after stereotactic radiotherapy for stage I lung cancer.* J Thorac Oncol. *2011;6(7):1221–1228.) GGO,* Ground-glass opacities.

treatment isodose.[107] A standardized classification system for benign changes has been proposed, with changes classified as acute (within 6 months after treatment) or late (more than 6 months after treatment) (Fig. 37.5). Acute changes include diffuse consolidation, patchy consolidation, diffuse ground-glass opacities, and patchy ground-glass opacities; late changes include a modified conventional pattern, defined as volume loss, traction bronchiectasis, consolidation similar to changes after conventional radiotherapy (but less extensive), mass-like fibrosis, and scar-like fibrosis. Such changes often continue to evolve more than 2 years after SABR, with late changes occasionally showing mass-like effects.[106] Multidisciplinary teams should recognize this finding in order to avoid unnecessary diagnostic procedures.

In a systematic review of the literature, so-called high-risk radiographic features associated with tumor recurrences on CT were identified.[108] These features were (1) an enlarging opacity at the primary site, (2) sequential enlarging opacity, (3) enlarging opacity after 12 months, (4) bulging margins of the opacity, (5) loss of a linear margin, and (6) loss of air on bronchograms. The review also suggested that a maximum standard uptake value of more than 5 on FDG-PET carried a high predictive value of recurrence.

Subsequently, a blinded assessment of serial CT images of 12 patients with pathology-proven local recurrence, which were matched 1:2 to images of 24 patients without recurrence, demonstrated that all previously identified high-risk features were significantly associated with local recurrence ($p < 0.01$). One additional high-risk feature—craniocaudal growth—was identified.[109] The best individual predictor of local recurrence was opacity enlargement after 12 months (100% sensitivity, 83% specificity, $p < 0.001$). The odds of recurrence increased fourfold for each additional

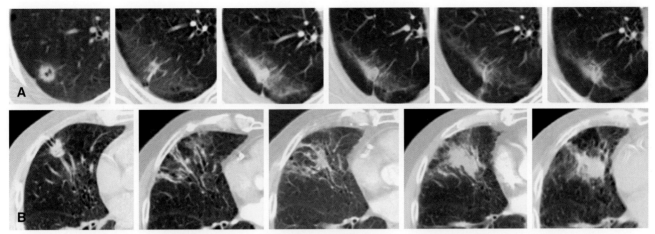

Fig. 37.6. Serial computed tomography images of patients (A) without or (B) with pathology-proven recurrence. Panel B shows the development of a mass in the radiated field that persists. *(Reprinted with permission from Huang K, Senthi S, Palma DA, et al. High-risk CT features for detection of local recurrence after stereotactic ablative radiotherapy for lung cancer. Radiother Oncol. 2013;109(1):51–57.)*

high-risk feature detected (Fig. 37.6). The presence of three or more high-risk features was highly sensitive and specific (greater than 90%) for recurrence. These findings suggest that assessment of CT images after SABR for the presence of high-risk features may enable an accurate prediction of local recurrence. This information has been incorporated into an imaging follow-up algorithm for patients who are candidates for salvage therapy (Fig. 37.7) in order to allow for the timely administration of curative salvage therapy.[109]

SALVAGE THERAPIES

The use of salvage surgery for suspected recurrence after SABR has been reported by some investigators.[110–112] The limited experience thus far suggests that this procedure is safe in experienced hands, even for some patients who were initially considered to be inoperable. The limited literature on the use of SABR for repeat radiation of local failure following initial SABR suggests that toxicity may be increased, particularly for centrally located lesions.[113]

REPRODUCIBILITY OF SABR RESULTS

A favorable therapeutic ratio of high local control and simultaneous low toxicity has been maintained even after a more widespread adoption of SABR outside of clinical trials and specialized radiotherapy centers.[82] Despite relevant variability and time trends in SABR practice, this reproducible therapeutic ratio suggests that clinical outcomes after SABR are fairly robust. Implementation of modern imaging, treatment planning, and image-guidance technology in recent years may not have increased local tumor control directly but may have improved outcomes on a population-based level by contributing to the rapid adoption of SABR in the radiotherapy community as a result of a streamlined SABR workflow and improved confidence of the treatment team.

ALTERNATIVES TO SABR FOR EARLY-STAGE NSCLC

The three prospective clinical trials comparing surgery and SABR in stage I NSCLC have been prematurely closed because of poor accrual.[114] In the absence of data from randomized trials, propensity score-matched pair analysis can be used to obtain two comparison groups with similar known prognostic factor characteristics. A propensity score-matched pair analysis comparing local–regional control after video-assisted thoracoscopic surgery lobectomy and SABR demonstrated superior local–regional control after SABR, but no differences in overall survival.[115]

In contrast, a propensity matched analysis of the SEER and Medicare databases comparing SABR to thoracoscopic sublobar resection or lobectomy in elderly patients showed that surgical resection may be associated with improved cancer-specific survival, particularly for larger tumors.[116] These conflicting results highlight the limitations of retrospective analyses and the need for strong randomized data.

It has been suggested that in patients who are borderline surgical candidates, a segmentectomy or extended wedge resection with adequate margins and evaluation of hilar and mediastinal nodes is a safe and effective alternative to lobectomy.[91] However, a recent propensity-matched analysis of the NCDB showed worse overall survival with segmentectomy and wedge resection compared with lobectomy for clinical stage IA NSCLC.[117] Additionally, considerably higher rates of morbidity and mortality are associated with surgical procedures in such patients in unselected populations, and mortality from competing risks is considerable.[118] Furthermore, compliance with guideline-specified mediastinal node staging is often poor in surgical populations, with SEER data demonstrating that the mediastinal lymph nodes were not examined in 62% of patients with a diagnosis of pathologic N0 or N1 NSCLC.[119] Another analysis of SEER data showed that no lymph nodes were examined in 51% of sublobar resections performed between 1998 and 2009.[120] The results of European studies also suggest poor compliance with node staging in fit patients who had surgery,[121] thereby minimizing any potential benefits of surgery. A Markov model analysis comparing the cost-effectiveness of SABR with wedge resection and lobectomy for patients with stage I NSCLC who are borderline surgical candidates concluded that SABR was almost always the most cost-effective treatment strategy.[122] In contrast, the same analysis for patients who were deemed to be fit for surgery for early-stage disease suggested that lobectomy may be the more cost-effective option.

Radiofrequency ablation (RFA) involves the image-guided percutaneous placement of one or more probes in the tumor, to which thermal energy is applied. In a 2012 literature review, the rates of local progression in early-stage NSCLC were lower after SABR than after RFA (3.5% to 14.5% vs. 23.7% to 43%).[123] Similarly, the 5-year survival rates were higher with SABR (47%) than with RFA (20.1% to 27%). The most common complication following RFA was pneumothorax, which occurred in 19.1% to 63% of patients. Guidelines from the American College of Chest Physicians and Society of Thoracic Surgeons recommend that, among high-risk patients with stage I NSCLC, use of RFA should be limited to patients who are not candidates for SABR or a sublobar resection.[91]

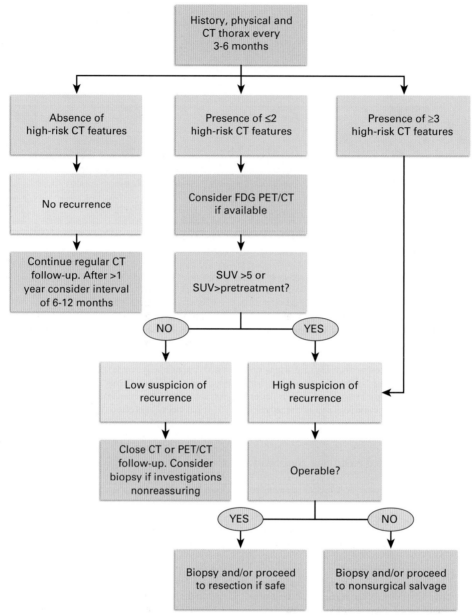

Fig. 37.7. Proposed algorithm for follow-up imaging after stereotactic ablative radiotherapy. *CT,* Computed tomography; *FDG-PET,* ^{18}F-2-deoxy-D-glucose-positron emission tomography; *SUV,* standard uptake value. *(Reprinted with permission from Huang K, Dahele M, Senan S, et al. Radiographic changes after lung stereotactic ablative radiotherapy (SABR)—can we distinguish recurrence from fibrosis? A systematic review of the literature. Radiother Oncol. 2012;102(3):335–342.)*

OLIGOMETASTASES FROM LUNG CANCER

The current clinical staging of lung cancer separates patients rather dichotomously into two groups: patients with and without distant metastases. Patients with overt metastases at the time of diagnosis are primarily treated with palliative systemic treatments. In the spectrum of patients who have no metastases and patients with overt diffuse disseminated systemic disease, an intermediate state exists when metastases are limited in number. This state is referred to as oligometastatic,[124] and patients in this subgroup may have longer overall survival, provided that all detectable tumor deposits are treated radically with surgery and/or radiotherapy. In a systematic review of 49 studies (2176 patients) of oligometastatic NSCLC, survival outcomes varied, with half of the patients having disease progression within approximately 12 months.[125] However, there are long-term survivors, and favorable subgroups have been identified in some—but not all—studies. The interest in oligometastases has grown because of the availability of molecular targeted therapies that have resulted in considerably longer treatment responses and median survival in subgroups of patients with metastatic NSCLC.

The oligometastatic subgroup lacks a precise definition, but a common clinical cut-off point between oligometastases and polymetastases is the number of distant metastases, currently defined as one to five, in two or fewer organs. Eradication of all tumors with less invasive surgical and nonsurgical ablative techniques is becoming increasingly more feasible, thus leading to a growing interest in the incorporation of these techniques into the management of metastatic NSCLC.[126] Nevertheless, the only level I evidence that supports the existence of the oligometastatic state, and the value of aggressively managing the metastases, pertains only to patients presenting with a single brain metastasis.[127,128] Despite the common surgical management of isolated liver and lung metastases in colorectal cancer, this approach has never been prospectively evaluated and proven superior to systemic treatment only for lung cancer.

IMMUNE EFFECTS OF SABR FOR OLIGOMETASTASES

The biologic mechanisms of radiation-induced tumor cell death at fractions greater than 8 Gy to 10 Gy appear to be different from the classical radiobiology paradigms applied to conventionally fractionated radiotherapy.[129] Hypofractionated high-dose radiotherapy is associated with the activation of the innate and adaptive immune responses, enhancing the surface expression of major histocompatibility complex class I molecules and promoting the priming of antigen-specific dendritic cells.[130] High-dose radiotherapy can also increase the number of antigen-presenting cells.[131] The CD8 T-cell response appears to be essential for the antitumor effects of radiotherapy and contributes to the effect of radiotherapy on distant macroscopic disease, also termed an abscopal effect. The so-called abscopal effect is illustrated by preclinical data demonstrating T-cell–dependent antitumor effects in tumors that develop outside of treatment fields.[132]

CLINICAL RESULTS OF SABR FOR OLIGOMETASTASES

In an emerging body of nonrandomized data, SABR has been found to be a relatively nontoxic approach to controlling disease at multiple metastatic sites.[133] In general, patient selection criteria for SABR are broadly similar to those applied to surgical management of oligometastases, but without the requirement of fitness for surgical candidates.

Three distinct cohorts of patients with oligometastases can be identified: patients with oligometastatic disease at the time of diagnosis, patients with oligoprogressive disease after cytoreductive therapy, and patients with oligorecurrent disease after curative local–regional therapy.[134] However, varying criteria used for selecting patients with oligometastases hampers effective comparison, as does the wide range of dose–fractionation schedules used.[135] Clinical data on SABR outcomes in the three oligometastatic categories are mainly derived from retrospective or prospective phase I and II studies, which were not limited to patients with NSCLC. A common approach identifies oligometastatic as being fewer than five lesions, and occurring in no more than two or three different organs, as more extensive disease is associated with a poorer prognosis.[136,137]

The majority of patients with brain metastases from NSCLC have a poor prognosis if unfavorable factors such as extensive extracranial disease and/or poor performance status (Karnofsky score of less than 70) are present. In these patients with a poor prognosis, palliative treatments, including a short course of whole-brain radiotherapy (WBRT), are most appropriate. Several classification systems using prognostic factors such as performance status, control of primary tumor, activity of extracranial disease, and age have been developed in order to identify subsets of patients who may have long-term survival. These classification systems identify patients who are suitable for aggressive treatment of brain metastases; the recursive partitioning analysis classification and disease-specific graded prognostic assessment score are the most widely used for patient prognosis.[138,139]

As demonstrated in smaller studies, prolonged survival is possible for patients with a primary lung cancer with a limited number of synchronous brain metastases if both the brain and the primary tumor are treated aggressively.[136,140] Survival may be further improved in patients with oligometastases limited to the brain only.[141]

Radiosurgery refers to single-fraction stereotactic radiotherapy, and high-precision delivery of a single fraction of 18 Gy to 20 Gy to brain metastases results in local control rates of 60% to 90%. The introduction of so-called frameless radiosurgery, where dedicated mask systems replace use of invasive frames, has improved procedural logistics and lowered the threshold for performing radiosurgery. The role of adjuvant WBRT in addition to local ablative therapies for patients who have one to three brain metastases was addressed in a European Organisation for Research and Treatment of Cancer study. In this study, planned WBRT following either surgery or radiosurgery was reported to reduce intracranial events and neurologic death but failed to improve the duration of functional independence and overall survival.[142] These findings were corroborated in another randomized trial comparing stereotactic radiosurgery (SRS) alone with SRS and WBRT in patients with one to three brain metastases that showed less cognitive deterioration at 3 months with SRS alone and no difference in overall survival.[143] In select patients with as many as five brain metastases, a good performance score, and absence of progressive extracranial disease, advanced techniques integrating simultaneous treatment of WBRT and stereotactic radiosurgery may prolong local control.[144]

There is a considerable amount of literature on the use of SABR for treatment of lung metastases, with results of high rates of tumor control and limited toxicity.[145] A literature review showed that the number of synchronous lung metastases in most trials was between one and three, with limited experience in up to five lesions.[146] Regardless of the use of either single- or multiple-fraction SABR, the 2-year weighted rate of local control was approximately 78%, with a corresponding overall survival rate of 50% to 53%. Grade 3 or higher toxicities were seen in fewer than 4% of all patients. For patients with a single lung metastasis, surgical data from the International Registry of Lung Metastases showed an overall survival rate of 70% at 2 years and 36% at 5 years.[147] Comparable results for surgery and SABR in terms of local control and progression-free survival were found in a retrospective study, despite the fact that fitter patients, in general, were operated on.[148] Overall toxicity after SABR was scored as grade 3 to 5 for 0% to 15% of patients. A pooled analysis of 700 patients in Germany receiving SABR demonstrated 2-year local control and overall survival of 81% and 54%, respectively. There was grade 2 or worse pulmonary toxicity in 6.5% of patients.[149]

Adrenal Gland

Isolated adrenal metastases are not uncommon in NSCLC. Better median and overall survival rates were reported in a systematic review of outcomes after adrenalectomy.[150] Data on the use of SABR suggest that 1-year local control rates range from 55% to 66% with little toxicity, even though most studies have a limited sample size and short follow-up. The risk of adrenal insufficiency should be considered, especially if both glands need to be treated.[151–153]

Liver

A variety of ablative techniques, including RFA, transarterial chemoembolization, percutaneous ethanol injection, and SABR have been used to treat liver metastases from all primary tumors. Reported experience with isolated liver metastases from NSCLC is limited; several prospective studies of SABR have shown that local control rates of approximately 90% are possible, but follow-up in these studies is generally limited.[154–161]

Lymph Nodes

Safety and efficacy data on the use of SABR for hilar and mediastinal nodes are limited, and patients with lymph node metastases should preferably be treated in clinical trials. The available data suggest that SABR may achieve tumor control in cases of isolated and well-defined nodal recurrences, mainly from abdominal tumors, with out-of-field relapse developing in most patients.[133]

Vertebrae

The vertebrae are commonly involved in metastatic lung cancer, and this can result in spinal cord compression or cauda equina involvement. Although the use of SABR is growing for the management of vertebral oligometastasis, radioresistant spinal metastasis, and previously radiated but progressive spinal metastasis (Fig. 37.8), American College of Radiology appropriateness criteria state that more research is needed to validate the findings of the available phase I and II studies.[162] Phase II studies have been performed with either pain control or radiographic response as

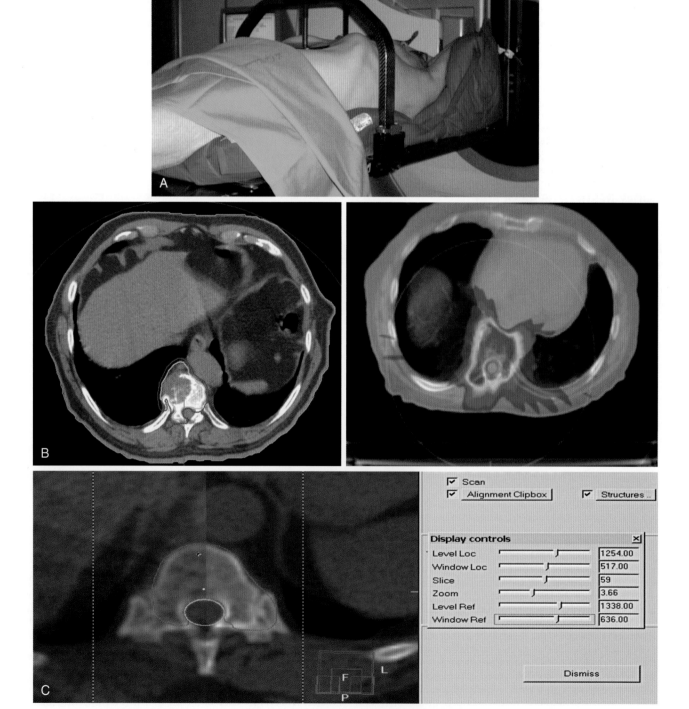

Fig. 37.8. Stereotactic ablative radiotherapy delivery for vertebral metastases, showing patient immobilization (A), highly conformal dose distribution with noticeable reduction in spinal cord (B), and delivery based on daily image guidance through cone-beam computed tomography (C).

study end points, but no randomized comparisons between conventionally fractionated radiotherapy and SABR have yet been published. The fractionation schedules used have varied widely, but local control and/or pain control rates of nearly 80% have been suggested by clinical evidence.[163]

Multiple Organs

Few studies have evaluated outcomes of local ablative strategies in selected patient cohorts with oligometastatic disease at the time of diagnosis, when only one of many metastases progresses during systemic treatment (oligoprogression), or when recurrence manifests in only one of multiple sites that had responded to initial therapy (oligorecurrence).

Two prospective pilot trials of SABR in limited oligometastatic disease enrolled 121 patients with five or fewer metastases.[164] Prior chemotherapy and radiotherapy were allowed, and most sites treated with SABR were in the lung, thoracic lymph nodes, and liver, with few brain metastases. For patients with cancer other than that of the breast, the 2-year overall survival and local control rates were 39% and 74%, respectively. Factors strongly associated with prolonged survival included the presence of one metastasis (compared with more than one) and smaller tumor volume.[164] Similarly, results from a prospective dose-escalation trial of SABR for patients with one to five lesions from various primary tumors have been reported.[165] Patients were included only if they had no brain metastases or had controlled brain disease, if they had no prior radiotherapy, or of if they had tumors smaller than 10 cm or more than 500 mL in volume. Toxicity was uncommon, and the maximum-tolerated dose was not reached in any cohort until a dose level of 48 Gy in three fractions. Patients with lung tumors comprised 26% of the 61 included patients, who had a total of 113 metastases. At a median follow-up of 20.9 months, the 2-year progression-free survival was 22%, with an overall survival of 56.7%. The authors did not find differences in outcomes between patients who had oligometastatic disease after induction therapy and patients who had de novo oligometastases. Patients with one to three metastases tended to have better outcomes than patients with four to five lesions, and disease progression after SABR mainly consisted of a limited number of new metastases.

In a prospective phase II study, which included 39 evaluable patients who had NSCLC with five or fewer metastases,[136] 87% had a single metastasis, and brain metastasis represented 44% of disease localizations. Thoracic disease was classified as stage IIIA in 23.1% of patients and as stage IIIB in 51.3%, and 95% received chemoradiotherapy for local–regional disease. Surgery or radiotherapy was permitted as local ablative treatment. The median overall survival was 13.5 months, and the median progression-free survival was 12.1 months.

Strategies for integrating systemic therapies with SABR have been reported for NSCLC and are based on the hypothesis that acquired resistance to tyrosine kinase inhibitors (TKIs) occurs in only a limited number of sites, the treatment of which may result in prolonged disease control.[166] A study was designed to investigate the effect of local therapies plus continuation of a TKI on the time to second progression. The study included 51 patients who had NSCLC with either anaplastic lymphoma kinase (*ALK*) gene rearrangement or epidermal growth factor receptor (*EGFR*) mutation, and who had oligoprogressive disease after first-line therapy with a TKI.[166] Among 25 patients treated with either crizotinib (15 patients) or erlotinib (10 patients) plus local surgery and/or radiotherapy to sites of progression, the median time to second progression was 6.2 months.

Another single-arm phase II analysis that showed promising results with the use of systemic therapy and SABR for oligometastatic disease included patients with stage IV NSCLC who failed early systemic therapy and had no more than six sites of extracranial disease. Patients were treated with erlotinib and concurrent SABR. Median progression-free survival was 14.7 months, and median overall survival was 20.4 months, both substantially higher than historical values for patients receiving systemic therapy alone.[167] These preliminary findings suggest that local ablative therapies may allow select patients to continue with the same systemic therapy. Comparable results were seen in another group of 18 patients with *EGFR* mutations and extracentral nervous system oligoprogression, treated either with surgery, RFA, or stereotactic radiosurgery plus continuation of a TKI.[168]

Given that the only randomized data to guide radiographic ablative management pertain to patients with brain metastases, more prospective controlled studies are needed to gain an understanding of the real effect of this strategy on clinical outcomes. Some clinical trials were ongoing at the time of publication (ClinicalTrials.gov identifiers: NCT01446744, NCT01345552, NCT01345539, NCT01565837, and NCT01185639). Advances in tumor biology and improved clinical knowledge on the oligometastatic state through improvements in imaging and molecular diagnostics are likely to be needed before progress can be made in treating patients with this disease presentation.

CONCLUSION

The recent advances in SABR have led to new treatment options for both early-stage NSCLC and oligometastatic disease. High-level population data are now available to support the role of SABR as the preferred treatment modality in early-stage NSCLC when patients are unfit for surgery or refuse to undergo the procedure. New randomized trials are underway to evaluate SABR versus surgery. When current SABR guidelines are adhered to, the results appear to be generalizable across centers. For oligometastatic NSCLC, more prospective data are required in order to establish the role of SABR in this setting.

KEY REFERENCES

3. Vansteenkiste J, De Ruysscher D, Eberhardt WE, et al. Early and locally advanced non-small-cell lung cancer (NSCLC): ESMO Clinical Practice Guidelines for diagnosis, treatment and follow-up. *Ann Oncol*. 2013;24(suppl 6):vi89–vi98.
17. Potters L, Kavanagh B, Galvin JM, et al. American Society for Therapeutic Radiology and Oncology (ASTRO) and American College of Radiology (ACR) practice guideline for the performance of stereotactic body radiation therapy. *Int J Radiat Oncol Biol Phys*. 2010;76(2):326–332.
18. Sahgal A, Roberge D, Schellenberg D, et al. The Canadian Association of Radiation Oncology scope of practice guidelines for lung, liver and spine stereotactic body radiotherapy. *Clin Oncol (R Coll Radiol)*. 2012;24(9):629–639.
19. Kirkbride P, Cooper T. Stereotactic body radiotherapy. Guidelines for commissioners, providers and clinicians: a national report. *Clin Oncol (R Coll Radiol)*. 2011;23(3):163–164.
20. Guckenberger M, Andratschke N, Alheit H, et al. Definition of stereotactic body radiotherapy: principles and practice for the treatment of stage I non-small cell lung cancer. *Strahlenther Onkol*. 2014;190(1):26–33.
30. Guckenberger M, Kestin LL, Hope AJ, et al. Is there a lower limit of pretreatment pulmonary function for safe and effective stereotactic body radiotherapy for early-stage non-small cell lung cancer? *J Thorac Oncol*. 2012;7(3):542–551.
38. Underberg RW, Lagerwaard FJ, Cuijpers JP, Slotman BJ, van Sörnsen de Koste JR, Senan S. Four-dimensional CT scans for treatment planning in stereotactic radiotherapy for stage I lung cancer. *Int J Radiat Oncol Biol Phys*. 2004;60(4):1283–1290.
41. Haasbeek CJ, Lagerwaard FJ, Cuijpers JP, Slotman BJ, Senan S. Is adaptive treatment planning required for stereotactic radiotherapy of stage I non-small-cell lung cancer? *Int J Radiat Oncol Biol Phys*. 2007;67(5):1370–1374.

54. Guckenberger M, Wilbert J, Krieger T, et al. Four-dimensional treatment planning for stereotactic body radiotherapy. *Int J Radiat Oncol Biol Phys*. 2007;69(1):276–285.

61. Senthi S, Haasbeek CJ, Slotman BJ, Senan S. Outcomes of stereotactic ablative radiotherapy for central lung tumours: a systematic review. *Radiother Oncol*. 2013;106(3):276–282.

65. Rieber J, Tonndorf-Martini E, Schramm O, et al. Establishing stereotactic body radiotherapy with flattening filter free techniques in the treatment of pulmonary lesions—initial experiences from a single institution. *Radiat Oncol*. 2016;11:80.

66. Haasbeek CJ, Lagerwaard FJ, Slotman BJ, Senan S. Outcomes of stereotactic ablative radiotherapy for centrally located early-stage lung cancer. *J Thorac Oncol*. 2011;6(12):2036–2043.

67. Network NCC: Non-Small Cell Lung Cancer (Version 4.2016).

68. Guckenberger M, Meyer J, Wilbert J, et al. Cone-beam CT based image-guidance for extracranial stereotactic radiotherapy of intrapulmonary tumors. *Acta Oncol*. 2006;45(7):897–906.

72. Nanda RH, Liu Y, Gillespie TW, et al. Stereotactic body radiation therapy versus no treatment for early stage non-small cell lung cancer in medically inoperable elderly patients: A National Cancer Data Base analysis. *Cancer*. 2015;121:4222–4230.

79. Timmerman R, Paulus R, Galvin J, et al. Stereotactic body radiation therapy for inoperable early stage lung cancer. *JAMA*. 2010;303(11):1070–1076.

81. Senthi S, Lagerwaard FJ, Haasbeek CJ, Slotman BJ, Senan S. Patterns of disease recurrence after stereotactic ablative radiotherapy for early stage non-small-cell lung cancer: a retrospective analysis. *Lancet Oncol*. 2012;13(8):802–809.

83. Chang JY, Senan S, Paul MA, et al. Stereotactic ablative radiotherapy versus lobectomy for operable stage I non-small-cell lung cancer: a pooled analysis of two randomised trials. *Lancet Oncol*. 2015;16:630–637.

92. Hunninghake GM, Hatabu H, Okajima Y, et al. MUC5B promoter polymorphism and interstitial lung abnormalities. *N Engl J Med*. 2013;368(23):2192–2200.

104. Scagliotti GV, Pastorino U, Vansteenkiste JF, et al. Randomized phase III study of surgery alone or surgery plus preoperative cisplatin and gemcitabine in stages IB to IIIA non-small-cell lung cancer. *J Clin Oncol*. 2012;30(2):172–178.

117. Khullar OV, Liu Y, Gillespie T, et al. Survival after sublobar resection versus lobectomy for clinical stage IA lung cancer: an analysis from the National Cancer Data Base. *J Thorac Oncol*. 2015;10:1625–1633.

127. Patchell RA, Tibbs PA, Walsh JW, et al. A randomized trial of surgery in the treatment of single metastases to the brain. *N Engl J Med*. 1990;322(8):494–500.

132. Demaria S, Kawashima N, Yang AM, et al. Immune-mediated inhibition of metastases after treatment with local radiation and CTLA-4 blockade in a mouse model of breast cancer. *Clin Cancer Res*. 2005;11(2 Pt 1):728–734.

136. De Ruysscher D, Wanders R, van Baardwijk A, et al. Radical treatment of non-small-cell lung cancer patients with synchronous oligometastases: long-term results of a prospective phase II trial (Nct01282450). *J Thorac Oncol*. 2012;7(10):1547–1555.

140. Lind JS, Lagerwaard FJ, Smit EF, Postmus PE, Slotman BJ, Senan S. Time for reappraisal of extracranial treatment options? Synchronous brain metastases from nonsmall cell lung cancer. *Cancer*. 2011;117(3):597–605.

143. Brown PD, Jaeckle K, Ballman KV, et al. Effect of radiosurgery alone vs radiosurgery with whole brain radiation therapy on cognitive function in patients with 1 to 3 brain metastases: a randomized clinical trial. *JAMA*. 2016;316:401–409.

See Expertconsult.com for full list of references.

38 Ablation Options for Localized Nonsmall Cell Lung Cancer

Carole A. Ridge and Stephen B. Solomon

SUMMARY OF KEY POINTS

- Since the initial identification of radiofrequency ablation (RFA) as the prototypical thermal ablation technique, it has been joined by microwave ablation, cryoablation, and, more recently, irreversible electroporation as potential options for tumor ablation.

- Factors that influence size of the ablation zone can be divided into probe and tissue characteristics. Probe characteristics can vary by the number of probes used, the use of internal cooling, and their configuration (linear or curved array). Tissue characteristics greatly influence the ablation zone size; lung tissue is prone to tissue dehydration when heat is applied. RFA in the lung can be impeded by tissue dehydration with resultant decreased electrical conductivity. Microwave energy, by contrast, can penetrate charred tissues, thus allowing continuous power application for the duration of the treatment and generation of very high temperatures in the lung.

- Thermal ablation can be offered to patients with medically inoperable stage I nonsmall cell lung cancer (NSCLC). Patients should be selected by an interdisciplinary team, and the maximum tumor diameter should probably not exceed 3 cm to 3.5 cm.

- Aside from its use in stage I lung cancer, RFA is useful for the treatment for patients with a solitary pulmonary nodule remaining after standard therapy of a stage IIIa or IV NSCLC; for salvage therapy of residual or recurrent disease after resection, chemotherapy, and/or radiation; and for pulmonary metastases where the primary disease is controlled in a patient who is a poor surgical candidate.

- Major complications from RFA are rare. The reported rate of major complications is 9.8% and comprises pleuritis, pneumonia, lung abscess, hemorrhage, and pneumothorax requiring pleurodesis.

- Reported 3-year and 5-year survival rates after RFA range from 36% to 88% and from 19% to 27%, respectively. Estimated 3-year cancer-specific survival ranges from 59% to 88%.

- The expected postablation findings on computed tomography include a residual nodule, fibrosis, atelectasis, and cavitation.

Radiofrequency ablation (RFA) was first described with use of a modified Bovie knife in the liver in animal studies published in 1990.[1,2] Subsequent descriptions of successful ablation of liver tumors in the mid-1990s elicited interest in using the technique in other organs.[3,4] RFA in the lung was first found to be safe and efficacious in animal studies in both healthy lung and VX2 sarcomas in the lungs of rabbits.[5,6] Successful use of RFA for lung tumors in humans was described in 2000 in a study of patients with inoperable NSCLC.[7] RFA has since been adopted as a treatment alternative for patients with early stage NSCLC who are unable to undergo surgical resection. Since the initial identification of RFA as the prototypical thermal ablation technique, it has been joined by microwave ablation, cryoablation, and, more recently, irreversible electroporation as potential options for tumor ablation.

MECHANISM OF ACTION OF ABLATION TECHNIQUES

Radiofrequency Ablation

Radiofrequency refers to the portion of the electromagnetic spectrum from 3 Hz to 300 GHz.[8] Thermal ablation using RFA occurs as a result of delivery of an electrical current to tumor cells surrounding the RFA probe tip. Molecules adjacent to the tip are forced to vibrate rapidly, thus creating frictional energy loss between adjacent molecules (Fig. 38.1). These energy losses are manifested as a rise in tissue temperature, known as the Joule effect. Tissues nearest to the electrode are heated most effectively, whereas more peripheral areas are heated by thermal conduction.

Thermal ablation with RFA results in coagulative necrosis. Once cytotoxic temperatures are achieved in the ablation zone, denaturation of intracellular proteins and destruction of the cell-membrane lipid bilayer result in irreversible cell death.[9,10] Heat is transferred from cells immediately adjacent to the electrode tip away from the electrode by thermal conduction. A temperature at the electrode tip above 60°C is needed to achieve cell death.[11,12] Tissue conductivity can, however, be impaired at temperatures above 95°C. Such overheating leads to boiling of the water-predominant tissues, causing steam formation, tissue charring, and a sharp rise in tissue impedance, thereby limiting the effectiveness of RFA.[13,14] Therefore the aim of thermal tumor ablation is to achieve a temperature range of 50°C to 100°C throughout the entire target volume for 4 minutes to 6 minutes without charring or vaporizing tissues.[15] Multiapplicator ablation is possible by rapidly switching from one electrode to another during electrode activation. The radiofrequency circuit requires a return path from the ablation probe tip. This return path consists of two to four grounding pads applied to the patient's skin. The grounding pads disperse current over a much wider surface area than the probe tip, which is therefore the only site of tissue damage.

Microwave Ablation

When an electromagnetic frequency of either 915 MHz or 2.45 GHz is applied to tissue, some of the energy forces molecules with an intrinsic dipole moment, such as water molecules, to continuously realign with the applied field. This rotation of molecules increases kinetic energy and local tissue temperatures in a process known as dielectric hysteresis (Fig. 38.2).[16] Tissue destruction occurs when tissues are heated to lethal temperatures, which can reach up to 150°C. Microwave power does not rely on electrical conductivity and can therefore penetrate tissues of low electric conductivity, such as lung and desiccated or charred tissue. The high temperatures achievable at the probe tip improve ablation efficacy by increasing thermal conduction into the surrounding tissues. Because it is not part of an electrical circuit, microwave ablation does not require grounding pads. Multiapplicator ablation is possible with microwave energy, and, unlike with RFA, this can be powered continuously without switching from one electrode to another during electrode activation. Also unique to microwave ablation is the ability to use multiple antennas, which are positioned and phased to exploit overlap of the electromagnetic field.[17]

Cryoablation

Cryoablation involves rapid cooling of the tissues by means of the Joule–Thompson effect, whereby rapid expansion of a high-pressure gas results in a change in the temperature of the gas.[18,19] When the gas, typically argon, reaches the distal tip of the cryoablation probe, it is forced through a narrow opening and rapidly expands at atmospheric pressure, leading to rapid cooling. This process occurs inside the needle so that the patient is not directly exposed to the emitted gas. The probe is then sequentially warmed and cooled again, to augment cellular damage. Warming is performed by the release of high-pressure helium through the probe tip, which increases in temperature when released into the atmosphere.[19,20]

During rapid tissue cooling, water is trapped within the cellular membrane, resulting in intracellular ice formation. When the temperature is maintained below the freezing point of water, intracellular ice formation can cause recrystallization and extension of the ice within the intracellular matrix. Alternatively, if gradual cooling occurs, extracellular ice crystals form, which sequester extracellular water. During the thawing cycle, water returns to the intracellular space and causes cellular lysis and enzymatic and membrane dysfunction (Fig. 38.3). As a secondary effect in the adjacent tissues, intracellular ice crystal formation in blood vessels causes damage to the vascular endothelial cells. Reperfusion in the post-thaw period recruits platelets, which contact the damaged endothelium, resulting in thrombosis and ischemia.[21,22] With each successive freeze–thaw cycle, tissue cooling is faster, and the volume of frozen tissue and extent of tissue destruction are enlarged.[15] The optimal temperature to ensure tumor death is around –50°C. Cryoablation has an advantage over other thermal ablation modalities in that the ice ball created during cryoablation is visible on computed tomography (CT) images, allowing the operator to monitor the extent of ablation.[23]

Irreversible Electroporation

Irreversible electroporation is a nonthermal technique for tumor ablation that causes irreversible damage to the cell membrane by applying pulsed electric fields of up to 3 kV/cm to the ablation target, thereby inducing cell death.[24,25] The cellular lipid bilayer is disrupted by these high-voltage electrical currents because of the formation of permanent nanopores, which in

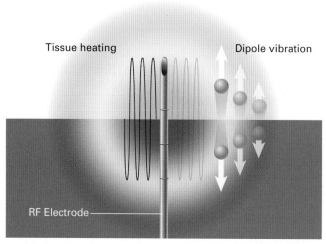

Fig. 38.1. Mechanism of action of radiofrequency (RF) ablation. Molecules adjacent to the tip are forced to vibrate rapidly, thus creating frictional energy loss between adjacent molecules that is manifested as a rise in tissue temperature. *(Reprinted with permission from Hong K, Georgiades C. Radiofrequency ablation: mechanism of action and devices. J Vasc Interv Radiol. 2010;21(8 Suppl):S179–S186.)*

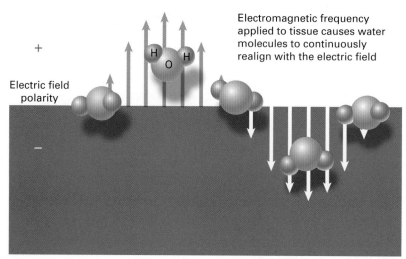

Fig. 38.2. Mechanism of action of microwave ablation. Electromagnetic frequency is applied to the target tissue, forcing water molecules to continuously realign with the applied field. This rotation of molecules increases kinetic energy and local tissue temperatures in a process known as dielectric hysteresis. *(Reprinted with permission from Brace CL. Radiofrequency and microwave ablation of the liver, lung, kidney, and bone: what are the differences? Curr Probl Diagn Radiol. 2009;38(3):135–143.)*

turn disrupt cellular homeostasis (Fig. 38.4).[26] Irreversible electroporation has two theoretical advantages over thermal ablation: (1) because it is nonthermal, the heat-sink phenomenon is not observed; and (2) irreversible electroporation theoretically preserves tissue interfaces and therefore is thought to spare sensitive structures such as the airways and nerve sheaths.[16] Its use in the lung has not been fully studied in humans, but its potential for preserving airways and mediastinal vessels makes it an attractive future option for the treatment of unresectable lung tumors in anatomically sensitive locations. Irreversible electroporation must be performed using general anesthesia with complete neuromuscular blockade, to avoid generalized muscle contractions. High-voltage pulses are delivered with electrocardiographic gating to minimize the risk of cardiac arrhythmias.[26] Further research is needed before the clinical application of this interesting technology can be optimized.

TECHNICAL FACTORS INFLUENCING SIZE OF THE ABLATION ZONE

Factors that influence size of the ablation zone can be divided into probe and tissue characteristics.

Probe Characteristics

Probe characteristics include electrode exposure length, number of probes, treatment duration, maximum temperature reached, type of energy used, and energy pulsing and cooling (in the case of RFA). Length of the RFA zone has been shown to increase proportionally using exposure lengths of up to 3 cm in the liver. Above this tip size, however, a cylindric ablation zone is not achieved and heterogeneity is more often observed, leading to a dumbbell-shaped ablation zone.[27] To offset this limitation, more than one probe can be used to produce overlapping ablation zones in larger or nonspherical lesions.[28] Umbrella-configuration RFA probes with multiple hooked arrays have also allowed the creation of larger ablation zones.[29] In addition, the size of the ablation zone increases linearly in proportion to the probe gauge size from 24G to 18G. Treatment duration is proportional to ablation zone volume up to a maximum of 6 minutes using RFA in the liver, but no additional benefit is achieved by using ablation times beyond 6 minutes.[27,30]

To avoid the deleterious effects of tissue vaporization and charring and to increase the size of the ablation zone, internally cooled probe tips have been devised, whereby chilled saline is pumped through the shaft of the needle.[31] Saline infusion of microwave ablation probes has also been shown to produce larger ablation zones in the lung and liver.[32] However, the viscosity of water can limit flow and cooling capacity in small-diameter microwave antennas,[33] and therefore compressed gas may be used to cool the microwave probe.[34] Similar advantages have been described using a pulsed RFA system, whereby cyclic periods of low-current deposition are alternated with higher peak currents; this strategy allows the tissues to rehydrate during the ablation, thus reducing tissue impedance and charring.[35] High levels of impedance at the ablation probe tip (e.g., >1000 ohm) can also be fed back to the radiofrequency generator and inhibit RFA impulse generation. As mentioned earlier, radiofrequency technology allows the combination of multiple probes to achieve a larger, more confluent ablation zone over a shorter treatment duration than with sequential ablation.[36]

The type of energy applied influences the size of the ablation zone and the time required to reach an ablative temperature. Radiofrequency relies on both electrical and thermal conductivity. Heating a tissue to temperatures near or above 100°C causes water to boil and evaporate, leading to tissue dehydration and altered electrical conductivity (e.g., charred tissue), which inhibits the flow of electrical current. Microwave energy, by contrast, can penetrate charred or desiccated tissues, thus allowing continuous power application for the duration of the treatment, generation of very high temperatures, and less susceptibility to heat-sink effects than radiofrequency energy. These high temperatures can be reflected along the probe shaft, raising concerns about fistula formation and skin burns at the needle entry site; these complications can be avoided by using shorter ablation sessions and cooled antenna devices.[33,37,38]

Tissue Characteristics

The electrical, thermal, and mechanical properties of the ablated tissue are largely dependent on water content and cellular makeup. Normal lung tissue, when compared with the liver, has lower electrical and thermal conductivity, relative permittivity, and effective conductivity. A low level of electrical and thermal

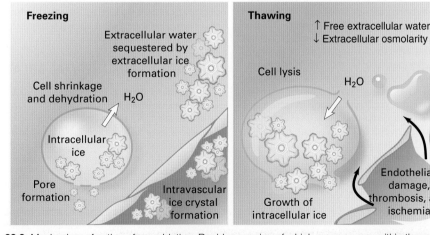

Fig. 38.3. Mechanism of action of cryoablation. Rapid expansion of a high-pressure gas within the cryotherapy probe tip results in rapid cooling within the ablation target; water is trapped within the cellular membranes, resulting in intracellular ice formation. If gradual cooling occurs, extracellular ice crystal formation sequesters extracellular water. During the thawing cycle, water returning to the intracellular space causes cellular lysis and cellular enzymatic and membrane dysfunction. Intracellular ice crystal formation in adjacent blood vessels causes damage to endothelial cells. *(Reprinted with permission from Erinjeri JP, Clark TW. Cryoablation: mechanism of action and devices. J Vasc Interv Radiol. 2010;21(8 Suppl):S187–S191.)*

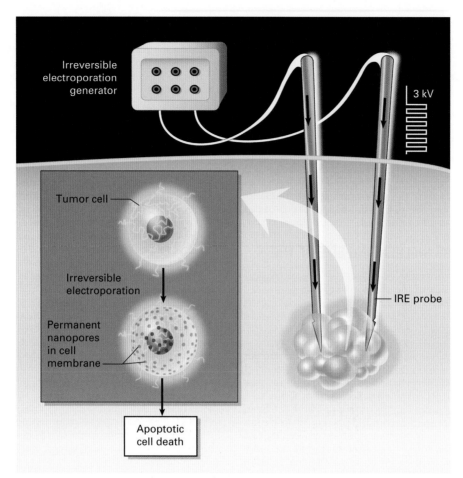

Fig. 38.4. Mechanism of action of irreversible electroporation (IRE). Pulsed electric fields are applied to the ablation target, thereby creating permanent nanopores in the cellular lipid bilayer, which in turn disrupt cellular homeostasis.

conductivity limits the flow of radiofrequency energy.[39] Lung tumors have relatively densely packed cells and therefore behave similar to solid organs, with higher conductivity than adjacent lung tissue. Enhanced heating has been observed in experimental models at the interface between these tissues (e.g., tumor and aerated lung), but the clinical application of this feature has not been elucidated.[40] Microwave ablation takes advantage of the low relative permittivity and effective conductivity of the lung and as a result leads to deeper penetration than in solid organs. Cryoablation relies on thermal conductivity and ice-ball formation, and because most tissues have a high water content, thermal conductivity is usually good. However, cryoablation in the lung is limited by its inherently low thermal conductivity. Nevertheless, this drawback is progressively overcome as ice-ball formation progresses, which increases the thermal conductivity of the ablation target.[41] Cryoablation in the lung produces an ablation zone slightly smaller than that produced in the kidney but larger than that produced in the liver.[42]

Heat Sink

Blood vessels within the target tissue provide a source of convective tissue cooling (or heating in the case of cryoablation) known as heat sink. Heat sink theoretically applies to all methods of thermal ablation, but is clinically observed in varying degrees. Vessel size within the target tissue is a major determinant of this effect. The presence of vessels larger than 3 mm in diameter in direct contact with the ablation target was reported to be associated with decreased coagulation necrosis in RFA and an increased rate of local recurrence in the liver and lung, respectively.[43,44] Microwave ablation appears to be less sensitive to the heat-sink effect because of a greater magnitude of heating and better tissue penetration than with RFA.[45] Cryoablation, which relies on thermal conductivity, has not shown a measurable heat-sink effect in the lung or liver.[22,46]

INDICATIONS FOR THERMAL ABLATION

The standard of care for stage I NSCLC is surgical resection. However, only one-third of patients are eligible for surgical intervention.[47] Thermal ablation can be offered to patients with medically inoperable stage I NSCLC using standards described by the Society of Interventional Radiology.[48] Patients should be selected by an interdisciplinary team, and the maximum tumor diameter should probably not exceed 3 cm to 3.5 cm.[49]

Because the duration of clinical experience and the volume of published data are greater for RFA than for other ablation modalities, RFA has received endorsement by means of clinical guidelines.[50] However, microwave ablation is likely to be increasingly used for NSCLC because of its theoretical advantages over RFA, including a less severe heat-sink effect and faster, greater heating. Cryoablation and irreversible electroporation have not yet been formally recommended for use in lung tumor ablation outside of a research setting.[23,51]

Aside from its use in stage I lung cancer, RFA has been identified as useful for the following: treatment for patients with a solitary pulmonary nodule remaining after standard therapy of a stage IIIa or IV NSCLC; salvage therapy of residual or recurrent disease after resection, chemotherapy, and/or radiation;[52] and pulmonary metastases where the primary disease is controlled in a patient who is a poor surgical candidate.[53] Combined RFA therapy and inhibition of the epidermal growth factor receptor (EGFR) receptor may also confer a benefit in the treatment of patients who have NSCLC with an EGFR mutation and acquired resistance to EGFR tyrosine kinase inhibitors in one or more metastases.[54]

COMPLICATIONS OF THERMAL ABLATION

Pneumothorax is the most commonly reported complication for all thermal modalities.[55] Self-limited pneumothorax had a reported incidence of 22.4% after RFA, and pneumothorax requiring chest tube insertion (but not pleurodesis) had a similar incidence (22.1%) in a retrospective study of 1000 patients.[55] Major complications from RFA are rare. The reported rate of major complications is 9.8% and comprises aseptic pleuritis, pneumonia, lung abscess, hemorrhage, and pneumothorax requiring pleurodesis.[55] Rarer major complications include bronchopleural fistula, tumor seeding, and nerve or diaphragmatic injury (<0.5% incidence). The reported mortality rate after RFA for lung tumors is 0.4%. Nerve injury has an incidence of 0.2% to 0.3%, affecting the phrenic, brachial, left recurrent laryngeal, and intercostal nerves and the stellate ganglion.[56]

The literature on microwave ablation includes reports of similar complication rates, including self-limited pneumothorax (27%), pneumothorax requiring chest tube insertion (12%), and skin burns (3%).[32] Although not commonly reported in the literature on RFA, skin burns have been described in two patients who had microwave ablation, one of whom required debridement and chest wall reconstruction, presumably due to shaft heating.[32] Intraprocedural or periprocedural death has not been described after microwave ablation. One death was reported from a delayed infectious complication at 6 months after microwave ablation.[57] Bronchopleural fistula has also been reported as a rare complication of microwave ablation, although endobronchial valve insertion is reported to be a potential therapy for fistulas.[58,59]

Complications from cryotherapy of lung tumors are similar to those of previously described ablation modalities. The risk of hemorrhage with cryotherapy is theoretically greater because this procedure lacks the cautery effect of heat-based ablation. Two studies of cryoablation-related complications reported hemoptysis in 36.8% to 55.4% and massive hemoptysis in 0% to 0.6%.[60,61] Pneumothorax and pleural effusion are the most common complications, with incidence rates of 61.7% and 70.5%, respectively. Less common complications include phrenic nerve palsy, frostbite, and empyema (0.5% each), and tumor seeding (0.2%).

Pulmonary function testing after RFA has been described in the literature. One study reported impairment of vital capacity and forced expiratory volume at 1 second at both 1 month and 3 months after ablation. In this study, severe pleuritis and ablation of a large volume of adjacent parenchyma were shown to be independently associated with a decline in pulmonary function. However, two other studies reported no deterioration in pulmonary function at 3 months, 6 months, or 24 months, which suggests that the functional impact of RFA may be transient.[62–64]

Careful patient selection may minimize the risk of complications. For example, in the largest case series that included a report of complications after RFA, previous systemic chemotherapy was a significant risk factor for aseptic pleuritis, and prior external-beam radiotherapy and advanced age were significant risk factors

for pneumonia. Patients with emphysema had a greater predilection for lung abscess and pneumothorax requiring pleurodesis. Finally, serum platelet count (≤180,000 cells/µL) and tumor size (>3 cm) are significant predictors of hemorrhage ($p < 0.002$ and 0.02, respectively).[65]

REPORTED OUTCOMES OF THERMAL ABLATION

Survival and Recurrence

The literature analyzing outcomes after RFA as a therapy for stage I primary NSCLC is limited by study size and population heterogeneity in terms of concomitant treatments administered (e.g., chemotherapy and in-field radiation) and selection bias.[66,67] The latter relates to the fact that long-term survival data are strongly influenced by medical comorbidity. For example, the all-cause mortality rate for patients with inoperable early stage lung carcinoma (19.1%) is substantially higher than that of operable patients (3.4%).[68] Therefore, lung cancer–specific survival and disease-free intervals may be better measures of treatment outcome. With allowance for these limitations, recurrence rates after RFA of stage I NSCLC were reported in 11 studies; the aggregate rate of local progression was 24% (95 of 403 patients)[63,64,67,69–74] and the rate of metastasis at any site was 31% (42 of 137; Table 38.1).[63,67,69,71,72] Reported 3-year and 5-year survival rates ranged from 36% to 88%[67,70,72–74] and from 19% to 27%, respectively.[63,67,75] Estimated 3-year cancer-specific survival ranged from 59% to 88%.[63,67,70,73] Patients with synchronous and metachronous primary NSCLCs were also reported to have similar local control rates and survival outcomes.[76] The cellular subtype previously called bronchioloalveolar carcinoma (now referred to as adenocarcinoma in situ or minimally invasive adenocarcinoma) may have a better prognosis after RFA. Lanuti et al.[72] described a 90% local control rate of bronchioloalveolar carcinoma after RFA, compared with 68.5% for all cell types.

Most of the literature on microwave ablation and cryoablation includes patients with both primary lung and metastatic lesions who were treated for varied indications (for both local control and palliation). The outcomes of patients with early stage lung cancer are not uniformly reported separately from those of patients with metastases; therefore firm data on long-term survival for stage I NSCLC treated with microwave ablation and cryoablation are currently lacking. Three retrospective studies report an aggregate local recurrence rate of 30% (27/90). Reported 3-year and 5-year survival rates were 43% to 48% and 28%, respectively. Estimated 3-year cancer-specific survival is reported in one study to be 65%.[77,78] Two small studies included reports of outcomes for patients with stage I lung cancer treated with cryoablation and described local recurrence rates of 3% and 11%, respectively, overall 3-year survival rates of 77% and 88%, respectively,[66,79] and a 3-year cancer-specific survival of 90.2%.[67]

Surveillance

CT is the most common modality used for surveillance after ablation of lung cancer. After an initial increase in size due to inflammation during the first 2 months, the ablation zone is expected to decrease in size. The expected findings on CT include the following: (1) a residual nodule; (2) fibrosis, which usually has an elongated linear appearance; (3) atelectasis; and (4) cavitation (Fig. 38.5). Cavitation occurs more frequently in patients with NSCLC near the chest wall or with emphysema.[81] Complete disappearance of the opacity at the ablation site is rarely observed.[82] Positron emission tomography (PET)–CT at 24 hours and at 1 month after ablation can demonstrate tracer activity at the ablation site, despite adequate treatment,

TABLE 38.1   Outcomes of Patients With Stage I Primary Nonsmall Cell Lung Cancer After Thermal Ablation as a Primary Therapy

Author	Year of Publication	Modality	No. of Tumors	Median Size (range), mm	2-Y Survival, %	3-Y Survival, %	5-Y Survival, %	3-Y CSS, %	No. of Tumors With Local Progression, %	No. of Tumors With Any Metastasis, %
Pennathur et al.[69]	2007	RFA	19	26[a] (16–38)	68	NR	NR	NR	3 (16)	NR
Hiraki et al.[70]	2007	RFA	20	20 (13–60)	84	83	NR	83	7 (35)	4 (20)
Simon et al.[74]	2007	RFA	80	30[a] (10–75)	57	36	27	NR	NR	NR
Hsie et al.[71]	2009	RFA	12	NR	NR	NR	NR	NR	1 (8)	4 (33)
Lanuti et al.[72]	2009	RFA	34[a]	20[a] (8–44)	78	47	NR	NR	12 (35)	15 (44)
Zemlyak et al.[67]	2010	RFA	12	NR	NR	87.5	19	87.5	4 (33)	3 (25)
Hiraki et al.[73]	2011	RFA	52	21[a] (7–60)	86	74	NR	80	16 (31)	NR
Ambrogi et al.[63]	2011	RFA	59[a]	26 (11–50)	NR	NR	25	59	13 (22)	16 (27)
Dupuy et al.[64]	2013	RFA	52	NR	70	NR	NR	NR	19 (37)	NR
Liu et al.[76]	2013	MWA	15	24 (8–40)	NR	NR	NR	NR	5 (33)	NR
Zemlyak et al.[67]	2010	Cryoablation	27	NR	NR	77	77	90.2	3 (11)	2 (7)
Yamauchi et al.[79]	2011	Cryoablation	34	14 (5–30)	88	88	NR	NR	1 (3)	6 (18)

[a]Mean value.
CSS, cancer-specific survival; *MWA*, microwave ablation; *NR*, not reported; *RFA*, radiofrequency ablation.

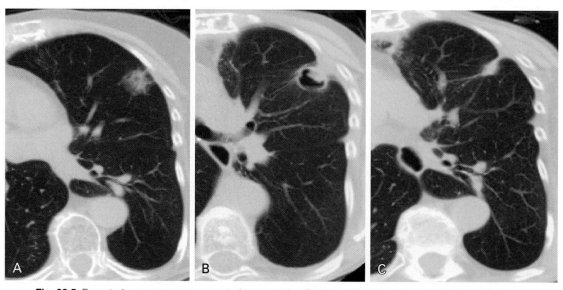

Fig. 38.5. Expected appearance on computed tomography after thermal ablation. At 1 month after radiofrequency ablation of a stage I adenocarcinoma in the left upper lobe (A), the ablation zone exhibits perilesional ground-glass opacity; cavitation can then develop within 6 months (B), followed by fibrosis, which has an elongated linear appearance (C).

as a result of inflammation. This is expected to resolve by 3 months after ablation.[83] The absence of tracer activity at the site of ablation on PET–CT at 6 months after ablation has been shown to correlate better with clinical outcome at 1 year than does PET–CT performed 4 days after ablation.[84] The expected appearance on early PET–CT is that of a ring or halo of low peripheral activity in the ablation zone with central photopenia, which may persist until 6 months but should resolve by 12 months (Fig. 38.6).[85]

Residual disease or recurrence of disease should be considered if imaging shows increasing uptake of contrast material in the ablation zone, growth of peripheral nodules, a change within the ablation zone from ground-glass opacity to solid opacity, enlargement of regional or distant lymph nodes, new sites of intrathoracic disease, or new extrathoracic disease. Other signs include increased metabolic activity on PET–CT more than 3 months after ablation (Fig. 38.7) or residual metabolic activity centrally or in a nodular pattern.[10]

TREATMENT CONSIDERATIONS

Identifying the Ideal Candidate for Ablation

Characteristics of the patient and lung lesion are important factors in selecting the ideal candidate for ablation. Ablation of stage I primary NSCLC can be considered for patients who are not candidates for curative surgical resection as a result of cardiorespiratory comorbidity or insufficient vital lung function. Patients being considered for ablation should have an Eastern Cooperative Oncology Group performance status of less than

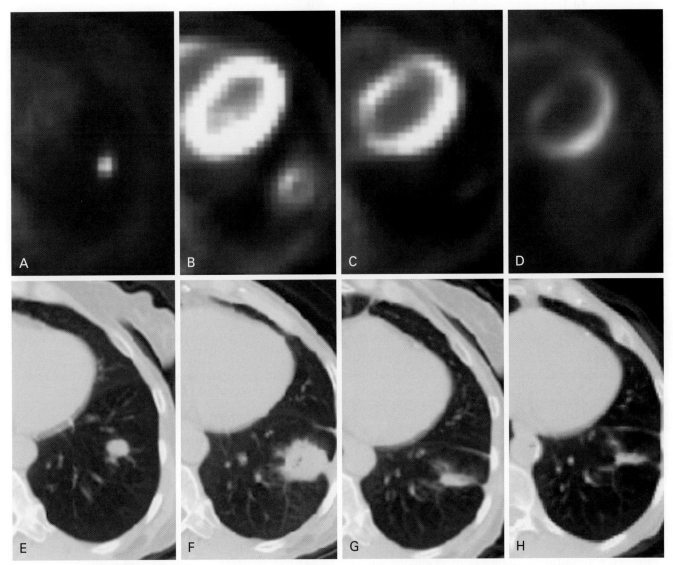

Fig. 38.6. Expected appearance on positron emission tomography–computed tomography after thermal ablation. (A–D) Nonfused PET images and (E–H) CT images of a left lower lobe adenocarcinoma before (A and E) and after radiofrequency ablation at surveillance periods of 4 months, 9 months, and 42 months exhibit a halo of low peripheral activity in the ablation zone with central photopenia at 4 months, which resolves by 9 months and remains photopenic at 42 months, indicating successful ablation.

3 and a life expectancy of more than 1 year.[86,87] Lesions larger than 3 cm have a higher incidence of tumor recurrence.[88] Lesions within 1 cm of sensitive structures such as the trachea, main bronchi, esophagus, and central vessels are associated with a higher risk of complications and may often receive incomplete ablation because of the heat-sink effect.[47]

Immunologic Effects

Spontaneous regression of untreated prostate and liver tumors has been reported after thermal ablation.[89–91] Damaged cells are thought to trigger an alarm to the immune system, which protects against self-damage, for example, in the setting of cell death due to necrosis. In particular, heat-shock proteins chaperone antigenic peptides of the cells from which they are derived and stimulate the maturation of dendritic cells, inducing the production of antigen-specific T cells.[92,93] Thermal ablation therefore represents an opportunity to induce antitumor immunity. This immunity is weak, however, and would not eradicate established

tumors if used as a sole therapy. Thermal ablation may be used in the future in combination with chemotherapeutic or immunotherapeutic agents to treat tumors.[94] Serologic evidence of an immune response has been documented after ablation of renal, lung, liver, soft tissue, and bone tumors, and this leads to an elevation of serum cytokine interleukin-6 and interleukin-10 levels, which are attractive potential targets for immunotherapy.[95]

Thermal Ablation in Combination With Adjunctive Therapies

Combined therapy using thermal ablation and radiotherapy may act synergistically to improve survival compared with either modality alone. In one study, thermal ablation followed by external-beam radiotherapy was given to 41 patients with inoperable stage I or II NSCLC. The local recurrence rate was 11.8% for tumors smaller than 3 cm and 33.3% for larger tumors, with an acceptably low complication rate of combined therapy.[96] A smaller series of 24 patients treated with a combination of RFA

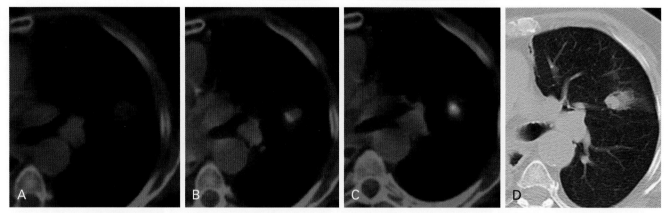

Fig. 38.7. Positron emission tomography–computed tomography (PET–CT) appearance of local recurrence after thermal ablation. This patient with left upper lobe squamous cell carcinoma after right pneumonectomy had radiofrequency ablation followed by PET–CT immediately after ablation (A) and 3 months after ablation (B, C). Residual tumor is demonstrated in the medial aspect of the lesion, where increasing metabolic activity and peripheral nodular opacity are shown (C, D).

and adjuvant external-beam radiotherapy resulted in a local recurrence rate of 9%.[96] However, the use of external-beam radiotherapy with RFA increases the potential for toxicity to normal lung tissue by ionizing radiation. A potential solution to this problem may be the use of brachytherapy to optimize local control while also sparing normal lung tissue. RFA followed by high-dose-rate brachytherapy, delivered via a catheter, yielded good local control in 82% of treated patients while lowering the risk of pulmonary toxicity.[98] The synergistic effect is thought to be due to the fact that thermal ablation is most effective in the central portion of the tumor, whereas radiation is better at treating tumor margins; in addition, thermal ablation causes neovascularity, whereby superoxide anions and free radicals form and cause DNA damage; this process is also thought to enhance the effect of radiotherapy.[87]

CONCLUSION

The field of ablation is evolving because of improved devices and greater operator experience. Ablation offers an effective way to treat localized NSCLC while limiting damage to the adjacent normal lung. Ablation options for the treatment of localized NSCLC include RFA, microwave ablation, and cryotherapy. Irreversible electroporation is a novel ablation method with potential application to lung tumors in sensitive locations and merits further research. The mechanism of action of each ablation technique differs based on the ablation modality used and the tissue to which it is applied. Understanding these aspects for each modality is essential for their effective and safe use. Selection of appropriate candidates is based on patient and lesion characteristics and influences clinical outcomes in terms of local recurrence, survival, and complication rates. Thermal ablation can be offered to patients with medically inoperable stage I NSCLC. Suitable lesions are selected based on a size of less than 3 cm to 3.5 cm and a location that avoids sensitive structures and minimizes the heat-sink effect. Clinical outcomes after RFA of stage I NSCLC are good in terms of local recurrence rate and cancer-specific survival. Thermal ablation therefore offers a therapeutic alternative for patients who are ineligible for surgical intervention. Long-term data after treatment

with microwave ablation and cryotherapy are awaited. Imaging surveillance after ablation of lung tumors includes both anatomic and metabolic imaging. The ablated lesion exhibits typical features on CT and PET, which evolve over time. Future directions for lung tumor ablation include combined approaches using thermal ablation and other therapies, which may synergistically improve clinical outcomes compared with either therapy alone.

KEY REFERENCES

1. McGahan JP, Browning PD, Brock JM, Tesluk H. Hepatic ablation using radiofrequency electrocautery. *Invest Radiol.* 1990;25(3): 267–270.
5. Goldberg SN, Gazelle GS, Compton CC, McLoud TC. Radiofrequency tissue ablation in the rabbit lung: efficacy and complications. *Acad Radiol.* 1995;2(9):776–784.
10. Abtin FG, Eradat J, Gutierrez AJ, Lee C, Fishbein MC, Suh RD. Radiofrequency ablation of lung tumors: imaging features of the post-ablation zone. *Radiographics.* 2012;32(4):947–969.
11. Goldberg SN, Gazelle GS, Mueller PR. Thermal ablation therapy for focal malignancy: a unified approach to underlying principles, techniques, and diagnostic imaging guidance. *AJR Am J Roentgenol.* 2000;174(2):323–331.
32. Wolf FJ, Grand DJ, Machan JT, Dipetrillo TA, Mayo-Smith WW, Dupuy DE. Microwave ablation of lung malignancies: effectiveness, CT findings, and safety in 50 patients. *Radiology.* 2008;247(3): 871–879.
49. Pereira PL, Masala S. Cardiovascular and Interventional Radiological Society of Europe (CIRSE). Standards of practice: guidelines for thermal ablation of primary and secondary lung tumors. *Cardiovasc Intervent Radiol.* 2012;35(2):247–254.
50. National Institute for Health and Care Excellence. http://www.nice.org.uk/nicemedia/live/11206/52082/52082.pdf.
65. Kashima M, Yamakado K, Takaki H, et al. Complications after 1000 lung radiofrequency ablation sessions in 420 patients: a single center's experiences. *AJR Am J Roentgenol.* 2011;197:W576–W580.
66. Belfiore G, Moggio G, Tedeschi E, et al. CT-guided radiofrequency ablation: a potential complementary therapy for patients with unresectable primary lung cancer—a preliminary report of 33 patients. *AJR Am J Roentgenol.* 2004;183(4):1003–1011.

See Expertconsult.com for full list of references.

39 Radiotherapy for Locally Advanced Nonsmall Cell Lung Cancer Including Combined Modality

Paul Van Houtte, Hak Choy, Shinji Nakamichi, Kaoru Kubota, and Francoise Mornex

SUMMARY OF KEY POINTS

- Concerning radiotherapy, higher physical or biologic dose (altered fractionation) is associated with better local control and, in some trials, with better survival. Current evidence favors a schedule of 60 Gy to 66 Gy in 6 weeks to 7 weeks, with no benefit for doses beyond that.
- Concurrent chemoradiation therapy is the optimal treatment strategy with curative intent for fit patients not candidates for surgery.
- Currently, there is no place for adding a molecularly targeted agent to the combined-modality regimens outside a clinical trial, which should select patients based on the relevant biomarker.
- The choice between surgery and chemoradiotherapy should be discussed within a multidisciplinary tumor board based on patient comorbidity and preferences, and prognostic factors.
- Prophylactic cranial radiation is not recommended as a standard therapy.

Stage III disease accounts for one-third of all lung cancers and comprises the most heterogeneous group of tumors in terms of clinical presentation and treatment options.[1,2] Two articles published in 2012 highlight the debate and controversy about managing stage IIIA nonsmall cell lung cancer (NSCLC).[3,4] Among thoracic surgeons surveyed, 84% of thoracic surgeons favored neoadjuvant therapy followed by surgery for microscopic N2 disease.[4] For grossly involved N2, 62% of these surgeons favored neoadjuvant therapy followed by surgery in the context of mediastinal downstaging but only 32% choose this approach for bulky disease.[4] In a survey of oncologists, 92% favored a neoadjuvant approach followed by surgery for minimal N2 and 52% chose chemoradiation therapy for bulky disease.[3] Treatment options for NSCLC range from aggressive use of a single modality through to trimodality treatment that includes surgery, chemotherapy, and radiotherapy.

Significant advances in treatment have improved outcomes for patients with locally advanced NSCLC since the 1980s. Active areas of research include determining the appropriate sequence of systemic treatments, discovering novel agents, and improving delivery of radiotherapy through technologic advances. Current treatment paradigms extend beyond age, performance status, and nonsmall cell histology and incorporate an expanding list of factors in the decision-making process. In the near future, therapeutic strategies will be individualized based on the identifiable molecular characteristics of a tumor,[5] leading to better patient outcomes and more effective clinical trial design. Technologic improvements in radiotherapy enable oncologists to target tumors with more precision and effectiveness, thus making it an option for patients who previously might have not been candidates for this treatment modality.

Definitive radiotherapy had been the standard of care for patients with locally advanced NSCLC until results from clinical trials showed that chemoradiation therapy improved survival. (When considering the trials reviewed in this chapter, it is important to remember that the old tumor, node, metastasis [TNM] classification system—the sixth edition—was usually used.)

Radiation alone is the definitive treatment for patients with locally advanced NSCLC who are not candidates for chemoradiation therapy. Radiotherapy also has a role in the treatment of select patients with isolated thoracic recurrence. Benefits of radiotherapy include palliation of tumor-related symptoms, local control of tumor growth, and a potential survival advantage.

RADIOTHERAPY DOSE AND FRACTIONATION

Dose

When radiotherapy alone is used to treat locally advanced NSCLC, the median survival is approximately 10 months and the 5-year survival rate is 5%.[6–9] In the 1970s, the Radiation Therapy Oncology Group (RTOG) conducted a phase III trial (RTOG 73-01) to evaluate the effect of radiotherapy dosage on local control rates and overall survival.[10] Patients were randomly assigned to treatment with 40 Gy, 50 Gy, or 60 Gy in 2-Gy daily fractions or to a split-course schedule. Local control rates were significantly better with the highest dose (52% vs. 62% vs. 73%, respectively; p = 0.02), although median survival rates were similar (10.6 months vs. 9.5 months vs. 10.8 months, respectively). The split-course schedule was associated with inferior local control and survival. This trial established 60 Gy in 30 fractions as the standard radiotherapy dose-fractionation scheme for decades.

Early radiotherapy portals were designed to cover the primary tumor, ipsilateral hilum, ipsilateral and contralateral mediastinum, and ipsilateral supraclavicular nodes, leading to a large irradiated volume. This approach was called elective nodal irradiation. As the toxicity of this approach and the relation between local failure occurring mainly at the level of the gross tumor volume and poor patient outcomes became more apparent, treatment planning shifted toward involved field radiation.[11] Concern about the potential for nodal recurrence has slowed the adoption of involved field radiation; however, a prospective randomized trial from China showed promising results. Patients with locally advanced NSCLC were treated with 68 Gy to 74 Gy involved field radiation or 60 Gy to 64 Gy elective nodal irradiation.[12] At 5 years, patients who received involved field radiation had significantly better overall response rates (90% vs. 79%, p = 0.032), local control (51% vs. 36%, p = 0.032), and fewer cases of pneumonitis (17% vs. 29%, p = 0.044). Treatment with involved field radiation significantly improved overall survival at 2 years (39.4% vs. 25.6%, p = 0.048). Despite several limitations of this study, the results are intriguing and suggest that involved field radiation is unlikely to compromise clinical outcomes. Furthermore, several studies have clearly demonstrated that the number of isolated nodal failures outside the involved field radiation remains very low.[13,14]

Technologic advances have enabled researchers to determine the optimal volume and explore the role of dose escalation in improving local control rates. The introduction of positron emission tomography (PET)–computed tomography (CT) imaging has enhanced treatment planning. The addition of cone-beam CT on linear accelerators has led to new radiotherapy such as intensity-modulated radiotherapy (IMRT)—either static or rotational—and image-guided radiotherapy, which improves the accuracy of daily radiotherapy delivery.[15] Because of these improvements, the classical safety margins can be decreased, allowing researchers to increase the total dose either physically or biologically.

In early phase I/II trials, increasing the radiotherapy dose to 74 Gy or more improved the median survival times to 24 months.[16–18] Given the promising results of these trials and a pooled analysis of Cooperative Group studies, a phase III randomized trial (RTOG 06-17 trial) was designed to compare concurrent chemoradiotherapy and dose-escalated radiotherapy with standard radiotherapy dosage. There was a second randomization to evaluate the role of cetuximab. Patients with locally advanced NSCLC were randomized to a standard-dose radiotherapy (60 Gy in 30 daily fractions) or a high-dose radiotherapy (74 Gy in 37 fractions) concurrently with weekly paclitaxel and carboplatin followed by two cycles of consolidation and to cetuximab or not. The 2-year survival rates were 58% for the standard dose and 45% for the high radiation dose.[19] The local failure rate was also higher in the experimental arm: 38.6% versus 30.7%, respectively, at 2 years. Planning target volumes were very similar between the two arms as well as the use of IMRT. However, although 10 patients died in the 74-Gy arms compared with two in the 60-Gy arms, the toxicity rates were not different between the two groups. Several explanations have been put forward to explain these worse outcomes in the higher dose arm, including heart toxicity and the loss of efficacy through longer overall treatment time and accelerated repopulation. It is important to note that the outcomes in the low-dose arm are among the best ever observed in a population with stage III NSCLC. A subsequent analysis examined the role of IMRT as patients were stratified according to the radiation technique: the planning target volume was larger for patients treated by IMRT compared with three-dimensional conformal radiation therapy (486 mL vs. 427 mL), but the outcomes were similar for the two techniques.[20] Less grade 3 pneumonitis, lower heart dose, and less dose reduction for chemotherapy were observed for patients treated by IMRT. There was a concern that IMRT could result in very low doses of radiation to large volumes of normal lung with increased pneumonitis risk, but an increased incidence of radiation pneumonitis was not observed.

Altered Fractionation Schedules

Multiple trials have tested the use of altered dose-fractionation schedules to improve the therapeutic index of radiotherapy. These approaches have included hyperfractionation (two or three fractions per day with a lower dose per fraction over the standard treatment duration), accelerated fractionation (use of a standard fraction size and total radiation dose, given over a shorter overall time), or a combination of these approaches. Compared with standard chemoradiation therapy, hyperfractionated radiotherapy with concurrent chemotherapy, delivered continuously or as a split course, has not been shown to increase survival in randomized studies.[21,22] However, studies have demonstrated improved outcomes with hyperfractionated accelerated radiotherapy (HART). In one randomized trial, the 2-year survival rate was better with continuous HART, delivering 54 Gy in 36 fractions of 1.5 Gy over 12 days, than with conventional radiotherapy alone, 60 Gy in 30 fractions (29% vs. 20%).[23] In Eastern Cooperative Oncology Group (ECOG) 2597, patients were given two cycles of carboplatin and paclitaxel and then randomly assigned to HART (1.5 Gy three times per day for 2.5 weeks) or standard radiotherapy (64 Gy in 2-Gy daily fractions). There was

a nonsignificant improvement in median survival (20.3 months vs. 14.9 months, $p = 0.28$) and 3-year overall survival (23% vs. 14%) for patients in the HART arm.[24]

The most informative results come from a meta-analysis of data from 2000 patients (eight trials) who had been randomly assigned to an altered regimen or conventional fractionation.[25] The analysis was limited to trials in which the chemotherapy was identical in both treatment arms. Modified fractionation resulted in a small, but significant, improvement in 5-year overall survival (10.8% vs. 8.3%; hazard ratio, 0.88; 95% confidence interval [CI], 0.80 to 0.97; $p = 0.009$). Severe esophageal toxicity was more frequent in the modified fraction group (19% vs. 9%).

Widespread adoption of modified radiotherapy schedules instead of conventional once-daily treatments has been limited by the logistical challenges of HART for the patient and treatment centers, as well as the higher rates of toxicity.

Hypofractionation

Hypofractionated radiotherapy is the delivery of fewer, larger (>2 Gy) doses of radiotherapy and is another potential strategy for improving dose intensity. This approach has become more feasible as a result of decreasing radiotherapy volumes, which allow for more conformal radiotherapy delivery and limit the dose delivered to normal tissue. Few studies have evaluated hypofractionation with modern radiotherapy techniques for locally advanced NSCLC. Two prospective phase II studies evaluating concurrent platinum-based chemotherapy with radiotherapy (2.4 Gy/d to 2.75 Gy/d) have reported an encouraging median survival of 20 months.[26,27] In the sequential or concurrent cancer radiation (SOCCAR) trial, 55 Gy was delivered in 20 fractions over 4 weeks with sequential or concurrent chemotherapy (cisplatin [DDP]–vinorelbine). In this limited phase II trial, 2-year survival rates were similar (50% vs. 46%) with 8% experiencing grade 3 esophagitis.[27] Additional studies using modern radiotherapy techniques are currently being conducted within a cooperative group setting as well as in single institutions. One study of interest is a phase III trial comparing a hypofractionated course of 60 Gy in 15 fractions over 3 weeks with conventional radiotherapy (60–66 Gy in 30–33 fractions over 6 weeks to 7 weeks) without concurrent chemotherapy for patients with stage II–III NSCLC and poor performance status (NCT01459497).

Ongoing research is examining isotoxic dose escalation based on normal tissue tolerance or using the stereotactic body irradiation therapy technique to increase the dose to ^{18}F-2-deoxy-D-glucose-avid portions of the tumor based on intratreatment PET–CT. Currently, a randomized trial is comparing a homogeneous dose distribution to the primary tumor or a heterogeneous dose distribution based on the metabolic image provided by a PET–CT (Fig. 39.1).[28] Last but not least, protons are under investigation in stage III NSCLC to take advantage of better dose distribution, especially allowing better sparing of the heart,[29] but the results of a randomized trial were disappointing.

In summary, higher physical or biologic dose (altered fractionation) is associated with better local control and, in some trials, with better survival, but the optimal dose and fractionation are yet to be defined. Currently, 60 Gy to 66 Gy in daily fractions of 2 Gy remains the most common schedule.

CHEMORADIATION THERAPY

Chemoradiation therapy is now the standard treatment for stage III NSCLC classified as N2 or N3. Results from meta-analyses of patients with unresectable stage III locally advanced NSCLC have demonstrated the benefits of platinum-based chemoradiation therapy given concurrently or sequentially in comparison with radiation alone.[30–33] Furthermore, a third meta-analysis has clearly demonstrated the superiority of a concurrent approach to sequential treatment.[34]

Role of Chemotherapy

For patients with medically inoperable or technically unresectable locally advanced NSCLC, thoracic radiotherapy alone, which is potentially curative, was regarded as a standard therapy in the 1980s; however, the treatment results were unsatisfactory due to a high rate of relapse and distant metastases. It was thought

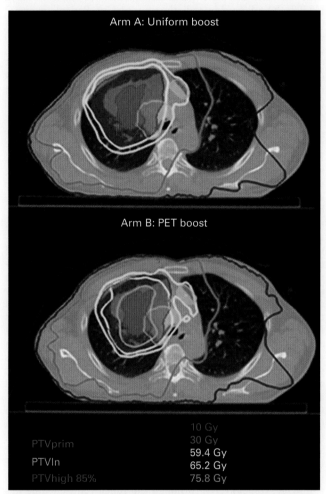

that chemotherapy with radiosensitizing anticancer drugs might improve survival by controlling remote metastases and increasing tumor sensitivity to radiotherapy, and several trials tested this hypothesis. Results from meta-analyses showed that survival after sequential or concurrent chemoradiation therapy that included a platinum agent was better than survival after radiotherapy alone.[30–33] The important role of chemotherapy was demonstrated with an absolute benefit of 3% at 2 years and 2% at 5 years. Furthermore, a third meta-analysis has clearly demonstrated the superiority of a concurrent to a sequential approach.[34]

Nevertheless, these findings were still not satisfactory, and subsequent investigations aimed to establish the optimal timing and type of chemotherapy needed to control micrometastases, increase the effects of radiotherapy, and improve local control and survival.

Sequential and Concurrent Therapy

Sequential chemoradiation therapy has been compared with concurrent chemoradiation therapy in several studies[21,35–37] (Table 39.1). The first published trial was from Furuse et al.:[35] radiotherapy (56 Gy using a split-course schedule) was given either concurrently or after an induction with mitomycin, vindesine, and DDP in unresectable locally advanced NSCLC. Median survival was significantly superior in patients receiving concurrent therapy (16.5 months), as compared with those receiving sequential therapy (13.3 months; $p = 0.03998$). The 5-year survival in the concurrent group (15.8%) was better than that in the sequential group (8.9%). The three other trials showed a trend in favor of the concurrent arm. RTOG 9410 was a randomized three-arm phase III trial comparing sequential with concurrent chemoradiation therapy.[21] The sequential arm consisted of DDP (100 mg/m^2) on days 1 and 29 and vinblastine (5 mg/m^2) per week for 5 weeks with chest radiotherapy (60 Gy) starting on day 50. One of the concurrent arms used the same chemotherapy regimen as the sequential arm with thoracic radiotherapy (60 Gy) starting on day 1. This concurrent arm had a significantly better 5-year survival rate compared with the sequential arm (16% vs. 10%, $p = 0.046$).

The NSCLC Collaborative Group performed a meta-analysis of six randomized trials and was based on individual patient data.[34] Compared with sequential chemoradiation therapy, concurrent chemoradiation therapy significantly improved overall survival (hazard ratio, 0.84; 95% CI, 0.74 to 0.95; $p = 0.004$) with an absolute benefit of 5.7% (23.8% vs. 18.1%) at 3 years and 4.5% (15.1% vs. 10.6%) at 5 years (Fig. 39.2). This benefit was mainly due to less locoregional progression without any difference in the rate of distant metastases. Concurrent chemoradiation therapy increased acute esophageal toxicity (grade 3–4) from 4% to 18% with a relative risk of 4.9 (95% CI, 3.1 to 7.8; $p < 0.001$). There was no significant difference in acute pulmonary toxicity.

Fig. 39.1. Positron emission tomography (PET) boost trial: the boost is either (A) homogeneous or (B) heterogeneous based on the ^{18}F-2-deoxy-D-glucose uptake. *(From van Elmpt W, De Ruysscher D, van der Salm A, et al. The PET-boost randomised phase II dose-escalation trial in non-small cell lung cancer. Radiother Oncol. 2012;104:67–71.)*

TABLE 39.1 Selected Randomized Trials of Sequential Versus Concurrent Chemoradiotherapy

Investigators	No. of Patients	RT, Gy	Chemotherapy Regimen	Median Survival Time (Mo)	2-Year Survival Rate, %	5-Year Survival Rate, %
Furuse et al.[35]	156	56	Conc RT DDP + MIT + VDS × 2	16.5	34.6	15.8
	158	56	DDP + MIT + VDS × 2 → Seq RT	13.3	27.4	8.9
Fournel et al.[36]	100	66	Conc RT DDP + ETP × 2 DDP + VNR × 2	16.3	39	21[a]
	101	66	DDP + VNR × 3 → Seq RT	14.5	26	14[a]
Zatloukal et al.[37]	52	60	DDP + VNR → Conc RT DDP + VNR × 2 → DDP + VNR	16.6	34.2	18.6
				12.9	14.3	9.3
	50	60	DDP + VNR × 4 → Seq RT	15.2	34	13
Curran et al.[21]	193	69.6	Conc RT DDP + ETP × 2	17.0	35	16
	200	63	Conc RT DDP + VLB × 2	14.6	32	10
	199	63	DDP + VLB × 2 → Seq RT			

[a]4 years.

Conc, concurrent; *DDP,* cisplatin; *ETP,* etoposide; *MIT,* mitomycin C; *RT,* radiotherapy; *Seq,* sequential; *VDS,* vindesine; *VLB,* vinblastine; *VNR,* vinorelbine.

In summary, concurrent DDP-based chemoradiation therapy has been consistently shown to improve survival at the cost of manageable increased toxicity. Concurrent chemoradiation therapy that includes DDP is recommended as the standard therapy for patients with inoperable locally advanced NSCLC who are eligible for radiotherapy. Sequential chemoradiation therapy or radiotherapy alone is appropriate for frail patients who are unable to tolerate concurrent chemoradiation therapy.

Chemotherapy Drug Combinations

Several phase III trials of chemoradiation therapy with platinum (especially DDP) and second-generation anticancer agents, such as vindesine, mitomycin, etoposide, and vinblastine, have produced strong evidence of the effectiveness of these drugs, as described earlier. The evidence for combination therapy with platinum and third-generation agents for the treatment of locally advanced NSCLC has been less conclusive, although some trials have shown

that such a combination produces significant response and survival when used to treat stage IV NSCLC. Additional data are needed to determine the optimal regimen. Several randomized trials are reviewed in the following sections (also see Tables 39.2 and 39.3).

Belani et al.[24] enrolled patients with unresectable locally advanced NSCLC in a three-arm phase II trial. Patients in arm 1 (sequential arm) received two cycles of induction chemotherapy with paclitaxel (200 mg/m^2) and carboplatin (area under the curve [AUC] = 6) followed by radiotherapy (63 Gy). Patients in arm 2 (induction and concurrent) received two cycles of induction chemotherapy with paclitaxel (200 mg/m^2) and carboplatin (AUC = 6) followed by weekly paclitaxel (45 mg/m^2) and carboplatin (AUC = 2) with concurrent radiation (63 Gy). Patients in arm 3 (concurrent and consolidation) received weekly paclitaxel (45 mg/m^2), carboplatin (AUC = 2), and radiotherapy (63 Gy) followed by two cycles of paclitaxel (200 mg/m^2) and carboplatin (AUC = 6). The median overall survival was 13.0 months, 12.7 months, and 16.3 months for arms 1, 2, and 3, respectively. The proportions of survivors in arm 1 at 1 year, 2 years, and 3 years were 57%, 30%, and 17%, respectively; in arm 2, 53%, 25%, and 15%, respectively; and in arm 3, 63%, 31%, and 17%, respectively. In this study, concurrent weekly paclitaxel, carboplatin, and thoracic radiotherapy followed by consolidation was associated with the best outcome but with greater toxicity.

Reduced (lower-dose) DDP and vinorelbine combination therapy is widely used as a standard treatment, but few prospective trials have been conducted. Zatloukal et al.[37] demonstrated the safety and efficacy of this combination in a trial of concurrent and sequential chemoradiation therapy for patients with locally advanced NSCLC. Fifty-two patients were randomly assigned to concurrent treatment and 50 patients to sequential treatment. The chemotherapy consisted of up to four cycles of DDP (80 mg/m^2) on day 1, and vinorelbine (25 mg/m^2 in the 1st and 4th cycles; 12.5 mg/m^2 during the 2nd and 3rd cycles) on days 1, 8, and 15, of a 28-day cycle. Radiotherapy (60 Gy) was given as five fractions per week for 6 weeks. In the concurrent arm, radiotherapy began on day 4 of cycle 2; in the sequential arm, it was started 2 weeks after completion of chemotherapy. Overall survival was significantly better in the concurrent arm (median survival, 16.6 months) than in the sequential arm (median survival, 12.9 months; p = 0.023, hazard ratio = 0.61; 95% CI, 0.39–0.93). The proportions of survivors were greater in the concurrent arm than in the sequential treatment arm at years 1, 2, and 3 (69.2%, 34.2%, and 18.6% vs. 53.0%, 14.3%, and 9.5%, respectively). Although the concurrent schedule was

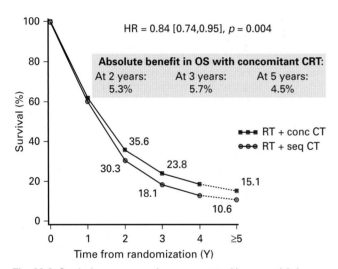

Fig. 39.2. Survival curve comparing concurrent with sequential chemoradiotherapy (CRT). *CT*, chemotherapy; *HR*, hazard ratio; *OS*, overall survival; *RT*, radiotherapy. (*Modified from Auperin A, Le Péchoux C, Rolland E, et al. Meta-analysis of concomitant versus sequential radiochemotherapy in locally advanced non-small-cell lung cancer. J Clin Oncol. 2010;28:2181–2190.*)

TABLE 39.2 Selected Randomized Trials of Concurrent Chemotherapy With Third-Generation Anticancer Agents or Molecular Targeted Agents

Investigators	No. of Patients	RT, Gy	Chemotherapy Regimen	Median Survival Time (Mo)	2-Year Survival, %
Belani et al.[24]	91	63	CBDCA + PTX × 2 → Seq RT	13	30
	74	63	CBDCA + PTX × 2 → Conc RT CBDCA + PTX × 2	12.7	25
	92	63	Conc RT CBDCA + PTX × 2 → CBDCA + PTX × 2	16.3	31
Zatloukal et al.[37]	52	60	DDP + VNR → Conc RT DDP + VNR × 2 → DDP + VNR	16.6	34.2
	50	60	DDP + VNR × 4 → Seq RT	12.9	14.3
Yamamoto et al.[38]	146	60S	Conc RT DDP + VDS + MIT × 2 DDP + VDS + MIT × 2	20.5	17.5
	147	60	Conc RT CBDCA + IRIN × 2 DDP + IRIN × 2	19.8	17.8
	147	60	Conc RT CBDCA + PTX × 2 CBDCA + PTX × 2	22.0	19.5
Segawa et al.[39]	101	60	Conc RT MIT + VDS + DDP × 2	23.7.	48.1
	99	60	Conc RT DOC + DDP × 2	26.8	60.3
Wang et al.[40]	33	60	Conc DDP + ETP × 2	20.2	36.4
	32	66	Conc CBDCA + PTX weekly	13.5	16.2
Senan et al.[41]	301	66	Conc RT DDP + PEM → PEM × 4	26.8	52
	297	66	Conc RT DDP + ETP → DDP + X × 2 Conc RT DDP + PEM × 4 + Cetux → PEM × 4	25	52

CBDCA, Carboplatin; *Conc*, concurrent; *DDP*, cisplatin; *DOC*, docetaxel; *ETP*, etoposide; *IRIN*, irinotecan; *MIT*, mitomycin C; *PEM*, pemetrexed; *PTX*, paclitaxel; *RT*, radiotherapy; *S*, split course; *Seq*, sequential; *VDS*, vindesine; *VNR*, vinorelbine; *X*, a second drug.

associated with a higher toxicity, the adverse event profile was acceptable in both arms.

Two phase III trials comparing second-generation to third-generation chemotherapy in combination with concurrent thoracic radiotherapy were conducted in Japan. The West Japan Oncology Group conducted a three-arm randomized trial comparing a combination of mitomycin, vindesine, and DDP with irinotecan and carboplatin in one experimental arm and paclitaxel and carboplatin in the other.[38] The Okayama Lung Cancer Study Group also used mitomycin, vindesine, and DDP as a control regimen, which they compared with docetaxel and DDP.[39] No difference was noted among the regimens in terms of survival, but febrile neutropenia occurred more often in the control arm.

Lastly, a small trial was conducted in China to compare the DDP and etoposide combination with that of carboplatin and paclitaxel and concurrent radiotherapy (60 Gy). Results from this trial showed that 3-year survival was better after treatment with DDP and etoposide (33% vs. 13%).[40]

Pemetrexed has commonly been used recently in advanced nonsquamous NSCLC with a better outcome. The PROCLAIM study is a phase III trial of pemetrexed and DDP chemotherapy combined with concurrent radiotherapy, followed by consolidation pemetrexed or two additional cycles of a platinum-based regimen. Because pemetrexed can be given in full doses with radical radiotherapy, there was hope that it might result in lower rates of distant metastasis. However, the 2-year survival rates for the two arms were 52% without any significant difference regardless of the end points.[41]

Induction and Consolidation Therapy

Even with concurrent chemoradiation therapy for locally advanced NSCLC, local and distant disease recurrences are a common event, and most patients die of progressive lung cancer. Early administration of full-dose systemic chemotherapy has the potential to improve survival by treating micrometastases early and downstaging the primary tumor before chemoradiation therapy.

A Cancer and Leukemia Group B (CALGB) study randomized 366 patients with stage III NSCLC to immediate chemoradiation therapy (carboplatin, paclitaxel, and 66 Gy of radiotherapy) or induction chemotherapy with two cycles of carboplatin and paclitaxel before chemoradiation therapy.[42] Survival differences were not significant ($p = 0.3$), with a median survival of 12 months (95% CI, 10 months to 16 months) and 14 months (95% CI, 11 months to 16 months), respectively. The 2-year survival was 29% (95% CI, 22% to 35%) for immediate chemoradiation therapy and 31% (95% CI, 25% to 38%) for induction chemotherapy. The addition of induction chemotherapy to concurrent chemoradiation therapy added toxicity and provided no survival benefit compared with concurrent chemoradiation therapy alone. Similarly, a meta-analysis of individual patient data from six small randomized phase II trials did not show any difference between induction and adjuvant chemotherapy given before or after definitive chemoradiation therapy.[43] A recent trial randomized patients after concurrent chemoradiotherapy to two additional cycles of oral vinorelbine and DDP or best supportive care alone and failed to show any benefit of additional chemotherapy.[44] The Hoosier Oncology Group randomly assigned patients who had already received treatment with DDP, etoposide, and definitive thoracic radiotherapy to consolidation docetaxel or observation.[45] This trial was terminated early because of increased toxicity during docetaxel administration: 5.5% of patients died as a result of this drug. The median survival was 21.2 months in the docetaxel arm compared with 23.2 months in the observation arm ($p = 0.883$).

In summary, induction chemotherapy, adjuvant chemotherapy, and/or maintenance therapy currently are not recommended for patients with unresectable locally advanced NSCLC.

Chemoradiation Therapy for Older Individuals

Clinical trials rarely provide data on chemoradiation therapy for individuals older than 70 years. Atagi et al.[46] randomly assigned patients older than 70 with a good performance status to radiotherapy (60 Gy) and concurrent low-dose carboplatin (30 mg/m² per day, 5 days a week for 20 days) or to radiotherapy alone. Although greater hematologic toxicity was reported in the combined arm, late toxicities and treatment-related deaths were similar in both arms. Chemoradiation therapy produced a clear survival benefit: the 2-year survival rates were 46% and 35%, respectively (Fig. 39.3). For carefully selected older patients without severe comorbidities, chemoradiation therapy may be considered with careful management of toxicities.

TABLE 39.3 Clinical Trials Utilizing Molecular Compounds With Combined Chemoradiotherapy for Locally Advanced Nonsmall Cell Lung Cancer

Study	Agent	Study design	Findings
RTOG 0324[52] Phase II	Cetuximab	Carboplatin/paclitaxel/cetuximab/RT → carboplatin/ paclitaxel × 2 cycles	Median OS 27.7 mo; 2-y OS 49.3%
CALGB 30407[51] Phase II	Cetuximab	Carboplatin/pemetrexed/RT ± cetuximab	Without cetuximab: 18 mo; OS 58% With cetuximab: 18 mo; OS 52%
SWOG 0023[54] Phase III	Gefitinib	Chemo/RT → docetaxel × 3 cycles → gefitinib versus placebo	Gefitinib: median OS 23 mo Placebo: median OS 35 mo
CALGB 30106[55] Phase II	Gefitinib	Poor risk group: carboplatin/paclitaxel → RT/gefitinib → gefitinib	Poor risk group: PFS 13.4 mo, median OS 19 mo
		Good risk group: carboplatin/paclitaxel → RT/gefitinib/ carboplatin/paclitaxel → gefitinib	Good risk group: PFS 9.2 mo, median OS 13 mo
University of Chicago[56] Phase I	Erlotinib	Group 1: carboplatin/paclitaxel → carboplatin/paclitaxel/RT/ erlotinib	Group 1: median OS 13.7 mo
		Group 2: cisplatin/etoposide/RT/erlotinib → docetaxel	Group 2: median OS 10.2 mo
Spigel et al.[59] Phase II	Bevacizumab	Carboplatin/pemetrexed/bevacizumab/RT → carboplatin/ pemetrexed/bevacizumab → bevacizumab	2/5 patients developed tracheoesophageal fistulae
ECOG 3598[61] Phase III	Thalidomide	Carboplatin/paclitaxel/RT ± thalidomide	1-y survival, 57% carboplatin/paclitaxel; 67% on the thalidomide arm 2-y survival, 34% and 33%
RTOG 0617[19] Phase III	Cetuximab	Carboplatin/palictaxel/RT ± cetuximab	Median overall survival with cetuximab 23.1 mo; 23.5 mo in those not receiving cetuximab

CALGB, Cancer and Leukemia Group B; *OS,* overall survival; *PFS,* progression-free survival; *RT,* radiotherapy; *RTOG,* Radiation Therapy Oncology Group; *SWOG,* Southwest Oncology Group.

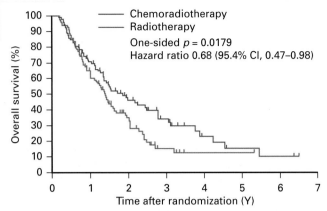

Fig. 39.3. Survival curve comparing concurrent chemoradiotherapy with radiotherapy alone for elderly patients. *(From Atagi S, Kawahara M, Yokoyama A, et al. Thoracic radiotherapy with or without daily low-dose carboplatin in elderly patients with non-small-cell lung cancer: a randomised, controlled, phase 3 trial by the Japan Clinical Oncology Group (JCOG0301). Lancet Oncol. 2012;13;671–678.)*

In summary, for most patients with unresectable locally advanced NSCLC, concurrent chemoradiation therapy is the optimal treatment strategy with curative intent. Combination therapy with platinum and second-generation anticancer agents effectively prolongs survival. The superiority or noninferiority of third-generation anticancer drugs has not been shown in phase III trials. Results from smaller studies show that these drugs may modestly increase median survival and 5-year survival. Furthermore, it is difficult to translate the results observed in stage IV to stage III patients treated with a combined approach.

MOLECULARLY TARGETED THERAPEUTIC AGENTS

Recent discoveries in molecular biology have led to the identification of numerous molecular pathways that may be responsible for cancer cell development, progression, and growth; these pathways may also have a role in cancer cell resistance to radiotherapy or other cytotoxic agents. Therefore, these pathways are being explored as potential targets for augmentation of radiotherapy or chemotherapy response. Since the 1990s, there has been an explosion of new molecularly targeted agents for use in lung cancer treatment.

The expanding list of molecular targets for NSCLC includes epidermal growth factor (EGF) and its receptor (EGFR), vascular endothelial growth factor (VEGF) and its receptor (VEGFR), the fusion of echinoderm microtubule-associated protein-like 4 and anaplastic lymphoma kinase (*EML4–ALK*), *B-Raf*, *PIK3CA* gene, *ErbB2* (*Her2*) amplification or mutant genes, mammalian target of rapamycin, and various other molecules that regulate different steps in their signal transduction pathways.[47] Although preclinical data would indicate that these molecules are viable targets that could be exploited to improve therapeutic efficacy, not all agents have produced clinical benefits. A handful of targeted agents have been approved for cancer treatment. Clinical trials of other agents are being conducted to determine their efficacy in combination with other cytotoxic agents, including ionizing radiotherapy. Some potential agents target a single molecular signaling pathway, whereas others are able to target multiple molecular signaling pathways. The most clinically advanced agents target the EGFR, VEGF/VEGFR, and ALK1 pathways.

Epidermal Growth Factor Receptor

EGFR targeting exemplifies the approach of combining radiotherapy with molecularly targeted therapy. EGFR plays an important role in tumor growth and response to cytotoxic agents, including ionizing radiotherapy. Upregulation of EGFR expression occurs in many types of cancer and is often associated with more aggressive tumors, poor prognosis, and tumor resistance to treatment with cytotoxic agents including radiotherapy.[48,49] Preclinical data provide a strong rationale for combining EGFR inhibitors with radiotherapy.

Cetuximab is a chimeric mouse anti-EGFR monoclonal antibody. Although it was a study of patients with head and neck squamous cell carcinoma that confirmed the benefit of cetuximab with radiotherapy, the agent has also been studied extensively in patients with NSCLC.[50] In 2011, CALGB and RTOG reported the results from phase II studies.[51,52] In the CALGB study, two novel chemotherapy regimens in combination with concurrent radiotherapy were evaluated. Patients in the first group received concurrent carboplatin and pemetrexed with thoracic radiotherapy (70 Gy). In the second group, patients received the same regimen plus cetuximab. Patients in both groups received four cycles of pemetrexed as consolidation therapy. The overall survival at 18 months was 58% without cetuximab and 54% with cetuximab. Treatment of NSCLC with the combination of thoracic radiotherapy, pemetrexed, carboplatin, and with or without cetuximab was shown to be feasible and fairly well tolerated.[51]

In the RTOG study, patients were treated with a combination of paclitaxel, carboplatin, and cetuximab with radiotherapy (63 Gy). All patients received a loading dose of cetuximab (400 mg/m^2) 1 week before radiotherapy, and patients received carboplatin, paclitaxel, and cetuximab for two additional cycles after completion of radiotherapy. The median survival was 22.7 months, and the 2-year survival rate was 49.3%.[52] Because of these very promising results, cetuximab was studied in the RTOG 0617 trial in which patients were randomly assigned to receive or not receive cetuximab in addition to concurrent chemoradiotherapy; however, no difference in survival was observed between the two arms. In a separate planned retrospective analysis, the EGFR expression could be evaluated on 203 patients; for patients expressing the EGFR, there was a statistical benefit with a higher survival rate, whereas for those not expressing EGFR, a negative trend was observed.[19] In the Raditux trial, patients received 66 Gy in 24 fractions plus daily DDP with or without cetuximab. The survival rates were very similar but the EGFR expression was not evaluated. More grade 3 lung toxicity was seen in the cetuximab arm (0% vs. 10%).[53]

Gefitinib and erlotinib are two tyrosine kinase inhibitors (TKIs) that are especially active in case of mutation and have been tested with radiotherapy. The Southwest Oncology Group (SWOG) performed a large phase III trial in which patients with stage III NSCLC were treated with standard chemoradiation therapy, and after consolidation with docetaxel for three cycles, the patients were randomly assigned to maintenance therapy with placebo or gefitinib. At interim analysis, overall survival was worse in the gefitinib maintenance arm (23 months vs. 35 months), and therefore the study was closed.[54] It is clear from this study that maintenance therapy with TKI after definitive chemoradiation therapy should be avoided in an unselected patient population.

CALGB 30106 was a phase II study designed to evaluate the addition of gefitinib to sequential or concurrent chemoradiation therapy in patients with unresectable NSCLC.[55] Patients were categorized as poor risk (performance status of 2 or higher, weight loss of 5% or more) or good risk (performance status of 0 or 1, weight loss less than 5%). All patients received induction chemotherapy with two cycles of carboplatin and paclitaxel plus gefitinib. (Gefitinib was removed from induction regimen in May 2004 when the SWOG trial did not demonstrate a benefit to adding gefitinib to chemotherapy.) Patients in the poor risk group received thoracic radiotherapy (66 Gy) with concurrent gefitinib. Patients in the good risk group received the same radiotherapy and gefitinib, but also received weekly carboplatin and paclitaxel. Consolidation gefitinib was given until disease progression. In the poor risk group, progression-free survival was 13.4 months, and median survival was 19 months. In the good risk group, progression-free survival was 9.2 months, and median survival was 13 months.

As many as 13 of 45 tumors had activating *EGFR* mutations, and 2 of 13 had T790M mutations. Seven of 45 tumors had *KRAS* mutations. When the results were analyzed by these molecular phenotypes, no significant difference in outcome was noted. Given the promising results for patients at poor risk, further studies will investigate the effectiveness of treating such patients with radiotherapy and gefitinib after induction chemotherapy; however, this regimen may not be beneficial for patients at good risk.

The findings from CALGB 30106 are consistent with studies of erlotinib and chemoradiation. Choong et al.[56] reported on a phase I study of erlotinib with chemoradiation. Patients in one group received induction chemotherapy with carboplatin and paclitaxel followed by carboplatin, paclitaxel, radiotherapy, and erlotinib. The second group of patients received DDP, etoposide, radiotherapy, and erlotinib followed by docetaxel. In both arms, the erlotinib dose was increased from 50 mg to 150 mg in three stages. The median survival in each group was 13.7 months and 10.2 months, respectively. Overall survival and progression-free survival were improved for patients in whom a rash developed. This study demonstrated the tolerability of such a regimen, but given the disappointing survival data, the need for improved patient selection criteria for EGFR-based treatments is clear.

Patient selection is likely to play an important role in the design of future studies of EGFR-targeted agents. For example, these agents have shown benefits for patients with *EGFR* mutations and studies may need to separate patients with activating *EGFR* mutations from patients with the general wild-type *EGFR*. A repeat evaluation of biomarkers after chemoradiation therapy may help to determine which subset of patients would benefit from additional therapy with anti-EGFR agents. Therefore molecular profiling, along with patient selection based on criteria such as *EGFR* mutation status, has become an important factor in predicting efficacy of anti-EGFR regimens. Future studies of anti-EGFR treatments used in combination with radiotherapy should also incorporate stringent patient selection criteria to maximize treatment benefit. The efficacy of combined treatment with EGFR inhibitors and radiotherapy may vary by tumor type and molecular profile, as well as the sequencing of the treatments.

Antiangiogenesis Agents

Inhibitors of angiogenesis have undergone extensive preclinical testing and some agents have been tested in clinical trials. Despite concerns that an antiangiogenic agent would enhance hypoxia, thereby impairing the efficacy of radiotherapy, the first preclinical study with a specific inhibitor of angiogenesis, angiostatin, showed a synergistic effect with radiotherapy.[57] Jain[58] proposed a model of tumor vasculature normalization that explains this effect. In this model, proangiogenic factors from tumors can cause abnormal neovascularization, and inhibition of tumor angiogenesis transiently normalizes the tumor vasculature. This has the counterintuitive effect of decreasing tumor hypoxia and improving the effectiveness of radiotherapy. Preclinical studies support this hypothesis, as have results from a phase I study with locally advanced rectal cancer.

Similar to the EGFR inhibitors, antiangiogenic compounds can be broadly classified as monoclonal antibodies directed against antiangiogenic molecules or their receptors (e.g., bevacizumab) or TKIs with narrow or broad-spectrum activity against one or more of these receptors (e.g., sorafenib, sunitinib, pazopanib). Studies of bevacizumab for the treatment of NSCLC have also included radiotherapy.

Efforts to improve the therapeutic ratio by adding bevacizumab to chemoradiation therapy have failed in multiple studies of patients with both small cell lung cancer (SCLC) and NSCLC. This regimen was associated with increased incidence of tracheoesophageal fistula in both SCLC and NSCLC.[59] Therefore patient selection factors such as location of the tumor and tumor histology, as well as the timing of bevacizumab integration with radiotherapy, need to be considered in the design of future studies.

Thalidomide has also been found to have potent immunomodulatory effects and antiangiogenic properties.[60] ECOG 3598 was a randomized study comparing chemoradiation therapy with or without thalidomide for patients with locally advanced NSCLC. Patients received carboplatin and paclitaxel, with or without thalidomide for two cycles, followed by weekly carboplatin and paclitaxel with radiotherapy, with or without thalidomide. In the thalidomide group, patients could be treated with adjuvant thalidomide for up to 2 years. There was no difference in progression-free survival or overall survival with addition of thalidomide.[61] Although this outcome might suggest that this treatment combination is not effective, the negative studies may also indicate the need for better patient selection when using specific agents.

Anaplastic Lymphoma Kinase Inhibitors

The *EML–ALK* fusion oncogene has become a very important potential biomarker for patients with NSCLC. Several ALK inhibitors have been identified; crizotinib is the most developed and has produced impressive responses. However, data have not indicated that ALK inhibitors have a radiosensitizing or synergistic effect when administered concurrently in combination with radiotherapy

Immune Checkpoint Inhibitors (PD-1/PD-L-1)

Interesting observations were made with the use of nivolumab and ipilimumab in stage IV patients or in experimental work with an abscopal response after radiotherapy using stereotactic radiotherapy to a metastatic site.[62] Currently, phase III trials are ongoing to evaluate the safety (the concern is risk of radiation pneumonitis) and the efficacy.[63]

In summary, as of 2016, no trial has proven the benefits of adding a molecularly targeted agent to the combined modality regimens in an unselected patient population. Currently, studies adding erlotinib or crizotinib for treatment of patients who are known to have EGFR mutation or ALK translocation are underway by NRG/Alliance in the United States.

The discovery of new biomarkers, advances in molecular therapeutics and imaging technology, and a better understanding of effective integration of chemotherapy and radiation treatments are making personalized medicine for NSCLC feasible. As more precise biomarkers are identified, the use of such personalized strategies will become routine. In addition, immunomodulatory therapy may play a larger role in the treatment of NSCLC. Initial studies of immunomodulatory agents in combination with cytotoxic agents have provided promising early results. Incorporation of such agents into a concurrent chemoradiation therapy is being investigated.

LOCOREGIONAL TREATMENT WITH SURGERY OR RADIOTHERAPY

The role of surgery in the multimodality treatment of stage III NSCLC is an open question and the subject of much discussion. In some cases, surgery has been performed after induction chemotherapy, whereas in some other cases it is an initial approach for minimal stage IIIA NSCLC followed by adjuvant chemotherapy, with or without postoperative radiotherapy. As survival outcomes following chemoradiation therapy have improved, the role of surgery has been challenged.

Randomized Trials of Surgery

Three large randomized trials conducted in North America and in Europe have compared surgery with radiotherapy (Table 39.4).[64–66] The selection criteria and the design of these trials differed: in the North American and German trials, patients had proven N2 that was considered to be resectable at the time of enrollment, whereas

TABLE 39.4 Results of Selected Phase III Trial Looking to the Role of Surgery or the Type of Induction Treatment[a]

Authors	Treatment	No. of Patients	R0 Resection, %	Pathologic CR, %	5-Year Survival, %	Local Progression, %
Thomas et al.[67]	CT→Surg→RT	260	54.5	11	16	62
	CT + RT→Surg	264	69	41	14	50
Pless et al.[68]	CT→RT	117	91	16	38	15
	CT	115	81	12	41	28
Albain et al.[64]	RT + CT→S→CT	202	71.3	17.7	27.2	10
	RT + CT→	194			20.3	22
van Meerbeeck et al.[65]	CT→Surgery	167	50	5	15.7	45
	CT→RT	165			14	62
Eberhardt et al.[66]	CT→RT + CT→S	81	94	33	44	
	CT→RT + CT	80			40	

[a]Differences may be partially explained by different definitions of pathologic complete response or the pattern of failure (first site, local with or without distant metastases).
CR, chemoradiation; *CT*, chemotherapy; *RT*, radiotherapy; *S*, surgery.

N2 disease was considered to be unresectable in the European Organisation for Research and Treatment of Cancer (EORTC) trial. The terms "resectable" or "unresectable" may be partially subjective and depend on the surgeon's judgment.

In the EORTC trial, 579 patients with a stage IIIA disease were treated first by three cycles of a platinum-based chemotherapy before being randomly assigned to surgery or 6 weeks of radiotherapy (60 Gy).[65] Only 332 patients with an objective response to chemotherapy were included in the trial. Among the surgical patients, 40% received additional postoperative radiotherapy. Pneumonectomy was performed in 47% of patients. The 30-day postoperative mortality rate was 4% for the whole series and 7% after a pneumonectomy, with no significant difference between right-sided or left-sided procedures. A complete resection was achieved in 50% of the surgical patients and a pathologic complete response occurred in 5%; downstaging to ypN0 or N1 was achieved in 41% of patients. In the radiotherapy arm, 80% of the patients received a dose of 60 Gy in 30 fractions to 32 fractions over 40 days to 46 days. Overall compliance with radiotherapy was 55%. Eighty-six percent of patients started radiotherapy within 10 weeks of the 1st day of the final chemotherapy. No difference was observed between the two arms in terms of survival; the 5-year survival rate was approximately 15%. With regard to the first site of progression, locoregional relapse was more frequent after radiotherapy than after surgery (55% vs. 32%).

In the US Intergroup trial, individuals were enrolled if they had T1–T3 tumors and pathologically confirmed N2 disease, if resection seemed technically feasible, and if they were good surgical candidates.[64] Patients were randomly assigned to preoperative chemoradiation therapy or an exclusive schedule of chemoradiation therapy. The chemotherapy regimen consisted of DDP (50 mg/m²) on days 1, 8, 29, and 36 and etoposide (50 mg/m²) on days 1–5 and 29–33 delivered concurrently with thoracic radiotherapy (45 Gy delivered over 5 weeks). CT images of the chest were evaluated 2 weeks to 4 weeks after the induction regimen in the surgical arm and during the 5th week in the radiotherapy arm. If disease had not progressed, surgery was performed or radiotherapy was pursued to 61 Gy. Two additional cycles of chemotherapy were planned for after surgery or radiotherapy.

Of the 202 patients in the surgical arm, 177 patients were eligible for thoracotomy; 144 had a complete resection and 121 began the consolidation chemotherapy. The operative mortality was high, especially after a right-side pneumonectomy (26%). Compliance with the additional two cycles of chemotherapy was 55% in the surgical arm and 74% in the radiotherapy arm, rates that are similar to those reported in adjuvant chemotherapy trials. No significant difference in survival was found between the two arms: the 5-year survival rate was 20.3% and 27.2% for the radiotherapy and surgical arms, respectively. In a retrospective unplanned exploratory analysis, a matched pair analysis was performed: compared with radiotherapy, lobectomy led to significantly better survival but pneumonectomy did not.

The German trial was closed after enrolling half of the patients; 246 patients with proven N2 disease in either stage IIIA or B received three cycles of induction chemotherapy with DDP and paclitaxel followed by concurrent chemoradiotherapy, 45 Gy, two times a day with DDP and vinorelbine.[66] In the last week of radiotherapy, patients were reevaluated and those deemed resectable were randomized between surgery and additional chemoradiotherapy to receive 65 Gy to 71 Gy. The majority of patients had stage IIIB disease (171 patients). After induction, 65% of patients were found to present a resectable tumor and were randomized. An R0 resection for cure was performed in 81%. No difference in survival was observed between the two arms with 5-year survival rates of 44% for the trimodality and 40% for the chemoradiotherapy.

The last two important phase III trials addressed the issue of the induction treatment, radiochemotherapy, or chemotherapy only. In the trial by Thomas et al.,[67] 524 patients were randomly assigned to induction chemotherapy followed by surgery and postoperative radiotherapy (chemotherapy arm) or induction chemotherapy followed by an accelerated course of chemoradiation and then surgery (chemoradiation therapy arm). This trial included more than 500 patients with stage IIIA or B disease. The number of complete resections was similar between the groups: 84 patients in the chemotherapy arm and 98 in the chemoradiation therapy arm. Of the patients assigned to a treatment group, operations were performed on fewer than 60%. Complete pathologic response was achieved in 17 patients in the chemotherapy arm and in 59 in the chemoradiation therapy arm but this outcome did not translate to a survival benefit: 5-year survival rate was approximately 15% in both arms. A biased interpretation of these results might be that radiotherapy produces no benefit; however, it should be noted that the chemotherapy arm did include postoperative radiotherapy and that this trial was designed to compare thoracic radiotherapy as part of the induction treatment and as adjuvant treatment. The Swiss trial included 232 patients with stage IIIA and compared induction with three cycles of chemotherapy (DDP and docetaxel) with the same induction followed by sequential radiotherapy (44 Gy in 22 fractions for 3 weeks) prior to surgery.[68] No statistical difference was observed between the two arms; however, there was a lower rate of pathologic complete response in the chemotherapy arm.

Authors of a meta-analysis of seven phase III trials comparing preoperative chemotherapy with surgery alone for stage IIIA disease found that chemotherapy produced a 6% absolute increase in survival, increasing 5-year survival from 14% to 20%.[69] Nevertheless, local failure remains a key issue: in the Swiss Group for Clinical Research phase II trial, local relapse subsequently developed in 60% of patients.[70] All the trials included in the meta-analysis were conducted in the 1990s, using the staging procedure and radiotherapy techniques available at that time; nevertheless, they provide interesting information on the possible role of surgery and radiotherapy.

Advantages and Disadvantages of Surgery

The discussion of the advantages of surgery assumes that N2 disease has been identified before the operation through a complete staging procedure and careful evaluation of mediastinum using PET–CT, endobronchial ultrasound, or mediastinoscopy if needed. The discussion does not apply to positive nodes discovered at the time of thoracotomy.

In addition to increasing survival, surgery can improve local control. In both the US Intergroup and the EORTC trials, surgery led to a 50% improvement in local control. Theoretically, the bulk of the disease is less an issue with surgical resection than with radiotherapy, with larger tumor volume being a limitation on the efficacy of radiotherapy. Unfortunately, the report from the Intergroup trial provided no information on the tumor volume. An incomplete resection is a futile thoracotomy because salvage treatments have limited efficacy. When a complete resection cannot be performed, salvage radiotherapy is delayed and toxicity increases.

Surgery enables a complete pathologic evaluation of tumor extent. The choice to add adjuvant or neoadjuvant chemotherapy is already known very often at the time the treatment decision is made. For patients with severe emphysema or chronic obstructive pulmonary disease, an operative procedure may allow for lung parenchyma expansion, leading to better lung functions: patients with chronic obstructive pulmonary disease have greater forced expiratory volume (FEV_1) after lobectomy.[71] Because complications, including hemorrhage or abscess, occur frequently after radiotherapy, surgery may be beneficial in cases of infection or cavitations inside the tumor.[72]

A major drawback of surgery is its association with substantial morbidity and mortality, especially in the case of pneumonectomy because of its association with lower pulmonary function and high rate of complications. The mortality rate after neoadjuvant treatment has ranged from 0% to 26%, and postoperative mortality rises from 7% at 30 days to 12% at 90 days. The 90-day mortality is 9% for left pneumonectomy and 20% for right pneumonectomy,[73] although some teams report lower mortality rates even for right-sided pneumonectomy, especially after a careful functional evaluation. Nevertheless, pneumonectomy impairs quality of life and can lead to late complications.[74] Planning to include an operative procedure in a multimodality treatment approach could lead to a delay in starting radiotherapy. For example, if a restaging procedure is performed 2 weeks to 4 weeks after two or three cycles of induction chemotherapy and a decision is then made not to perform surgery, the long delay between the last chemotherapy and the start of thoracic radiotherapy could allow tumor regrowth.[75]

The preoperative chemotherapy regimens currently available lead to a low rate of pathologic complete response and downstaging in less than half of patients. Induction chemoradiation therapy has produced better rates of pathologic complete response and downstaging. However, this did not change the survival outcomes reported in the German study, a meta-analysis, or two other trials.[67,68,76,77] There is consensus that preoperative chemoradiation therapy is reasonable for superior sulcus tumors if there is no evidence of mediastinal node involvement.[78,79] Furthermore, a radiologic response after induction with concurrent chemoradiation therapy does not always correlate with the pathologic response, as some residual mass may be fibrosis.

Considerations for Choosing Surgery or Radiotherapy

Use of radiotherapy is less restricted by comorbidities and tumor extent than is the use of surgery, and surgical morbidity is avoided. However, radiotherapy is associated with acute toxicity such as radiation-induced acute esophagitis, especially with concurrent chemoradiation therapy. Limitations of radiotherapy include limited organ tolerance in the lung, spinal cord, and heart and lower

TABLE 39.5 Survival Rates According to the Type of Nodal Involvement in Selected Surgical Series

	Classification	N	5-Year Survival, %
Albain et al.[64]	ypN0	45	41
	ypN1–3	85	24
van Meerbeeck et al.[65]	ypN0–1	64	29
	ypN2	86	7
Decaluwé et al.[82]	ypN0–1	38	49
	ypN2 single level	33	37
	ypN2 multilevel	11	0
Casali et al.[81]	Single cN2		23.8
	Multiple cN2		14.7
Andre et al.[80]	Single cN2	118	8
	Multiple cN2	122	3

efficacy for patients with bulky disease. The choice between radiotherapy and surgery for an individual patient should be based on several factors. A primary consideration is the extent of N2 disease and the clinical presentation. Andre et al.[80] identified four negative prognostic factors: clinical N2 diagnosed on CT before surgery, involvement of multiple station levels, a pT3 or T4 classification, and the lack of induction chemotherapy. The 5-year survival rate dropped from 34% for patients with one-level N2 discovered at surgery to 3% for multiple-level clinical N2. Similarly, Casali et al.[81] reported that the 5-year survival rate decreased from 24% to 15% when N2 nodes were diagnosed before surgery. When induction chemotherapy is used, mediastinal downstaging and the number of positive nodal stations are crucial factors: Decaluwé et al.[82] reported that the 5-year survival rate decreased from 37% for patients with single-level persistent disease to 7% for patients with multilevel persistent disease (Table 39.5).

Good survival outcomes in surgery trials are often attributed to the operation. When interpreting these results, however, it is important to remember that only a small proportion of patients are candidates for surgery, and not all patients who receive an induction treatment subsequently have surgery. Indeed, factors such as tumor response and mediastinal downstaging are generally evaluated after induction treatment to decide whether surgery should be performed. Results are better for patients with a tumor that responds to induction than for patients with a tumor that does not respond, which has been shown for other types of tumor as well. In the EORTC trial,[65] only patients who had a response were included in the study and no difference was observed between surgery and radiotherapy. Prognostic factors such as tumor response and downstaging are often confused with predictive factors used to select a course of, for example, surgery or radiotherapy. Because the prognosis is poor for patients with unfavorable tumor response and a greater number of involved stations, the risk of surgery should be avoided.

When selecting a treatment approach, other factors to consider are the patient's overall condition including comorbidities, cardiovascular function, and the available clinical expertise in both fields. For surgeons, the key issue is the ability to perform a complete resection; as noted previously, any result other than complete resection is a futile thoracotomy. All attempts should be made to avoid a pneumonectomy as this procedure decreases short- and long-term quality of life. The risk of death after this procedure increases with time and strongly depends on the side of surgery; the 6-month mortality rate is as high as 24% for right pneumonectomy.[83] For the radiation oncologist, the primary issue is the ability to deliver an effective dose of radiotherapy, taking into consideration the tolerance of organs at risk.

Tumor bulk is an interesting parameter to consider. The tendency is to consult a surgeon if the tumor is small and a radiation oncologist if the tumor is large. However, the efficacy of radiotherapy is directly correlated with the number of cells in the tumors, and results are better for a lower number of cells than for

TABLE 39.6   PCI for NSCLC in Retrospective and Prospective Studies

Study	Year	Design	No. of Patients	Primary Therapy	PCI, Dose Gy/ Fraction	Brain No. PCI	Failures (%) PCI	p
Jacobs et al.[105]	1987	Retro	78	NA	30/15	24	5	0.06
Skarin[94]	1989	Retro	34	Trimodality	36/18	26	14	
Strauss et al.[106]	1992	Retro	54	Trimodality	30/15	12	0	
Albain et al.[89]	1995	Retro	126	Trimodality	36/18	16	8	0.44
Stuschke et al.[91]	1999	Prosp	75	Trimodality	30/15	54	13	<0.001
Cox et al.[107]	1981	Prosp	281	RT only	20/10	13	6	0.038
Umsawasdi et al.[108]	1984	Prosp	97	Multimodality	30/10	27	4	0.002
Russell et al.[92]	1991	Prosp	187	RT only	30/10	19	9	0.10
Pottgen et al.[109]	2007	Prosp	106	Multimodality	30/15	34.7	7.8	0.02
Gore et al.[110]	2011	Prosp	340	Multimodality	30/15	18	7.7	0.004
Li et al.[112]	2015		156	Multimodality	30/10	38.6	12.3	0.001

NA, not applicable; *NSCLC*, nonsmall cell lung cancer; *PCI*, prophylactic cranial irradiation; *Prosp*, prospective; *Retro*, retrospective; *RT*, radiotherapy.

a larger tumor with hypoxic regions. Another unanswered question is the role of surgery when the volume of normal tissue to be irradiated is too large and the risk of radiotherapy-induced toxicity is too high. For patients who are not candidates for surgery, concurrent chemoradiation therapy is the favored approach, raising the question of optimal treatment for fragile or an older individual. Last, the search continues for a biomarker to help with selecting the most appropriate locoregional treatment.

The guidelines from the American College of Chest Physicians include the following statement: "neoadjuvant therapy followed by surgery is neither clearly better nor clearly worse than definitive chemoradiation therapy."[84] The authors obviously favored a multidisciplinary approach but the heterogeneity of patients in trials limits the strength of the recommendation.

BRAIN METASTASES AND PROPHYLACTIC CRANIAL RADIATION

Brain metastases in patients with NSCLC are frequent complications that affect survival and quality of life, especially for patients with locally advanced disease. Chemoradiation therapy has been associated with increased frequency of brain metastases, causing relapse to occur first in the brain.[88–89]

The incidence of relapse with brain metastases in patients with locally advanced NSCLC after locoregional treatment ranges from 12% to 54%.[86,89–96] The risk of brain metastases has been associated with stage,[95] tumor size,[96] histology,[92] length of survival from diagnosis,[94–97] female sex,[98] age less than 60 years,[93,99] and type of locoregional therapy.[88,92,97,100] The authors of several studies of multimodality therapy for locally advanced NSCLC have reported an excellent median survival of 20 months to 43 months and a 3-year survival rate of 34% to 37%.[88,93,100–104] The brain was a common site of metastases in these studies. Overall, brain metastases have occurred in 22% to 55% of patients, and the frequency of brain as first site of relapse has ranged from 16% to 43%.

Prophylactic cranial irradiation has been evaluated for the treatment of locally advanced NSCLC in several retrospective and prospective studies.[86,88,89,91,104–110] The results have demonstrated that prophylactic cranial radiation reduces the incidence or delays the onset of brain metastases (Table 39.6). In a phase III trial, Cox et al.[107] randomly assigned 281 patients to receive prophylactic cranial radiation (20 Gy in 10 fractions) or no prophylactic cranial radiation. Prophylactic cranial radiation reduced the frequency of brain metastases in patients with NSCLC from 13% to 6% (p = 0.038), but there was no significant difference in median survival between the groups. Umsawasdi et al.[108] reported results from 97 patients with locally advanced NSCLC treated with chemoradiation therapy who were randomly assigned to

prophylactic cranial radiation (30 Gy in 10 fractions) or no prophylactic cranial radiation. Prophylactic cranial radiation significantly decreased the incidence of brain metastases compared with not receiving the treatment (4% vs. 27%, p = 0.002). No survival benefit was observed for the treated group due to adverse effects from other relapses. An RTOG prospective randomized study compared prophylactic cranial radiation (30 Gy in 10 fractions) and no brain treatment in patients with nonsquamous NSCLC.[89] Brain metastases developed in 18 (19%) of 94 patients randomly assigned to no prophylactic cranial radiation with eight (9%) of 93 patients who received the treatment (p = 0.10). No survival difference was found between the treatment arms. Pottgen et al.[109] randomly assigned 106 patients with stage IIIA NSCLC to prophylactic cranial radiation (30 Gy in 15 fractions) or no prophylactic cranial radiation and found that the treatment significantly reduced the probability of brain metastases as the first site of metastases (7.8% at 5 years vs. 34.7%; p = 0.02). There was no significant difference in neurocognitive performance between the groups.

The largest prospective study on prophylactic cranial radiation is the RTOG 0214, which involved 340 patients with stage III NSCLC who had definitive locoregional treatment.[110] Patients were randomly assigned to prophylactic cranial radiation (30 Gy in 2 Gy per fractions) or no prophylactic cranial radiation. This study was closed early because of slow accrual. Although the 1-year overall survival rate was similar between the groups (75.6% vs. 76.9% in the treatment and observation groups, respectively), the 1-year incidence of brain metastases was significantly different (7.7% vs. 18.0% for the treatment and observation groups, respectively, p = 0.004). There were no significant differences in global cognitive function measured with the Mini-Mental Status Examination or quality of life after prophylactic cranial radiation, but memory had declined significantly at 1 year as measured with the Hopkins Verbal Learning Test.[111] A last recent phase III trial included 156 patients operated on for a stage III–N2 NSCLC. After postoperative adjuvant chemotherapy, the patients were randomly allocated between prophylactic cranial radiation (30 Gy in 10 fractions) and observation. A reduction in brain metastases (10 in the treatment arm and 29 in the observation arm) and longer progression-free survival were observed without any difference in survival.[112]

In summary, prevention of symptomatic relapse with brain metastases in patients with locally advanced NSCLC may improve quality of life and overall survival. Studies have shown that prophylactic cranial radiation significantly decreases brain metastases among patients with locally advanced NSCLC. However, prophylactic cranial radiation is not recommended as a standard therapy, because available data do not provide evidence of survival benefit or sufficient information about late toxicity.

TABLE 39.7 Survival According to the Treatment From Selected Series

Authors	Study	N	Treatment	5-Year Survival
Koshy et al.[114]	National database	564	Neoadj C-RT lobectomy	33.5
		188	Neoadj C-RT Pneum.	20.7
		510	Lob. Adj C	20.3
		123	Pneum. Adj C	13.3
		9857	Conc Chemo RT	10.9
Albain et al.[64]	Phase III	202	RT + CT and surgery	27.2
		194	RT + CT	20.3
van Meerbeeck et al.[65]	Phase III	167	CT→Surgery	15.7
		165	CT→RT	14
Thomas et al.[67]	Phase III	260	CT→Surgery→RT	16
		264	CT + RT→Surgery	14
Auperin et al.[34]	Meta-analysis	602	CT→RT	11
		603	RT + CT	15

CT, chemotherapy; *RT,* radiotherapy.

OUTCOME MEASUREMENTS

Although various metrics can be used to evaluate treatment outcomes, overall survival is the most relevant end point. The wide range of reported survival outcomes within the stage III group reflects differences in prognostic characteristics and comorbidities as well as variations in treatments. The International Association for the Study of Lung Cancer collects data from trials, registries, and cases series in which patients have been treated with different modalities. When the data were analyzed, the 5-year survival rate was 19% for clinical stage IIIA, 7% for stage IIIB, 24% for pathologic stage IIIA, and 9% for stage IIIB.[113] The 5-year survival rate has also been reported in several influential trials (Table 39.7).[34,64,65,67,114] We should highlight the ongoing improvement in survival seen in trials over the last decades leading to 2-year survival rates over 50% with chemoradiation therapy.[19,41]

Progression-free survival and pattern of failures are less accurate end points. After chemoradiation therapy, it is often difficult to assess the tumor response because of radiotherapy-induced fibrosis; therefore, what researchers call local control is actually the lack of tumor progression. In a meta-analysis by Auperin et al.,[34] the proportion of patients with local and distant progression at 3 years after concurrent chemoradiation therapy was 28% and 40%, respectively. Thus more effective treatments are necessary to address two important problems: unsatisfactory locoregional control and high risk of development of distant metastases.

Another important end point is quality of life in terms of physical and mental health. Currently available treatments have a major effect on patients' ability to function, particularly after a pneumonectomy. Studies should be designed to better evaluate the toxicity related to surgery, radiotherapy, and chemotherapy. The quality of mental and physical health does not always change in parallel: emotional well-being may improve after treatment, despite declines in physical functioning. Deterioration is usually observed during and after treatment. Fatigue, dyspnea, coughing, and pain may last for months or even years. A correlation has been observed between quality-of-life scores and tumor response or even tumor extent. Comorbidities, extent of surgery, multimodality treatment, and continued smoking have a negative effect on the quality of life.[74,115] Smoking cessation should be encouraged in conjunction with any form of treatment with curative aim.

CONCLUSION

The treatment of clinical stage III locally advanced NSCLC should be carried out by a multidisciplinary team that includes medical oncologists, pulmonologists, surgeons, imaging specialists, and radiation oncologists. Multimodality therapy should be selected based on the patient's performance status, age, histology, tumor size and location, pulmonary and other organ function, and comorbidities.

Novel anticancer agents and new molecularly targeted drugs, as well as advances in radiation technology, are expected to improve outcomes in the near future. Despite substantial advances in the treatment of locally advanced NSCLC, it remains a deadly disease for most patients. Future treatment success depends on developing and improving therapeutic strategies.

KEY REFERENCES

10. Perez CA, Bauer M, Edelstein S, Gillespie BW, Birch R. Impact of tumor control on survival in carcinoma of the lung treated with irradiation. *Int J Radiat Oncol Biol Phys.* 1986;12:539–547.
12. Yuan S, Sun X, Li M, et al. A randomized study of involved-field irradiation versus elective nodal irradiation in combination with concurrent chemotherapy for inoperable stage III nonsmall cell lung cancer. *Am J Clin Oncol.* 2007;30:239–244.
15. De Ruysscher D, Faivre-Finn C, Nestle U, et al. European Organisation for Research and Treatment of Cancer recommendations for planning and delivery of high-dose, high-precision radiotherapy for lung cancer. *J Clin Oncol.* 2010;28:5301–5310.
19. Bradley JD, Paulus R, Komaki R, et al. Standard-dose versus high-dose conformal radiotherapy with concurrent and consolidation carboplatin plus paclitaxel with or without cetuximab for patients with stage IIIA or IIIB non-small-cell lung cancer (RTOG 0617): a randomised, two-by-two factorial phase 3 study. *Lancet Oncol.* 2015;16:187–199.
34. Auperin A, Le Péchoux C, Rolland E, et al. Meta-analysis of concomitant versus sequential radiochemotherapy in locally advanced non-small-cell lung cancer. *J Clin Oncol.* 2010;28:2181–2190.
41. Senan S, Brade A, Wang LH, et al. PROCLAIM: randomized phase III trial of pemetrexed-cisplatin or etoposide-cisplatin plus thoracic radiation therapy followed by consolidation chemotherapy in locally advanced nonsquamous non-small-cell lung cancer. *J Clin Oncol.* 2016;34:953–962.
42. Vokes EE, Herndon 2nd JE, Kelley MJ, et al. Induction chemotherapy followed by chemoradiotherapy compared with chemoradiotherapy alone for regionally advanced unresectable stage III non-small-cell lung cancer: Cancer and Leukemia Group B. *J Clin Oncol.* 2007;25:1698–1704.
51. Govindan R, Bogart J, Stinchcombe T, et al. Randomized phase II study of pemetrexed, carboplatin, and thoracic radiation with or without cetuximab in patients with locally advanced unresectable non-small-cell lung cancer: Cancer and Leukemia Group B trial 30407. *J Clin Oncol.* 2011;29:3120–3125.
53. Walraven I, van den Heuvel M, van Diessen J, et al. Long-term follow-up of patients with locally advanced non-small cell lung cancer receiving concurrent hypofractionated chemoradiotherapy with or without cetuximab. *Radiother Oncol.* 2016;118:442–446.
63. Johnson DB, Rioth MJ, Horn L. Immune checkpoint inhibitors in NSCLC. *Curr Treat Options Oncol.* 2014;15:658–669.
64. Albain KS, Swann RS, Rusch VW, et al. Radiotherapy plus chemotherapy with or without surgical resection for stage III non-small-cell lung cancer: a phase III randomised controlled trial. *Lancet.* 2009;374:379–386.
66. Eberhardt W, Pöttgen C, Gauler T, et al. Phase III study of surgery versus definitive concurrent chemoradiotherapy boost in patients with resectable stage IIIA(N2) and selected stage IIIB non-small-cell lung cancer after induction chemotherapy and concurrent chemoradiotherapy (ESPATUE). *J Clin Oncol.* 2015;33:4194–4201.
68. Pless M, Stupp R, Ris HB, et al. Induction chemoradiation in stage IIIA/N2 non-small-cell lung cancer: a phase 3 randomised trial. *Lancet.* 2015;386:1049–1056.
110. Gore EM, Bae K, Wong SJ, et al. Phase III comparison of prophylactic cranial irradiation versus observation in patients with locally advanced non-small-cell lung cancer: primary analysis of radiation therapy oncology group study RTOG 0214. *J Clin Oncol.* 2011;29:272–278.

See Expertconsult.com for full list of references.

40 Radiotherapy in the Management of Small Cell Lung Cancer: Thoracic Radiotherapy, Prophylactic Cranial Irradiation

Sara Ramella and Cécile Le Péchoux

SUMMARY OF KEY POINTS

- In patients with clinically nonmetastatic small cell lung cancer (SCLC), positron emission tomography–computed tomography (PET–CT) as well as brain imaging is suggested to classify tumor stage.
- To classify stage, it is recommended to use the Veterans Administration system (limited disease [LD] vs. extensive disease [ED]) as well as the International Union for International Cancer Control TNM Classification of Malignant Tumors seventh edition (2009), which recommended tumor, node, and metastasis (TNM) staging based on analysis of the International Association for the Study of Lung Cancer database. The prognostic value of clinical and pathologic T and N staging in patients with SCLC is confirmed in the eighth edition. For the M descriptors, more research is warranted.
- In patients with nonmetastatic SCLC or LD, combined chemoradiation is the standard. Concomitant chemoradiotherapy gives the best results and is preferred to sequential chemoradiotherapy, but the latter can be an option in fragile patients. Compliance with alternating regimens may be difficult, but promising results have been published.
- In fit, nonmetastatic SCLC patients, early chemoradiotherapy is recommended. In more fragile patients, for whom good compliance with early concomitant chemoradiotherapy cannot be expected, there is no survival advantage with early chemoradiation.
- A randomized phase III trial showed no difference between once-daily (66 Gy/33 fractions per 6.6 weeks) and twice-daily radiation (45 Gy/30 fractions per 3 weeks) given along with chemotherapy for patients with LD-SCLC.
- In patients with nonmetastatic SCLC who achieve a complete or partial response to initial therapy, prophylactic cranial irradiation (PCI) at the dose of 25 Gy in 10 daily fractions is recommended. It should not be administered concomitantly with chemotherapy.
- In metastatic SCLC, PCI is also recommended among patients with any response to chemotherapy based on a randomized trial and the meta-analysis. The same regimen (25 Gy/10 fractions per 2 weeks) or a more hypofractionated regimen (20 Gy/5 fractions per 1 week) may be administered. A recent Japanese study showed a decrease in brain metastasis rate but failed to demonstrate survival advantage with PCI in patients with extensive stage SCLC, but mature data are awaited.

- Patients should be informed of potential adverse effects on neurocognitive functioning that may be caused by PCI especially in elderly patients to balance the benefit of PCI on survival and risk of brain metastases.
- In patients with ED-SCLC who have completed chemotherapy and achieved a response, a course of consolidative thoracic radiotherapy (TR) is suggested by the results of a randomized trial. A subgroup analysis has shown that among patients with partial response in the chest, but not complete response, consolidation TR had an impact on survival.

Small cell lung cancer (SCLC) represents less than 20% of all lung cancers. It is an aggressive tumor, and only a third of patients have limited stage disease at diagnosis. As SCLC has a high propensity for early metastatic dissemination, chemotherapy has been and still is the cornerstone of treatment, but SCLC is also very sensitive to radiotherapy (RT).

Patients often have bulky mediastinal disease at presentation.[1] After staging procedures, SCLC was classically presented as LD or ED according to the Veterans Administration Lung Cancer Study Group Classification.[2] LD was defined as confined to a hemithorax and the regional lymphatic nodes (mediastinum, ipsilateral, and contralateral hilar regions, and supraclavicular fossa), thus theoretically encompassable with an RT field. Although this classification has been used for many years, the International Association for the Study of Lung Cancer has recommended the use of the new TNM classification for nonsmall cell lung cancer (NSCLC) for SCLC as well.[3] The seventh and the future eighth TNM classifications split patients into a larger number of prognostically homogeneous subgroups, which could better define those patients for whom thoracic RT (TR) might be beneficial.[3,4] Recent advances in the management of SCLC are principally attributed to the improved knowledge of the indications for RT, both in nonmetastatic (or limited) and in metastatic (or extensive) diseases. By contrast, in the last two decades, chemotherapy progress has reached a plateau. The integration of TR with systemic chemotherapy in SCLC as well as PCI is really a "unique success story in the field of radiation oncology and highlights the potential for effective local therapy to impact overall outcomes."[5]

This relative "success story" started with the publication in the early 1990s of an individual patient data-based meta-analysis of randomized trials comparing combined chemoradiotherapy with chemotherapy alone, which demonstrated an absolute overall survival (OS) benefit of 5.4% in favor of combination therapy (3-year OS of 8.9% vs. 14.3% in the chemoradiation arm). Pignon and colleagues[6] collected and analyzed individual data from 13 trials involving 2140 patients with LS-SCLC: the relative risk of death in the chemoradiation group, as compared with the chemotherapy alone group, was 0.86 (95% confidence

CHAPTER 40 Radiotherapy in the Management of Small Cell Lung Cancer: Thoracic Radiotherapy, Prophylactic Cranial Irradiation **375**

40

interval [CI], 0.78–0.94; $p = 0.001$). This equated to a 14% reduction in death with the addition of radiation. Warde and Payne[7] published similar findings in a literature-based analysis of 11 randomized trials. They showed that the addition of TR to chemotherapy led to an overall benefit of 5.4% on 2-year survival, and an improved 2-year intrathoracic tumor control (from 16.5% in the chemotherapy arm alone to 34.1% in the combined modality arm), resulting in a benefit in local control of about 25%. The combination of chemotherapy and RT became a standard in the early 1990s after the publication of these two meta-analyses. Subsequently, these benefits have been confirmed by other studies. The current state-of-the-art treatment for SCLC patients with nonmetastatic disease involves cisplatin (or carboplatin in more fragile patients)–etoposide chemotherapy combined with chest RT, as reported in guidelines worldwide.[8–10]

It is possible, however, that the two reported meta-analyses underestimate the results that can be obtained with platinum-based chemotherapy and contemporary RT as only a few studies included in the meta-analyses used platinum-based chemotherapy and concurrent chemoradiation, which are considered nowadays as part of the optimal treatment approach.

There are indeed different ways of combining chemotherapy and TR: they can be administered concurrently, sequentially, or in an alternating fashion. Furthermore, the issue of timing of RT has also been addressed in randomized trials: whether radiation should be given early or late in the overall course of treatment has long been a subject of debate.[11] Sequential schedules allow the delivery of full-dose chemotherapy followed by full-dose RT; tumor shrinkage can be observed after systemic therapy, but repopulation and selection of resistant cellular clones may lead to treatment failure.[1] The alternating schedule has a good toxicity profile, although from a practical point of view, it may be a complicated approach; the good results obtained in a French Study group randomized trial could not be reproduced by a larger European Organization for Research and Treatment of Cancer (EORTC) study.[12,13] The concomitant approach has the radiobiologic advantage of reducing the overall treatment time, which is a particularly relevant issue in SCLC treatment, although it is associated with an increased risk of acute toxicity, especially esophagitis. Even so, this latter approach has now become the standard of care.

Two phase III trials have studied alternating schedules: an EORTC study, which compared an alternating chemoradiation regimen with a sequential regimen,[13] and the "Petites Cellules" study,[14] which compared an alternating regimen with a concomitant chemoradiation approach. It should be noted that none of these trials used platinum-based chemotherapy. Results were poor in both trials, with no difference in terms of OS between the two arms (median 15 months vs. 14 months in the first study; 13.5 months vs. 14 months in the second one).

The Japan Clinical Oncology Group (JCOG) performed a phase III trial comparing a sequential and concurrent chemoradiation approach.[15] A total of 231 patients with LD-SCLC were randomly assigned to receive four cycles of cisplatin plus etoposide every 3 weeks followed by accelerated hyperfractionated TR at the dose of 45 Gy in 3 weeks (sequential arm) or the same four cycles of chemotherapy administered every 4 weeks with the same modality of TR starting on day 2 of the first cycle of chemotherapy (concurrent arm). The results favored the concurrent schedule with a median survival of 27.2 months versus 19.7 months of the sequential arm, even if the difference was not significant ($p = 0.097$).

TIMING QUESTION

Several phase III trials have examined the question of timing, that is, administration of early versus late RT during the course of combined chemotherapy and RT; however, the issue

remains controversial.[16–21] To try to clarify the issue, several meta-analyses were conducted between 2004 and 2007.[22–26] The definition of early and late TR differs in these literature-based meta-analyses. The first two meta-analyses were published in 2004 by Fried et al.[22] and Huncharek and McGarry[23] on more than 1500 patients each. Both studies showed an advantage for early RT. In the first study, late TR was defined as beginning 9 weeks after initiation of chemotherapy or after completion of the third cycle of chemotherapy.[22] This meta-analysis showed a statistically significant benefit of 5% of early TR over late TR in terms of 2-year OS (relative risk [RR], 1.17; $p = 0.03$). Moreover, both studies reported that the best results could be achieved if platinum and etoposide were administrated concomitantly with early RT. In a meta-analysis published by De Ruysscher et al.,[24] early RT was defined as beginning within 30 days after the start of chemotherapy. The 2-year and 5-year OS rates were not significantly different (odds ratio [OR], 0.84; 95% CI, 0.56–1.28 vs. OR, 80; 95% CI, 0.47–1.38). However, when the only trial that delivered concurrent nonplatinum-based chemotherapy was excluded, the results were significantly in favor of early RT, with a 5-year survival rate of 20.2% for early versus 13.8% for late RT (OR, 0.64; 95% CI, 0.44–0.92; $p = 0.02$). Based on the same published data of four randomized trials, De Ruysscher et al.[25] hypothesized that the start of any treatment until the end of RT (SER) was important to consider in SCLC, taking into account both overall duration of RT and timing of TR. They concluded that a shorter time between the initiation of chemotherapy and the subsequent completion of RT was prognostic for survival. There was a significantly higher survival rate in the shorter SER arms; a 5-year OS rate of 20% was reached when the SER was less than 30 days (RR, 0.62; 95% CI, 0.49–0.80; $p = 0.0003$). Moreover, each additional week of the SER resulted in an overall absolute decrease in the 5-year survival rate of 1.8%. Acute toxicity, and particularly severe esophagitis, is related to timing and SER with a higher incidence in case of early RT and shorter time between start and end of therapy (OR, 0.63; 95% CI, 0.40–1.00; $p = 0.05$ and OR, 0.55; 95% CI, 0.42–0.73; $p = 0.0001$, respectively). This SER concept should certainly be further evaluated and considered in designing future studies as repopulation of cells seems to be a major cause of failure. As emphasized by Brade and Tannock[1] in an editorial, repopulation of cells between dose fractions is important for recovery in normal tissue, but repopulation of surviving tumor cells also occurs and offsets tumor cell kill. Repopulation triggered by neoadjuvant chemotherapy may inhibit the effectiveness of subsequent RT.

The same team published an update of their literature-based meta-analysis including 11 trials; there was no difference in 2-year survival, but once again excluding the only nonplatinum-based trial, the benefit of early RT became statistically significant (OR, 0.73; 95% CI, 0.57–0.94; $p < 0.05$).[26]

Another interesting observation that emerges from these studies is related to treatment compliance. Two studies with the same design and therapeutic regimen have been included in this meta-analysis: the NCI-C trial and the London trial.[20,21] The survival advantage observed for the early RT group in comparison with the late one (21 months vs. 16 months; $p < 0.05$, respectively) reported by the NCI-C trial was not confirmed by the London trial (14 vs. 15 months, respectively). However, in the latter study, patients randomized to early chest radiation received significantly less chemotherapy than in the late arm (69% in the early group and 80% in the late one, $p = 0.03$). In the NCI-C study, the percentage of intended total dose completed was the same for the early and late groups (both 86%). Similar disappointing survival results have also been reported by the Hellenic trial;[17] when analyzing compliance, a significant reduction in completion of planned chemotherapy was reported in patients who had early RT (71% in the early group and 90% in the late group, $p = 0.01$). Hence, it would seem that only patients who can receive early RT as planned according to the protocol benefit from it. This issue has been thoroughly addressed in an individual data-based meta-analysis that concluded that there was no difference in terms of OS between "earlier or shorter" versus "later or longer" TR when all trials were analyzed together.[11] However, "earlier or shorter" delivery of TR with planned chemotherapy significantly improved 5-year OS at the expense of more acute toxicity, especially esophagitis. The authors highlight that the hazard ratio (HR) for OS is significantly in favor of "earlier or shorter" RT where there was a similar proportion of patients who were compliant with chemotherapy in both arms (HR, 0.79; 95% CI, 0.69–0.91) and in favor of "later or longer" RT among trials with different compliance to chemotherapy (HR, 1.19; 95% CI, 1.05–1.34; interaction test, $p < 0.0001$). Thereby, the absolute gain between "earlier or shorter" and "later or longer" TR in 5-year OS for similar compliance trials was 7.7% (95% CI, 2.6% to 12.8%) and was –2.2% (–5.8% to 1.4%) for different compliance trials. As expected, "earlier or shorter" TR was associated with a higher incidence of severe acute esophagitis.

Finally, a large retrospective study examined the National Cancer Database to assess practice patterns and survival for TR timing in relation to chemotherapy in 8391 nonmetastatic SCLC patients. This study suggested that early initiation of TR was associated with improved survival (5-year survival rate of 21.9%) compared with late initiation (5-year survival rate of 19.1%, $p = 0.01$), particularly when hyperfractionated radiation was utilized (28.2% vs. 21.2%, $p = 0.004$).[27]

Sun et al.[28] published a randomized trial of 219 patients, who were allocated to receive four cycles of cisplatin and etoposide with radiation beginning with the first cycle or the third cycle. It was not included in any of the meta-analyses. Patients received a total dose of 52.5 Gy in 25 daily fractions of 2.1 Gy over 5 weeks. Late RT was not inferior to early RT in terms of complete response rate, which was the main end point (early vs. late: 36.0% vs. 38.0%, respectively). After a median follow-up of 59 months, OS was similar in the two groups (rates at 2 years and 5 years after randomization in the early vs. late radiation arms were 50.7% vs. 56.0% and 24.3% vs. 24.0%, respectively). Thus as recommended by European and North American guidelines, patients with nonmetastatic disease, with good performance status (PS) and good compliance should be treated with concurrent chemoradiotherapy.[8–10] TR should be administered early in the course of treatment, in fit patients, for whom a good compliance may be expected, preferably beginning with cycle one or two of chemotherapy. According to the study of Sun et al.,[28] TR could be administered concomitantly to the third cycle with equivalent results. Nevertheless, this observation should be confirmed in another study because one should be cautious when extrapolating results issued from Asian population studies to non-Asian patients in lung cancer. Chemotherapy should consist of four cycles of a platinum agent and etoposide.

FRACTIONATION AND DOSE

Historically, modest total doses of daily fractionated radiation (1.8–2 Gy daily to 40–50 Gy) were used because of the observed responsiveness of SCLC to radiation. Although the clinical response rates with these total doses are high, durable local control is poor.[29–31] The hypothesis that hyperfractionated radiation therapy might be more effective than normofractionated schedules is based on in vitro marked radiosensitivity even to small doses of radiation, and on the high kinetics of SCLC proliferation and its repopulation between two fractions of treatment.[32] The in vitro observation of the lack of a shoulder on the cell survival curve for SCLC cell lines provides some of the rationale for

the hyperfractionated schedule, in which the dose per fraction is 1.5 Gy. Two phase III trials comparing conventional RT with hyperfractionated accelerated twice-daily RT schemes have been published.[33,34] In both trials, concomitant cisplatin plus etoposide chemotherapy was delivered with twice-daily RT; however, in the first trial RT was delivered after three cycles of chemotherapy, whereas in the second one RT started upfront during the first cycle of chemotherapy. In the NCCTG study,[33] the overall treatment time was similar in the conventional and hyperfractionated arms because of a 2.5-week split at the midpoint of treatment, and this could be the cause of the lack of difference in local progression (33% in the once-daily arm vs. 35% in the twice-daily arm) and OS (20.6 months in both arms). In the Intergroup trial 0096/ECOG 3588,[34] 417 patients were randomly assigned to receive a total of 45 Gy of concurrent TR, given either 1.5 Gy twice daily over a 3-week period or the conventional once daily over a period of 5 weeks. A significant difference in OS was reported in the last trial (19 months in the once-daily arm vs. 23 months in the twice-daily arm, $p = 0.04$) with a benefit in 2-year and 5-year survival rates (41% vs. 47% and 16% vs. 26%, respectively). As expected, grade III esophagitis was more frequent in the investigational arm (27% vs. 11%). An individual patient data meta-analysis on hyperfractionated and accelerated regimens in lung cancer has been conducted, which included trials comparing conventional fractionation with altered fractionation schedules in both SCLC and NSCLC.[35] This meta-analysis showed a significant OS benefit from accelerated or hyperfractionated RT in patients with NSCLC. The effect of altered fractionation on OS was similar among patients with SCLC, but not statistically significant (HR, 0.87 [95% CI, 0.74–1.02, $p = 0.08$]). The absolute benefit on OS was 1.7% at 3 years (from 29.6% to 31.3%) and 5.1% at 5 years. An interesting interaction between modified regimen and PS was reported (PS 0: HR, 0.81; PS 1: HR, 0.86; PS 2: HR, 2.22), underlining once again the correlation between survival benefit derived from altered fractionation regimens and the importance of patients being fit enough to undergo a more intensive regimen.

Despite the results of the Intergroup trial, showing that the 45-Gy twice-daily regimen could improve survival, accelerated hyperfractionated RT has not been widely adopted in general clinical practice. The reasons are possibly related to the logistical difficulties of delivering twice-daily RT, the increase in acute toxicity (especially esophageal), and possibly to the fact that the control arm used rather low doses of RT. However, the most important lesson that came from INT 0096 is the demonstration that intensified RT with concomitant chemotherapy could have an impact on survival.

A recent randomized phase II Norwegian trial compared two schedules, one using twice-daily fractionation (45 Gy in 30 fractions) and the other once-daily (42 Gy in 15 fractions) so that the overall radiation treatment time was the same. Although survival favored the twice-daily regimen in this small trial, it was not statistically significant (median 25.1 months vs. 18.8 months, $p = 0.61$). Response rates were significantly higher with the twice-daily regimen, with no difference in severe toxicities between schedules.[36] The way to intensify local therapy can be summarized in two strategies: total dose escalation and further exploration of altered fractionation schedules (i.e., applying concomitant boost).

Modern data on RT dose escalation come from several Cancer and Leukemia Group B (CALGB) studies starting with a phase I trial to determine the maximum tolerated dose of the twice-daily regimen and of the once-daily treatment delivered concomitantly to the fourth cycle of platinum-based chemotherapy.[37] The total recommended dose was 45 Gy for twice-daily RT, and 70 Gy for conventional fractionation. These promising results led to several phase II trials, which all confirmed the feasibility of delivering 70 Gy with concomitant chemotherapy.[38]

CHAPTER 40   Radiotherapy in the Management of Small Cell Lung Cancer: Thoracic Radiotherapy, Prophylactic Cranial Irradiation   **377**

40

The concomitant regimen (carboplatin and etoposide based) was administered after two cycles of chemotherapy with paclitaxel and topotecan. The median survival was 23 months in patients who had a weight loss over 5% compared with 31 months in patients with weight loss less than 5% before diagnosis. In a pooled analysis of limited-stage SCLC patients treated with two cycles of induction chemotherapy followed by concurrent platinum-based chemotherapy and RT, the authors analyzed 200 patients from three consecutive CALGB L-SCLC phase II trials (39808, 30002, and 30206) using high-dosage once-daily RT with concurrent chemotherapy.[39] The median follow-up was 78 months. Grade 3 or greater esophagitis was 23%. The median survival for pooled population was 19.9 months, and the 5-year rate was 20%. The 2-year progression-free survival was 26%. The authors concluded that 2-Gy daily RT to a total dosage of 70 Gy is well tolerated, and with similar outcome to twice-daily RT administered with chemotherapy. However, this hypothesis should be confirmed in a randomized trial, which is ongoing (NCT00433563).

The second method for intensifying local treatment was applied by Radiation Therapy Oncology Group (RTOG) researchers conducting some clinical studies with a hybrid approach, consisting of once-daily RT at standard fractionation in the first part of treatment followed by twice-daily RT to counter repopulation. The RTOG applied this dose escalation method from a total dose of 50.4 Gy to 64.8 Gy.[40] The esophagitis rate was lower than in the INT 0096 trial (18% in comparison with 27%), and so were the median and 2-year survival rates (19 months and 36.6% in comparison with 23 months and 47%, respectively).

To establish the optimal dose and fractionation, two phase III trials have been undertaken comparing two modalities of concurrent chemoradiation: hyperfractionated accelerated RT (45 Gy in 3 weeks as given in the INT 0096 study) and once-daily RT at higher dosage (66–70 Gy in 6.5 weeks) corresponding to a higher biologic effective dose but with superior overall treatment time.

The Intergroup trial CALGB 30610/RTOG 0538 (NCT00632853) started as a three-arm study. It was decided that the experimental arm with the higher rate of toxic events would be discontinued. Arm B was then closed in 2013. This trial is continuing as a two-arm study comparing arm A (twice-daily RT of 45 Gy) with arm C (once-daily RT of 70 Gy).

- Arm A: twice-daily RT up to a total dose of 45 Gy delivered concurrently to the first cycles of four cisplatin and etoposide chemotherapy regimens;
- Arm B: hybrid approach applied concurrently to the same chemotherapy regimen (this arm has been discontinued after a preplanned interim analysis);
- Arm C: once-daily RT at standard fractionation up to a total dose of 70 Gy with the same chemotherapy regimen.

The second phase III trial is the CONVERT intergroup study (concurrent once-daily vs. twice-daily RT; NCT00433563), which is a United Kingdom–led study comparing twice-daily and once-daily RT. The results of the CONVERT study were presented at the American Society of Clinical Oncology Annual Meeting, in 2016.[41] The study enrolled 547 patients with proven SCLC from 73 centers in seven European countries and Canada between 2008 and 2013. Patients were randomized to receive either concurrent twice-daily radiation therapy (45 Gy in 30 twice-daily fractions over 3 weeks) or concurrent once-daily radiation therapy (66 Gy in 33 once-daily fractions over 6.5 weeks), both starting with the second cycle of chemotherapy on day 22. Four or six cycles of cisplatin–etoposide were given according to the investigator's prespecified choice. Patients with any response were offered prophylactic cranial radiation. At a median follow-up of 45 months, 2-year and 3-year survival

rates and median survival were 56%, 43%, and 30 months, respectively, for the twice-daily radiation therapy versus 51%, 39%, and 25 months for the once-daily radiation therapy (HR, 1.17; 95% CI, 0.95–1.45; $p = 0.15$). Toxicities were comparable; grade 3/4 esophagitis rate was 19% in the twice-daily arm and 18% in the once-daily arm. The results of CONVERT support the use of either regimen for standard-of-care treatment of nonmetastatic SCLC with good PS. The authors insisted that survival in both arms was higher than previously reported probably because of better patient selection.

To summarize, the evidence strongly supports concurrent chemotherapy and RT for patients with LS-SCLC. The available data also suggest that RT should begin early in good performance patients; the RT fractionation programs that satisfy these parameters have been associated with better survival.

RADIATION TREATMENT VOLUMES

The two major issues regarding treatment volume in SCLC can be summarized as follows:

- Is it appropriate to use the postchemotherapy target volume after induction chemotherapy in cases where RT is delayed?
- Do we need to electively treat clinically uninvolved regional lymph nodes?

An evolution in target volume definition can be recognized over the last two decades. In the early 1990s, emerging evidence demonstrated that smaller radiation target volumes did not adversely affect tumor control in the management of LD-SCLC.[42,43] In fact, more than 80% of failures occurred in-field, suggesting that inadequate radiation doses rather than inadequate volumes were the primary cause of intrathoracic recurrence.[44] Therefore the prevailing issue of recent research has been to reduce the treatment field size while increasing the radiation dose and sparing surrounding organs at risk. The analysis of the site of recurrence after chemoradiation may help define the optimal treatment volume. In the randomized study by Kies et al.[42] published in 1987, patients achieving a partial response or stable disease after induction chemotherapy were randomized to receive RT either to the prechemotherapy volume or to the postinduction reduced tumor volume. The local recurrence rate was not significantly different in the two arms (32% vs. 28%). Liengswangwong et al.[43] and Arriagada et al.[30] came to the same conclusions in their studies. Consequently, treating the residual tumor after induction chemotherapy may be sufficient. However, it should be underlined that most patients treated in these older studies had no chemotherapy-based treatment planning. More recent trials have explored the role of involved-field RT. In 2008, a report from the International Atomic Energy Agency explored whether one should electively treat all mediastinal nodes, or selectively include those with some clinical risk for harboring disease, or perhaps omit elective nodal irradiation (ENI) altogether.[45] This review revealed how limited the evidence was for defining the place of ENI in SCLC at that time. The authors suggested the need for prospective clinical trials and recommended that, given the lack of strong evidence regarding ENI in LD-SCLC, the use of ENI should be considered on a case-by-case basis.

More recently, prospective clinical trials have explored this issue and have reported on isolated mediastinal relapse, defined as failure in an initially uninvolved lymph node region in the absence of local recurrence or distant metastasis. A small prospective study (37 patients) from the Netherlands Cancer Institute reported only two out-of-field isolated nodal failures (5.3%) with an excellent 5-year survival of 27% using involved-field RT as part of combined modality treatment.[46] In another small study from the United Kingdom (38 patients), where patients were treated omitting ENI based on CT imaging,[47] no isolated nodal failure was reported. Eight patients were found to have an intrathoracic recurrence: two within the planning target volume only, four within the planning target volume and distantly. There were only two cases of thoracic nodal relapse (6.5%), and both were accompanied by distant metastases. The Maastricht group outlined the possible importance of PET–CT in defining treatment volumes in SCLC. In the first prospective study,[48] with the gross tumor and nodal volume being defined by CT imaging, they reported an isolated nodal failure in 3 of 27 patients (11%), all in the supraclavicular region. Thus the omission of ENI on the basis of CT scan resulted in a higher-than-expected rate of isolated nodal failure in the ipsilateral supraclavicular fossa. However, the authors stated that because of the small sample size, no definitive conclusion could be drawn, and recommended to continue use of ENI outside of clinical trials. However, they started a small prospective trial evaluating selective nodal irradiation based on ^{18}F-2-deoxy-D-glucose (FDG)-PET for LD-SCLC.[49] Of the 60 patients enrolled, 39 (65%) developed a recurrence, but only two patients (3%) experienced isolated nodal failure. These findings are in contrast with the previous experience of CT-based selective nodal irradiation.[46]

In 2012, Xia et al.[50] examined the pattern of failures in 108 patients included in two successive trials and treated with combined involved-field RT and chemotherapy. They reported an isolated nodal failure rate in 5 patients (4.6%) treated with involved-field RT and chemotherapy using CT imaging for target definition, all in the ipsilateral supraclavicular area. Moreover, another four supraclavicular nodal failures with simultaneous distant metastases were also observed. To try to clarify the role of prophylactic irradiation of the supraclavicular area, a retrospective analysis on 239 patients has been conducted by Feng et al.[51] The supraclavicular metastasis incidence was 34.7%; multivariate analysis showed that upper mediastinal involvement (level 2 or 3) was significantly associated with supraclavicular metastasis. Thus such patients with upper mediastinal involvement could theoretically benefit from prophylactic irradiation of the supraclavicular lymph nodes. The lesions located in the right upper lobe had a higher incidence of supraclavicular involvement. In patients with supraclavicular involvement, 36% had bilateral or contralateral lymph node metastases and the frequency of contralateral involvement was higher for left-sided tumors than for those on the right.

The available data suggest that FDG-PET scans are more accurate than CT in the primary staging of SCLC and subsequently may lead to a reduction in the rate of isolated nodal failure.[9,52–55] A systematic review suggests that compared with conventional staging, PET can alter management in at least 28% of SCLC patients, resulting in the addition of life-prolonging RT in 6% and averting unnecessary RT with associated toxicity in 9%.[52] The cost analysis revealed that the PET-based strategy and the conventional methods do not seem significantly different, but PET may reduce health-care costs through avoidance of inappropriate TR.[53] A planning study on FDG-PET–based selective mediastinal node irradiation in 21 LD-SCLC patients showed a change in the PET treatment plan compared with the CT-based plan in 24% of cases.[54]

In a retrospective study by Shirvani et al.[55] examining the role of FDG-PET–based treatment planning before intensity-modulated RT combined with chemotherapy in 60 patients with SCLC and omitting ENI, a low rate of isolated nodal failure was found (2%). The authors concluded that ENI could be safely omitted in patients who underwent staging with PET–CT and treatment with intensity-modulated RT. Recently, a continuation of the work by Van Loon et al.[49] has been published by Reymen and colleagues,[56] expanding the initial series of 59 patients to 119 patients treated with concomitant chemotherapy and accelerated hyperfractionated RT, with only CT-PET–positive

or pathologically proven nodal sites being included in the target volume. Isolated elective nodal failure occurred only in two patients (1.7%) as in other studies using PET–CT for treatment planning. Median follow-up was 38 months, median OS was 20 months (95% CI, 17.8–22.1 months), and 2-year survival was 38.4%. In multivariate analysis, only total gross tumor volume (corresponding to postchemotherapy tumor volume and prechemotherapy nodal volume) and PS significantly influenced survival ($p = 0.026$ and $p = 0.016$, respectively).

A comparison of treatment outcomes between involved field and ENI in LS-SCLC was conducted retrospectively in a Korean study of 80 patients.[57] The two groups had similar overall and progression-free survival; however, for patients who had no PET scan, survival was significantly longer in patients who had ENI. All the isolated nodal recurrences were observed in patients who had no PET scan in their initial workup.

In a retrospective study of 253 patients treated in one institution over more than 10 years, the authors focused on locoregional failures. The cumulative locoregional failure rate was 29% and 38% at 2 years and 5 years, respectively. About 30% of local and regional failures were in-field, so most failures were marginal or out-of-field. Thus, according to these authors, it may be possible to prevent locoregional failure with improved RT target definition and careful consideration of the initial extent of disease.[58]

In conclusion, if patients do not have PET staging, the extension of the initial disease should be carefully evaluated to reduce the risk of isolated nodal failure and impaired survival outcome, and elective irradiation of the supraclavicular region should be considered. Subsequently, involved-field irradiation for limited stage SCLC can be considered with pretreatment PET–CT scan implementation. The two phase III trials investigating once-daily versus twice-daily RT will hopefully contribute to clarify volume issues. They do not recommend ENI, but require that both FDG-PET–avid lymph nodes and enlarged regional lymph nodes by CT criteria (regardless of FDG-PET activity) are included in the radiation treatment volume.

CHEMOTHERAPY REGIMEN COMBINED WITH RADIOTHERAPY

Since the early 80s, etoposide combined with cisplatin or carboplatin has been the cornerstone treatment of SCLC. Several new chemotherapy combinations have been explored in LD, with some of them seeming promising, especially paclitaxel and irinotecan.[59–64] However, none has shown superiority in terms of efficacy or tolerance compared with the platin-based and etoposide regimen, which remains the widely accepted standard. The JCOG published a randomized trial investigating the efficacy of irinotecan plus cisplatin in patients with nonmetastatic disease (JCOG0202).[63] The hypothesis that irinotecan and cisplatin could improve OS compared with etoposide plus cisplatin as demonstrated in ED by the same group could not be confirmed.[65] Of 281 patients enrolled, 272 received induction etoposide plus cisplatin and accelerated hyperfractionated RT (45 Gy) and 258 were randomly assigned to consolidation chemotherapy with etoposide–cisplatin or irinotecan–cisplatin (3 cycles). However, even if there was no significant difference in terms of survival between the two arms—35.8% in the etoposide–cisplatin arm and 33.7% in the investigational irinotecan plus cisplatin arm, respectively (HR, 1.09 [95% CI, 0.80–1.46]; $p = 0.70$)—the 5-year OS rate was among the best reported so far in phase III studies. Median survival was 3.2 years in the etoposide–cisplatin arm and 2.8 years in the irinotecan plus cisplatin arm. As outlined by the authors, this result might be partly attributable to selection of patients, but also to quality control of RT that may have an impact on outcome, as shown in a recent meta-analysis.[66] A phase II trial was also performed in the United States, with a different design consisting of two cycles with cisplatin and irinotecan followed by once-daily chest irradiation (70 Gy) administered concurrently with carboplatin etoposide (CALGB 30206). The 2-year survival was 31%, so it did not meet the survival target for further development.[64]

If many therapeutic strategies have been disappointing in SCLC, there are promising strategies such as immunotherapy. Several studies in patients with lung cancer have suggested a possible favorable association between the increased presence of immunologically active cells in the tumor and survival, suggesting that immunotherapy may be a viable approach for patients with SCLC. Early clinical trials with nivolumab and ipilimumab have shown activity in a broad range of cancers, including SCLC.[67]

There is an ongoing randomized phase II study (NCT02046733) investigating the efficacy and tolerability of the standard treatment (chemotherapy and RT) alone, compared with the standard treatment followed by immunotherapy (nivolumab and ipilimumab) in patients with limited SCLC, and more trials are ongoing in ED.

EXTENSIVE DISEASE: THORACIC RADIOTHERAPY

The majority of metastatic (or ED) SCLC patients respond to induction chemotherapy, but more than 50% of patients will eventually experience intrathoracic failure.[8,9,68,69] The hypothesis to add RT to chemotherapy is based on possible improvement in local control and survival benefits by controlling residual disease that is resistant to chemotherapy. Moreover, in a patient population with incurable malignancy, maintenance of local control to minimize/delay symptoms as long as possible may be considered as an important clinical objective. The role of radiation therapy in extensive SCLC was traditionally reserved for patients who required local palliation, and typically was not considered part of the standard of care in the absence of mediastinal symptoms. In 1999, Jeremic et al.[70] published a randomized study to evaluate whether TR as consolidation treatment could improve the poor results observed in ED-SCLC. Patients were randomized to either six cycles of chemotherapy of cisplatin–etoposide or six cycles of the same chemotherapy with 54 Gy of hyperfractionated TR. Patients who had a complete response outside the thorax after three cycles of chemotherapy and an at least partial response in the thorax benefited from subsequent concurrent chemotherapy and radiation. Median survival time (17 months vs. 11 months, $p = 0.041$), 5-year survival rate (9.1% vs. 3.7%, $p = 0.041$), and median time to local recurrence (30 months vs. 22 months, $p = 0.062$) were all improved in the RT group. This trial was conducted in a single institution and underpowered so the issue remained controversial.

There are two very recent trials that have investigated the role of extracranial RT in addition to PCI following platinum-based chemotherapy in patients with ED-SCLC. The Dutch Lung Cancer Study Group has activated an international randomized controlled trial of TR versus observation for patients with ED-SCLC who responded to chemotherapy. The trial coordinated by Slotman et al.[71] accrued 483 patients (Chest Radiotherapy in Extensive Stage SCLC Trial [CREST]). In CREST, patients were randomized to receive TR (30 Gy in 10 fractions within 2 weeks) plus PCI or PCI only. While there was no difference between groups in the primary end point of 1-year OS, a significant difference was observed in OS at 2 years in a secondary analysis (13% vs. 3%, with and without chest radiation, respectively, $p = 0.004$). The HR for OS was 0.84 with a 95% CI just passing through 1.00 (0.69–1.01; $p = 0.066$). The study also showed that TR led to a significant improvement in progression-free survival ($p < 0.001$) and a nearly 50% reduction in the risk of intrathoracic progression ($p < 0.001$). A subsequent analysis has shown that TR

improved OS significantly as well as progression-free survival in patients who had residual intrathoracic disease after chemotherapy.[72] In these patients, the difference in OS was statistically significant ($p = 0.03$; HR, 0.81; 95% CI, 0.66–0.98; stratified). In patients who achieved a complete intrathoracic response, no benefit of TR was observed. Within the RTOG, a randomized phase II trial was activated to determine the role of consolidation extracranial RT (thoracic and other extracranial metastatic sites) plus PCI after a response to systemic chemotherapy (RTOG 0937; clinical trials.gov NCT01055197).[73] Extensive stage SCLC patients with up to three extrathoracic sites were randomized to PCI only or PCI plus consolidative RT to the thorax and residual distant metastases to a total dose of 45 Gy in 15 fractions within 3 weeks. The primary end point was 1-year survival, and a total of 154 patients were to be enrolled. However, as the planned interim analysis seemed to show that the study crossed the futility boundary, the trial was closed to accrual after inclusion of 91 patients. Observed 1-year OS was 60.1% (95% CI, 41.2% to 74.7%) in the PCI arm and 50.8% (95% CI, 34% to 65.3%) in the PCI plus consolidative RT arm ($p = 0.21$). The authors concluded that the observed OS exceeded predicted OS in both arms, and consolidative RT to the thorax and extracranial metastases delayed progression of disease but did not improve 1-year OS.

PROPHYLACTIC CRANIAL IRRADIATION

Brain metastases are frequent in SCLC and responsible for serious impairment of patients' survival and quality of life.[74] Approximately 15% of patients have brain metastasis at the time of diagnosis, and this rate is even higher with more accurate imaging, such as magnetic resonance imaging (MRI). Moreover, about half of patients in complete remission after treatment for LD-SCLC will develop brain relapse.[75] In the early 1980s, PCI was therefore introduced to prevent brain metastasis. Most of the randomized trials testing PCI showed a significant decrease of brain metastasis incidence in favor of PCI; however, none of them individually could demonstrate a significant improvement in OS. Thus a meta-analysis was undertaken, based on individual data of almost 1000 patients in complete remission included in seven randomized phase III studies.[76] Thoracic complete remission corresponded to at least normalization of chest x-ray in most trials. In this meta-analysis, 85% of the patients had LD- and 15% had ED-SCLC; administered PCI dose ranged from 8 Gy in one fraction to 40 Gy in 20 fractions. At 3 years, there was an absolute decrease of 25.3% in the cumulative incidence of brain metastasis (59% in the control arm vs. 33% in the PCI arm, $p < 0.001$) and an absolute increase in survival of 5.4% from 15.3% in the control group to 20.7% in the treatment group ($p = 0.01$). Interestingly, an indirect comparison of four total dose groups (8 Gy, 24–25 Gy, 30 Gy, and 36–40 Gy) showed a significant trend ($p = 0.02$) toward a decrease in the risk of brain failure with higher PCI dose. The authors also identified a trend ($p = 0.01$) toward a lower risk of brain metastasis with earlier administration of PCI after start of the treatment. Therefore PCI became part of the standard of care for complete and good responders based on CT scan evaluation. More recently, in a retrospective study based on the National Cancer Institute's Surveillance, Epidemiology, and End Results (SEER) Program, which involved almost 8000 patients, Patel et al.[77] have reported similar results, with a significant improvement in both overall and cause-specific survival in favor of PCI. The 5-year OS rate was 19% among patients who had PCI versus 11% among patients who had no PCI ($p \leq 0.001$).

Other challenges raised by the meta-analysis are optimal timing and optimal dose for PCI. The PCI Collaborative Group has published an intergroup trial addressing the question of dose–effect to prevent the development of brain metastases in patients with LD who achieved a complete response (i.e., at least a normal chest radiograph).[78] It compared a standard dose of 25 Gy in 10 fractions with a higher dose of 36 Gy (36 Gy/18 fractions or 36 Gy in 24 twice-daily fractions). It is noteworthy that to evaluate a possible increased neurologic toxicity, quality of life and neurologic assessments both before and after PCI were performed. Toxicities and treatment delivery were not different between the two arms. Patients who received the high-dose had a nonsignificant decrease in brain metastases compared with patients who received the standard dose. The rate of brain metastasis at 2 years was 29% and 23% in the high-dose and standard-dose groups, respectively ($p = 0.18$). For unclear reasons, OS was significantly decreased among patients in the high-dose PCI group (HR for death, 1.2 [95% CI, 1.00–1.44]). The importance of fractionation in terms of efficacy, tolerance, and possible neurologic sequelae could be determined by a phase II/III trial (RTOG 0212), which compared three schedules: 25 Gy in 10 fractions; conventional fractionation (36 Gy in 18 fractions); and hyperfractionated accelerated RT (36 Gy in 24 twice-daily fractions).[79] At 1 year after PCI there was a significant increase in the occurrence of neurotoxicity in the 36-Gy cohort ($p = 0.02$). Logistic regression analysis revealed increasing age to be the most significant predictor of chronic neurotoxicity ($p = 0.005$).

Another important issue is whether elderly people should have PCI, as the rate of elderly patients with SCLC is increasing, and about 50% of nonmetastatic patients are 70 years or older. Using the same SEER database, the authors identified 1926 patients aged 70 years or older who were diagnosed with LD between 1988 and 1997; amongst them, 138 patients (7.2%) received PCI. Median age was 75 years, ranging from 70 years to 94 years; in this group of patients, 2-year and 5-year OS rates (33.3% and 11.6%, respectively) were significantly better among patients who received PCI than in patients who did not receive PCI (23.1% and 8.6%, respectively; $p = 0.028$). On multivariate analysis, PCI was found to be an independent predictor of OS in patients aged 80 years or less.[80] However, this potential benefit has to be balanced against the potential neurocognitive sequelae of PCI that are known to increase with age.[74] PCI at 25 Gy in 10 fractions is now recommended for LD-SCLC good responders.[8–10] A recent review has also examined the role of PCI in SCLC in specific subgroups such as resected or elderly patients.[74]

PROPHYLACTIC CRANIAL IRRADIATION IN EXTENSIVE DISEASE

Even if the PCI meta-analysis, which included 15% of patients with ED, supported PCI in ED for complete responders, the question remained unanswered for patients with partial response.[76] Furthermore, most clinicians were reluctant to administer PCI in metastatic patients. The EORTC thus decided to undertake a phase III trial randomizing exclusively patients with ED who had partial or complete response to first-line treatment. They would be randomly assigned PCI (20–30 Gy) or no PCI.[81] Patients in the PCI arm were mostly treated with a short-course schedule: among the 143 irradiated patients, 89 received 20 Gy in 5 fractions, and the others were treated with various fractionation schedules (30 Gy in 10 fractions, 30 Gy in 12 fractions, or 25 Gy in 10 fractions). The results of this study were strongly in favor of PCI: not only did PCI significantly reduce the risk of symptomatic brain failure, but it also significantly improved OS. The cumulative risk of symptomatic brain metastases at 1 year was 14.6% in the PCI arm and 40.4% in the control arm ($p < 0.001$), and the 1-year survival rate was 13.3% in the control arm and 27.1% in the PCI arm ($p = 0.003$). Because of the low median survival in this setting, long-term toxicity is not of major concern, and the short-course schedule (20 Gy in 5 fractions) should

be favored. However, less hypofractionated schedules (such as the schedule applied to LD) could be offered to patients with higher life expectancy. This study has had major implications and contributed to the modification of the standard of treatment for patients with metastatic SCLC.[8–10]

However, preliminary results of a Japanese phase III trial are in disagreement with the findings of the EORTC study.[82] The design was quite similar, but the inclusion criteria as well as the main objective differed. In the Japanese study, all patients had brain MRI before randomization and had follow-up with brain MRI every 3 months. The primary end point of the Japanese study was OS, and the study investigated whether PCI (25 Gy in 10 fractions) could affect survival compared with no PCI, as reflected by an HR of 0.45. The secondary end point was time to brain metastasis (assessed every 3 months by brain MRI). The planned sample size was 330 patients, but after a planned interim analysis, patient enrollment was stopped because of futility. Of the 224 patients enrolled from 2009 to 2013, 163 patients were analyzed. The cumulative risk of developing brain metastases at 1 year was significantly lower in the PCI group (32.2%) than in the control group (58.0%; $p < 0.001$). Median survival was 10.1 months in the PCI group compared with 15.1 months in the control group ($p = 0.091$). Therefore the results of this trial confirmed once again that PCI reduced the risk of developing brain metastases, whether symptomatic or asymptomatic. However, it did not show a benefit in terms of survival. The researchers concluded that PCI did not confer any survival benefit for patients with extensive SCLC when absence of brain metastases was confirmed by MRI before enrollment and asymptomatic brain metastases were detected early and treated. There was a nonsignificant trend for longer survival in patients who did not receive PCI compared with those who did. The fully published results of this trial are awaited, so in the meantime some guidelines recommend PCI for all patients who respond to treatment, while others say that close surveillance may also be proposed in metastatic patients.

Even if there are strong data showing that PCI reduces the incidence of brain metastasis and improves OS in SCLC, its indications should also be considered in the light of its potential neurotoxicity.

In the 1980s, several studies had reported neurologic and intellectual impairment or abnormalities on brain CT scan potentially related to PCI that were of concern to clinicians.[74,83–85] Acute toxicity is generally manageable and mostly involves alopecia, headache, fatigue, nausea, and vomiting. Long-term toxicity is of concern, because irreversible sequelae such as severe memory loss, intellectual impairment, or even dementia, ataxia, or seizures have been reported in retrospective studies and attributed to PCI. However, most of these studies were small, retrospective, and of questionable methodology. For example, baseline evaluations were lacking in most of them. Since then, it has been clearly demonstrated that many patients with SCLC have neurologic and cognitive impairments prior to the administration of PCI.[75,86–88] They may be due to effects of chemotherapy on the brain, a paraneoplastic syndrome, aging, an immunologic dysfunction, or even microscopic cranial metastases leading to frontal–subcortical cognitive abnormalities. Other factors related to treatment have been implicated in increasing the risk for chronic neurotoxicity, including a daily fraction size over 3 Gy per fraction and concomitant administration of chemotherapy during PCI. In a retrospective study with no neurologic baseline evaluation, Shaw et al.[89] found that the actuarial risk of severe or worse brain toxicity was 2% at 2 years and 10% at 5 years posttreatment and only occurred in those who received daily fraction sizes of PCI of at least 3 Gy. It should be outlined that in two randomized trials,[75,87] a prospective evaluation was performed in the group of patients treated with PCI and in patients who had no PCI. They did not show any significant difference in neurologic functions between the PCI and no-PCI groups, with a follow-up limited to 30 months. However, these neurologic evaluations did not focus on neurocognitive functions. Quality of life was evaluated in one of the larger studies,[87] and there was no significant difference between the PCI and no-PCI groups, at baseline, at 6 months, and at 1 year; however, compliance was not optimal. More recently, in a retrospective study, so as to evaluate the benefits and the possible risks of PCI, Lee et al.[90] developed a model taking into account the OS and the quality of life, which is related to the frequency and the severity of PCI-related late neurotoxicity, in patients who have achieved complete response. The authors were then able to determine the quality-adjusted life expectancy. They concluded that quality-adjusted life expectancy was greater with PCI, but, as the OS increases, frequency and severity of neurotoxicity should be as low as possible to keep this benefit.

In the Intergroup study evaluating the optimal PCI dose in patients with nonmetastatic SCLC, a mild deterioration was observed across time of communication deficit, fatigue, intellectual deficit, and memory (all $p < 0.005$).[91] This study also confirmed the importance of age as a cofactor of neurocognitive decline. All patients included in the RTOG 0212 study had a thorough neurocognitive assessment in their follow-up, similar to the one used in another RTOG randomized trial (RTOG 0214) evaluating PCI in NSCLC. Gondi et al.[92] thus evaluated tested and self-reported cognitive functioning after PCI for lung cancer among 410 patients who had PCI and 173 patients who had no PCI. PCI was associated with a higher risk of decline in self-reported cognitive functioning at 6 months (OR, 3.60; $p < 0.0001$) and 12 months (OR, 3.44; $p < 0.0001$). Memory was evaluated with the Hopkins Verbal Learning Test-Recall, which is a well-validated assessment of list-learning memory, including encoding, retrieval, and retention of new information. A decline over time at 6 months and 12 months was also associated with PCI ($p = 0.002$) but was not closely correlated with decline in self-reported cognitive functioning, so the authors concluded that these tests may evaluate distinct elements of the cognitive spectrum.

Because alteration of the limbic circuit, and more specifically the hippocampus, may contribute to memory and neurocognitive deficit, recent studies have analyzed the precise location of brain metastases to explore whether whole-brain irradiation with hippocampal avoidance could be envisaged in the future.[93–95] Very few patients with SCLC brain metastases were included in these studies, so further research is needed to evaluate whether brain irradiation with hippocampal avoidance might be effective in patients with SCLC brain metastases. Several studies have now been launched, evaluating PCI with hippocampus sparing.[74] Another approach that is being explored is close surveillance with MRI and administration of stereotactic RT to new brain metastases.[96] More data are needed, and the fully published results of the trial of Seto et al.[82] will bring us further information concerning this approach in ED-SCLC.

Thus in conclusion, patients should be informed of these potential adverse effects on neurocognitive functioning that have to be put in balance with the benefit of PCI on survival and brain metastasis.[74,76,78,81,90,97] Median age of patients included in the meta-analysis and patients included in the Intergroup study and EORTC RTOG studies was 60 to 62.[76,78,81,92] Therefore for elderly patients, this balance of benefit to risk should be highlighted.

PCI remains the standard of care in all SCLC patients who have a good response to treatment. The optimal dose is 25 Gy/10 fractions in patients with nonmetastatic disease; for patients with metastatic SCLC, the same PCI dose or a dose of 20 Gy/5 fractions can be delivered.

KEY REFERENCES

6. Pignon JP, Arriagada R, Ihde DC, et al. A meta-analysis of thoracic radiotherapy for small-cell lung cancer. *N Engl J Med.* 1992;3;327(23):1618–1624.

11. De Ruysscher D, Lueza B, Le Péchoux C, et al. Impact of thoracic radiotherapy timing in limited-stage small-cell lung cancer: usefulness of the individual patient data meta-analysis. *Ann Oncol.* 2016;27(10):1818–1828.

15. Takada M, Fukuoka M, Kawahara M, et al. Phase III study of concurrent versus sequential thoracic radiotherapy in combination with cisplatin and etoposide for limited-stage small-cell lung cancer: results of the Japan Clinical Oncology Group Study 9104. *J Clin Oncol.* 2002;20:3054–3060.

26. Pijls-Johannesma M, De Ruysscher D, Vansteenkiste J, Kester A, Rutten I, Lambin P. Timing of chest radiotherapy in patients with limited stage small cell lung cancer: a systematic review and meta-analysis of randomised controlled trials. *Cancer Treat Rev.* 2007;33(5):461–473.

34. Turrisi 3rd AT, Kim K, Blum R, et al. Twice-daily compared with once-daily thoracic radiotherapy in limited small-cell lung cancer treated concurrently with cisplatin and etoposide. *N Engl J Med.* 1999;340:265–271.

35. Mauguen A, Le Péchoux C, Saunders MI, et al. Hyperfractionated or accelerated radiotherapy in lung cancer: an individual patient data meta-analysis. *J Clin Oncol.* 2012;30(22):2788–2797.

41. Faivre-Finn C, Snee M, Ashcroft L, et al. *CONVERT: an international randomised trial of concurrent chemo-radiotherapy comparing twice-daily (BD) and once-daily (OD) radiotherapy schedules in patients with limited stage small cell lung cancer (LS-SCLC) and good performance status (PS). 2016 ASCO Annual Meeting.* Alexandria, VA: American Society of Oncology; 2016. [abstr 8504].

71. Slotman BJ, van Tinteren H, Praag JO, et al. Use of thoracic radiotherapy for extensive stage small-cell lung cancer: a phase 3 randomised controlled trial. *Lancet.* 2015;385:36–42.

74. Péchoux CL, Sun A, Slotman BJ, De Ruysscher D, Belderbos J, Gore EM. Prophylactic cranial irradiation for patients with lung cancer. *Lancet Oncol.* 2016;17(7):e277–e293.

76. Aupérin A, Arriagada R, Pignon JP, et al. Prophylactic cranial irradiation for patients with small-cell lung cancer in complete remission. Prophylactic Cranial Irradiation Overview Collaborative Group. *N Engl J Med.* 1999;341:476–484.

78. Le Pechoux C, Dunant A, Senan S, et al. Standard-dose versus higher-dose prophylactic cranial irradiation (PCI) in patients with limited-stage small-cell lung cancer in complete remission after chemotherapy and thoracic radiotherapy (PCI 99-01, EORTC 22003-08004, RTOG 0212, and IFCT 99-01): a randomised clinical trial. *Lancet Oncol.* 2009;10:467–474.

81. Slotman B, Faivre-Finn C, Kramer G, et al. Prophylactic cranial irradiation in extensive small-cell lung cancer. *N Engl J Med.* 2007;357:664–672.

91. Le Péchoux C, Laplanche A, Faivre-Finn C, et al. Prophylactic Cranial Irradiation (PCI) Collaborative Group. Clinical neurological outcome and quality of life among patients with limited small-cell cancer treated with two different doses of prophylactic cranial irradiation in the intergroup phase III trial (PCI99-01, EORTC 22003-08004, RTOG 0212 and IFCT 99-01). *Ann Oncol.* 2011;22(5):1154–1163.

See Expertconsult.com for full list of references.

41 Palliative Radiotherapy for Lung Cancer

Andrea Bezjak, Alysa Fairchild, and Fergus Macbeth

SUMMARY OF KEY POINTS

- Palliative radiotherapy is an effective and well tolerated treatment for palliation of thoracic and other symptoms in patients with lung cancer (both nonsmall cell lung cancer and small cell lung cancer).
- There is ample high-quality evidence from many randomized trials that short courses (one or two fractions only) of thoracic radiation provide high rates of symptomatic relief.
- There is ongoing controversy about whether moderate dose radiation schedules are superior to shorter courses in terms of symptom control or survival benefit; they do result in more toxicity.
- Single-fraction palliative radiation is recommended for uncomplicated bone metastases, with high rates of pain relief.
- Dexamethasone at a low dose administered on the day of single-fraction radiation for bone metastases and for 4 subsequent days significantly reduces the incidence of pain flare with tolerable side effects.
- Stereotactic radiotherapy is emerging as an option for management of patients with vertebral body metastases; trials are in progress to compare it with conventional palliative radiation.
- Brain metastases are common in patients with lung cancer; options for management include whole-brain radiotherapy, stereotactic radiation, surgical resection, observation, or best supportive care. Prediction tools can be helpful in identifying patients who have better versus poorer prognosis, in order to guide most appropriate therapy.

Despite substantial advances in earlier diagnosis, with prompt staging and management, and with the improved results of lung cancer treatment, metastatic disease is either present at the time of diagnosis or will develop after initial curative treatment in many patients with lung cancer. A minority of patients with metastases outside the thorax may be candidates for more aggressive multimodality treatment, such as patients with a solitary brain metastasis. However, virtually all patients with stage IV disease and indeed the majority with stage III disease will not be cured, despite the increase in therapeutic options including targeted therapy and systemic chemotherapy that may indeed extend survival and improve or control their cancer for a period of time.

For most patients with metastases, success would be defined as prolonged survival with good quality of life; good performance status; few symptoms of disease; and then, when all options have been exhausted, a peaceful and comfortable death. As a result, the aims in treating patients with incurable disease are prolonging survival, maintaining or improving quality of life, and controlling any cancer-related symptoms with minimum toxicity and inconvenience. Palliative radiotherapy was one of the first treatments to provide symptom improvement

for patients with either locally advanced thoracic or metastatic disease, and it continues to have a favorable therapeutic index. The side effects are often minor, and the benefit in terms of symptom improvement is substantial. This finding has been well documented for patients with symptomatic intrathoracic disease and for patients with bone metastases. The evidence for the effectiveness of palliative radiotherapy for patients with lung cancer with brain metastases has been debated in the literature, but it is still the mainstay of treatment for these patients. Palliative radiotherapy is also widely used for metastases at other sites, such as lymph nodes, skin or subcutaneous nodules, adrenal metastases, liver metastases, and orbital or retinal metastases, although there is little formal evidence, other than clinical experience, for its use. Local symptoms may be improved regardless of the histologic subtype of tumor. Small cell lung cancer (SCLC) responds quite rapidly to radiotherapy, and symptoms will improve in most patients. Even though the biology of SCLC, with its tendency to grow rapidly and metastasize, means that chemotherapy is usually the treatment of choice, palliative radiotherapy undoubtedly has a place in treatment management and should not be overlooked. In patients with nonsmall cell lung cancer (NSCLC), the response to palliative radiation is more variable, although symptom response does not directly correlate with radiographic responses and can be seen quite early; e.g., hemoptysis can resolve 12 hours to 24 hours after large-dose-per-fraction radiotherapy, and similarly bone pain may respond in that time frame as well, particularly after single-fraction radiotherapy. Whether response is related to radiation effect on cancer cells, or tumor vasculature, or the surrounding cell matrix with apocrine and metacrine effects or other factors, is far from understood. Elucidating the precise mechanism by which palliative radiotherapy leads to symptom palliation would be a major advance in management of patients with incurable cancers.

This chapter covers the indications for palliative radiotherapy, dose fractionation, planning issues, outcomes including symptoms, quality-of-life benefits and potential effects on prolonging survival, toxicity, and potential repeat treatment issues in patients with lung cancer with either thoracic (lung or mediastinal lymph nodes) or metastatic disease, specifically bone, brain, and other symptomatic sites. Most of the evidence relates to NSCLC, but as mentioned, SCLC would be expected to have a greater symptomatic response to palliative radiotherapy, although a less certain overall benefit in terms of length of disease control.

PALLIATIVE RADIOTHERAPY FOR THORACIC SYMPTOMS

The aim of palliative radiotherapy is to relieve symptoms as completely and as durably as possible. But, as with any palliative treatment, there is a trade-off between the burden of the treatment itself—inconvenience and acute and potentially long-term side effects—and the benefits in terms of symptom relief, quality of life, and, perhaps, improved survival. Evidence-based clinical practice guidelines published in 2012 detail the evidence and recommendations for the role of radiotherapy in thoracic symptom palliation; there is also evidence that international patterns of practice differ.[1,2]

Indications

Palliative thoracic radiotherapy is indicated whenever a patient has disease that is not potentially curable and has troublesome symptoms that can be attributed to growth of the primary tumor and/or mediastinal node disease. These findings need to be integrated into the whole care of the patient and any systemic therapy that is ongoing or being planned. Thoracic palliative radiotherapy is most often used when a patient is unfit for chemotherapy because of poor performance status or comorbidities and there is no appropriate targeted therapy, or when symptoms persist or recur during or after systemic therapy. Additionally, for patients with NSCLC, because the response to radiotherapy is faster and more reliable than to chemotherapy, there are often occasions when local symptoms mean that it is better to treat patients with radiotherapy first and consider systemic treatment later. For patients with SCLC, palliative radiotherapy is probably only indicated as a first-line treatment in emergency situations such as severe stridor or if the patient is considered too unwell to tolerate systemic chemotherapy, but is often useful when there is symptomatic recurrence and resistance to chemotherapy.

Most of the common symptoms from intrathoracic disease are well palliated by radiotherapy. These include cough, hemoptysis, and chest pain. The response rates range from 50% to 90%,[3] with the highest complete response rates seen for hemoptysis. Breathlessness appears to be less well palliated as it may be also caused by a number of other factors, such as obstructive airways disease, cardiac disease, lymphangitis carcinomatosa, or pleural effusion. Moreover, when there is a tumor in an airway causing lung, lobar, or sublobar atelectasis, the lung may not always reexpand even if the tumor shrinks and the airway is opened up, especially if there has been infection or a coexisting pleural effusion. However, any patient who presents with stridor or computed tomography (CT) evidence of a tumor threatening a major airway should be considered for urgent radiotherapy, as even modest shrinkage of a tumor causing obstruction of a large airway can provide considerable symptom relief. Superior vena cava obstruction (when due to tumor compression rather than thrombus) may also be relieved by palliative radiotherapy, although when severe, more rapid improvement may follow a stenting procedure. However, if a patient has both superior vena cava obstruction and airway compromise, the placement of a superior vena cava stent would not palliate the airway compromise, whereas palliative radiotherapy could improve both; thus, the pros and cons regarding placement of a stent followed by radiotherapy rather than palliative radiotherapy alone need to be carefully considered.

Sometimes it may be considered appropriate to treat patients prophylactically before symptoms develop. There no good evidence that this approach improves outcomes. The authors of one randomized clinical trial carried out in the United Kingdom before widespread use of chemotherapy for patients with NSCLC found that in a group of asymptomatic patients randomly assigned to no immediate palliative radiotherapy, 56% died without having had radiotherapy and that there was no substantial difference in symptom control or survival between patients who received immediate or as required palliative radiotherapy, neither at an early time point nor a later 6-month time point.[4]

Palliative radiotherapy may be delivered either by external beam or as intracavitary; i.e., endobronchial brachytherapy.

External-Beam Radiotherapy

Most palliative radiotherapy to the chest can be delivered simply with uncomplicated fields and short courses of mega-voltage radiotherapy. Because this treatment is palliative and the aim is to improve the patient's symptoms and improve quality of life, unnecessarily complex and prolonged courses of treatment should be avoided, especially in patients with a poor performance status and limited life expectancy.

Radiotherapy Planning

Usually simple parallel opposed anterior/posterior beam arrangements are sufficient, and although recent CT images are useful to assess the extent of disease, complex CT planning should not be needed. The fields should be designed to cover the extent of the tumor causing the troublesome symptoms, but should be kept as small as possible to minimize toxicity (Fig. 41.1), especially as many patients with advanced lung cancer have coexisting chronic obstructive pulmonary disease and therefore already compromised pulmonary function. Widespread sites of disease that are unlikely to be causing symptoms, such as involved but relatively small nodes in the mediastinum, should not necessarily be included. More complex field arrangements may occasionally be needed if there is a risk of overlap with previously treated areas or it is considered essential to minimize the dose to the spinal cord (see later).

Radiotherapy Regimens

The regimens for palliative radiotherapy evolved pragmatically over the past 20 years before they were subjected to any rigorous evaluation in randomized controlled trials (Table 41.1). A number of randomized controlled trials have compared various regimens for palliation and these have been summarized and reviewed in two systematic reviews.[3-5] These reviews included 14 randomized controlled trials meeting the selection criteria (more than 3000 patients) but use different approaches to incorporating different dose/fractionation regimens in a meta-analysis. For patients with a poor performance status (2–4) there is no evidence that longer, more fractionated regimens provide better palliation or longer survival than shorter regimens, such as 10 Gy in a single fraction or 16 or 17 Gy in two fractions over 1 week. For patients with a good performance status (0 or 1) the evidence is more uncertain, but it is possible that higher dose, more fractionated regimens (such as 36 to 39 Gy in 12 or 13 fractions) provide more durable symptom control and longer survival than lower dose regimens, but at the expense of more toxicity, especially esophagitis (see later). However, the increase in 1-year survival is likely to be modest—assuming a 1-year survival of 45% in this group of patients with better prognosis, the increase is likely to be around 10%, similar to that achieved with cisplatin-based chemotherapy.

However, although shorter courses of palliative radiotherapy are almost certainly as effective as more prolonged ones for most patients, especially patients who are less well, there appears to be a reluctance to use such regimens in many parts of the world.[1] This reluctance may be because of unfamiliarity, lack of exposure during training, concerns about the risks associated with using large fractions (see later) and the ability to retreat after larger doses per fraction, or unrealistic expectations about the anticipated life expectancy of the patient and possible survival benefits from longer courses. But this reluctance is also influenced by departmental policy and a widespread belief that what is commonly prescribed is indeed the best, and sometimes is also influenced by financial considerations. It is therefore important to consider the burden placed on patients and their families or caregivers from a prolonged course of treatment with repeated hospital visits, when useful palliation can be provided by only one or two fractions.

Side Effects

Typically, palliative thoracic radiotherapy is well tolerated with few toxicities, none of which is likely to be life-threatening. This

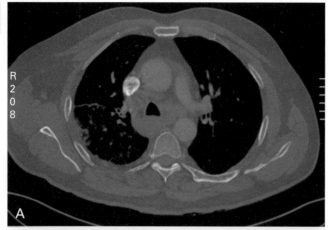

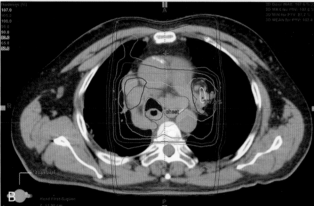

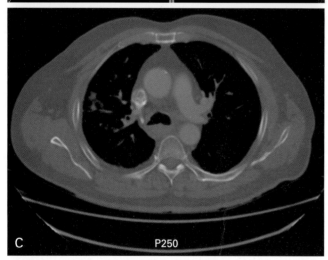

Fig. 41.1. Illustration of thoracic palliative radiotherapy plan. (A) Baseline diagnostic CT scan. (B) CT simulation image of palliative radiotherapy plan delivering 20 Gy in five daily fractions via a four-field technique (*red,* GTV; *turquoise,* PTV; *orange,* spinal canal; *dark blue,* esophagus). (C) Diagnostic CT scan 7 weeks after completing radiotherapy and two cycles of carboplatin/pemetrexed. *CT,* computed tomography; *GTV,* gross tumor volume; *PTV,* planning tumor volume.

TABLE 41.1 Commonly Used Palliative Radiotherapy Regimens for Thoracic Radiation

Dose (Gy)	No. of Fractions	No. of Days	BED (Gy10)
10	1	1	20
16	2	8	29
17	2	8	31
20	5	5–7	28
30	10	12–14	39
36	12	14–16	47
39	13	15–17	51

BED (Gy10), biologically effective dose in gray for alpha/beta ratio of 10 (i.e., effect on tumor and acutely responding tissues).

to normal lung in those circumstances. In cases of symptomatic radiotherapy pneumonitis, corticosteroids may improve the symptoms of cough and dyspnea, but need to be tapered gradually in order to prevent relapse.

Larger fraction palliative radiotherapy may be associated with specific side effects that have been described by a number of authors.[6–8] In the first 24 to 48 hours after treatment, up to 50% of patients may experience nausea, brief episodes of acute chest pain, or fever and rigors. These side effects are rarely severe and usually do not last long, but may cause patients anxiety and distress unless they are warned and given appropriate medication. Acute changes in peak expiratory flow rate have also been described, and caution is needed in patients with substantial airway obstruction.[9] A short course of corticosteroids such as prednisolone given for a few days during radiotherapy may be helpful.

Spinal cord damage (radiation myelopathy) was recorded in a few cases in the clinical trials following the use of 17 Gy in 2 fractions and 39 Gy in 13 fractions.[10] Care should therefore be exercised when using these regimens, and steps should be taken to avoid the spinal cord or reduce the dose, especially in patients with a relatively good prognosis and when lower energy radiation (e.g., from cobalt 60) with a less favorable dose distribution is used.

Repeat Radiation

Occasionally, recurrent tumor in the chest causes symptoms in patients who had a good response to palliative radiotherapy. The patient may have had systemic treatment in the meantime, but disease has progressed despite treatment or subsequently after treatment. The clinical question then arises as to whether it is safe and appropriate to consider a further course of palliative radiotherapy. The major risk from repeat radiation is radiation myelitis, possibly leading to paraparesis, if the spinal cord is included in both treatment volumes and the total dose exceeds tolerance. A further risk is radiation pneumonitis if large volumes of the residual normal lung are included in the retreatment fields.

Repeat radiotherapy is never an easy decision and several factors need to be considered:

- clinical benefit gained (degree of improvement and duration) with the first treatment and the likelihood of substantial tumor and symptomatic response from repeat radiotherapy
- patient's likely prognosis
- risk of radiation myelitis, given the original dose fractionation and the proposed second dose to the spinal cord
- volume of lung in the proposed retreatment field, especially if the beams are arranged to avoid the spinal cord.

Inherent in all these considerations is great uncertainty, and, in particular, little is known about the cumulative risk to the spinal cord and whether recovery takes place following initial treatment. However it is reasonable to make some pragmatic judgments

finding is in marked contrast with the potentially severe and persistent toxicity caused by chemotherapy. The most common side effects of palliative thoracic radiotherapy are fatigue and esophagitis. The severity of esophagitis is generally dose-related, and in most patients it is easily managed and resolves within a week or so. Radiation pneumonitis may occur if large fields and higher doses are used, and care should be taken to minimize the dose

TABLE 41.2 Commonly Used Palliative Radiotherapy Regimens for Radiotherapy for Bone Metastases

Indication	Recommended Schedule	Select References
Uncomplicated bone metastases	8 Gy/1 fraction	D'Addario 2010[49]; Lutz 2011[48]; Vassiliou 2009[61]; Macbeth 2007[100]; Kvale 2007[30]
Impending pathologic fracture, radiotherapy alone	20 Gy/5 fractions, 30 Gy/10 fractions, or	Agarawal 2006[31]; Kvale 2007[30];
Established pathologic fracture, radiotherapy alone	40 Gy/15 fractions	Townsend 1994[34]
Impending/pathologic fracture, postoperative radiotherapy		
Neuropathic pain	8 Gy/1 fraction or 20 Gy/5 fractions	Roos 2005[36]
Associated soft-tissue mass	20 Gy/5 fractions or 30 Gy/10 fractions	NCCN[59]
Hemibody radiation	6–8 Gy/1 fraction	Salazar 1986[45]
Highly conformal radiation, stereotactic ablative radiotherapy	20 Gy/1 fraction	Gerszten 2006[47]
Repeat radiation	8 Gy/1 fraction or 20 Gy/5 fraction	Chow 2013[69]
Impending spinal cord compression, radiotherapy alone	Multifraction	NICE 2008[66]
Established spinal cord compression, radiotherapy alone	8–30 Gy/1–10 fractions[a]	Prewett 2010[70]; Rades 2010[75]; Maranzano 2009[79]; NICE 2008[66]; Maranzano 2005[79]
Spinal cord compression, postoperative radiotherapy	20–30 Gy/5–10 fractions	NICE 2008[66]; Patchell 2005[77]

[a]Depending on performance status.

about the balance of risk and benefit and to discuss these openly with the patient and his or her relatives. If after being fully informed, the patient is prepared to accept what is probably for most patients with a limited prognosis a quite small risk of myelitis, versus an uncertain but likely symptomatic benefit, then repeat radiotherapy may be appropriate. Clearly, the health-care provider should only proceed with repeat radiotherapy once clear consent processes have been completed.

Brachytherapy

Endobronchial brachytherapy using iridium-192 is an established method of treating tumors in the main bronchi. It involves bronchoscopy and insertion of a small catheter, which is connected to a device that sends the radioactive source to prespecified positions along the tube that correspond to the location of the tumor; the radioactive sources remain in prespecified positions for a few minutes, as needed to deliver the prescribed dose of radiation. The advantage of this technique is that a high dose can be delivered locally to the tumor but it is not effective if there is bulky extraluminal tumor or complete obstruction of the bronchus.

The authors of a Cochrane review summarized the clinical trial evidence and concluded that brachytherapy is less effective than external-beam palliative radiotherapy as first-line treatment.[11] Its use should therefore be restricted to patients who have symptomatic recurrent tumor, which is mainly within the lumen of the bronchus.

Palliative Chemoradiation Therapy

Many patients with symptomatic incurable NSCLC may be candidates for both palliative chemotherapy and radiotherapy; the usual approach is to sequence the therapy, typically starting with palliative radiotherapy for local symptoms, as the expected symptomatic response rates are overall higher than with palliative chemotherapy. This finding has been confirmed in a randomized phase III study of palliative radiotherapy with or without chemotherapy; toxicity was greater and patient outcomes were not better with the addition of concurrent chemotherapy (fluorouracil [5FU]).[12] In 2013, Strøm et al.[13] published the results of a randomized trial that compared chemotherapy alone (cisplatin and vinorelbine) with concomitant chemoradiation in which 45 Gy in 15 fractions was given along with cycle 2, in patients with "poor prognosis" stage III NSCLC. Survival was significantly better in the patients receiving chemoradiation, (1-year survival 53.2% vs. 34.0%; $p < 0.01$), even those aged over 70 years and with bulky disease,[14-16] but with increased toxicity. The survival benefit was

not, however, seen in those with World Health Organization Performance Status.[2] Although these results are interesting, they come from only one underpowered trial and should be treated with caution. It would certainly not be appropriate to extrapolate them to the management of those with stage IV disease.

BONE METASTASES

Bone metastases will develop in as many as 40% of patients with lung cancer at some point.[17] The prevalence of bone metastases has increased because of longer survival related to advances in systemic therapy, but the median survival of 13 weeks in patients with lung cancer with bone metastases is poor in comparison to that of other tumors.[18] Bone metastases are the most common cause of cancer-related pain,[19] and up to 75% of patients experience symptoms that impair their quality of life. As patients with lung cancer and bone metastases have incurable disease, treatment intent is palliative; treatment goals are pain relief, preservation of mobility and function, prevention of skeletal-related events, and optimized quality of life.

Bone metastases can be described as complicated or uncomplicated; complicated generally refers to impending or established pathologic fracture, previous surgery, impending or established spinal cord compression, impending or established nerve-root compression, neuropathic pain, previous radiotherapy, or associated soft-tissue mass. Skeletal-related events are usually defined as pathologic fracture, spinal cord compression, hypercalcemia, or the need for surgery or radiotherapy.[20] Management costs of bone metastases secondary to lung cancer are substantial and primarily driven by treating skeletal-related events.[20]

The selection of the optimal method of palliative radiotherapy depends on symptom burden, extent of disease, life expectancy, performance status, comorbidities, toxicity, risk of skeletal-related events, prior treatment, whether metastases are (un)complicated, and patient wishes and would be best assessed and determined by an interdisciplinary team. Table 41.2 lists the indications and the usual fractionation schedules recommended.

International Bone Metastases Consensus End Points

Although many phase III trials assessed the palliative benefit of radiotherapy in patients with painful bone metastases, caution is required when interpreting and generalizing the results of older studies because of variable definitions of response, including what constitutes complete and partial relief.[21,22] The International Bone Metastases Consensus Working Party has defined a uniform set of eligibility criteria, end point measurements, repeat

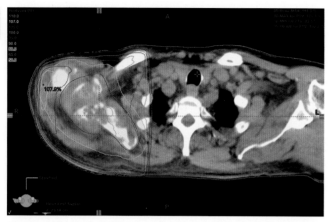

Fig. 41.2. Example of parallel-opposed pair technique delivering 8 Gy in one fraction to a painful right scapular metastasis (*red,* gross tumor volume; *turquoise,* planning tumor volume).

radiation guidelines, and statistical analysis for clinical trials to increase consistency in reporting.[21]

Indications for External-Beam Radiotherapy: Uncomplicated Bone Metastases

External-beam radiotherapy provides durable and timely symptom relief while minimizing toxicity, resource utilization, and the number of visits to the cancer center, but would not be expected to confer a survival benefit. Tumors do not have to be completely eradicated in order to improve symptoms, and therefore doses lower than that required for lesion ablation are used for palliation. Moreover, the treatment of asymptomatic bone metastases may be deferred unless there is a risk of a serious adverse event such as spinal cord compression.

Authors and investigators of more than 20 randomized controlled trials, two systematic reviews, and four meta-analyses have shown that single-fraction palliative external-beam radiotherapy provides equivalent pain relief to multiple fractions in patients with a variety of tumors (up to 25% in lung cancer).[22–25] The most recent meta-analysis included 25 studies comprising 2818 patients who were randomly assigned to single-fraction radiotherapy and 2799 to multiple-fraction radiotherapy.[22] The overall response rate to single-fraction radiotherapy was 60%, and the complete response rate was 23% (intent-to-treat), which was comparable to the 61% and 24% rates for patients who received multiple-fraction radiotherapy. There were no differences in acute toxicity, pathologic fracture (3%), or spinal cord compression (2% to 3%). None of the meta-analyses separated out treatment effects by histology, and there is no convincing evidence that outcomes differ by primary site.[22] Single-fraction radiotherapy has been repeatedly recommended as the standard of care for uncomplicated bone metastases (Table 41.2) Fig. 41.2 demonstrates a radiotherapy plan using an anterior and posterior beam to deliver 8 Gy in one fraction to a painful right scapular metastasis.

Despite this strong evidence, there has so far been reluctance to adopt single-fraction schedules as standard practice in many countries.[26] In a large prospective study conducted in the United States,[25] in 1574 patients with lung cancer and metastatic disease who received palliative bone radiotherapy, only 6% received single-fraction radiotherapy. Patients who were younger than age 55 years, had had surgery at a metastatic site, or had received chemotherapy were more likely to receive radiotherapy. Patients treated in integrated networks (e.g., health maintenance organizations) received on average 3.4 fewer fractions ($p = 0.001$) and 4 Gy less dose ($p = 0.049$), although the overall rates of

radiotherapy delivery were similar.[27] Suggested reasons for this reticence include country of training, membership affiliation, institutional structure, available pain management teams, wait times for radiotherapy consultation or delivery, reimbursement levels, and departmental policy.[20,26–28]

Indications for External-Beam Radiotherapy: Complicated Bone Metastases

Impending Pathologic Fracture

An impending pathologic fracture is defined as a bone metastasis that has a substantial likelihood of fracture under normal physiologic loads. Patients with an impending pathologic fracture may benefit from surgery, radiotherapy, or both, but no randomized trials have reported a comparison of these modalities. Provided that the surrounding bone can support the implanted hardware,[29] prophylactic stabilization reduces pain and avoids the serious consequences of fracture, although postoperative recovery may delay continuation of systemic therapy.[28] Generally, postoperative radiotherapy follows. A proportion of patients will not be candidates for operative intervention or will refuse. In that case, radiotherapy alone can be delivered.[30]

Established Pathologic Fracture

If a pathologic fracture has occurred, surgery with suitable reconstruction is indicated, especially for lower limb bones in patients with a good prognosis.[31] Surgery cannot prolong survival but improves stability, activities of daily living, function, pain, and quality of life.[31,32] Most guidelines recommend fractionated radiotherapy if surgery is not indicated (Table 41.2), although goals of care and expected lifespan may result in the decision to prescribe single-fraction radiotherapy. In an apparently solitary, histologically confirmed metastasis, especially after a long disease-free interval, doses on the higher end of the spectrum (e.g., 30 Gy in 10 fractions) may be prescribed, although there is no conclusive evidence that this improves local control.

Postoperative Radiotherapy

Postoperative radiotherapy is used to promote bone healing by suppressing tumor growth, preventing destabilization of the prosthesis by maintaining the structural integrity of the bone in which the implant is fixed.[33] Postoperative radiotherapy decreases pain, increases the frequency of normal use of the extremity, prevents disease progression, minimizes the need for revision procedures, and reduces the risk of refracture.[34] Following intramedullary nailing, all implanted hardware should be included in the radiation portal to decrease the risk of seeding (Fig. 41.3). Treatment is generally started within 2 to 4 weeks after surgery, once the wound has healed satisfactorily. Although commonly a multiple-fraction schedule is prescribed (Table 41.2),[34] patients with postoperative clinical deterioration may be considered for single-fraction radiotherapy.[33]

Neuropathic Pain

Although neuropathic pain from bone metastases does not usually respond well to standard analgesics,[35] it does respond to radiotherapy.[36] Roos et al.[36] compared 8 Gy in a single fraction with 20 Gy in five fractions for 245 patients with any primary site; 31% had lung cancer. Pain relief was seen in 53% of patients who had single-fraction radiotherapy and in 61% of patients who had multiple-fraction radiotherapy (intent-to-treat) at 2 months. The median time to treatment failure was longer in the fractionated arm (3.7 vs. 2.4 months), but did not reach significance. The authors recommended 20 Gy in five fractions; however, patients

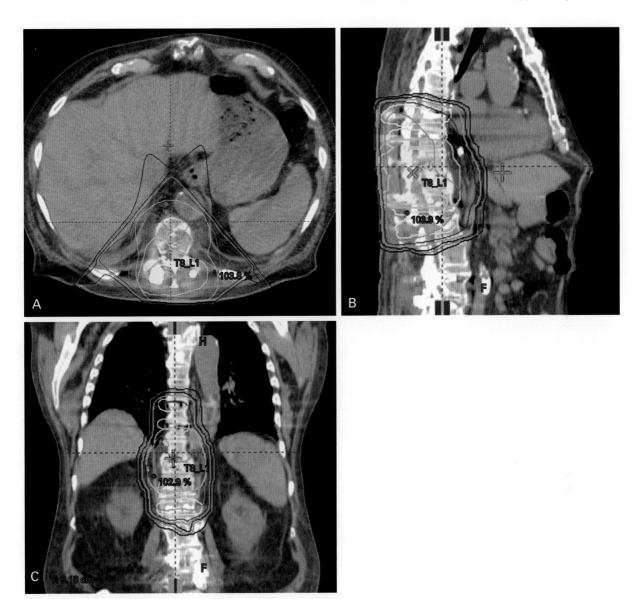

Fig. 41.3. Example of postoperative radiotherapy delivered after surgical decompression, vertebrectomy, tumor resection, and stabilization for a T11 pathologic fracture secondary to nonsmall cell lung cancer. Using a five-field technique, 20 Gy was delivered over five daily fractions to encompass a planning tumor volume *(turquoise)*, which included the pathologic fracture, adjacent involved T10 vertebral body, and surgical bed including hardware *(yellow contour)*. (A) axial image; (B) sagittal image; and (C) coronal image.

with decreased performance status, shorter expected survival, or substantial comorbidities should receive single-fraction radiotherapy (Table 41.2).

Quality of Life

As the main treatment goal of radiotherapy is symptom control, the most appropriate way to assess response (pain, other quality-of-life aspects) is by patient-reported outcomes.[37] Measuring quality of life was recommended for all bone metastases clinical trials by 91% of experts in an international survey.[21] Authors of many recent studies have reported health-related quality of life and functional interference after palliative radiotherapy for bone metastases. In general, patients whose pain improves after radiotherapy also experience substantially improved physical and role function.[38–40] Improvements extend to associated symptoms, such as insomnia and constipation, and responders describe

better emotional functioning, general activity, normal work, and overall quality of life by 2 months.[38–41] Neither anatomic location nor radiotherapy dose predicts the degree of improvement.[40,41] Differences in the likelihood of functional response by primary site have been suggested; in one study, 27% of patients with lung cancer had responded by 2 months, compared with 70% of patients with breast and prostate cancer.[40]

Indications for Hemibody External-Beam Radiation

Hemibody radiation is an effective treatment for widespread symptomatic bone metastases,[42] particularly for patients with poor performance status, although it used to be practiced more often in the past. It may be delivered to the upper half (base of skull to iliac crest; 6 Gy in one fraction), lower half (iliac crest to ankles; 8 Gy in one fraction), or middle of the body (diaphragm to pubic symphysis; 6 Gy in one fraction). Hemibody radiation provides pain relief in 70% to 80% of patients, often within 24 to 48 hours, and may decrease future requirements for opioids and local external-beam radiotherapy.[43–45]

Indications for Stereotactic Radiosurgery

Stereotactic radiosurgery is administered as a radioablative dose to a lesion in a highly conformal manner, typically in a single or a few fractions. It is presently being investigated for certain clinical circumstances, such as repeat treatment of bone metastases near the spinal cord.[46] There are possible advantages with stereotactic radiosurgery:[47]

- Smaller volumes of normal tissue radiated
- Higher degree of preservation of organ function
- Radiobiologic benefits due to the high dose per fraction
- Improved local control

However, these advantages may be outweighed by cost, need for specialized equipment, and laborious set-up and treatment. Randomized trials comparing conventional external-beam and stereotactic radiotherapy for bone metastases are ongoing. Gerszten et al.[47] prospectively evaluated outcomes of single-fraction radiosurgery delivered to 87 patients with spinal bone metastases secondary to lung cancer. Of the 87 patients, 70 patients had previous maximum external-beam radiotherapy. The mean tumor dose was 20 Gy in one fraction, delivered over an average of 90 minutes. No patient experienced radiotherapy-related neurologic deficits. A total of 65 of 73 patients were treated primarily for pain and had long-term improvement.[47] Enrollment of fit patients in clinical trials at centers with sufficient experience should be encouraged.[47-49]

Side Effects of External-Beam Radiotherapy

Acute side effects are generally mild and self-limiting or controllable by conservative measures. Most begin 1 to 2 weeks after treatment, although some, such as nausea, begin within hours. They may not peak until after the end of radiotherapy and usually resolve in 2 to 3 weeks. As radiotherapy is a localized treatment, all the potential side effects except fatigue are site-specific. Late effects, which may appear months or years after treatment, are uncommon, usually permanent, and should be managed by a radiation oncologist. Although the possibility of late toxicity in patients with incurable malignant disease must be considered, many patients will not live long enough to be at risk. Side effects and recommended management strategies have been reviewed.[50]

Pain flare is a common side effect in patients who have undergone external-beam radiotherapy for bone metastases. Pain flare is a short-lived worsening of pain in the treated area, can occur in up to 44% of patients within a week after starting radiotherapy, and lasts for a median of 3 days.[51,52] It is not clear whether pain flare is more common after single fractionation. In one study, the authors found that patients with lung cancer were less likely to experience pain flare (23%) compared with patients with breast and prostate cancers.[53] In a recently reported double-blind, placebo-controlled randomized trial, dexamethasone 8 mg orally starting on the day of single-fraction radiotherapy and for 4 consecutive days afterward significantly decreased the rate of pain flare with tolerable side effects.[54]

Integration of External-Beam Radiotherapy With Other Modalities

External-Beam Radiotherapy and Minimally Invasive Techniques

Percutaneous vertebroplasty and kyphoplasty are minimally invasive outpatient surgical techniques for restoring stability to lytic spinal bone metastases, as well as improving pain and mobility and preserving quality of life, functional independence, and performance status; when used in the pelvis and elsewhere, the technique is referred to as osteoplasty.[55,56] These treatments are an option for patients with medical comorbidities, mechanical component to their pain, even if multilevel spinal disease but cannot be used in the setting of a soft-tissue mass.[57] There is no evidence that adding external-beam radiotherapy improves clinical outcomes,[48] although both can decrease pain refractory to other modalities.[55,58]

External-Beam Radiotherapy and Systemic Therapy

Chemotherapy addresses systemic as well as bone disease. It can improve pain and quality of life and prolong survival in patients with bone metastases, but may be hazardous for heavily pretreated patients with extensive bone marrow disease. Response rates and duration are usually lower than that of radiotherapy, drugs can be expensive, there may be a long interval before onset of relief, and side effects are also systemic. Concurrent radiotherapy and chemotherapy have not been extensively investigated in patients with bone metastases although it is common for patients with bone metastases to receive these modalities sequentially.

Bisphosphonates may prevent or delay skeletal-related events in lung cancer.[59,60] Because bisphosphonates and external-beam radiotherapy have different dose-limiting toxicities, bisphosphonates could provide background control alongside acute local pain relief provided by radiotherapy.[61,62] Vassiliou et al.[63] published their experience of concurrent radiotherapy (30–40 Gy) and monthly intravenous ibandronate in 45 evaluable patients with multiple primary sites; 29% had lung cancer. All groups had substantial reductions in pain and opioid requirements, and improved performance status and physical functioning. At 3 months, the complete response rate was 69% and the partial response rate was 31%. Radiographic bone density and lesion healing were substantially increased at all time points. No patient required repeat treatment, and only one pathologic fracture occurred in a patient with lung cancer. Other studies evaluating the combination have been reviewed by Vassiliou et al.;[63] no randomized data are available.[61] External-beam radiotherapy and concurrent bisphosphonates have been recommended by one guideline.[30] They are also a consideration where radiotherapy is contraindicated.[62]

Denosumab is a fully human monoclonal antibody, which specifically targets the receptor activator of nuclear factor kappa B ligand, an osteoclast regulatory factor. It may delay the onset of bone metastases and treat established bone destruction.[64] In patients with bone metastases due to NSCLC, denosumab may increase median overall survival compared with zoledronic acid (9.5 vs. 8 months).[65] Denosumab is recommended as an option for preventing skeletal-related events in adults with bone metastases from solid tumors if bisphosphonates would otherwise be prescribed or after bisphosphonates have become ineffective.[17,59,66] However, there is no high-quality evidence available on combined denosumab and radiotherapy.

Repeat Radiotherapy

Repeat radiotherapy may be considered when other treatments are either ineffective or not indicated.[67,68] Rates of repeat treatment in the most recent meta-analysis were 20% after 8 Gy in one fraction compared with 8% after multiple-fraction radiotherapy ($p < 0.00001$).[22] One reason more patients receive repeat treatment after SF radiation is because they can; many radiation oncologists are reluctant to deliver repeat treatment after ≥30 Gy, particularly if the spinal cord is in the volume.[52] An intergroup study randomly assigned 850 patients who had received previous radiotherapy and had painful bone metastases to receive radiotherapy at 8 Gy in one fraction or 20 Gy in five fractions. The intention-to-treat response rate at 2 months after 8 Gy (28%) was no lower than that after 20 Gy (32%); by per-protocol analysis, rates were 45% and 51%, respectively. There were no differences in rates of pathologic fracture, spinal cord compression, or quality of life, but adverse events at day 14 were substantially worse after multiple fractions.[69] Studies that report time to maximum response after external-beam radiotherapy have found it commonly takes 4 to 6 weeks. Therefore, repeat treatment should be delayed until this time, which also allows response to the first course to be assessed and pain flare to have resolved.[21]

Spinal Cord Compression

Spinal cord compression will develop in 5% of all patients with cancer, and lung cancer is ultimately diagnosed in 15% to 30% of patients with spinal cord compression as their presenting event.[70–72] The median survival from diagnosis of spinal cord compression due to lung cancer is poor: it is less than 2 months in one study.[73] Urgent magnetic resonance imaging (MRI) of the entire spine should be undertaken on the least suspicion of neurologic symptoms or signs, especially in a patient with known vertebral metastases.

Definitive treatment (surgery or radiotherapy) within 24 hours is recommended to optimize symptom control, preserve neurologic function and ambulation, decrease tumor bulk, and maximize quality of life.[74] The spinal service should be consulted for an opinion if a tissue diagnosis is required; there is a solitary level of compression; there is spinal instability or bony fragments within the spinal canal; the patient cannot have radiation (e.g., because of previous radiation at that level); neurologic deterioration occurs during or after maximal dose radiotherapy; there is radiotherapy-resistant histology; there is rapid symptom progression; or there is acute onset paraplegia.[74]

In general, factors associated with a better prognosis include longer time to development of motor deficits, ambulatory ability before and after therapy, radiotherapy-sensitive histology, and a single site of compression, treated in a timely fashion.[30,75]

Best supportive care including opioids, venous thromboembolism prophylaxis, and rehabilitation are reviewed in a 2008 United Kingdom guideline.[74] There is good evidence that corticosteroids are effective. Unless contraindicated, all patients should receive a loading dose of 10 mg to 16 mg of dexamethasone, followed by 16 mg daily in divided doses thereafter.[74] After radiotherapy, the dose can be tapered. If neurologic function deteriorates, the dose should be increased temporarily.[74]

Impending Spinal Cord Compression

Retrospective studies suggest that radiotherapy may preserve neurologic function in patients with spinal metastases with radiographic signs that suggest the spinal cord is at risk.[76] In the absence of good evidence on dose, fractionated radiotherapy should probably be offered (Table 41.1).[21,76]

Established Spinal Cord Compression

Surgery and postoperative radiotherapy is superior to radiotherapy alone for symptomatic patients with an expected survival of more than 3 months and a single level of compression, resulting in significantly better ambulation rates, retention of ambulation and continence, maintenance of functional and motor scores, and lower doses of steroids and analgesics.[77] This combined-modality approach has therefore been recommended for spinal cord compression or spinal instability (compression fracture, dislocation, or retropulsed bone fragments), in patients with sufficient performance status and life expectancy, by many international bodies.[30,52,74] Because patients with SCLC often have

a short lifespan, surgery is less often considered.[78] If surgery is not indicated or declined, radiotherapy alone should be offered,[49] which is still the most common treatment for epidural spinal cord compression.[49,73] The most appropriate radiotherapy schedule is still being debated (Table 41.1). This debate is likely due to the scarcity of good data exploring dose schedules in common use. Patients with spinal cord compression were excluded from most clinical trials investigating radiotherapy for uncomplicated bone metastases. Two randomized Italian phase III trials investigated short-course and single-fraction treatment in patients with poor prognosis.[79,80] No significant differences were found for relief of back pain, ability to walk after radiotherapy, bladder function, duration of motor improvement, toxicity, or survival between short-course regimens.[80] There were no differences between short-course and single-fraction radiotherapy except for median duration of response, which was longer for 8 Gy in two fractions.[79] The authors of a series of retrospective studies from a large multicenter database have reported similar immediate functional and neurologic outcomes and survival with short- and longer-course radiotherapy. However, longer-course radiotherapy is probably associated with better local control and less in-field recurrence.[75] Although a patient with a poor prognosis who is paraplegic will not benefit from radiotherapy in terms of neurologic status, delivery of external-beam radiotherapy for pain control should be considered. Postoperative radiotherapy should be offered to all patients with a satisfactory surgical outcome once the wound has healed.[74]

Repeat Radiotherapy for Spinal Cord Compression

Recurrent spinal cord compression in a previously radiated region may be treated with further radiotherapy, provided the patient responded well to the previous course and the interval has been greater than 3 months. Highly conformal radiotherapy techniques such as stereotactic radiosurgery provide a method of salvage treatment in patients with limited metastases and good performance status and can be considered to reduce the cumulative spinal cord dose.[74,75,81] Although stereotactic radiosurgery could be undertaken for patients who have recurrent pain at a previously radiated spinal segment, it cannot be used in an emergency setting such as frank spinal cord compression.[81] Surgical decompression could be undertaken in the setting of maximal previous radiotherapy.[70]

BRAIN METASTASES

Brain metastases are a common site of metastatic disease in patients with lung cancer, whether occurring at the time of diagnosis (as neurologic symptoms are frequently the presenting symptoms that prompt testing that leads to a diagnosis of lung cancer) or later. Some patients are living longer because of better systemic therapy and increasing recognition of treatable mutations, but many chemotherapeutic agents do not penetrate the blood–brain barrier well enough to eradicate micrometastatic disease. Thus, the incidence and prevalence of brain metastases in patients with lung cancer are increasing. There is also a subgroup of asymptomatic patients with a low burden of brain metastatic disease found during routine MRI, as part of staging or restaging. They may have only one or a few small metastases and may be candidates for stereotactic brain radiotherapy (gamma-knife or linac-based treatment) or surgical resection for larger lesions that are surgically accessible, especially if the lesions are symptomatic and causing mass effect. However, management of patients with a good performance status who have a relatively low burden of disease and a solitary brain metastasis is not truly palliative in its intent, but is aimed at eradicating intracranial metastatic disease and prolonging life. Admittedly, there is only anecdotal evidence that such aggressive treatment leads to permanent eradication of all cancer. This section covers palliative management, such as, management of symptomatic patients who have multiple brain metastases.

Brain metastases that are found because of symptoms of raised intracranial pressure, such as headaches and nausea, or because of seizures or focal neurologic deficits usually cause substantial morbidity and affect the patients' physical and mental functioning and performance status. The presence of multiple symptomatic brain metastases is a sign of poor prognosis. The most appropriate management of symptomatic patients will depend on a number of patient and tumor factors. Many options are available:

- End-of-life care alone
- Corticosteroids alone
- Corticosteroids and a short course of whole-brain radiotherapy (WBRT)
- A combination of WBRT and focal stereotactic brain radiotherapy
- Surgical resection of the symptomatic lesion for palliation, usually followed by WBRT

The important clinical decision is to identify the most favorable group, such as, patients who might benefit from a more aggressive approach, with the aim of prolonged neurologic control, and the unfavorable group, patients who have poor prognosis for whom the goal might be short-term palliation and end-of-life care. Most patients will fall into an intermediate prognosis group, for whom WBRT and corticosteroids are the mainstay of management.

Selection of Patients Who Are More Likely to Benefit From Treatment

Several methods have been developed to aid clinicians and clinical trialists for identifying patients who are likely to have a better prognosis and might benefit from a more aggressive treatment. The best known method is the Radiotherapy Oncology Group (RTOG) Recursive Partitioning index (RPA), developed from pooling of data from several RTOG phase III trials.[82] These trials did not include only patients with lung cancer, although in most trials of brain metastases, lung cancer is the most common primary tumor. The best group, RPA class I, consisted of patients who had reasonable performance status (Karnofsky score greater than 70), a controlled primary tumor, age younger than 65 years, and brain as the only site of metastases. Further analyses of the RTOG clinical trials have led to the development of the Graded Prognostic Assessment (GPA),[83] which considers more categories of age and performance status and includes the number of brain metastases (1, 2–3, greater than 3), with the best prognosis in patients that are younger, with excellent performance status and a solitary brain metastasis.

Further publications by the same group have refined the GPA and have created disease-specific (DS)-GPAs.[83] To illustrate, the lung cancer DS-GPA includes performance status, age, presence of extracranial metastases, and the number of brain metastases, whereas the melanoma and renal cell carcinoma DS-GPA only includes performance status and the number of brain metastases. Several authors have compared the various prognostic indices for brain metastases. Rodrigues et al.[84] performed a systematic review of nine published and validated brain metastases prognostic indices including the RTOG RPA, the GPA and DS-GPA, Rotterdam, Basic Score for bone metastases, Golden Grading System, and RADES I and II. These authors compared the indices with respect to a range of characteristics and reported that although none is ideal, all had some clinical usefulness. The authors concluded that RTOG RPA was the best validated to date. In another report, these prognostic

indices were used on two institutional databases of 500 patients treated either with stereotactic radiotherapy (381 patients) or WBRT (120 patients).[85] Comparisons were made using novel metrics (net reclassification improvement index, integrated discrimination improvement index, and decision curve analysis). Different indices performed better on different metrics; overall best results were with RTOG RPA, Golden Grading system, RADES I, and Rotterdam, but the GPA was best in identifying poor prognosis patients. Thus, any of these indices could and should be used in clinical practice and clinical trials to identify a subgroup of patients with good prognosis who would benefit from a more aggressive approach to their brain metastases, a subgroup with a poor prognosis, and an intermediate group who should be considered for whole-brain radiotherapy.

Whole-Brain Radiotherapy: Dose Fractionation and Planning

Palliative radiotherapy for patients with multiple brain metastases, where the goal is palliation, consists of WBRT, with two parallel opposed lateral fields, covering the entire brain but sparing the eye and minimizing dose to the salivary glands and oropharyngeal mucosa, in order to reduce the toxicity. Traditionally, planning was not CT-based but used clinical mark-up, relying on the anatomic landmarks of the superior orbital ridge and the external auditory canal to delineate the inferior border of the WBRT field as they are appropriate surrogates for the base of skull; a field that cleared the scalp in all other borders would encompass the entire content of the intracranial fossa while avoiding the eyes and other organs at risk. However, the anterior- and inferiormost parts of the brain and especially the meninges were being underdosed or not covered, and the precise level of cervical spine that was included in the radiotherapy field was hard to evaluate and especially hard to match with any future cervical spine radiotherapy fields. Thus, many centers have moved to CT-based planning, where those issues, including dose delivered to the lens, the most radiation-sensitive structure in the eye, could be better estimated, although this may not be of relevance to many patients who have short life expectancies and will not live long enough for radiotherapy-induced cataracts to develop. This finding led to an appreciation of the dose inhomogeneity with traditional planning, and attempts to create more homogeneous doses, with segments, or even with intensity modulated radiotherapy. Intensity modulated radiotherapy is a sophisticated radiotherapy technique, frequently used for high-dose radiotherapy planning, which can allow sparing of particularly sensitive structures such as the hippocampus in an attempt to reduce the risk of memory impairment after WBRT,[86] or sparing of the scalp to avoid the otherwise universal (albeit temporary) side effect of alopecia. However, whether the use of these sophisticated and typically more expensive technologic advances is appropriate for palliative radiotherapy is debatable; it hinges on the goals of care and a realistic estimate of the patient's life expectancy.

There have been many randomized trials in which the authors have attempted to define the most appropriate dose and fractionation of palliative WBRT, and others in which the authors have investigated the addition of chemotherapy or radiosensitizers to improve the therapeutic ratio of WBRT. The standard radiotherapy schedules are considered to be 30 Gy in 10 daily fractions over 2 weeks and 20 Gy in 5 fractions over 1 week. Although the five fractions over 1 week is a biologically lower dose (although it is not one-third less, as the fraction size is higher and overall duration lower, which increases its biologic potency), head-to-head comparisons have not shown better outcomes with the higher dose. In a Cochrane review on WBRT for multiple brain metastases, the authors summarized 39 randomized trials (more than 10,000 patients), some of which were studies on altered fractionations (e.g., hyperfractionated or accelerated radiotherapy), WBRT with and without radiosensitizers, WBRT with or without radiosurgery boost, or radiosurgery with or without WBRT.[87] Their conclusion was that no alternative regimen was better than standard radiotherapy (30 Gy in 10 fractions or 20 Gy in fractions) in terms of overall survival, neurologic function, or symptom control.

Outcomes

One of the challenges in assessing the effectiveness of palliative management of patients with brain metastases is the lack of consensus on what constitutes palliation. The investigators of many clinical trials have focused on overall survival, even though that may be influenced by the presence of extracranial disease. Others have tried to assess neurologic progression-free survival and neurologic control, most frequently through radiographic response rates rather than the patients' actual symptoms or functioning. There have been attempts to measure palliation, by assessing control of the presenting neurologic symptoms, steroid dose, and the patient's performance status—all factors probably most relevant to assessing whether patients have actually benefited from radiotherapy.[88] Using those criteria, only a minority of patients in clinical practice appear to derive palliative benefit from WBRT.[89] This finding is partly due to the fact that a proportion of patients with a poor prognosis die within 6 to 8 weeks of a diagnosis of brain metastases and thus do not live long enough to derive a clear palliative benefit,[90] and partly because neurologic symptoms improve with corticosteroids, a fact that is well recognized but poorly documented.[91] There is clear evidence that corticosteroids themselves cause toxicity, especially with prolonged use[92]; but there is no good evidence for the use of high doses, such as dexamethasone 16 mg per day, when lower doses, such 4 or 8 mg per day, may be as effective and less toxic.[93] One approach to mitigate corticosteroid-related side effects is to personalize the starting dose depending on the degree of edema and symptom response; to taper rapidly to a low dose, such as 2 mg or 4 mg of dexamethasone per day; and then consider whether a complete wean is appropriate, depending on the patient's prognosis and symptom burden. To answer the question of how best to manage the palliation of patients with brain metastases who have a poorer prognosis, investigators in the United Kingdom have completed a phase III, multicenter randomized controlled trial in which patients with optimal supportive care with or without WBRT (20 Gy in five fractions) are compared. The primary outcome was quality-adjusted life years, with survival, performance status, and symptoms as the secondary outcomes. This study has recently been reported as not showing a benefit to WBRT over best supportive care.[94,95]

Toxicity of WBRT

The main acute side effects of WBRT are fatigue and, sometimes, headaches, nausea, and vomiting, related to an increase in intracranial pressure presumably due to the cytotoxic and other effects of radiotherapy causing edema; these side effects are usually prevented by giving adequate doses of corticosteroids. Occasionally, patients will have swelling of the parotid gland, usually after the first or second fraction. Subacute side effects include ongoing fatigue, as well as alopecia, skin reaction (dryness, redness, hyperpigmentation), and possibly transient reduced hearing due to a combination of middle ear fluid accumulation and dry wax in the auditory canal. With the usual palliative dose regimens, there should be no permanent effect on hearing, as the radiotherapy doses delivered are well within tolerance of nerves.

The main late effect of concern is impaired cognitive function. For a long time, this effect was not appreciated, probably because of the poor prognosis of those who are treated with palliative WBRT. Studies have brought attention to this important quality-of-life issue, demonstrating impairments in memory and other cognitive function using standardized tests, although data have been debated in terms of their generalizability and have led to divergent conclusions. Reduction of delayed neurotoxicity is an area of active investigation.[95] The use of pharmacologic agents such as memantine or hippocampal sparing radiotherapy to preserve cognitive function[96,97] are covered in more detail in Chapter 43.[96,97]

Alternative Management Approaches

As outlined at the beginning of the section on brain metastases, if the goal of treatment is eradication of neurologic disease in a patient with minimal or no extracranial disease, stereotactic radiotherapy or surgical resection, with or without WBRT, may be considered. Authors of studies and practice patterns in some areas of the world, notably the United States, have championed the avoidance of WBRT in order to reduce the negative cognitive impact. Small randomized trials of stereotactic radiotherapy for brain metastases demonstrated better neurologic and cognitive outcomes and improved survival in patients randomly assigned to stereotactic radiotherapy.[98] It was not clear whether the differences were indeed due to the therapeutic benefit of stereotactic radiosurgery, given that additional brain metastases developed in patients who were treated with stereotactic radiosurgery initially but continued to be treated aggressively, typically with further stereotactic radiosurgery. In contrast, patients randomly assigned to initial WBRT were deemed to be closer to the end of life and were not offered further therapy upon progression. Thus, a larger proportion of patients in that arm were closer to the last months of their life when the primary outcome of this trial, cognitive function at 4 months after randomization, was assessed. Their poor performance on that test may have been a reflection of the terminal state of disease, rather than the direct effect of WBRT.

Additional larger randomized studies are being conducted to try to determine whether withholding of WBRT will indeed lead to better overall neurologic outcomes, when taking into account both tumor recurrence, further therapy, and neurologic and functional outcomes. Until then, countries and centers are quite divided in their opinions on what is the best strategy; it would not be unusual if the controversy were to continue even after data from randomized controlled trials are available. Unfortunately, it is hard to completely separate the views of what is the most important end point from training and local practice, financial incentives and disincentives, and, in some jurisdictions, patient expectations and demands; these findings further fuel the current debate, which of course extends to management of patients with brain metastases well beyond lung cancer.

Repeat Treatment

In the past, patients with brain metastases had a short life expectancy, and repeat treatment was rarely contemplated. Investigators from several centers have reported that repeat WBRT may be considered for patients who have shown a good and prolonged response to previous radiotherapy, although what is considered a prolonged response is not well defined. Current practice is to consider stereotactic radiotherapy for progression in solitary metastases, and although there is no randomized level evidence for that approach, stereotactic radiotherapy is a relatively well-tolerated treatment that might provide better local control. Whether this finding will result in overall clinical benefit is largely dependent on other patient selection factors and needs to be balanced against the risks of short- and long-term toxicity. There may indeed be a role for repeat WBRT,[98,99] but the toxicity of such a second course, especially in terms of cognitive function, should be considered.

PALLIATIVE RADIOTHERAPY TO OTHER AREAS

Palliative radiotherapy is also widely used for SCLC and NSCLC metastases to other sites, such as lymph nodes, skin or subcutaneous nodules, adrenal metastases, liver metastases, and orbital or retinal metastases. There are virtually no formal studies evaluating the effectiveness of palliative radiotherapy for those sites, as it would take a long time for any center to accrue patients with those specific metastatic sites to a study. However, principles of palliative radiotherapy apply—if one can identify with reasonable confidence which site of tumor involvement is causing a symptom, and can target that tumor with a radiation field that delivers a certain dose with minimal/modest toxicity, one should expect a therapeutic benefit, typically within days or a few weeks at most, especially if large doses per fraction are employed. With some application of clinical judgment, good history taking, physical examination, and judicious use of tests, symptom improvement should be possible to attain in a large proportion of patients. Thus, only patients who have multiple symptoms from multiple areas of involvement or an overall life expectancy of less than 3–4 weeks may be too far progressed to benefit from palliative radiotherapy. Many other patients with SCLC and NSCLC may indeed derive a considerable palliative benefit from short courses of palliative radiotherapy directed to sites of symptomatic disease.

CONCLUSION

Palliative thoracic radiotherapy is an extremely valuable option in the management of patients with both SCLC and NSCLC. There is good evidence for its effectiveness in controlling most symptoms and for its relative lack of toxicity and it can be used safely in patients who are frail and unwell. Many patients can be treated safely with one or two large fractions and do not need to travel daily to the hospital for treatment.[100] For some patients with a good performance status, an option that may give more durable symptom control and the possibility of a modest survival benefit at the expense of more esophagitis is a higher dose regimen, such as 36 Gy to 39 Gy in 12 or 13 fractions.

Although there has in the past been well-conducted research into the most effective dose regimens of palliative radiotherapy, there has been little if any research into the most effective way of integrating palliative radiotherapy with systemic treatments to ensure that patients whose disease is almost certainly incurable get the most durable and least toxic symptom control. For instance, if a patient has metastatic disease and symptomatic intrathoracic disease, what sequence of treatments is most effective? Or, if a patient has major intrathoracic disease, does palliative radiotherapy given before or immediately after systemic treatment improve the degree and duration of the palliation of thoracic symptoms?

Ideally, the care of patients with advanced symptomatic lung cancer should be managed by a multidisciplinary team so that all relevant treatments can be used to their best effect. Such teamwork is increasingly common, especially in well-organized oncology centers. However, with the increasing use of a variety of systemic treatments in patients with advanced disease, the value of palliative thoracic radiotherapy may be underestimated and patients denied a useful and relatively nontoxic treatment option.

KEY REFERENCES

1. Rodrigues G, Macbeth F, Burmeister B, et al. International practice survey on palliative lung radiotherapy: third international consensus workshop on palliative radiotherapy and symptom control. *Clin Lung Cancer*. 2012;13(3):225–235.
2. Rodrigues G, Videtic GM, Sur R, et al. Palliative thoracic radiotherapy in lung cancer: an American Society for Radiation Oncology evidence-based clinical practice guideline. *Pract Radiat Oncol*. 2011;1(2):60–71.
4. Falk SJ, Girling DJ, White RJ, et al. Immediate versus delayed palliative thoracic radiotherapy in patients with unresectable locally advanced non-small cell lung cancer and minimal thoracic symptoms: randomised controlled trial. *BMJ*. 2002;325:465.
5. Stevens R, Macbeth F, Toy E, Coles, Lester JF. Palliative radiotherapy regimens for patients with thoracic symptoms from non-small cell lung cancer. *Cochrane Database of Systematic Reviews*. 2015; (Issue 1). Art.No:CD002143.
21. Chow E, Hoskin P, Mitera G, et al. Update of the international consensus on palliative radiotherapy endpoints for future clinical trials in bone metastases. *Int J Radiat Oncol Biol Phys*. 2012;82(5):1730–1737.
26. Fairchild A, Barnes E, Ghosh S, et al. International patterns of practice in palliative radiotherapy for painful bone metastases: evidence-based practice? *Int J Radiat Oncol Biol Phys*. 2009;75(5):1501–1510.
36. Roos D, Turner S, O'Brien P, et al. Randomized trial of 8Gy in 1 versus 20Gy in 5 fractions of radiotherapy for neuropathic pain due to bone metastases (TROG 96.05). *Radiother Oncol*. 2005;75:54–63.
48. Lutz S, Berk L, Chang E, et al. Palliative radiotherapy for bone metastases: an ASTRO evidence-based guideline. *Int J Radiat Oncol Biol Phys*. 2011;79(4):965–976.
54. Chow E, Meyer R, Ding K, et al. Dexamethasone versus placebo in the prophylaxis of radiation-induced pain flare following palliative radiotherapy for bone metastases: a double-blind randomized, controlled, superiority trial. *Lancet Oncol*. 2015;16(15):1463–1472.
69. Chow E, van der Linden Y, Roos D, et al. Single versus multiple fractions of repeat radiation for painful bone metastases: a randomised, controlled, non-inferiority trial. *Lancet Oncol*. 2014;15(2):164–171.
77. Patchell R, Tibbs P, Regine W, et al. Direct decompressive surgical resection in the treatment of spinal cord compression caused by metastatic cancer: a randomized trial. *Lancet*. 2005;366:643–648.
82. Gaspar L, Scott C, Rotman M, et al. Recursive partitioning analysis (RPA) of prognostic factors in three Radiation Therapy Oncology Group (RTOG) brain metastases trials. *Int J Radiat Oncol Biol Phys*. 1997;37(4):745–751.
83. Sperduto PW, Kased N, Roberge D, et al. Summary report on the graded prognostic assessment: an accurate and facile diagnosis-specific tool to estimate survival for patients with brain metastases. *J Clin Oncol*. 2012;30(4):419–425.
84. Rodrigues G, Bauman G, Palma D, et al. Systemic review of brain metastases prognostic indices. *Pract Radiat Oncol*. 2013;25(4):227–235.
85. Rodrigues G, Gonzalez-Maldonado S, Bauman G, Senan S, Lagerwaard F. A statistical comparison of prognostic index systems for brain metastases after stereotactic radiosurgery or fractionated stereotactic radiation therapy. *Clin Oncol (R Coll Radiol)*. 2013;25(4):227–235.
86. Gondi V, Tomé WA, Mehta MP. Why avoid the hippocampus? A comprehensive review. *Radiother Oncol*. 2010;97(3):370–376.
87. Tsao MN, Rades D, Wirth A, et al. Radiotherapeutic and surgical management for newly diagnosed brain metastasis(es): an American Society for Radiation Oncology evidence-based guideline. *Pract Radiat Oncol*. 2012;2(3):210–225.

See Expertconsult.com for full list of references.

42 Acute and Late Toxicities of Thoracic Radiotherapy: Pulmonary, Esophagus, and Heart

José Belderbos, Laurie Gaspar, Ayse Nur Demiral, and Lawrence B. Marks

SUMMARY OF KEY POINTS

- The acute and late toxicity of radiotherapy (RT) for lung cancer usually involves the lungs, esophagus, and heart.

Lung

- Post-RT, there are multiple biochemical and molecular events involving type II pneumocytes, surfactant protein transudation into alveolar spaces, with subsequent inflammation with associated capillary obstruction, and then much later tissue fibrosis.
- The risk for clinical lung injury has been associated with various dosimetric factors (e.g., mean lung dose), clinical factors (e.g., preexisting pulmonary comorbidities), and cytokines (e.g., IL-6, IL-8, and TGF-β1).
- Prednisone is typically effective in treating patients with troublesome symptoms of radiation peumonitis.

Esophagus

- Acute esophageal injury is common and is manifest by pain with swallowing, reflecting mucosal injury. Late injury is typically manifest as partial obstruction or fistula.
- Various dosimetric and clinical factors (e.g., concurrent chemotherapy) have been associated with acute and late injury.
- Acute symptoms are treated with dietary changes, proton pump inhibitors, analgesics, local anesthetics, promotility agents, intravenous fluids, and/or nasogastric tube or gastrostomy tube insertion. Late esophageal stenosis or fistulae may require repeated dilatations or stents.

Heart

- Radiation can accelerate atherosclerosis of "large vessels" (often seen only many years/decades post-RT) and/or cause subclinical microvascular injury (within months of RT). Pericardial inflammation and thickening may also occur.
- Additional work is needed to better understand the radiation dose/volume/risk relationships and clinical relevance of heart injury in patients with lung cancer.

The organs most commonly at risk of injury during and shortly after thoracic radiotherapy for lung cancer are the lungs and esophagus. Injury to the heart is usually a late effect and is conditional on the patient living long enough for it to become clinically evident.

PULMONARY TOXICITY

Pathophysiology

Radiation pneumonitis (RP) can be divided into three stages—latent, acute, and late.[1] Following radiation there is a latent phase in which there is no apparent symptomatic or radiologic changes. However, microscopically there is degranulation and loss of type II pneumocytes, loss of surfactant, swelling of the basement membrane, and protein transudation into the alveolar spaces. Due to an influx of macrophages and fibroblasts, there is a release of cytokines such as transforming growth factor-beta (TGF-β), interleukin (IL)-2, fibronectin and growth factors such as IGF-1, platelet-derived growth factor, and tumor necrosis factor-alpha (TNF-α). During the acute phase there can be imaging changes and clinical symptoms. The chest x-ray or computerized tomography (CT) scan may show the typical changes of a diffuse infiltrative process corresponding to the radiation field (Fig. 42.1). The symptoms are classically a nonproductive cough, fatigue, shortness of breath, and/or fever. This acute phase occurs within 6–7 months of the delivery of radiation, with a peak incidence of 2–3 months. Microscopically there is a continued inflammatory response with capillary obstruction and an increase in leukocytes, plasma cells, macrophages, fibroblasts, and collagen fibers. The alveolar septa appear thickened and the alveolar space smaller. In the late phase of RP, the imaging will show dense consolidation and volume loss of lung tissue. Some of the acute symptoms such as fever, cough, and fatigue often resolve although it would not be uncommon to have chronic shortness of breath. Pathologically, there is fibrosis of the endothelium and an increase in the thickness of the alveolar septa with obliteration of many alveolar spaces.

The trachea and bronchi are lined with pseudostratified ciliated columnar epithelial cells and mucus-producing goblet cells. A mild to moderate dry cough is common during the acute phase of lung radiation due to depletion of the mucosa. This cough usually resolves shortly after 60–66 Gy radiation therapy, and severe late complications are relatively unusual. In 88 stage III nonsmall cell lung cancer (NSCLC) patients treated to 66 Gy or higher, Lee et al.[2] observed bronchial stenosis in three patients between 2–7 months, representing 11% of all late complications. Miller et al.[3] reported an actuarial rate of treatment-related bronchial stenosis at 1 and 4 years of 7% and 38%, respectively. Radiation dose was suspected to be a factor, with bronchial stenosis observed in 4% and 25% of patients treated to 74 Gy and 86 Gy, respectively. The correlation of mainstem bronchial stenosis with doses of 73 Gy or more was confirmed in a further study by Kelsey et al.[4] This narrowing of the bronchi occurred as early as 3 months following radiation. The caliber of the trachea on the other hand was unchanged following even high doses of radiation.

Grading of Lung Toxicity

Radiation-induced pulmonary toxicity after radical radiotherapy or chemoradiation is complex to score in lung cancer patients because it is difficult to distinguish from tumor progression and exacerbation of preexisting pulmonary comorbidities. The Common Terminology Criteria for Adverse Events (CTCAE) grading system, in common use worldwide for scoring of toxicity, has been modified over the years (http://www.eortc.be/services/doc/ctc/).

The Radiation Therapy Oncology Group (RTOG) had its own grading system initially but has adopted the CTCAE over the last 10 years. An important difference between the RTOG and CTCAE grading system is that the RTOG differentiates between acute (pneumonitis) and late (fibrosis) toxicity based upon the time interval (90 days) after treatment. The choice of

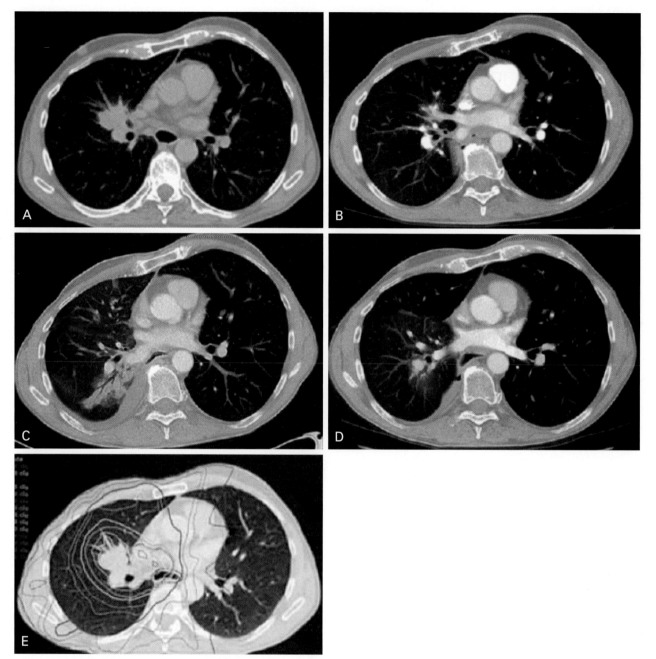

Fig. 42.1. CT scan before irradiation of a stage III NSCLC tumor in the right lung. The corresponding CT slices at 1, 3, and 6 months after 66 Gy in 24 fractions using IMRT and the dose distribution. At 3 months a lung volume reduction and infiltrative changes are seen corresponding to the delivered dose. At 6 months these changes disappeared. (A) CT scan before irradiation of a stage III NSCLC tumor in the right lung; (B) 1 month posttreatment; (C) 3 months posttreatment; (D) 6 months posttreatment; and (E) the dose distribution showing isodose lines of the radiation treatment plan. *CT,* computed tomography; *IMRT,* intensity-modulated radiation therapy; *NSCLC,* nonsmall cell lung cancer. *(Reprinted with permission from José Belderbos.)*

90 days is somewhat arbitrary as the active inflammatory phase of pneumonitis can persist beyond 90 days. Tables 42.1 and 42.2 summarize the RTOG grading systems as well as the CTCAE version for pneumonitis and pulmonary fibrosis.[4,5] In all these grading systems grade 5 toxicity is death (http://ctep.cancer.gov/protocolDevelopment/electronic_applications/ctc.htm#ctc_40).

Changes in Pulmonary Function Tests

The RTOG grading system was heavily dependent on the prescription of drugs or oxygen, which varies greatly from physician

to physician. The CTCAE grading systems did away with that in the later versions, but still require subjective assessment of symptom severity, its effect on activities of daily living, and the indication for oxygen. More objective criteria to measure pulmonary toxicity have been sought such as changes in pulmonary function tests (PFTs).

Miller et al.[6] summarized the changes in PFTs in 13 patients who had been treated definitively with radiation therapy and were thought to have no tumor recurrence for 2 years or longer. These patients had been followed prospectively with PFTs approximately every 6 months. PFTs included spirometry with forced expiratory volume in 1 second (FEV_1) and forced vital

TABLE 42.1 Pneumonitis Grading Criteria

	Grade 1	Grade 2	Grade 3	Grade 4
RTOG	Mild symptoms of dry cough or dyspnea on exertion.	Persistent cough requiring narcotic or antitussive agents. Dyspnea with minimal effort but not at rest.	Severe cough, unresponsive to narcotic antitussive agent or dyspnea at rest. Clinical or radiologic evidence of acute pneumonitis. Intermittent oxygen or steroids may be required.	Severe respiratory insufficiency. Continuous oxygen or assisted ventilation.
CTCAE v4.0 2009	Asymptomatic; clinical or diagnostic observations only; intervention not indicated.	Symptomatic; medical intervention indicated; limiting instrumental activities of daily living.	Severe symptoms; limiting self-care ADL; oxygen indicated.	Life-threatening respiratory compromise; urgent intervention indicated (e.g., tracheotomy or intubation).

CTCAE, Common terminology criteria for adverse events; *RTOG,* Radiation Therapy Oncology Group.

TABLE 42.2 Pulmonary Fibrosis

	Grade 1	Grade 2	Grade 3	Grade 4
CTCAE v4.0 2009	Mild hypoxemia; radiologic pulmonary fibrosis <25% of lung volume.	Moderate hypoxemia; evidence of pulmonary hypertension; radiographic pulmonary fibrosis 25–50%.	Severe hypoxemia; evidence of right-sided heart failure; radiographic pulmonary fibrosis >50–75%.	Life-threatening consequences (e.g., hemodynamic/pulmonary complications); intubation with ventilatory support indicated; radiographic pulmonary fibrosis >75% with severe honeycombing.

CTCAE, Common terminology criteria for adverse events.

capacity (FVC), diffusing capacity for carbon monoxide (DLCO), and lung volumes. There was a decline in the 6-month median FEV_1, FVC, and DLCO that reverted to baseline by 1 year. This improvement at 1 year following radiation therapy was attributed to tumor response. However, there was then a yearly reduction in the median FEV_1, FVC, and the DLCO of 7%, 9.5%, and 3.5%, respectively. The changes in FEV1 and FVC were significant. Ten of these 13 patients developed some new respiratory symptoms that developed at 6 weeks to 21 months following treatment, with a median of 6 months. The authors attributed this progressive decline in PFTs to progressive/evolving radiation-induced lung injury, possibly due to the continuous cycle of tissue hypoxia resulting in an influx of proinflammatory cells that release cytokines that perpetuate the process.[7]

Observations such as this of progressive decline in lung function have resulted in a reluctance of some clinicians to prescribe high-dose radiotherapy to patients with poor pulmonary reserve. However, there is evidence that the extent of decline is linked to pretreatment function such that patients with poor PFTs pretreatment are at less risk of symptomatic lung toxicity or reduction in FVC or FEV_1 compared with patients with good spirometry.[8,9] These somewhat paradoxic observations suggest that poor PFTs should not by themselves be a contraindication to high-dose radiotherapy.

One prospective study of 185 patients given PFTs before and after thoracic RT found that the median maximal percentage reductions in FEV_1, uncorrected DLCO (not corrected for hemoglobin levels), and DLCO were 11.5%, 14.9%, and 15.3%, respectively.[10] Reductions in corrected and uncorrected DLCO were larger than that observed for FEV1. Reductions in uncorrected DLCO were associated with the mean lung dose (MLD) and percentage of perfused lung (measured by SPECT) receiving 30 Gy or more (V30). However, the changes in the SPECT scans were relatively smaller than the observed changes in PFTs in many patients. In a later analysis in an expanded group of patients, the correlation between the predicted drop in DLCO and subsequent pneumonitis was not considered high enough to be very clinically useful.[11]

Others have found a significant correlation between preradiation and postradiation therapy DLCO and pulmonary toxicity. In one large institutional retrospective study 85% of patients with

NSCLC had a postradiation reduction of DLCO.[12] The mean reduction in pretreatment and posttreatment DLCO was 20%. The proportional drop in DLCO differentiated between patients who developed RP grade 1 versus grade II (common toxicity criteria [CTC] v3). This reduction in DLCO correlated with RP grade ≤1 versus ≥2 in patients who were age 65 years or more, had advanced stage (III–IV vs. I–II), were smokers, received chemotherapy, had V20 Gy ≥ 30% (the percentage of normal lung receiving 20 Gy or more), and had baseline DLCO or FEV_1 equal to or more than 60% of predicted. Patients who had higher proportional reductions in DLCO had significant higher rates of severe RP. However, the reductions in DLCO still varied widely between the grades of RP, making it less useful to use in routine clinical practice.

RADIATION PNEUMONITIS

RP typically presents between 1 to 7 months after treatment of external-beam radiotherapy. Clinical symptoms range from shortness of breath, unproductive cough, and occasionally mild fever to death from respiratory failure. RP is diagnosed in approximately 30% of the patients irradiated with radical intent.[13] In patients with respiratory comorbidity such as chronic obstructive pulmonary disease it is often difficult to distinguish whether an acute episode of cough and dyspnea is related to RP or an (postobstructive) infection, disease progression, or preexisting lung disease. RP has a considerable impact on the patient morbidity (quality of life) and less on mortality.

Cooperative group studies of concurrent chemoradiation therapy in stage III NSCLC using 2-dimensional (2-D) or 3-D CT planning have demonstrated grade 3 or higher RP rates in the range of 8% to 18% (Table 42.3).[14–18] The lack of clarity as to how toxicity was calculated or graded makes it difficult to compare rates of RP from study to study. The RTOG designed its dose escalation studies with an upper limit of 15% grade 3 or higher toxicity, most of which were pulmonary.[19,20] Other studies have accepted higher rates of toxicity.[2] In a large institutional experience in patients with stage III disease treated with concurrent chemoradiation with 3-D planning technique, where the incidence of pneumonitis was calculated on an actuarial basis, the risk of symptomatic pneumonitis was more than 30%.[21]

TABLE 42.3 Cooperative Studies Stage III NSCLC Concurrent Chemoradiation

Study Author (Y)	Treatment	Toxicity Grading	Pneumonitis
SWOG 0023 Kelly et al. (2008)[14]	61 Gy qd Cisplatin/etoposide	Pulmonary CTCv2 >Gr 3	8.3% Overall
RTOG 9410 Curran et al. (2011)[15]	60 Gy qd or 69.6 bid Gy Cisplatin/vinblastine or cisplatin/etoposide	Pulmonary RTOG >Gr 3	14% Sequential 15% Concurrent
HOG/US Oncology Hanna et al. (2008)[16]	59.4 Gy Cisplatin/etoposide	Pneumonitis CTCv3 >Gr 3	1.4% Concurrent with no consolidation 9.6% Concurrent with consolidation docetaxel
CALGB 39801 Vokes et al. (2007)[17]	66 Gy Carboplatin/paclitaxel	Pneumonitis CTCv2 >Gr 3	10% Induction and concurrent 4% Concurrent
EORTC 08972-22973 Belderbos et al. (2007)[18]	66 Gy/24 fx qd	Pneumonitis RTOG/EORTC >Gr 3	14% Sequential (gemcitabine-cisplatin) 18% Concurrent (daily dose cisplatin)

CALGB, Cancer and Leukemia Group B; *HOG,* Hoosier Oncology Group; *NSCLC,* nonsmall cell lung cancer; *qd,* once daily; *RTOG,* Radiation Therapy Oncology Group.

Dosimetric Factors

Estimation of the probability of developing RP after treatment with high-dose RT is important for patients with inoperable lung cancer.[22] An important question is could the lung toxicity be predicted from the delivered dose and historical toxicity models? The total dose for an organ-at-risk after conventional fractionated radiotherapy is calculated as the biologic effective dose or normalized total dose in 2 Gy per fraction (NTD2Gy) according to the linear–quadratic model. Studies of the risk of RP relative to the radiation dose received to a certain volume of "normal" lung have used various theoretic models. These studies were only possible with the adoption of CT planning. In two of these models the dose–volume histogram is first reduced to a single parameter, which is subsequently related to the incidence of radiation pneumonitis. Single parameters are the MLD and the volume of the lung receiving more than a certain threshold dose (Vx). The MLD is defined as the average dose throughout the lungs (minus the gross tumor volume). One of the seminal articles by Graham et al.[23] that studied the risk for 99 lung cancer patients with the incidence of RP found that it was correlated with the percent of normal lung receiving 20 Gy or more (V20). In this analysis Graham subtracted the planning target volume (PTV) from the total bilateral lung volume. The PTV is the volume that contains the gross disease, areas thought to represent microscopic extension with an additional margin to account for daily set-up variation. This method of calculating the V20 was continued in several RTOG radiation dose escalation studies.[19,20] However, RTOG 0617, which is a phase III study comparing 60 Gy with 74 Gy with concurrent carboplatin/paclitaxel, calculated normal irradiated lung as the total lung minus the clinical target volume, i.e., the volume thought to contain only gross tumor and microscopic extension.[24] Wang et al.[24] demonstrated that the differences in the calculated mean lung dose or other dosimetric parameters varied greatly depending on which formula was used to define "normal lung." The choice of which of the various formulas to use can lead to significant variation in the prediction of subsequent pulmonary toxicity. The most conservative approach is to subtract only the gross tumor volume (or the internal target volume if using 4-D CT simulation technique). Multiple authors have recommended this approach since the choice of the clinical target volume or PTV margin is more variable from physician to physician.[24,25]

Marks et al.[25] reviewed over 70 articles that correlated dose–volume parameters with subsequent RP following conventionally fractionated radiation therapy of NSCLC. This review, part of the Quantitative Analyses of Normal Tissue Effects in the Clinic (QUANTEC) initiative, cautioned that there was no MLD below which there was no risk of RP. There is also the issue of overestimating RP in these patients due to exacerbation of preexisting pulmonary comorbidities, or tumor progression producing similar complaints. The correlation of MLD and the risk of RP was not linear but had a mildly exponential increase that was more pronounced with increasing MLD. The risk of symptomatic RP with MLD of 20 Gy and 30 Gy was approximately 20% and 40%, respectively. A significant variation in the risk of RP with increasing normal lung volumes, i.e., V20, V30, etc., was reported within the 14 studies summarized by QUANTEC. For example, for V20 of 30% the reported symptomatic RP varied from less than 10% to approximately 50%. There was less variation among the 10 studies that correlated MLD and subsequent symptomatic RP.

In addition to looking at the radiation dose to the total normal lung, there may also be an association between the ipsilateral normal lung dose and the risk of RP. Ramella et al.[26] found that if the V20, V30, and MLD of the total lung volume did not exceed 31%, 18%, and 20 Gy, respectively, there was additional predictive value to the ipsilateral (affected) lung constraints. For example, if the ipsilateral V20 was 52% or less, the risk of RP was 9%, whereas if it was greater than 52%, the risk of RP was 46%. These dosimetric values were calculated by subtracting the PTV from the ipsilateral affected lung.

The use of intensity modulated radiation therapy (IMRT) has been reported to be associated with less pneumonitis compared with 3-D conformal radiotherapy, but it is difficult to understand why if normal lung parameters such as MLD or V20 are similar.[27] IMRT plans are characterized by a more conformal dose distribution and steeper dose fall off and result in a decrease of the V20 and MLD,[28] although the volume of lung receiving a low dose (V5) will be higher. It has been recommended that contralateral lung V5 be kept below 60% to reduce the risk of potentially fatal pneumonitis.[29]

RTOG 0617, a phase III study comparing 60 Gy versus 74 Gy for locally advanced NSCLC, stratified patients according to 3-D CT or IMRT treatment planning. Preliminary results of this study indicate that quality of life was superior in patients treated with IMRT.[30] There is unlikely to be a phase III study directly comparing 3-D CT and IMRT treatment planning. A population-based study of comparative effectiveness found similar rates of early and late pulmonary toxicity for both techniques.[31]

Fewer studies have been done to predict the risk of RP following treatment of limited SCLC. However, there is likely a similar correlation between the dosimetric factors and subsequent RP. For example, Tsujino et al.[32] looked at the risk of RP in patients with limited small cell lung cancer (SCLC) who were treated with cisplatin-based chemotherapy and concurrent thoracic radiation of 45 Gy given two fractions daily, over 15 treatment days. The 12-month cumulative incidence of symptomatic RP was 0%, 7.1%, 25%, and 42.9% in patients with a V20 of <20%, 21% to 25%, 26% to 30%, and >31%, respectively.

Clinical Factors

The impact of nondosimetric factors in predicting the risk of RP has been an area of intense study. Appelt et al.[33] analyzed the patient data used to make the QUANTEC recommendations to look for

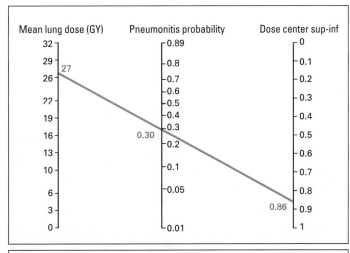

Fig. 42.2. Nomogram to predict incidence of radiation pneumonitis. *(Reprinted with permission from Bradley JD, Hope A, El Naqa I, et al. A nomogram to predict radiation pneumonitis, derived from a combined analysis of RTOG 9311 and institutional data.* Int J Radiat Oncol Biol Phys. *2007;69(4):985–992.)*

clinical risk factors.[25] Factors found to significantly increase the risk of RP were preexisting pulmonary comorbidity, mid or inferior tumor location, current smoking, age older than 63 years, and sequential (as opposed to concurrent) chemotherapy.

Other studies have found that sequential or concurrent chemotherapy involving cisplatin/etoposide does not appear to increase the risk of RP.[17,34,35] RTOG 8808/ECOG 4588 was a three-arm phase III study comparing radiation only, 60 Gy in 2 Gy daily fractions (considered "standard"), or 69.6 Gy in 1.2 Gy fractions twice daily, or sequential cisplatin/vinblastine chemotherapy and standard radiation therapy.[35] The 18-month cumulative incidence of toxicity, primarily pulmonary, was almost 30% in the combined modality arm, as compared with 20% to 25% incidence in the radiation therapy–only arms. The statistical significance between the pulmonary toxicity in the various arms is not stated although the authors said the toxicity was acceptable. Most of the toxicity occurred within the first 3 to 6 months in all treatment arms, with a relative flattening of the incidence after 9 months.

Given the difference from study to study in the nondosimetric variables predicting the risk of pneumonitis, meta-analyses have been done. Vogelius et al.[36] reviewed the English language lung cancer literature between 1990–2010 in which RP was correlated with some patient or treatment variables. In the 31 studies analyzed, the statistically significant risk factors for increased RP were older age, mid-lower lung disease location, and presence of pulmonary comorbidity. The use of sequential rather than concurrent chemotherapy was found to increase the risk of RP

but the authors suspected this was likely due to patient selection rather than a "real" predictive factor. Interestingly, smoking at the time of treatment was found to protect against RP. Even a prior history of smoking was associated with a decreased risk of RP, although this did not reach statistical significance.

Patients with collagen vascular diseases (CVD) are likely at increased risk of RP. In an excellent review by Lee et al.[37] it appears that cytokines such as TGF-β are chronically elevated in such patients. There is often preexisting lung fibrosis. Radiation therapy may cause a patient with quiescent CVD to develop active CVD. These patients are also noted to have increased late toxicity as compared with patients without CVD. Lung fibrosis may extend outside of the high-dose region, so treatment volumes should be reduced when possible, although there is no reason to omit radiation therapy if it is indicated. Interestingly, tumors developing in patients with CVD may be more radiosensitive, prompting consideration of a radiation dose reduction of at least 10%.

Combined Dosimetric and Clinical Factors

Dosimetric and nondosimetric factors can be combined to increase the ability to predict RP. Bradley et al.[38] proposed a nomogram to predict RP based on mean lung dose and the tumor location, superior to inferior (Fig. 42.2).

Taking it one step further, Palma et al.[13] performed a meta-analysis of both dosimetric and nondosimetric factors based on individual patient data. The authors did a search of articles published between 1993 and 2010, in which clinical and dosimetric factors of patients treated with concurrent chemoradiation therapy were available to be correlated with RP. These data were then utilized to conduct a recursive partitioning analysis (RPA) from a 557-patient dataset, and then the RPA was validated using another 279-patient dataset. Factors predicting greater risk of pneumonitis were carboplatin/paclitaxel chemotherapy (vs. cisplatin/etoposide), age greater than 65 years, V20, and MLD (Fig. 42.3).

Biomarkers

Inflammatory cytokines are made by many cells within the lung, including the alveolar macrophages, type II pneumocytes, T lymphocytes, and lung fibroblasts. The blood levels of these cytokines pre-RT, during, and post-RT have been an area of intense interest. For example, Chen et al.[39] found that circulating IL-6 levels pre-RT, during, and post-RT have been correlated with an increased risk of RP. In that study, TNF, another inflammatory cytokine, was not associated with an increased risk of RP.

TGF-β1 is a cytokine that has been extensively studied as a marker predictive of RP.[40,41] It was noted that patients with NSCLC have increased pretreatment levels of TGF-β1 and that increased levels were associated with a higher MLD and a higher incidence of RP. Several studies showed that the absolute levels of TGF-β1 were not as predictive of RP as the observation of an increasing ratio of pretreatment to intratreatment TGF-β1 for stage III NSCLC treated with definitive radiation, with or without chemotherapy.[42] The predictive value of the TGF-β1 ratio was even higher when combined with the MLD. The combination of a MLD of more than 20 Gy and a TGF-β1 ratio of more than 1 was associated with a 66% incidence of RP. Similarly, IL-8 levels pretreatment and then at weeks 2 and 4 of radiation therapy were associated with RP.[43] Patients with RP grade 2 or higher tended to have higher baseline IL-8 levels and these had a slight downward trend during radiation therapy, as opposed to low and stable IL-8 levels in patients without RP. Combining IL-8, TGF-β1, and MLD into a single model led to an improved ability to predict RP as compared with either variable alone.

Certain polymorphisms of the VEGF gene have been correlated with the incidence and severity of RP.[44]

Recall Radiation Pneumonitis

Recall RP is when symptoms of RP are activated by administration of a drug sometime after completion of radiotherapy, with worse than expected RP. Recall RP has been associated with multiple chemotherapy drugs such as taxanes, gemcitabine, vinca alkaloids, doxorubicin, and epirubicin.[45–48] Tyrosine kinase inhibitors such as erlotinib and sunitinib have also been associated with radiation recall pneumonitis and increased risk of severe RP following palliative or definitive radiation therapy.[45,47,49,50]

Prevention and Management

Amifostine

Amifostine, a thiol derivative, is a scavenger of free radicals generated during radiation therapy.[51] Other possible mechanisms of action include increasing the consumption of oxygen within the cells and condensation of DNA, making the strands more resistant to free radicals.[52] A small phase III study in stage III NSCLC patients given radiation and concurrent chemoradiation therapy (paclitaxel or carboplatin) found a significant decrease in the rate of symptomatic RP.[53] The rate of grade 3 or higher (RTOG grading system) in the amifostine versus nonamifostine arms was

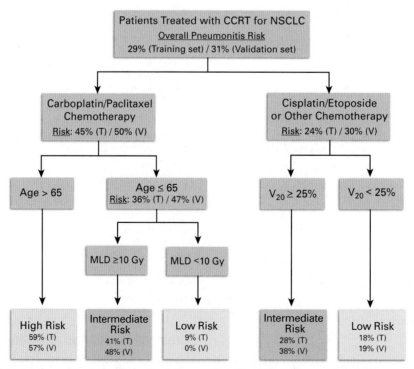

Fig. 42.3. Recursive partitioning analysis of radiation pneumonitis risk in patients undergoing concurrent chemoradiation therapy (CCRT) for nonsmall cell lung cancer (NSCLC). Patients were randomly divided into a training set (T) and validation set (V). *MLD*, mean lung dose; *V20*, volume of lung receiving equal to or greater than 20 Gy. *(Reprinted with permission from Palma DA, Senan S, Tsujino K, et al. Predicting radiation pneumonitis after chemoradiotherapy for lung cancer: an international individual patient data meta-analysis. Int J Radiat Oncol Biol Phys. 2013;85(2):444–450.)*

56.3% and 19.4%, respectively (*p* = .002). However, a larger phase III study, RTOG 9801, investigated the ability of amifostine to reduce chemoradiation-induced esophagitis.[54] Amifostine did not reduce treatment-related esophagitis in that study when it was given daily with carboplatin/paclitaxel and concurrent thoracic radiation for stage III NSCLC. A subsequent report indicated that amifostine also did not reduce either median survival or late toxicities, including RP.[55]

Pentoxifylline and Vitamin E

The combination of pentoxifylline and vitamin E has been shown to decrease radiation-related soft-tissue fibrosis of the breast and extremities.[56-58] Pentoxifylline is a methylxanthine derivative developed and prescribed for impaired microcirculation. It improves blood perfusion by erythrocyte deformability and decreased blood viscosity. Pentoxifylline appears to decrease fibroblast, cellular matrix, and collagen production by blocking the activity of TNF, decreasing IL and oxygen radicals, and stimulating collagenase activity.[59] Vitamin E, a tocopherol, acts as an antioxidant and protects membrane phospholipids from oxidative damage by scavenging reactive oxygen species generated during oxidative stress. Vitamin E also inhibits TGF and collagen production.[59,60]

A small randomized study of pentoxifylline 400 mg versus placebo three times a day during radiation therapy for either lung or breast cancer demonstrated superiority in the pentoxifylline arm in the posttreatment patient-reported breathing function, DLCO, and imaging studies.[61] Larger studies should be done to validate this finding.

Steroids

Surprisingly, there has been little clinical research into the use of prophylactic steroids to reduce the incidence and severity of RP. A rodent study found that small doses of steroids three times a week for 15 weeks starting 10 to 11 weeks from delivery of thoracic radiation significantly delayed the onset of and death due to RP.[62] A prospective study in humans would be clinically relevant.

Angiotensin-Converting Enzyme Inhibitors

Angiotensin-converting enzyme (ACE) inhibitors have been studied in both animals and humans. The mechanism of its protective effect is not clear but may have something to do with the reduction in pulmonary arterial pressure, resulting in less severe edema.[63] Rodent studies established the rationale for angiotensin-converting enzyme inhibitors, such as captopril, in the reduction of acute pneumonitis following radiation therapy.[64] This effect was most notable at moderate doses of radiation therapy. Following very high doses of hemithoracic radiation, i.e., 80 Gy in 10 fractions, captopril had no significant protective effect. Retrospective studies also confirmed the apparent protective effect of ACE inhibitors on pulmonary toxicity following concurrent chemoradiation for stage III NSCLC.[65] A phase II cooperative group study (RTOG 0213) was initiated to test this hypothesis but closed due to poor accrual. The study was designed to test the ability of captopril to alter the incidence of pulmonary damage at 12 months from completion of radiation treatment in SCLC or NSCLC patients receiving at least 45 Gy.

TGF-β Tyrosine Kinase Inhibitors

There are no human clinical studies of inhibitors of TGF-β to reduce RP, but preclinical studies suggest potential utility. Flechsig et al.[66] found that a 4-week course of a tyrosine kinase inhibitor to TGF-β improved the survival of rodents following whole thoracic radiation.

Treatment of Radiation Pneumonitis

There are no prospective studies evaluating the effectiveness of treatment of RP. Most cases are self-limiting. Patients with troublesome symptoms from presumed RP are usually started on prednisone 50–60 mg per day for 1–2 weeks and then decreased slowly by 10 mg per week, assuming the symptoms are improved or stable.[19,30] Oxygen may be needed and a referral to a pulmonologist should be considered if the symptoms are severe or do not improve as anticipated.

ESOPHAGUS TOXICITY

Pathophysiology

Radiation-induced esophagitis is an inflammation of the esophagus, which develops 2 to 3 weeks after the initiation of radiation therapy. Radiation affects the part of the esophagus within the irradiated area. The normal esophageal mucosa undergoes continuous cell turnover and renewal. These mucosal cells are sensitive to irradiation-induced damage. Acute radiation esophagitis is primarily due to effects on the basal epithelial layer. This causes a thinning of the mucosa, which can progress to denudation.

In 1960, the onset of radiation effects in the esophagus was first studied in rats and displayed timelines and clinical findings.[67] Four days after radiation a submucosal infiltration of leucocytes was seen, mucosal necrosis was seen at 7 days, and a moderate inflammation of the muscularis of the esophagus and some submucosal telangiectasia was seen 10 days after radiation. By 20 days most of the rats showed reepithelization of the esophagus. However, in animals killed more than 3 months after exposure, defects in the muscle walls and atrophy of the epithelium were seen.[67]

Grading of Esophagus Toxicity

Esophagus toxicity is scored using the CTCAE (version 4.0). Grade 2 is scored in case of symptomatic dysphagia and altered eating and intravenous fluids may be indicated for a period shorter than 24 hours. Grade 3 esophagus toxicity is scored in case of symptomatic and severely altered eating/swallowing and the use of intravenous fluids, tube feedings, or total parenteral nutrition equal to or more than 24 hours. Grade 4 esophagus toxicity includes life-threatening consequences for the patients, and grade 5 is scored in case of death. The CTC scoring system, however, does not differentiate between early and late symptoms. The RTOG/EORTC scoring system differentiates between acute esophagus toxicity (AET), symptoms within 3 months after concurrent chemoradiation therapy, and late esophagus toxicity (LET), symptoms persisting or occurring more than 3 months after the end of treatment (Table 42.4). AET influences the quality of life of the patient and may result in treatment interruption, but generally resolves after treatment. Patients who develop esophagus stenosis, perforation, or fistula are categorized as severe LET (grade 3–5). Severe LET seriously affects the patients' quality of life or even leads to death. Although several models are available to predict the incidence and severity of AET, for LET

TABLE 42.4 Late Esophagus Toxicity Scoring From 3 Months After Treatment According to TOG/EORTC

Grade 0–1	Mild fibrosis; slight difficulty in swallowing solids; no pain on swallowing.
Grade 2	Unable to take solid food normally; swallowing semisolid food; dilatation may be indicated.
Grade 3	Severe fibrosis; able to swallow only liquids; may have pain on swallowing; dilatation required.
Grade 4	Necrosis/perforation fistula.
Grade 5	Death.

predictive models are sparse. So far, several studies have reported the incidence of severe LET using 3-D–conformal-radiotherapy (3DCRT) and IMRT (Table 42.5).[17,68–76] Using 3DCRT, the reported crude incidence of severe LET in concurrent RCT varies from 5% to 16%. Without solid evidence, several implications can be drawn from previous studies: severe AET is associated with severe LET.

Radiation Esophagitis

The improved survival of patients with locally advanced NSCLC who are treated with concurrent radiochemotherapy comes at a price of increased esophagus toxicity.[75,77–80] Due to overlap with the target volume because of involvement of mediastinal lymph nodes or mediastinal tumor invasion a part of the esophagus is often irradiated in lung cancer. Acute toxicity is manifested clinically as dysphagia, odynophagia, and substernal discomfort and usually occurs within 2 to 3 weeks after the initiation of radiation therapy. Patients may describe a sudden, sharp, severe chest pain radiating to the back. Patients with insufficient intake due to radiation esophagitis are at risk for premature discontinuation of therapy. Predicting the risk of esophagus toxicity makes it possible to take appropriate precautions, such as preventive medication or tube feeding. Identifying the low-risk patients for radiation esophagitis gives the opportunity to escalate the dose of radiotherapy to improve tumor control.

Dosimetric Factors

Estimation of the probability and severity of esophagus toxicity after concurrent chemoradiation treatment is crucial. This allows the individual prescription of tumor doses based on normal tissue complication probabilities. Several prediction models have been reported to estimate the risk of AET based on the planned dose distributions. Currently used models to predict AET in

lung cancer patients after intensity IMRT and concurrent chemotherapy were mainly derived from patients treated with 3-D chemoradiation.

When using IMRT and concurrent chemoradiation in patients with NSCLC, reported were a dose–effect relationship of AET in 185 patients,[81] severe LET in 171 patients,[68] and dose–volume parameters of the esophagus. Severe LET was defined as grade equal to or greater than 3 RTOG/EORTC (Table 42.6).[17,82–92] In these Dutch studies,[81,68] hypofractionated IMRT treatment up to 66 Gy in 24 fractions and concurrent daily low-dose cisplatin (6 mg/m² with a maximum of 12 mg) was administered in consecutive patients. Cisplatin was administered as a bolus injection 1 hour to 2 hours before each fraction. The dose distributions were first converted to normalized total doses to account for fractionation effects with an α/β-ratio of 10 Gy for AET and α/β-ratio of 3 Gy for LET. Equivalent uniform dose (EUD) to the esophagus and the volume percentage receiving more than x Gy (Vx) were evaluated by the Lyman-Kutcher-Burman model. A total of 22% patients with NSCLC developed AET toxicity greater than or equal to grade 3, and 6% severe LET was observed. The median time to AET grade 3 was 30 days, with a median duration of >80 days. The median onset time of severe LET was 5 months (range 3~12). All 11 patients expressed LET within 1 year. Eight patients developed esophagus stenosis (grade 3), which could be treated by dilatation. A fistula was diagnosed in three patients, and these patients were treated with intraluminal stent. All three patients with fistulae died from respiratory insufficiency caused by pneumonia shortly after the stent was placed (up to 3 months). Pathologically proven tumor progression was the cause of esophageal fistulae in three other patients (28, 31, and 31 months) and not scored as LET. Severe LET occurred in 7% of the patients (4 of 61) with grade 2 AET and 19% of the patients (7 of 37) with grade 3 AET. Severe LET was significantly ($p = 0.002$) associated with the maximum grade of AET. Patients with unrecovered AET had a significantly ($p < 0.001$) higher risk of developing

TABLE 42.5 Crude Incidence of Reported Severe LET in Patients With NSCLC Treated With Sequential and Concurrent Radiochemotherapy Regimens[7]

Author (Y)	Patients	Radiotherapy	Chemotherapy	Criteria	Median Follow-Up (Mo)	Median Overall Survival (Mo)	Crude Incidence LET
Byhardt et al. (1998)[69]	Stage II, IIIA/B N = 136	3DCRT 60 Gy/6 wk (QD)	Sequential	RTOG	—	13.6	2% ≥G3 LET
	N = 82	3DCRT 63 Gy/6.5 wk	Sequential/Concurrent	RTOG	—	16.3	4% ≥G3 LET
	N = 170	3DCRT 69.6 Gy/6 wk (BID)	Concurrent	RTOG	—	15.8	8% ≥G3 LET
Maguire et al. (1999)[70]	Stage I–IIIA/B N = 66	3DCRT 64.2~85.6 Gy (QD/BID)	None/Sequential/Concurrent	RTOG	—	—	3% ≥G3 LET
Uitterhoeve et al. (2000)[71]	T1~T4, N0~N2 N = 40	3DCRT 60.5~66 Gy/30~32 d (Hypo)	Concurrent	RTOG	21	13.5	5% ≥G3 LET
Rosenman et al. (2002)[72]	Stage IIIA/B N = 62	3DCRT 60~74 Gy (QD)	Sequential + Concurrent	RTOG	43	24	6% ≥G3 LET
Komaki et al. (2002)[73]	Stage II, IIIA/B N = 81	3DCRT 63 Gy/7 wk (QD)	Sequential + Concurrent	RTOG	—	16.4	4% ≥G3 LET
	N = 82	3DCRT 69.6 Gy/6 wk (BID)	Concurrent	RTOG	—	15.5	16% ≥G3 LET
Singh et al. (2003)[74]	N2/N3, T3/T4 N = 207	3DCRT 60~74 Gy (QD)	None/Sequential/Concurrent	RTOG	24	—	6% ≥G3 LET
Bradley et al. (2004)[75]	Stage I–IIIA/B N = 166	3DCRT 60~74 Gy (QD)	None/Sequential/Concurrent	RTOG	—	—	3% ≥G3 LET
Belderbos et al. (2007)[18]	Stage I–IIIA/B N = 76	3DCRT 66 Gy/30~32 d (Hypo)	Sequential	RTOG	39	16.2	4% ≥G3 LET
	N = 66	3DCRT 66 Gy/30~32 d (Hypo)	Concurrent	RTOG	39	16.5	5% ≥G3 LET
van Baardwijk et al. (2012)[76]	Stage III N = 137	3DCRT 51~69 Gy (BID + QD)	Concurrent	CTCAE	30.9	25.0	7.3% ≥G3 LET
Chen et al. (2013)[68]	Stage II–IIIA/B N = 171	IMRT 66 Gy/30~32 d (Hypo)	Concurrent	RTOG/EORTC	33	24	6% ≥G3 LET

BID, Twice daily; *CTCAE,* cancer and Leukemia Group B; *3DCRT,* 3-D–conformal-radiotherapy; *IMRT,* intensity modulated radiation therapy; *LET,* late esophagus toxicity; *QD,* once daily; *RTOG,* Radiation Therapy Oncology Group.

severe LET, compared with patients without AET or with a recovered AET. In the EUD, $n = 0.03$ model, all severe LET patients had a NTD greater than 70 Gy on the esophagus. In the EUDn-LKB model, the fitted values and 95% confidence intervals (CIs) were TD50 = 76.1 Gy (73.2~78.6), $m = 0.03$ (0.02~0.06) and $n = 0.03$ (0~0.08). In the Vx-LKB model, the fitted values and 95% CIs were Tx50 = 23.5% (16.4~46.6), $m = 0.44$ (0.32~0.60) and $x = 76.7$ Gy (74.7~77.5).

The V50 was identified as the most accurate predictor of grade ≥3 AET.[81] Werner-Wasik et al.[80] described in their review on esophagus toxicity that a higher dose, even on a small part of the esophagus, might be a risk factor for AET. They described several dosimetric parameters to be predictive in univariate analysis for grade 2 and grade 3 AET: V20 through V80. But most at risk for AET were esophagus volume doses receiving greater than 40 Gy to 50 Gy. The systematic review by Rose et al.[79] demonstrated that the Dmean, V20, V30, V40, V45, and V50 were the best-studied dosimetric predictors with high levels of association with AET. The dosimetric predictors of AET in Rose and colleagues' review are consistent with the predictor advocated by Kwint et al.,[81] namely, the V50.

A large multiinstitutional study on 1082 patients treated with 3DCRT, or IMRT concurrent with chemotherapy, analyzed acute radiation esophagitis.[93] The median radiotherapy dose was 65 Gy, and median follow-up was 2.2 years. Most patients (92%) received platinum-containing concurrent chemoradiation therapy regimens. The development of radiation esophagitis was common, scored as grade 2 in 348 patients (32.2%), grade 3 in 185 patients (17.1%), and grade 4 in 10 patients (0.9%). The high-dose volumes were the most important predictors for radiation esophagitis.[93] The V60 emerged as the best predictor for both moderate and severe AET. A low-risk subgroup was identified with a very low V60 of less than 0.07%, an intermediate-risk subgroup with a V60 of 0.07% to 16.99%, and a high-risk subgroup with a V60 of equal to or greater than 17% (Fig. 42.4).

Clinical Factors

In the meta-analysis of Auperin et al.,[94] which demonstrated the superiority of concurrent over sequential chemoradiation for NSCLC, the incidence of grade 3 or grade 4 esophagitis increased from 4% in the sequential group to 18% in patients randomized to concomitant chemotherapy. The type of chemotherapy may be important, as a strong association was found between maximum grade of neutropenia and severity of dysphagia by de Ruysscher et al.[95]

A systematic review of the literature was published comparing acute and late toxicities and to determine which concurrent

TABLE 42.6   Toxicity Results ≥Grade 3 of NSCLC Patients on Concurrent RCT Used in Phase II and Phase III Study Arms Treated Between 1992 and 2010; Combinations with Cisplatin[81]

Author (Y)	Chemotherapy Scheme	Nausea/ Vomiting (%)	Esophagitis (%)	Leukopenia (%)	Anemia (%)	Thrombocytopenia (%)	Grade 5 Toxicity (%)
Belderbos et al. (2007)[18]	ML	6	17	3	0		1
Pradier et al. (2005)[83]	ML			5			0
Schaake-Koning et al. (1992)[84]	ML	24	4	3		0	0
Schaake-Koning et al. (1992)[84]	ML	21	1	1		0	2
Trovo et al. (1992)[85]	ML	5	2		0		1
Trovo et al. (1992)[85]	ML	1	16	0	0		
Blanke et al. (1995)[86]	MH	5	3	5			2
Cakir et al.[a] (2004)[87]	MH	24 (2)	10	15 (3)	8		
Furuse et al. (1999)[88]	PH	23	2.6	98.7	10.3	52.6	
Furuse et al. (1995)[89]	PH	16	6	95	28	45	2
Ichinose et al. (2004)[90]	PH	4	3	16	6	1	0
Kim et al. (2005)[91]	PH		4	b	b	b	0.7
Schild et al.[c](2002)[92]	PH	26	18 (2)	38 (40)		26 (3)	3

[a]Exact toxicity grade unknown, probably < grade 2 (grade 3).
[b]19% hematologic toxicity not further specified.
[c]Grade 4 toxicity.
H, high-dose; *L*, daily low-dose; *M*, monochemotherapy; *NSCLC*, nonsmall cell lung cancer; *P*, polychemotherapy.

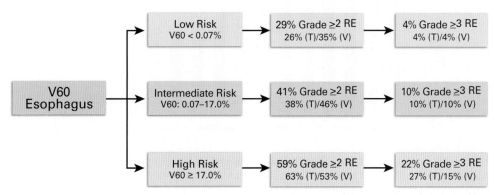

Fig. 42.4. V60 as predictor for both moderate and severe radiation esophagitis (RE). *T*, training set; *V*, validation set. Based on data reported by Palma et al.[93]

chemoradiation scheme should preferably be offered to patients with locally advanced nonmetastatic NSCLC.[82] In all 17 selected papers (phase II and phase III trials published between 1992 and 2010) on concurrent concurrent chemoradiation, acute toxicity consisting of esophagitis equal to or greater than grade 3 was reported. AET incidence varied from 1% up to 18% of the patients. In three studies the incidences of AET grades ≥3 were similar: 17% and 18% (Table 42.6). In most studies late toxicity was not reported, however. In the low-dose cisplatin studies, LET grade 3 to grade 4 was reported in 5% of the patients. The conclusion of Koning's systematic review was that concurrent RCT with monochemotherapy consisting of daily cisplatin resulted in favorable acute and late toxicity compared with concurrent chemoradiation with single high-dose chemotherapy, doublets or triplets.[82]

Modified fractionation is also associated with a greater risk of esophagitis as demonstrated in the meta-analysis by Mauguen et al.[96] The risk of grade 3 or 4 esophagitis was 9% for conventional treatment and 19% with modified fractionation, with very accelerated fractionation being the most toxic.

Combined Dosimetric and Clinical Factors

Several groups analyzed the relation of clinical parameters and radiation esophagitis. No evidence, however, for increased acute toxicity in older patients treated with concurrent chemoradiation using IMRT or in patients with severe comorbidity was found in the analysis by Uyterlinde et al.[97] In a total of 35% of the patients acute toxicity grade greater than or equal to 3 was reported. Grade 5 toxicity was scored in 1% of the patients. Similar toxicity was observed between older patients (equal to or greater than 70 years) and younger patients (less than 70 years, $p = 0.26$). No significant association was found among prior weight loss, high Charlson Comorbidity Index of ≥5, and acute severe toxicity ($p = 0.36$). V50 esophagus (odds ratio [OR], 1.33 per 10% increase; $p = 0.01$) and patients with PS ≥2 (OR, 3.45; $p = 0.07$) were at risk to develop acute toxicity grade 3.

Esophageal FDG uptake using 18FDG-PET postconcurrent chemoradiation was investigated and correlated with AET grade.[98] A total of 82 patients treated with 66 Gy in 24 fractions were selected on the presence of a post-RT positron emission tomography (PET) scan acquired within 3 months after concurrent RCT. The value of PET(post) in relation to AET was evaluated by comparing the mean esophageal standard uptake value of the highest 50% between grade less than 2 and grade greater than or equal to 2 AET. The local dose on the esophagus wall was correlated to the standard uptake value and modeled using a power-law fit. The Lyman-Kutcher-Burman model was used to predict grade ≥2AET. The local dose–response relation was used in the Lyman-Kutcher-Burman model to calculate the EUD. Resulting prediction accuracy was compared to D(mean), V(35), V(55), and V(60). The LKB parameters (95% CI) were $n = 0.130$ (0.120 to 0.141), $m = 0.25$ (0.13 to 0.85), and TD(50) = 50.4 Gy (37.5–55.4), which resulted in improved predictability of AET compared with other predictors.[98]

Prevention and Management

Elective nodal irradiation has been associated with increased esophageal dose, resulting in a two-fold increase in the esophageal V50 compared with treatment plans treating involved lymph nodes only.[99] Due to the steep dose fall-off of IMRT compared with 3DCRT and the ability to shape the dose around organs at risk, it is possible to reduce the volume of the esophagus irradiated, so a lower incidence of AET is expected. One planning study in node-positive patients achieved a decrease in esophageal V50 from 26% to 28% with 3DCRT to 19% using IMRT while maintaining the same tumor control probability.[99] In order to investigate the differences between AET and the use of 3DCRT or IMRT, the AET incidences for patients treated with the same concurrent RCT regimen were compared.[81] The AET incidences were not significantly different between 3DCRT-based and IMRT-based concurrent RCT patients. In order to illustrate the differences between 3DCRT and IMRT, the Vx (α/β-ratio = 10) in steps of 5 Gy derived for 36 patients treated with concurrent RCT (EORTC 08972-22973 trial) and the AET study by Kwint et al.[81] are depicted in Fig. 42.5. From this figure it can be appreciated that with IMRT the volume of esophagus receiving a dose from 5 Gy to 40 Gy was significantly smaller, while at 70 Gy it was increased. Moreover, the LKB model based on the V50 was not significantly different between IMRT and 3DCRT. In clinical practice, high-dose volumes to the esophagus (V50 to V60) and the use of concurrent chemotherapy are the most important predictors for AET and LET.[13,68,81] The NTD-corrected esophagus EUD less than 70 Gy could be a dose constraint to minimize

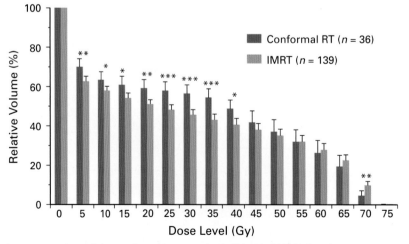

Fig. 42.5. Average esophageal dose–volume histogram for the historical NSCLC patients planned with concurrent chemotherapy and 3DCRT, and the IMRT dataset. The error bars denote the 95% standard error. Both groups were compared for each dose level using a 2-sided t-test (* $p < 0.05$, ** $p < 0.01$, *** $p < 0.001$). *(Reprinted with permission from Kwint M, Uyterlinde W, Nijkamp J, et al. Acute esophagus toxicity in lung cancer patients after intensity modulated radiation therapy and concurrent chemotherapy. Int J Radiat Oncol Biol Phys. 2012;84(2):e223–e228.)*

severe LET.[99] Another way to prevent esophagus toxicity was reported by Uyterlinde et al.:[97] daily prehydration was associated with a reduced rate of both renal and acute esophageal toxicity and an increased chemotherapy adherence in patients receiving a daily dose of cisplatin and concurrent radiotherapy for locally advanced NSCLC.

Management

Acute esophagitis is treated with dietary changes, proton pump inhibitors, analgesics (including opiates), local anesthetics (lignocaine viscous), promotility agents, intravenous fluids, and/or nasogastric tube or gastrostomy tube insertion. Dietary changes are focused on keeping the patient comfortable and maintaining nutrition, body weight, and fluid intake. High-calorie food and liquids are good choices. Softening the patient's diet, avoiding extremely hot or cold foods, and refraining from alcohol and spicy food are important in alleviating the discomfort of esophagitis. Patients with complaints of esophagus stenosis are generally treated by (repeated) dilatation procedures. Some patients will develop a perforation or fistula, which can be treated with intraluminal stenting.

HEART

Much of what is known about radiation injury to the heart, especially effects on mortality, has been derived from studies in patients with breast cancer, in whom the heart is irradiated incidentally, and the majority of whom are long-term survivors after treatment.

Pathophysiology

Evidence from rodent models suggests that radiation can cause both microvascular and macrovascular cardiac pathology.[100] The microvascular pathology is characterized by a decrease in capillary density, causing chronic myocardial ischemia and fibrosis. Macrovascular disease occurs through an accelerated development of age-related atherosclerosis.[100]

Based on these experimental findings, Darby et al.[100] suggested two hypotheses for the biologic mechanisms that lead to increased morbidity and mortality from coronary artery disease after radiation exposure in humans. The first hypothesis is that radiation increases the frequency of MI by accelerated atherosclerosis of "large vessels." The macrovascular injury is often manifest only many years/decades post-RT. The second hypothesis is that radiation causes microvascular injury that is largely subclinical (this is consistent with the imaging changes observed in clinical studies). If and when the patient experiences some macrovascular injury, the latent subclinical microvascular injury may synergistically increase the risk/clinical severity by reducing the heart's reserve[100] (Fig. 42.6).

Heart Imaging Data From Irradiated Patients

In order to study heart injury in a prospective manner, surrogate markers such as imaging have been used to assess cardiac injury.[101–105] In a large prospective study conducted at Duke University, tangential RT to the left breast/chest wall was found to be associated with reductions in regional perfusion as assessed by SPECT scans.[101] A representative pre-RT and post-RT image from one patient is shown in Fig. 42.7.[101] The perfusion defects were typically seen on the anterior heart, that is, limited to and within the RT field. The frequency of observing new perfusion defects was related to the volume of the left ventricle within the RT beam (Fig. 42.8).

The functional consequence of these perfusion defects is unknown. There were higher rates of wall motion abnormalities in patients with (versus without) perfusion defects in this study, i.e., 12% to 40% versus 0% to 9%, respectively, depending on the post-RT interval ($p = 0.007–0.16$).[101]

Similarly, Gyenes et al.[106] noted myocardial perfusion defects at about 1 year post-RT. Several other authors also reported myocardial perfusion imaging abnormalities post-RT, but the majority of these studies considered patients treated many years post-RT.[107]

Gayed et al.[108] assessed myocardial perfusion imaging results before and after chemoradiotherapy in 16 patients with esophageal cancer and 25 patients with lung cancer.[108] Seven of the 25 (29%) patients with lung cancer developed myocardial ischemia in the radiation field at a mean of 8.4 months after radiotherapy. Considering the combined group, myocardial perfusion imaging result was not a statistically significant predictor of future cardiac complications after chemoradiotherapy. A history of congestive heart failure or arrhythmia was a significant predictor of cardiac morbidity.[108]

Umezawa et al.[109] evaluated subclinical radiation-induced myocardial changes using scintigraphy with a new agent, iodine-123 β-methyl-iodophenyl pentadecanoic acid (I-123

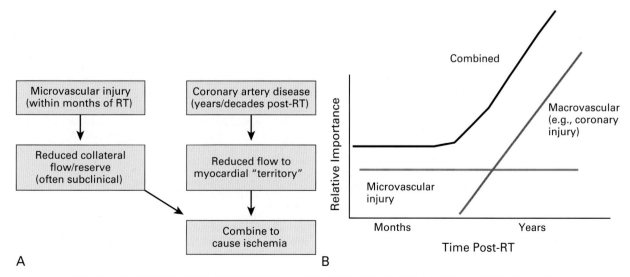

Fig. 42.6. (A) Interaction of two mechanisms to produce clinical heart disease; and (B) hypothesis of the combined effect of these two mechanisms over time.

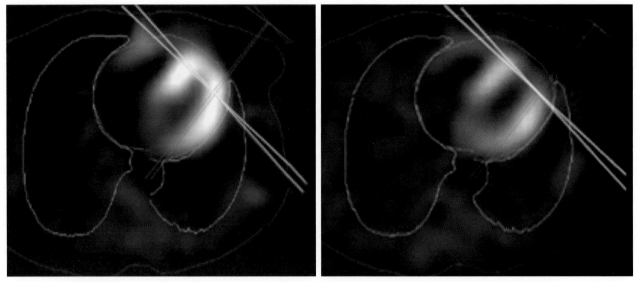

Fig. 42.7. A representative pre-RT and post-RT image from one patient treated with tangential RT to the left breast/chest wall with RT-associated reductions in regional perfusion as assessed by single photon emission computed tomography (SPECT) scans. *RT,* radiation therapy. *(Reprinted with permission from Marks LB, Xiaoli Y, Prosnitz RG, et al. The incidence and functional consequences of RT-associated cardiac perfusion defects.* Int J Radiat Oncol Biol Phys. *2005;63(1):214–223.)*

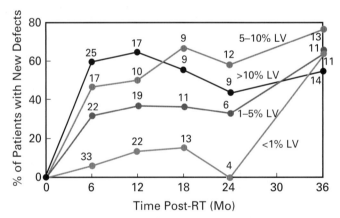

Fig. 42.8. The incidence of new perfusion defects in subgroups of patients with different volumes of left ventricle (LV) included within the radiation therapy (RT) field (i.e., those areas receiving greater than 50% of prescribing dose). *(Reprinted with permission from Marks LB, Xiaoli Y, Prosnitz RG, et al. The incidence and functional consequences of RT-associated cardiac perfusion defects.* Int J Radiat Oncol Biol Phys. *2005;63(1):214–223.)*

BMIPP), in 34 patients who maintained complete response to curative radiation therapy for esophageal cancer. I-123 BMIPP evaluates myocardial fatty acid metabolism. Reduced uptake was detected in 13%, 43%, and 68% of the myocardial segments that received 0 Gy, 40 Gy, and 60 Gy, respectively. These investigators suggested that I-123 BMIPP myocardial scintigraphy may be useful to identify RT-induced myocardial damage.[109]

In conclusion, these imaging data demonstrate that there are acute physiologic changes in the heart post-RT (i.e., within a few years of RT) and that these changes are correlated with dose and might reflect subclinical injury.

Grading of Heart Toxicity

Types of Cardiovascular Toxicity

Radiation-associated heart disease includes a wide spectrum of cardiac diseases, which are listed in Table 42.7. Early effects include pericarditis and pericardial effusion (months to a few years postradiation). Late effects include disease of the coronary arteries, the heart valves, the myocardium, and the conductive system (10 to 15 years after radiation). Both chemotherapy and radiotherapy may cause cardiovascular toxicity. This has been clearly demonstrated in patients irradiated for Hodgkin disease, breast cancer, esophageal cancer, and medulloblastoma.

Scoring of Cardiac Toxicity

Cardiac toxicity is scored using the CTCAE (version 4.0) including all types of adverse events related to pericardium, myocardium, valves, coronary arteries, and cardioelectrical activity. The CTC scoring system, however, does not differentiate between early and late symptoms. The RTOG/EORTC scoring system differentiates between acute and late cardiac toxicity (Table 42.8).

TABLE 42.7 Radiation Effects on the Heart[a]

	Acute	Late
Pericarditis	Acute exudative pericarditis is rare and often occurs during radiotherapy as a reaction to necrosis/inflammation of a tumor located next to the heart. Delayed acute pericarditis occurs within weeks after radiotherapy and can be revealed by either an asymptomatic pericardial effusion or a symptomatic pericarditis. Cardiac tamponade is rare. Spontaneous clearance of this effusion may take up to 2 years.	Delayed chronic pericarditis appears several weeks to years after radiotherapy. In this type, extensive fibrous thickening, adhesions, chronic constriction, and chronic pericardial effusion can be observed. It is observed in up to 20% of patients within 2 years following irradiation. Constrictive pericarditis can be observed in 4–20% of patients and appears to be dose–dependent and related to the presence of pericardial effusion in the delayed acute phase.
Cardiomyopathy	Acute myocarditis related to radiation induced inflammation with transient repolarization abnormalities and mild myocardial dysfunction.	Diffuse myocardial fibrosis (often after a >30-Gy radiation dose) with relevant systolic and diastolic dysfunction, conduction disturbance, and autonomic dysfunction. Restrictive cardiomyopathy represents an advanced stage of myocardial damage due to fibrosis with severe diastolic dysfunction and signs and symptoms of heart failure.
Valve disease	No immediate apparent effects.	Valve apparatus and leaflet thickening, fibrosis, shortening, and calcification predominant on left-sided valves (related to pressure difference between the left and right side of the heart). Valve regurgitation more commonly encountered than stenosis. Stenotic lesions more commonly involving the aortic valve. Reported incidence of clinically significant valve disease: 1% at 10 years; 5% at 15 years; 6% at 20 years after radiation exposure. Valve disease incidence increases significantly after >20 years following irradiation: mild AR up to 45%, > moderate AR up to 15%, AS up to 16%, mild MR up to 48%, mild PR up to 12%.
CAD	No immediate apparent effects. (Perfusion defects can be seen in 47% of patients 6 months after radiotherapy and may be accompanied by wall-motion abnormalities and chest pain. Their long-term prognosis and significance are unknown.)	Accelerated CAD appearing at a young age. Concomitant atherosclerotic risk factors further enhance the development of CAD. Latent until at least 10 years after exposure. (Patients younger than 50 years of age tend to develop CAD in the first decade after treatment, while older patients have longer latency periods.) Coronary ostia and proximal segments are typically involved. CAD doubles the risk of death; relative risk of death from fatal myocardial infarction varies from 2.2 to 8.8.

[a]Adapted from Lancellotti P et al.[138]
AR, Aortic regurgitation; *AS*, aortic stenosis; *CAD*, coronary artery disease; *MR*, mitral regurgitation; *PR*, pulmonary regurgitation.

TABLE 42.8 Acute and Late Cardiac Toxicity Scoring According to RTOG/EORTC

A. ACUTE CARDIAC TOXICITY SCORING ACCORDING TO RTOG/EORTC

Grade 0	Grade 1	Grade 2	Grade 3	Grade 4	Grade 5
No change over baseline	Asymptomatic but objective evidence of EKG changes or pericardial abnormalities without evidence of other heart disease	Symptomatic with EKG changes and radiologic findings of congestive heart failure or pericardial disease/no specific treatment required	Congestive heart failure, angina pectoris, pericardial disease responding to therapy	Congestive heart failure, angina pectoris, pericardial disease, arrhythmias not responsive to nonsurgical measures	Death

B. LATE CARDIAC TOXICITY SCORING ACCORDING TO RTOG/EORTC

Grade 0	Grade 1	Grade 2	Grade 3	Grade 4	Grade 5
None	Asymptomatic or mild symptoms Transient T wave inversion & ST changes Sinus tachycardia >110 (at rest)	Moderate angina on effort Mild pericarditis Normal heart size Persistent abnormal T wave and ST changes Low QRS	Severe angina Pericardial effusion Constrictive pericarditis Moderate heart failure Cardiac enlargement EKG abnormalities	Tamponade/severe heart failure/severe constrictive pericarditis	Death

EKG, Electrocardiogram; *RTOG*, Radiation Therapy Oncology Group.

Data From Lung Cancer Patients

The data for patients with lung cancer are more sparse. Historically, radiotherapy-associated cardiac toxicity has generally not been considered a significant clinical issue in patients with lung cancer. This has been due, at least in part, to the fact that many patients with lung cancer have limited survival duration and that radiation-induced cardiotoxicity has been considered a "late effect." In the postoperative setting, there have been several studies noting decreased overall survival with the addition of postoperative RT in lung cancer patients.[110–112] In a meta-analysis of randomized trials, there was a 6% absolute reduction in overall survival at 2 years for NSCLC patients irradiated postoperatively.[113] The causes of death in these studies are not uniformly reported. In the Dautzenberg et al.[110] trial (which randomized 728 patients with NSCLC who had undergone complete surgical resection to receive either postoperative RT at a total dose of 60 Gy or observation only), the RT patients had a rate of cardiac mortality that was approximately three times the rate seen in the control group (an estimated 5.1% versus 1.7%, or an absolute excess 3.4% rate).[110]

Data From Breast Cancer Patients

One of the earliest recognitions of radiation-associated cardiac injury was in patients radiated for breast cancer. In 1987 and 1989, Cuzick et al.[114,115] published a series of articles based on meta-analysis studies comparing treatment with surgery, with or without postmastectomy radiation therapy. This seminal analysis clearly demonstrated the potential negative cardiotoxic effects of radiation treatment. In a classic figure (Fig. 42.9), there is a detriment in overall survival for the irradiated patients that is clinically manifest between 10 to 15 years postrandomization. A similar finding is well illustrated in a review by Demirci et al.[116]

On the other hand, the recently published study from Darby et al.[117] notes excess radiation-associated cardiac events very soon post-RT. How do we reconcile this finding with the apparent delayed cardiac toxicity observed in the earlier studies, such as those from Cuzick et al.[114,115] This simply is an issue of competing risks. The observed impact of RT on overall survival reflects the competing improvements in breast cancer–specific mortality, and reductions in overall survival due to cardiac disease. If there are indeed early post-RT excess ≥ cardiac deaths, there must be counterbalancing reductions in breast cancer specific mortality

during the first approximate 0–10 years post-RT, accounting for the net "no change" in overall survival seen by Cuzick et al.[114,115] and others.[118,119] Therefore, there likely was an improvement in breast cancer–specific mortality in the short term that was negated by the toxic effects of the radiation (Fig. 42.10).

Data From Patients With Hodgkin Disease

A retrospective series from Stanford including 2332 patients with Hodgkin disease treated in 1960 to 1991 compared cardiac event rate with that of the general population.[120] In that series, the mean age was 29 years and treatment varied: 1183 received radiation therapy alone, and 1119 received radiation + chemotherapy. The mean follow-up was 9.5 years and there were 88 deaths attributed to heart disease. Relative risks of posttreatment death from acute myocardial infarction according to years after initial Hodgkin disease treatment are shown in Table 42.9. Note that the relative risk of cardiac events is increased within just a few years of RT.

Dosimetric Factors

The Darby study in breast cancer patients noted a 7.4% increased risk for ischemic heart disease per Gy (for mean heart dose).[117] In a series of patients with NSCLC that were treated postoperatively with external-beam radiation, the mean heart dose was 18

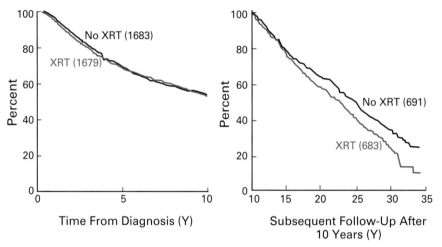

Fig. 42.9. The overall impact on overall survival is the summation of the effects on breast cancer–specific survival and for radiation-induced cardiac mortality, as shown. *XRT (Adapted from Cuzick J. Overview of adjuvant radiotherapy for breast cancer. Recent Results Cancer Res. 1989;115:220–225.)*

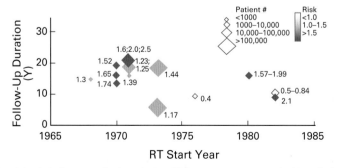

Fig. 42.10. Relative risk of cardiac mortality in patients with breast cancer treated with radiotherapy as a function of both treatment era (x-axis) and follow-up duration (y-axis). *(Reprinted with permission from Demirci S, Nam J, Hubbs JL, Nguyen T, Marks LB. Radiation-induced cardiac toxicity after therapy for breast cancer: interaction between treatment era and follow-up duration. Int J Radiat Oncol Biol Phys. 2009;73(4): 980–987.)*

Gy. As a gross estimation, the product of these two values would suggest a 133% increased risk of cardiac injury in these patients. That corresponds to a relative risk (RR) of 2.33, which is similar to the ≈3 RR reported in the study by Dautzenberg et al.[110]

In RTOG 0617, a randomized, two-by-two factorial phase 3 study, standard-dose (60 Gy) versus high-dose (74 Gy) conformal radiotherapy with concurrent and consolidation carboplatin plus paclitaxel with or without cetuximab for patients with stage IIIA or IIIB NSCLC was investigated.[137] The high-dose arm was associated with a lower overall survival rate due to (at least in part) more toxicity. Multivariate analysis revealed heart V5 as an independent prognostic factor affecting overall survival (p = 0.0035). While several heart dose–volume constraints have been suggested, additional work is needed to better understand the dose/volume/risk relationships.

Combined Modality Therapy

Hardy et al.[121] reported a SEER-based study of 34,209 patients with stages I–IV NSCLC treated from 1991 to 2002. Their data are summarized in Table 42.10 and perhaps suggest an increased risk of cardiac injury with RT and/or CT.[121]

TABLE 42.9 Relative Risks of Posttreatment Death From Acute Myocardial Infarction According to Years After Initial Hodgkin Disease Treatment[a]

Years After Initial HD Treatment	Relative Risk of Acute MI Death	95% Confidence Interval
0–4	2.0	1.1–3.3
5–9	3.6	2.2–4.5
10–14	3.0	1.6–5.2
15–19	5.0	2.6–8.7
>20	5.6	1.8–13.6

[a]Adapted from Hancock SL, Tucker MA, Hoppe RT. Factors affecting late mortality from heart disease after treatment of Hodgkin's disease. *JAMA.* 1993;270(16):1949–1955.
HD, Hodgkin disease; *MI,* myocardial infarction.

Pneumonitis Versus Cardiac Injury

Given the uncertainties in scoring radiation pneumonitis it has been suggested that some patients considered to have radiation pneumonitis might really have cardiac injury (or perhaps both).[122,123] Several authors have looked for a relationship between cardiac dosimetric parameters and radiation pneumonitis, with inconsistent findings.[124–126] Huang et al.[124] and van Luijk et al.[125] noted cardiac parameters to be associated, while Tucker et al.[126] did not. The most compelling dataset is from Washington University. In a study of 209 patients receiving definitive radiation therapy for NSCLC, the risk of radiation pneumonitis was most related to the heart D10 (minimum dose to the hottest 10% of the heart), lung D35, and maximum lung dose (Spearman Rs = 0.268, p < 0.0001).[124] Similarly, some studies,[127,128] but not all, have noted radiation pneumonitis to be more common in patients with tumors located in the inferior (versus superior) aspects of the lung.[129] Thus, the human data are unclear as to the role of cardiac irradiation in the genesis of radiation pneumonitis.

In an elegant study performed in rats using protons, the addition of cardiac irradiation to lung irradiation has been demonstrated to influence the post-RT respiratory rate.[125] While this can be interpreted to suggest that cardiac irradiation influences radiation pneumonitis, respiratory rate is a somewhat nonspecific end point.

Prevention and Management

In cases where the heart can be spared, it is recommended to limit the dose to the heart as much as possible. However, limiting the dose to the heart usually results in excess dose to other neighboring structures. In weighing the risks to the various organs, we typically follow the QUANTEC guidelines. Additional suggested dose–volume limits for the heart from other reports, listed in Table 42.11, should also be taken into consideration. Various techniques exist for achieving heart sparing in the RT of patients with lung cancer. When using 3-D conformal RT for lower lobe lung tumors, the dose to the heart can be reduced by using nonaxial beams.[130] IMRT can also be effectively used to reduce cardiac doses.[131,132] In general, in the curative setting, under-dosing the target to limit cardiac dose should be avoided since local failure is usually the greater problem.

TABLE 42.10 Cardiac Toxicity Related to Treatment for Nonsmall Cell Lung Cancer Patients 65 Years or Older[a]

	Relative Risk of Ischemic Heart Disease	Relative Risk of Cardiac Dysfunction	Relative Risk of Conduction Disorders	Relative Risk of Cardiomyopathy	Relative Risk of Heart Failure
No treatment	1	1	1	1	1
Chemotherapy only	1.2	1.6	1.02	0.82	1.3
Radiotherapy only	0.85	1.5	1.01	0.46	1.06
Chemoradiotherapy	1.1	2.4	1.4	0.49	1.2

[a]Adapted from Hardy D, Liu CC, Cormier JN, Xia R, Du XL. Cardiac toxicity in association with chemotherapy and radiation therapy in a large cohort of older patients with non-small-cell lung cancer. *Ann Oncol.* 2010;21(9):1825–1833.

TABLE 42.11 Suggested Dose–Volume Limits for the Heart

Author (Y)	Center	End Point	Suggestion for Limit
Schytte et al. (2010)[133]	Odense University Hospital, Denmark	Survival	Mean left ventricle dose <14.5 Gy
Konski et al. (2012)[134]	Fox Chase Cancer Center, USA	Symptomatic cardiac toxicity	Whole heart V20 <70% Whole heart V30 <65% Whole heart V40 <60%
Fukada et al. (2013)[135]	Keio University, Japan	Symptomatic pericardial effusion	Mean pericardial dose <36.5 Gy Pericardial V45 <58%
Wei et al. (2008)[136]	MD Anderson Cancer Center, USA	Pericarditis/Pericardial effusion	Mean pericardial dose <26 Gy Pericardial V30 <46%
Bradley et al. (2013)[137]	RTOG 1308 (tentative)		V30 ≤50%; V 45 ≤35% Max dose to 0.03 cc ≤70 Gy

RTOG, Radiation Therapy Oncology Group.

CONCLUSION

The toxicities of thoracic radiation described in this chapter can result in significant patient discomfort and reduced quality of life, especially with esophagitis. Occasionally these toxicities can result in death. The only existing and effective preventive strategy is to limit the dose–volume metrics of the organ at risk. Treatment of esophagitis and pneumonitis is essentially supportive as in most cases the toxicities are self-limiting. There is therefore a pressing need for the development of prophylactic treatments that can selectively protect normal tissues without impairing the anticancer effects of full-dose radiotherapy.

Acknowledgment

Supported in part by US NIH grant CA 69579, the Department of Defense, and the Lance Armstrong Foundation (LBM).

KEY REFERENCES

1. Abratt RP, Morgan GW. Lung toxicity following chest irradiation in patients with lung cancer. *Lung Cancer*. 2002;35(2):103–109.
13. Palma DA, Senan S, Tsujino K, et al. Predicting radiation pneumonitis after chemoradiation therapy for lung cancer: an international individual patient data meta-analysis. *Int J Radiat Oncol Biol Phys*. 2013;1;85(2):444–450.
15. Curran WJ, Paulus R, Langer CJ, et al. Sequential vs. concurrent chemoradiation for stage III non-small cell lung cancer: randomized phase III trial RTOG 9410. *J Natl Cancer Inst*. 2011;103(19):1452–1460.
21. Wang S, Liao ZX, Wei X, et al. Analysis of clinical and dosimetric factors associated with treatment related pneumonitis (TRP) in patients with non-small-cell lung cancer (NSCLC) treated with concurrent chemotherapy (CCT) and three-dimensional conformal radiotherapy (3D-CRT). *Int J Radiat Oncol Biol Phys*. 2006;66:1399–1407.
23. Graham MV, Purdy JA, Emami B, et al. Clinical dose-volume histogram analysis for pneumonitis after 3D treatment for non-small cell lung cancer (NSCLC). *Int J Radiat Oncol Biol Phys*. 1999;45(2):323–329.
25. Marks LB, Bentzen SM, Deasy JO, et al. Radiation dose-volume effects in the lung. *Int J Radiat Oncol Biol Phys*. 2010;76(suppl 3):S70–S76.
32. Tsujino K, Hirota S, Kotani Y, et al. Radiation pneumonitis following concurrent accelerated hyperfractionated radiotherapy and chemotherapy for limited-stage small-cell lung cancer: dose-volume histogram analysis and comparison with conventional chemoradiation. *Int J Radiat Oncol Biol Phys*. 2006;64(4):1100–1105.
33. Appelt AL, Vogelius IR, Farr KP, Khalil AA, Bentzen SM. Towards individualized dose constraints: adjusting the QUANTEC radiation pneumonitis model for clinical risk factors. *Acta Oncol*. 2014;53(5):605–612.
36. Vogelius IR, Bentzen SM. A literature-based meta-analysis of clinical risk factors for development of radiation induced pneumonitis. *Acta Oncol*. 2012;51(8):975–983.
43. Stenmark MH, Cai XW, Shedden K, et al. Combining physical and biologic parameters to predict radiation-induced lung toxicity in patients with non-small-cell lung cancer treated with definitive radiation therapy. *Int J Radiat Oncol Biol Phys*. 2012;84(2):e217–e222.
82. Koning C, Wouterse SJ, Daams JG, et al. Toxicity of concurrent radiochemotherapy for locally advanced non-small-cell lung cancer: a systematic review of the literature. *Clin Lung Cancer*. 2013;14(5):481–487.
93. Palma DA, Senan S, Oberije C, et al. Predicting esophagitis after chemoradiation therapy for non-small cell lung cancer: an individual patient data meta-analysis. *Int J Radiat Oncol Biol Phys*. 2013;87(4):690–696.
94. Auperin A, Le Pechoux C, Rolland E, et al. Meta-analysis of concomitant versus sequential radiochemotherapy in locally advanced non-small-cell lung cancer. *J Clin Oncol*. 2010;28:2181–2190.
96. Mauguen A, Le Péchoux C, Saunders MI, et al. Hyperfractionated or accelerated radiotherapy in lung cancer: an individual patient data meta-analysis. *J Clin Oncol*. 2012;30(22):2788–2797.
100. Darby SC, Cutter DJ, Boerma M, et al. Radiation-related heart disease: current knowledge and future prospects. *Int J Radiat Oncol Biol Phys*. 2010;76(3):656–665.
108. Gayed I, Gohar S, Liao Z, McAleer M, Bassett R, Yusuf SW. The clinical implications of myocardial perfusion abnormalities in patients with esophageal or lung cancer after chemoradiation therapy. *Int J Cardiovasc Imaging*. 2009;25(5):487–495.
121. Hardy D, Liu CC, Cormier JN, Xia R, Du XL. Cardiac toxicity in association with chemotherapy and radiation therapy in a large cohort of older patients with non-small-cell lung cancer. *Ann Oncol*. 2010;21(9):1825–1833.
137. Bradley JD, Paulus R, Komaki R, et al. Standard-dose versus high-dose conformal radiotherapy with concurrent and consolidation carboplatin plus paclitaxel with or without cetuximab for patients with stage IIIA or IIIB non-small-cell lung cancer (RTOG 0617): a randomised, two-by-two factorial phase 3 study. *Lancet Oncol*. 2015;16(2):187–199.

See Expertconsult.com for full list of references.

43 Neurotoxicity Related to Radiotherapy and Chemotherapy for Nonsmall Cell and Small Cell Lung Cancer

Thomas E. Stinchcombe and Elizabeth M. Gore

SUMMARY OF KEY POINTS

- Radiation-induced brachial plexopathy (RIBP) occurs with treatment of apical tumors and is frequently complicated by tumor-related brachial plexopathy (TRBP). Stereotactic ablative radiotherapy (SABR) of apical tumors, which employs a higher dose per fraction, can cause RIBP as well.

- RIBP symptoms include upper extremity paresthesias, motor weakness, muscle atrophy, and neuropathic pain. The peak incidence is 1–2 years, and the onset is often insidious over months to years.

- The most common side effect of radiation to the spinal cord is Lhermitte sign, which is caused by reversible demyelination of the ascending sensory neurons. Lhermitte sign is a shock-like sensation in the spine and extremities exacerbated by neck flexion, almost always symmetrical, and not associated with a dermatomal distribution. Radiation-induced Lhermitte sign begins 3 months and subsides within 6 months of the completion of radiotherapy.

- Radiation myelopathy can be devastating, and the clinical presentation depends on the level of the spinal cord affected. In general it begins with paresthesia and muscle weakness, and as the syndrome progresses gait disturbance and paraparesis appear. Radiation myelopathy is a diagnosis of exclusion, and patients must be evaluated for tumor progression and paraneoplastic syndromes with magnetic resonance imaging (MRI) of the cord.

- Assessment of the neurotoxic effects of radiation therapy can be confounded by the impact of brain metastases on neurologic function. Long-term outcome data are limited as a result of the short survival, and pretreatment and posttreatment neurologic testing has not been routine.

- Chemotherapy induced peripheral neuropathy (CIPN) is associated with taxanes (e.g., paclitaxel, docetaxel, nanoparticle albumin-bound paclitaxel), platinum agents (e.g., cisplatin and carboplatin), and vinca alkaloids (vinorelbine). Neuropathy associated with microtubule-targeting agents (vinca alkaloids and taxanes) is dependent on the length of the nerves, and patients frequently present with numbness and paresthesias of the feet and fingertips.

- The rate and severity of CIPN depends on the dose, duration and combination of chemotherapy agents used. Patients with a history of nerve damage from diabetes, alcohol use, and inherited neuropathy are at increased risk for the development of CIPN.

Chemotherapy and radiotherapy are routinely used for the treatment of nonsmall cell lung cancer (NSCLC) and small cell lung cancer (SCLC). Both types of treatment can cause acute and chronic neurotoxicities, which may affect the health-related quality of life of the patient and his or her ability to tolerate therapy. Management of the toxicities varies depending on the patient's prognosis. In the palliative setting, acute toxicities may result in dose reduction, treatment delay, or treatment discontinuation, thus offsetting the potential benefits of palliative treatment. In the potentially curative setting, chronic treatment-related toxicities may be more clinically relevant. Unfortunately, the assessment of acute neurotoxicities has been variable, and the prospective collection of data on chronic neurotoxicities has been limited. Selected neurotoxicities are addressed in the National Cancer Institute (NCI) Common Terminology Criteria for Adverse Events (CTCAE) version 4.0 (Table 43.1);[1] however, many of these toxicities are based on physician assessment, and the determination of a grade 2 or grade 3 toxicity can be patient- and/or physician-dependent. When neurotoxicities do develop, management is often based on the patient's symptoms. Current research is investigating methods of identifying patients who are at increased risk for neurotoxicity, as well as prevention strategies and improved treatment options.

NEUROTOXICITY FROM RADIOTHERAPY

Neurotoxic effects of radiotherapy for lung cancer, predominantly to the brachial plexus, spinal cord, and brain, are important in the curative and palliative setting. Understanding the neurotoxic effects of radiotherapy is increasingly important, as patients with lung cancer are living longer and radiotherapy techniques are evolving. Intensity-modulated radiotherapy (IMRT) and image-guided radiotherapy (IGRT) allow for delivery of increasing total doses of radiation to the tumor while potentially resulting in a high total dose of radiation to small volumes of normal tissues and inhomogeneous doses across large volumes. SABR is a special consideration because it can potentially result in a very high dose per fraction to small volumes of the lung. As patients are living longer with more aggressive local treatment and more effective systemic therapy, the effects of late toxicity are more likely. It is imperative that current and future studies and clinical practice include long-term follow-up with appropriate documentation of dose, grading, and resulting toxicity.

Brachial Plexus

Data regarding RIBP in patients with lung cancer are limited because of the perceived lack of clinical significance. High-dose radiation to the brachial plexus is limited to cases of apical tumors and is frequently complicated by TRBP. However, RIBP may increase in incidence because of improved therapy for advanced lung cancer and treatment of earlier-stage lung cancer, with SABR resulting in longer survival. The risk of RIBP is associated with increased radiation dose and higher dose per fraction,

TABLE 43.1 National Cancer Institute Common Terminology Criteria for Adverse Events Version 4.0, Grades 1–4

Adverse Event	Grade 1	Grade 2	Grade 3	Grade 4
Brachial plexopathy	Asymptomatic; clinical or diagnostic observations only; intervention not indicated	Moderate symptoms, limiting instrumental ADL	Severe symptoms; limiting self-care ADL	NA
Cognitive disturbance	Mild cognitive disability; not interfering with work, school, life performance; specialized educational services, devices not indicated	Moderate cognitive disability; interfering with work, school, life performance but capable of independent living; specialized resources on part-time basis indicated	Severe cognitive disability; significant impairment of work, school, life performance	NA
Concentration impairment	Mild inattention or decreased level of concentration	Moderate impairment in attention or decreased level of concentration; limiting instrumental ADL	Severe impairment in attention or decreased level of concentration; limiting self-care ADL	NA
Memory impairment	Mild memory impairment	Moderate memory impairment; limiting instrumental ADL	Severe memory impairment; limiting self-care ADL	NA
Neuralgia	Mild pain	Moderate pain; limiting instrumental ADL	Severe pain; limiting self-care	NA
Paresthesia	Mild symptoms	Moderate symptoms; limiting instrumental ADL	Severe symptoms; limiting self-ADL	NA
Peripheral motor neuropathy	Asymptomatic; clinical or diagnostic observations only; intervention not indicated	Moderate symptoms; limiting instrumental ADL	Severe symptoms; limiting self-care ADL; assistive device indicated	Life-threatening consequences; urgent intervention indicated
Peripheral sensory neuropathy	Asymptomatic; loss of deep tendon reflexes or paresthesia	Asymptomatic; loss of deep tendon reflexes or paresthesia	Severe symptoms; limiting self-care ADL	Life-threatening consequences; urgent intervention indicated

ADL, activities of daily living; *NA,* not applicable.

as well as with the volume of the brachial plexus treated and the concomitant use of chemotherapy.[2] Appropriate radiation dose to the brachial plexus and acceptable risk of RIBP varies depending on the stage of disease and intent of therapy. In many cases, avoiding high radiation dose to the brachial plexus results in undertreating the tumor. When disease is potentially curable or long-term survival is anticipated, the high risk of RIBP may be unavoidable and an understanding of the risks is important for counseling patients.

The diagnosis of RIBP is often complicated by tumor involvement, surgery, and/or unrelated trauma or injury. Symptoms include upper extremity paresthesias, motor weakness, muscle atrophy, and neuropathic pain. The latency period for the onset of symptoms can be a few months to as many as 20 years; the peak incidence is around 1 to 2 years.[3–5] The onset of RIBP is often insidious, occurring over 6 months to as long as 5 years and progressing in intensity, eventually resulting in paralysis of the upper extremity.[3] RIBP is almost always chronic and progressive, although there are rare reports of early transient RIBP. Symptoms reported and attributed to early transient RIBP include pain, paresthesias, and weakness occurring in 2 to 14 months following therapy with regression and often complete resolution of symptoms.[6] MRI and/or computed tomography (CT) are important diagnostic tools to rule out progressive or metastatic disease. Electromyography can be used to support a diagnosis of RIBP.[7]

Most information regarding the effects of radiation on the brachial plexus is from the literature on breast cancer. The brachial plexus is at least partially treated in almost all cases of breast or chest wall radiotherapy and is frequently involved in regions of matching fields, leading to high doses as a result of unintended field overlap. In addition, patients who receive radiotherapy for breast cancer tend to have relatively long follow-up, increasing the likelihood that late reactions will manifest. Over the past 50 years, different radiation techniques have been used to treat breast cancer, resulting in varying incidences of RIBP. In the 1950s and 1960s, RIBP was diagnosed in more than 50% of patients treated with 50 Gy to 60 Gy at 5 Gy per fraction; currently, RIBP develops in less than 1% to 2% of patients treated with less than 55 Gy at 1.8 Gy to 2 Gy per fraction.[8]

RIBP in patients with head and neck cancer is an increasing area of interest because of the use of IMRT for treatment of the disease. In an attempt to restrict radiation dose to organs at risk while maximizing dose to treatment target volumes with the use of IMRT, there is a relatively inhomogeneous dose distribution, and the implications may not be completely understood. If organs at risk are not appropriately contoured, these hot spots could be inadvertently in a high-risk area. Proper anatomic definition of the brachial plexus is necessary for understanding potential side effects and complying with dose–volume constraints. The development of a brachial plexus contouring atlas by the Radiation Therapy Oncology Group (RTOG) has facilitated and encouraged the consistent and routine evaluation and reporting of radiation effects to the brachial plexus in the treatment of head and neck cancers. RTOG guidelines recommend a maximum dose of 60 Gy to 66 Gy or less to the brachial plexus. Truong et al.[9] retrospectively contoured and reviewed doses to the brachial plexus in 114 patients treated with IMRT for head and neck cancer with 69.3 Gy in 33 fractions. There were no reports of RIBP, despite a maximum dose of more than 66 Gy to the brachial plexus in 20% of patients, with a median follow-up of 16.2 months. Longer follow-up is needed to assess the true incidence of RIBP in patients with head and neck cancer. Chen et al.[10] prospectively evaluated the incidence of clinically significant peripheral neuropathies in patients undergoing radiotherapy for head and neck malignancies and reported an incidence of 12% for all patients and 22% for patients who were followed for more than 5 years. The investigators also suggested that RIBP symptoms in patients with head and neck cancer are underreported. Their data suggested a threshold dose of more than 70 Gy to the brachial plexus, although RIBP was also reported in some patients treated with doses less than 60 Gy, suggesting other contributing factors. Prior neck dissection and higher maximum dose of radiotherapy were associated with an increased risk of RIBP.[10]

Eblan et al.[2] evaluated RIBP in 80 patients treated to 50 Gy or more of conventionally fractionated radiotherapy for apical NSCLC; the median follow-up was 17.2 months. RIBP developed in five patients, which was more common among patients who had prior TRBP. The 3-year competing risk-adjusted rate of RIBP was 12%, whereas the 3-year estimated rate of TRBP as a

CHAPTER 43 Neurotoxicity Related to Radiotherapy and Chemotherapy for Nonsmall Cell and Small Cell Lung Cancer **411**

43

result of treatment failure was 13%. The median onset of TRBP was 4 months compared with 11 months for RIBP, and symptom severity was greater for patients in whom TRBP developed. RIBP did not develop in any of the patients who received less than a maximum dose of 78 Gy to the brachial plexus, and for patients in whom RIBP did develop, considerable volumes were irradiated to doses above 66 Gy.[2] Amini et al.[11] identified 90 patients treated with definitive radiotherapy and concurrent chemotherapy and more than 55 Gy to the brachial plexus. The median dose to the brachial plexus was 70 Gy and the median follow-up was only 14 months; grade 1 to grade 3 RIBP developed in 16% of patients. The median time to symptoms was 6.5 months. Independent predictors of RIBP were a median dose to the brachial plexus of more than 69 Gy, a maximum dose of more than 75 Gy to 2 cm,[3] and the presence of plexopathy before radiation.

The brachial plexus receives a considerably higher dose per fraction with SABR and therefore is susceptible to greater risk of late complications. Maximum dose of SABR, as well as dose–volume tolerance and clinical presentation with high dose per fraction, is uncertain. Forquer et al.[12] evaluated the risk of brachial plexopathy in 37 lesions treated with SABR for apical lung tumors; RIBP developed in 7 of 37 patients treated.[12] Five patients had neuropathic pain alone, one patient had pain and weakness, and one patient had pain, numbness, and paralysis of the hand and wrist. At a median follow-up of 7 months, the absolute risk of RIBP was 32% with a dose to the brachial plexus of more than 26 Gy and 6% with a maximum dose of 26 Gy or less in three to four fractions. The median time to development of RIBP was 13 months. In contrast to RIBP reported in other series, symptoms improved in six of seven patients over 3 to 10 months, including improvement of neuropathic pain. One patient who had received a maximum dose of 76 Gy to the brachial plexus had onset of pain and tingling at 9 months of follow-up, with progression to muscle wasting and weakness at 42 months.

Consistent contouring and dose–volume analyses in symptom reporting in the literature will continue to improve the clinical understanding of radiation tolerance of the brachial plexus. Currently, for apical lung tumors adjacent to or contiguous with the brachial plexus, restricting the dose to the brachial plexus may not be possible without compromising tumor control. A better understanding of dose–volume constraints and symptoms will assist in determining the risk of RIBP and proper patient counseling.

Spinal Cord

Radiation myelitis is a rare complication of radiotherapy for lung cancer because, in most cases, the spinal cord can be avoided without compromising disease coverage. This avoidance is particularly true for lung cancer in an era of smaller treatment fields directed at gross disease, three-dimensional conformal radiotherapy planning, IMRT, and IGRT. IMRT plans can shape the high-dose lines around the cord, and with IGRT, high doses adjacent to the spinal cord can be delivered with relative confidence that the set-up is reproducible and accurate.

The most common side effect of radiation to the spinal cord is Lhermitte sign, which is caused by reversible demyelination of the ascending sensory neurons as a result of inhibition of oligodendrocyte proliferation.[13] Lhermitte sign was first described in relation to injury to the cervical spinal cord; is associated with other demyelinating disorders, including multiple sclerosis; and can be induced by radiotherapy or chemotherapy.[14–16] Lhermitte sign is a shock-like sensation in the spine and extremities exacerbated by neck flexion; it is almost always symmetrical, is not associated with a finite dermatomal distribution, and is transient, subsiding with oligodendrocyte recovery and remyelination. Radiation-induced Lhermitte sign begins at about 3 months and subsides within 6 months of the completion of

radiotherapy. The incidence of Lhermitte sign is reported to be between 3.6% and 13% in large patient groups receiving radiotherapy for head and neck and thoracic malignancies. Risk factors associated with the development of Lhermitte sign are total radiation doses above 50 Gy to the cervical spinal cord and daily radiation fraction doses above 2 Gy.[14] Pak et al.[13] found a relatively high incidence of Lhermitte sign (21%) with IMRT for head and neck cancer and concurrent chemotherapy. The strongest predictors of Lhermitte sign were higher percentage and cord volumes receiving 40 Gy or more. The investigators suggested that the higher incidence of Lhermitte sign in their series might have been related to higher reporting in a prospective setting and the chemotherapeutic agents. Lhermitte sign appearing in the context of transient radiation myelopathy is not associated with chronic progressive myelitis; however, delayed radiation myelopathy, which is irreversible and results in paralysis, may be preceded by Lhermitte sign.[16] Lhermitte sign that predates delayed radiation myelopathy is found later in onset than the usual latency period of Lhermitte sign found in transient radiation myelopathy.

Because delayed radiation myelopathy can be a devastating side effect, radiation oncologists take every precaution to avoid it. Although glial cells and vascular endothelium are proposed to be the main targets for radiation and play a role in the pathogenesis of radiation myelopathy, experimental data support that radiation-induced vascular damage resulting in vascular hyperpermeability and venous exudation is a basic process.[17] The clinical presentation of radiation myelopathy depends on the area of the affected spinal cord and the extent of the lesion. Generally, paresthesia and muscle weakness, which begins in the legs, are the main early symptoms. As the lesion progresses, various symptoms present, such as gait disturbance and paraparesis.[17] Schultheiss and Stephens[18] emphasized that radiation myelopathy is a diagnosis of exclusion, and patients should be evaluated for tumor progression and paraneoplasia. In almost all cases of radiation myelopathy, the latency period is longer than 6 months, and MRI may show tumor swelling or atrophy, and the level of protein in cerebrospinal fluid may be slightly elevated, with lymphocytes present.[18] Radiation myelopathy is irreversible, although some interventions, including corticosteroids, heparin or warfarin, and hyperbaric oxygen, have been suggested to have benefit.[19]

The maximum dose considered safe for spinal cord tolerance and for the prevention of delayed radiation myelopathy is 45 Gy to 50 Gy delivered with conventional fractionation (1.8–2 Gy daily). Schultheiss[20] combined reported data from the literature to establish the parameters of the dose–response function for clinical radiation myelopathy. He used data from 18 reported series that included the number of patients treated with a consistent dose regimen, dose, number of fractions, number of myelopathy cases resulting from the dose regimen, and information about the survival experience of patients at risk. At a 45-Gy dose, the probability of myelopathy is 0.03%; at 50 Gy, the probability is 0.2%. The dose for a 5% myelopathy rate is 59.3 Gy. Quantitative Analyses of Normal Tissue Effects in the Clinic (QUANTEC) analysis demonstrated that, when conventional fractionation of 1.8–2 Gy/fraction is delivered to the full-thickness cord, the estimated risk of myelopathy is less than 1% at 54 Gy and less than 10% at 61 Gy.[21]

Data are limited regarding the risk of radiation myelopathy and repeat radiation to the spinal cord. Data on repeat radiation in animals and humans suggest partial repair of radiotherapy-induced subclinical damage becoming evident about 6 months after radiotherapy and improving over the next 2 years. Follow-up data for spinal cord injury after repeat radiation for recurrent disease is limited and few cases of radiation myelopathy are reported. In general, attempts should be made to avoid the spinal cord if repeat treatment is indicated.

The understanding of spinal cord tolerance with SABR is evolving. The acceptable maximum dose is dependent on dose per fraction. Gibs et al.[22] reported six cases of radiation myelopathy among 1075 patients treated for benign and malignant spinal cord tumors. They recommended limiting the volume of spinal cord treated above an 8-Gy equivalent dose in one fraction. Delayed radiation myelopathy developed at a mean of 6.2 months (range, 2 to 9 months). Saghal et al.[23] evaluated five cases of radiation myelopathy following spine SABR and compared dosimetric data with those in a larger series of patients treated with spine SABR in which no radiation myelopathy occurred. The investigators concluded that the maximum point dose to the thecal sac should be respected for spine SABR. For single-fraction SABR, 10 Gy to a maximum point is safe, and up to five fractions and biologic estimated dose of 30 Gy to 35 Gy secondary to the thecal sac also poses a low risk of radiation myelopathy.[23] This finding was supported by data reported by Macbeth et al.,[24] showing no radiation myelopathy at 10 Gy in a single fraction. Based on extensive literature review, QUANTEC for spine radiosurgery demonstrated that a maximum cord dose of 13 Gy in a single fraction or 20 Gy in three fractions appeared to be associated with a less than 1% risk of injury.[21]

Brain

Neurotoxic effects of radiation to the brain are variably assessed in the setting of lung cancer. Data are available, primarily in the absence of controls, for patients with inoperable brain metastases treated palliatively with whole-brain radiation therapy (WBRT), local therapy with surgery or stereotactic radiosurgery for patients treated with and without WBRT, and with prophylactic cranial radiation for either SCLC or NSCLC. The neurotoxic effects of radiation therapy to the brain are difficult to assess because of several factors: most patients with lung cancer who are treated with WBRT have neurologic deficits from brain metastases, long-term follow-up is limited as a result of short survival, and neurologic testing has not been routine.

Series that evaluated neurotoxic effects of radiation for brain metastases have consistently shown that the risk of neurocognitive deficits as a result of WBRT is outweighed by the benefits of treatment. In 1989, De Angelis et al.[25] evaluated 12 patients with neurologic complications attributed to WBRT for brain metastases and reported an incidence of 1.9% to 5.1% for WBRT-induced dementia. All 12 patients, who were treated with total doses of 25 Gy to 39 Gy at 3 Gy to 6 Gy per fraction, had cortical atrophy and hypodense white matter on CT images. The authors concluded that more protracted schedules should be used for the safe and efficacious treatment of good-risk patients with brain metastases.

In RTOG 91-04, a phase III trial designed to assess overall survival of patients with unresectable brain metastases treated with 54.4 Gy/1.6 Gy twice daily or 30 Gy/3 Gy once daily, no difference in overall survival was found between radiation doses; the median survival in both arms was only 4.5 months.[26] A secondary analysis of this study was conducted to evaluate the importance of a Mini-Mental Status Exam (MMSE) before treatment on long-term survival and neurologic function of patients treated with 30 Gy/3 Gy once daily. Both pretreatment MMSE ($p = 0.0002$) and Karnofsky performance status ($p = 0.02$) were significant factors for survival. WBRT appeared to be associated with an improvement in MMSE score and a lack of decline to below 23 on the MMSE in long-term survivors.[27] Additional analysis of both arms of this trial showed that the use of 30 Gy/3 Gy once daily as compared with 54.4 Gy/1.6 Gy twice daily was not associated with a significant difference in neurocognitive function as measured by MMSE. Control of brain metastases had a noticeable effect on the MMSE score.[28]

Neurocognitive function with a neuropsychometric battery before and after WBRT (30 Gy/3 Gy once daily) was assessed prospectively in a phase III trial of WBRT with or without motexafin gadolinium.[29] Impairment was found in more than 90% of patients at baseline, and the results suggested that only tumor control correlated with neurocognitive function.[30] Li et al.[31] evaluated 135 of 208 patients in the control arm of the study who were available for evaluation at 2 months.[31] The authors found that WBRT-induced tumor shrinkage correlated with better survival and preservation of neurocognitive function. Neurocognitive function was stable or improved in long-term survivors, and tumor progression adversely affected neurocognitive function more than WBRT.

Studies in which patients treated with and without WBRT after local therapy for a limited number of brain metastases are evaluated have also routinely included assessment of neurotoxic effects. This setting provides an opportunity to review neurocognitive effects of radiotherapy in a patient population with a relatively good performance status and less extensive systemic disease. In general, these studies have shown that WBRT can be delivered safely without substantial changes in neurocognitive function and that it improves local control but not overall survival. Chang et al.[32] conducted a phase III trial comparing stereotactic radiosurgery with and without WBRT for patients with one to three brain metastases, with the primary end point being a change in neurocognitive function at 4 months as measured by the Hopkins Verbal Learning Test (HVLT). The investigators found that patients treated with stereotactic surgery plus WBRT had noticeable impairment in learning and memory function by HVLT compared with the patients who were treated with stereotactic radiosurgery alone. This study, however, has been controversial because of unexpected survival differences favoring the stereotactic radiosurgery arm and for the timing of the neurocognitive assessment to one time point.

The European Organisation for Research and Treatment of Cancer (EORTC) conducted a phase III trial assessing whether adjuvant WBRT (30 Gy/3 Gy once daily) increases the duration of functional independence after surgery or stereotactic radiosurgery for brain metastases.[33] Adjuvant WBRT reduced intracranial relapses (surgery: 59% to 27%, $p = 0.001$; stereotactic radiosurgery: 31% to 19%; $p = 0.040$) and neurologic deaths. WBRT did not affect the rate of decline in performance status. The median time to World Health Organization performance status higher than 2 was 10.0 months after observation and 9.5 months after WBRT ($p = 0.71$).

Aoyama et al.[34] prospectively evaluated WBRT after local therapy for brain metastases and did not find a difference in survival or in neurocognitive function. Intracranial relapse occurred considerably more frequently among patients who did not receive WBRT and, consequently, as demonstrated in other studies, salvage treatment was frequently needed when upfront WBRT was not used. Neurocognitive function was scored 0 to 4 based on the degree of functional impairment and level of assistance required. Neurocognitive function assessment using the MMSE was optional. MMSE data for at least one time point were available for 28 of 44 patients who lived 12 months or longer (16 patients in the WBRT plus stereotactic radiosurgery group and 12 in the stereotactic radiosurgery-alone group) at a median follow-up of 30.5 months (range, 13.7 to 58.7 months). The median MMSE scores before and after treatment were 28 and 27, respectively, in the WBRT plus stereotactic radiosurgery group and 27 and 28 in the stereotactic radiosurgery-alone group. The investigators also evaluated MRI for leukoencephalopathy, and radiographic findings consistent with leukoencephalopathy were found in seven patients in the WBRT plus stereotactic radiosurgery group and in two patients in the stereotactic radiosurgery-alone group ($p = 0.09$). Three of these

CHAPTER 43 Neurotoxicity Related to Radiotherapy and Chemotherapy for Nonsmall Cell and Small Cell Lung Cancer **413**

43

nine patients also had symptomatic leukoencephalopathy; the other six patients were asymptomatic.

Prophylactic Cranial Radiation

Prophylactic cranial radiation is a superior setting to assess the effects of radiotherapy on the whole brain, although it comes with some challenges. Even with the use of prophylactic cranial radiation, survival is limited for patients with lung cancer, routine use of neuropsychologic testing in this patient population is limited, and frequently, patients have baseline neuropsychologic deficits before prophylactic cranial radiation, partially as a result of prior chemotherapy and possibly also because of paraneoplastic effects from the underlying malignant process.

Historically, high rates of toxicity with prophylactic cranial radiation were reported when it was given concurrently with chemotherapy or when it was given at high dose per fraction to patients with SCLC.[35] After low-dose concurrent chemotherapy and prophylactic cranial radiation, 44% of patients with SCLC had abnormal neuropsychologic tests at a median follow-up of 6.2 years.[35] Unexpected neurocognitive deficits have been detected in patients with SCLC after combination chemotherapy, with no noticeable change in those deficits after prophylactic cranial radiation.[36] The authors suggest that neuropsychologic abnormalities associated with SCLC may be secondary to the disease itself (paraneoplasia) and systemic therapy.

Le Péchoux et al.[37] published the results of an international phase III study (PCI99-01, EORTC 22003-08004, RTOG 0212, and IFCT 99-01) comparing 25-Gy and 36-Gy prophylactic cranial radiation for patients with limited-disease SCLC.[37] Over 3 years, the authors found no significant difference between the two groups in any of the 17 selected items assessing quality of life and neurologic and cognitive functions. However, in both groups, there was mild deterioration in communication, memory, intellectual capacity, and leg strength ($p < 0.005$ for all).

RTOG 0212 was a randomized phase II trial designed to evaluate the incidence of chronic neurotoxicity and changes in quality of life among patients who received prophylactic cranial radiation for limited-disease SCLC; some patients from this study were also involved in the international phase III prophylactic cranial radiation trial. Patients in RTOG 0212 were treated to 25 Gy/2.5 Gy once daily, 36 Gy/2 Gy once daily, or 36 Gy/1.2 Gy twice daily. There were no significant baseline differences among the treatment groups in terms of quality-of-life measures, and one of the neuropsychologic tests, namely the HVLT. However, at 12 months after prophylactic cranial radiation, there was a significant increase in the occurrence of chronic neurotoxity in the 36-Gy cohort ($p = 0.02$). According to logistic regression analysis, increasing age was found to be the most significant predictor of chronic neurotoxicity ($p = 0.005$).

RTOG 0214 evaluated the use of prophylactic cranial radiation for patients with locally advanced NSCLC. Prophylactic cranial radiation was shown to considerably decrease the risk of brain metastasis from 18% to 7.7% at 1 year. However, there was no significant difference in overall survival or disease-free survival.[38] A secondary end point of this study was to evaluate the neuropsychologic impact of prophylactic cranial radiation. There were no significant differences at 1 year between the two arms in any component of the EORTC Quality of Life Questionnaire (EORTC-QLQ) C30 or EORTC-QLQ BN20 studies, although a trend for greater decline in patient-reported cognitive functioning was noted with prophylactic cranial radiation. There were no significant differences in MMSE score or activities of daily living. However, for HVLT, there was a significantly greater decline in immediate recall ($p = 0.03$) and delayed recall ($p = 0.008$) in the prophylactic cranial radiation arm at 1 year.

Gondi et al.[39] reported a pooled secondary analysis of tested and self-reported cognitive functioning of patients treated with prophylactic cranial radiation in RTOG 0212 and RTOG 0214.[39] Among patients with lung cancer in whom brain relapse did not develop, prophylactic cranial radiation was associated with decline in HVLT-tested and self-reported cognitive functioning; however, decline in HVLT and self-reported cognitive functioning were not closely correlated, suggesting that they may represent distinct elements of the cognitive spectrum.

Radiographic Imaging Studies

WBRT is one of the most effective modalities for the treatment and prevention of brain metastases, although it can result in neurocognitive deficits. WBRT is associated with the development of delayed white matter abnormalities or leukoencephalopathy and has been correlated with cognitive dysfunction. The effects of WBRT have been studied in the setting of treatment for intracranial disease and prophylactic cranial irradiation. Prophylactic cranial irradiation is ideal for studying the effect of WBRT, as patients do not have baseline neurologic effects from metastatic or primary tumors in the brain.

Stuschke et al.[40] studied neuropsychologic function and MRI of the brain in patients with locally advanced NSCLC after prophylactic cranial radiation. T2-weighted MR images demonstrated white matter abnormalities of higher grade in patients who received prophylactic cranial radiation than in those patients who did not. Two of nine patients treated with prophylactic cranial radiation and none of four patients not treated with prophylactic cranial radiation had grade 4 white matter abnormalities. A trend toward impaired neuropsychologic functioning was also found in patients with white matter abnormalities of higher degree. Impairments in attention and visual memory in long-term survivors were found among patients in both prophylactic cranial radiation and nonprophylactic cranial radiation groups.

In prophylactic cranial radiation studies, MR images have not been prospectively evaluated before and after therapy for radiation effects and correlation with clinical toxicity. Johnson et al.[35] evaluated CT and MR images of patients 6 to 13 years after receiving prophylactic cranial radiation for SCLC. Findings on CT were abnormal (i.e., demonstrated ventricular dilation, cerebral atrophy, and/or cerebral calcification) in 12 of 15 patients, and white matter abnormalities were present on MR images for seven of 15 patients. Anatomic abnormalities documented by CT and MRI were more frequent among patients with abnormal neuropsychologic function.

Little is known about the factors that predispose patients to white matter changes that occur with WBRT. Sabsevitz et al.[41] used MRI volumetrics to prospectively evaluate the effect of white matter health before treatment on the development of white matter changes after WBRT. Age at the time of treatment and volume of abnormal fluid-attenuated inversion recovery before treatment were significantly associated with white matter changes following WBRT; however, pretreatment fluid-attenuated inversion recovery volume was the strongest predictor of white matter changes after treatment. No significant relationships were found between dose of WBRT, total glucose, blood pressure, or body mass index and development of white matter changes. Szerlip et al.[42] retrospectively reviewed serial MR images and measured volumetric white matter changes over time for patients treated with WBRT and who survived more than 1 year. Following WBRT, white matter changes accumulated at an average rate of 0.07% of total brain volume per month. On multivariate analysis, greater rates of accumulation were associated with older age, poor levels of glycemic control, and the diagnosis of hypertension.

Routine use of MRI before and after therapy and correlation with neuropsychologic assessment are necessary to better understand the neurotoxic effects of brain radiation. Additionally, factors predicting neurologic change or faster rate of neurologic change are important to understand. Paying careful attention to mitigating risk, such as through control of hyperglycemia or hypertension or possibly avoiding or delaying WBRT for patients at high risk of complications, is vital for individualizing care.

PREVENTION OF NEUROCOGNITIVE COMPLICATIONS

Recent clinical efforts to minimize toxicity of radiotherapy have focused on modifying radiotherapy techniques and using neuroprotectants. Memantine is a clinically useful drug for many neurologic disorders, including Alzheimer disease. The principal mechanism of action of memantine is believed to be the blockade of current flow through channels of N-methyl-D-aspartate receptors. Memantine has been associated with a moderate decrease in clinical deterioration of cognition, mood, behavior, and the ability to perform daily activities in patients with Alzheimer disease. In RTOG 0614, a trial that studied the neuroprotective effects of memantine in patients treated with palliative WBRT,[43] memantine was found to be well tolerated, with a toxicity profile very similar to placebo. Overall, patients treated with memantine had better cognitive function over time; specifically, memantine delayed time to cognitive decline and reduced the rate of decline in memory, executive function, and processing speed of patients who received WBRT. The primary end point was delayed recall at 24 weeks; although less decline of delayed recall was found with the use of memantine, this decline lacked significance, possibly due to substantial patient loss. Follow up in this patient population is challenging secondary to death and noncompliance related to disease progression.

According to emerging evidence, the pathogenesis of radiation-induced neurocognitive function deficit may involve radiation-induced injury to proliferating neuronal progenitor cells in the subgranular zone of the hippocampi.[44] IMRT allows for sparing of the hippocampus while otherwise treating the whole brain with radiation therapy. In RTOG 0933, a single-arm phase II study, hippocampal avoidance WBRT for brain metastases with a primary cognitive end point was evaluated in comparison to a historic control of WBRT without hippocampal avoidance (RTOG 9801).[45] Conformal avoidance of the hippocampus during WBRT was associated with memory preservation at 4 and 6 months of follow-up. These phase II results compared favorably with those in historic series.[39]

Chemotherapy-Induced Peripheral Neuropathy

Agents commonly used in the treatment of NSCLC and SCLC that are associated with CIPN include the taxanes, (e.g., paclitaxel, docetaxel, nanoparticle albumin-bound paclitaxel [nabpaclitaxel]), platinum agents (e.g., cisplatin and carboplatin), and vinca alkaloids (e.g., vincristine, vinorelbine, vinblastine). The mechanism, incidence, and symptoms of CIPN vary with the class of agent. Neuropathy induced by microtubule-targeting agents (e.g., vinca alkaloids and taxanes) is dependent on the length of the nerves, and patients frequently present with symptoms in their fingertips and feet. The vinca alkaloids can cause autonomic neuropathy as well as peripheral neuropathy, symptoms of which can present as abdominal cramping, ileus and constipation, and, rarely, cranial nerve neuropathies.[46] Cisplatin-related sensory neuropathy usually becomes clinically detectable after a cumulative dose of 300 mg/m², carboplatin has a lower rate of neurotoxicity than does cisplatin.[47] Oxaliplatin is associated with cold dysesthesias, paresthesias, and CIPN, but is not a standard agent used in the treatment of NSCLC or SCLC.

The rate and severity of CIPN depends on the dose, duration, and combination of agents used. Patients with a history of nerve damage from diabetes, alcohol-use, or an inherited neuropathy are at increased risk for the development of CIPN, and symptomatic neuropathy may develop with lower doses or earlier in treatment.[46] Initial symptoms of CIPN are often symmetric sensory and motor impairment of the extremities causing tingling (paresthesias) or numbness (hypoesthesia) of the fingertips or feet. The loss of proprioception may cause unsteady gait, ataxia, or a tendency to fall. Other common symptoms are pain or motor neuropathy resulting in muscle weakness. In general, NCI-CTCAE grade 2 or grade 3 sensory neuropathy is thought to be clinically significant and requires an intervention such as dose delay and/or reduction or, potentially, discontinuation of the offending agent. Physicians often underestimate the frequency and severity of symptoms, and so patient-reported outcomes may be a more accurate assessment of the frequency and severity of this toxicity.[48,49]

Chemotherapy Treatments Associated With CIPN

The selection of chemotherapy combinations is frequently influenced by patients' preexisting conditions and their risk for the development of CIPN. Patients with a preexisting neuropathy or with conditions that predispose them to CIPN often will receive a chemotherapy combination that is associated with a lower rate of CIPN (e.g., a platinum agent and pemetrexed or a platinum agent and gemcitabine). Cisplatin or carboplatin and paclitaxel, docetaxel, vinorelbine, and nab-paclitaxel are used in the treatment of NSCLC, and all are associated with CIPN. The combination of cisplatin and vincristine is a standard combination for adjuvant therapy and for metastatic disease. Two different schedules of cisplatin and vinorelbine have been investigated in phase III trials of adjuvant therapy, and the rate of CIPN was evaluated with the use of these agents (Table 43.2).[50,51] The rate of all-grade constipation and grade 3 constipation—a symptom of autonomic neuropathy—found in these trials was approximately 45% and 5%, respectively. Given the significant improvement in overall survival and long-term survival in the adjuvant setting, the rate of neurotoxicities is acceptable, but diligent surveillance and symptom management are required. In a three-arm phase III trial, docetaxel plus cisplatin and docetaxel plus carboplatin were compared with vinorelbine plus cisplatin for advanced-stage NSCLC,[52] and patients could receive a maximum of six cycles. The rate of grade 3 or grade 4 sensory neuropathy was numerically lower in the docetaxel plus carboplatin arm (Table 43.2). These trials provide an estimate of the rate of CIPN with commonly used chemotherapy combinations.

The relationship between CIPN and single-agent paclitaxel and the combination of carboplatin and paclitaxel has been extensively studied in clinical trials. In a prospective study of patients receiving weekly paclitaxel (70–90 mg/m²) who completed the EORTC-CIPN instrument, 20% of patients had a clinically significant pain score with the first dose of paclitaxel.[53] The rate of chronic neuropathy was higher among patients with higher paclitaxel-acute pain syndrome pain scores with the first dose of paclitaxel.[53] Common symptoms of paclitaxel-acute pain syndrome include a diffuse aching of the legs, hips, and lower back 1 to 3 days after the paclitaxel administration. Numbness and tingling were more prominent chronic neuropathic symptoms than shooting or burning pain. Longer duration of treatment with carboplatin and paclitaxel has been associated with a higher rate of CIPN. A phase III trial of carboplatin and paclitaxel every 3 weeks for four cycles compared with carboplatin and paclitaxel until disease progression or unacceptable toxicity revealed similar efficacy.[54] However, the rate of grade 2 to grade 4 sensory neuropathy increased from 19.9% (95% CI, 13.6–26.2%) at cycle 4 to 43% (95% CI, 28.6–57.4%) at cycle 8. An association between cumulative paclitaxel dose and development of sensory neuropathy has been demonstrated in other studies as well.[55] In a phase III trial that compared cisplatin and paclitaxel every 3 weeks to carboplatin and paclitaxel every 3 weeks, patients continued therapy until disease progression or a maximum of 10 cycles.[56] Rates for all-grade and grade 3 peripheral neuropathy were similar for the two combinations.

TABLE 43.2 Rate of Chemotherapy-Induced Neuropathy Reported in Phase III Trials of Platinum Agent Doublets

Author	Chemotherapy	No. of Patients	Rate of Sensory Neuropathy (all grades) (%)	Rate of Grade 3 or 4 Sensory Neuropathy (%)
Winton et al.[50]	Cisplatin 50 mg/m^2 days 1 and 8 every 28 days Vinorelbine 25 mg/m^2 weekly for 16 weeks	242[b]	48	2[a]
Douillard et al.[51]	Cisplatin 100 mg/m^2 day 1 Vinorelbine 30 mg/m^2 days 1, 8, & 15 (cycle: every 28 days)	367[b]	28	3
Fossella et al.[52]	Cisplatin 75 mg/m^2 & docetaxel 75 mg/m^2 every 21 days	1218	NR	3.8
	Carboplatin AUC of 6 & docetaxel 75 mg/m^2 every 21 days		NR	3.9
	Cisplatin 100 mg/m^2 day 1 every 28 days & vinorelbine 25 mg/m^2 weekly		NR	0.7
Rosell et al.[56]	Cisplatin 80 mg/m^2 & paclitaxel 200 mg/m^2 every 21 days	618	58	9
	Carboplatin AUC of 6 & paclitaxel 200 mg/m^2 every 21 days		59	8
Bonomi et al.[58c]	Cisplatin 75 mg/m^2 & paclitaxel 135 mg/m^2 every 21 days	399	NR	23
	Cisplatin 75 mg/m^2 & paclitaxel 250 mg/m^2 every 21 days		NR	40
Belani et al.[59]	Carboplatin AUC of 6 & paclitaxel 225 mg/m^2 every 3 days	440	NR	18[d]
	Carboplatin AUC of 6 on day 1 & paclitaxel 100 mg/m^2 on days 1, 8, & 15 every 28 days		NR	12
Socinski et al.[60]	Carboplatin AUC of 6 on day 1 & nab-paclitaxel 100 mg/m^2 on days 1, 8, & 15 every 21 days	1052	46	3
	Carboplatin AUC of 6 & paclitaxel 200 mg/m^2 every 21 days		62[d]	11[e]

[a]The rate of all-grade and grade 3 motor neuropathy observed was 15% and 3%, respectively.
[b]Numbers represent patients receiving cisplatin and vinorelbine.
[c]This trial included three arms, and the two arms containing paclitaxel are included in the table. The results are reported as grade 3 neurologic toxicity.
[d]The results represent the rate of grade 2 or grade 3 neuropathy, and the difference is significant ($p = 0.05$).
[e]Significant differences in the rates of all grades of sensory neuropathy ($p < 0.001$) and grade 3 or grade 4 sensory neuropathy ($p < 0.05$) were noted.
AUC, area under the curve; NR, not reported.

A lower-dose weekly schedule compared with every-3-week paclitaxel has been investigated in several trials to improve efficacy or reduce toxicity, and higher and lower doses of paclitaxel have been researched as well. Paclitaxel sensory neuropathy is also dose-related, and it rarely occurs below doses of 170 mg/m^2.[55,57] In a phase III trial of cisplatin and low-dose paclitaxel (135 mg/m^2) every 3 weeks or high-dose paclitaxel (250 mg/m^2) every 3 weeks, a significantly higher rate of grade 3 neurologic toxicity was found in the high-dose paclitaxel arm (40% vs. 23%);[58] however, the low and high doses of paclitaxel investigated in this trial are not currently used in the treatment of NSCLC. In another phase III trial, carboplatin and paclitaxel every 3 weeks was compared with carboplatin on day 1 and paclitaxel on days 1, 8, and 15 every 4 weeks for four cycles; treatment was given for up to four cycles.[59] The rate of grade 2 and grade 3 neuropathy was significantly lower in the weekly arm compared with the every-3-week arm (12% vs. 18%; $p = 0.05$). In a smaller phase II trial, carboplatin every 3 weeks was compared with either paclitaxel 225 mg/m^2 every 3 weeks or 75 mg/m^2 weekly for 12 weeks;[60] the rate of sensory neuropathy was not significant between the two arms ($p = 0.27$). These data are suggestive of a lower rate of CIPN with a lower dose of paclitaxel used on a weekly schedule.

Standard formulation paclitaxel uses a Cremophor-base, and nab-paclitaxel formulation does not. In a phase III trial, carboplatin and nab-paclitaxel 100 mg/m^2 on days 1, 8, and 15 every 3 weeks was compared with carboplatin and standard formulation paclitaxel 200 mg/m^2 every 3 weeks.[61] Treatment was continued for at least six cycles and was allowed to continue in the absence of disease progression or unacceptable toxicity. The median cumulative dose of paclitaxel in the nab-paclitaxel and standard paclitaxel formulation arms was 1325 mg/m^2 and 1125 mg/m^2, respectively.

The rate of all-grade sensory neuropathy in the nab-paclitaxel and standard paclitaxel formulation arms was 46% and 62% ($p < 0.001$) respectively, the rate of grade 3 or grade 4 sensory neuropathy was 3% and 11% ($p < 0.05$), respectively, and the median improvement of grade 3 or higher sensory neuropathy to grade 1 in the nab-paclitaxel and paclitaxel arms was 38 and 104 days, respectively. It is important to note that the dose, schedule, and formulation of paclitaxel were different between the two arms, and it is unclear if one or a combination of these factors contributed to the difference in CIPN found in this trial. Infusion of nab-paclitaxel over 2 hours instead of the standard 30 minutes was compared with nab-paclitaxel 125 mg/m^2 on days 1, 8, and 15 every 4 weeks in a single-arm phase II trial.[62] A significant decrease was found in the grade of the average peripheral neuropathy, as well as in the rate of grade 2 or higher peripheral neuropathy compared with historic controls, which suggests that a longer infusion time with nab-paclitaxel may reduce the rate of clinically significant CIPN.

In summary, the rate of clinically relevant grade 2 or grade 3 sensory neuropathy found with platinum and taxane or vinorelbine combination therapy for the treatment of NSCLC is approximately 10% to 20%, and the rate of severe grade 3 sensory neuropathy is approximately 5%. Limiting the duration of carboplatin and paclitaxel to four cycles reduces the risk of clinically significant neuropathy, and the lower dose weekly schedule of paclitaxel may be associated with a lower rate of CIPN.

Prevention of CIPN

A number of agents have been investigated for the prevention of CIPN. Amifostine, an organic thiophosphate that acts as a scavenger of free radicals, was investigated as a cytoprotective agent for chemotherapy-induced and radiotherapy-induced toxicities. This agent was investigated in several small trials of various chemotherapy regimens, and a definitive improvement in clinical symptoms of CIPN was not found.[47] Glutathione is thought to prevent the accumulation of platinum adducts in the dorsal root ganglia, and to date, the trials in which glutathione is being researched for prevention of CIPN have been inconclusive.[47] In a phase III placebo-controlled, double-blinded clinical trial glutathione was investigated for the prevention of CIPN in patients with ovarian cancer treated with carboplatin and paclitaxel (ClinicalTrials. gov identifier: NCT02311907). Acetyl-L-carnitine (ALC) is a natural compound involved in the acetylation of tubulin, a process that provides neuronal protection.[63,64] ALC was investigated in a randomized, double-blind, placebo-controlled trial of 409 women treated with paclitaxel for breast cancer.[65] CIPN was assessed using the Functional Assessment of Cancer Therapy-Taxane scale at 12 and 24 weeks (a lower score indicates worse CIPN); patients who were assigned to ALC compared with placebo had a 0.9-point lower score at 12 weeks than patients who received placebo (95% CI, –2.2 to 0.4; $p = 0.17$) and a 1.8-point lower score at 24 weeks (95% CI, –3.2 to –0.04; $p = 0.01$). Grade 3 or grade 4 neurotoxicity was more frequent in the ALC arm than in the placebo arm (8 vs. 1). The worsening of CIPN with this nutritional supplement is discouraging and illustrates the need to perform randomized controlled trials of nutritional supplements. Alpha-lipoic acid (ALA) may improve nerve blood flow by antioxidant action and has been investigated as a treatment of diabetic peripheral neuropathy.[66,67] Accrual has been completed for a placebo-controlled phase III trial to evaluate alpha-lipoic acid (given for at least 24 weeks) for the prevention of CIPN in patients receiving cisplatin or oxaliplatin (ClinicalTrials.gov identifier: NCT00112996).

Pharmacologic Therapy for CIPN

When clinically significant CIPN develops, often defined as grade 2 or higher, treatment options are limited. The most problematic symptom for many patients is pain associated with the paresthesias, and a number of therapies have been investigated with variable success (Table 43.3). The primary end point for these trials is generally assessment of the grade of toxicity and patient-reported outcomes. In 2013, duloxetine was investigated in a randomized, double-blind, placebo-controlled, cross-over trial with the primary end point of reduction in average pain score.[68] Patients were required to have at least grade 1 sensory pain based on the NCI-CTCAE version 3.0 (reported as 4 or higher on a 10-point pain scale) and have neuropathic pain for 3

months or longer after completing chemotherapy. To be considered eligible for the trial, patients could have received treatment with paclitaxel, oxaliplatin, single-agent docetaxel, nab-paclitaxel, or cisplatin; however, none of the patients enrolled had received cisplatin. The majority of the patients enrolled had breast cancer (38%) or gastrointestinal cancer (56%). Eligible patients were randomly assigned to receive either duloxetine daily during the initial treatment period and placebo at cross-over period, or to receive placebo as initial treatment and duloxetine as cross-over treatment. The initial treatment period was week 1 to week 5, followed by a 2-week washout period, and cross-over (weeks 8 to 12); treatment consisted of either placebo or duloxetine 30 mg daily for the first week, and placebo or duloxetine 60 mg daily for 4 weeks. Patients reported the pain severity and functional interference weekly using the Brief Pain Inventory Short Form, in which 0 indicates no pain and 10 indicates pain "as bad as you can imagine." The minimal clinically important difference in pain severity was determined to be a 0.98 difference in average pain score. CIPN was also assessed using the NCI-CTCAE version 3.0 on a weekly basis. Patients assigned to duloxetine as their initial 5-week treatment reported a decrease in average pain of 1.06 (95% CI, 0.72–1.40), and patients assigned to placebo reported a decrease in average pain of 0.34 (95% CI, 0.01–0.66; $p = 0.003$). The effect size was moderately large at 0.513, and the percentage of patients reporting a decrease in pain with duloxetine and placebo first was 59% and 38%, respectively. Patients treated with duloxetine reported a greater decrease in the amount of pain that interfered with daily function ($p = 0.01$) and greater improvement in pain related to quality of life using the Functional Assessment of Cancer treatment, Gynecological Oncology Group Neurotoxicity subscale ($p = 0.03$). The most common adverse events were fatigue (7%), insomnia (5%), and nausea (5%). In an exploratory analysis, patients who received oxaliplatin experienced more benefit from duloxetine than patients who received taxanes ($p = 0.13$).

Other agents that have been investigated in double-blind, placebo-controlled trials for the treatment of CIPN include gabapentin and venlafaxine (Table 43.3).[69,70] In a phase III trial of gabapentin (target dose of 2700 mg daily) compared with placebo, patients with either a numeric score of 4 or higher on the numeric rating scale or 1 or higher on the Eastern Cooperative Oncology Group neuropathy scale had a 2-week washout and then crossed over to the other therapy. Changes in symptom severity were similar between the two groups, and this study did not suggest any benefit for gabapentin for the treatment of CIPN. In a smaller study, venlafaxine 50 mg 1 hour before the oxaliplatin infusion and venlafaxine 37.5 mg twice a day from day 2 to

TABLE 43.3 Select Phase III Trials of Therapies for Treatment of Chemotherapy-Induced Peripheral Neuropathy

Author	Agent	No. of Patients	Trial Design	Primary End Point	Outcome[a]
Smith et al.[68]	Duloxetine	231	Randomized, double-blind, placebo-controlled, cross-over	Average pain assessed using BPI-SF	Significant improvement ($p = 0.003$)
Rao et al.[69]	Gabapentin	115	Randomized, double-blind, placebo-controlled, cross-over	Average pain assessed using NRS & ENS	No significant difference
Durand et al.[70]	Venlafaxine	48	Double-blind, placebo-controlled	NRS, NPSI, & oxaliplatin-specific neurotoxicity	Full relief according to NRS significantly more common in venlafaxine arm (31.3% vs. 5.3%, $p = 0.03$)
Barton et al.[71]	Topical BAK-PLO	208	Double-blind, placebo-controlled	EORTC QLQ-CIPN20 at 4 weeks	Sensory neuropathy ($p = 0.053$); motor neuropathy ($p = 0.021$)

[a]A trend toward improvement in sensory neuropathy and a significant improvement in motor neuropathy was observed with BAK-PLO compared to placebo.

BAK-PLO, baclofen 10 mg, amitriptyline 40 mg, ketamine 20 mg in a pluronic lecithin organogel; *BPI-SF*, Brief Pain Inventory-Short Form; *ENS*, Eastern Cooperative Oncology Group neuropathy scale; *EORTC QLQ-CIPN20*, European Organisation for Research and Treatment of Cancer 20-item quality-of-life chemotherapy-induced peripheral neuropathy questionnaire; *NRS*, numerical rating scale; *NPSI*, neuropathic pain symptom inventory.

day 11 or placebo was investigated. The primary end point was the percentage of patients reporting 100% relief while receiving treatment as assessed by a numeric rating scale; in the venlafaxine and placebo arms, this end point was reached in 31.3% and 5.3%, respectively ($p = 0.03$).

In a double-blind, placebo-controlled trial a compounded gel containing 10 mg of baclofen, 40 mg of amitriptyline, and 20 mg of ketamine (BAK-PLO) was investigated compared with an identical-appearing placebo gel.[71] The primary end point was change in sensory neuropathy subscale as measured by the EORTC QLQ-CIPN20 instrument, which includes sensory, motor, and autonomic subscales from baseline to 20 weeks. A trend toward improvement was found in the sensory subscale ($p = 0.053$) as well as in the motor subscale ($p = 0.021$). The improved symptoms included tingling and shooting or burning pain in the fingers and hands and the ability to a hold a pen. A significant difference between the two treatment arms in the Brief Pain Inventory score and the CTCAE grade was not found.

CONCLUSION

Historically the acute and chronic toxicities of radiotherapy and chemotherapy for patients with NSCLC and SCLC were not considered to be clinically relevant. Consequently the majority of the data on the frequency and severity of neurotoxicity was retrospective. However, with improved survival and an increased number of treatment options for lung cancer patients the impact of these toxicities has become more apparent and relevant. This has led to the development of clinical trials that prospectively assess neurologic toxicity. Many chemotherapy and radiotherapy trials are investigating treatment agents or radiotherapy techniques that may reduce the risk of neurologic toxicity. Several prospective studies have investigated preventive agents and assessed the efficacy of symptomatic treatments for neurologic toxicity.

KEY REFERENCES

2. Eblan MJ, Corradetti MN, Lukens JN, et al. Brachial plexopathy in apical non-small cell lung cancer treated with definitive radiation: dosimetric analysis and clinical implications. *Int J Radiat Oncol Biol Phys*. 2013;85(1):175–181.
17. Okada S, Okeda R. Pathology of radiation myelopathy. *Neuropathology*. 2001;21(4):247–265.
30. Meyers CA, Smith JA, Bezjak A, et al. Neurocognitive function and progression in patients with brain metastases treated with whole-brain radiation and motexafin gadolinium: results of a randomized phase III trial. *J Clin Oncol*. 2004;22(1):157–165.
37. Le Péchoux C, Laplanche A, Faivre-Finn C, et al. Clinical neurological outcome and quality of life among patients with limited small-cell cancer treated with two different doses of prophylactic cranial irradiation in the intergroup phase III trial (PCI99-01, EORTC 22003-08004, RTOG 0212 and IFCT 99-01). *Ann Oncol*. 2011;22(5):1154–1163.
38. Gore EM, Bae K, Wong SJ, et al. Phase III comparison of prophylactic cranial irradiation versus observation in patients with locally advanced non-small-cell lung cancer: primary analysis of radiation therapy oncology group study RTOG 0214. *J Clin Oncol*. 2011;29(3):272–278.
53. Loprinzi CL, Reeves BN, Dakhil SR, et al. Natural history of paclitaxel-associated acute pain syndrome: prospective cohort study NCCTG N08C1. *J Clin Oncol*. 2011;29(11):1472–1478.
68. Smith EM, Pang H, Cirrincione C, et al. Effect of duloxetine on pain, function, and quality of life among patients with chemotherapy-induced painful peripheral neuropathy: a randomized clinical trial. *JAMA*. 2013;309(13):1359–1367.
69. Rao RD, Michalak JC, Sloan JA, et al. Efficacy of gabapentin in the management of chemotherapy-induced peripheral neuropathy: a phase 3 randomized, double-blind, placebo-controlled, crossover trial (N00C3). *Cancer*. 2007;110(9):2110–2118.

See Expertconsult.com for full list of references.

44

Frontline Systemic Therapy Options in Nonsmall Cell Lung Cancer

Suresh S. Ramalingam, Rathi N. Pillai, Niels Reinmuth, and Martin Reck

SUMMARY OF KEY POINTS

- The determination of tumor histology in nonsmall cell lung cancer (NSCLC) has become essential in treatment decision-making due to differential efficacy and toxicities seen with newer therapies.
- International Association for the Study of Lung Cancer (IASLC) guidelines recommend testing all patients with lung adenocarcinoma for both *EGFR* mutations and *ALK* rearrangements.
- Further molecular profiling of both adenocarcinoma and squamous cell lung cancers has identified novel driver mutations that are being investigated as potential targets of new therapies.
- Platinum doublet chemotherapy is the established standard first-line therapy in patients with advanced or metastatic NSCLC.
- The duration of platinum-based first-line therapy should be four to six cycles.
- Triple drug chemotherapy in NSCLC does not improve survival and often results in increased toxicity.
- *ERCC1* and *RRM1* have not been useful as predictive biomarkers for selection of chemotherapy based on prospective randomized clinical trials.
- Bevacizumab has been approved in combination with chemotherapy for the first-line therapy of patients with advanced NSCLC with nonsquamous histologies. Other antiangiogenic therapies in NSCLC have been disappointing.
- Patients with activating mutations in *EGFR* benefit from upfront therapy with EGFR tyrosine kinase inhibitors.
- Patients with *ALK* rearrangements can be successfully treated with ALK inhibitors, such as crizotinib.
- For patients with tumor PDL-1 expression >50%, pembrolizumab, an immune checkpoint inhibitor, is superior to platinum-based chemotherapy.
- Elderly patients with advanced NSCLC benefit from combination chemotherapy; selection of appropriate patients is vital.
- Patients with borderline performance status can also benefit from combination chemotherapy; patient selection requires careful consideration of comorbidities.

Lung cancer presents at an advanced stage at the time of diagnosis in the majority of patients. The overall goals of treatment for advanced stage disease are palliation and improvement in survival. Local treatment modalities such as radiotherapy and surgery play a limited role and are implemented primarily for symptom control. Systemic therapy remains the principal therapeutic modality for advanced stage nonsmall cell lung cancer (NSCLC). Until the late 1990s, treatment of advanced lung cancer followed the straightforward algorithm of platinum-based combination therapy, irrespective of histologic subtype, without any option for further lines of treatment. With the introduction of so-called third-generation cytotoxic drugs, the treatment of NSCLC changed and overall survival improved to approximately 8 months for patients with a good performance status. In the past two decades, there has been a gradual shift in therapy from the use of systemic chemotherapy in all patients, to the current approach in which histology and molecular status play a key role in treatment selection (Fig. 44.1). This has been made possible by greater insights into lung cancer biology, the availability of novel therapeutic agents, and the increasing focus on identification of biomarkers to guide therapy.[1] As a result, while a cure from advanced NSCLC still remains elusive, a significant subset of patients has long-term survival and an improved quality of life.

PROGNOSTIC FACTORS IN NONSMALL CELL LUNG CANCER

The assessment of prognosis is an important factor affecting the selection of appropriate treatment for each individual patient. The variables that are associated with prognosis can be grouped into categories: tumor-related, such as primary site, histology, and extent of disease; patient-related, such as performance status, comorbidity, and sex; and environmental factors, such as nutrition and the choice and quality of treatment.

Clinical Factors

Performance status and comorbid conditions are amongst the most important prognostic factors. Moreover, these determinants are also of utmost importance for the selection of therapy, as outlined later. The systematic determination of comorbidities is an essential component to preselect appropriate chemotherapy regimens and to provide the best supportive care.

In addition to noncancer-related comorbidities, patients also suffer from symptoms related to the primary tumor, mediastinal spread, or paraneoplastic syndromes. Moreover, lung cancer commonly produces systemic effects such as anorexia, weight loss, weakness, and profound fatigue. In a study of 12,428 NSCLC patients in the international staging database of the International Association for the Study of Lung Cancer (IASLC), performance status, age, and gender appeared to be independent prognostic factors for survival in addition to clinical stage.[2] In advanced NSCLC, some routine laboratory tests (mainly white blood cells and hypercalcemia) were also found to be significant prognostic variables. Nowadays, the clear majority of lung cancer cases are diagnosed in patients aged >65 years.[3] Age at diagnosis is another important factor that needs to be considered for therapy decision making. Often, increasing age is accompanied by multiple comorbidities, which further limit therapeutic options and outcome of the patient.

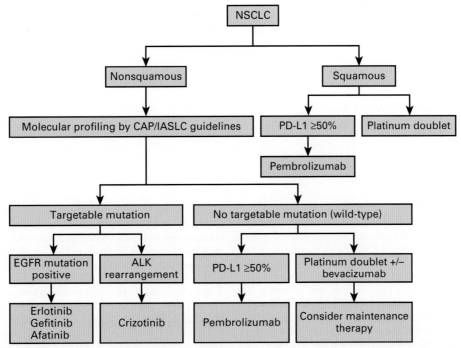

Fig. 44.1. Treatment algorithm for treatment-naive NSCLC. *ALK,* anaplastic lymphoma kinase; *EGFR,* epidermal growth factor receptor; *IASLC,* International Association for the Study of Lung Cancer; *NSCLC,* nonsmall cell lung cancer.

Ethnicity

While lung cancer remains a leading cause of mortality for all races, recent research has focused on ethnic variations in this disease. One of the most striking disparities seen is the difference in lung cancer risk and survival for African and Asian ethnicities. For example, the epidermal growth factor receptor (*EGFR*) mutation rate differs considerably between various ethnicities. Epidemiologic research has focused on behavioral, cultural, and socioeconomic factors that may influence risk, although no clear link has been established.[4] Access to care is also variable among various ethnic groups and remains an important barrier to the delivery of optimal therapy.

Tumor Stage

The anatomic extent of the disease, as described by the TNM classification, is the most important prognostic factor in NSCLC. The seventh edition of the TNM classification that came into effect in 2010 derived from the analysis of the largest database ever generated for this purpose, with data from 46 sources in more than 19 countries around the world and with information about patients treated with all modalities of care.[5,6] An important change involved the recognition that patients with extrathoracic disease have a slightly less favorable outcome compared with patients with metastatic spread confined to the thorax, even within the stage IV category. This has resulted in the division of stage IV to M1a and M1b based on the presence or absence of extrathoracic metastasis. It has also been recognized that malignant pleural or pericardial effusions portend a particularly poor prognosis among those with stage IV disease. In recognition of the importance of this, malignant effusions were moved from stage IIIB to IV disease in the seventh edition.

With additional cases analyzed in this international database, there will be further changes to the TNM classification system forthcoming in the eighth edition.[7] The increased importance of T stage in prognosis has resulted in upstaging of tumors greater than 5 cm to T3 and those greater than 7 cm to T4. There will also be a new staging grouping, IIIC, created for patients with N3 nodal involvement and T3 or T4 primary tumors, to reflect the worse prognosis of these most locally advanced tumors. Finally, within metastatic disease, patients with a solitary metastasis in a single extrathoracic organ will be classified as M1b. Presence of oligometastases merits consideration of local therapies in addition to systemic therapy. These patients have similar survival to patients classified as M1a with lung, pleural or pericardial involvement and will share the stage IVA designation. The majority of metastatic patients who present with multiple metastatic lesions will be considered M1c disease and will be characterized as stage IVB.

Histology

The distinction between squamous and nonsquamous histology was the first step in the personalized treatment of patients with advanced NSCLC. Hence, accurate diagnosis of tumor histology has become essential in treatment decision-making and can impact considerations of both toxicity and potential efficacy of selected agents used in the management of this disease. For example, the use of the anti–vascular endothelial growth factor (VEGF) antibody bevacizumab is associated with a higher risk of pulmonary bleeding when used in patients with predominantly squamous cell histology. Also, the cytotoxic drug pemetrexed was found to be inactive in patients with squamous NSCLC. Therefore, the classification of NSCLC into the major categories of squamous cell carcinoma, adenocarcinoma, and large cell carcinoma is critical for treatment decisions. However, histologic subclassification of NSCLC remains a challenge for many reasons. The tumor is very heterogeneous in every aspect: pathology, presence of molecular alterations, radiographic appearance, clinical presentation, and response to systemic therapy. The initial diagnostic biopsies often have a limited amount of material that is inadequate to conduct necessary tests to identify histology and genotype. The availability of immunostains such as TTF-1, p63, and p40 has greatly improved the accuracy of histologic subclassification.

TABLE 44.1 Single-Agent Activity of Chemotherapy in Randomized Trials Comparing Monotherapy With Combination Chemotherapy

Cytotoxic Agent	Patients (n)	Response Rate (%)	Median Survival (months)	Reference (year)
Vinorelbine	206	14	7.2	Le Chevalier (1994)[11]
Irinotecan	129	21	10.6	Negoro (2003)[12]
Cisplatin	206	17	8.1	Gatzemeier (2000)[13]
Cisplatin	262	11	7.6	Sandler (2000)[14]
Cisplatin	219	14	6.4	Von Pawel (2000)[15]
Cisplatin	209	12	6	Wozniak (1998)[16]
Gemcitabine	84	20	6.7	Vansteenkiste (2001)[17]
Gemcitabine	170	12	9	Sederholm (2002)[18]
Docetaxel	152	22	8	Georgouilas (2004)[19]
Paclitaxel	277	17	6.7	Lilenbaum (2005)[20]

Modified from Milton and Miller, Seminars in Oncology 2005.[21]

Molecular Markers

NSCLC tumors often harbor mutations in a number of critical genes such as p53, K-RAS, and LKB-1. The prognostic relevance of these mutations continues to be defined for patients with advanced NSCLC. Certain markers have gained attention because they also harbor predictive value. For example, the presence of an activating *EGFR* mutation translates into both predictive and prognostic information. Patients with *EGFR* mutation have overall better outcomes compared with those with wild-type *EGFR*, and also derive robust benefits from specific therapeutic inhibitors of the EGFR pathway. Similarly, limited early evidence indicates that patients with abnormal anaplastic lymphoma kinase (*ALK*) gene rearrangement have higher risk of recurrence following surgery for early-stage disease and a higher clinical benefit with pemetrexed therapy. The prognostic role of *K-Ras* mutations in lung adenocarcinoma has been debated extensively. Earlier evidence suggested poor sensitivity to chemotherapy and overall prognosis with *K-Ras* mutation, but emerging recent data have failed to confirm this. *K-Ras* mutated patients appear to have a very low likelihood of objective response with *EGFR* inhibitors. The knowledge of the prognostic and predictive potential of various molecular markers is bound to increase significantly in the coming years as molecular testing is adopted to routine practice settings.

TREATMENT OF ADVANCED NONSMALL CELL LUNG CANCER

Systemic Chemotherapy

Systemic chemotherapy prolongs survival and leads to symptom palliation compared with best supportive care alone for patients with advanced NSCLC.[8] Similar to therapeutic developments for other solid tumors, the efficacy of a variety of cytotoxic agents has been tested in both preclinical and clinical studies in NSCLC in the last decades. Initial results on single-agent therapy, including cisplatin (CDDP), ifosfamide, vinblastine, vindesine, etoposide, and mitomycin-C, indicated limited activity leading to objective response rates of ≤15% and median response durations of 2 months to 3 months. However, complete responses after these treatments were rare, and their benefit on median survival, with the exception of cisplatin, was inconsistent.[9] The relatively modest efficacy and the considerable toxicity of these cytotoxic agents led to considerable nihilism regarding the use of chemotherapy for NSCLC for many years. Starting in the mid-1980s, several novel cytotoxic drugs were evaluated in NSCLC, such as vinorelbine, paclitaxel, docetaxel, irinotecan, gemcitabine, and oxaliplatin, which showed response rates of 20% to 25% (Table 44.1).[10]

Combinations of various agents have also been evaluated in patients with NSCLC. Two meta-analyses showed a clear significant survival advantage for a two-drug regimen versus monotherapy, but on the other hand also demonstrated a significant increase in hematologic and nonhematologic side effects.[22,23]

Among several combinations, platinum-based chemotherapy was shown to lead to higher response rates and prolonged survival in comparison with monotherapy, albeit with the cost of increased toxicity.[8] Given the limited availability of supportive care for chemotherapy-related toxicities in the early 1990s, the use of chemotherapy in patients with metastatic NSCLC was still under debate despite the consistent evidence for its modest activity.

Platinum Compounds

Platinum compounds form DNA adducts, which ultimately result in activation of p53-dependent and p53-independent apoptosis.[24] As monotherapy, cisplatin has anticancer activity comparable with that of other single agents, leading to response rates of approximately 15% and a median survival of 6 to 8 months.[21] In order to increase the efficacy of systemic treatment, several combination regimens have been extensively studied (Table 44.2). Several randomized trials as well as meta-analyses provided scientific evidence that platinum-based combination therapy prolonged the survival of patients with advanced NSCLC. In 1995, a meta-analysis using updated data on 1190 patients with advanced NSCLC from 11 randomized clinical trials was published. The results, updated in 2008, demonstrated a 27% reduction in the risk of death for patients treated with cisplatin-containing regimens compared with supportive care alone, which translated to an absolute improvement in survival of 10% (5% to 15%) at one year.[8]

Compared with older regimens such as cisplatin with vindesine or vinblastine, cisplatin and mitomycin-C with vinblastine or vindesine, or cisplatin with etoposide, combinations of cisplatin with newer drugs (referred to as third-generation drugs: gemcitabine, taxanes, vinorelbine, topoisomerase I inhibitors) seem to exert somewhat higher efficacy and improved tolerability. For example, compared with platinum–gemcitabine combinations, several studies indicated inferior response rates, time to progression, and median overall survival (OS) for cisplatin, ifosfamide and mitomycin,[30] cisplatin and vindesine,[31] or cisplatin and etoposide regimens.[32] Hematologic toxicity, especially thrombocytopenia, was pronounced in the gemcitabine-platinum groups whereas nonhematologic side effects appeared more frequently in the "classic" arms.[30–32] Moreover, Le Chevalier et al.[33] showed a significantly better response rate and survival for cisplatin–vinorelbine compared with cisplatin–vindesine.

The choice of the newer agent (gemcitabine, paclitaxel, or vinorelbine) that is combined with cisplatin does not seem to significantly affect the treatment efficacy (see Table 44.2). For instance, phase III studies (e.g., Southwest Oncology Group [SWOG] 9509) failed to demonstrate superiority of carboplatin–paclitaxel over cisplatin–vinorelbine in 408 patients.[25] Similarly, the Italian Lung Cancer Study Group failed to detect any significant difference in outcome for cisplatin–gemcitabine, carboplatin–paclitaxel, and cisplatin–vinorelbine in 612 patients with previously untreated advanced NSCLC.[26] However, both studies

TABLE 44.2 Phase III Trials Comparing Platinum-Based Combinations

Regimen	Patients	Response Rate (%)	Median Survival	p	Reference (year)
Cisplatin/vindesine	200	19	7.4	0.04	Le Chevalier
Cisplatin/vinorelbine	206	30	9.2		(1994)[11]
Cisplatin/vinorelbine	202	28	8	NS	Kelly (2001)[25]
Carboplatin/paclitaxel	206	25	8		
Carboplatin/paclitaxel	201	32	9.9	NS	Scagliotti
Cisplatin/vinorelbine	201	30	9.5		(2002)[26]
Cisplatin/gemcitabine	205	30	9.8		
Cisplatin/paclitaxel	305	21	7.8	NS	Schiller (2002)[27]
Cisplatin/gemcitabine	288	22	8.1		
Cisplatin/docetaxel	289	17	7.4		
Carboplatin/paclitaxel	290	17	8.1		
Cisplatin/vinorelbine	404	25	10.1		Fossella (2003)[28]
Cisplatin/docetaxel	408	32	11.3	0.04[a]	
Carboplatin/docetaxel	406	24	9.4	NS[a]	
Cisplatin/vindesine	151	21	9.6	0.01	Kubota (2004)[29]
Cisplatin/docetaxel	151	37	11.3		
Cisplatin/vindesine	122	32	10.9	0.12	Negoro (2003)[12]
Cisplatin/irinotecan	129	44	11.5		

[a]In comparison to the cisplatin/vinorelbine arm.
NS, not significant.
Modified from Milton and Miller, Seminars in Oncology 2005.[21]

demonstrated differences between these regimens regarding their toxicity profiles. In the largest study that included 1207 patients (Eastern Cooperative Oncology Group [ECOG] 1594), Schiller et al.[27] found no significant efficacy differences among the regimens cisplatin–paclitaxel, cisplatin–gemcitabine, cisplatin–docetaxel, and carboplatin–paclitaxel regarding response rates (17% to 22%) and median survival (7.4–8.1 months).[27] Differences were only noted in toxicity profiles, with cisplatin–gemcitabine causing more thrombocytopenia, cisplatin–docetaxel causing more neutropenia, and the carboplatin–paclitaxel arm experiencing the lowest rate of potentially life-threatening toxicities. Another phase III study (TAX 326) randomized 1218 patients to receive cisplatin–docetaxel, carboplatin–docetaxel, or the control arm of cisplatin–vinorelbine. Patients treated with cisplatin–docetaxel had a higher response rate (31.6% vs. 24.5%, $p = 0.029$) and median survival (11.3 vs. 10.1 months, $p = 0.044$).[28] Based on these observations, platinum-based chemotherapy remains the standard therapy in advanced or metastatic NSCLC. With the current combination partners, a plateau of efficacy has been reached.

Cisplatin Versus Carboplatin

Carboplatin is another platinum derivate with a tenfold longer half-life than cisplatin. Due to structural differences from cisplatin, it exhibits lower reactivity and slower DNA binding kinetics in vitro. In clinical studies, the nonhematologic tolerability of carboplatin is superior to that of cisplatin, making it a more convenient platinum analog for palliative chemotherapy.

Several studies have compared the efficacy of cisplatin with carboplatin in the management of advanced NSCLC. Rosell et al.[34] reported a significantly improved survival for cisplatin–paclitaxel compared with carboplatin–paclitaxel with a higher rate of nonhematologic side effects in the cisplatin arm and a higher rate of neutropenia and thrombocytopenia in the carboplatin arm.[34] In the TAX 326 trial, there was a nonsignificant trend toward improved survival for the combination of cisplatin–docetaxel over carboplatin–docetaxel.[28] In contrast, the ECOG 1594 trial noted similar survival duration between the cisplatin and carboplatin-based treatment arms. However, there was a lower incidence of nonhematologic events such as nausea, vomiting, nephrotoxicity, and neurotoxicity with carboplatin-based therapy.[27] This observation has also been made in other smaller trials[21] with carboplatin-based regimens.

A meta-analysis using data from eight trials demonstrated that cisplatin-based chemotherapy offered a significantly higher objective response rate compared with carboplatin-based chemotherapy (odds ratio [OR], 1.36; 95% confidence interval [CI], 1.15 to 1.61; $p = 0.001$) and a nonsignificant improvement in survival (hazard ratio [HR], 1.050; 95% CI, 0.907 to 1.216; $p = 0.515$).[35] In this meta-analysis, a subgroup analysis of the five trials that incorporated cisplatin or carboplatin with a new agent identified a significantly superior median survival for cisplatin-treated patients (HR, 1.106; 95% CI, 1.005–1.218; $p = 0.039$). These data were confirmed by another meta-analysis including 2968 patients from nine trials.[36] Cisplatin-treated patients experienced a significantly higher response rate (OR, 1.37; 95% CI, 1.16–1.61; $p < 0.001$). Moreover, cisplatin-based treatment was associated with an improved median OS relative to treatment with carboplatin (9.1 versus 8.4 months; HR, 1.07; 95% CI, 0.99–1.15; $p = 0.1$) that was significant in subgroup analyses for patients with nonsquamous tumors (HR, 1.12; 95% CI, 1.01–1.23) and those treated with third-generation chemotherapy (HR, 1.11; 95% CI, 1.01–1.21). However, cisplatin-based chemotherapy was associated with more severe nausea, vomiting, and nephrotoxicity while severe thrombocytopenia was more frequent during carboplatin-based chemotherapy.[36] Hence, the selection of the platinum compound should be made based on the regimen most likely to result in the best therapeutic index. In recent years, the availability of effective antiemetic agents has improved the therapeutic index of cisplatin-based regimens.

Triplets for Advanced NSCLC

To further increase the efficacy of systemic therapy in advanced NSCLC, a series of studies have evaluated the potential role for the use of three-drug regimens. These studies have consistently demonstrated that three-drug regimens are associated with higher toxicity, have at times higher objective response rates, but offer no statistically significant improvement in survival as compared with that offered by standard doublets (Table 44.3). For example, a phase III trial of 557 stage IIIB/IV NSCLC randomized patients to receive cisplatin–gemcitabine for six cycles, cisplatin–gemcitabine–vinorelbine for six cycles, or three cycles of gemcitabine–vinorelbine followed by three cycles of vinorelbine–ifosfamide.[37] Response rates were inferior for the nonplatinum sequential doublet while no differences in median survival or time to progression were observed. Predictably, toxicity was

TABLE 44.3 Two Drugs Compared With Three Drugs in NSCLC

Doublet Chemotherapy	Triplet Chemotherapy	Response Rate (%)	Grade 3–4 Neutropenia	Grade 3–4 Thrombocytopenia	Grade 3–4 Nausea/ Vomiting
Cisplatin/ gemcitabine[37]	Cisplatin/gemcitabine/ ifosfamide	42 vs. 41	32 vs. 57	4 vs. 19	22 vs. 32
Cisplatin/gemcitabine or gemcitabine/ vinorelbine[38]	Cisplatin/ifosfamide/ gemcitabine or gemcitabine/ifosfamide/ vinorelbine	29 vs. 28	36 vs. 44	16 vs. 20	8 vs. 7

NSCLC, Nonsmall cell lung cancer.

significantly higher for the triplet regimen. Similarly, a recent phase II study found no statistically significant difference between doublet (cisplatin–gemcitabine or gemcitabine–vinorelbine) and triplet (cisplatin–ifosfamide–gemcitabine, or gemcitabine–ifosfamide–vinorelbine) combinations; however, grade 3–4 leukopenia was significantly more common in triplets.[38]

In a systematic overview, third generation triplet therapy had a significantly higher response rate (OR, 1.33; 95% CI, 1.50–2.23; $p < 0.001$) compared with standard doublet therapy;[39] however, median survival (MR, 1.10; 95% CI, 0.91–1.35; $p = 0.059$) was not statistically different and the incidence of grades 3–4 hematologic toxicity, neuropathy, and diarrhea was significantly increased with triplet therapy. Based on these results, platinum-based doublet chemotherapy remains the standard first-line treatment for patients with metastatic NSCLC.

Platinum-Free Versus Platinum-Based Chemotherapy

In daily practice, several types of patients with advanced NSCLC are not optimal candidates to receive platinum-based chemotherapy due to the presence of certain comorbid conditions such as renal insufficiency, borderline performance status (PS), or preexisting sensory neuropathy. Hence, studies were conducted to evaluate whether the combination of two newer chemotherapeutic agents may be better suited for first-line therapy. In some earlier studies, a trend toward a higher survival was observed in patients treated with platinum-based combinations compared with those treated with platinum-free regimens.[21,40,41] In a recent phase II study, a total of 433 stage IIIB–IV NSCLC patients received cisplatin–gemcitabine, gemcitabine–vinorelbine, cisplatin–ifosfamide–gemcitabine, or gemcitabine–ifosfamide–vinorelbine.[38] Platinum-based regimens had a significantly longer overall survival (11.3 vs. 9.7; $p = 0.044$) compared with the other treatment arms but also resulted in higher incidence of grade 3–4 toxicity. In a meta-analysis based on abstracted data from randomized phase II and III studies, D'Addario et al.[42] observed a significantly higher 1-year survival rate for platinum-based combinations compared with the nonplatinum regimens (34% vs. 29%; OR, 1.21; 95% CI, 1.09–1.35; $p = 0.0003$). However, when single-agent trials were excluded and platinum-based therapies were compared with third-generation–based combination regimens only, no statistically significant difference could be found (1-year survival, 36% for platinum regimens vs. 35% for nonplatinum regimens). In a more recent systematic review of randomized controlled trials comprising 4920 patients, the use of cisplatin-based doublet regimens was associated with a higher 1-year-survival rate (Hazard Ratio (HR), 1.16, 95% CI, 1.06–1.27; $p = 0.001$) compared with nonplatinum regimens, but also with an increased risk of anemia, neutropenia, neurotoxicity, and nausea.[43] Conversely, carboplatin-based doublet regimens were associated with a similar 1-year survival rate (HR = 0.95, 95% CI, 0.85–1.07; $p = 0.43$) to that of nonplatinum doublets. Taken together, nonplatinum regimens do not have a clearly defined role in NSCLC and are only considered appropriate for patients that are not candidates for platinum agents.

Duration of Chemotherapy

The commonly used NSCLC chemotherapy regimens are administered in 3- or 4-week cycles. Imaging studies are recommended every two to three cycles to assess response to therapy. For patients that achieve an objective response or stable disease, the number of cycles of therapy has been a subject of several randomized studies. Socinski et al.[44] randomized advanced NSCLC patients to treatment with the combination of carboplatin and paclitaxel for either four cycles or to continuation of therapy until disease progression. Interestingly, the median number of treatment cycles administered in both arms was four. There was no statistically significant improvement in OS for the extended chemotherapy approach. Predictably, toxicity was more common with administration of chemotherapy beyond four cycles. Another study by Smith et al.[45] that compared three cycles of chemotherapy with six cycles also found no improvement in OS with the latter. In a systematic meta-analysis including 13 randomized control trials, 3027 patients receiving first-line (largely platinum-based) chemotherapy for three to four cycles were compared with patients with continuation of the same chemotherapy for six cycles or until disease progression.[46] While extending chemotherapy substantially improved progression-free survival (PFS; HR, 0.75; 95% CI, 0.69–0.81; $p < 0.00001$), there was a statistically significant, but clinically only modest reduction in the hazard for death as compared with standard duration of chemotherapy over three to four cycles (HR, 0.92; 95% CI, 0.85–0.99; $p = 0.03$). Moreover, extension of chemotherapy was associated with higher toxicity and impaired quality of life. These findings were confirmed in a recent systematic review and meta-analysis of randomized trials comparing six versus fewer cycles of only platinum-based chemotherapy that had individual patient data available for analysis.[47] While an improvement in PFS was observed in the four eligible studies with 1139 patients (HR 0.79; 95% CI, 0.68–0.90; $p = 0.0007$), there was no overall survival benefit to receipt of six cycles of platinum-based chemotherapy (median 9.54 months versus 8.68 months with fewer cycles; HR 0.94; 95% CI, 0.83–1.07; $p = 0.33$). This was independent of histology, sex, performance status, and age. Hence, most guidelines recommend limiting the duration of platinum-based first-line therapy to four to six cycles and prefer considering the induction of maintenance therapy.

Maintenance Therapy

After four to six cycles of first-line or induction chemotherapy, approximately two-thirds of patients have nonprogressive disease. Continuation of first-line platinum-based combination regimens beyond four to six cycles results in heightened toxicities and diminished quality of life without providing a major survival advantage.[44,46] Thus, the standard therapeutic approach has entailed stopping treatment at that point, close clinical and radiographic surveillance, and initiation of second-line treatment at the time of progression. This "wait and watch" approach is frequently chosen after achieving maximal response to initial therapy. However, a "drug holiday" is often associated with patient anxiety about disease recurrence or progression coupled with concerns for clinical deterioration and the inability to receive subsequent therapy.

The availability of effective newer cytotoxic and molecularly targeted agents with overall good tolerability and low toxicity profile has led to the concept of maintenance therapy in order to maintain or improve the disease burden after completion of first-line therapy. Maintenance therapy involves either switching to a different compound (switch maintenance) or continuation of one drug partner of the induction regimen (continuation maintenance) in patients with a response or at least stabilization of disease.[48] The role of maintenance therapy is discussed extensively in Chapter 46.

IMPORTANCE OF HISTOLOGY IN THE TREATMENT OF NSCLC

NSCLC includes many histologic subtypes including adenocarcinoma, squamous cell carcinoma, and large cell carcinoma, all of which have diverse clinical behaviors. Until a few years ago, all histologic subtypes of NSCLC were treated with similar systemic therapy regimens. Though distinct differences in sites of metastasis, OS, and smoking behavior were recognized, there was no specific reason to use histology for selection of systemic therapy. The importance of distinguishing histology of NSCLC was realized with the development of new therapies that resulted in different toxicities and outcomes based on the histology. This effect was first realized in the phase II study of bevacizumab; the risk of pulmonary hemorrhage was predominantly seen in patients with squamous histology.[49] Bevacizumab was subsequently restricted to patients with predominant nonsquamous histology. Several other antiangiogenic agents have also demonstrated a higher risk of bleeding with squamous histology, thus defining this as a class effect.

Pemetrexed was the first cytotoxic agent that has shown a clear correlation between histology and efficacy. Scagliotti et al.[1] conducted a phase III study to compare the efficacy of cisplatin and pemetrexed with that of cisplatin and gemcitabine for patients with advanced NSCLC. The OS and PFS were similar for the study population, which included approximately 1700 patients. A preplanned subset analysis was conducted to study the outcomes for patients with nonsquamous histology. This revealed a significant improvement in survival for nonsquamous patients with the cisplatin-pemetrexed regimen (11.8 months vs. 10.4 months). Conversely, the cisplatin–gemcitabine regimen was superior in patients with squamous cell histology. Based on this study, and similar observations from other studies with pemetrexed, this agent is not considered appropriate for the treatment of squamous cell lung cancer.

In contrast, nab-paclitaxel, an albumin-bound formulation of paclitaxel, benefits patients with squamous cell lung cancer preferentially over nonsquamous tumors. In a phase III study of weekly nab-paclitaxel with carboplatin compared with standard paclitaxel and carboplatin given every 3 weeks, comparable OS was noted for the two regimens.[50] The response rate was superior with nab-paclitaxel regimen for the overall patient population (32% vs. 25%). The response rate was higher with nab-paclitaxel in patients with squamous histology (response rate ratio 1.6890, 95% CI, 1.271–2.221, $p < 0.001$). There was no difference in overall response rate (ORR) in patients with nonsquamous histology between the two regimens (26% with nab-paclitaxel versus 25% with paclitaxel, $p = 0.808$). Nab-paclitaxel is a Food and Drug Administration approved therapy for advanced NSCLC in combination with carboplatin. It has the advantage of not requiring premedications needed with the standard formulation of paclitaxel. It is also associated with a lower incidence of grades 3–4 neuropathy compared with paclitaxel. The biologic reasons behind the correlation between histology and efficacy of pemetrexed and nab-paclitaxel are not known, and some exploratory hypotheses are described in a subsequent section of this chapter.

MANAGEMENT OF ELDERLY PATIENTS

In the United States, patients aged more than 65 years represent two-thirds of the lung cancer cases, and the median age at diagnosis is >70 years. Furthermore, nearly 15% of patients are over the age of 80 years at diagnosis.[51] A number of physiologic functions, especially renal and hematopoietic functions, are altered with ageing that impact on chemotherapy tolerance and toxicity.[51] Furthermore, elderly patients have more comorbid conditions compared with younger ones and are more likely to take prescription medications for other ailments, which may interfere with the pharmacokinetic disposition of anticancer agents.[52–54] Comorbid conditions can be evaluated using the Charlson Comorbidity Index,[55] or by the more detailed Cumulative Illness Rating Scale-Geriatric.[56] In a Veterans Affairs Central Cancer Registry containing 20,511 NSCLC cancer patients from 2003 to 2008, the percentage of patients receiving guideline-recommended chemotherapy treatment decreased with increasing age.[57] In an analysis of the SEER-Medicare database in the United States, only about 25% of the older patients received systemic chemotherapy for advanced stage disease.[58] Furthermore, platinum-based regimens were given to less than 25% of the patients that received chemotherapy.

Until recently, the majority of the treatment recommendations for chemotherapy in elderly NSCLC patients were based on subset analyses of outcomes for elderly patients included in clinical trials for all patient age-groups. Elderly patients in these studies were likely to be highly selected based on functional status and might not be representative of the older patient population "at-large." Moreover, there is a wide variation between studies regarding the definition of older patients across clinical trials. In earlier studies, age >65 years was often used to define older patients. In recent trials, >70 years has become the threshold for elderly patient-specific trials. Another noteworthy aspect is that many studies in the general lung cancer population limit entry to patients <75 years of age. For all these reasons, treatment decisions for older patients should be made based on available data, patient preferences, comorbid illness, and molecular status.

The role of chemotherapy exclusively in older patients was established in a phase III study that demonstrated superiority for vinorelbine over best supportive care (ELVIS study).[59] The survival improvement was observed despite early closure of the study due to slow accrual and the fact that the necessary sample size had not been met. This was the first elderly patient–specific study in lung cancer to define the role for chemotherapy in advanced stage disease. Subsequently, a study that compared the combination of gemcitabine with vinorelbine versus both revealed no therapeutic advantage for the combination.[60] These studies led to the adoption of single-agent chemotherapy as the standard approach for older lung cancer patients.

The role of combination regimens in older patients was not defined until recently. Subset analysis from a number of randomized trials demonstrated that outcomes for older patients enrolled in clinical trials were similar to that of younger individuals.[61–63] In a study reported by Lilenbaum et al.,[20] treatment with carboplatin and paclitaxel was associated with an increase in response and survival compared with single-agent therapy with paclitaxel, but the differences did not reach statistical significance. A benefit of similar magnitude was observed for the combination compared with monotherapy in a subgroup analysis of patients >70 years, and there was no significant difference in survival between elderly patients and younger patients with carboplatin–paclitaxel. However, in a combined analysis of two SWOG trials, elderly patients (above 70 years) treated with platinum-based combinations had a

TABLE 44.4 Phase III Trials Including Elderly Patients With Advanced NSCLC

Author (year)	Number of Patients	Median Age (y)	Drugs	Response Rate (%)	Median Survival (Months)	1-Year Survival Rate (%)	p
ELVIS (1999)[59]	76	74	Vinorelbine	19.7	6.5	32	0.03
	85		BSC	–	4.9	14	
Frasci (2000)[68]	60	74	Vinorelbine	22	7	13	<0.01
	60		Gemcitabine + vinorelbine	15	4.5	30	
Gridelli (2003)[60]	700	74	Vinorelbine	21	8.5	42	NS
			Gemcitabine	16	6.5	28	
			Gemcitabine + vinorelbine	18.1	7.4	34	
Kudoh (2006)[69]	182	76	Vinorelbine	9.9	9.9	NR	NS
			Docetaxel	22.7	14	NR	
Quoix (2011)[65]	226	77	Vinorelbine or gemcitabine	10	6.2	25.4	0.0004
	225		Carboplatin + weekly paclitaxel	27	10.3	44.5	

BSC, Best supportive care; *NR*, not reported; *NS*, not significant; *NSCLC*, nonsmall cell lung cancer.
Adapted from Quoix et al.[52]

shorter survival (7 months versus 9 months; (*p* = 0.04) and experienced more frequent grade 3–5 neutropenias compared with younger patients.[64]

Most studies addressing directly the benefit of chemotherapy to elderly patients demonstrated a survival benefit to some extent for patients treated with the more aggressive therapy arm (Table 44.4).[52] In a recent phase III study by Quoix et al.,[65] 451 patients aged 70–89 years with locally advanced or metastatic NSCLC and WHO performance status scores of 0–2 received either four cycles of carboplatin/paclitaxel or five cycles of vinorelbine or gemcitabine monotherapy.[65] Second-line treatment was defined to be erlotinib for both arms. The study population had a median age of 77 years. The median OS was significantly superior for doublet chemotherapy (10.3 versus 6.2 months; HR 0.64, 95% CI, 0.52–0.78; *p* < 0.0001). The combination regimen was also associated with more hematologic and nonhematologic toxicity including neutropenia (48.4% vs. 12.4%) and asthenia (10.3% vs. 5.8%). This is the first prospective trial for elderly patients that demonstrated a survival benefit for combination chemotherapy. It is noteworthy that the study utilized a weekly schedule of paclitaxel with administration of carboplatin every 4 weeks, which appears to have a slightly favorable tolerability over the standard 3-weekly schedule. It is evident from this cumulative evidence that elderly patients with a good performance status are appropriate candidates for platinum-based chemotherapy. Also, consideration for primary prophylaxis with granulocyte colony stimulating factor might be appropriate for certain combination regimens in elderly patients.[66] Given the potential detrimental effects of cisplatin on the kidneys and other end organs in older subjects, carboplatin-based regimens are preferred for the treatment of advanced NSCLC. For less fit patients, monotherapy might be suitable;[67] however, one needs to balance possible benefits and risk followed by discussion with the patients about the role of chemotherapy.

MANAGEMENT OF PATIENTS WITH A POOR PERFORMANCE STATUS

The performance status (PS) of the patient is an important prognostic factor in lung cancer. An ECOG PS of 2, alternatively termed "marginal PS" or "poor risk," is defined as being "ambulatory and capable of all self-care but unable to carry out any work activities; up and about more than 50% of waking hours."[70] The designation of PS remains subjective, as evidenced by the discordance between physician assessments of performance status versus self-assessment by patients.[71] Physicians tend to overestimate the performance status of patients in general.

Subset analyses of trials for patients with advanced NSCLC with eligibility ranging from PS 0 to 2 have historically shown

that PS 2 patients experience a much shorter survival.[65,72,73] Some studies have pooled PS 2 patients with the elderly, most commonly defined as being older than 70 years of age. Though decline in PS is often related to high disease burden related to lung cancer, it should be distinguished from poor PS related to comorbid illness. Until now, studies conducted in older patients have not adequately made this distinction, which makes it difficult to recommend aggressive therapies for those with poor PS. In recent years, several studies have been conducted exclusively for patients with a poor PS. The combination of carboplatin and paclitaxel was superior to single-agent paclitaxel (median survival of 4.7 vs. 2.4 months) in PS 2 patients in a prospectively specified subgroup analysis for patients with poor PS that were enrolled in the Cancer and Leukemia Group B (CALGB) trial.[20] In another study for patients with a poor PS, the combination of carboplatin and paclitaxel was superior to single-agent therapy with erlotinib (9.7 months compared with 6.5 months with erlotinib).[20,74] In a recent phase III trial for advanced NSCLC patients, patients with PS 2 were randomly assigned to a combination therapy of carboplatin–pemetrexed or pemetrexed alone.[75] PS was determined by the treating physician and verified by another physician at each participating site. There was a statistically and clinically significant improvement with the doublet in response rate (23.8% vs. 10.3%; *p* = 0.032), progression-free survival (median, 5.8 vs. 2.8 months; HR, 0.46; 95% CI, 0.35–0.63; *p* < 0.001), and OS (median, 9.3 vs. 5.3 months; HR, 0.62; 95% CI, 0.46–0.83; *p* = 0.001). However, toxicity was also higher in the combination arm, with more treatment-related deaths (3.9% vs. 0%). This was the first prospective study to demonstrate benefit from platinum-based therapy in patients with poor PS. Future trials should address the impact of comorbid conditions versus cancer burden as the reason behind decline in PS for patients and its correlation to outcome with combination therapies.

Taking the recent data into account, patients with heavy disease burden and poor PS may also be offered combination therapy. As with any clinical decision, therapy selection is utterly dependent on the patient preference and physician judgment throughout the process of selecting palliative chemotherapy in the setting of advanced NSCLC. Molecular testing is strongly recommended even in patients with a poor PS, since the use of appropriate targeted therapy in selected patients has been reported to result in robust responses and improved physical function.[76]

BIOMARKERS FOR SELECTION OF CHEMOTHERAPY

The use of biomarkers to select appropriate chemotherapy regimens has long been a focus of research. Lung cancer cells have a relative deficiency of DNA repair machinery compared with normal cells; this makes them more sensitive to the DNA damaging effects of cytotoxic chemotherapy.[77] Somatic excision repair cross-complementing gene 1 (*ERCC1*) has been evaluated as a prognostic and predictive biomarker of response to treatment with platinum agents. Ribonucleotide reductase M1 (*RRM1*) is the catalytic subunit of ribonucleotide reductase, which converts ribonucleoside diphosphates into deoxyribonucleosides in DNA synthesis.[78] Since RRM1 is the primary target of gemcitabine, it has been studied as a predictive biomarker for efficacy of gemcitabine.

A randomized phase III study was conducted to utilize *ERCC1* expression to personalize therapy in NSCLC.[79] The hypothesis was to treat patients with *ERCC1*-overexpressing tumor with nonplatinum regimens and those with low *ERCC1* expression with platinum-containing regimens; 82.4% of patients randomized had adequate tissue for *ERCC1* mRNA expression analysis; 444 patients with stage IIIB or IV NSCLC were then randomized in a 2:1 ratio to the genotypic arm, where patients were treated according to their *ERCC1* status (*ERCC1* low patients with cisplatin and docetaxel and *ERCC1* high patients with gemcitabine and docetaxel) or to the control arm, where all patients received cisplatin and docetaxel irrespective of biomarker status. The study achieved its primary end point of improvement in response rate with 50.7% in the genotypic arm compared with 39.3% in the control arm ($p = 0.02$). However, since there was no significant improvement in survival in the genotype arm, this limited the utility of *ERCC1* as a predictive biomarker. In another recently published phase III study, treatment was assigned based on tumoral expression of ERCC1 and RRM1 for patients with chemotherapy-naive advanced NSCLC. ERCC1 and RRM1 expression were determined by an automated quantitative analysis (AQUA) based on immunohistochemistry.[80] Out of 275 eligible patients, 183 were randomized to the customized approach and 92 patients to control. There was no difference between the two groups in the primary end point of PFS, or the secondary outcomes of OS or response rate (11 months and 36.5% with customized therapy vs. 11.3 months and 38.8% in control arm, $p = 0.66$ for survival). In addition to these disappointing results, problems regarding the sensitivity of the antibodies used for detection of ERCC1 expression have recently been observed.[81]

Pemetrexed exerts anticancer effects by inhibiting thymidylate synthase (TS), dihydrofolate reductase, and glycinamide ribonucleotide formyl transferase.[82] TS is an enzyme that converts deoxyuridylate to deoxythymidylate that is necessary for DNA synthesis. Since TS is the main target of pemetrexed, low levels of TS have been hypothesized to predict increased response rate to pemetrexed therapy. In a study of 56 patients with NSCLC, TS mRNA and protein levels were higher in patients with squamous cell carcinoma.[83] TS levels may explain why patients with squamous cell histology are resistant to pemetrexed compared with adenocarcinoma histology, though this remains to be confirmed.

Taxanes bind to β-tubulin and lead to stabilization of microtubules, resulting in apoptosis. High levels of β-tubulin have been associated with resistance to treatment with docetaxel and paclitaxel in cell lines.[84] In 91 patients with advanced NSCLC who were treated with paclitaxel (47) or nontaxane regimens (44), those with low expression of class III β-tubulin by immunohistochemistry (IHC) had improved response rates, PFS, and OS when treated with paclitaxel.[85] In a meta-analysis of 552 patients in 10 studies examining either paclitaxel or vinorelbine containing regimens, decreased expression of class III β-tubulin was associated with improved OS (HR, 1.40; $p < 0.00001$).[86] These observations have not been confirmed in prospective studies and the role of β-tubulin as a predictive marker for taxanes still remains unproven.

COMBINATION OF TARGETED AGENTS WITH PLATINUM-BASED CHEMOTHERAPY

The development of molecularly targeted agents has led to the evaluation of several novel compounds in combination with platinum-based chemotherapy for first-line treatment of advanced NSCLC. These studies were usually supported by supra-additive or synergistic preclinical interactions between these agents. However, the vast majority of these studies failed to demonstrate an improvement in survival with the addition of a targeted agent to standard chemotherapy. These studies were typically conducted in unselected patient populations and did not include efforts to identify predictive biomarkers. More recently, studies with novel combinations are focused on identifying a subset of patients that might derive robust benefits. The first combination strategy to demonstrate survival benefit was the addition of bevacizumab, a monoclonal antibody against the VEGF, to standard chemotherapy.

ANTIANGIOGENIC THERAPY

It has been widely observed that for tumor development and growth to proceed beyond a defined volume, the development of a new blood supply is necessary.[87,88] Therefore, most solid tumors need the formation of new blood vessels for continued growth and metastasis, which may be achieved by the induction of endothelial cell sprouting from the preexisting vasculature (so-called angiogenesis).[87,89,90] The monoclonal anti-VEGF antibody bevacizumab, which blocks the binding of VEGF to its high-affinity receptors, was the first angiogenesis inhibitor to complete clinical development and is currently the only antiangiogenesis agent approved for the treatment of lung cancer.

In a phase II trial in 99 unselected NSCLC patients, a higher response rate (31.5% vs. 18.8%), longer median time to progression (7.4 vs. 4.2 months), and a modest increase in survival (17.7 vs. 14.9 months) was observed for treatment with carboplatin and paclitaxel plus bevacizumab (15 mg/kg) compared with the chemotherapy control arm.[49] However, 9% of the patients treated with bevacizumab experienced life-threatening pulmonary hemorrhage (PH), which was fatal in four patients. Since the majority of the patients with hemoptysis had squamous cell histology, tumor cavitation, and disease location close to major blood vessels, these clinical situations were excluded in subsequent studies.

Two large clinical trials demonstrated efficacy of bevacizumab in combination with a platinum containing chemotherapy in patients with advanced NSCLC of nonsquamous histology, resulting in the FDA approval for this setting (Table 44.5).[91,92] In the ECOG 4599 study, a substantial clinical benefit for NSCLC patients treated with 15 mg/kg bevacizumab plus carboplatin and paclitaxel versus chemotherapy alone was seen (HR, 0.66 for PFS with a median of 6.2 vs. 4.5 months; HR, 0.79 for OS with a median of 12.3 vs. 10.3 months).[91] These results were partly confirmed by another large phase III trial where NSCLC patients had an improved PFS with the addition of low-dose bevacizumab (7.5 mg/kg; HR, 0.75 (0.64–0.87); $p = 0.0003$) or high-dose bevacizumab (15 mg/kg; HR, 0.85 (0.73–1.00); $p = 0.0456$) to a standard chemotherapy of cisplatin and gemcitabine.[92] In the later study, however, the median net gain of PFS was relatively modest with bevacizumab, and, more importantly, there was no improvement in OS (HR, 0.93; 95% CI, 0.78–1.11; $p = 0.42$ and HR, 1.03; 95% CI, 0.86–1.23; $p = 0.761$ for the 7.5 and 15 mg/kg groups, respectively).[93] As a result of these phase III trials in chemotherapy-naive NSCLC patients, bevacizumab has been approved for the treatment of advanced NSCLC, excluding predominantly squamous cell histology, in combination with platinum containing chemotherapy.

Bevacizumab and other antiangiogenic agents are associated with a low, but significant risk of grade ≥3 or fatal (grade 5) pulmonary hemorrhage. Two meta-analyses have found that the use of bevacizumab in combination with chemotherapy for the treatment of various tumor types conferred a significantly increased risk of severe and fatal bleeding events and treatment-related mortality versus chemotherapy alone.[94,95] However, patients

TABLE 44.5 Comparison of Phase III Studies of Platinum Doublet Therapy With Bevacizumab

	ECOG 4599[79]	AVAiL[92,93]
Regimen	Carboplatin/paclitaxel/± bevacizumab	Carboplatin/gemcitabine/± bevacizumab
Bevacizumab Dose	15 mg/kg	Low dose: 7.5 mg/kg
		High dose: 15 mg/kg
Response Rate	35% vs. 15%	34% (low) vs. 30% (high) vs. 20%
Median Progression-Free Survival	6.2 months vs. 4.5 months	6.7 months (low) vs. 6.5 months (high) vs. 6.1 months
Median Overall Survival	12.3 months vs. 10.3 months	13.6 months (low) vs. 13.4 months (high) vs. 13.1 months
Hazard Ratio Death	0.79 (95% CI, 0.67–0.92), $p = 0.003$	0.93 (95% CI, 0.78–1.11), $p = 0.42$ (low)
		1.03 (95% CI, 0.86–1.23), $p = 0.76$ (high)

CI, Confidence interval.

with NSCLC are at an increased risk of pulmonary hemorrhage owing to the underlying disease process, with non–life-threatening bleeds occurring in 16% of 877 patients with lung cancer.[96] Nearly 3% of these were fatal. Massive pulmonary hemorrhage was significantly associated with squamous cell tumors, cavitation, and with bronchial (vs. peripheral) tumors.[96] Recently, an expert panel recommended that patients with squamous histology and/or a history of grade ≥2 hemoptysis (≥2.5 mL per event) should not receive bevacizumab.[97] However, no clinical or radiologic features (including cavitation and central tumor location) reliably predict severe pulmonary hemorrhage in bevacizumab-treated patients. Major blood vessel infiltration and bronchial vessel infiltration, encasement, and abutting may increase the risk of pulmonary hemorrhage; however, standardized radiologic criteria for defining infiltration have not been established. In all these studies, patients received maintenance therapy with bevacizumab after completion of chemotherapy; still, the benefit of this maintenance has not been prospectively addressed in large clinical trials for NSCLC, so far.

Other Antiangiogenic Agents

The therapeutic success achieved with bevacizumab in NSCLC has prompted the evaluation of several other antiangiogenic agents. Various small-molecule tyrosine kinase inhibitors (TKIs) have been tested in clinical studies in advanced NSCLC. As a common feature of these agents, the spectrum of inhibited receptors is not limited to VEGF receptor (VEGFR) but comprises various further growth factors and signaling pathways. While the broader activity was considered likely to improve the therapeutic benefit, the spectrum of side effects is also expanded, and it renders difficult conclusions regarding the relevance of targeting VEGFR. To date, no drug in this class has demonstrated survival improvement in randomized studies. Phase II studies addressing monotherapy with multi-TKIs have demonstrated modest activity with response rates ranging from 7% to 10% and median time to progression from 2.4 months to 5.8 months in pretreated NSCLC patients. Moreover, several phase III trials have recently been completed that have assessed multikinase antiangiogenic TKIs in a second-, third-, and/or fourth-line setting such as sunitinib (in combination with erlotinib),[98] vandetanib (in combination with docetaxel or pemetrexed),[99,100] and sorafenib monotherapy.[101] Unfortunately, the outcome of these trials was disappointing; despite an improvement in response rates and PFS in most trials, these antiangiogenic TKIs had no impact on OS. Some additional phase III trials are ongoing to assess novel newer agents that have shown promising activity in phase II trials such as pazopanib and apatinib.[102]

In a recent meta-analysis of 15 randomized controlled trials investigating multitargeted antiangiogenic TKIs (vandetanib, sunitinib, cediranib, sorafenib, motesanib) in combination with chemotherapy or as monotherapy in advanced NSCLC, treatment with multi-TKIs was associated with a significantly longer PFS (HR, 0.824; 95% CI, 0.759–0.895; $p < 0.001$) and superior response rate (OR, 1.27; 95% CI, 1.13–1.42; $p < 0.0001$) compared with the control arm.[103] However, OS was not significantly different (HR, 0.962; 95% CI, 0.912–1.015; $p = 0.157$). Other VEGFR inhibitors currently under development include pazopanib, apatinib, and nintedanib.

Two phase III trials (LUME-Lung 1 and 2) were presented investigating nintedanib, a TKI targeting VEGF-, PDGF-, and FGF-receptors. After failure of first-line chemotherapy, 1314 stage IIIB–IV NSCLC patients were randomized to treatment with docetaxel with or without nintedanib (LUME-1).[104,105] The primary end point, PFS, was significantly improved by the addition of nintedanib (3.4 vs. 2.7 months; HR, 0.79; 95% CI, 0.68–0.92; $p = 0.0019$) while OS was not significantly different (10.1 vs. 9.1 months; HR, 0.94; 95% CI, 0.83–1.05; $p = 0.2720$). However, in a prespecified subgroup analysis, patients with adenocarcinoma had both a significant and clinically meaningful improved PFS (4.0 vs. 2.8 months; HR, 0.77; 95% CI, 0.62–0.96; $p = 0.0193$) and OS (12.6 vs. 10.3 months; HR, 0.83; 95% CI, 0.70–0.99; $p = 0.0359$). Also, there was a significant improvement in disease control rate with the nintedanib plus docetaxel combination (adenocarcinoma 60.2% vs. 44%; OR, 1.93; $p < 0.0001$; squamous cell carcinoma 49.3% vs. 35.5%; OR, 1.78; $p < 0.0009$). These data were somewhat confirmed by another phase III trial investigating the second-line combination of pemetrexed with or without nintedanib in patients with advanced or recurrent, non-squamous NSCLC after treatment with first-line chemotherapy (LUME-2).[106] Despite stopping the trial after recruitment of 713 of the 1300 intended patients, the primary end point was still met as PFS was significantly superior after treatment with nintedanib plus pemetrexed (4.4. vs. 3.6 months; HR, 0.83; 95% CI, 0.70–0.99; $p = 0.0435$). Collectively, the LUME-1 study is the first phase III study demonstrating a survival benefit of adding a multi-TKI to chemotherapy in a prespecified subgroup.

Ramucirumab is a monoclonal antibody that binds to VEGFR-2 and blocks ligand binding and activation. A phase III study (REVEL) investigated ramucirumab in combination with docetaxel as second-line therapy after failure of platinum-based therapy ($n = 1253$ patients including those with squamous histology).[107] The addition of ramucirumab to docetaxel resulted in a significant improvement in median OS (10.5 months vs. 9.1 months; HR, 0.86; 95% CI, 0.75–0.98; $p = 0.023$) and PFS (4.5 months vs. 3.0 months; HR, 0.76; 95% CI, 0.68–0.86; $p < 0.0001$). Notable toxicities with ramucirumab were neutropenia, febrile neutropenia, fatigue, leukopenia, and hypertension. The combination of docetaxel with ramucirumab has gained approval by the United States FDA for salvage therapy of advanced NSCLC. Aflibercept is an investigational recombinant protein composed of epitopes of the extracellular domains of human VEGFR fused to the constant region (Fc) of human immunoglobulin G1 (IgG1) functioning as a soluble decoy receptor. The addition of aflibercept to second-line docetaxel in NSCLC patients was associated with improved ORR, but there was no improvement in OS.[108] Vascular disrupting agents that cause destruction of existing tumor vasculature have also been studied in lung

TABLE 44.6 EGFR TKI Versus Platinum Doublet Chemotherapy in *EGFR*-Mutated NSCLC

Platinum Doublet	EGFR TKI	Response Rate	HR Progression (95% CI)	HR Death (95% CI)
Carboplatin/paclitaxel[118]	Gefitinib	31% vs. 74%	0.30 (0.22–0.41) $p < 0.001$	Not reported $p = 0.31$
Cisplatin/docetaxel[119]	Gefitinib	32% vs. 61%	0.489 (0.336–0.71) $p < 0.0001$	1.638 (0.749–3.582) $p = 0.211$
Carboplatin/gemcitabine[120]	Erlotinib	36% vs. 83%	0.16 (0.10–0.26) $p < 0.0001$	Not reported
Cisplatin/docetaxel or gemcitabine[121]	Erlotinib	18% vs. 64%	0.37 (0.25–0.54) $p < 0.0001$	1.04 (0.65–1.68) $p = 0.87$
Cisplatin/pemetrexed[122]	Afatinib	23% vs. 56%	0.58 (0.43–0.78) $p = 0.001$	1.12 (0.73–1.73) $p = 0.60$

CI, confidence interval; *EGFR*, epidermal growth factor receptor; *HR*, hazard ratio; *TKI*, tyrosine kinase inhibitor.

cancer without much success.[109] There are no proven biomarkers to select patients for antiangiogenic agents in NSCLC. This has undoubtedly limited the utilization of these agents in the clinic.

EPIDERMAL GROWTH FACTOR BLOCKADE IN NSCLC

EGFR Tyrosine Kinase Inhibitors

EGFR is a member of the ErbB family of transmembrane tyrosine kinase receptors, which bind ligands such as epidermal growth factor. Upon ligand-binding, the receptor undergoes either homo- or hetero-dimerization with another member of the ErbB family, resulting in activation of downstream signaling cascades that lead to cell proliferation and survival.[110] The determination that many cancers, including NSCLC, have aberrant EGFR signaling led to the development of EGFR-blocking therapies. Gefitinib and erlotinib are small molecule EGFR TKIs that have activity in NSCLC, particularly in patients with activating mutations in EGFR.

EGFR TKIs were first studied in unselected NSCLC patients in the second- and third-line setting. Erlotinib was found to benefit patients with previously treated metastatic disease in the BR.21 study.[111] Initial phase II studies with gefitinib were also conducted in unselected patients and observed response rates of approximately 10% to 19%. With both of these agents, there was a greater likelihood for response in females, never-smokers, patients with Asian ethnicity, and those with adenocarcinoma histology. The biologic rationale for these observations came to light with the discovery of mutations in the EGFR in 2004.[100,101] Patients that derived robust responses to EGFR TKIs were likely to harbor an activating mutation in the tyrosine kinase-binding pocket of the *EGFR* gene. The mutations were primarily localized to two "hot" spots on exons 19 and 21. The prevalence of the activating mutations was more frequent in the clinical subset of patients that experienced a higher response rate with EGFR TKIs. Following this landmark discovery, a number of phase II studies were conducted exclusively for patients with EGFR mutation. Treatment with either gefitinib or erlotinib resulted in response rates of 50% to 80% with median PFS of 8 to 12 months.

Before the description of EGFR activating mutations, phase III studies were conducted to combine erlotinib and gefitinib with standard chemotherapy for the first-line therapy of advanced NSCLC. None of these studies demonstrated an improvement in OS.[112–115] Subsequent trials included clinical enrichment to identify patients that might benefit from EGFR TKI given alone or in combination with chemotherapy. The CALGB conducted a randomized phase II study in never-smokers with advanced NSCLC.[116] Patients received erlotinib alone or in combination with carboplatin and paclitaxel. Overall, there was no difference in efficacy for the entire patient population in the two treatment arms. However, in the 40% of patients with EGFR mutation, the response rate and OS were higher than in those with wild-type EGFR. There was no suggestion of improvement in efficacy

with the addition of chemotherapy to erlotinib in patients with an EGFR mutation. This study suggested that clinical selection is unlikely to help identify patients appropriate for EGFR TKI therapy.

This issue was definitively addressed by the Iressa Pan-Asia Study (IPASS) that enrolled Asian patients with adenocarcinoma of the lung and never or light cigarette smoking history. Patients were randomized to treatment with gefitinib or carboplatin and paclitaxel for frontline therapy of advanced stage disease.[117] There was a significant improvement in PFS with gefitinib compared with carboplatin/paclitaxel with a HR of 0.74 (95% CI, 0.65–0.85; $p < 0.001$). In 261 patients found to have *EGFR* mutations, treatment with gefitinib achieved an ORR of 71.2% compared with only 47.3% with chemotherapy, with an increase in PFS (HR, 0.48; 95% CI, 0.36–0.64; $p < 0.001$). The response rate in the 176 patients who tested negative for *EGFR* mutation with gefitinib was only 1.1% versus 23.5% with chemotherapy; in contrast, the mutation negative patients derived a PFS benefit with carboplatin and paclitaxel (HR, 2.85; 95% CI, 2.05–3.98; $p < 0.001$). These results demonstrated that EGFR TKIs only benefit patients with *EGFR* mutations in the frontline setting. Therefore, molecular selection, and not clinical selection, should be used to identify patients that will benefit from frontline use of EGFR TKIs.

Several studies have compared gefitinib or erlotinib with different chemotherapy regimens in *EGFR*-mutated patients treated in the first-line setting; all these studies have shown an ORR from 60% to 80% with PFS benefit (Table 44.6).[118–121] Maemondo et al.[118] published the results of the first study of EGFR TKI versus carboplatin and paclitaxel in the frontline setting in patients with activating EGFR mutations. Patients were selected by the presence of activating *EGFR* mutation; patients with the resistant T790M mutation were ineligible. This study randomized 230 patients to treatment with either gefitinib or carboplatin and paclitaxel. Patients who received EGFR TKI achieved an ORR of 73.7% compared with only 30.7% with chemotherapy ($p < 0.001$). Patients with *EGFR* mutations treated with gefitinib also achieved a longer PFS with median of 10.8 months versus 5.4 months with chemotherapy (HR, 0.30; 95% CI, 0.22–0.41; $p < 0.001$). This was consistent with the results seen in the subgroup analysis of EGFR-mutated patients in the IPASS study. Although there was a trend toward longer OS with TKI (30.5 months vs. 23.6 months), this was not statistically significant ($p = 0.31$). Similar to other EGFR TKI studies, almost all (94.6%) of the patients treated in the chemotherapy arm went on to receive EGFR TKI at the time of disease progression. In a subgroup analysis by *EGFR* mutation type, there was no difference in PFS or response rate between patients with exon 19 deletions compared with point mutations in L858R on exon 21. This study helped confirm that *EGFR* activating mutations are predictive of therapeutic benefit from treatment with EGFR TKIs.

The majority of studies demonstrating the success of EGFR TKI in EGFR-mutated patients have been conducted in predominantly Asian populations. The EURTAC study was a randomized phase III study comparing the efficacy of erlotinib with chemotherapy (cisplatin and docetaxel or cisplatin and gemcitabine) in European patients with activating *EGFR* mutations. This study achieved its primary end point of PFS benefit at the first interim efficacy analysis with only 174 patients enrolled: patients treated with erlotinib achieved a median PFS of 9.7 months compared with 5.2 months in the chemotherapy arm (HR, 0.37; 95% CI, 0.25–0.54; $p < 0.0001$). Interestingly, patients with exon 19 deletions seemed to derive a greater PFS benefit than those with L858R mutations, which was also observed in the IPASS study. Again, similar to previous studies of EGFR TKI versus chemotherapy, ORR with erlotinib was 64% compared with only 18% with chemotherapy, and there was no survival benefit seen (HR, 1.04; 95% CI, 0.65–1.68; $p = 0.87$). This was the first study examining the efficacy of EGFR TKI therapy in a non-Asian population, and its findings were similar to the PFS advantages seen in Asian populations with *EGFR* mutations treated with EGFR TKI. These studies substantiate the evidence that patients should be tested for the presence of activating *EGFR* mutations at the time of diagnosis of lung cancer, as they derive robust therapeutic gains from EGFR TKI therapy.

Afatinib, an irreversible inhibitor of EGFR, HER2, and ErbB4 receptors, was first studied in advanced NSCLC patients who failed prior EGFR TKI therapy after previous chemotherapy in the LUX-Lung 1 study.[123] In EGFR-mutated patients who were EGFR TKI naive, afatinib was associated with a response rate of over 60%.[124] Patients were initially treated with the maximum tolerated dose of 50 mg of afatinib; however, the higher dose resulted in severe rash and diarrhea, and consequently 40 mg/day was used thereafter. A phase III study was conducted to compare the efficacy of afatinib with standard chemotherapy in patients with an *EGFR* mutation. In the frontline setting, *EGFR*-mutated patients treated with afatinib had a longer PFS (11.1 months) than those treated with cisplatin and pemetrexed (6.9 months) (HR, 0.58; 95% CI, 0.43–0.78; $p < 0.001$); those with exon 19 deletions and L858R mutations achieved an even greater benefit, with PFS of 13.6 months (HR, 0.47; 95% CI, 0.34–0.65; $p < 0.001$).[122] On the basis of these results, the FDA approved afatinib for the treatment of *EGFR*-mutated NSCLC. Afatinib is associated with a higher incidence of skin rash, diarrhea, and mucositis compared with the first-generation EGFR TKIs. Dacomitinib, another irreversible EGFR inhibitor, also demonstrated favorable efficacy in a randomized phase II study when compared with erlotinib.[125] Based on these observations, phase III studies are presently underway to compare irreversible inhibitors with first generation compounds in patients with advanced NSCLC. The LUX-Lung 7 study randomized 319 patients with EGFR activating mutations to afatinib 40 mg daily or gefitinib 250 mg daily.[126] The primary end points of PFS (11.0 months with afatinib vs. 10.9 months with gefitinib; HR, 0.73; 95% CI, 0.57–0.95; $p = 0.017$) and time to treatment failure were more favorable with afatinib (13.7 months vs. 11.5 months; HR, 0.73; 95% CI, 0.58–0.92; $p = 0.0073$), though there was no difference in survival. The toxicity profile was less favorable with afatinib, though discontinuation rate of treatment due to toxicity was similar in both groups.

Combining EGFR-blockade with angiogenesis inhibition may be a strategy to improve outcomes in patients with activating *EGFR* mutations. In a phase II study in Japan, 154 patients were randomized to erlotinib 150 mg daily or erlotinib plus bevacizumab 15 mg/kg IV every 3 weeks.[127] The study achieved the primary end point with improvement in median PFS of 9.7 months with erlotinib to 16 months with combination therapy (HR, 0.54; 95% CI, 0.36–0.79; $p = 0.0015$). The addition of bevacizumab resulted in a higher incidence of grade 3 or higher adverse events (AEs) with 91% of patients in the combination arm compared with only 53% in the erlotinib arm, with the most common AEs including rash, hypertension, and proteinuria. This

combination has recently been approved for use in Europe. Confirmatory trials are underway in the United States.

Monoclonal Antibody Against EGFR

Cetuximab is a chimeric monoclonal antibody that binds and inhibits the EGFR. Cetuximab has been tested in combination with chemotherapy in patients with metastatic NSCLC in phase III studies. The First-Line ErbituX in lung cancer (FLEX) study randomized 1125 patients with chemotherapy naive advanced NSCLC (stage IIIB/IV) with EGFR expression by IHC to chemotherapy consisting of cisplatin and vinorelbine given with or without cetuximab.[128] This study demonstrated a superior OS with the addition of cetuximab to chemotherapy (11.3 months vs. 10.1 months, HR 0.871 [0.762–0.996, $p = 0.044$]). However, the median PFS was similar for the two arms, at 4.8 months (HR, 0.943; $p = 0.39$). Cetuximab increased ORR from 29% with chemotherapy alone to 36% ($p = 0.01$). Another phase III study (BMS099) failed to detect a survival benefit with the addition of cetuximab to first-line chemotherapy in the metastatic setting.[129] This trial randomized 676 patients with metastatic NSCLC to treatment with chemotherapy consisting of carboplatin and a taxane (either paclitaxel or docetaxel) with or without cetuximab. Unlike the FLEX study, this study did not select patients based on EGFR expression status. There was an improvement in ORR (25.7% with cetuximab versus 17.2% without, $p = 0.007$) but this did not result in a difference in median PFS, which was the primary end point, with a HR of 0.902 (0.761–1.069; $p = 0.236$). The lack of benefit remained consistent in analysis of OS: median OS with cetuximab was 9.69 months versus 8.38 months with chemotherapy alone but was not statistically significant (HR, 0.89 [0.754–1.051; $p = 0.169$]). In an exploratory post-hoc analysis, the development of a rash prior to day 21 with cetuximab was correlated with an OS benefit: median OS with early rash was 10.4 months compared with only 8.9 months in those without early rash (HR, 0.76; 95% CI, 0.59–0.98).

The SWOG S0819 study randomized 1333 patients to carboplatin and paclitaxel (with bevacizumab if appropriate) with or without cetuximab.[130] The primary end points of the study were OS and PFS in patients who were EGFR positive by fluorescence in situ hybridization (FISH). The addition of cetuximab did not increase median OS (HR, 0.94; $p = 0.34$). However, in the EGFR positive patients (by FISH), median OS improved from 9.8 months in the control arm to 13.4 months in the cetuximab arm (HR, 0.83; $p = 0.10$). In the squamous patients who were EGFR positive by FISH, the median OS benefit with cetuximab was more dramatic: 11.8 months versus 6.4 months (HR, 0.56; $p = 0.06$). These results suggest that EGFR FISH testing may help select patients who are the most likely to benefit from adding cetuximab to combination chemotherapy in the frontline setting.

Other novel EGFR-targeted antibody therapies have also been studied in NSCLC. Matuzumab, a humanized IgG1 monoclonal antibody against EGFR, was tested in a phase II study in combination with pemetrexed in the second-line treatment of NSCLC.[131] This study failed to achieve its primary end point of increase in ORR (11% with matuzumab compared with 5% pemetrexed, $p = 0.332$) with a trend toward an increase in survival with the addition of matuzumab (7.9 months with pemetrexed, 5.9 months with matuzumab every 3 weeks, and 12.4 months with weekly matuzumab); 87% of tumors had EGFR expression by IHC; in a subgroup analysis, all but one of the responses was seen in EGFR positive tumors. Panitumumab, a fully human IgG2 monoclonal anti-EGFR antibody, was tested in combination with multiple different chemotherapy regimens in phase I and II trials in patients with metastatic NSCLC in first-line and beyond, with modest results.[132] Finally, necitumumab (IMC-11F8), a recombinant human antibody with a similar structure to cetuximab, was studied in the SQUIRE trial in combination with cisplatin and gemcitabine in squamous cell lung cancer. The addition of necitumumab to chemotherapy resulted in a modest but statistically significant improvement in median OS from 9.9 months to 11.5 months (HR, 0.84; 95% CI, 0.74–0.96; p = 0.01).[133] These findings have led to regulatory approval of this regimen for the frontline therapy of patients with metastatic squamous cell carcinoma of the lung in both the United States and Europe.

Biomarkers for EGFR Blockade

Many different biomarkers have been assessed in patients treated with EGFR-targeted therapies. Biomarker analyses of early studies have demonstrated no consistent association with EGFR IHC, copy number by FISH, or Kirsten rat sarcoma (KRAS) mutations.[134–137] The cytosine-adenine (CA) dinucleotide repeat, a polymorphism present in intron 1 of EGFR that modulates its transcription, has also been studied as a potential biomarker for EGFR-targeted therapies. There have been conflicting data about the utility of short CA repeats as a biomarker, as this was correlated with response and PFS in a Korean study but not in a retrospective analysis of the BR.21 study.[138,139] Given the challenges of obtaining adequate tumor tissue for analysis of EGFR mutations, there has been interest in utilizing serum proteomics to develop a predictive algorithm with matrix-assisted laser desorption ionization mass spectrometry (MALDI MS).[140] Patients can be stratified into good and poor prognosis subgroups by MALDI MS, which has been commercially developed as the VeriStrat assay (Biodesix, Boulder, CO, USA). The utility of the VeriStrat assay has been evaluated in retrospective patient cohorts.[141,142] More recently, VeriStrat was tested prospectively in the phase III PROSE study, which randomized patients with metastatic NSCLC to treatment with erlotinib or chemotherapy with either pemetrexed or docetaxel.[143] VeriStrat was able to identify patients that benefited from erlotinib in the second-line setting. The utility of this test in the frontline therapy setting has not been studied.

In 2004, two groups independently described sensitizing mutations in EGFR in patients with NSCLC that achieved objective responses with gefitinib.[144,145] The predictive potential of EGFR mutations was confirmed in the IPASS study that demonstrated improved ORR and PFS benefit in patients treated with gefitinib.[117] In an updated analysis of the IPASS study, there was no OS benefit seen in patients treated with gefitinib versus carboplatin and paclitaxel, with a HR of 0.90 (95% CI, 9.79–1.02; p = 0.109), irrespective of EGFR mutation status.[146] These results suggest that the presence of an EGFR mutation is the strongest predictor of ORR and PFS in patients treated with EGFR TKIs. The lack of association of EGFR mutation with predicting OS benefit is likely due to the crossover design of the IPASS study and subsequent EGFR TKI studies in the frontline setting.[118–121] Multiple studies have proven the value of utilizing activating EGFR mutations as the selection criterion for first-line therapy with EGFR TKI.[118–121]

On the basis of these studies, new guidelines have been created to guide testing of NSCLC tissue for EGFR mutations in pathology labs.[147] These guidelines confirm that molecular testing should be performed to select patients with adenocarcinoma of the lung for EGFR TKI therapy. All patients with adenocarcinoma histology should be tested for EGFR mutations, irrespective of clinical characteristics or the presence of other histologies mixed with adenocarcinoma histology. Testing should be performed at the time of diagnosis for patients with metastatic disease and can be performed on resection specimens based on institutional preferences. Specimens that can be used for testing include fresh, frozen, or formalin-fixed, paraffin embedded tissue. There are multiple acceptable methodologies available for detection of EGFR mutations (Sanger sequencing, polymerase chain reaction [PCR]-based assays, single-base extension genotyping, high performance liquid chromatography assays). It is recommended that the assay used should be able to detect mutations in samples with at least 50% tumor content. Based on the studies discussed above, it is not recommended to routinely test for EGFR IHC, copy number by FISH, or Kirsten rat sarcoma (KRAS) mutations to select patients for EGFR TKI therapy.

Resistance to EGFR TKIs

The efficacy of EGFR TKIs in EGFR-mutated NSCLC is eventually overcome by the development of acquired resistance, with a median PFS ranging from approximately 10 to 14 months. The Jackman criteria were developed to clearly define patients with acquired resistance to help guide future studies for this patient population.[148] The Jackman criteria define acquired resistance as the development of disease progression while on EGFR TKI for at least 30 days with no other intervening systemic therapy in patients treated with single-agent EGFR TKI with either a known sensitizing EGFR mutation or documented disease stabilization or response by Response Evaluation Criteria in Solid Tumors (RECIST) criteria for at least 6 months while on EGFR TKI if mutation status is unknown.

Various strategies have been studied in the clinic to overcome resistance to EGFR inhibitors. One strategy has been to continue EGFR TKI beyond progression. The ASPIRATION study investigated the efficacy of this approach in an Asian population.[149] Patients received erlotinib 150 mg daily until disease progression and could be continued on therapy postprogression at the investigator's discretion. The median time to initial progression (PFS1) was 10.8 months; of these 176 patients, 93 continued on TKI postprogression. The PFS2 (time to discontinuation of erlotinib after initial progression) was 14.1 months with a median OS of 31 months. This prospective study shows that treatment beyond progression may help delay initiation of second-line therapy, although this should be limited to patients who do not have rapid disease progression or clinical deterioration.

The IMPRESS study examined the utility of continuing EGFR inhibition with the initiation of platinum doublet chemotherapy following the development of acquired resistance.[150] This international study randomized 265 patients to cisplatin and pemetrexed with gefitinib 250 mg daily or placebo for up to six cycles. There was no difference in the primary end point of PFS: median PFS was 5.4 months in both arms (HR, 0.86; 95% CI, 0.65–1.13; p = 0.27). These results confirm that there is no role for combining EGFR TKI with salvage platinum doublet chemotherapy in patients who develop acquired resistance to frontline EGFR inhibition.

Multiple mechanisms of resistance have been described by studying tumor tissue from patients who develop resistance on EGFR-targeted therapy. The most common is the development of the T790M mutation in nearly 50% of patients: T790M is a gatekeeper mutant, which hinders the binding of the TKI to the enzyme active site, similar to the T315I mutation in CML.[151,152] Surprisingly, T790M mutants have a slower rate of growth compared with the parent mutated EGFR. New TKIs that can overcome the steric hindrance of the T790M are being developed. The FDA recently approved a third-generation T790M inhibitor, osimertinib, dosed at 80 mg daily for the treatment of patients with T790M resistant EGFR-mutated NSCLC after progression on first-line TKI. The approval was on the basis of a phase I dose expansion study that showed an ORR of 61% (95% CI, 52–70) and median PFS of 9.6 months (95% CI, 8.3 to not reached [NR]) in patients with T790M mutation.[153] Those without T790M had a more modest ORR of 21% (95% CI, 12–34) with PFS of 2.8 months (95% CI, 2.1–4.3). The most common AEs with osimertinib were diarrhea, rash, and nausea;

the incidence of grade 3 or higher AEs was only 32%. Osimertinib is now being studied in the first-line setting for patients with EGFR mutation.

Combination strategies such as afatinib and cetuximab have shown some promise in the lab in overcoming EGFR resistance.[152,154] This combination can also overcome HER2 overexpression, which is another resistance pathway seen in close to 10% of patients with acquired resistance.[155] Another resistance mechanism is amplification of the hepatocyte growth factor receptor (MET) oncogene, which has been described in 5% to 20% of EGFR TKI resistant patients and can occur in the presence or absence of the T790M mutation.[156,157] Other mechanisms of resistance include phenotypic transformation to small cell lung cancer (14%), PIK3CA mutations (5%), and epithelial to mesenchymal transformation.[158] These varied resistance mechanisms highlight the importance of obtaining biopsies at the time of disease progression on EGFR TKI in order to guide subsequent therapies.

Although T790M is a common mechanism of acquired resistance to EGFR TKI, it has also been described as a de novo mutation in the absence of exposure to EGFR TKI. Inukai and colleagues[159] first described 9 patients with de novo T790M in a cohort of 280 patients when testing with a mutant enriched PCR assay; none of these patients responded to gefitinib, even the 4 patients with concurrent activating EGFR mutations. The IPASS study also had a low incidence of de novo T790M mutants (4.2% or 11 patients), seven of whom had either L858R mutation or exon 19 deletion as well; however, treatment responses for these patients were not reported.[117] In the iTARGET study, only one patient had a de novo T790M mutation and was resistant to treatment with gefitinib.[160] In a study of detection of EGFR mutations by sequencing of circulating tumor cells or plasma free DNA, low levels of T790M were detected in pretreatment samples in over a third of patients (10 of 26 patients); this resulted in a shorter PFS of 7.7 months compared with 16.5 months in EGFR-mutated patients treated with EGFR TKIs.[161] Recently a small series of patients with de novo T790M patients was reported.[162] The clinical features of these patients were similar to those of patients with activating EGFR mutations; however, the patients with de novo T790M had very low response rates to erlotinib with a much shorter median PFS and OS (1.5 months and 16 months, respectively) compared with patients with activating EGFR mutations (median OS 3 years). In this cohort, all patients had concurrent activating EGFR mutations (80% L858R and 20% exon 19 deletions). These studies suggest that de novo T790M mutations may exist subclinically in certain patients and are selected as a dominant clone with EGFR TKI therapy, leading to poor response rates and survival outcomes with TKI therapy. Interestingly, the presence of germline T790M mutations has been linked with familial lung adenocarcinoma cancer risk.[163,164] In an evaluation of 10 patients with de novo T790M mutations, 50% of the cases carried germline T790M alterations. There is an ongoing perspective trial (INHERIT-EGFR) to better characterize the lung cancer risk in carriers of germline T790M mutations.[165]

ALK-REARRANGED NSCLC

The EML4-ALK translocation in NSCLC was first described in 2007. This genetic abnormality induces the transformation of lung cancer cells by constitutive activation of ALK.[166] The EML4-ALK translocation is present in 1% to 5% of NSCLC cases and tends to occur more frequently in younger NSCLC patients who are never-smokers, with median age at diagnosis of 52 years.[167] Crizotinib is a dual inhibitor of ALK and MET, which was found to have activity in patients with ALK rearrangements, with an ORR of 57% in the initial phase I study.[168] In a recent update of the expanded phase I study, the ORR was reported at 60.8% with a median PFS of 9.7 months;[169] on the basis of these results, the

FDA approved crizotinib for the treatment of ALK-rearranged NSCLC. Patients treated with crizotinib in the second-line setting have an ORR of 65% and also derive a benefit of increased PFS of 7.7 months compared with 3 months with pemetrexed or docetaxel (HR, 0.49; 95% CI, 0.37–0.64; p < 0.001).[170] Crizotinib is generally well tolerated; the most frequently seen adverse events include gastrointestinal toxicities, vision changes that usually subside with continued therapy, and peripheral edema.

Unfortunately, similar to EGFR inhibition with EGFR TKIs, the benefits of crizotinib are frequently overcome by the development of resistance. A secondary mutation in the EML4-ALK gene, at C1196M, which is a gatekeeper mutant similar to T790M in EGFR, was observed in an initial report.[171] Amplification of the ALK gene also contributes to acquired resistance to crizotinib.[172] Evaluation of patients who developed crizotinib resistance has also shown other novel mutations in the ALK kinase, autophosphorylation of EGFR, KRAS mutation, and amplification of KIT as other mechanisms of resistance.[173,174]

Newer ALK inhibitors are in development to overcome some of these resistance mechanisms. Ceritinib is a potent ALK inhibitor that has shown impressive activity in a phase I study of 131 patients with ALK-rearranged NSCLC: the ORR was 58% (95% CI, 48–67) in patients who received at least 400 mg daily with median PFS of 7 months.[175] Clinical activity was seen in patients who had previously failed on crizotinib; the ORR was 56% in patients who were crizotinib failures. Ceritinib was mainly associated with gastrointestinal toxicities and fatigue.

Another novel ALK inhibitor, CH5424802, now known as alectinib, was tested in a phase I/II study in Japan for ALK-rearranged NSCLC patients: the maximum tolerated dose was defined as 300 mg twice a day though no dose limiting toxicities were observed.[176] The ORR was 93.5% with two complete responses, and the median PFS had not been reached at the time of the report. The most frequent grade 3 adverse events were neutropenia and elevated creatine phosphokinase (CPK). In a phase I/II study of alectinib in patients who progressed or were intolerant of crizotinib, dose limiting toxicities of grade 3 headache and elevated Gamma-Glutamyl Transpeptidase (GGT) were seen in two patients at a dose level of 900 mg twice daily.[177] The ORR was 55%, with a 52% response rate seen in central nervous system (CNS) metastases. This study determined the recommended phase II dose of alectinib to be 600 mg twice a day. Alectinib's activity in crizotinib resistant patients was confirmed in a phase II study of 87 patients who received alectinib 600 mg twice daily after disease progression on crizotinib.[178] The ORR was 48% (95% CI, 36–60) with median PFS of 8.1 months (95% CI, 6.2–12.6); 100% intracranial disease control was seen in the 16 patients with measurable CNS disease. The most common AEs were constipation, fatigue, myalgia, and peripheral edema. These results have led to approval of alectinib in patients who have progressed on or are intolerant of crizotinib.

Alectinib has also shown efficacy in treatment-naive ALK-positive NSCLC patients compared with the current standard crizotinib as reported in the J-ALEX study.[179] This study randomized 200 patients with centrally confirmed ALK-positive metastatic disease (by IHC, FISH, or reverse transcription-PCR) to alectinib 300 mg twice daily or crizotinib 250 mg twice daily in the frontline setting. The patients in the alectinib arm had an improved ORR of 91.6% (95% CI, 85.6–97.5%) compared with the crizotinib arm with only 78.9% (95% CI, 70.5–87.3%). More impressively, the primary end point of improved median PFS with alectinib was achieved with a HR of 0.34 (95% CI, 0.17–0.71; p < 0.0001). The improved efficacy of alectinib also came with reduced toxicity: the rate of grade 3–4 AEs was 26.2% compared with 51.9% in the crizotinib arm. Based on these impressive results, the FDA has designated breakthrough status for alectinib as first-line therapy in ALK-positive advanced disease. Finally, heat shock protein 90 inhibition with IPI-504[180] and STA-9090[181] has shown promise in patients with *ALK*-rearranged NSCLC and may provide alternative approaches to overcome crizotinib resistance.

There are various diagnostic assays for the detection of ALK rearrangement, including FISH and IHC. A break-apart FISH assay was used to select patients for the initial phase I and II studies of crizotinib; the commercially available Vysis ALK Break Apart FISH probe kit (Abbott Molecular Probes, Abbott Park, Illinois, USA) was approved as a companion diagnostic for selection of ALK-rearranged patients to be treated with crizotinib by the FDA.[182] A positive result is the presence of at least 15% split red and green signals or isolated red signals.[183] IHC is a cheaper testing methodology and is more readily available in most pathology labs compared with the more technically challenging FISH test. The sensitivity and specificity of ALK detection of IHC has ranged between 90% to 100% and 95.8% to 99%, respectively, when correlated with ALK FISH in multiple studies.[184–186] Recent guidelines from the College of American Pathologists and IASLC recommend the use of ALK FISH for the diagnosis of ALK rearranged NSCLC to select patients for treatment with crizotinib; IHC may be used as an initial screening assay.[147]

MOLECULAR CHARACTERIZATION OF NSCLC

A number of genetic alterations beyond EGFR mutations and ALK rearrangements have been discovered in lung adenocarcinoma through the efforts of the Lung Cancer Mutation Consortium (LCMC).[187,188] More than 1000 adenocarcinomas were characterized for the presence of 10 driver mutations in LCMC-1 and more recently another 875 patient cases were analyzed for 14 driver mutations in LCMC-2.[189] Almost 60% of patients had at least one mutation: the most frequently found mutations were in *KRAS*, *EGFR*, *EML4-ALK*, and *MET* amplification (Table 44.7). Based on the testing, 28% of patients received a targeted therapy directed to the driver mutation, including several in ongoing clinical trials. Patients treated with targeted therapy in LCMC-1 achieved a longer median survival (3.5 years) compared with patients who did not receive targeted therapy or were identified as wild-type and had no targeted therapy options (2.4 years and 2.1 years, respectively, *p* < 0.0001). Similarly in LCMC-2, patients with driver mutations that received targeted therapy had prolonged survival (2.7 years) compared with those who did not receive targeted therapy (1.5 years) and wild-type patients (1.7 years). In *EGFR*-mutated patients who received targeted therapy, the presence of a secondary *TP53* mutation results in median survival of 2.9 years compared with NR in those without mutation, suggesting that p53 function may modulate response to targeted therapy. The results of both LCMC-1 and LCMC-2 demonstrate that expanded molecular profiling of lung adenocarcinomas and resultant targeted therapy improves survival in patients with advanced stages of disease.

Based on the efforts of the LCMC, there are multiple early phase studies of novel targeted therapies in lung adenocarcinoma patients. In fact, *BRAF*, which is a serine threonine kinase in the RAS-RAF-MEK pathway, is mutated in NSCLC in 2% to 5% of patients. Similar to melanoma and colon cancer, NSCLC can harbor activating mutations in *BRAF*, such as V600E, which accounts for at least half of *BRAF* mutations in NSCLC, and non-V600E mutations, which can be activating or inactivating.[190–192] Patients with *BRAF* mutations tend to have a smoking history in contrast to patients with *EGFR*-mutations and *ALK* rearrangements. As in *BRAF*-mutated melanoma, dual inhibition of the MAP kinase pathways with dabrafenib and trametinib has shown activity in *BRAF*-mutated NSCLC. In a single-arm phase II study of 57 patients with V600E *BRAF* mutations who have progressed on platinum doublet therapy, the ORR was 63.2% (95% CI, 49.3–75.6) with a median duration of response of 9.0 months

TABLE 44.7 Prevalence of Common Molecular Targets in Adenocarcinoma and Squamous Cell NSCLC

Molecular Target	Frequency (%)
ADENOCARCINOMAS (LCMC-2)	
KRAS	25
EGFR: sensitive to EGFR TKI (deletion 19, L858R, L861Q, G719X)	10
ALK rearrangement	4
MET amplification	3
V600E BRAF	2
EGFR: not sensitive to EGFR TKI (exon 20 insertions, T790M)	2
RET translocation	2
ROS1 translocation	2
HER2	1
PIK3CA	1
SQUAMOUS CELL (TCGA)	
TP53	81
MLL2	20
PIK3CA	16
CDKN2A	15
NFE2L2	15
KEAP1	12
NOTCH1	8
PTEN	8
RB1	7
HLA-A	3

ALK, anaplastic lymphoma kinase; *BRAF*, v-raf murine sarcoma viral oncogene homolog B; *CDKN2A*, cyclin dependent kinase inhibitor 2A; *EGFR*, epidermal growth factor receptor; *HER2*, human epidermal growth factor receptor 2; *HLA-A*, human leukocyte antigen-A; *KEAP1*, Kelch-like ECH-associated protein 1; *KRAS*, Kirsten rat sarcoma viral oncogene homolog; *LCMC-2*, lung cancer mutation consortium-2; *MET*, hepatocyte growth factor receptor; *MLL2*, myeloid/lymphoid or mixed lineage leukemia protein 2; *NFE2L2*, nuclear factor, erythroid 2 like 2; *NOTCH1*, Notch1; *NSCLC*, nonsmalll cell lung cancer; *PIK3CA*, phosphatidylinositol-4,5-biphosphate 3 kinase catalytic subunit alpha; *PTEN*, phosphatase and tensin homolog; *RB1*, retinoblastoma; *RET*, proto-oncogene tyrosine-protein kinase receptor; *ROS1*, ROS proto-oncogene 1, receptor tyrosine kinase; *TCGA*, The Cancer Genome Atlas; *TKI*, tyrosine kinase inhibitor; *TP53*, tumor protein 53.

(95% CI, 6.9–19.6).[193] *ROS1* fusions have been described in 1% to 2% of adenocarcinomas, which have been successfully targeted with crizotinib based on an expansion cohort of 50 patients from the phase I crizotinib study.[194] The use of crizotinib resulted in an ORR of 72% (95% CI, 58–84) with a median duration of response of 17.6 months (95% CI, 14.5–NR) and median PFS of 19.2 months (95% CI, 14.4–NR). These results have led to the approval of crizotinib for patients with *ROS1* translocations. *MET* exon 14 splicing variants result in MET amplification and are found in about 4% of lung adenocarcinomas and in a high number of sarcomatoid lung carcinomas; there are a growing number of reports of the success of using MET inhibitors like crizotinib and cabozantinib in patients with *MET* exon 14 mutations.[195–198] These studies emphasize the importance of routine genetic testing of lung adenocarcinomas to select patients who may benefit from new therapies.

In contrast, squamous cell lung cancers have lagged behind adenocarcinomas with targeted treatments, although a major breakthrough came as a result of the efforts of The Cancer Genome Atlas (TCGA).[199] The TCGA data have shown that squamous cell lung cancers, similar to other smoking-related cancers, have a high rate of somatic mutations. Multiple pathways are altered in these tumors (see Table 44.7), but up to 70% of squamous cell lung tumors have alterations in receptor tyrosine kinase pathways, which may be developed as targets for therapy.

IMMUNOTHERAPY IN NSCLC

Recent developments in the use of agents that modify immune checkpoints are finally realizing the promise of immune modulation in patients with NSCLC. Ipilumumab is a monoclonal antibody that blocks the binding of a T-cell inhibitory receptor CTLA-4 to its ligands and results in activation of T cells that can infiltrate and attack tumors. Another immune checkpoint that has been targeted with initial success in NSCLC is the programmed death-1 (PD-1) receptor, which is an inhibitory receptor on tumor infiltrating lymphocytes.[200] Its ligand, PD-L1, is overexpressed in many tumors, including NSCLC; blockade of this pathway with monoclonal antibodies against either PD-1 or PD-L1 has shown promising activity in NSCLC. The PD-1 inhibitors nivolumab and pembrolizumab have been shown to be superior to docetaxel in patients with squamous and nonsquamous histologies in the salvage setting.[201–203] PD-L1 expression by tumor proportion score has been highly correlated with efficacy of pembrolizumab;[204] regulatory approval of pembrolizumab in both the United States and Europe has been tied to high expression of PD-L1 by tumor proportion score, defined as 50% or higher expression.

Recent data with pembrolizumab have prompted a major shift in the treatment paradigm for first-line therapy of advanced NSCLC. The KEYNOTE-024 study screened 1934 treatment-naive advanced stage NSCLC patients who were *EGFR* and *ALK* negative to enroll 305 patients with at least 50% PD-L1 expression by tumor proportion score (30.2%).[205] These patients were randomized to pembrolizumab 200 mg every 3 weeks for up to 35 cycles or investigators' choice platinum doublet chemotherapy for up to 6 cycles. Patients with nonsquamous histology who received pemetrexed could receive continuation maintenance therapy. The primary end point of median PFS was superior with pembrolizumab (10.3 months vs. 6.0 months; HR, 0.50; 95% CI, 0.37–0.68; $p < 0.001$). The overall survival was also improved with a HR of 0.60 (95% CI, 0.41–0.89; $p = 0.005$). Compared with chemotherapy, pembrolizumab resulted in better ORR (44.8% vs. 27.8%) and duration of response (NR vs. 6.3 months), with less toxicity. The rate of overall treatment-related AEs and grade 3–5 AEs was 73.4% and 53.3% with pembrolizumab versus 90.0% and 26.6% with chemotherapy, respectively. These results show that PD-1 inhibition with pembrolizumab in patients with high PD-L1 staining is superior to the current standard of platinum doublet chemotherapy and will likely be reviewed favorably by regulatory agencies in the near future.

Combination immunotherapy strategies to overcome both CTLA4 and PD-1 inhibition have been successful in metastatic melanoma and are also being studied in NSCLC. The Checkmate 012 trial evaluated the safety of new dosing combinations of nivolumab and ipilimumab including nivolumab 1 mg/kg with ipilimumab 1 mg/kg every 3 weeks for four cycles followed by nivolumab maintenance 3 mg/kg every 2 weeks compared with various nivolumab dosing regimens (1 mg/kg and 3 mg/kg) every 2 weeks with longer interval ipilimumab dosing (every 12 weeks and every 6 weeks) until disease progression.[206] Interestingly, the longer interval ipilimumab dosing resulted in a numerically higher ORR (25% to 39% vs. 13%) with similar TRAE rates (69% to 73% vs. 77%). The rate of treatment adverse effects (TRAEs) (11% to 13%) leading to discontinuation in the longer ipilimumab interval arms was similar to nivolumab monotherapy. There was a trend toward higher response rate in patients with higher PD-L1 staining. On the basis of the promising results from this trial, the efficacy of nivolumab 3 mg/kg every 2 weeks plus ipilimumab 1 mg/kg every 6 weeks is being studied in multiple later stage trials.

CONCLUSION

The treatment of NSCLC has evolved dramatically from the early use of alkylating agents, to the use of cisplatin doublet therapy, to the development of newer more tolerable drugs that can be utilized beyond the frontline setting and in maintenance strategies, and more recently to targeted therapies against pathways activated in NSCLC such as VEGF, EGFR, and ALK. There are now novel immunotherapies that show promise in patients with advanced NSCLC. Future studies will better characterize patients likely to derive benefit from these targeted strategies by the identification of predictive biomarkers. Assessment of tumor tissue, both pretreatment and at the time of disease progression, will become more integral to the development of targeted therapies for specific genetic aberrations that drive metastasis and treatment resistance. The genomics revolution will ultimately lead to the realization of personalized therapy for NSCLC and improved outcomes for these patients.

KEY REFERENCES

1. Scagliotti GV, Parikh P, von Pawel J, et al. Phase III study comparing cisplatin plus gemcitabine with cisplatin plus pemetrexed in chemotherapy-naive patients with advanced-stage non-small-cell lung cancer. *J Clin Oncol.* 2008;26(21):3543–3551.
5. Goldstraw P, Crowley J, Chansky K, et al. The IASLC Lung Cancer Staging Project: proposals for the revision of the TNM stage groupings in the forthcoming (seventh) edition of the TNM classification of malignant tumours. *J Thorac Oncol.* 2007;2(8):706–714.
6. Rami-Porta R, Ball D, Crowley J, et al. The IASLC Lung Cancer Staging Project: proposals for the revision of the T descriptors in the forthcoming (seventh) edition of the TNM classification for lung cancer. *J Thorac Oncol.* 2007;2(7):593–602.
7. Goldstraw P, Chansky K, Crowley J, et al. The IASLC Lung Cancer Staging Project: proposals for revision of the TNM stage groupings in the forthcoming (eighth) edition of the TNM classification for lung cancer. *J Thorac Oncol.* 2016;11(1):39–51.
15. von Pawel J, von Roemeling R, Gatzemeier U, et al. Tirapazamine plus cisplatin versus cisplatin in advanced non-small-cell lung cancer: a report of the international CATAPULT I study group. Cisplatin and tirapazamine in subjects with advanced previously untreated non-small-cell lung tumors. *J Clin Oncol.* 2000;18(6):1351–1359.
25. Kelly K, Crowley J, Bunn Jr PA, et al. Randomized phase III trial of paclitaxel plus carboplatin versus vinorelbine plus cisplatin in the treatment of patients with advanced non–small-cell lung cancer: a Southwest Oncology Group trial. *J Clin Oncol.* 2001;19(13):3210–3218.
26. Scagliotti GV, De Marinis F, Rinaldi M, et al. Phase III randomized trial comparing three platinum-based doublets in advanced non-small-cell lung cancer. *J Clin Oncol.* 2002;20(21):4285–4291.
27. Schiller JH, Harrington D, Belani CP, et al. Comparison of four chemotherapy regimens for advanced non-small-cell lung cancer. *N Engl J Med.* 2002;346(2):92–98.
28. Fossella F, Pereira JR, von Pawel J, et al. Randomized, multinational, phase III study of docetaxel plus platinum combinations versus vinorelbine plus cisplatin for advanced non-small-cell lung cancer: the TAX 326 study group. *J Clin Oncol.* 2003;21(16):3016–3024.
30. Rudd RM, Gower NH, Spiro SG, et al. Gemcitabine plus carboplatin versus mitomycin, ifosfamide, and cisplatin in patients with stage IIIB or IV non-small-cell lung cancer: a phase III randomized study of the London Lung Cancer Group. *J Clin Oncol.* 2005;23(1):142–153.
32. Cardenal F, Lopez-Cabrerizo MP, Anton A, et al. Randomized phase III study of gemcitabine-cisplatin versus etoposide-cisplatin in the treatment of locally advanced or metastatic non-small-cell lung cancer. *J Clin Oncol.* 1999;17(1):12–18.
37. Alberola V, Camps C, Provencio M, et al. Cisplatin plus gemcitabine versus a cisplatin-based triplet versus nonplatinum sequential doublets in advanced non-small-cell lung cancer: a Spanish Lung Cancer Group phase III randomized trial. *J Clin Oncol.* 2003;21(17):3207–3213.
45. Smith IE, O'Brien ME, Talbot DC, et al. Duration of chemotherapy in advanced non-small-cell lung cancer: a randomized trial of three versus six courses of mitomycin, vinblastine, and cisplatin. *J Clin Oncol.* 2001;19(5):1336–1343.
46. Soon YY, Stockler MR, Askie LM, Boyer MJ. Duration of chemotherapy for advanced non-small-cell lung cancer: a systematic review and meta-analysis of randomized trials. *J Clin Oncol.* 2009;27(20):3277–3283.

66. Repetto L, Biganzoli L, Koehne CH, et al. EORTC Cancer in the Elderly Task Force guidelines for the use of colony-stimulating factors in elderly patients with cancer. *Eur J Cancer.* 2003;39(16):2264–2272.

75. Zukin M, Barrios CH, Pereira JR, et al. Randomized phase III trial of single-agent pemetrexed versus carboplatin and pemetrexed in patients with advanced non-small-cell lung cancer and Eastern Cooperative Oncology Group performance status of 2. *J Clin Oncol.* 2013;31(23):2849–2853.

80. Bepler G, Williams C, Schell MJ, et al. Randomized international phase III trial of ERCC1 and RRM1 expression-based chemotherapy versus gemcitabine/carboplatin in advanced non-small-cell lung cancer. *J Clin Oncol.* 2013;31(19):2404–2412.

81. Friboulet L, Olaussen KA, Pignon JP, et al. ERCC1 isoform expression and DNA repair in non-small-cell lung cancer. *N Engl J Med.* 2013;368(12):1101–1110.

106. Hanna NH, Kaiser R, Sullivan RN, et al. Lume-lung 2: A multicenter, randomized, double-blind, phase III study of nintedanib plus pemetrexed versus placebo plus pemetrexed in patients with advanced nonsquamous non-small cell lung cancer (NSCLC) after failure of first-line chemotherapy. *J Clin Oncol.* 2013;31(suppl): [Abstract 8034].

108. Ramlau R, Gorbunova V, Ciuleanu TE, et al. Aflibercept and docetaxel versus docetaxel alone after platinum failure in patients with advanced or metastatic non-small-cell lung cancer: a randomized, controlled phase III trial. *J Clin Oncol.* 2012;30(29): 3640–3647.

109. Lara Jr PN, Douillard JY, Nakagawa K, et al. Randomized phase III placebo-controlled trial of carboplatin and paclitaxel with or without the vascular disrupting agent vadimezan (ASA404) in advanced non-small-cell lung cancer. *J Clin Oncol.* 2011;29(22):2965–2971.

145. Lynch TJ, Bell DW, Sordella R, et al. Activating mutations in the epidermal growth factor receptor underlying responsiveness of non-small-cell lung cancer to gefitinib. *N Engl J Med.* 2004;350(21): 2129–2139.

147. Lindeman NI, Cagle PT, Beasley MB, et al. Molecular testing guideline for selection of lung cancer patients for EGFR and ALK tyrosine kinase inhibitors: guideline from the College of American Pathologists, International Association for the Study of Lung Cancer, and Association for Molecular Pathology. *J Thorac Oncol.* 2013;8(7):823–859.

153. Janne PA, Yang JC, Kim DW, et al. AZD9291 in EGFR inhibitor-resistant non-small-cell lung cancer. *N Engl J Med.* 2015;372(18):1689–1699.

170. Shaw AT, Kim DW, Nakagawa K, et al. Crizotinib versus chemotherapy in advanced ALK-positive lung cancer. *N Engl J Med.* 2013;368(25):2385–2394.

171. Choi YL, Soda M, Yamashita Y, et al. EML4-ALK mutations in lung cancer that confer resistance to ALK inhibitors. *N Engl J Med.* 2010;363(18):1734–1739.

175. Shaw AT, Kim DW, Mehra R, et al. Ceritinib in ALK-rearranged non-small-cell lung cancer. *N Engl J Med.* 2014;370(13):1189–1197.

194. Shaw AT, Ou SH, Bang YJ, et al. Crizotinib in ROS1-rearranged non-small-cell lung cancer. *N Engl J Med.* 2014;371(21):1963–1971.

203. Herbst RS, Baas P, Kim DW, et al. Pembrolizumab versus docetaxel for previously treated, PD-L1-positive, advanced non-small-cell lung cancer (KEYNOTE-010): a randomised controlled trial. *Lancet.* 2016;387(10027):1540–1550.

See Expertconsult.com for full list of references.

45 Systemic Options for Second-Line Therapy and Beyond

Glenwood Goss and Tony Mok

SUMMARY OF KEY POINTS

- There are a growing proportion of patients who are candidates for second-line therapy and beyond.
- Treatment choices are dictated by tumor histology, molecular phenotype (e.g., *EGFR, ALK, ROS1*, etc.), and components of frontline chemotherapy including also the use of maintenance and bevacizumab.
- In patients with no actionable molecular targets, several options are available that include chemotherapy (docetaxel, pemetrexed), epidermal growth factor receptor (EGFR)-targeted therapies (erlotinib and afatinib for squamous cell carcinoma), and ramacirumab (an anti-vascular endothelial growth factor receptor [VEGFR] 2 monoclonal antibody) in combination with docetaxel and immune checkpoint inhibitors.
- Recent studies comparing EGFR tyrosine kinase inhibitors (TKIs) with single-agent chemotherapy for patients with known wild-type *EGFR* tumors have cast doubts on the clinical efficacy of second-line EGFR TKIs.
- Patients with actionable molecular targets such as *EGFR* sensitizing mutations, *ALK*, and *ROS1* translocation, who did not receive the appropriate targeted therapy in front line, must receive it in a second line strategies.
- Third-generation EGFR TKI such as osimertinib for patients with tumors positive for T790 resistant mutation and second-generation anaplastic lymphoma kinase (ALK) inhibitors (ceritinib, alectinib and brigatinib) showed relevant clinical activity when tested in the second-line setting.
- In the second-line setting immune checkpoint inhibitors (nivolumab, pembrolizumab, and atezolizumab) showed an overall response rate of 5% to 40% in patients with durable responses, but at the present time there are no reliable biomarkers predicting the subgroup of patients who would most benefit. Candidate biomarkers include PDL-1 expression, mutational load, and neoantigen expression.
- Although erlotinib is approved for third-line therapy, the strength of the evidence is limited and a new wave of clinical trials is needed.
- Studies comparing EGFR TKIs with single-agent chemotherapy for patients with known wild-type *EGFR* tumors have cast doubts on the clinical efficacy of second-line EGFR TKIs.

In order to discuss the systemic options for the management of patients in whom first-line chemotherapy has failed, it is necessary to revisit certain aspects of the disease that are covered elsewhere in this text in greater detail. Lung cancer is the most common cancer worldwide and it accounts for approximately 28% of all cancer deaths.[1] For therapeutic purposes, nonsmall cell lung cancer (NSCLC), which includes 85% of all lung cancers, is divided into squamous and nonsquamous histology, for which there are differing approaches to treatment.[2] Substantial advances in our understanding of the biology and molecular pathology of NSCLC have allowed us to identify oncogenic drivers and molecular biomarkers predictive of efficacy with targeted therapies, which further divides NSCLC into smaller therapeutic subgroups.[3] However, even in the case of the most intensively studied of these oncogenic drivers, the *EGFR* gene, there are still many unanswered questions. For example, at a histologic level, the mechanism of the evolution of NSCLC to small cell lung cancer is unknown and our knowledge of the genetic evolution of NSCLC between the first- and second-line settings is scanty.[4] Large studies evaluating the genetics of lung cancer in primary and metastatic sites sequentially across first, second, and subsequent lines of therapy have not been reported in the literature. In the setting of first-line treatment, controversy exists about treating patients with maintenance chemotherapy or waiting until disease progression. In the second-line setting, the appropriate treatment is unresolved and the number of patients eligible for second-line therapy following maintenance chemotherapy is uncertain, as there are conflicting data in the literature.[5,6] A study by Fidias et al.[5] comparing early maintenance chemotherapy with treatment at the time of progression demonstrated that only 37% of patients received second-line treatment at the time of progression compared with 95% who were treated with immediate maintenance.[5] Overall survival favored the maintenance arm (median overall survival, 12.3 vs. 9.7 months; $p = 0.853$), suggesting that immediate maintenance chemotherapy was the treatment of choice. However, the authors noted that the median overall survival for patients in the deferred-treatment arm who received second-line therapy (37%) was 12.5 months, equivalent to that for patients in the maintenance arm. In contrast, Bylicki et al.,[6] in a three-arm randomized study that enrolled 464 patients, found that with careful observation, 95% of patients in the observation arm were eligible for second-line chemotherapy at the time of disease progression (84% received study-defined second-line treatment) and that there was no difference in survival between the maintenance arm and the observation arm. The close observation required to establish eligibility for second-line treatment, however, may not be feasible outside of a clinical trial. In an older retrospective review by Murillo and Koeller[7], published in 2006, among patients with stage IIIb and IV NSCLC treated at 10 community centers in the United States, 84% received first-line, 56% received second-line, 26% received third-line, 10% received fourth-line, and 5% received fifth-line chemotherapy.[7] Further questions have recently been generated by the addition of the immune checkpoint inhibitors to our second-line armamentarium. These agents are by no means the universal panacea with overall only 5% to 40% of patients responding to treatment and our ability to identify the benefiting group mediocre at best.[8,9] With preliminary data suggesting intriguing signals of efficacy of immune checkpoint inhibitor monotherapy in certain treatment-naive subgroups and additional activity in combination with chemotherapy in the upfront management of unselected patients with advanced NSCLC,[9–13] the role of immune checkpoint inhibitors as second-line agents is uncertain.

HISTORY

It was not until 1995 that a large meta-analysis of eight randomized studies comparing cisplatin-based combination chemotherapy with best supportive care for advanced NSCLC demonstrated with certainty that chemotherapy had a modest impact on survival, with a median survival improvement from 4 to 7 months and a 1-year survival rate of 5% to 15%.[14] The result of the meta-analysis was subsequently confirmed in a four-arm randomized phase III study evaluating response and survival rates between third-generation chemotherapies (e.g., paclitaxel, docetaxel, and gemcitabine) when combined with a platinum agent (either cisplatin or carboplatin). This study demonstrated a modest survival improvement, with a median survival of 7.9 months and a 1-year survival rate of 33%.[15] However, it should be noted that platinum-doublet chemotherapy control arms of recent trials have been associated with better median overall survival than chemotherapy arms in earlier trials, most likely because of better performance status of the study population and some stage migration.[16]

Until the two publications by Shepherd et al.[17] and Fossella et al.[18] in 2000, the role of second-line chemotherapy was uncertain. The literature consisted of phase I and phase II trials, most of which were small and consisted of fewer than 30 patients; in addition, details about prior treatment and patient performance status were frequently not included in the publication. Furthermore, although response rates were reported, very few studies provided median survival or 1-year survival rates. A review of the literature demonstrated disappointing results for clinical trials in a second-line setting, with most studies showing response rates of less than 10% and median survival times of 4 months or less.[19] The agents most frequently evaluated in phase II studies included the vinca alkaloids vindesine and vinorelbine, the taxanes (paclitaxel and docetaxel), and gemcitabine. Variable and conflicting results were reported with second-line vinorelbine and in two trials in which vinorelbine, 25 mg/m^2 or 20 mg/m^2, was administered weekly, no responses were seen.[20,21] However, in a small trial of vinorelbine 30 mg/m^2 that included only 10 patients a 20% response rate was reported by Sandora et al.[22] Several studies that tested paclitaxel also produced conflicting results, perhaps in part because of the variability in both the dose and administration time.[19] No responses were seen in a small study in which paclitaxel 140 mg/m^2 was administered over 96 hours.[23] In another trial, paclitaxel 200 to 250 mg/m^2 was administered over 24 hours and 2 (14%) confirmed partial responses were noted, with two additional responses that lasted less than 4 weeks.[24] In two trials in which varying doses of paclitaxel were given over 1 hour, 1 (2.5%) of 13 patients in the first study had a response,[25] whereas 26 responses (25%) occurred in the second study.[26] Gemcitabine was also investigated, and Gridelli et al.[27] noted partial responses in 6 (20%) of 30 patients treated with gemcitabine 1000 mg/m^2 weekly for 3 weeks of a 4-week cycle. However, the most extensively studied agent was docetaxel. In phase II trials, docetaxel was administered at 100 mg/m^2 every 3 weeks, with objective response rates ranging from 15% to 22%.[19] These promising results led to two randomized studies of second-line docetaxel for patients previously treated with cisplatin-based chemotherapy. (These studies will be discussed in more detail later in the chapter.)

SECOND-LINE CHEMOTHERAPY

Only one randomized phase III trial has compared chemotherapy plus best supportive care to best supportive care alone for patients with advanced NSCLC previously treated with platinum-based chemotherapy.[17] Patients with a performance status of 0 to 2, stage IIIb or IV disease with either measurable or evaluable tumor who had received one or more platinum-based chemotherapy regimens were randomly assigned to docetaxel 100 mg/m^2 or 75 mg/m^2 plus best supportive care every 3 weeks or best supportive care only. The primary outcome of the study was overall survival, and the secondary end points included objective tumor response, duration of response, and change in quality of life. All patients in the docetaxel arms were assessed every 3 weeks. Of the 204 patients randomized, 104 patients were assigned to the docetaxel arm, 84 had measurable lesions, and 6 (7.1%) of the 84 had a partial response. Time to progression was longer for patients treated with docetaxel than for patients who received best supportive care only (10.6 vs. 6.7 weeks; $p < 0.001$), as was the median survival (7.0 vs. 4.6 months; log-rank test, $p = 0.047$). The difference was more significant for the 75-mg/m^2 dose of docetaxel compared with the best supportive care arm (median survival, 7.5 vs. 4.6 months; log-rank test, $p = 0.010$; and 1-year survival rate, 37% vs. 11%; $p = 0.003$). Adverse events included febrile neutropenia, which occurred in 11 patients treated with docetaxel at 100 mg/m^2, 3 of whom died, and in 1 patient treated with docetaxel, 75 mg/m^2. Grade 3 or grade 4 nonhematologic toxicity with the exception of diarrhea occurred at a similar rate in both the docetaxel and best supportive care arms. In this study, the 100-mg/m^2 dose was associated with five reported toxicity-related deaths. Three of the deaths were docetaxel-related, and an association with docetaxel treatment could not be ruled out for the other two deaths. At this dose, the median number of cycles delivered was only two and this, combined with a 10% early death rate, probably accounted for the lack of improved survival in the 100-mg/m^2 treatment arm. When the docetaxel dose was reduced to 75 mg/m^2 in the second half of the trial, dose delivery improved, with a median of four cycles, and the rate of febrile neutropenia decreased from 22% to 2%, with no toxicity-related deaths. This high rate of toxicity-related death had not been seen in other phase II studies involving a dose of 100 mg/m^2,[18,19,28] but led the authors to conclude that only docetaxel at a dose of 75 mg/m^2 is associated with significant prolongation of survival. Of note, clinical benefit in this study could be demonstrated by end points other than response and survival. A significant positive effect of docetaxel was evident in the analysis of both the usage of narcotics and nonnarcotics for pain and in the need for radiotherapy. In summary, this was the first trial to document that in patients with advanced NSCLC and good performance status, second-line chemotherapy with docetaxel 75 mg/m^2 after platinum-based chemotherapy is justified, with a significant prolongation of survival and reduced pain.

The above findings were supported by a three-arm multicenter, open-label randomized phase III trial of patients with stage IIIb or IV NSCLC who progressed on platinum-based therapy.[18] The trial was designed to compare docetaxel 100 mg/m^2 every 3 weeks and docetaxel 75 mg/m^2 every 3 weeks to a control arm of vinorelbine 30 mg/m^2 administered intravenously on days 1, 8, and 15 of the 3-week cycle or ifosfamide 2 g/m^2 on days 1–3 of a 3-week cycle (with the choice of drug left to the investigator's discretion). Patients had to have either measurable or assessable lesions and an Eastern Cooperative Oncology Group (ECOG) performance status of 0 to 2. No restriction was based on the number of prior regimens or the amount of prior chemotherapy. A total of 373 patients were randomly assigned, and the three treatment groups were well-balanced for key patient characteristics. The overall response rates were 10.8%, 6.7%, and 0.8% for the docetaxel 100 mg/m^2, docetaxel 75 mg/m^2, and the vinorelbine or ifosfamide arms, respectively. Patients who received docetaxel had a longer time to disease progression ($p = 0.046$) and a greater progression-free survival (PFS) at 26 weeks ($p = 0.05$). Although the overall survival was not significantly different between the three arms, the 1-year survival was significantly greater for the docetaxel 75 mg/m^2 arm when compared with the control arm (32% vs. 19%; $p = 0.025$). Prior exposure to paclitaxel did not decrease the likelihood of response to docetaxel nor did it impact survival. The authors concluded that clinical benefit as determined by objective response, PFS, and 1-year survival favored patients who received docetaxel. Grade 4 neutropenia and fever were higher in the two docetaxel arms than in the control arm; however, other treatment-related adverse events were similar across the three arms.

These two studies, supported by data from multiple phase II studies, resulted in docetaxel being registered with the US Food and Drug Administration (FDA) and the European Medicines Agency as an approved chemotherapy agent for second-line treatment for advanced NSCLC. However, despite the prolongation in 1-year survival by 10% to 20% and improved quality of life when compared with ifosfamide, vinorelbine, or best supportive care alone, these gains were modest, which led to the evaluation of pemetrexed, a novel multitargeted, antifolate in the second-line setting. This compound inhibits the enzyme thymidylate synthase, resulting in decreased thymidine necessary for pyrimidine synthesis.[29] As a drug that also inhibits dihydrofolate reductase and glycinamide ribonucleotide formyl transferase, vitamin supplementation with folate and vitamin B12 is required to limit hematologic and nonhematologic toxicity associated with pemetrexed, including neutropenic fever. Therefore, supplementation with folic acid at 0.35 mg to 1 mg orally daily and vitamin B12 at 1000 µg intramuscularly every 9 weeks is essential to control the toxicity of this drug and has been used in most trials investigating this agent.[30] Phase II studies of pemetrexed in previously untreated patients with NSCLC demonstrated single-agent response rates of 17% to 23%.[31,32] In a phase II study of pemetrexed for patients with advanced NSCLC who had disease progression within 3 months after completing first-line chemotherapy, the response rate was 8.9% and the median survival was 5.7 months.[33] Based on the similar overall survival found for pemetrexed and docetaxel and the expected lower toxicity with pemetrexed, a multinational phase III study comparing these two agents in the second-line treatment of NSCLC was undertaken. The primary objective of this noninferiority study was to compare overall survival between the two treatment groups on an intent-to-treat basis. Secondary objectives were to compare toxicities, response rate, PFS, time to progression, time to treatment failure, time to response, duration of response, and quality of life between the two treatment groups. Eligible patients had to have a performance status of 0 to 2 and have received previous treatment with one chemotherapy regimen for advanced NSCLC. The study included 571 patients who were randomly assigned to receive pemetrexed 500 mg/m^2 intravenously on day 1 plus vitamin B12, folic acid, and dexamethasone every 21 days or to receive docetaxel 75 mg/m^2 intravenously on day 1 plus dexamethasone every 21 days.[34] The overall response rate was 9.1% and 8.8% for pemetrexed and docetaxel, respectively ($p = 0.105$). The PFS was 2.9 months in both arms, and the median survival was 8.3 months and 7.9 months, respectively. The 1-year survival rate in each arm was 29.7%. Patients receiving docetaxel were more likely to have grade 3 or 4 neutropenia ($p < 0.001$), febrile neutropenia ($p < 0.001$), and neutropenia with infection ($p = 0.004$); hospitalization for neutropenic fever was more frequent in the docetaxel arm (13.4% vs. 1.5%; $p < 0.001$). Use of granulocyte colony-stimulating factor support was also greater in the docetaxel arm (19.2% vs. 2.6%; $p = 0.001$) than pemetrexed. The authors concluded that, in patients with advanced NSCLC in whom one line of previous chemotherapy had failed, pemetrexed was equivalent to docetaxel in terms of clinical efficacy but with fewer side effects and should therefore

be considered a standard treatment option in the second-line NSCLC setting.

Despite good overall clinical efficacy in these trials, not all patients benefit from pemetrexed. In a retrospective analysis of phase III pemetrexed studies Scagliotti et al.[35,36] found significant treatment-by-histology interaction for overall survival and PFS. Specifically, patients with nonsquamous tumors treated with pemetrexed had a significantly longer overall survival (hazard ratio [HR]: 0.78; 95% confidence interval [CI], 0.61–1.00; $p = 0.48$) and PFS (HR: 0.82; 95% CI, 0.66–1.02; $p = 0.076$) than patients treated with docetaxel. Conversely, patients with squamous tumors treated with pemetrexed appeared to have a worse overall survival and PFS (overall survival: HR: 1.56; 95% CI, 1.08–2.26; $p = 0.018$ and PFS: HR: 1.40; 95% CI, 1.01–1.96; $p = 0.004$) compared with docetaxel. The treatment-by-histology interaction test for overall survival and PFS was $p = 0.001$ and $p = 0.004$, respectively. This finding, confirming the benefit of pemetrexed for nonsquamous histology, has been supported by the findings of studies with pemetrexed in the first-line and maintenance settings.[16,37]

While a number of questions have been answered in trials, reviews, or meta-analyses of the literature,[38–42] a number of questions remain. Is a combination of two or more drugs superior to single-agent chemotherapy, and is a weekly schedule better than an every 3-week schedule?

CHOICE OF CHEMOTHERAPY AGENT

A review of multiple randomized phase II trials comparing docetaxel to single-agent paclitaxel, gemcitabine, ifosfamide, vinorelbine, and pemetrexed demonstrated that none of these agents was superior to docetaxel in the second-line setting.[40] In this review, two-drug combinations, both platinum and nonplatinum, were also compared with docetaxel in multiple phase II randomized studies. Among platinum-based doublets, none was found to be superior to docetaxel in the second-line setting. Four randomized studies compared a single-agent with a two-drug nonplatinum-based regimen, and three trials compared docetaxel to a combination of docetaxel plus gemcitabine or docetaxel plus irinotecan. Of note, in all trials reviewed, none of the two-drug regimens was shown to improve survival. Furthermore, toxicities were more common among combination regimens, sometimes leading to toxicity-related deaths or negative outcomes related to symptom relief, prolongation of survival, and improved quality of life for patients with incurable disease, which are the primary aims of second-line treatment.[43] Similarly, doublet therapy that includes pemetrexed does not appear to improve survival compared with single-agent pemetrexed in the second-line setting, based on the findings of a meta-analysis.[41] The comparable efficacy of single-agent and doublet chemotherapy in the second-line setting has been supported by four meta-analyses in the literature.[39–42]

SCHEDULING OF CHEMOTHERAPY

Three randomized trials (one phase II and two phase III studies) compared weekly docetaxel delivery to the classic schedule of every 3 weeks.[44–46] In the phase II study,[44] response, median survival, and 1-year survival were not significantly different but favored the every 3 weeks regimen. Similarly, the two phase III studies did not show a difference in overall survival or quality of life.[45,46]

The number of cycles of chemotherapy that a patient should receive in the second-line setting is a matter of debate. This question has not been answered, as it has not been formally addressed in a randomized trial. In the trials of both Shepherd et al.[17] and Hanna et al.,[34] patients were treated until disease progression and the mean number of cycles was four. The reason leading to treatment discontinuation has been inconsistently reported in the literature, but it is most likely due to drug-related toxicity and disease progression. Given that time to progression in randomized phase III trials ranges from 2 to 3 months, corresponding with three or four cycles of chemotherapy, progression may be considered the main reason for discontinuation of second-line treatment. In conclusion, following reviews of four large meta-analyses of second-line trials in the literature, single-agent docetaxel or single-agent pemetrexed administered every 3 weeks remains the gold standard for good performance status patients (without a known treatable oncogenic driver) eligible for chemotherapy. This is detailed in guidelines from both the National Comprehensive Cancer Network and the American Society of Clinical Oncology.[47,48]

THIRD- AND SUBSEQUENT-LINE OF CHEMOTHERAPY

If patients treated with a targeted agent are excluded, there are scanty data regarding the outcomes of patients treated with chemotherapy following first- and second-line chemotherapy for advanced NSCLC. In a retrospective analysis, Massarelli et al.[49] reviewed 700 patient records and identified patients who had received at least two chemotherapy regimens, including at least one course of platinum-based chemotherapy and one course of docetaxel.[49] In this review, the response rate to first-line chemotherapy for all 700 patients was 20.9%; the rates were 16.3%, 2.3%, and 0% for second-line, third-line, and fourth-line chemotherapy, respectively.[49] The disease-control rate also decreased dramatically from first- to fourth-line treatment, although it was higher for second-line treatment (74.4%) than for first-line treatment (62.8%). The median overall survival time from the start of the last chemotherapy, either first- or fourth-line treatment, was 4 months. Patients with stage III disease at initial diagnosis had a longer overall survival from diagnosis than patients with stage IV disease ($p = 0.02$). These data suggest that treating patients with currently available chemotherapy regimens following two lines of chemotherapy should not be standard of care and that further chemotherapy should be explored in the context of a clinical trial.

SECOND-LINE TREATMENT WITH MOLECULARLY TARGETED AGENTS

Many of the molecularly targeted therapies were first investigated as second- or third-line therapy, especially at the time when a reliable biomarker was not available. Here, we review the role of a number of molecularly targeted therapies and their comparative data with single-agent chemotherapy.

Gefitinib

Gefitinib, an EGFR TKI, was the first molecularly targeted therapy investigated as second- or third-line therapy in an unselected population. Early studies were designed and initiated prior to the identification of the *EGFR* mutation. Two such trials, Iressa Dose Evaluation for Advanced Lung Cancer (IDEAL) I and IDEAL II, had as their primary objectives the assessment of tumor response (or tumor regression in IDEAL II) and improvement of lung cancer–related symptoms at two doses (250 mg and 500 mg daily) of gefitinib.[50,51] In these trials, there was no significant difference in treatment outcomes between the two doses. However, it was interesting to note in IDEAL I, in which a majority of patients were of Japanese descent, that tumor response rates were 18.4% and 19% for the two doses, respectively. In contrast, tumor response rates were 12% and 9% in IDEAL II, a predominantly North American–based study. This was the first observation of ethnic difference in treatment response to an EGFR TKI. Another interesting observation in these trials was that select patients had rapid and dramatic responses to gefitinib and this observation became the foundation for the eventual discovery of the *EGFR* mutation. Despite the relatively disappointing overall results of gefitinib in

TABLE 45.1 Randomized Studies That Compared Gefitinib With Single-Agent Docetaxel as Second-Line Therapy for an Unselected Population

Study	No. of Patients	Response Rate[a] (%)	Progression-Free Survival (Mo)	Overall Survival (Mo)
INTEREST[46]	1466	9.1 vs. 7.6	2.2 vs. 2.7	7.6 vs. 8.0
V-15-32[47]	489	22.5 vs. 12.8	2.0 vs. 2.0	11.5 vs. 14.0
ISTANA[49]	161	28.1 vs. 7.6	3.3 vs. 3.4	14.1 vs. 12.2
SIGN[48]	141	13.2 vs. 13.7	3.0 vs. 3.4	7.5 vs. 7.1

[a]Response given as the rate for gefitinib versus the rate for docetaxel.

the general unselected population, the drug was granted accelerated approval by the FDA in May 2003, allowing patients with advanced NSCLC to receive gefitinib if both a platinum-based doublet and single-agent docetaxel had failed. However, a subsequent large-scale randomized phase III study comparing gefitinib with placebo as second- or third-line therapy in an unselected population published in 2005 was negative.[52] This study enrolled 1692 patients in whom one or more lines of chemotherapy had failed. The primary end point of overall survival was 5.6 months for the gefitinib arm and 5.1 months for the placebo arm (HR: 0.89; $p = 0.087$). Only the preplanned subgroup analysis showed a survival benefit among nonsmokers compared with smokers (HR: 0.67; $p = 0.012$) and among Asian as compared with non-Asian study participants (HR: 0.66; $p = 0.01$). As a result of this negative trial, the FDA revoked its approval of gefitinib in this setting in 2005.

A number of randomized studies have compared gefitinib with docetaxel as second-line therapy in an unselected population (Table 45.1). The Iressa NSCLC Trial Evaluating Response and Survival versus Taxotere (INTEREST) was a noninferiority study of 1433 pretreated patients.[53] The primary objective of the study was overall survival, and the coprimary analysis was noninferiority between the two arms. The hazard ratio was 1.02 (95% CI, 0.905–1.150). Three other studies shared a similar trial design but investigated different ethnic populations. V-15-32 was also a noninferiority study but failed to meet the primary end point of overall survival.[54] The upper limit of the 95% CI was 1.40, and the preset limit was less than 1.25. The explanation for this negative finding was the high proportion of patients in the chemotherapy arm who had gefitinib as salvage therapy. Results from the Second-line Indication of Gefitinib in NSCLC (SIGN) study, which was conducted in a Caucasian population, were similar to those of INTEREST; the response rate was 13.2% and 13.7%, for gefitinib and docetaxel, respectively.[55] Overall survival, the primary end point of the study, was also similar (7.5 vs. 7.1 months). Another study from Korea (IRESSA as Second-line Therapy in Advanced NSCLC-Korea [ISTANA]) had a similar study design and sample size but demonstrated a significantly higher response rate for gefitinib (28.1%) compared with chemotherapy (7.6%).[56] This difference is best explained by the difference in the study populations, as the likelihood of tumors harboring *EGFR* mutations is much higher among Korean patients. However, the high tumor response rate did not translate into prolonged PFS or overall survival. These four studies demonstrated that in an unselected population gefitinib is not inferior to single-agent docetaxel; these trials, however, did not directly address the role of EGFR TKIs in patients with known wild-type *EGFR* tumors. Only in subsequent studies of patients with known wild-type *EGFR* tumors has the role of EGFR TKIs in this population become clear.

Erlotinib

BR.21 is the major study that supports the use of erlotinib as second- or third-line therapy in an unselected population.[57] In this randomized phase III study, 731 patients with tumors of unknown *EGFR* mutation status at enrollment were randomly

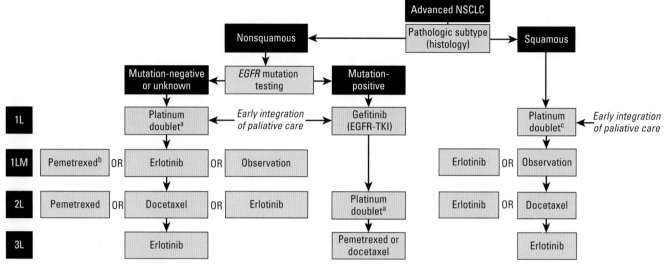

Fig. 45.1. Algorithm for first- (1L, 1LM [maintenance]), second- (2L), and third-line (3L) therapy in advanced nonsmall cell lung cancer (NSCLC). Subsequent lines of treatment assume no previous exposure to the agent about to be used. [a]Includes pemetrexed-based doublet. [b]As maintenance after nonpemetrexed-containing doublets only. [c]Excludes pemetrexed doublets. *EGFR*, epidermal growth factor receptor gene; *TKI*, tyrosine kinase inhibitor. *(Reprinted with permission from Leighl NB. Treatment paradigms for patients with metastatic non-small cell lung cancer: first-, second-, and third-line.* Curr Oncol. *2012;19(suppl 1):S52–58.)*

assigned to receive erlotinib or placebo. The tumor response rate in the erlotinib arm was low (8.9%), but the drug was associated with longer PFS (2.2 vs. 1.8 months) and overall survival (6.7 vs. 4.7 months). This study established erlotinib as a worldwide standard of care in second- or third-line therapy for NSCLC. Unfortunately, only 204 tumor samples from this study were available for biomarker analysis.[58] This analysis showed that patients with wild-type *KRAS* tumors had longer overall survival than patients with *KRAS*-mutant tumors, and patients with tumors that were positive for *EGFR* on fluorescent in situ hybridization (FISH) did better than patients with tumors that were negative on FISH. On the other hand, a sensitizing *EGFR* mutation was not a predictor of survival, but this finding could potentially be explained by the limited sample size (37 patients). The tumor response rate to second-line erlotinib was 27% and 7% for patients who had tumors with or without an *EGFR* mutation, respectively (HR: 0.55; 95% CI, 0.25–1.19), but the difference was not significant. However, due to the small number of patients with tumors with known *EGFR* mutations in this trial, these data are not robust and are not likely representative of the true efficacy of second-line erlotinib for patients with *EGFR* sensitizing mutation. A single-arm study of erlotinib for patients with *EGFR*-positive tumors demonstrated response rates of 73.5% and 67.4% as first- and second-line therapy, respectively.[59] For 104 patients receiving a second-line EGFR TKI, the median PFS was 13 months, which, again, was not different from that for first-line therapy. Overall survival was also similar for first- and second-line treatment (28 and 27 months). Therefore, it is fair to conclude that second-line erlotinib shares similar efficacy as first-line erlotinib for patients who have tumors with EGFR mutations.

Epidermal Growth Factor Receptor Tyrosine Kinase Inhibitors for Patients With Known Wild-Type *EGFR* Tumors

Although erlotinib was approved as a standard second- or third-line therapy for an unselected population, the role of EGFR TKIs for patients with wild-type *EGFR* tumors remains controversial. Until recently, despite the positive results

against placebo in BR.21, there were no direct comparative data against second-line chemotherapy in an unselected population. Recent studies comparing EGFR TKIs with single-agent chemotherapy for patients with known wild-type *EGFR* tumors have cast doubts on the clinical efficacy of second-line EGFR TKIs. An Italian study (TAILOR) randomly assigned 222 patients with documented wild-type *EGFR* tumors to either single-agent docetaxel or erlotinib. The overall survival was 8.2 months for patients receiving docetaxel and 5.4 months for patients receiving erlotinib (HR: 0.73; *p* = 0.05).[60] The difference in the median PFS was minimal (2.9 vs. 2.4 months), and the tumor response rate was 10% for docetaxel and 3% for erlotinib. The authors concluded that single-agent chemotherapy was superior to erlotinib for patients who had tumors with known wild-type *EGFR*.

A Japanese study randomly assigned 300 unselected patients to receive either erlotinib or docetaxel (at 60 mg/m²). The primary end point of PFS was similar between the two groups (2.0 vs. 3.2 months for erlotinib and docetaxel, respectively). However, the subgroup analysis on 199 patients with proven wild-type *EGFR* tumors showed that docetaxel was superior to erlotinib (median PFS, 2.9 vs. 1.3 months; HR: 1.45; *p* = 0.01).[61] However, overall survival was similar between the two groups (9.0 vs. 10.1 months). Another study compared gefitinib with pemetrexed in 157 patients with wild-type *EGFR* NSCLC.[62] The primary end point of superior PFS was met (HR: 0.54 favoring the pemetrexed arm). In summary, three randomized studies comparing EGFR TKIs with single-agent chemotherapy have consistently reported superiority of chemotherapy for patients with known wild-type *EGFR* tumors. However, these three studies are all much smaller and less robust than BR.21 and therefore have to be interpreted with circumspection. An algorithm for treatment has been developed on the basis of current guidelines (Fig. 45.1).

Vascular Endothelial Growth Factor Inhibitors

Addition of an antiangiogenic agent may potentially improve treatment outcomes of second-line therapy. The use of bevacizumab, a monoclonal antibody against the ligand of vascular endothelial growth factor (VEGF), was extensively investigated as first-line therapy. Limited data are available about the use of bevacizumab as second- or third-line therapy. Herbst et al.[63] conducted a small phase II three-arm study in which second-line chemotherapy with or without bevacizumab was compared with erlotinib plus bevacizumab in 120 unselected patients. A median PFS of 4.8, 3.0, and 4.4 months, respectively, was reported. There was also an improvement in overall survival in the subgroup of patients treated with bevacizumab and erlotinib. This study provided the foundation for a randomized phase III study in which investigators compared erlotinib alone with erlotinib plus bevacizumab (BeTa Study).[64] A total of 636 patients were enrolled, and the combination was associated with improved PFS but no significant difference in median overall survival (9.3 vs. 9.2 months). This study was considered to be negative, and no further randomized studies were done to evaluate this combination as second-line therapy.

Multiple VEGF receptor (VEGFR) TKIs were investigated as second- or third-line therapy for lung cancer with unknown biomarker status. Several of these VEGFR TKIs inhibit VEGFR-2 and/or VEGFR-3 and also target EGFR, ret proto-oncogene (RET), c-KIT, and others. Vandetanib, a small-molecule TKI, inhibits VEGFR, EGFR, and RET and was investigated as a single agent or in combination with chemotherapy in three phase III studies. In ZEST, vandetanib was compared with erlotinib as second- or third-line therapy, and progression-free and overall survival were similar for both agents.[65] However, greater toxicity was associated with vandetanib. A second study (ZODIAC) compared the combination of vandetanib plus docetaxel with docetaxel alone.[66] The combination was superior in terms of PFS (4.0 vs. 3.2 months; $p < 0.0001$) but not in overall survival. The third study (ZEAL) was similar to ZODIAC except that the cytotoxic agent was pemetrexed instead of docetaxel.[67] Interestingly, this study demonstrated improvement in the response rate but no difference in progression-free or overall survival. The collective data from these three studies were inconsistent, and this inconsistency may be explained by the largely heterogeneous study population and the lack of an informative biomarker for VEGF inhibition.

Other VEGFR TKIs, including sorafenib, sunitinib, and cediranib, were also investigated in randomized phase III studies. In the MISSION trial, sorafenib was compared with placebo as third- or fourth-line therapy. The improvement in overall survival, the primary end point of the study, was not met (8.2 vs. 8.3 months). However, there was a significant difference in PFS (2.8 vs. 1.4 months) and the subgroup analysis suggested that the small subgroup of patients with activating EGFR mutations had improved in progression-free and overall survival.[68] Sunitinib was investigated in a randomized phase III study that compared the combination of sunitinib plus erlotinib with erlotinib alone. Similarly, there was improvement in PFS (15.5 vs. 8.7 weeks) but not in overall survival (9 vs. 8.2 months).[69] The common finding, noted in many of these studies, of an improvement in PFS suggests that a small subgroup of patients may have benefited from a VEGFR TKI but the scale of benefit was not sufficient to have an impact on overall survival.

Aflibercept is an antiangiogenic fusion protein that prevents VEGF from binding to VEGFR. The protein is composed of VEGFR-1 and VEGFR-2 and a humanized immunoglobulin G1 (IgG1) monoclonal antibody. This drug essentially prevents angiogenesis by trapping the plasma VEGF, thus justifying its other name, VEGF Trap. A large phase III study (VITAL) compared the combination of docetaxel and aflibercept with docetaxel alone for patients in whom first-line chemotherapy had failed. The tumor response rate was 23.3% and 8.9% respectively, and PFS was also improved (HR: 0.82; $p = 0.0035$).[70] However, overall survival, the primary end point, was not significantly better and the drug was not approved for use in NSCLC.

To date, only a limited number of randomized phase III studies testing a VEGF TKI have met the primary end point of prolonged overall survival. The first study involved nintedanib, a multitarget inhibitor of VEGFR 1–3, fibroblast growth factor receptor 1–3, platelet-derived growth factor receptor (PDGFR)-α and PDGFR-β, and RET. The combination of docetaxel and nintedanib was compared with docetaxel alone in 1314 patients in LUME-1.[71] The median PFS was better for the nintedanib arm (3.4 vs. 2.7 months; HR: 0.79; 95% CI, 0.68–0.92; $p = 0.0019$). Benefit was found in both the squamous cell carcinoma and adenocarcinoma subgroups. However, improvement in overall survival was found only in patients with adenocarcinoma (12.6 vs. 10.3 months; $p = 0.03$). Another study with a similar study design using pemetrexed (LUME-2) was prematurely terminated. Despite the positive randomized phase III study, the role of nintedanib in combination with docetaxel remains controversial. A second randomized phase III trial of ramucirumab, an IgG1 monoclonal antibody targeting the VEGFR-2 extracellular domain, was shown to improve survival when combined with docetaxel 75 mg/m² in patients with advanced squamous and nonsquamous NSCLC who had progressed after a platinum-containing chemotherapy. In this placebo controlled trial (REVEL), ramucirumab was found to significantly improve both median overall survival (10.5 months vs. 9.1 months, HR: 0.86; 95% CI, 0.75–0.98) and PFS (4.5 months vs. 3.0 months, HR: 0.76; 95% CI, 0.68–0.86).[72] Based on these results, ramucirumab was approved for the treatment of advanced NSCLC in 2014.

NOVEL TARGETS

Second- and Third-Generation Epidermal Growth Factor Receptor Inhibitors

The second-generation EGFR TKIs include canertinib, neratinib, afatinib, and dacomitinib. These irreversible adenosine triphosphate (ATP) competitor inhibitors make covalent bonds with cysteine residues at position 797 in EGFR. They are more potent than gefitinib and erlotinib against EGFR (HER1) and also inhibit other EGFR family members (e.g., HER2 and HER4). They inhibit the common EGFR sensitizing mutations (exon 19 del and exon 21 L858R point mutation) at lower drug concentrations when compared with the T790M mutation and, therefore, eventually select for cancer cells with EGFR T790M. In humans, the concentration of the drug needed to overcome T790 mutation-mediated resistance may not be achievable in the absence of significant toxicity.[73] Among the four drugs, afatinib is the furthest along in development and was approved by the FDA in 2013 for the first-line treatment of patients with metastatic NSCLC with the EGFR exon 19 deletion or L858R point mutation, as detected by an FDA-approved test. The approval of afatinib was based on the demonstration of improved PFS in a multicenter international, open-label randomized trial.[74] As mentioned earlier, afatanib has been evaluated in the third- and fourth-line setting in a phase IIb/III randomized trial of afatinib compared with placebo for patients with advanced metastatic NSCLC after failure of erlotinib, gefitinib, or both, and one or two lines of chemotherapy (LUX-Lung 1) and in a phase II trial in patients with advanced NSCLC that progressed during prior treatment with erlotinib, gefitinib, or both (LUX-Lung 4).[75,76] The results of a recently completed trial comparing afatinib with erlotinib for patients with squamous cell carcinoma of the lung in whom four cycles of first-line platinum-doublet chemotherapy had failed (LUX Lung 8) have demonstrated significant improvement in median PFS (2.4 months vs. 1.9 months, HR: 0.82; 95% CI, 0.68–1.0) and overall survival (7.9 months vs. 6.8 months, HR: 0.81; 95% CI, 0.69–0.95) with afatinib compared with erlonitib in patients with squamous histology and resulted in afatinib's regulatory approval in 2016 for the treatment of squamous NSCLC in the second-line setting.[77]

Dacomitinib is a pan-erb inhibitor that irreversibly binds to the ATP domain of each of three kinase members of the HER family (EGFR/HER1, HER2, and HER4). In preclinical studies dacomitinib demonstrated higher potency of HER kinase inhibition and greater anticancer activity than gefitinib and erlotinib in sensitive and resistant cell lines and xenograft NSCLC models.[78] In phase I and phase II trials in patients with progressive NSCLC after treatment with an EGFR TKI and/or one or more chemotherapy regimens, dacomitinib showed antitumor activity.[79–81] Subsequently, a randomized phase II open-label study compared dacomitinib with erlotinib in patients with advanced measurable NSCLC who had an ECOG performance status of 0 to 2 and in whom one or two prior chemotherapy regimens for advanced disease had failed.[82] The primary end point of the study was the comparison of PFS between the two arms. Secondary end points included overall response rate, duration of response, overall survival, safety, and patient-reported outcomes of health-related quality of life and disease/treatment-related symptoms. In the study, 188 patients were randomly assigned, and the treatment arms were balanced for most clinical and molecular characteristics. The median PFS was 2.9 months for patients treated with dacomitinib and 1.9 months for patients treated with erlotinib (HR: 0.66; 95% CI, 0.47–0.91; two-sided $p = 0.012$). The median overall survival was 9.5 months for dacomitinib and 7.4 months for erlotinib (HR: 080%; 95% CI, 0.56–1.13; two-sided $p = 0.205$).[82] In exploratory analysis, the median PFS was 3.7 months for dacomitinib and 1.9 months for erlotinib (HR: 0.55; 95% CI, 0.35–0.85; two-sided $p = 0.006$) for patients with wild-type KRAS tumors. For patients with wild-type KRAS/wild-type EGFR tumors, the median PFS was 2.2 months for dacomitinib and 1.8 months for erlotinib (HR: 0.61; 95% CI, 0.37–0.99; two-sided $p = 0.43$). Common treatment-related adverse events were dermatologic and gastrointestinal and predominantly grade 1 and 2 but occurred more frequently with dacomitinib than with erlotinib.[82] Given these results a multinational, multicenter randomized double-blind phase III study comparing the efficacy and safety of dacomitinib with that of erlotinib as second- or third-line treatment for patients with advanced NSCLC previously treated with at least one prior regimen (the ARCHER study) was undertaken. Despite the encouraging early results, dacomitinib was not found to be superior to erlotinib in terms of PFS in unselected pretreated NSCLC or in those with known KRAS wild-type disease.[83] In a separate randomized phase III trial (BR.26) dacomitinib was also found not to improve overall survival compared with placebo (6.83 months vs. 6.31 months, HR: 1.00; 95% CI, 0.83–1.21) in third and subsequent lines of treatment in patients previously treated with chemotherapy and an EGFR TKI, despite delaying disease progression (2.66 months vs. 1.38 months, HR: 0.66; 95% CI, 0.55–0.79).[84] In molecular subgroup analysis, similar results were observed in both EGFR mutant and EGFR wild-type disease, however patients with KRAS mutant disease did worse in terms of overall survival from dacomitinib than did their wild-type counterparts (0.79 months vs. 2.1 months).[84]

The third-generation EGFR inhibitors most advanced in development include AZD9291 (osimertinib),[85] CO1686 (rociletinib),[86] and BI 1482694 (olmutinib).[87] These agents were designed to specifically inhibit the EGFR T790 mutation. AZD9291 and CO1686 have been investigated most extensively. Osimertinib (AZD9291) is a third-generation, oral, irreversible selective inhibitor that targets both the EGFR sensitizing and the T790M-resistant mutant forms of EGFR, while maintaining a margin of selectivity relative to wild-type EGFR. Ballard et al.[88] have investigated the metabolism of AZD9291 in a mouse model and have found that there are two active metabolites, AZ5104, which is approximately seven times more potent than parent AZD9291, and AZ7550, which has similar potency to AZD9291. Osimertinib has been investigated in a phase I, multicenter open-label study in a population with advanced NSCLC who had disease progression after treatment with an EGFR TKI. Among the first 60 patients enrolled to the study, 54 of whom were Asian, the median number of lines of prior therapy was three in the dose-escalation phase of the study and four in the expansion phase.[89] All patients received at least one prior EGFR TKI. The T790M mutation status was known in 28 of the 60 enrolled patients. Of the 26 evaluable patients, 12 had a response; of the 12 evaluable patients with the T790M mutation, 7 had response as measured by RECIST criteria. Grade 3 or greater adverse events occurred in 3 (5%) of 60 patients.[89] Diarrhea occurred in 8 patients (13%) and rash in 8 patients (13%). No dose-limiting toxicity was detected at doses up to 80 mg/day.[89] In updated pooled results from the AURA extension and the AURA phase II studies, which included 411 pretreated patients with EGFR T790M mutation-positive NSCLC, once-daily 80-mg osimertinib yielded an overall response rate of 66% (95% CI, 61% to 71%) with a median PFS of 11 months (95% CI, 9.6–12.4 months).[90] Based on these results, osimertinib has received regulatory approval in the treatment of patients with EGFR T790M positive NSCLC patients progressing after prior EGFR TKI therapy.[91] In an ongoing phase III trial comparing osimertinib with second-line platinum-based chemotherapy (AURA 3) in 419 patients with EGFR T790M mutation-positive NSCLC progressing after prior EGFR TKI, osimertinib has recently demonstrated improved PFS,[92] with full study results to be presented later this year.

In a preliminary report of the first-in-human phase I evaluation of rociletinib (CO1686), the investigators noted that among the first 42 patients enrolled (median number of previous regimens = 4) the T790M mutation was present in the tumors of 31 patients (74%), with an exon 19 deletion or L858R point mutation present in the tumors of 95% of patients.[93] At doses up to 900 mg twice daily and 400 mg three times per day, rociletinib was well tolerated and the maximum tolerated dose had not been reached. The minimum plasma concentration was greater than 200 mg/mL or more for at least 16 hours in 12 patients; 6 of these patients with a T790M mutation had tumor shrinkage of at least 10%.[93] In this initial study, the safety profile of CO1686 appeared to differ from that of the first- and second-generation EGFR inhibitors, with a mild transient rash developing in only 1 of 42 patients and grade 1 or 2 diarrhea occurring in 6 patients. However, hyperglycemia was reported as occurring in 21%.[93] Based on these results, rociletinib (CO1686) received breakthrough designation in mutant NSCLC with T790M mutations from prior EGFR TKI therapy. Updated data on 345 previously treated EGFR mutant NSCLC patients showed an overall response rate of 48% in T790M-positive NSCLC patients and 33% to 36% among T790M-negative patients.[94] However, despite these encouraging results, clinical development of rociletinib has been stopped, based on lower efficacy than projected and the side effect profile of the maturing data from the phase I and phase II trials.

Finally, olmutinib (BI 1482694) has also recently demonstrated clinical activity in a phase II trial of patients with EGFR TKI–resistant NSCLC with centrally confirmed T790M mutations.[95] In the 76 patients T790M+ patients who were treated with daily 800-mg olmutinib, AE grade ≥3 were limited to rash (5%) and pruritis (1%), with 3 patients (4%) discontinuing treatment due to abdominal pain ($n = 1$), interstitial lung disease ($n = 1$), and neuropathy peripheral ($n = 1$). Of the 71 patients evaluable for response, 44% had a confirmed objective response. The median duration of response was 8.3 months

(5.6–not reached) in these heavily pretreated patients, 75% of whom had received ≥2 prior lines of systemic therapy (including EGFR TKI).[95] Based on these promising results, the ELUXA trial program has been launched, aimed at investigating the therapeutic potential of olmutinib as a monotherapy, and in combination with program death 1 (PD1) pathway inhibitors, antiangiogenic agents and targeted agents, with larger phase III trials also being planned.

ANAPLASTIC LYMPHOMA KINASE

Advanced NSCLC harboring an *ALK* gene arrangement accounts for approximately 4% of cases.[96] Crizotinib is an oral small molecule inhibitor that targets *ALK, MET,* and *ROS1*.[97] Phase I and phase II trials have reported objective response rates of 60% in advanced ALK-positive NSCLC patients.[98,99] In randomized phase III trials, crizotinib has been shown to be superior to single-agent chemotherapy in the second-line setting.[100] In the upfront management of patients with *ALK*-positive NSCLC, improved PFS has recently been reported with crizotinib over platinum-based doublet chemotherapy (10.9 months vs. 7.0 months, HR: 0.45; 95% CI, 0.35–0.60) and has become the treatment of choice in the management of these patients.[101] As with most targeted therapies, drug resistance invariably develops in patients treated with crizotinib.

Second-generation ALK inhibitors have been developed, aimed at improving antitumor activity and providing treatment options for patients with acquired resistance to crizotinib. A selective novel oral ALK inhibitor, ceritinib (LDK378), provides a 20-fold greater potency than crizotinib in enzymatic assays. In a phase I trial, ceritinib demonstrated substantial clinical activity in patients with *ALK*-positive NSCLC. A total of 130 patients were enrolled to the trial, 68% of whom had been previously treated with crizotinib.[102] Fifty-nine patients were enrolled to the dose-escalation phase, where 750 mg daily was established as the maximum tolerated dose, with the remaining 71 patients being enrolled in the expanded cohort at a dose of 750 mg/day. Among the 114 patients with NSCLC who received ceritinib at doses from 400 to 750 mg/day, the response rate was 58%. In the 80 patients with crizotinib-resistant tumors, the response rate was 56%.[102] The median PFS in patients receiving at least 400 mg of ceritinib daily was 7.0 months (95% CI, 5.6–9.5). The most common adverse advents were nausea (82%), diarrhea (75%), vomiting (65%), and fatigue (47%). The most common grade 3 or 4 adverse advents were elevation of serum alanine aminotransferase levels (21%), elevation of serum aspartate aminotransferase (11%), and diarrhea (7%).[102] These results suggest that ceritinib is a potent and safe ALK inhibitor with activity in crizotinib-resistant ALK-positive NSCLC. Based on the emerging results from this trial, ceritinib was approved for the treatment of patients with *ALK*-positive NSCLC, progressing after crizotinib.[103] In a recent update of this phase I trial that reported on 255 patients enrolled to the study, the response rate was 72% among the 83 patients that had not previously received crizotinib and 56% in the 183 patients that had acquired resistance to crizotinib.[104] Importantly, in patients with confirmed brain metastases, intracranial disease control was 79% and 65%, in crizotinib-naive and crizotinib-resistant patients, respectively.[104] With these results as background, a number of phase I and phase II monotherapy and combination trials in *ALK*-positive biomarker select NSCLC with ceritinib are ongoing, both in patients with crizotinib resistance and in ALK-inhibitor naive populations, including those with brain metastases.

Alectinib, another selective second-generation ALK inhibitor, has demonstrated efficacy in *ALK*-rearranged NSCLC resistant to crizotinib. In a phase I dose-escalation trial of oral alectinib

(300–900 mg twice daily), an objective response was noted in 24 (55%) of the 44 patients evaluable for activity.[105] Among patients with baseline CNS metastases (n = 21), 52% had an objective response.[105] Overall, alectinib was well tolerated, with common adverse events being fatigue (30%), myalgia (17%), and peripheral edema (15%) almost all grade 1 to 2.[105] Based on activity, tolerability, and drug pharmacokinetics, 600 mg twice daily was established as the recommended dose for the subsequent phase II trials of alectinib.

In the first alectinib phase II single-arm trial, patients with *ALK*-positive NSCLC progressing after crizotinib were enrolled to the trial and treated with 600 mg twice daily until progression, death, or withdrawal. Among the first 87 patients enrolled to study, responses were observed in 33/69 (48%) patients with measurable disease.[106] Adverse events were similar to the phase I trial, with constipation (36%), fatigue (33%), myalgia (24%), and peripheral edema (23%) noted as the most common adverse events. Grade 3 and 4 were primarily limited to changes in blood parameters, including increases in blood creatine phosphokinase (8%), alanine aminotransferase (6%), and asparate aminotransferase (4%).[106] In a second larger phase II trial in crizotinib-refractory *ALK*-positive NSCLC, 138 patients received 600 mg twice-daily oral alectinib, 84 (61%) of whom had baseline CNS metastases.[107] Among the 122 patients evaluable for response, the overall response rate was 50% (95% CI, 41% to 59%), with a median duration of response of 11.2 months. The CNS control rate was 83% and the CNS overall response rate was 57% among the 35 patients with baseline measurable CNS lesions.[107] Common adverse events with alectinib were similar to those previously reported. Based on the combined data from these phase II trials, alectinib received regulatory approval in 2014 for the treatment of crizotinib-resistant *ALK*-positive NSCLC. Alectinib is currently being compared with crizotinib in a randomized phase III head to head trial as first-line therapy in the management of *ALK*-positive NSCLC (NCT02075840), which has recently closed to accrual, with results expected early in 2017.

Finally, brigatinib (AP26113) has also demonstrated substantial antitumor activity in phase I/II trials of *ALK*+ NSCLC, including patients with crizotinib-resistant disease.[108–110] In an ongoing open-label phase I/II trial in advanced NSCLC, enriched for *ALK*+ NSCLC, in patients receiving daily oral brigatinib (30–300 mg) the objective response rate among crizotinib-resistant *ALK*+ NSCLC patients was 72% (51/71).[108] In the phase II component of this trial, response was found to differ by dosing regimen, with objective response rates of 77%, 80%, and 65% for the 90 mg daily, 90 mg daily for 7 days followed by 180 mg daily (90 mg to >180 mg), and 180 mg total daily regimens, daily.[108] As a result of these findings, a randomized phase II trial comparing the 90 mg daily to the 90 mg daily for 7 days followed by 180 mg dosing regimens is currently underway (ALTA), preliminary results of which have recently been reported.[110] Among the 222 *ALK*+ crizotinib-resistant NSCLC patients enrolled to the trial, investigators assessed overall response rate in ARM A (90 mg qd) was 46% with a PFS of 8.8 months and in ARM B (90 mg qd to >180 mg qd) was 54% with a PFS of 11.1 months.[110] In this trial, dose reductions and adverse events for ARM A versus B were 3% versus 6% and 7% versus 18%, respectively.[110] Given its greater efficacy and acceptable safety profile, the escalating dose of brigatinib (90 mg qd to >180 mg qd) is being brought forward in a planned head-to-head trial against crizotinib in the upfront management of *ALK*+ NSCLC.[110] Unlike the newer generation EGFR inhibitors where response depends on the presence of induced *EGFR* T790M mutations, brigatinib activity in crizotonib-resistant *ALK*+ NSCLC has subsequently been established as independent of secondary ALK mutations.[109]

ROS1

Approximately 2% of lung cancers harbor ROS fusion proteins.[111] Several different ROS proto-oncogene 1, receptor tyrosine kinase (*ROS1*) rearrangements have been described in NSCLC, and FISH detects the presence of *ROS1* rearrangement with a ROS1 break-apart probe. *ROS1* rearrangements are nonoverlapping with other oncogenic mutations found in NSCLC.[112] Preclinical data suggest that NSCLC tumors harboring *ROS1* rearrangements may be sensitive to crizotinib. Crizotinib has been shown to bind with high affinity to both ALK and ROS1, and cell-based assays of target inhibition of different kinase targets have demonstrated sensitivity of both ALK and ROS1 to crizotinib.[113,114] Patients whose tumors harbored the ROS1 gene rearrangement were enrolled in an expansion cohort in the original dose-escalation trial of crizotinib (ClinicalTrials.gov identifier: NCT00585195). Most patients were heavily pretreated and received crizotinib 250 mg twice daily. A total of 50 patients were enrolled to the *ROS1* expansion cohort. The majority of patients were never-smokers (78%), and most patients had been treated with at least one line of standard cytotoxic therapy prior to receiving crizotinib.[115] For the full study population, the overall objective response was 72% (95% CI, 58–84%), with a median duration of response of 17.6 months. The safety profile of crizotinib in patients with ROS1-rearrangment was similar to the previously reported trials in ALK-positive NSCLC, with most treatment-related adverse events being mild, of grade 1 or 2.[115] Based on these results, crizotinib received breakthrough therapy designation and regulatory approval in the treatment of ROS1-rearranged NSCLC in 2016, thus defining a second molecular subgroup benefiting from the multitargeted agent, crizotinib.

B-Raf Kinase

v-Raf murine sarcoma viral oncogene homolog B1 (*B-RAF*) is a gene that codes a protein B-Raf, which is a serine/threonine-protein kinase. Activating *BRAF* V600E mutations in NSCLC are present in less than 2% of adenocarcinomas of the lung.[116] A number of B-Raf inhibitors are in development, including vemurafenib,[117] sorafanib,[118] dabrafenib,[119] and AZD628. The United States FDA has already approved both dabrafenib and vemurafenib for the treatment of metastatic melanoma. Dabrafenib 150 mg twice daily has recently been evaluated in a phase II open-label single-arm study in *BRAF*-positive NSCLC, most of whom (78/84) had received prior systemic treatment.[120] Among the pretreated patients, the overall response rate was 33% (95% CI, 23–45%) and 4/6 treatment-naive patients had a treatment response.[120] Despite these encouraging preliminary results, a high frequency of serious adverse events was reported in this trial 35/84 (42%) including pyrexia (6%), decreased ejection fraction (2%), and pneumonia (2%).[120] The toxicity profile, combined with the low mutation rate of *B-raf* in NSCLC, may therefore limit the clinical utility of this compound in NSCLC.

KRAS

Kirsten rat sarcoma (*KRAS*) mutations are the most common oncogenic alterations in NSCLC, occurring in approximately 20% to 30% of adenocarcinomas of the lung.[121] It has been difficult to target and inhibit the KRAS receptor, and, therefore, recent efforts have concentrated on inhibiting downstream pathways.[122] One such pathway is the mitogen activated protein kinase (MAPK) pathway, and MEK is a member of the MAPK kinase-signaling cascade.[123] A number of MEK inhibitors are in development,[124] including selumetinib (AZD6244, ARRY142866), which inhibits MEK1 and MEK2 signaling

downstream of KRAS.[125] This drug has been evaluated in the second-line setting in combination with docetaxel in a randomized phase II study of patients with stage IIIB and IV *KRAS*-mutant NSCLC who had received prior chemotherapy.[125] The patients were randomly assigned to receive docetaxel 75 mg/m² intravenously every 3 weeks with either selumetinib 75 mg twice daily or placebo twice daily. The primary end point was overall survival, and secondary end points include PFS, response rate, duration of response, change in tumor size, proportion of patients alive and free of progression at 6 months, and safety and tolerability. Of 422 patients who were screened, 103 were documented as having *KRAS*-mutant NSCLC, and 87 were randomly assigned to treatment. Baseline characteristics, which included performance status, gender, and *KRAS* codon 12 mutations, were balanced between the arms. The median number of cycles was four in the docetaxel plus placebo arm and five in the docetaxel plus selumetinib arm. The most frequent grade 3 or 4 hematologic toxicities were neutropenia, occurring in 54% of patients treated with placebo and in 67% treated with selumetinib, and febrile neutropenia, occurring in 0% and 16% of patients treated with placebo and selumetinib, respectively. The most common nonhematologic toxicities include dyspnea (11% and 2.3%), acneiform dermatitis (0% and 7%), and respiratory failure (5% and 7%) in the placebo versus selumetinib arms respectively. Overall survival was longer in the selumetinib plus docetaxel arm (9.4 vs. 5.2 months) but this difference was not significant (HR: 0.8; 80% CI, 0.56–0.14; one-sided $p = 0.2$). All secondary end points were significantly improved in the selumetinib plus docetaxel compared with the docetaxel plus placebo arm, including response rate (0% vs. 37%; $p > 0.0001$) and PFS (2.1 vs. 5.3 months; HR: 0.58; 80% CI, 0.42–0.79; one-sided $p = 0.013$).[125] A multicenter open-label nonrandomized phase I and phase II study of selumetinib in combination with gefitinib 250 mg daily in patients who failed an EGFR TKI is open for accrual at the time of writing (ClinicalTrials.gov identifier: NCT02025114). Also, a phase III double-blind randomized placebo-controlled study (SELECT-1) is underway to assess the efficacy and safety of selumetinib in combination with docetaxel for patients receiving second-line treatment for *KRAS*-mutant locally advanced or metastatic NSCLC (NCT01933932). Lastly, the results of two substudies in a randomized phase II study comparing selumetinib with selumetinib plus erlotinib in patients who had either wild-type *KRAS* or *KRAS*-mutant tumors have recently been published. In the first substudy, previously treated patients with *KRAS* wild-type NSCLC were randomized to erlotinib (150 mg daily) or a combination of erlotinib (100 mg daily) without selumetinib (150 mg daily), and the primary outcome was PFS. In the second substudy, pretreated patients with *KRAS* mutant NSCLC were randomized to selumetinib (75 mg BID) alone or the combination of erlotinib (100 mg) and selumetinib (150 mg), and the primary outcome was objective response rate in the second study.[126] In both substudies, selumetinib failed to improve treatment outcomes, with comparable PFS noted in the first trial (2.4 months vs. 2.1 months) and overlapping objective response rates between treatment arms noted in the latter trial (0% [95% CI, 0–33.6%] vs. 10% [95% CI, 2.1% to 26%]).[126] Given these findings, selumetinib does not appear to enhance the erlotinib sensitivity, irrespective of KRAS status.

MET

c-MET is a gene that encodes a transmembrane tyrosine kinase receptor, the hepatocyte growth factor receptor, which is commonly altered in NSCLC tumor tissue.[127] *MET* activation increases the expression of some EGFR ligands, and coactivation of *EGFR* and *MET* has been reported in a distinct subset of NSCLCs.[128] *MET* overexpression is one of the potential mechanisms of acquired resistance to EGFR TKIs in tumors with

EGFR activating mutations, and resistance to erlotinib has been noted in wild-type *EGFR* NSCLC cell lines through MET activation. Thus, *EGFR* and *MET* may cooperate in driving tumor carcinogenesis. *MET* is activated on binding hepatocyte growth factor, also known as scatter factor, which is the only ligand for the MET receptor.[129]

A number of small-molecule TKIs and monoclonal antibodies are in development,[130] and tivantinib, a selective small-molecule MET inhibitor, and onartuzumab, a Met monoclonal antibody, have been evaluated in a phase III study. Onartuzumab was initially explored in a double-blind, placebo-controlled, randomized trial in which patients with advanced NSCLC received oral erlotinib 150 mg daily continuously plus onartuzumab 15 mg/kg intravenously every 3 weeks or erlotinib plus placebo intravenously every 3 weeks. Eligibility requirements included advanced stage IIIB or IV NSCLC, an ECOG performance status of 2 or less, and failure of one or two previous systemic regimens (including platinum-based chemotherapy). The trial enrolled 137 patients who were randomly assigned to the onartuzumab plus erlotinib arm (69 patients) or to the erlotinib plus placebo arm (68 patients).[131] Baseline characteristics were well-balanced between the treatment arms in the intent-to-treat population, with the exception of EGFR mutation status. The coprimary end points of the study were PFS in the intent-to-treat population and in the subgroup of patients with MET-positive tumors; additional end points included overall survival, response rate, and safety. There was no improvement in PFS or overall survival in the intent-to-treat population. However, patients with tumors that were strongly positive for MET on immunohistochemistry (IHC) who were treated with erlotinib plus onartuzumab had improved PFS (HR: 0.53; *p* = 0.04) and overall survival (HR: 0.37; *p* = 0.002). Conversely, clinical outcomes were worse for patients with MET-negative tumors (as defined by weakly staining or absent staining on IHC) who were treated with onartuzumab plus erlotinib.[131] These findings led to a randomized double-blind phase III study of onartuzumab plus erlotinib compared with placebo plus erlotinib for patients with advanced MET-positive NSCLC (METLung). At least one, but no more than two, prior lines of platinum-based chemotherapy for advanced NSCLC must have failed. With a sample size of 490, the trial was designed to detect an improvement in overall survival of 41% with the addition of onartuzumab to erlotinib. This trial was stopped early for futility following an interim analysis after 244 deaths had occurred, which showed no improvement in overall survival (6.8 months vs. 9.2 months, HR: 1.27; *p* = 0.068), PFS (2.7 months vs. 2.6 months, HR: 0.99; *p* = 0.63), or response rate (8.4% vs. 9.6%, *p* = 0.63) with the addition of onartuzumab.[132] Ongoing exploratory analysis based on molecular subgroups may elucidate why these results did not support phase II trial findings.

Tivantinib has been explored in a randomized phase III study in combination with erlotinib (MARQUEE trial). This trial enrolled 1048 patients who were randomly assigned to receive tivantinib and erlotinib or placebo and erlotinib.[133] In order to be eligible, patients had to have nonsquamous NSCLC and previous treatment with at least one line of platinum-based chemotherapy. The study failed to meet its primary end point of overall survival (median 8.5 months for tivantinib and erlotinib vs. 7.8 months for placebo and erlotinib; HR: 0.98; *p* = 0.81). Subset analysis demonstrated that, among patients who had tumors with at least 2+ positive MET immunostaining in more than 50% of tumor cells, PFS favored the tivantinib and erlotinib arm (3.6 vs. 1.9 months; HR: 0.74; *p* < 0.0001).[133]

Recently, *MET* exon 14 skipping (*METex14*) has been described as a potential driver alteration in lung cancer targetable by MET TKIs.[134,135] In a retrospective analysis on 11,205 formalin fixed paraffin embedded (FFPE) lung cancer specimens, hybrid-capture–based comprehensive genomic profiling revealed *METex14* alterations in 298 (2.7%) lung carcinoma samples including sarcomatoid (7.7%), adenosquamous (7.2%), histology not otherwise specified (3.0%), adenocarcinoma (2.9%), squamous cell (2.1%), large cell (0.8%), and small cell (0.2%). Acinar features were present in 24% of the *METex14* samples. The median age of *METex14* patients was 73 years (range: 43–95) and 60% were female. No obvious difference in these patient characteristics was observed among *METex14* patients with varying histologies, and overall *METex14* alterations were found in 2.7% of all lung cancer samples examined.[136]

Crizotinib, an oral small molecule inhibitor that targets ALK, MET, and ROS1 that is currently approved in the treatment of *ALK*-positive and *ROS1*-positive NSCLC, has recently also demonstrated antitumor activity in patients with *MET exon 14*–altered NSCLC. In an ongoing phase I trial (PROFILE 1001) among the first 15 patients treated at a dose of 250 mg who were evaluable for response there were 10 patients with antitumor activity by RECIST.[137] Common treatment-related adverse events were edema (35%), nausea (35%), vision disorder (29%), brachycardia (24%), and vomiting (24%), which were comparable with previous reports in ALK-positive and ROS1-rearranged NSCLC.[137] These results support earlier clinical case reports of off-label crizotinib in patients harboring *MET exon 14* splice site mutations[138] and suggest the need for further evaluation of crizotinib in this patient population.

In summary, while MET inhibition appears to be a promising therapeutic strategy in several malignancies, including lung cancer, it is unclear which of several biomarkers of efficacy is the most appropriate and which patients should be considered for anti c-MET therapy

HEAT SHOCK PROTEIN 90 INHIBITORS

Heat shock protein 90 (HSP90) is a molecular chaperone for multiple proteins that are considered important oncogenic drivers in NSCLC and recognized as a key facilitator of cancer cell growth and survival.[139] There are a number of second-generation, nongeldanamycin HSP90 inhibitors currently in clinical development, including AUY922[140] and ganetespib.[141] A phase I study of AUY922 in advanced solid tumors established a recommended phase II dose of 70 mg/m^2.[140] AUY922 was explored in a phase II study in patients with previously treated advanced NSCLC stratified by molecular status.[142] Patients in whom at least two prior lines of chemotherapy had failed received AUY922 at a dose of 70 mg/m^2 by a 1-hour infusion once weekly. Four strata were considered in enrolling patients: tumors with *EGFR* activating mutations, tumors with *KRAS* mutations, tumors with *ALK* rearrangements, and wild-type *EGFR/KRAS/ALK* tumors. The study included 112 patients, 35 with *EGFR*-mutant tumors (31%), 14 with *ALK*-positive tumors (12%), and 31 with wild-type *EGFR/KRAS/ALK* tumors (28%); most had already received three or more prior systemic regimens. Diarrhea, visual disturbances, and nausea were the most common side effects. Six (18%) of 33 *EGFR*-positive tumors, 2 of 8 *ALK*-positive tumors, 4 of 30 wild-type *EGFR/KRAS/ALK* tumors, and none of 26 *KRAS*-positive tumors responded to treatment according to RECIST criteria.[142]

In phase I studies, ganetespib has demonstrated a favorable safety profile and single-agent activity in previously treated patients with advanced NSCLC.[141] Based on synergistic preclinical interactions between docetaxel and ganetespib, a randomized open-label phase II study of docetaxel with or without ganetespib was undertaken. Eligible patients with good performance status had advanced adenocarcinoma of the lung and had received one prior systemic therapy. Docetaxel was given at 75 mg/m^2 on day 1 every 3 weeks, and, in the experimental arm, ganetespib was given intravenously on days 1 and 15 at a dose of 150 mg/m^2 in a 3-week cycle.[143] Coprimary end points of the study were PFS for patients with an elevated serum lactate dehydrogenase level or for patients with tumors harboring *KRAS* mutations. In the first 225 patients enrolled, the median number of cycles in the docetaxel plus ganetespib arm was five, compared with four in the docetaxel arm. Neutropenia, fatigue, diarrhea, and fever were the most frequent adverse events. According to a preliminary report, overall survival was better in the docetaxel plus ganetespib arm (HR: 0.69; 90% CI, 0.48–0.99; p = 0.093), as was PFS (HR: 0.7; 90% CI, 0.93–0.94; p = 0.012).[143] Because of an increased risk of hemoptysis in nonadenocarcinoma noted early in the trial, the trial was subsequently limited to patients with adenocarcinoma. In the final analysis, while no improvement was noted in the patients with an elevated lactate dehydrogenase (eLDH) (HR: 077; p = 0.1134) or the *KRAS*+ (HR: 1.11; p = 0.3384) subgroups, there was a PFS trend favoring combination therapy (HR: 0.82; p = 0.078) in the intent-to-treat population (n = 253) and a statistically nonsignificant improvement in overall survival (HR: 0.84; p = 0.11).[144] A phase III combination trial of docetaxel and ganetespib is being planned for patients with adenocarcinoma NSCLC diagnosed >6 months prior to study enrollment, based on added benefit of combination therapy noted in this predefined subgroup in GALAXY-1. Given these results and others, preliminary and encouraging data suggest that second-generation HSP90 inhibitors are worthy of further investigation in advanced NSCLC.

IMMUNE CHECKPOINT INHIBITORS

Several genetic and epigenetic alterations are inherent to most cancer cells and provide tumor-associated antigens that the immune host system can recognize, thereby requiring tumors to develop specific immune-resistant mechanisms. An important immune-resistant mechanism involves immune inhibitory pathways termed immune checkpoints that normally mediate immune tolerance and mitigate collateral tissue damage.[145]

CYTOTOXIC T-LYMPOCYTE ASSOCIATED ANTIGEN 4

Ipilimumab is a fully humanized monoclonal antibody that specifically blocks the binding of the T-cell receptor cytotoxic T-lymphocyte associated antigen 4 (CTLA-4) to its ligands, CD80 (B7-1) and CD86 (B7-2).[146,147] This blockade augments T-cell activation and proliferation, which leads to tumor infiltration by T cells and tumor regression.[148] Early clinical trials with ipilimumab have shown activity in a broad range of cancers.[149,150] Ipilimumab has been the first agent of this class to demonstrate a significant improvement in overall survival in patients with previously treated as well as previously untreated metastatic melanoma.[151,152] To assess the activity of ipilimumab in patients with lung cancer Lynch et al.[153] undertook a randomized phase II three-arm study in chemotherapy-naive patients with NSCLC. Patients were randomly assigned to receive either carboplatin and paclitaxel with placebo or ipilimumab at two different doses. The first was concurrent ipilimumab (four doses of ipilimumab plus paclitaxel and carboplatin followed by two doses of placebo plus paclitaxel and carboplatin) or phased ipilimumab (two doses of placebo plus paclitaxel and carboplatin followed by four doses of ipilimumab plus paclitaxel and carboplatin). Treatment was administered intravenously every 3 weeks for 18 weeks. Eligible patients continued on ipilimumab or placebo every 12 weeks as maintenance therapy. Response was assessed using immune related response criteria and modified World Health Organization (WHO) criteria. The primary end point was immune-related PFS. The study met its primary end point of improved PFS for phased ipilimumab compared with the control (HR: 0.72; p = 0.05) but not for concurrent ipilimumab (HR: 0.81; p = 0.13).[153] Phased ipilimumab also improved PFS according to modified WHO criteria (HR: 0.69;

p = 0.02). Overall rates of grade 3 and 4 immune-related adverse events were 15%, 20%, and 6% for phased ipilimumab, concurrent ipilimumab, and control, respectively.[153] These results have led to a randomized multicenter, double-blind phase III trial comparing the efficacy of ipilimumab plus paclitaxel and carboplatin versus placebo plus paclitaxel and carboplatin in patients with stage IV chemotherapy-naive or recurrent squamous NSCLC (ClinicalTrials.gov identifier: NCT01285609). Tremelimumab, an IgG2 antibody with high affinity to CTLA-4, in an open-label phase II study in advanced NSCLC has also achieved an objective response of 5%.[154] Tremelimumab is being developed in combination with other targeted agents and immunotherapies, including the checkpoint inhibitors listed below.

Anti-Program Death 1 and Program Death 1 Ligand

PD1 is a key immune checkpoint receptor expressed by activated T cells, and it mediates immunosuppression. PD1 functions primarily in peripheral tissue were T cells may encounter immune suppressive PD1 ligand (PDL1) that is expressed by tumor cells, stromal cells, or both.[155,156] Inhibition of the interaction between PD1 and PDL1 can enhance T-cell responses in vitro and mediate preclinical antitumor activity.[157,158] There are a number of PD1 and PDL1 inhibitors in preclinical and clinical development, including the PD1 inhibitors nivolumab and pembrolizumab (MK 3475) and the PDL1 inhibitors durvalumab (MEDI4736), atezolizumab (MPDL3280A), amplimmune (AMP-224), and BMS-936559. In a dose-escalation study, the anti-PD1 monoclonal antibody nivolumab (BMS936558) was administered as a single dose in 39 patients with advanced solid tumors demonstrating a favorable safety profile and provided preliminary evidence of clinical activity.[159] This led to a multidose study where nivolumab was administered intravenously every 2 weeks of an 8-week treatment cycle and patients received treatment for up to 2 years. Objective responses were observed in a substantial proportion of patients with NSCLC, melanoma, or renal cell cancer, and they were seen at all dose levels. In the patients with lung cancer, 14 objective responses were observed at doses of 1.0, 3.0, or 10.0 mg/kg with a response rate of 6%, 32%, and 18% respectively. Objective response rates were observed across all NSCLC histologic types including 6 (33%) of 18 patients with squamous cell tumors, 7 (12%) of 56 with nonsquamous tumors, and 1 of 2 with lung tumors not otherwise specified. Sixty-one pretreatment tumor specimens from 42 patients were analyzed for PDL1 expression, and 25 were positive for PDL1 expression by IHC. Of these 25 patients, 9 had an objective response whereas none of the 17 patients with PDL1-negative tumors had an objective response suggesting that PDL1 expression by IHC may be a biomarker of efficacy. In the phase I dose-escalation and expansion study, 127 NSCLC patients were treated with nivolumab and 122 were evaluable for response, with 20 (16%) patients demonstrating a response by RECIST criteria. While responses were noted across all histologic subtypes, they were more common in patients with squamous NSCLC. Specifically, objective responses were observed in 6 out of 18 patients (33%) with squamous tumors and 7 out of 56 (12%) with nonsquamous tumors. Across all NSCLC histologies and doses evaluated, the response rate was 26% at 2 years, suggesting that there are durable responses in this heavily pretreated population.[160] In a subsequent open-label phase III trial in squamous NSCLC patients who had progressed following first-line chemotherapy (Checkmate 017), nivolumab was shown to improve overall survival compared with docetaxel (9.2 months vs. 6.0 months, HR: 0.59 months; 95% CI, 0.44–0.79), with 1-year response rates of 42% and 24% for nivolumab and docetaxel, respectively.[161] In addition, nivolumab had greater tolerability than docetaxel, with grade 3 and 4 treatment-related adverse events being 7% and 55% for nivolumab and docetaxel, respectively.[161] Similar results were obtained in an open-label randomized phase III trial of nivolumab versus docetaxel in patients with nonsquamous histology progressing after up front chemotherapy.[162] The median overall survival was better with nivolumab as compared with docetaxel (12.2 months vs. 9.4 months, HR: 0.73; 95% CI, 0.59–0.89) and 1-year survival for patients treated with nivolumab or docetaxel was 51% and 39%, respectively. As in patients with squamous histology, nivolumab was more tolerable than docetaxel in the second-line setting, with lower rates of grade 3 and 4 treatment-related toxicity reported as compared with docetaxel (10% vs. 54%).[162] Based on the results of Checkmate 017 and Checkmate 057, nivolumab has received regulatory approval in patients with both squamous and nonsquamous histology.

Pembrolizumab (MK3475), a humanized IgG4 anti-PD1 monoclonal antibody, has demonstrated safety and efficacy in an ongoing phase I trial (KEYNOTE-001, NCT01295827). Early clinical and safety data of the first 38 patients with squamous or nonsquamous NSCLC treated with pembrolizumab demonstrated an overall response rate of 24% (9 patients). Patients with a high level of PDL1 expression had an overall response rate of nearly 70% while patients with lower rates of expression experienced a lower response rate.[163] With the aim to define and validate PDL1 expression levels associated with response to pembrolizumab, the phase I trial was expanded to include a training group (n = 182) or a validation cohort (n = 313) treated with either 2 mg/kg or 10 mg/kg every 3 weeks or 10 mg/kg every 2 weeks. PDL1 expression was assessed in all tumor samples and reported as the percentage of cells staining for PDL1 (proportion score). The overall response rate to pembrolizumab in all the NSCLC patients was 19.4%.[8] In the training group, a proportion score of 50% was identified as the threshold that defined pembrolizumab sensitivity. In the validation cohort, 45.2% of patients with a proportion score of at least 50% responded to pembrolizumab, supporting high PDL1 protein expression as a biomarker of pembrolizumab sensitivity. Pembrolizumab has since received regulatory approval in patients with advanced NSCLC whose tumors express PDL1, based on the companion diagnostic, the PDL1 IHC 22C3 pharmDx test.

Atezolizumab is an IgG1 antibody PDL1 inhibitor that in a phase I trial of 85 patients with NSCLC reported a 23% best overall response rate, with only 11% drug-related grade 3 or 4 adverse events. The majority of responses were observed within 14 weeks and all patients who had a response completed 1 year of treatment without disease progression.[164,165] Atezolizumab was subsequently investigated in phase II trials in patients with previously treated advanced NSCLC, in a single-arm trial in PDL1 expression–positive select patients (NCT01846416), and against docetaxel in a randomized controlled trial irrespective of PDL1 status (POPLAR), which was assessed prospectively and used as a stratification factor (NCT01903993). In 205/1009 patients preselected by PDL1 status enrolled to the single-arm trial (BIRCH), the highest response rates were noted in previously untreated patients (n = 142), with the highest score of PDL1 expression on tumor cells (TC3) or tumor infiltrating immune cells (IC3) in patients receiving second-line atezolizumab after failing chemotherapy (n = 271) and in patients receiving third-line atezolizumab (n = 254) with response rates of 29%, 27%, and 25%, respectively.[9] In the randomized trial, compared with second-line docetaxel, atezolizumab has found improved overall survival in the full study cohort (12.6 months vs. 9.7 months, HR:

0.73; 95% CI, 0.53–0.99).[166] In this trial, the efficacy of atezolizumab was associated with PDL1 expression, with greater efficacy noted in patients with higher PDL1 expression (HR: 0.49 in TC3/IC3, HR: 0.54 in TC2/TC3 and IC2/IC3 vs. HR: 0.59 in TC1/TC2/TC3 or IC1/IC2/IC3).[166] In both phase II trials, atezolizumab was well tolerated with safety profiles comparable with other checkpoint inhibitors. Atezolizumab received a breakthrough therapy designation in 2015 for the treatment of PDL1 expression–positive NSCLC progressing after first-line chemotherapy. Atezolizumab is currently being evaluated as a monotherapy against docetaxel in the second-line setting in a phase III randomized trial and in phase I trials in combination with targeted agents such as erlotinib and alectinib (NCT02013219) and in combination with chemotherapy (NCT02813785). Finally, durvalumab, MEDI4736, an IgG4 antibody to PDL1, has also been evaluated in patients with advanced solid malignancies, including NSCLC. In a phase I dose escalation trial, 0.1–10 mg/kg doses of durvalumab every 2 weeks and 15 mg/kg doses every 3 weeks were evaluated in patients with advanced solid malignancies.[167] No dose-limiting toxicities or maximum tolerated doses for either regimen were identified. Treatment-related adverse events in the first 26 patients enrolled to the trial were 34%, which were all of grade 1 and 2. In the 26 heavily pretreated patients, 4 partial responses were observed (3 NSCLC, 1 melanoma).[167] Among 198 NSCLCs (82 squamous, 116 nonsquamous) enrolled to an expansion cohort using a 10 mg/kg dose every 2 weeks, drug-related adverse events occurred in 48% and included fatigue (14%), decreased appetite (9%), and nausea (8%).[168] In the 149 patients evaluable for response (>24 weeks follow-up), the overall response rate was 14% among all patients and 23% in patients whose tumors were PDL1-positive using the Ventana PDL1 IHC (SP263) assay. Notably, the overall response rate was higher in patients with squamous histology (21%) than in patients with nonsquamous histology (10%).[168] A single-arm phase II trial (ATLANTIC) limited to patients with PDL1-positive NSCLC is currently ongoing (NCT02087423) evaluating durvalumab in the third-line setting. Durvalumab is also being evaluated in a randomized phase III trial alone and in combination with the anti-CTLA-4 agent tremelimumab (ARCTIC) against standard of care in PDL1-positive NSCLC patients who have failed two prior lines of therapy (NCT02352948)[169] and in a phase I study in combination with gefitinib in previously treated *EGFR* mutation-positive NSCLC (NCT02088112).[170]

CONCLUSION

Many ongoing phase II and phase III clinical trials are directly comparing or combining a host of these novel therapies. In particular the immune checkpoint inhibitors are being combined with chemotherapy, other targeted molecules, and as immune checkpoint doublets (Table 45.2). As a consequence the evaluation of new therapies in the second-line setting has become both extremely competitive and complex. The results of these trials will contribute to our understanding of the molecular etiology of lung cancer and the biology of progression and resistance and provide us with the next generation of targets. Ultimately, this plethora of activity will lead to significant improvement in patient survival and outcomes.

Acknowledgment

Dr. Goss thanks his research associate Johanna Spaans and his administrative assistant Valerie Smaglinskie for their support in drafting this chapter.

TABLE 45.2 Selection of Ongoing Phase II and Phase III Clinical Trials Directly Comparing or Combining Novel Therapies With Standard Platinum-Based Chemotherapy in Patients With Nonsmall Cell Lung Cancer

Phase	Study Design	Treatment Line	Treatments	Sponsor	ClinicalTrials.gov Identifier
Phase II	Randomized, open-label, two-arm	Second-line (Mandated first line of docetaxel, carboplatin, and bevacizumab)	Bevacizumab + pemetrexed vs. pemetrexed alone	Milton Hershey Medical Center	NCT00735891
Phase III	Randomized, double-blind, two-arm	Second-line	Docetaxel + ramucirumab vs. docetaxel + placebo	Eli Lilly and Co.	NCT01168973
Phase III	Randomized, open-label, two-arm	Second-line	Pemetrexed vs. erlotinib	NCI	NCT00738881
Phase II	Randomized, open-label, three-arm	Second-line	Pemetrexed vs. sunitib vs. pemetrexed + sunitib	NCI	NCT00698815
Phase Ib/II	Randomized, open-label	Second-line	Eribulin mesylate + pemetrexed vs. pemetrexed	NCI	NCT01126736
Phase II (TARGET)	Randomized, open label, three-arm	Second-line (pts must be folate-receptor positive ++)	EC145 vs. EC145 + docetaxel vs. docetaxel alone	Merck Sharp and Dohme Corp	NCT01577654
Phase II (TASLISMAN)	Randomized, open-label, two-arm	Second-line (pts must be male former smokers)	Erlotinib vs. intermittent dosing of erlotinib + docetaxel	Hoffman-La Roche	NCT01204697
Phase II	Randomized, open-label, two-arm	Second-line	Suramin + docetaxel vs. docetaxel	University of Wisconsin	NCT01671332
Phase III	Randomized, open-label, two-arm	Second-line	Polyglutamate paclitaxel (CT-2103) vs. docetaxel	Cell Therapeutics	NCT00054184
Phase III (SUNRISE)	Randomized, double-blind, two-arm	Second-line	Bavituximab + docetaxel vs. docetaxel + placebo	Peregrine Pharmaceuticals	NCT01999673
Phase III	Randomized, open-label, two-arm	Second-line	Custirsen (TV-1011/OGX-011) vs. docetaxel	Teva Pharmaceuticals	NCT01630733
Phase II	Randomized, open-label, two-arm	Second-line (pts must have KRAS, NRAS, BRAF, or MEK1 mutations)	GSK1120212 vs. docetaxel	GlaxoSmithKline	NCT01362296
Phase II	Randomized, open-label, two-arm	Second-line	Gefitinib vs. pemetrexed	Gachon University Gil Medical Center	NCT01783834
Phase III	Randomized, open-label, two-arm	Second- or third-line	Paclitaxel + bevacizumab vs. docetaxel	Intergroupe Francophone de Cancerologie Thoracique	NCT01763671
Phase II	Randomized, open-label, two-arm	Second-line	Pemetrexed + (carboplatin or cisplatin) + erlotinib vs. pemetrexed + (carboplatin or cisplatin)	Vanderbilt-Ingram Cancer Center	NCT01928160
Phase II	Nonrandomized, open-label, two-arm	Third-line	Vorinostat (SAHA, Zolinza) vs. bortezomib (PS341, Velcade)	University of Wisconsin	NCT00798720

BRAF, v-Raf murine sarcoma viral oncogene homolog B; *KRAS,* V-Ki ras2 Kirsten rat sarcoma viral oncogene homolog; *MEK1,* dual-specificity mitogen-activated protein kinase 1; *NRAS,* neuroblastoma RAS viral oncogene homolog; *pts,* patients.

KEY REFERENCES

8. Garon EB, Rizvi NA, Hui R, et al. Pembrolizumab for the treatment of non-small cell lung cancer. *N Eng J Med.* 2015;372:2018–2028.
10. Gettinger S, Rizvi N, Chow LQ, et al. Nivolumab monotherapy for first-line treatment of advanced non-small cell lung cancer. *J Clin Oncol.* 2016;34(25):2980–2987.
17. Shepherd FA, Dancey J, Ramlau R, et al. Prospective randomized trial of docetaxel versus best supportive care in patients with non–small-cell lung cancer previously treated with platinum-based chemotherapy. *J Clin Oncol.* 2000;18:2095–2103.
34. Hanna N, Shepherd FA, Fossella FV, et al. Randomized phase III trial of pemetrexed versus docetaxel in patients with non–small-cell lung cancer previously treated with chemotherapy. *J Clin Oncol.* 2004;22(9):1589–1597.
37. Ciuleanu T, Brodowicz T, Zielinski C, et al. Maintenance pemetrexed plus best supportive care versus placebo plus best supportive care for non-small cell lung cancer: a randomised, double-blind, phase 3 study. *Lancet.* 2009;374:1432–1440.
57. Shepherd FA, Rodrigues PJ, Ciuleanu T, et al. Erlotinib in previously treated non-small-cell lung cancer. *N Engl J Med.* 2005;353:123–132.

71. Reck M, Kaiser R, Mellemgaard A, et al. Nintedanib (BIBF 1120) + docetaxel in NSCLC patients progressing after one prior chemotherapy regimen: LUME-Lung 1, a randomized, double-blind, phase III trial. ASCO; 2013. abstr # LBA 8011.
72. Garon EB, Ciuleanu TE, Arrieta O, et al. Ramucirumab plus docetaxel versus placebo plus docetaxel for second-line treatment of stage IV non-small-cell lung cancer after disease progression on platinum-based therapy (REVEL): a multicentre, double-blind, randomised phase 3 trial. *Lancet.* 2014;384(9944):665–673.
77. Soria JC, Felip E, Cobo M, et al. Afatinib versus erlotinib as second-line treatment of patients with advanced squamous cell carcinomas of the lung (LUX-lung8): an open-label randomised controlled phase 3 trial. *Lancet Oncology.* 2015;16:897–907.
83. Ramalingham SS, Janne PA, Mok T, et al. Dacomitinib versus erlotinib in patients with advanced-stage, previously treated non-small cell lung cancer (ARCHER 1009): a randomized double-blind, phase 3 trial. *Lancet Oncology.* 2014;15(12):1369–1378.
100. Shaw AT, Kim DW, Nakagawa K, et al. Crizotinib versus chemotherapy in advanced *ALK*-positive lung cancer. *N Engl J Med.* 2013;368:2385–2394.

111. Bergethon K, Shaw AT, Ou SHI, et al. ROS1 rearrangements define a unique molecular class of lung cancers. *J Clin Oncol.* 2012;30(8):863–870.

115. Shaw AT, Ou SHI, Bang YJ, et al. Crizotinib in ROS1-rearranged non-small cell lung cancer. *N Engl J Med.* 2014;371(21):1963–1971.

120. Planchard D, Kim TM, Mazieres J, et al. Dabrafenib in patients with BRAF v600e–positive advanced non-small cell lung cancer: a single-arm, multicentre, open-label, phase 2 trial. *Lancet Oncol.* 2016;17:642–650.

135. Awad MM, Oxnard GR, Jackman DM, et al. MET exon 14 mutations in non-small cell lung cancer are associated with advanced age and stage-dependent MET genomic amplification and c-MET overexpression. *J Clin Oncol.* 2016;34(7):721–730.

136. Ou SHI, Frampton GM, Suh J, et al. Comprehensive genomic profiling of 298 lung cancer of varying histologies harbouring MET exon 14 alterations. *J Clin Oncol.* 2016;34(suppl 15). [abstr 9021].

137. Drilon AE, Camidge DR, Ou SHI, et al. Efficacy and safety of crizotinib in patients (pts) with advanced MET exon 14-altered non-small cell lung cancer. *J Clin Oncol.* 2016;34(suppl). [abstr:108].

161. Brahmer J, Reckamp KL, Bass P, et al. Nivolumab versus docetaxel in advanced squamous-cell non-small cell lung cancer. *N Engl J Med.* 2015;373:123–135.

162. Borghaei H, Paz-Ares L, Horn L, et al. Nivolumab versus docetaxel in advanced nonsquamous non-small cell lung cancer. *N Engl J Med.* 2015;373(17):1627–1639.

See Expertconsult.com for full list of references.

46 | Maintenance Chemotherapy for Nonsmall Cell Lung Cancer

Maurice Perol, Heather Wakelee, and Luis Paz-Ares

SUMMARY OF KEY POINTS

- Maintenance therapy offers the possibility of continued active treatment to delay disease progression and symptom deterioration and, more importantly, improved overall survival of patients with advanced nonsmall cell lung cancer (NSCLC) already treated with induction chemotherapy.
- The target population for maintenance are patients who achieved objective response or disease stabilization with induction chemotherapy with minimal cumulative toxicity.
- Meta-analyses and patients' preference support the use of maintenance in advanced NSCLC.
- Maintenance chemotherapy doesn't impair quality of life nor generate an additional cost compared with the benefits achieved.
- Excluding targeted agents with known driver mutations, no predictive biomarkers are available to select better candidates for maintenance therapy with chemotherapy.
- In this setting new treatment opportunities with immunotherapy and other agents represent a research priority.

The quest to control NSCLC has been long and remains frustrating, but since the 2000s, substantial advances have been made in therapeutic options for patients with this disease. The most striking advances have been in treatments linked to the identification of molecular changes acting as so-called drivers of malignancy for many patients, but optimization of the delivery of chemotherapy, particularly with maintenance therapy, has also led to improved survival for patients.

The concept of maintenance therapy was initially rejected after several studies published in the early 2000s demonstrated that continuation of a platinum-based doublet beyond four cycles did not result in a significant survival advantage but did cause progressive toxicity.[1,2] Around the same time, studies demonstrated the efficacy of second-line chemotherapy, most notably with docetaxel.[3,4] The overall interpretation of these results led to the standard treatment paradigm of treatment with a platinum-based doublet for four cycles (six for patients who had response) followed by a so-called treatment holiday until the time of progression, at which point standard second-line chemotherapy was offered. The widespread belief was that patients benefited from a break from chemotherapy and that close surveillance would provide the opportunity for patients to receive beneficial future treatments.

This approach began to be questioned, however, with the development of new agents. For example, some new chemotherapy drugs, such as pemetrexed, could be given on a continuous basis with a lower risk of long-term toxicities such as neuropathy, which had limited the long-term use of other agents, such as the taxanes.[5] In addition, the era of targeted agents began, and almost all of these agents (such as bevacizumab, erlotinib, and gefitinib) are administered continuously until progression.

The maintenance approach is currently defined as continuation or switch maintenance treatment. With continuation maintenance, one or two of the agents administered as part of a first-line combination regimen are continued beyond the four to six cycles. This concept is not completely new because it was extensively investigated in several trials starting in the 1980s, but it was only in 2006, with the licensing of bevacizumab, that an approved drug was available in a continuous maintenance setting.[6] More recently, strongly positive data with pemetrexed given as continuation maintenance therapy after four cycles of a platinum-based doublet further contributed to a change in the treatment paradigm.[7] Less compelling data support the use of gemcitabine as continuous maintenance therapy.

The concept of switch maintenance is more recent and is based on switching to an alternative agent (i.e., one that was not part of the first-line regimen) after completion of four to six cycles of doublet chemotherapy in the absence of disease progression. Definitive data support the use of pemetrexed and erlotinib,[8,9] and less robust data are available for docetaxel.[10] It could be argued that such an approach may be simply considered early initiation of second-line treatment. Although the agents investigated in this setting, namely pemetrexed, erlotinib, and docetaxel, are indeed all approved agents for standard second-line therapy, their use for patients who had an objective response or disease stabilization after completion of first-line chemotherapy is biologically different from their use after disease progression. The term early second-line treatment is therefore inaccurate and should not be used.

The results of the Sequential Tarceva in Unresectable NSCLC (SATURN) and JMEN trials were the true impetus for maintenance therapy, which led to guidelines in support of maintenance therapy, issued in 2011,[11,12] and increased awareness about the benefits of this approach. Clinical investigations in this area have helped demonstrate that second-line chemotherapy is subsequently given to about two-thirds of patients who have a treatment holiday after disease stabilization with four to six cycles of chemotherapy.[10,14] Maintenance therapy, either as continuation or switch, leads to improved survival for patients with NSCLC.

HISTORICAL MAINTENANCE TRIALS

In 1989, a study to evaluate the effect of prolonging chemotherapy for patients with stable disease beyond two or three cycles of a four-drug regimen (methotrexate, doxorubicin, cyclophosphamide, and lomustine) found no benefit for a longer duration.[15] The study was small, with 74 patients randomly assigned to maintenance chemotherapy or to discontinuation of chemotherapy, and the results showed a nonsignificant trend toward longer overall survival of nearly 4 months for maintenance chemotherapy, but cast doubt on the use of prolonged first-line chemotherapy or maintenance therapy.[15] Despite this uncertainty, patients and physicians seemed to favor continued therapy, as evidenced by difficulty in recruiting to a randomized trial of six courses of mitomycin-C, vinblastine, and cisplatin compared with observation after three cycles of the same regimen. The authors noted that most patients who declined to enroll in the study said they refused because they preferred to continue treatment.[16] However, despite this challenge, the trial was completed and it showed no improvement in survival for prolonged chemotherapy and demonstrated an increase in fatigue and other types of toxicities, further supporting the idea that less is better when considering the continuation of combination cytotoxic regimens.[2] At that time, the number of treatment cycles varied, as did the regimens used for first-line therapy.

Socinski et al.[1] published the results of a practice-changing trial in 2002. The backbone regimen for this trial was carboplatin and paclitaxel, based on the findings of multiple phase III studies performed in the United States and Europe that had demonstrated the tolerability and efficacy of this regimen.[17–20] All patients received four cycles of carboplatin (area under the curve [AUC] of 6) and paclitaxel (200 mg/m^2) on a 21-day regimen, with disease assessment after every two cycles. Patients in one arm of the trial had a break from treatment after four cycles, with assessments for progression done every 6 weeks, and patients in the other arm received chemotherapy every 3 weeks until disease progression or until the decision was made to end treatment. It was planned that all patients were to receive second-line therapy with weekly paclitaxel (80 mg/m^2) given at the time of progression. A total of 230 patients were enrolled, predominantly between 1998 and 1999. Response rates were 22% and 24%, respectively, in the two arms, with no additional responses after four cycles for patients who had received continued chemotherapy. The median survival times were 6.6 and 8.5 months, respectively, but the difference was not significant ($p = 0.63$). Of note, 45% of patients received second-line chemotherapy, and more patients received continued chemotherapy than were given a treatment holiday. Toxicities, particularly neuropathy, were higher among patients who received continued chemotherapy, but there was no clear difference in quality of life between the two treatment arms. The conclusion drawn from this trial was that treatment beyond four cycles of a platinum-based doublet did not lead to improved survival and could lead to increased toxicity.[1] Thus, the standard practice shifted toward this approach, with an additional two cycles offered to patients who had a response, such that four to six cycles of a platinum-based doublet, followed by a treatment holiday, was the standard approach. Two subsequent studies addressed the question of four versus six cycles of first-line chemotherapy, and both failed to show a clear benefit with the additional two cycles, thus supporting four cycles of first-line doublet therapy as the standard of care.[21,22]

Another contemporary phase III study compared three cycles with six cycles of carboplatin (equivalent to AUC of 5) given on day 1 and vinorelbine (25 mg/m^2) on days 1 and 8 every 3 weeks. A total of 297 patients were enrolled, and the median survival was 28 weeks for three cycles and 32 weeks for six cycles (hazard ratio [HR], 1.04; 95% confidence interval [CI], 0.82–1.31; $p = 0.75$), casting further doubt on the additional benefit of prolonged cycles of first-line chemotherapy.[23]

All of these studies evaluated continuation of the initial regimen beyond four to six cycles compared with a true maintenance approach assessing prolongation of chemotherapy only in patients benefiting from platinum-based chemotherapy. An early maintenance study comparing a continuation and a switch approach enrolled 493 patients in 2000–2004 to receive three cycles of a triplet regimen (gemcitabine, ifosfamide, and cisplatin) on an every-3-week schedule. After three cycles, the 281 patients who did not have disease progression were randomly assigned to receive continued chemotherapy until disease progression or intolerability, or to receive switch maintenance therapy with paclitaxel (225 mg/m^2) every 3 weeks, also continued until disease progression or intolerability. The progression-free survival was similar in both arms (4.4 vs. 4.0 months; $p = 0.56$). Although numerically the median overall survival favored continued chemotherapy (11.9 vs. 9.7 months), the difference was not significant ($p = 0.17$). The 1-year survival rate was 49% for continued chemotherapy and 42% for switch therapy. Putting this trial into context with other maintenance studies is challenging, as patients in both arms continued with treatment until disease progressed, the randomization occurred after only three cycles of a platinum-based combination, and a substantial number of patients in each arm received the opposite regimen at the time of disease progression (69 of the 140 patients in the continued chemotherapy arm subsequently received paclitaxel).[24]

One of the first true maintenance studies evaluated switch maintenance therapy with vinorelbine after four cycles of mitomycin, ifosfamide, and cisplatin.[25] The study registered 573 patients with advanced stage NSCLC treated either with chemoradiation therapy for stage III disease or chemotherapy for stage IV disease, but only 181 were randomly assigned to the treatment arms of maintenance therapy with vinorelbine or no maintenance therapy. Of the 91 patients in the maintenance therapy arm, 7 died as a result of toxicity. No survival advantage was noted, which dampened enthusiasm for this approach.[26]

A randomized phase II trial demonstrated more robust activity with continuation maintenance therapy with paclitaxel. The trial included 401 patients who were randomly assigned to one of three treatment groups: weekly paclitaxel with every-4-week carboplatin or weekly paclitaxel with weekly carboplatin according to two different schedules.[26] Patients who did not have disease progression at week 16 were further randomly assigned to maintenance therapy with weekly paclitaxel (70 mg/m^2) for 3 of 4 weeks or to observation (65 patients in each group). The every-4-week carboplatin regimen was superior in terms of response, and the maintenance therapy resulted in a 9-week longer time to progression, a 15-week improvement in median survival, and improvements in 1- and 2-year survival rates. This study was conducted to determine the optimal weekly regimen of paclitaxel and carboplatin, and the efficacy of maintenance therapy was not a key question. However, these results led to adoption of maintenance therapy in the subsequent phase III trial, in which 444 patients were randomly assigned to weekly paclitaxel (100 mg/m^2) for 3 of 4 weeks plus carboplatin (AUC of 6) on day 1 of an every-4-week cycle or to standard every-3-week paclitaxel (225 mg/m^2) on day 1 with carboplatin (AUC of 6).[25] Patients in both treatment groups subsequently received maintenance therapy with paclitaxel (70 mg/m^2) for 3 of 4 weeks until disease progressed. Although the toxicity profiles differed, the efficacy outcomes did not. Because maintenance therapy with paclitaxel was given to patients in both groups, its contribution is not clear.[27]

Positive results with a continuation maintenance approach were found in a trial evaluating gemcitabine.[28] Of the 352 patients enrolled who received cisplatin (80 mg/m^2) on day 1 and gemcitabine (1250 mg/m^2) on days 1 and 8 every 3 weeks, 206 patients had no disease progression and were eligible for random assignment to continuation with gemcitabine or to no further treatment (2:1 randomization). Maintenance therapy with gemcitabine was associated with a significantly improved time to progression and a trend in favor of overall survival that did not reach statistical significance (median, 13.0 vs. 11.0 months; $p = 0.195$). Because of the lack of a significant improvement in overall survival, the results did not have a major impact on clinical practice.

Although study findings suggested a benefit with maintenance therapy, particularly continuation maintenance with paclitaxel or gemcitabine,[26,28] additional positive results were not reported until 2008. The tolerability of docetaxel, gemcitabine, and, more recently, pemetrexed, led to continued exploration of the concept of maintenance therapy.

TABLE 46.1 Recent Trials of Switch Maintenance Treatment With Chemotherapy

Author/Trial	Induction Treatment[a] Regimen	Maintenance Treatment Regimen	Median Age (Y)	PS 2 (%)	SCC Histology (%)	Never-Smokers (%)	Women (%)
Fidias et al.[10]	Carboplatin AUC 5 on day 1; gemcitabine 1000 mg/m² on days 1 & 8, every 3 wk × 4	Docetaxel 75 mg/m² every 3 wk × 6 (n = 153) Observation (n = 156)	65.4 65.5	5.9 10.3	16.3 18.8	NR NR	37.9 37.8
JMEN[8]	Platinum-based doublet (without pemetrexed) every 3 wk × 4	Pemetrexed 500 mg/m² every 3 wk + best supportive care (n = 441) Placebo + best supportive care (n = 226)	60.6 60.4	0 0	26 30	26 28	27 27

[a]In the trial by Fidias et al. 566 patients received induction treatment, and 309 (54.6%) were randomly assigned to maintenance therapy; the number of patients in JMEN who received induction treatment was not recorded.

AUC, area under the curve; HR, hazard ratio; NR, not recorded; PS 2, performance status of 2; SCC, squamous cell carcinoma.

MODERN MAINTENANCE TRIALS

Switch Maintenance With Chemotherapy (Table 46.1)

Fidias et al.[10] pioneered the modern use of the switch maintenance approach in a clinical trial in which 309 (54.6%) of 566 patients with nonprogressive disease after four cycles of first-line gemcitabine and carboplatin were randomly assigned to second-line treatment with docetaxel (maximum of six cycles) either immediately or at the time of disease progression. The median progression-free survival was longer for patients treated with immediate docetaxel than for patients treated with delayed docetaxel (5.7 vs. 2.7 months; HR, 0.71; p = 0.0001). The difference in median overall survival between the two treatment approaches did not reach significance (12.3 vs. 9.7 months; HR, 0.84; p = 0.0853) in this undersized trial. Overall survival was the primary end point of the trial, which lessened the impact of the other results. Approximately 37% of the patients assigned to receive delayed docetaxel never received it because of substantial symptomatic deterioration, death, or the investigator's decision. A subanalysis restricted to patients who did receive docetaxel in both arms showed that overall survival was identical in both arms (12.5 months), suggesting that the trend toward improved outcomes was associated with more patients in the immediate group receiving docetaxel. The toxicity profiles were similar for the two treatment approaches, and no differences in quality-of-life factors were found.

The JMEN trial evaluated pemetrexed as single-agent switch maintenance therapy. The trial design did not incorporate mandatory poststudy therapy, randomization was 2:1, and progression-free survival was the primary end point, which drew criticisms compared with the trial by Fidias et al.,[8] in which overall survival was the primary end point. However, the advantages of the JMEN trial were that its statistical assumptions were more realistic and the sample size allowed for more robust comparisons. In this trial, 663 patients with stage IIIB or IV disease who did not have disease progression during four cycles of platinum-based chemotherapy (without pemetrexed) were randomly assigned to receive best supportive care with or without pemetrexed until disease progression. Maintenance therapy with pemetrexed significantly improved the median progression-free survival (4.3 vs. 2.6 months; HR, 0.50; 95% CI, 0.42–0.61; p < 0.0001) and overall survival (13.4 vs. 10.6 months; HR, 0.79; 95%

CI, 0.65–0.95; p = 0.012) (Fig. 46.1A). Of note, relatively fewer patients in the pemetrexed group received systemic postdiscontinuation therapy (51% vs. 67%; p = 0.0001), and 19% of patients in the control group received salvage treatment with pemetrexed. A prespecified analysis showed a significant interaction between treatment and histology, consistent with the findings in similar prior trials in different NSCLC settings.[28] For patients who had tumors with nonsquamous cell histology, pemetrexed was associated with a greater benefit in terms of both progression-free survival (4.4 vs. 1.8 months; HR, 0.47; 95% CI, 0.37–0.60; p < 0.00001) and overall survival (median, 15.5 vs. 10.3 months; HR, 0.70; 95% CI, 0.56–0.88; p = 0.002), compared with patients who had tumors with squamous cell histology (Fig. 46.1B). In a subgroup analysis, the overall survival advantage with pemetrexed was greater for patients with stable disease at the end of induction chemotherapy (HR, 0.61) than for patients who had a partial or complete response (HR, 0.81). Treatment discontinuations due to drug-related toxic effects were more frequent with pemetrexed than with placebo (5% vs. 1%), as were drug-related grade 3 or 4 adverse events (16% vs. 4%; p < 0.0001), particularly fatigue (5% vs. 1%; p = 0.001) and neutropenia (3% vs. 0%, p = 0.006). No pemetrexed-related deaths occurred. Quality-of-life evaluations showed no global differences but a significant delay in worsening of pain and hemoptysis.[29] As a result of this trial, both the Food and Drug Administration (FDA) and the European Medicines Association (EMA) approved pemetrexed as switch maintenance therapy for metastatic NSCLC, specifically for patients with nonsquamous cell tumors in whom disease has not progressed after first-line platinum-based chemotherapy.

Continuation Maintenance With Chemotherapy (Table 46.2)

Since the 2006 publication of a phase III trial of continuation maintenance with gemcitabine,[28] this approach has been evaluated in two additional studies.[31,32] In the first of these studies, patients with stable or responsive disease after carboplatin plus gemcitabine were assigned to either gemcitabine with best supportive care or best supportive care alone (control). The study closed after 6 years because of slow accrual, with 225 patients randomly assigned instead of the planned 332. Of note, most patients had a performance status of 2 at study entry (64%) and of 2 or 3 at the time of randomization (57%). Maintenance treatment with gemcitabine was generally well tolerated,

TABLE 46.1 (Continued)

| Poststudy Treatment (%) | | Progression-Free Survival | | | Overall Survival | | | | |
Study Drug	Any	HR (95% CI)	Median (Mo)	p	HR (95% CI)	Median (Mo)	p	Toxicity	Quality of Life
NR 63	NR NR	0.71 (0.55–0.92)	5.7 2.7	0.0001	0.84 (0.65–1.08)	12.3 9.7	0.0853	Neutropenia: 27.6%; febrile neutropenia: 3.5%; fatigue: 9.7% Neutropenia: 28.6%; febrile neutropenia: 2%; fatigue: 4.1%	No differences (LCSS)
<1 18	51 67	0.50 (0.42–0.61)	4.3 2.6	0.0001	0.79 (0.65–0.95)	13.4 10.6	0.012	Total: 16% Fatigue: 5%; anemia: 3%; infection: 2% Total: 4% Fatigue: 1%; anemia: 1%; infection: 0%	No overall differences; better control of pain & hemoptysis

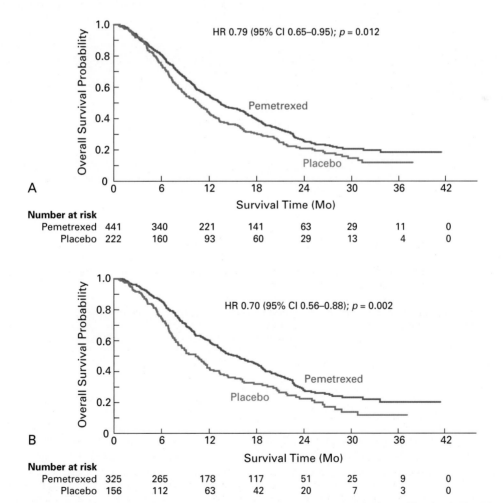

Fig. 46.1. Overall survival in all patients (A) and in patients with nonsquamous cell tumors (B) in the JMEN trial of switch maintenance therapy with pemetrexed. *CI*, confidence interval; *HR*, hazard ratio. *(Reprinted with permission from Ciuleanu T, Brodowicz T, Zielinski C, et al. Maintenance pemetrexed plus best supportive care versus placebo plus best supportive care for non-small cell lung cancer: a randomised, double-blind, phase 3 study. Lancet. 2009;374(9699):1432–1440.)*

TABLE 46.2 Recent Trials of Continuation Maintenance Treatment With Chemotherapy

	Induction Treatment		Maintenance Treatment					
Author/Trial	Regimen	No. of Patients Randomized (%)	Regimen	Median Age (Y)	PS 2 (%)	SCC Histology (%)	Never-Smokers (%)	Women (%)
Belani et al.[112]	Carboplatin AUC 5 on day 1; gemcitabine 1000 mg/m² on days 1 & 8, every 3 wk × 4 (n = 519)	255 (49.1)	Gemcitabine 1000 mg/m² on days 1 & 8, every 3 wk + best supportive care (n = 128)	67.2 67.5	64 76	NR NR	NR NR	40 33
			Best supportive care alone (n = 127)					
IFCT[31]	Cisplatin 80 mg/m² on day 1; gemcitabine 1250 mg/m² on days 1 & 8, every 3 wk × 4 (n = 834)	464 (55.6)	Gemcitabine 1250 mg/m² on days 1 & 8, every 3 wk (n = 154)	57.9 59.8	2.6 1.2	22.1 19.4	11 7.7	26.6 27.1
			Observation (n = 155)					
Zhang et al.[32]	Cisplatin 75 mg/m² on day 1; docetaxel 60 or 75 mg/m² on day 1, every 3 wk × 4 (n = 378)	184 (48.7)	Docetaxel 60 mg/m² day 1, every 3 wk × 6 + best supportive care (n = 123)					
			Best supportive care alone (n = 61)					
PARAMOUNT[33]	Cisplatin 75 mg/m² on day 1 + pemetrexed 500 mg/m² on day 1, every 3 wk × 4 (n = 939)	539 (57.4)	Pemetrexed 500 mg/m² every 3 wk + best supportive care (n = 359)	60 62	0 0	0 0	223 19	44 38
			Placebo + best supportive care (n = 180)					
AVAPERL[35]	Cisplatin 75 mg/m² & pemetrexed 500 mg/m² + bevacizumab 7.5 mg/kg on day 1, every 3 wk × 4 (n = 376)	253 (67.3)	Pemetrexed 500 mg/m² + bevacizumab 7.5 mg/kg on day 1, every 3 wk (n = 128)	60 60	1.9 5.8	0 0	24.8 26.1	42.4 43.3
			Bevacizumab 7.5 mg/kg on day 1, every 3 wk (n = 125)					
PointBreak[37]	Carboplatin AUC 6 + pemetrexed 500 mg/m² + bevacizumab 15 mg/kg on day 1, every 3 wk × 4 Carboplatin AUC 6 + paclitaxel 200 mg/m² + bevacizumab 155 mg/kg on day 1, every 3 wk × 4	590 (62.8)	Pemetrexed 500 mg/m² + bevacizumab 15 mg/kg on day 1, every 3 wk (n = 292)	63.8 64.3	0 0	0 0	13.4 11.8	49.3 46.6
			Bevacizumab 15 mg/kg on day 1, every 3 wk (n = 298)					
PRO-NOUNCE[40]	Carboplatin AUC 6 + pemetrexed 500 mg/m² on day 1, every 3 wk (n = 182) Carboplatin AUC 6 + paclitaxel 200 mg/m² + bevacizumab 15 mg/kg on day 1 every 3 wk × 4 (n = 179)	193 (52.4)	Pemetrexed 500 mg/m² on day 1 every 3 wk (n = 98)	65.8 65.4	0 0	0 0	32.2 3.9	7.7 34.1
			Bevacizumab 15 mg/kg on day 1 every 3 wk (n = 95)					

AUC, area under the curve; *FACT-G*, functional assessment of cancer therapy-general; *FACT-GOG*, functional assessment of cancer therapy-gynecologic group; *FACT-Ntx*, functional assessment of cancer-neurotoxicity; *HR*, hazard ratio; *NR*, not recorded; *PS 2*, performance status of 2; *SCC*, squamous cell carcinoma.

Poststudy Treatment (%)		Progression-Free Survival			Overall Survival				
Study Drug	Any	HR (95% CI)	Median (Mo)	p	HR (95% CI)	Median (Mo)	p	Toxicity	Quality of Life
2 3	16 17	1.04 (0.81–1.45)	3.9 3.8	0.58	0.97 (0.72–1.30)	9.3 8.0	0.84	Neutropenia: 15%; anemia: 9%; fatigue: 5% Neutropenia: 2%; anemia: 5%; fatigue: 2%	NR
0 0	77.2 90.9	0.56 (0.44–0.72)	3.8 1.9 5.4 2.8	0·001 0·002	0.89 (0.69–1.15)	12.1 10.8	0.3867	Neutropenia: 20.8%; anemia: 2.6%; fatigue: 1.9% Neutropenia: 0.6%; anemia: 0.6%; fatigue: 0%	No differences NR
2 4	64 72	0.62 (0.40–0.79)	4.1 2.8	0·0001	0.78 (0·64–0.96)	13.9 11.0	0.0195	Neutropenia: 5.8%; anemia: 6.4%; fatigue 4.7% Neutropenia: 0%; anemia: 0.6%; fatigue: 1.1%	No differences (EQ-5D)
NR	69.6 70.8	0.48 (0.35–0.66)	7.4 3.7	0·001	0.87 (0·63–1.21)	17.1 13.2	0.29	Any: 37.6% Neutropenia: 5.6%; anemia: 3.2%; fatigue: 2.4% Any: 21.7% Neutropenia: 0%; anemia: 0%; fatigue: 1.7%;	No differences
13.4 39.9	57.2 64.8	NR	8.6 6.9	NR	NR	17.7 15.7	0.84	Neutropenia: 14%; anemia: 11%; fatigue: 9.6% Neuropathy: 0%; hypertension: 3.1% Neutropenia: 11.4%; anemia: 0.3%; fatigue: 1.7% Neuropathy: 4.7%; hypertension: 6.0%	No differences except less neurotoxicity was reported in the pemetrexed arm (FACT-G, FACT-L FACT & GOG-Ntx)
47.3 52.5	77.2 90.9	1.06 (0.84–1.35)	4.4 5.5	0–610	1.07 (0.83-1.36)	10.5 11.7	0.615	Neutropenia: 25%; anemia: 19%; thrombopenia: 24%; fatigue: 6.4%; vomiting: 1.8% Neutropenia:49%; anemia: 5%; thrombopenia: 10%; fatigue 5.4%; vomiting: 5.48%	No differences

however there was a higher incidence of grade 3 or 4 toxicity, namely, anemia, neutropenia, thrombocytopenia, or fatigue. The treatment arms did not differ in terms of progression-free survival (HR, 1.09; 95% CI, 0.89–1.45) or overall survival (HR, 0.97; 95% CI, 0.72–1.30). The trial outcomes appeared to have been influenced by the unfitness of the study population; for example, the rate of poststudy treatment was 16% in the gemcitabine arm and 17% in the control arm. Indeed, patients with a poor performance status had a significantly worse outcome than patients with a performance status of 1 (HR, 1.50; 95% CI, 1.10–2.03; $p < 0.009$). Based on these and similar results, there is agreement that maintenance treatment should not be recommended to patients with a poor performance status. The implications of these results on the adoption of continuation maintenance with gemcitabine for other patients are less clear, as it is likely the negative findings were based more on the general fitness of the enrolled patients than on a lack of effectiveness of gemcitabine per se.

In the second of the studies, the IFCT-GFPC 0502 trial, patients were randomly assigned to observation or one of two different drugs for maintenance therapy, gemcitabine or erlotinib, if they did not have disease progression after four courses of induction therapy with cisplatin plus gemcitabine.[32] Progression-free survival was the primary end point, and no comparison between the two maintenance arms was planned. The study design imposed the same second-line treatment (pemetrexed) in all three arms to avoid bias in the survival analysis as a result of an imbalance in subsequent treatments. Independently assessed progression-free survival was almost 2 months longer in the gemcitabine arm than in the observation arm (HR, 0.55; 95% CI, 0.54–0.88; $p = 0.003$), and the benefit was consistent across all clinical subgroups, including different histologies. Preliminary survival analysis did not show any meaningful differences among the study arms, but patients who received second-line pemetrexed or who had a performance status of 0 appeared to derive greater benefit. Exploratory analysis showed that the magnitude of response to induction chemotherapy may affect the overall survival benefit of maintenance therapy with gemcitabine. Among patients with an objective response to induction chemotherapy, the median overall survival was 15.2 months with gemcitabine compared with 10.8 months with observation (HR, 0.72; 95% CI, 0.51–1.04). Maintenance with gemcitabine was well tolerated, with grade 3 or 4 treatment-related adverse events (mostly neutropenia and thrombocytopenia) reported more commonly in the gemcitabine arm (27%) than in the observation arm (2%).

The TFINE study evaluated the role of docetaxel in the continuation maintenance setting. In this study, 378 patients were initially randomly assigned (1:1) to receive cisplatin (75 mg/m^2) plus docetaxel (75 mg/m^2 or 60 mg/m^2) for four cycles.[32] Patients with stable disease after first-line treatment were subsequently randomly assigned (1:2) to best supportive care or maintenance therapy with docetaxel (60 mg/m^2) for up to six cycles. The two docetaxel doses yielded similar response rates as induction treatment, but the higher dose was associated with higher rates of diarrhea and neutropenia. Continuation maintenance therapy with docetaxel significantly prolonged progression-free survival at a magnitude similar to that in the switch setting (median, 5.4 vs. 2.8 months; $p = 0.002$).

The PARAMOUNT trial was designed to determine if maintenance therapy with pemetrexed would improve efficacy compared with placebo after four courses of cisplatin and pemetrexed in patients with advanced nonsquamous cell NSCLC.[33] Of the 939 patients enrolled, 57% were randomly assigned (2:1) after the induction phase to continuation maintenance therapy with pemetrexed plus best supportive care or placebo plus best supportive care. The primary objective of this study, progression-free survival, was improved in the maintenance therapy arm compared with the placebo arm (median, 4.1 vs. 2.8 months, HR, 0.62; p

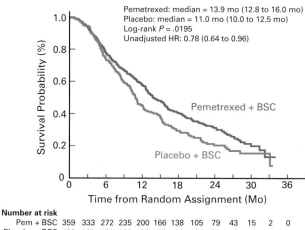

Fig. 46.2. Overall survival from date of randomization to maintenance therapy in the PARAMOUNT trial of continuation maintenance therapy with pemetrexed. *BSC,* best supportive care; *HR,* hazard ratio. *(Reprinted with permission from Paz-Ares LG, de Marinis F, Dediu M, et al. PARAMOUNT: Final overall survival results of the phase III study of maintenance pemetrexed versus placebo immediately after induction treatment with pemetrexed plus cisplatin for advanced nonsquamous non-small cell lung cancer. J Clin Oncol. 2013;31(23):2895–2902.)*

= 0.0001). An independent review of progression-free survival (88% of patients) confirmed the investigator-assessed results. The mature survival analysis confirmed the superiority of maintenance therapy with pemetrexed (median overall survival, 13.9 vs. 11.0 months; HR, 0.78; $p = 0.0195$; Fig. 46.2).[7] Pemetrexed improved survival consistently, including response to induction therapy (HR, 0.81) and stable disease (HR, 0.76). Use of postdiscontinuation therapy was similar: 64% and 72% in the maintenance therapy arm and placebo arm, respectively. Pemetrexed remained tolerable for the vast majority of patients, even in the long-term; however, the rates of anemia, fatigue, and neutropenia were higher in the maintenance therapy arm than in the placebo arm. No significant differences in health status were found during maintenance therapy between the arms, as assessed with the EQ-5D questionnaire.[34] The EMA approved pemetrexed as continuation maintenance therapy based on the findings of this study.

Another trial (AVAPERL) analyzed the contribution of pemetrexed maintenance in combination with bevacizumab in patients exposed to both drugs in a cisplatin-based triplet as induction therapy.[36] The trial included 376 patients with nonsquamous cell NSCLC, 253 of whom were randomly assigned to maintenance therapy. Compared with bevacizumab alone, pemetrexed plus bevacizumab significantly prolonged progression-free survival from the time of induction therapy (median, 10.2 vs. 6.6 months; HR, 0.50; 95% CI, 0.37–0.69; $p < 0.001$) and from the time of randomization (median, 7.4 vs. 3.7 months; HR, 0.48; 95% CI, 0.35–0.66; $p < 0.001$). This benefit was confirmed in all major subgroups analyzed, including patients with stable disease or response after induction therapy. An updated evaluation on overall survival, a secondary end point, showed a nonsignificant 4-month advantage in favor of the combined maintenance treatment (median, 13.1 vs. 17.2 months; HR, 0.87; $p = 0.29$).[36] More severe toxicity occurred in the pemetrexed plus bevacizumab arm, including grade 3–5 hematologic events (10.4% vs. 0%) and nonhematologic events (31.2% vs. 21.7%). A smaller trial assessed the same experimental arm with the combination of pemetrexed and bevacizumab as maintenance therapy after a carboplatin-pemetrexed-bevacizumab induction regimen in comparison with the same induction regimen followed by pemetrexed alone; the primary end point was the progression-free survival rate at 1 year.[38] The study was clearly underpowered and 1-year progression-free survival did not significantly differ between the two arms. However, there was a trend favoring the combined maintenance arm with a median progression-free survival measured from enrollment of 11.5 months compared with 7.3 months in the pemetrexed maintenance arm (HR, 0.73; 95% CI, 0.44–1.19; *p* = 0.198). Two other trials have provided further information on the role of continuation maintenance therapy with pemetrexed, one with bevacizumab and one without. The PointBreak trial randomly assigned 939 patients with advanced nonsquamous cell NSCLC to receive induction treatment with pemetrexed, carboplatin, and bevacizumab followed by maintenance therapy with pemetrexed and bevacizumab or to induction treatment with paclitaxel, carboplatin, and bevacizumab followed by bevacizumab.[39,40] In contrast to expectations, this trial showed superimposable survival curves for both treatment arms (HR, 1.00; *p* = 0.949), with a modest benefit in progression-free survival (HR, 0.83; 95% CI, 0.71–0.96; *p* = 0.012) favoring the pemetrexed and bevacizumab arm. It must be noted, however, that the induction phase of the study is important to the final overall analysis, as when the analysis is restricted to the 590 patients who were followed up after maintenance therapy (292 who received pemetrexed and bevacizumab and 298 who received bevacizumab alone), the separation of the progression-free survival curve (median, 8.6 vs. 6.9 months) as well as the overall survival curve (median, 15.7 vs. 17.7 months) is more apparent, although not of the magnitude seen in the AVAPERL study.

The toxicity was as expected based on the known profiles of the agents, including more anemia and fatigue for patients who received pemetrexed as part of induction therapy, and more neuropathy and hypertension for patients who received paclitaxel. Patient-reported changes in quality of life did not differ according to treatment, with the exception of neurotoxicity and alopecia, which were less frequently associated with pemetrexed.[41]

The PRONOUNCE study also compared two combined induction plus maintenance strategies in advanced nonsquamous NSCLC. The primary end point, progression-free survival without grade 4 toxicity, has controversial clinical relevance.[42] Patients were assigned to receive four courses of pemetrexed and carboplatin followed by pemetrexed (182 patients) or paclitaxel, carboplatin, and bevacizumab followed by bevacizumab (179 patients). There were no differences in progression-free survival (HR, 1.06; *p* = 0.610) or overall survival (HR, 1.07; *p* = 0.616). Therefore, this undersized trial did not demonstrate a difference in efficacy between the two approaches, but equivalence cannot be claimed, as the trial did not robustly rule out differences of moderate or small magnitude. There were no unexpected findings in terms of safety profile for either regimen.

Another trial, ERACLE (NCT00948675), compared cisplatin and pemetrexed with pemetrexed maintenance to carboplatin, paclitaxel, and bevacizumab with bevacizumab maintenance.[43] This trial is similar to PRONOUNCE, with three exceptions: the platinum agent used (cisplatin vs. carboplatin), the number of induction chemotherapy cycles (6 vs. 4), and the primary end point (differences in quality of life between the two arms vs. progression-free survival without grade 4 toxicity). This underpowered randomized study only showed a nonsignificant trend favoring the pemetrexed arm for EuroQoL 5 Dimensions-Index.

We await a large phase III trial of continuation versus switch maintenance therapy. Two small phase II trials have addressed this debate, but neither was large enough to provide conclusive findings. In one of these studies,[50] patients were randomly assigned to four cycles of either carboplatin and paclitaxel or carboplatin and gemcitabine; patients in both arms who had no disease progression subsequently received gemcitabine (1000 mg/m²) on days 1 and 8 every 3 weeks.[44] The progression-free

survival was 4.6 months in the paclitaxel (switch) arm and 3.5 months in the gemcitabine (continuation) arm, and there was no difference in the median overall survival (approximately 15 months in both arms; HR, 0.79; *p* = 0.60). In the other study, conducted in Japan, patients who had disease control after four cycles of induction chemotherapy with carboplatin and pemetrexed were randomly assigned to receive either continuation therapy with pemetrexed or switch therapy with docetaxel.[45] The study enrolled 85 patients, 51 of whom subsequently received maintenance therapy. The median progression-free survival from the time of randomization was 4.1 months for continuation therapy with pemetrexed compared with 8.2 months for switch therapy with docetaxel (HR, 0.56; 95% CI, 0.28–1.08; *p* = 0.084). The overall survival from the time of randomization was 20.6 months for continuation therapy compared with 19.9 months for switch therapy (HR, 0.79; 95% CI, 0.3–2.00; *p* = 0.622). Although no firm conclusions can be drawn from such a small study, the results are intriguing and do not make a clear argument in favor of switch versus continuation maintenance. It is interesting to note that more than 30% of patients in the switch therapy arm received pemetrexed as second-line therapy and 45% of patients in the continuation therapy arm subsequently received docetaxel as second-line therapy.[43] Larger trials of this nature are needed to help resolve this question.

Maintenance With Noncytotoxic Agents

Epidermal Growth Factor Receptor Inhibitors (Table 46.3)

Maintenance therapy with cytotoxic drugs evolved in parallel with the development of targeted therapy agents with mechanisms of action and toxicity profiles supporting long-term use. The use of these agents tended to continue until disease progression rather than be stopped after a predefined number of cycles. Many targeted therapy agents are taken daily by mouth.

The original approval of the epidermal growth factor receptor (EGFR) tyrosine kinase inhibitor erlotinib was for once daily oral administration in the second- or third-line setting, with treatment continued until disease progression.[46] The question of duration of therapy was not addressed, as the toxicity profile did not necessitate discontinuation. Initial trials with the EGFR inhibitor gefitinib were similar. Trials to address duration of therapy in patients with stable disease have not been conducted, nor are such studies likely in the future. The questions surrounding duration of therapy now focus on the concept of continuation beyond disease progression. A discussion of EGFR inhibitor therapy must address its use for patients who have tumors with EGFR-activating mutations (EGFR mutation-positive tumors) compared with patients who have EGFR wild-type tumors. Studies of continuation of EGFR inhibitor therapy beyond disease progression have centered on patients with EGFR mutation-positive tumors. The use of EGFR inhibitors as first-line therapy is now considered standard for patients with EGFR mutation-positive NCSLC, and three agents have been approved for use in the United States: erlotinib, afatinib, and more recently gefitinib. In all trials that have evaluated EGFR inhibitors, the agent was continued until disease progression.

Continuation maintenance with an EGFR inhibitor after first-line concurrent use with doublet chemotherapy was evaluated in four large placebo-controlled phase III global trials (two with erlotinib and two with gefitinib): TRIBUTE, TALENT, INTACT1, and INTACT 2.[46–48] In these early trials, the EGFR inhibitor was given concurrently with a first-line platinum-based doublet and then continued until disease progression, with cessation of chemotherapy after a maximum of six cycles. None of these trials demonstrated a survival benefit for the combination arm, even with the maintenance approach.[46–48] Concern was raised about antagonism when the chemotherapy

TABLE 46.3 Recent Phase III Trials of Switch Maintenance Treatment With EGFR-TKIs

Induction Treatment			Maintenance Treatment					
Author/Trial	Regimen	No. of Patients Randomized (%)	Regimen	Median Age (Y)	PS 2 (%)	SCC Histology (%)	Never-Smokers (%)	Women (%)
SATURN[9]	Platinum-based chemotherapy × 4 cycles (n = 1949)	889 (45.6)	Erlotinib 150 mg daily (n = 458) Placebo (n = 451)	60 60	0 0	38 43	18 17	27 25
IFCT[31]	Cisplatin 80 mg/m^2 on day 1; gemcitabine 1250 mg/m^2 on days 1 & 8 every 3 wk × 4 (n = 834)	464 (55.6%)	Erlotinib 150 mg daily (n = 155) Observation (n = 155)	56.4 59.8	5.2 2.6	17.4 19.4	11 7.7	27.1 27.1
ATLAS[52,53]	Platinum-based chemotherapy + bevacizumab × 4 (n = 1160)	768 (66%)	Bevacizumab & erlotinib (150 mg) daily (n = 370) Bevacizumab & placebo (n = 373)	64 64	0 0	3 1.6	16.5 17.7	47.8 47.7
WJTOG 0203[48]	Carboplatin/paclitaxel OR 1 of 4 cisplatin doublets × 3 (n = 604)		Gefitinib 250 mg daily after 3 cycles of chemotherapy (n = 302, with 298 treated) Gefitinib 250 mg daily after up to 6 cycles of chemotherapy (n = 301, with 297 treated)	62 63	0 0	21 32	30 32	36 35
INFORM[54]	Platinum doublet (NP) × 4 (n = 296)		Gefitinib 250 mg (n = 148) Placebo (n = 148)	55 55	2 3	18 20	53 55	44 38
EORTC 08021[55]	Platinum doublet (NP) × 4 (n = 173)		Gefitinib 250 mg (n = 86) Placebo (n = 87)	61 62	7 5	17 22	21 23	22 24

[a]Twenty percent of the patients in the gefitinib arm and 32% of the patients in the placebo arm received an EGFR inhibitor.

[b]Thirteen patients in the gefitinib arm received erlotinib; 8 patients in the placebo arm received gefitinib, and 27 patients in the placebo arm received erlotinib.

[c]Twenty-one patients in the gefitinib arm received chemotherapy, and 13 received an EGFR inhibitor; 23 patients in the placebo arm received chemotherapy and 35 received an EGFR inhibitor.

EORTC, European Organisation for Research and Treatment of Cancer; HR, hazard ratio; NP, NR, not reported; PS 2, performance status of 2; SCC, squamous cell carcinoma. FACT-L, Functional assessment of cancer therapy-lung.

Poststudy Treatment (%)		Progression-Free Survival			Overall Survival				
Study Drug	Any	HR (95% CI)	Median	p	HR	Median (Mo)	p	Toxicity	Quality of Life
11	71	0.71 (0.62–0.82)	12.3 wk	<0.0001	0.81 (0.70–0.95)	12.0	0.0088	Any 3+: 12%	No differences (FACT-L)
21	72		11.1 wk			11.0		Rash: 60% (9% 3+); diarrhea: 18%	
								Any 3+: 1%	
								Rash: 8% (0% 3+); diarrhea: 3%	
5.8	79.9	0.69 (0.54–0.88)	2.9	0.003	0.87 (0.68-1.13)	11.4	0.3043	Rash: 63% (9% 3/4); diarrhea: 20%	No differences
0	90.9		1.9			10.8		Rash (3/4): 0%; diarrhea: <1%	
39.7	50.3	0.722 (0.59–0.88)	4.76	0.0012	0.90 (0.74–1.09)	15.9	0.2686	Rash (3/4): 10%; diarrhea (3/4): 9%	NR
39.7	55.5		3.75			13.9		Rash (3/4): <1%; diarrhea (3/4): <1%	
58	75	0.68 (0.57–0.80)	4.6	<0.001	0.86 (0.72–1.03)	13.7	0.11	Transaminitis (3/4) 11%	No differences (LCS v 4)
0	55 (gefitinib)		4.3			12.9		Transaminitis (3/4) 4%	
3[a]	51	0.42 (0.33–0.55)	4.8	<0.0001	0.84 (0.62–1.14)	18.7	0.26	Any rash: 50%; diarrhea: 25%; 3 toxicity-related deaths	FACT-L–time to worsening slowed on gefitinib arm (odds ratio, 3.41; 95% CI, 1.65–7.06; p = 0.0009)
8[a]	67		2.6			16.9		Rash: 9%; diarrhea: 9%	
15[b]	40[c]	0.61 (0.45–0.83)	4.1	0.002	0.81 (0.59–1.12)	10.9	0.204	Transaminitis (3/4): 10.6%; fatigue: 4.7%; rash (3): 1.2%	No differences
40[b]	67[c]		2.9			9.4		Transaminitis (3/4): 1.2%; fatigue: 1.2%; rash (3): 0%	

and EGFR inhibitor were given concurrently, and thus, later maintenance trials focused solely on a switch maintenance strategy.

Between 2003 and 2005, the phase III West Japan Thoracic Oncology Group Trial 0203 randomly assigned patients to either six cycles of a platinum-based doublet or three cycles of a platinum-based doublet followed by gefitinib (250 mg orally daily).[50] More than 600 patients were enrolled, and the study demonstrated a benefit in progression-free survival in the gefitinib arm (HR, 0.68; 95% CI, 0.57–0.80; $p < 0.001$), but no overall survival benefit for the trial as a whole (HR, 0.86; 95% CI, 0.72–1.03; $p = 0.11$). There was a significant overall survival benefit for patients with adenocarcinoma, but it must be noted that this study was conducted in Japan prior to routine EGFR mutation testing and likely included a large percentage of patients with EGFR-activating mutations. At final analysis, 54% of the patients in the chemotherapy-only arm subsequently received an EGFR inhibitor, compared with 75% in the chemotherapy followed by gefitinib arm. (Only 58% of patients in the gefitinib arm received the chemotherapy followed by maintenance with gefitinib.) It is noteworthy that of the entire study population, 68% were female, 78% had adenocarcinoma, and 30% had never smoked.[50]

The SATURN trial changed the use of EGFR inhibitors in the maintenance setting.[9] This study enrolled 1949 patients over 2.5 years, ending in May 2008, to a run-in of four cycles of platinum-based chemotherapy. The 889 patients who did not have disease progression after completion of the four cycles were then randomly assigned to receive erlotinib (150 mg orally daily) or placebo until disease progression or treatment-ending toxicity. Patients were stratified according to the results of EGFR expression on immunohistochemistry (IHC) but not by EGFR mutation status or response to induction chemotherapy

(objective response vs. stable disease). The primary end points were progression-free survival in all patients and in patients who had tumors with overexpression of EGFR. The progression-free survival was longer with erlotinib (12.3 vs. 11.1 weeks; HR, 0.71; 95% CI, 0.62–0.82; $p < 0.001$), and the difference was slightly greater among patients with tumors that overexpressed EGFR (12.3 vs. 11.1 weeks; HR, 0.69; 95% CI, 0.58–0.82; $p < 0.0001$). The largest benefit in progression-free survival was found in the small group of patients who had EGFR mutation-positive tumors (18 patients who received erlotinib and 22 who received placebo) (HR, 0.10; 95% CI, 0.04–0.25; $p < 0.0001$). The progression-free survival benefit associated with erlotinib was also significant for the group of patients who had EGFR wild-type tumors (165 who received erlotinib and 163 who received placebo) (HR, 0.78; 95% CI, 0.63–0.96; $p = 0.0185$). The benefit in progression-free survival translated into a benefit in overall survival for all patients in the trial (HR, 0.81; 95% CI, 0.7–0.95; $p = 0.088$) as well as for patients who had EGFR wild-type tumors (HR, 0.77; 95% CI, 0.61–0.97; $p = 0.0243$) (Fig. 46.3). Toxicity was as expected, with rash and diarrhea as the major toxicities reported with erlotinib maintenance.

In a subset analysis of SATURN, investigators sought to determine whether response to first-line chemotherapy could predict the effectiveness of maintenance erlotinb for individual patients. In this subset analysis, the progression-free survival benefit with erlotinib was more pronounced for patients who had stable disease as their best response to first-line chemotherapy. More significantly, an overall survival benefit was found only for patients with stable disease (HR, 0.72; 95% CI, 0.59–0.89; $p = 0.0019$) compared with patients who had had a previous response to chemotherapy (HR, 0.94; not significant).[51] This pattern, however, has not been consistently reported in other maintenance trials.

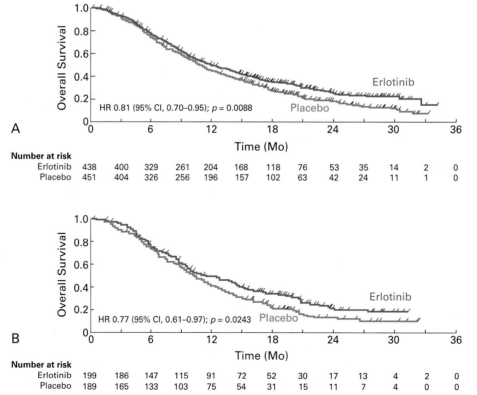

Fig. 46.3. Kaplan-Meier estimates of overall survival in the intention-to-treat population (A) and in patients with EGFR wild-type tumors (B) in the SATURN trial of switch maintenance therapy with erlotinib. *CI,* confidence interval; *HR,* hazard ratio. *(Reprinted with permission from Cappuzzo F, Ciuleanu T, Stelmakh L, et al. Erlotinib as maintenance treatment in advanced non-small cell lung cancer: a multicentre, randomised, placebo-controlled phase 3 study. Lancet Oncol. 2010;11(6):521–529.)*

All 889 patients randomly assigned in the SATURN trial provided tissue for biomarker testing.[50] Neither EGFR expression by IHC nor EGFR testing with fluorescent in situ hybridization (FISH) predicted for benefit in progression-free or overall survival. For the 49 patients with EGFR-mutation positive tumors, the progression-free survival favored erlotinib (HR, 0.10; 95% CI, 0.04–0.25; $p < 0.001$). Although the progression-free survival significantly favored maintenance therapy with erlotinib in the 388 patients with EGFR wild-type tumors (HR, 0.78; 95% CI, 0.63–0.98, $p = 0.0185$), the interactive $p < 0.001$ demonstrated that EGFR mutation status is predictive of a greater progression-free survival benefit. Despite the progression-free survival effect, the overall survival benefit was more pronounced in the group of patients with EGFR wild-type tumors, which was likely confounded by the fact that 67% of the patients with EGFR-mutation positive tumors in the placebo arm subsequently received treatment with an EGFR inhibitor. The progression-free survival was lower for the 90 patients who had tumors with V-Ki-ras2 Kirsten rat sarcoma viral oncogene homolog (KRAS) mutation compared with the 403 patients who had KRAS wild-type tumors, regardless of treatment (HR, 1.50; 95% CI, 1.06–2.12; $p = 0.02$), and there was a trend toward a shorter overall survival. However, the progression-free survival curves favored erlotinib for both the patients with KRAS wild-type tumors and patients with KRAS-positive tumors, although the benefit was significant for patients with KRAS wild-type tumors (HR, 0.70; 95% CI, 0.57–0.87; $p = 0.0009$) but not for patients with KRAS-positive tumors (HR, 0.77; not significant). In a subset analysis of 126 Asian patients in the SATURN trial, progression-free survival was significantly longer for patients in the erlotinib arm who had EGFR-positive tumors according to IHC (HR, 0.50; $p = 0.0057$) and there was a trend toward increased overall survival in the erlotinib arm, which was significant for the subgroup with EGFR-positive tumors on IHC ($p = 0.0233$).[51] The overall response rate was significantly higher in the erlotinib arm (24%) than in the placebo arm (24% vs. 5%; $p = 0.0025$).

The phase III ATLAS trial also randomly assigned patients who did not have disease progression after four cycles of a platinum-based doublet to maintenance erlotinib (150 mg orally daily) or placebo, but, unlike SATURN, bevacizumab was given during induction chemotherapy and was continued during the maintenance phase in both arms. The progression-free survival was significantly better in the bevacizumab and erlotinib arm (HR, 0.71; $p = 0.0012$), but this finding did not translate into an overall survival benefit (median, 14.4 vs. 13.3 months; not significant).[54] Similarly to the SATURN trial, EGFR IHC, EGFR FISH, and EGFR/KRAS mutation status were not predictive of outcome.[53]

As discussed in the section on chemotherapy, the IFCT-GFPC 0502 trial randomly assigned patients with stable disease after four courses of induction chemotherapy with cisplatin and gemcitabine to observation or to one of two different maintenance regimens: continuation gemcitabine or switch erlotinib.[31] The progression-free survival for the 155 patients assigned to switch erlotinib was significantly better than that for the 155 assigned to observation (HR, 0.69; 95% CI, 0.54–0.88; $p = 0.003$). However, overall survival was not significantly different between the 155 patients assigned to switch erlotinib and the 155 patients assigned to observation, given that the study was not powered to demonstrate a survival difference.[32] Unlike the SATURN trial, there was no differential benefit in progression-free or overall survival depending on whether patients had a response or stable disease with induction therapy; in fact, the overall survival trend was better for patients who had a response to chemotherapy.

On April 16, 2010, the US FDA approved erlotinib for use as maintenance therapy for patients who did not have disease progression after four cycles of platinum-based first-line chemotherapy. Overall survival was a secondary end point of the trial's sponsor but was the primary regulatory end point for this approval recommendation.[60] The European Medicines Agency gave an approval for erlotinib as maintenance agent restricted to patients with stable disease after induction chemotherapy. Nevertheless, the benefit of erlotinib maintenance therapy in patients with EGFR wild-type NSCLC was reassessed and questioned by the IUNO trial (NCT01328951), which was a randomized, double-blind, placebo-controlled, phase III study of maintenance erlotinib versus erlotinib at the time of disease progression in EGFR wild-type patients who have not progressed following 4 cycles of platinum-based chemotherapy. Detailed results of the trial are not known yet but overall survival (primary end point) was not superior in patients randomized to receive maintenance erlotinib compared with patients assigned to receive maintenance placebo followed by erlotinib upon progression (HR, 1.02; 95% CI, 0.85–1.22, $p = 0.82$). In the maintenance phase, erlotinib did not provide a progression-free survival benefit compared with placebo (HR, 0.94; 95% CI, 0.80–1.11, $p = 0.48$). Based on these results, the benefit-risk of erlotinib was reconsidered as negative for maintenance treatment in patients whose tumors do not have an EGFR activating mutation explaining that erlotinib approval for maintenance therapy was withdrawn by EMA.

Gefitinib has been evaluated in other maintenance studies. The largest of these studies, INFORM, enrolled 296 patients with stable disease after four cycles of cisplatin-based induction chemotherapy and randomly assigned them to receive gefitinib (250 mg orally daily) or placebo as switch maintenance treatment.[56] Toxicities were as expected, with one confirmed death from interstitial lung disease. The progression-free survival was 4.8 months for patients who received gefitinib compared with 2.6 months for patients who received placebo (HR, 0.42; 95% CI, 0.33–0.55; $p < 0.0001$). EGFR mutation testing was not required and was known only for 79 patients. Overall survival was similar for gefitinib and placebo arm in the intention to treat population (HR, 0.88; 95% CI, 0.68–1.14; $p = 0.335$) and in subgroups with wild-type EGFR (HR, 1.27; 95% CI, 0.7–2.3; $p = 0.431$) or unknown EGFR mutations (HR, 0.92; 95% CI, 0.68–1.25; $p = 0.603$). In the EGFR mutation–positive subgroup, the gefitinib arm showed a higher overall survival than the placebo arm (HR, 0.39; 95% CI, 0.15–0.97; $p = 0.036$).[57] A smaller phase III trial of maintenance therapy with gefitinib compared with placebo in patients with no disease progression after four cycles of a platinum-based doublet similarly demonstrated a significant benefit in progression-free survival with gefitinib, despite early closing of the trial due to low accrual.[55] EORTC 08021 closed after enrolling only 173 patients; it showed a significantly better progression-free survival for gefitinib than for placebo (HR, 0.61; 95% CI, 0.45–0.83; $p = 0.0015$), but only a trend toward better overall survival.

Another trial included compared pemetrexed plus cisplatin followed by maintenance gefitinib with gefitinib monotherapy in 236 East Asian patients with advanced nonsquamous NSCLC and unknown epidermal growth EGFR mutation status but did not reveal any significant progression-free or overall survival difference in the entire study population. Nevertheless, retrospectively, the pemetrexed-cisplatin followed by gefitinib arm provides a better survival for patients with wild-type EGFR while patients with EGFR activating mutations benefited from front-line gefitinib treatment.[59] All these data strongly support that the benefit coming from gefitinib maintenance treatment is restricted to patients with EGFR activating mutations.

EGFR targeted antibodies, such as cetuximab, have also been evaluated in NSCLC, always with a continuation maintenance approach after concurrent use in first-line therapy. In the best-known trial, FLEX, cetuximab was added to first-line cisplatin and vinorelbine for patients with advanced stage NSCLC that overexpressed EGFR on IHC. Although there was no clear response nor progression-free survival benefit, this large study of more than 1000 patients did show an approximately 1-month overall survival advantage for the cetuximab arm ($p = 0.044$).[61] Another randomized phase III trial explored platinum and taxane combinations with concurrent cetuximab followed by continuation maintenance cetuximab, and showed that the addition of cetuximab improved response but did not offer advantages in survival end points.[62] Cetuximab for NSCLC is still under investigation for continuation maintenance therapy. The largest ongoing trial has been conducted by the Southwest Oncology Group (SWOG 0819 trial) (NCT00946712) and includes concurrent and continuation maintenance cetuximab in the study arm, as well as concurrent and continuation maintenance bevacizumab for appropriate candidates of that drug in both the control and study arms. EGFR expression by FISH is used as a biomarker in the study.[63] This large phase III study failed to meet its two coprimary end points with no benefit in overall survival for the entire study population ($N = 1333$, HR, 0.94; 95% CI, 0.84–1.06; $p = 0.34$) and no significant progression-free survival improvement for patients with EGFR FISH positive tumors ($N = 400$, HR, 0.91; 95% CI, 0.74–1.12; $p = 0.37$). There was a trend toward an overall survival benefit in EGFR FISH positive patients (HR, 0.83; 95% CI, 0.67–1.04; $p = 0.10$) and for the subgroup of EGFR FISH positive patients who did not receive bevacizumab ($N = 234$, HR, 0.75; 95% CI, 0.57–0.998; $p = 0.048$). An exploratory analysis suggested a significant improvement of overall survival for patients with FISH positive squamous cell carcinoma ($N = 321$, HR, 0.56; 95% CI, 0.37–0.84; $p = 0.006$). However, the contribution of the maintenance part of cetuximab treatment cannot be assessed with this study design.

Another EGFR targeted antibody, necitumumab, has been assessed in squamous cell carcinoma given both concurrently and as continuation maintenance on a weekly basis with cisplatin and gemcitabine (maximum of six cycles) in a large open-label phase III study (SQUIRE trial, NCT00981058).[64] The addition of necitumumab to chemotherapy led to a significant improvement of overall survival (HR, 0.84; 95% CI, 0.74–0.96; $p = 0.01$), corresponding to a median survival of 11.5 months vs. 9.9 months in the control arm. Once again, the study was not designed to evaluate the role of the maintenance part of necitumumab treatment, given that 275 out of the 545 patients continued necitumumab after chemotherapy with a median of four additional cycles. EGFR expression as assessed by semiquantitative evaluation (H-score) was not predictive of survival benefit. An exploratory analysis in a subgroup of patients with available FISH testing suggested a larger survival benefit in patients with EGFR amplification ($N = 208$; HR, 0.70; 95% CI, 0.52–0.96).[65] The toxicity profile was similar to that of cetuximab, knowing that a parallel trial with pemetrexed and cisplatin plus necitumumab for patients with nonsquamous NSCLC, however, was stopped early for toxicity, primarily hypercoagulability.[66] An ongoing phase III trial (NCT01769391) is evaluating necitumumab with carboplatin and paclitaxel for patients with squamous cell NSCLC, and studies in Asia are investigating use of the agent in combination with cisplatin and gemcitabine for the same population of patients.

Vascular Endothelial Growth Factor Targeted Agents

Bevacizumab remains the only vascular endothelial growth factor (VEGF) targeted agent approved for the first-line treatment of NSCLC. Both registration trials in which bevacizumab was added to first-line chemotherapy involved continuation maintenance with bevacizumab for patients who did not have progressive disease after four to six cycles of a platinum-based doublet given concurrently with bevacizumab.[64–66] In the E4599 trial, 878 patients with newly diagnosed NSCLC were treated with carboplatin and paclitaxel with or without bevacizumab; there was a significant improvement in overall survival, the primary end point, for patients receiving bevacizumab (12.3 vs. 10.3 months; HR, 0.79; 95% CI, 0.67–0.92; $p = 0.003$). Additionally, the response rate and progression-free survival were significantly higher in the bevacizumab arm, whether the agent was

given concurrently with chemotherapy or as continuation maintenance therapy. The placebo-controlled AVAiL trial randomly assigned more than 1000 patients to receive first-line cisplatin and gemcitabine with bevacizumab or placebo, again given both concurrently with chemotherapy and as continuation maintenance therapy. This study also showed significant improvements in response and progression-free survival, but not in overall survival.

Thus, bevacizumab continues as maintenance therapy beyond completion of a platinum-based doublet in all standard treatment protocols. The contribution of the maintenance component, however, has not been established. A secondary retrospective landmark analysis of E4599 evaluated patients who were alive without progression for at least 21 days after completion of six cycles of chemotherapy. The progression-free survival after induction therapy was longer for patients in the bevacizumab arm (who were receiving bevacizumab maintenance) compared with patients in the chemotherapy arm (4.4 vs. 2.8 months; HR, 0.64; $p < 0.001$). The median overall survival after induction therapy was 12.8 months in the bevacizumab maintenance arm and 11.4 months in the chemotherapy arm (HR, 0.75; $p = 0.03$).[63] In a retrospective analysis of 272 patients with advanced NSCLC who were treated in community practices, 27% of patients had received maintenance bevacizumab. As expected, these patients tended to be younger and more fit. Landmark and propensity score analyses supported a reduced risk of death with bevacizumab maintenance (landmark: HR, 0.52; 95% CI, 0.37–0.73; propensity: HR, 0.70; 95% CI, 0.39–1.28). Thus, the maintenance therapy contributed to an overall benefit in this retrospective sample, even after statistical adjustments were made for selection bias.[71] Nonrandomized studies have been done in which bevacizumab was given with chemotherapy but not continued as maintenance therapy; however, the results of these trials have not advanced knowledge about the effectiveness of this approach because of the heterogeneity of patients enrolled and the various chemotherapy regimens, as well as the lack of randomization.[72,73]

In other disease settings, maintenance therapy with bevacizumab improves outcomes. For example, in a randomized phase III trial of ovarian cancer (GOG-0218), bevacizumab was added to carboplatin and paclitaxel either as concurrent therapy only or as concurrent and continuation maintenance therapy. The progression-free survival was significantly better for the arm with continuation maintenance therapy compared with the control arm (no bevacizumab) (HR, 0.72; 95% CI, 0.63–0.82; $p < 0.0001$). However, the progression-free survival did not differ between patients who received only concurrent bevacizumab and patients in the control arm.[74] Recent data have also suggested benefit with continuation maintenance therapy with bevacizumab beyond disease progression in colon cancer.[75] In that phase III trial, patients who had disease progression during first-line chemotherapy plus bevacizumab were randomly assigned at the time of progression to receive second-line chemotherapy with or without bevacizumab; bevacizumab was associated with a significantly longer overall survival (11.2 vs. 9.8 months; HR, 0.81; 95% CI, 0.69–0.94; $p = 0.0062$). These findings have led to an ongoing trial to evaluate the role of continuation bevacizumab beyond progression in combination with second-line therapy for patients with advanced stage NSCLC.[76]

There is uncertainty about whether bevacizumab is needed beyond the completion of chemotherapy. That question will be addressed by the E5508 trial, which is enrolling patients with EGFR wild-type NSCLC who have not had disease progression after four cycles of carboplatin, paclitaxel, and bevacizumab (E4599 regimen). The patients will be randomly assigned to receive continuation of the bevacizumab, pemetrexed in addition to bevacizumab, or pemetrexed alone. Other recent maintenance trials with bevacizumab (PointBreak, PRONOUNCE) have evaluated different chemotherapy regimens, but have included concurrent and continuation maintenance with bevacizumab in all arms.

Multiple VEGF receptor (VEGFR) inhibitors are being studied in NSCLC, several as concurrent therapy with a first-line platinum-based doublet and continuation maintenance therapy. Although many studies have shown an improvement in response and progression-free survival with this strategy, none have demonstrated an overall survival benefit compared with standard first-line chemotherapy without maintenance therapy with a VEGFR inhibitor. The usefulness of maintenance therapy with these agents has therefore not been clearly addressed, as the trials to date have evaluated VEGFR inhibitors in combination with chemotherapy and continued without a randomization to maintenance therapy or no maintenance therapy. In a phase III placebo-controlled study, sorafenib given concurrently with carboplatin and paclitaxel and as maintenance therapy after four cycles failed to improve overall survival and increased mortality among patients who had tumors with squamous cell histology.[77] Similarly, the phase III MONET1, which randomly assigned patients to carboplatin and paclitaxel, with or without motesanib (AMG 706) followed by continuation maintenance therapy with motesanib, did not meet its primary end point of improved overall survival (HR, 0.89; $p = 0.137$).[78] The findings of a randomized phase II study with vandetanib for advanced stage NSCLC hinted that maintenance with vandetanib was of benefit, but the results of the study were not conclusive. All patients received chemotherapy plus vandetanib, with randomization to maintenance vandetanib or placebo for patients who did not have disease progression after completion of four cycles; the progression-free survival was similar to that for historical controls for chemotherapy alone in both arms.[79]

Ongoing trials are evaluating other VEGFR inhibitors given concurrently and then as maintenance therapy for advanced NSCLC, including a trial in which axitinib is given with either cisplatin and pemetrexed (for nonsquamous cell NSCLC, NCT007687855) or cisplatin and gemcitabine (for squamous cell NSCLC). The combination of cisplatin, gemcitabine, and axitinib has been shown to be feasible, but without a control arm, it remains difficult to assess the role for axitinib in this schedule.[80] Because of the toxicity associated with sunitinib given with concurrent chemotherapy, this agent has been studied as true switch maintenance therapy. A phase II study in which sunitinib (50 mg/d orally for 4 weeks followed by 2 weeks off) was given after four cycles of carboplatin and paclitaxel was not randomized and did not meet its primary end point.[81] However, the phase III CALGB 30607 study comparing sunitinib given orally daily on a continuous schedule with placebo as maintenance therapy after four cycles of platinum-based first-line chemotherapy demonstrated an improvement of progression-free survival without prolongation of overall survival.[82] Two hundred and ten patients were randomized with a progression-free survival of 4.3 months for patients assigned to the sunitinib arm versus 2.8 months for the placebo arm (HR, 0.58; 95% CI, 0.42–0.79; $p = 0.0004$), irrespective of histology; overall survival was not different (HR, 1.08; $p = 0.64$).

Unfortunately, other efforts at maintenance therapy with vascular pathway agents have been disappointing. A large phase III placebo-controlled trial of carboplatin and paclitaxel with or without the vascular disrupting agent vadimezan (ASA404) included maintenance therapy with vadimezan as part of the study design. The outcomes did not differ between the two arms, so it is unclear whether maintenance therapy was of any benefit.[83] Thalidomide was also studied as a continuous maintenance agent given orally for 2 years after four cycles of induction chemotherapy with carboplatin and gemcitabine. All results favored the placebo arm, leading to abandonment of further exploration of maintenance therapy with thalidomide.[84] Another agent with antiangiogenic properties, tested as a maintenance therapy in a large phase III placebo-controlled trial, is the oral agent carboxyaminoimidazole (CAI), a carboxyamide-amino-triazole. Treatment with CAI or placebo was started after completion of first-line chemotherapy and, although the trial had accrual issues and included only 186

patients, the results indicated increased toxicity but no improvements in efficacy end points.[85]

Immunotherapy

Although none has demonstrated efficacy in NSCLC to date, vaccine and other immune-based strategies are being studied as a form of continuation maintenance therapy. Older trials focused on interferon gamma and interleukin-2, with encouraging preliminary results, but no further development.[86,87] The true vaccines studied in larger trials in NSCLC include belagenpumatucel-L and BLP-25, among others. In patients with stage IV NSCLC, these agents are often given as switch maintenance therapy, started after completion of chemotherapy. Encouraging results from a randomized phase II study of belagenpumatucel-L, a transforming growth factor beta-2 allogeneic tumor cell vaccine,[88] led to a recently completed randomized phase III trial of the vaccine as switch maintenance therapy for patients who had a response to six cycles of platinum-based chemotherapy for advanced stage NSCLC. The results of that trial were not available at the time of publication. L-BLP-25, a vaccine against MUC-1, also showed encouraging results as a maintenance approach for patients with stable or responding disease after first-line chemotherapy for advanced stage NSCLC. Although initial studies have focused on patients with inoperable stage III NSCLC, it is possible that future research will evaluate L-BLP-25 as maintenance treatment for stage IV NSCLC.[89] Other ongoing vaccine trials in the stage IV maintenance arena include a trial that has recently completed accrual (NCT00415818), in which TG4010, a MUC-1 and interleukin-2 vaccine, is being given to patients with MUC-1-expressing tumors during six cycles of a platinum-based doublet and continuing after that treatment. Another vaccine trial, ongoing in the United Kingdom (NCT01444118), seeks to validate work done in Cuba with a compound composed of an adjuvant plus humanized recombinant antigen EGF (cyclophosphamide and recombinant human rEGF-P64K/Montanide ISA 51) vaccine. In a phase III trial of the immunotherapy agent racotumomab, the agent will be studied in patients with advanced stage NSCLC who have had a response to standard first-line chemotherapy (NCT01460472). Although most of the patients will have stage III disease, approximately 30% of the more than 1000 patients in the trial will have stage IV disease.

Another ongoing phase III trial is evaluating the CTLA-4 targeted antibody ipilimumab in combination with carboplatin and paclitaxel, with continuation maintenance therapy with ipilimumab. This phase III trial was initiated based on a phase II trial of the combination that showed that the addition of ipilimumab as maintenance therapy to carboplatin and paclitaxel was superior to chemotherapy alone as well as to ipilimumab given concurrently with the first cycle of chemotherapy.[90]

Other key components of inhibitory immune checkpoints include PD-1 and its ligands PD-L1 and PD-L2. PD-1 mainly affects T-cell activity in peripheral tissues through interaction with PD-L1 and PD-L2. Targeting PD-1/PD-L1 interaction with PD-1 or PD-L1 antibodies can restore tumor-related immune responses, leading to tumor shrinkage and long-lasting responses in approximately 15% to 20% of pretreated NSCLC patients.[91] PD-1/PD-L1 inhibitors have been evaluated in a second-line setting in comparison with docetaxel. Twin phase III trials showed significantly improved survival for the PD-1 inhibitor nivolumab compared with docetaxel in squamous and nonsquamous carcinoma, respectively.[92] Pembrolizumab, another PD-1 inhibitor, also demonstrated a significant improvement of overall survival in comparison with docetaxel in patients with tumors expressing PD-L1 in at least 1% of tumor cells.[94] Similarly, the PD-L1 inhibitor atezolizumab showed an improvement of overall survival in a randomized phase II study with docetaxel as the control arm.[95] PD-L1 expression was correlated with improved survival in nonsquamous patients, but use of PD-L1 expression to guide therapy remains controversial. Optimal duration of anti-PD-1/PD-L1 therapy is actually unknown as most of these compounds are still continued as maintenance agents until toxicity or disease progression after obtaining maximal response.

At this point, PD-1 inhibitors are becoming the standard of care for second-line therapy of advanced NSCLC but they will soon move toward the frontline therapy. Many phase III studies are ongoing or have completed their accrual and have been published, which evaluate platinum based chemotherapy versus either anti-PD-1/PD-L1 as a single agent in PD-L1 positive tumors or in combination with chemotherapy or anti-CTLA4 for PD-L1 positive and PD-L1 negative tumors. All these studies are designed with the continuation of PD-1/PD-L1 inhibitors until toxicity or disease progression, in particular after cessation of chemotherapy or anti-CTLA4 in combination studies. None of these trials specifically address the role of anti-PD1/anti-PD-L1 inhibitors as maintenance treatment except for the SAFIR02 lung trial (NCT02117167) in which patients with disease control at the end of platinum-based induction chemotherapy and without targetable genetic alteration are randomized between standard maintenance treatment or durvalumab (anti-PD-L1 antibody). The role of immune checkpoints inhibitors is rapidly increasing in the treatment of advanced NSCLC, with many unresolved issues including the important question of the optimal duration of treatment.

META-ANALYSES

Over the last few years, several meta-analyses have been conducted in an effort to summarize the impact of maintenance treatment strategies on efficacy and toxicity and to analyze the value of the different approaches (continuation or switch) and treatment agents (chemotherapy or targeted agents).[29,82–85] Lima et al.[82] performed a meta-analysis of seven randomized controlled trials (1559 patients) comparing different durations of first-line treatment for advanced stage NSCLC. Patients receiving more chemotherapy had significantly longer progression-free survival (HR, 0.75; 95% CI, 0.60–0.85; $p < 0.0001$) than patients who had a shorter duration of treatment, but there were no differences in relative mortality (HR, 0.97; 95% CI, 0.84–1.11; $p = 0.65$). In addition, there was no difference in the overall response rate between the groups (odds ratio, 0.78; 95% CI, 0.60–1.01; $p = 0.96$). Longer treatment was associated with more severe leukopenia but with no significant increase in nonhematologic toxicities. Almost concurrently, Soon et al.[83] published their meta-analysis of 13 trials (3027 patients) that not only included studies with varying durations of combination first-line chemotherapy, but also available randomized controlled trials evaluating continuation and switch maintenance approaches with chemotherapy. Consistently, they found that extending chemotherapy improved progression-free survival significantly (HR, 0.75; 95% CI, 0.69–0.81; $p < 0.00001$) and also resulted in a modest but still clinically significant improvement in overall survival (HR, 0.92; 95% CI, 0.86–0.99; $p = 0.03$). Subgroup analysis demonstrated that effects on progression-free survival were greater with third-generation regimens and with switch maintenance strategies. Extending chemotherapy was again associated with more frequent adverse events, and impaired health-related quality of life in two of seven trials.

A third meta-analysis, which comprised eight trials and 3736 patients (three trials of continuation maintenance and five trials of switch maintenance) of chemotherapy or targeted agents, was published in 2011.[84] A clinically substantial and statistically significant improvement in progression-free survival was found with both maintenance strategies (switch maintenance therapy: HR, 0.67; 95% CI, 0.57–0.78; continuous maintenance therapy: HR, 0.53; 95% CI, 0.43–0.65; interaction $p = 0.128$). Switch maintenance therapy significantly improved overall survival compared with placebo or observation (HR, 0.85; 95% CI, 0.79–0.92; $p = 0.001$), and the continuation maintenance approach resulted in a similar

improvement in overall survival (HR, 0.88; 95% CI, 0.74–1.04; $p = 0.124$), despite lacking statistical significance, probably because of low statistical power (779 patients included in three trials; Fig. 46.4). Indeed, the interaction test suggested that the magnitude of the benefit from the two maintenance strategies was similar ($p = 0.777$). Subgroup analyses showed no significant differences in overall or progression-free survival between switch maintenance therapy with cytotoxic agents or tyrosine kinase inhibitors. In general, toxicity was greater with maintenance therapy.

Three further meta-analyses were reported in 2012 and 2013, with data from 10 randomized controlled trials (3451 patients) or 11 randomized controlled trials (3686 patients and 4790 patients), and the outcomes were comparable to those in the earlier meta-analyses.[30,99,100] In one analysis, Cai et al.[100] found a significant improvement in overall survival with switch maintenance (HR, 0.80; 95% CI, 0.72–090; $p = 0.0002$), but only a trend toward better overall survival with continuation maintenance (HR, 0.82; 95% CI, 0.66–1.01; $p = 0.06$). Both strategies improved progression-free survival, and the greatest benefit was found for tumors with nonsquamous cell histologies. A more recent meta-analysis did not alter these results: Zhou et al.[101] also reported a meta-analysis of 13 trials with 4960 patients showing a significant overall survival benefit for maintenance therapy (HR, 0.84; 95% CI, 0.78–0.89; $p < 0.001$) without significant differences for switch and continuation maintenance strategy (HR, 0.83 vs. 0.86; $p = 0.631$ [for interaction]). Another meta-analysis of 14 randomized control trials involving 5841 patients provided very similar results.[102] A recent systematic review of 14 randomized trials assessing systemic maintenance therapy confirmed the significant survival benefit related to pemetrexed maintenance treatment in nonsquamous lung carcinoma (HR, 0.74; 95% CI, 0.64–0.86; $p = 0.0003$), which was larger than that of EGFR tyrosine kinase inhibitors (HR, 0.84; 95% CI, 0.75–0.94; $p = 0.002$).[103] On the other hand, gemcitabine and docetaxel maintenance chemotherapy did not provide any significant survival advantage, which is consistent with the results of another meta-analysis dedicated to the role of pemetrexed and gemcitabine maintenance therapy.[104]

Several meta-analyses focused solely on the benefit of maintenance therapy with EGFR inhibitors have also been published recently. The three randomized trials with switch maintenance erlotinib (SATURN, Atlas, IFCT-GFPC 0502) were pooled (1942 patients), and the HR was 0.76 ($p < 0.00001$) for progression-free survival and 0.87 ($p = 0.003$) for overall survival, but the analysis did not include individual patient data.[105] Chen et al.[88] included five trials of either maintenance erlotinib or gefitinib (2436 patients) and found an increase in progression-free survival (HR, 0.63; 95% CI, 0.76–0.93) compared with placebo or observation; the HR for overall survival was 0.84 (95% CI, 0.76–0.93) regardless of stage, sex, ethnicity, performance status, smoking status, EGFR mutation status, or prior response to therapy.[88] Nevertheless, none of these meta-analyses include the recent data of the negative IUNO trial.

No large randomized trials have compared maintenance erlotinib with pemetrexed. There have been some efforts to carry out an indirect comparison, including one analysis that identified five randomized controlled trials that were then included in an indirect comparison meta-analysis. The findings suggested superiority of pemetrexed in terms of progression-free survival (HR, 0.71; 95% CI, 0.6–0.85; $p = 0.0001$). However, the difference in overall survival was not significant (HR, 0.88; 95% CI, 0.71–1.08; $p = 0.22$), although there was a trend in favor of pemetrexed.[107] Tan et al.[108] used a network meta-analysis to define the best maintenance option according to patients characteristics (EGFR status, performance status [PS], histology, and response to induction). This method allows comparing different therapeutic interventions across a trial's network sharing the same control arm (no maintenance treatment) and ranking the impact of different maintenance strategies. The meta-analysis confirmed the positive impact of a good PS on the survival benefit from maintenance therapy and that of a response to induction chemotherapy for

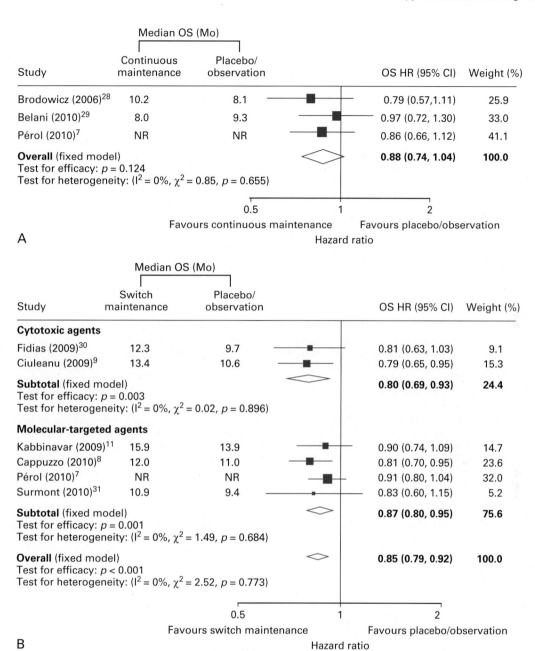

Fig. 46.4. Comparison of overall survival between continuous maintenance therapy and placebo or observation (A) and between switch maintenance therapy and placebo or observation (B). *CI,* confidence interval; *HR,* hazard ratio; *NR,* not recorded; *OS,* overall survival. *(Reprinted with permission from Zhang X, Zang J, Xu J, et al. Maintenance therapy with continuous or switch strategy in advanced non-small cell lung cancer: a systematic review and meta-analysis. Chest. 2011;140(1):117–126.)*

gemcitabine continuation maintenance. However, the heterogeneity of studies according to the proportion of patients receiving second-line treatments and the low level of EGFR testing in most of the maintenance trials may limit the scope of these results.

COST-EFFECTIVENESS

A discussion of maintenance therapy is incomplete without addressing financial implications. There have been multiple evaluations of costs of maintenance pemetrexed and erlotinib, some of which have been crucial to the approval or disapproval of maintenance therapy in many European countries. In the United Kingdom, the National Institute for Health and Clinical Excellence (NICE) standard willingness-to-pay range is approximately £20,000 to £30,000 per quality-adjusted life year (QALY).

Using the results from the JMEN trial, the incremental cost-effectiveness ratios for pemetrexed were more than £30,000 and, per NICE, were closer to £50,000 per QALY. Despite this assessment, NICE approved switch (but not continuation) maintenance with pemetrexed for nonsquamous NSCLC in 2010.[109] In the United States, researchers used a semi-Markov model utilizing Medicare reimbursement rates for drug costs estimates and found an incremental cost per life-year gained for nonsquamous cell NSCLC of US $133,371 for pemetrexed compared with observation and nearly US $150,000 for erlotinib maintenance.[110] Switch maintenance therapy with pemetrexed is approved in the United States. From a Swiss health-care system perspective, a Markov model was constructed based on the results of the JMEN trial, and the incremental cost-effectiveness ratio of adding pemetrexed until disease progression was calculated as cost per QALY gained. When an assumption was made for a reduction of the costs for best supportive care by 25% in the pemetrexed arm, the incremental cost-effectiveness ratio was €47,531 per QALY, which was below the Swiss cut point, but was considered by the authors as not cost-effective.[111] An analysis of estimated costs in China for continuation maintenance therapy with pemetrexed was estimated at more than US$100,000 per QALY gained.[112]

Maintenance therapy with erlotinib is also expensive, but a comprehensive analysis published in 2012 estimated that switch maintenance therapy with erlotinib had an incremental cost per life-year gained of €20,711 (UK) and €25,124 (Germany), which was considered to be cost-effective.[113] A separate analysis performed with a model based on the national health-care payers in France, Germany, and Italy, using a probabilistic sensitivity analysis, also concluded that this approach was cost-effective. The authors estimated that the cost per life-year gained with maintenance erlotinib was €39,783 in France, €46,931 in Germany, and €27,885 in Italy.[114] In the UK, for patients with stable disease after four cycles of first-line chemotherapy with a platinum-based doublet, the use of switch maintenance erlotinib was not thought to be cost-effective, with prices of more than £40,000 per QALY gained; NICE did not approve switch maintenance erlotinib.[115] From a US perspective, the additional costs of maintenance therapy with erlotinib were analyzed in the context of a health-care plan with 50,000 members, and the authors concluded that, assuming that a high number of patients would receive erlotinib as second- or third-line therapy, the costs of changing to a maintenance approach were minimal.[116] Few analyses have attempted to estimate the financial implications of pemetrexed versus erlotinib maintenance. One analysis limited to direct costs (drug acquisition, administration, and treatment of adverse events) that was conducted from the perspective of national health-care decision makers in France, Germany, Italy, and Spain estimated a total monthly per-patient treatment cost for erlotinib of €2140 in France, €2732 in Germany, €1518 in Italy, and €2048 in Spain; the corresponding per-patient treatment costs for pemetrexed were €3453, €5534, €2921, and €3164. The authors concluded that, given similar efficacy, erlotinib was more cost-effective.[117] Clearly, further similar analyses will be needed to fully assess the cost of maintenance therapy. The cost-utility analysis of the IFCT-GFPC 0502 French study showed that ICERS of gemcitabine- or erlotinib maintenance therapy varied as a function of histology, PS, and response to first-line chemotherapy.[118]

PATIENT SELECTION

The selection of patients to receive maintenance therapy remains controversial. Despite early support of the concept, prior response to chemotherapy does not seem to be an indicator of benefit from switch maintenance. In the trials by Fidias et al.[10] and Perol et al.,[32] which evaluated switch maintenance with docetaxel and continuation maintenance with gemcitabine, respectively, patients with a prior response appeared to have the greatest benefit from maintenance therapy. In contrast, in the erlotinib arm of the trial by Perol et al.,[32] the benefit was similar regardless of prior response and in the SATURN trial, the majority of benefit with switch maintenance erlotinib appeared to be in patients with stable disease during first-line chemotherapy.[9,32] Thus, although a few criteria are available to help select an agent (e.g., nonsquamous cell histology for pemetrexed and EGFR mutation status for erlotinib), little information is available to help guide the more important decision of whether to consider maintenance therapy or not for an individual patient. Perhaps the strongest caution comes from a trial of continuation maintenance with gemcitabine, which enrolled a substantial number of patients with a poor performance status and, unlike most other maintenance trials, was negative.[31]

Some experts have advocated imaging, including fluorode-oxyglucose-positron emission tomography, to help determine which patients are more likely to benefit from maintenance therapy,[119,120] and others have recommended that patients with a higher symptom burden are more likely to benefit from maintenance therapy.[14,121] In one retrospective analysis from a single institution, it was noted that socioeconomically disadvantaged patients were more likely to be lost to follow-up before initiation of second-line therapy and were therefore in greater need of maintenance therapy because they may not receive beneficial second-line treatment if there is a delay.[14]

Patient preferences for maintenance therapy have not been studied extensively. However, a pilot study was done with 30 patients who answered a 10-question survey about patient attitudes toward maintenance therapy before chemotherapy and after two and four cycles. Of the patients, 83%, 67%, and 43% considered maintenance therapy to be worthwhile for an overall survival benefit of 6, 3, or 1 month, respectively.[122] Another study conducted a thematic content analysis of focus groups for patients who were receiving, but had not completed, first-line chemotherapy. Patients discussed survival benefits, disease control, "buying time," and the importance of doing something as reasons to consider maintenance therapy.[123]

Based on available data, the choice for maintenance therapy remains an individual decision for each patient. Tolerance of first-line chemotherapy and performance status after completion of first-line chemotherapy must be weighed against competing patient desires for a treatment break and reluctance to be not receiving treatment. The 2015 American Society of Clinical Oncology (ASCO) updated guidelines on maintenance therapy state that for patients with stable disease or response after four cycles of a first-line pemetrexed-containing regimen, pemetrexed continuation maintenance may be used; if initial regimen does not contain pemetrexed, an alternative chemotherapy (switch) may be used, or a break from chemotherapy may be recommended until disease progression.[11] The European Society for Medical Oncology (ESMO) 2014 guidelines are similar to those of ASCO for switch maintenance strategy; however, continuing pemetrexed following completion of first-line cisplatin plus pemetrexed chemotherapy is recommended in patients with non-squamous histology.[12] Both ASCO and ESMO guidelines were anterior to the release of erlotinib IUNO trial results. In its 2011 guidelines, the Italian Association of Thoracic Oncology suggests that maintenance therapy be discussed with patients with no disease progression who have a good performance status and minimal toxicity after four to six cycles of first-line chemotherapy.[13]

REMAINING QUESTIONS AND FUTURE STUDIES

The current evidence supports the use of maintenance treatment—continuation and switch with chemotherapy or targeted agents—as a means to improve the outcomes of patients with advanced NSCLC. However, the evidence does not indicate that all patients are appropriate candidates or that all patients should receive maintenance therapy. Indeed, patient preferences, convenience, and cost are factors to be considered. In addition, toxicity and the robustness of the efficacy evidence vary across the different approaches and drugs used in the trials performed so far, as the design, sample size, and end points have also varied. This situation sets a number of remaining questions to be answered in ongoing and future research.

Many clinicians and investigators question whether the results of the maintenance trials would persist if six rather than four courses were given as induction treatment. Studies to date have failed to demonstrate a clear benefit of six cycles,[1,2] and it is unlikely that a new trial will be designed to answer the question. Some patients, especially those who have a response, benefit from additional platinum-based chemotherapy courses after four cycles, but the experimental data to support this clinical habit are scarce, if they exist at all.[1,97] An across-trial comparison of cisplatin and pemetrexed (JMDB and PARAMOUNT trials) suggests no additional benefit for the fifth and sixth induction courses in terms of efficacy but some increase in neurotoxicity and ototoxicity, toxicities that in fact may jeopardize the prolonged delivery of maintenance treatment.[7,29,124] Indeed, the shape of the curves in maintenance trials suggest the benefit is most obvious not in the first 2 months (as one would expect from continuation to six cycles), but after 6 to 12 months, suggesting most of the benefit occurs in patients who receive prolonged therapy.

The evidence on the efficacy of switch maintenance is solid in terms of delaying disease progression (30% to 50%) and in decreasing the risk of death (15% to 30%).[84,125] It is doubtful that this advantage would remain, at least in a clinically significant way, if all patients were treated at the time of disease progression after a treatment break as it has been shown in the negative IUNO study comparing switch maintenance with erlotinib to erlotinib at the time of disease progression for patients with wild-type EGFR tumors.[10,32] Following the suggested hypothesis that the amount and number of therapies are more important than the timing, progress in the early identification of disease reactivation in this context is needed.

A number of questions remain unresolved concerning the strategy of continuation maintenance therapy, as the only data on improved overall survival were found for pemetrexed in patients with nonsquamous cell tumors in the PARAMOUNT trial.[7] Indeed, the findings of this trial have been questioned, as only a small proportion of patients in the control arm, all with proven sensitivity to pemetrexed during induction chemotherapy, were rechallenged with the antifolate. This strategy is occasionally used in clinical practice, and data to support the approach are limited, although it is supported by some positive experiences with the reintroduction of EGFR inhibitors in patients initially sensitive to these therapies and in mesothelioma.[126,127] One must question whether other drugs such as gemcitabine and docetaxel would be equally effective for continuation maintenance. These drugs have been shown to improve progression-free survival but not overall survival in poorly powered trials. The most recent meta-analyses have provided some evidence, but larger trials are needed, particularly with squamous cell tumors. The CECOG and IFCT trials included a reasonable number of patients with tumors of this histology (40% and 21%, respectively), and the overall results did not differ by the pathologic subtype.[28,32]

As discussed earlier, there is a lack of data to guide decision making about continuation versus switch maintenance therapy. Pemetrexed has yielded superimposable effects when used as switch or continuation maintenance treatment.[7,8,10,128] Intuitively, continuation maintenance therapy should be superior, as it allows for all of the potential benefit from the current treatment before giving a second drug. A biologically plausible hypothesis is that patients with substantial remission during induction chemotherapy may further benefit from prolonged administration of the nonplatinum agent of the first-line regimen, whereas patients with less sensitive disease would be candidates for early switch maintenance with a non–cross-resistant agent. In fact, the SATURN, JMEN, and IFCT trials provided experimental support for continuation maintenance for patients who had a response to induction chemotherapy and preferential benefit for switch maintenance for patients with stable disease.[9,32] The PARAMOUNT trial, however, showed no influence in outcome dependent on the initial response to a platinum agent and pemetrexed followed by pemetrexed.[7] Similarly, the meta-analysis does not bring any additional data favoring the selection of the maintenance strategy (continuation vs. switch) according to the response to first-line chemotherapy.[101] The ongoing NCT01631136 trial from the IFCT group is comparing an overall treatment strategy of cisplatin plus pemetrexed followed by pemetrexed to a response-tailored approach of cisplatin plus gemcitabine followed by gemcitabine (objective response) or pemetrexed (stable disease).

There is general agreement on the need for useful tools to select patients who will benefit from maintenance therapy, to minimize the number of patients who are exposed to continuous treatment and its associated toxicities and costs. Unfortunately, few trials to explore predictive biomarkers have been done. Only EGFR mutation is an appropriate predictor, in this case for treatment with an EGFR inhibitor.[9,52] As mentioned, nonsquamous histology is predictive for benefit from pemetrexed, but with a relatively lower positive predictive value.[8] In future trials, investigators should further intensify their efforts in the molecular characterization of tumors for known prognostic and predictive indicators. For example, it may be helpful to know how many tumors had anaplastic lymphoma kinase translocations and EGFR-activating mutations in the pemetrexed studies; the outcome for these patients may have been different if they had not been included but instead treated with specific agents such as crizotinib, erlotinib, or gefitinib.[129]

Given the modest benefits provided at present by maintenance treatments, many efforts are concentrated on the search for new therapies and combinations to be tested in this setting. The days of four cycles of a platinum-based doublet, followed by a chemotherapy holiday until progression, are behind us, but many questions about how best to optimize maintenance therapy remain. It appears now clear that new approaches with immunotherapy will soon change the way of treating a significant proportion of advanced NSCLC patients in frontline and maintenance settings.

KEY REFERENCES

7. Paz-Ares LG, de Marinis F, Dediu M, et al. PARAMOUNT: final overall survival results of the phase III study of maintenance pemetrexed versus placebo immediately after induction treatment with pemetrexed plus cisplatin for advanced nonsquamous non-small-cell lung cancer. *J Clin Oncol.* 2013;31(23):2895–2902.
8. Ciuleanu T, Brodowicz T, Zielinski C, et al. Maintenance pemetrexed plus best supportive care versus placebo plus best supportive care for non-small-cell lung cancer: a randomised, double-blind, phase 3 study. *Lancet.* 2009;374(9699):1432–1440.
9. Cappuzzo F, Ciuleanu T, Stelmakh L, et al. Erlotinib as maintenance treatment in advanced non-small-cell lung cancer: a multicentre, randomised, placebo-controlled phase 3 study. *Lancet Oncol.* 2010;11(6):521–529.
10. Fidias PM, Dakhil SR, Lyss AP, et al. Phase III study of immediate compared with delayed docetaxel after front-line therapy with gemcitabine plus carboplatin in advanced non-small-cell lung cancer. *J Clin Oncol.* 2009;27(4):591–598.
28. Brodowicz T, Krzakowski M, Zwitter M, et al. Cisplatin and gemcitabine first-line chemotherapy followed by maintenance gemcitabine or best supportive care in advanced non-small cell lung cancer: a phase III trial. *Lung Cancer.* 2006;52(2):155–163.
32. Perol M, Chouaid C, Perol D, et al. Randomized, phase III study of gemcitabine or erlotinib maintenance therapy versus observation, with predefined second-line treatment, after cisplatin-gemcitabine induction chemotherapy in advanced non-small-cell lung cancer. *J Clin Oncol.* 2012;30(28):3516–3524.
34. Paz-Ares L, de Marinis F, Dediu M, et al. Maintenance therapy with pemetrexed plus best supportive care versus placebo plus best supportive care after induction therapy with pemetrexed plus cisplatin for advanced non-squamous non-small-cell lung cancer (PARAMOUNT): a double-blind, phase 3, randomised controlled trial. *Lancet Oncol.* 2012;13(3):247–255.
36. Barlesi F, Scherpereel A, Rittmeyer A, et al. Randomized phase III trial of maintenance bevacizumab with or without pemetrexed after first-line induction with bevacizumab, cisplatin, and pemetrexed in advanced nonsquamous non-small-cell lung cancer: AVAPERL (MO22089). *J Clin Oncol.* 2013;31(24):3004–3011.
38. Kayarama M, Inui N, Fujisawa T, et al. Maintenance therapy with pemetrexed and bevacizumab versus pemetrexed monotherapy after induction therapy with carboplatin, pemetrexed, and bevacizumab in patients with advanced non-squamous non small cell lung cancer. *Eur J Cancer.* 2016;58:30–37.

See Expertconsult.com for full list of references.

47 Pharmacogenomics in Lung Cancer: Predictive Biomarkers for Chemotherapy

George R. Simon, Rafael Rosell Costa, and David R. Gandara

SUMMARY OF KEY POINTS

- Discussed are tumor factors that affect treatment responses and outcome and host genetic elements that affect drug metabolism. Only pharmacogenomics elements that interact with chemotherapeutic agents are described.

- Prognostic biomarkers describe a specific tumor characteristic that allows for dichotomization of a cohort of patients into different groups based on an outcome that is independent of the treatment rendered.

- How biomarkers are measured and what is defined as positive or negative are crucial considerations pertinent to their use.

- At least 50% of patients with lung cancer have actionable driver mutations.

- Although the epidermal growth factor receptor (EGFR) signaling cascades are complex, tyrosine kinase in the EGFR intracellular domain is the key factor that triggers signaling.

- Anaplastic lymphoma kinase (ALK) activation occurs primarily via three different mechanisms: (1) fusion protein formation, (2) ALK overexpression, and (3) activating *ALK* point mutations.

- Crizotinib yields high response rates (exceeding 60%) and improves survival when used in patients with advanced nonsmall cell lung cancer who have *ALK* gene rearrangements and have progressed on previous therapy.

- The clinical uses of markers such as *ERCC1* and *RRM1* remain to be elucidated.

- *KRAS* mutational status is predictive of lack of therapeutic efficacy with EGFR tyrosine kinase inhibitors.

- MET and ROS1 genomic alterations are more rare driver mutations that, when detected, may enable more precise treatment for patients with lung cancer.

- Molecular biomarkers such as *ERCC1*, *RRM1*, *BRCA1*, thymidylate synthase, and others remain investigational.

Effective treatment strategies for advanced stage lung cancer continue to be elusive despite substantial advances in the treatment of specific subsets of patients. Over the past decade, however, our understanding of the molecular mechanisms that underlie cellular transformation and the development of lung cancer has increased greatly. This knowledge has led to the development of therapeutic agents targeted against specific intracellular or extracellular targets presumed to be critical in the molecular pathways of carcinogenesis. For example, tyrosine kinase inhibitors, which have demonstrated increased efficacy and tolerability compared with chemotherapy in patients with metastatic lung cancer and epidermal growth factor receptor (*EGFR*) mutations or anaplastic lymphoma kinase (*ALK*) translocations, are now first-line treatment for patients with these tumor markers.[1]

Host germline genetic variations can affect the pharmacokinetics and pharmacodynamics of individual drugs and thus affect patient outcomes.[2] Thus, genetically determined pharmacokinetic variations may affect both the antitumor efficacy and host toxicities. In addition to genetic determinants in the host, environmental factors can affect the way drugs are metabolized, which in turn can affect their efficacy. In lung cancer, the primary example is smoking. Smoking is reported to alter the metabolism of several chemotherapeutic drugs and targeted agents, such as erlotinib.[3] However, the extent of the effect smoking has on the pharmacokinetics of individual drugs may be determined by individual host genetics.[4,5]

Researchers in the field of pharmacogenetics seek to gain a better understanding of the association between human/host genetics and drug response and toxicity. Advances in knowledge about tumor genomics, afforded by the genome-wide integrative analysis possible in the postgenomic era, when integrated with the field of pharmacogenetics, provide a modern basis for the field of pharmacogenomics. Thus, pharmacogenomic research is designed to determine host genetic variations, the genomic make-up of a tumor, the interaction between host genetic variations and tumor make-up, and the net effect on treatment responses and outcome. This chapter discusses tumor factors that affect treatment responses and outcome and host genetic elements that affect drug metabolism and its implications for routine clinical practice. As the title of the chapter indicates, only pharmacogenomics elements that interact with chemotherapeutic agents are described.

TUMOR-RELATED FACTORS

Tumor-related molecular determinants are broadly divided into two categories: prognostic biomarkers and predictive biomarkers.[6] Each of these characteristics of a molecular determinant can have therapeutic implications. A prognostic biomarker is an indicator of the innate aggressiveness of the tumor and is indicative of patient survival independent of treatment, whereas a predictive biomarker is an indicator of therapeutic efficacy. A prognostic biomarker describes a specific tumor characteristic that allows for the dichotomization of a cohort of patients into different groups based on outcome that is independent of the treatment rendered; for example, overall survival is better for patients with biomarker-positive tumors compared with patients with biomarker-negative tumors. Predictive biomarkers, on the other hand, suggest benefit or lack of benefit for a specific treatment based on the presence, absence, or overexpression or underexpression of the predictive biomarker, and thus, these biomarkers directly affect treatment decision-making. Some biomarkers may have both a prognostic and predictive function. Such so-called panoramic biomarkers make interpretation of data in different settings nuanced, and the dual prognostic-predictive value of the biomarker must be taken into account. Prototypic examples of biomarkers with both prognostic and predictive functions are excision repair cross-complementing 1 (ERCC1) and ribonucleotide reductase M1

(RRM1). In stage I and II nonsmall cell lung cancer (NSCLC), the prognostic function of ERCC1 and RRM1 may predominate, suggesting that overall survival will be better for patients with tumors positive for these markers after surgical resection than for patients with tumors negative for the markers. However, in stage IV NSCLC, the predictive function is most relevant, suggesting that tumors positive for ERCC1 or RRM1 will have inferior responses to cisplatin or gemcitabine, respectively, compared with cancers that are ERCC1- or RRM1-negative. Stage III NSCLC presents a challenge, as the dual function of ERCC1 and RRM1 makes interpretation of their significance difficult in a setting in which cisplatin is typically used, potentially in combination with other drugs such as paclitaxel, pemetrexed, or etoposide, as well as radiotherapy. It is unclear whether the prognostic function or the predictive function predominate or if a predominant function is relevant when additional treatment modalities are used.[7] These issues have confounded and confused the interpretation of several studies done with these and other markers.[8]

Measurement of Molecular Biomarkers

Another crucial consideration pertinent to the use of biomarkers, whether prognostic, predictive, or panoramic, is how they are measured and what is defined as positive or negative. For some biomarkers, it can be clearly discerned whether the marker is present or absent in the tumor; classic examples of this type of biomarker are mutations of the *EGFR* gene or translocations of the echinoderm microtubule-associated protein-like 4 (*EML4*) and *ALK* genes. Because the molecular aberrations can be clearly and unambiguously measured, the effect of these mutations on patient outcomes is clear.

However, most biomarkers are present on a continuum in almost all tumors, and, as such, variations in measurement techniques and interpretation of values are more likely. Typically, a lower expression of these biomarkers is considered negative and a higher expression is considered positive. The challenge is that the level of expression corresponding to positive or negative is often arbitrary and, for ease of interpretation, the cutoff point is often the statistical median. This approach artificially renders a continuous variable into a discrete one, which potentially confounds the strength of the association being measured. The strength of the association may be particularly vulnerable around the median. Investigators have attempted to partially offset this problem by dichotomizing the results in a particular cohort into quartiles and examining the association between a marker and an outcome by comparing the highest quartile with the lowest quartile.[9]

The measurement technique is crucial to successful incorporation of biomarkers into clinical decision-making. Discrete biomarkers (i.e., those that are either present or absent) are best measured at the DNA level. Mutations, translocations, and copy number gains fall into this category. Mutations and translocations are best measured by sequencing the gene of interest, preferably in its entirety, and this technique will identify common and rare mutations, as well as mutations that are as yet unidentified. Multiplexed polymerase chain reaction (PCR)-based techniques will identify common mutations but will only detect mutations for which the primers are included in the multiplex panel.

Nondiscrete biomarkers are best measured at the RNA or protein level. As an example, most epithelial tissue expresses the EGFR protein, with the expression higher in some tissues than in others. Increased EGFR expression is not a consequence of an abnormality of the *EGFR* gene at the DNA level but is most likely a consequence of increased transcription of the normal *EGFR* gene to RNA and then eventual translation of the RNA to protein. Thus, the increased expression of a particular gene may be measured at the RNA or the protein level.

Measurement at the RNA or protein level each is associated with advantages and disadvantages. Measurement at the RNA level is more technically complex and thus could be more challenging to accomplish in the routine clinical setting. The expression of a gene is measured relative to the expression of a housekeeping gene and expressed as a unitless ratio. The values derived also depend on the use of specific standardization techniques and procedures, which can vary from laboratory to laboratory. Because of this potential variation, numerically similar values may not be congruent across different laboratories and platforms. Additionally, the cutoff values for high versus low must be individually established for each laboratory and validated by clinical data. Nevertheless, measuring RNA through quantitative PCR, if done with proper controls and standardization procedures, is precise, reproducible, and quantifiable. Hence, despite the technical difficulties, quantitative PCR has been the favored approach by several investigators. Controversy also exists as to the optimal sample for quantitative PCR. Most investigators consider a fresh frozen sample to be ideal, but it is not practical to obtain fresh frozen biopsy specimens in the clinical setting, especially from patients with advanced NSCLC. However, most investigators now believe that good-quality mRNA can be extracted from formalin-fixed paraffin-embedded (FFPE) tissue, and thus, such samples can be used for quantitative PCR. However, the process used to make the FFPE samples may potentially alter the message, which raises questions about the relevance of quantitative PCR measurements in FFPE samples.[10]

Immunohistochemistry (IHC) is most commonly used to measure protein levels in clinical samples. IHC has several advantages, including relative ease of use, widespread availability in most clinical pathology laboratories, and the capability of evaluating FFPE samples. The performance characteristics of IHC, however, are critically dependent on having a good antibody that effectively binds only to the antigen of interest. Additionally, the intensity of the staining is arbitrarily graded as 0 through 3 (0 = no staining, 1= weak staining, 2 = moderate staining, and 3 = strong staining) or by the H score (the H score is a product of staining intensity and the percent of cells stained; for example, if 50% of the slides show an intensity of more than 3, 20% show an intensity of more than 2, and 30% are negative, then the H score would be 150 + 40 = 190). Despite these scoring methods and the use of rigorous (positive and negative) controls, these techniques can still lead to variation in interpretation. The definition of positive is also arbitrary and if, for example, 2+ or higher is considered positive, the arbitrariness between a score of 1 or 2 thus jeopardizes the very definition of positive versus negative.

To partially counteract the arbitrary nature of IHC grading methods, the automated quantitative analysis of in situ protein expression (AQUA) method was developed.[11] The AQUA method involves the use of fluorescent microscopic technology that measures the expression of proteins of interest by quantifying the intensity of antibody-conjugated fluorophores within a specific cellular compartment (such as the nucleus or cytoplasm) in a tumor. A quantitative score is thus generated based on the intensity of immunofluorescence. The AQUA method thus provides a more continuous scoring of protein expression in tissue samples.[12] Even though the AQUA method eliminates some of the subjectivity in the interpretation of IHC, the method is still associated with some of the same challenges as IHC. For example, AQUA also depends on an antibody that binds only to the protein of interest and the cutoff point to define positive and negative is arbitrary.

Driver Mutations in Lung Adenocarcinomas

The recognition of *EGFR* and *ALK* oncogenes as predictive biomarkers in lung cancer has led an ongoing investigation to identify additional oncogenic drivers with predictive and prognostic importance. Certain subsets of NSCLC can now be further defined at a molecular level by driver mutations in multiple oncogenes that lead to constitutive activation of mutant signaling proteins, causing induction and sustaining tumorigenesis. Mutations can be detected in all NSCLC histologies, including adenocarcinoma, squamous cell carcinoma, and large cell carcinoma, and in current-, former-, and never-smokers (defined as individuals who smoked fewer than 100 cigarettes in a lifetime).[13]

It is estimated that at least 50% of patients with lung cancer have actionable driver mutations.[14,15] Actionable driver mutations are defined as molecular abnormalities with downstream effects that initiate or maintain the neoplastic process, which can be negated by agents directed against each genomic alteration.[19] Some of the evidence of the driver mutations of significance in lung cancer comes from research conducted by the 14-member Lung Cancer Mutation Consortium (LCMC), which has investigated metastatic lung adenocarcinomas since 2009 to identify and study driver genomic alterations. Between 2009 and 2012 more than 1000 patients underwent genotyping to determine the frequency of oncogenic drivers in lung cancer and demonstrate the practicality of using routine genetic analyses to inform treatment with targeted therapies.[16]

In the LCMC patient cohort actionable driver mutations were found in 64% of tumors from patients with lung adenocarcinomas.[16] Table 47.1 lists the driver mutations the LCMC investigators identified. Most of these driver mutations were found in a small percentage of patients. The most common driver mutations detected were in the *EGFR*, *KRAS*, and *ALK* genes.[16]

The *ALK* fusion oncogene and sensitizing *EGFR* mutations have become accepted predictive biomarkers in lung cancer. The National Comprehensive Cancer Network (NCCN) recommends genotyping for *EGFR* mutations and *ALK* rearrangements in its algorithm for patients with metastatic disease.[1]

Epidermal Growth Factor Receptor

EGFR (also known as HER1) is a transmembrane receptor for the epidermal growth factor with intrinsic tyrosine kinase activity. It is encoded by a gene located on chromosome 7.[17] EGFR belongs to a family of receptor tyrosine kinases, which upon activation result in stimulation of multiple downstream pathways within the cell, including those involved in cell survival, proliferation, and resistance to apoptosis.[18,19]

In normal cells the tyrosine kinase activity of the EGFR is strictly regulated, and therefore cell growth is controlled. Although the EGFR signaling cascades are complex, tyrosine kinase in the EGFR intracellular domain is the key factor that triggers signaling. If tyrosine kinase activity is blocked (i.e., via

TABLE 47.1 Driver Mutations in Lung Adenocarcinomas[16]

Mutation	Incidence (%)
ALK rearrangements	8
BRAF	2
EGFR, sensitizing	17
EGFR, other	4
ERBB2, formerly HER2	3
KRAS	25
MEK1	<1
MET amplification	<1
NRAS	<1
PIK3CA	<1

ALK, anaplastic lymphoma kinase; *BRAF*, v-raf murine sarcoma viral oncogene homolog B; *EGFR*, epidermal growth factor receptor; *ERBB2*, erb-B2 receptor tyrosine kinase 2; *HER2*, human epidermal growth factor receptor 2; *KRAS*, Kirsten rat sarcoma viral oncogene homolog; *MEK1*, mitogen-activated protein kinase kinase; *MET*, hepatocyte growth factor receptor; *NRAS*, neuroblastoma RAS viral oncogene homolog; *PIK3CA*, phosphatidylinositol-4,5-biphosphate 3 kinase catalytic subunit alpha.

a molecular targeted agent), EGFR is unable to transduce signals to the cell nucleus.[20] In cancer cells, various mechanisms of EGFR activation have been identified, including receptor overexpression, ligand overexpression, and *EGFR* gene amplification.

EGFR Overexpression

EGFR expression refers to measurement of levels of receptor protein (either normal [wild-type] protein or abnormal [meaning from the mutated gene]) by IHC and is distinct from detection of an actual EGFR mutation. EGFR expression is detectable in approximately 80% to 85% of patients with NSCLC, although the levels of expression vary widely on a continual scale.[21]

Approximately 40% to 80% of NSCLC tumors overexpress EGFR.[19] This wide range in the frequency of EGFR overexpression may be due to differences in the techniques used to determine EGFR overexpression, the criteria used to define overexpression levels, and the differences in study populations. Wild-type is the term used to describe EGFR that is overexpressed but not mutated. The result of overexpression is an overabundance of receptors that are available to interact with ligands. Wild-type EGFR becomes activated by binding to ligands. Ligand binding induces receptor dimerization, and the ligand-bound EGFR activates tyrosine kinase-mediated signaling pathways, leading to tumor proliferation, survival, and resistance to apoptosis.[18]

Tumor cells can overexpress EGFR as well as its ligands. Ligand overexpression increases EGFR dimerization, activation, and tyrosine kinase-mediated signaling, which can lead to uncontrolled tumor growth.[22]

EGFR overexpression is more common in squamous cell carcinoma and adenocarcinoma, and to a lesser extent in large-cell carcinoma.[19] Although the clinical significance of overexpression in NSCLC remains controversial, some investigators have found that overexpression of EGFR is associated with more aggressive tumors, a poor clinical prognosis, and, in certain tumor types, the development of resistance to radiation and cytoxic agents.[19]

Among patients with NSCLC, wild-type EGFR is more common than mutated EGFR. Compared with mutated EGFR, patients who harbor wild-type EGFR show reduced benefit for EGFR tyrosine kinase inhibitors such as erlotinib and gefitinib. This may be because the wild-type EGFR typically sends a downstream signal that ultimately stimulates the growth of tumor cells that are dependent on the receptor, and gefitinib or erlotinib can modestly inhibit this relatively weak signal. In contrast, the mutated EGFR is constitutively activated with a prominent downstream signal that can be dramatically inhibited by gefitinib and erlotinib.[18]

EGFR Mutations

Somatic mutations of *EGFR* genes can result in the production of mutated receptors.[23] About 10% to 15% of Caucasian patients with NSCLC and 30% to 40% of Asian patients have tumor-associated *EGFR* mutations.[17] These mutations occur within *EGFR* exons,[15-18] which encode a portion of the EGFR kinase domain.[19] The majority (about 90%) of these mutations are exon 19 deletions or exon 21L858R point mutations.[18,25] Regardless of ethnicity, *EGFR* mutations are more often found in tumors from women, never-smokers (defined as less than 100 cigarettes in a patient's lifetime), or former-smokers with adenocarcinoma histology.[17]

Mutant EGFR does not require a ligand for receptor dimerization and activation. Thus, EGFRs that harbor mutations remain constitutively activated without ligand binding. Although the mutated receptor needs no growth factor for signaling, ligand binding increases receptor activity. Cancer cells harboring *EGFR* gene mutations often become highly dependent on the EGFR pathway, a state referred to as "oncogene addiction."[27]

There are several consequences of EGFR mutations, including: (1) constitutive activation of the EGFR tyrosine kinase activity and resulting hyperactivation of downstream targets; (2) diminished affinity for ATP; (3) increased sensitivity to tyrosine kinase inhibitors; or, conversely, (4) development of resistance to tyrosine kinase inhibitors for certain types of mutations.[24]

EGFR-activating mutations are found to be favorable prognostic markers of survival and predictive markers of response in terms of tumor shrinkage.[19] EGFR mutation status correlates strongly with the probability of response to an EGFR tyrosine kinase inhibitor, as well as a more favorable prognosis in patients with advanced lung adenocarcinoma.[23,25]

This association between EGFR-activating mutations and increased clinical responses seen with EGFR tyrosine kinase inhibitors has been investigated in multiple clinical studies. Evidence shows that the growth and downstream signaling inhibition of cells with EGFR-activating mutations is consistently more sensitive to treatment with EGFR tyrosine kinase inhibitors than the signaling in cells with wild-type EGFR. Moreover, EGFR tyrosine kinase inhibitors bind with higher affinity to the mutant receptors compared with the wild-type receptor.[18]

The randomized, phase, open-label Iressa Pan-Asia Study marked a seminal moment in the treatment of patients with EGFR-activating mutations. In this study of previously untreated patients with NSCLC, a significant interaction was found between treatment and EGFR gene mutation with respect to progression-free survival. In the subset of 261 patients with EGFR gene mutations, progression-free survival was significantly longer among patients receiving the tyrosine kinase inhibitor gefitinib than among those receiving chemotherapy (hazard ratio [HR] for progression or death, 0.48; 95% CI, 0.36–0.64; $p < 0.001$). Conversely, in the subgroup of 176 patients who were negative for the mutation, progression-free survival was significantly longer among those who received carboplatin–paclitaxel (HR for progression or death with gefitinib, 2.85; 95% CI, 2.05–3.98; $p < 0.001$).[26]

Even though patients with lung cancer harboring EGFR gene mutations generally exhibit a favorable response to EGFR tyrosine kinase inhibitors, certain EGFR gene mutations are associated with resistance to tyrosine kinase inhibitors. The T790M mutation, which results in a substitution of methionine for threonine at position 790 of the EGFR tyrosine kinase domain, leads to biochemical and structural alteration that causes resistance to therapy with a tyrosine kinase inhibitor.[23] The T790M mutation has been reported in about 60% of patients with disease progression after initial response to erlotinib, gefitinib, or afatinib.[27–29] The T790M mutation also has been identified as an oncogenic mutation, promoting oncogenesis especially when the T790M mutation occurs in combination with other EGFR-activating mutations.[30]

Other, less-common EGFR gene mutations (approximately 10%) located in the kinase domain that may have significance with regard to sensitivity and resistance to EGFR tyrosine kinase inhibitors have been identified (Table 47.2).

TABLE 47.2 Less-Common EGFR Mutations in NSCLC[31,32]

Mutation	Frequency (%)	Clinical Significance
Exon 21 mutation (L861X[a])	2	TKI sensitivity
Exon 18 mutation (G719X)	3	TKI sensitivity
Exon 19 insertion	1	TKI sensitivity
Exon 20 insertion	4–9	TKI resistance

[a]The "X" is used to designate that several amino acid substitutions are possible at the site.

EGFR, Epidermal growth factor receptor; NSCLC, nonsmall cell lung cancer; TKI, tyrosine kinase inhibitor.

Anaplastic Lymphoma Kinase

The ALK gene encodes a tyrosine kinase receptor that is normally expressed in central and peripheral nervous systems, testes, skeletal muscle, basal layer keratinocytes, and the small intestine. ALK appears to function in neuronal development and differentiation during embryogenesis and its expression falls to low levels at age three weeks and remains low throughout adult life.[33]

ALK activation occurs primarily via three different mechanisms: (1) fusion protein formation, (2) ALK overexpression, and (3) activating ALK point mutations. In ALK translocations, the fusion partner regulates ALK expression levels, its subcellular location, and when it is expressed. Multiple different ALK gene rearrangements have been described in NSCLC. The majority of these ALK fusion variants are comprised of portions of the echinoderm microtubule-associated protein-like 4 (EML4) gene.[33] Dimerization of the ALK fusion product, which is mediated by the fusion partner, results in constitutive activation of the ALK tyrosine kinase. Signaling downstream of ALK fusions results in activation of cellular pathways known to be involved in cell growth and cell proliferation. An estimated 2% to 7% of patients with NSCLC have ALK gene rearrangements.[34]

ALK gene rearrangements tend to occur mutually exclusive of EGFR mutations. Thus, the presence of ALK gene rearrangements is associated with resistance to EGFR tyrosine kinase inhibitors. Patients with ALK gene rearrangements have similar clinical characteristics to those with EGFR mutations (including adenocarcinoma histology and nonsmoking or light smoking histories) except they are more likely to be men and may be younger.[35] Rarely are ALK gene rearrangements detected in patients with squamous cell carcinoma.[36]

Crizotinib is a dual ALK/MET tyrosine kinase inhibitor approved for ALK-positive and ROS1-positive NSCLC.[13] Crizotinib has been shown to yield very high response rates (exceeding 60%) and improve survival when used in patients with advanced NSCLC who have ALK gene rearrangements and have progressed on previous therapy, including those with brain metastases.[37–39] The NCCN recommends crizotinib for first-line and subsequent therapy in patients with ALK-positive NSCLC. Ceritinib and alectinib are newer ALK inhibitors recommended for use in patients who progress on crizotinib or are intolerant of crizotinib.[1]

KRAS

RAS binding proteins, including KRAS, are central mediators downstream of growth factor receptor signaling. In its mutated form, KRAS is constitutively active, able to transform immortalized cells and promote cell proliferation and survival.

KRAS gene mutations are detected in tumors from former-, current-, and never-smokers, although they are rarer in never-smokers. Approximately 25% of patients with lung adenocarcinoma in North America have KRAS mutations, making KRAS the most common mutation.[40,41] The exact role of KRAS as a predictive or prognostic biomarker in metastatic lung cancer remains undetermined as few prospective trials have examined the utility of using KRAS mutational status to inform treatment with targeted agents. Nevertheless, KRAS gene mutations are predictive of lack of therapeutic efficacy with tyrosine kinase inhibitors that target EGFR, such as erlotinib and gefitinib.[40,42] Moreover, patients with KRAS gene mutations appear to have a shorter survival than patients with wild-type KRAS.[43,44] EGFR and KRAS mutations appear to occur mutually exclusive of each other.[45,46]

MET

The MET gene encodes a receptor tyrosine kinase, which becomes activated upon binding of its ligand, hepatocyte growth factor. Consequently multiple downstream pathways within the cell become activated, including those involved in cell survival and proliferation. In cancer, aberrant signaling through the MET receptor promotes pleiotropic effects, including growth, survival, invasion, migration, angiogenesis, and metastasis.

In NSCLC, multiple mechanisms of MET activation have been reported, including both gene amplification and mutation. Overexpression of MET protein in tumor tissue relative to adjacent normal tissues occurs in 25% to 75% of NSCLC and is associated with a poor prognosis.[47] Data suggest MET protein expression and activation predict poor response to subsequent treatment with EGFR tyrosine kinase inhibitors, despite the presence of tyrosine kinase inhibitor–sensitizing mutations within the *EGFR* gene.[47]

ROS1

ROS1 is a receptor tyrosine kinase of the insulin receptor family that is involved in chromosomal translocations in lung cancer. ROS1 fusions, which have been found to be potential driver mutations in a NSCLC cell line, lead to constitutive kinase activity and are associated with sensitivity in vitro to tyrosine kinase inhibitors. Signaling downstream of ROS1 fusions results in activation of cellular pathways known to be involved in cell growth and cell proliferation. Approximately 2% of NSCLC tumors harbor alterations in the *ROS1* gene.[48] Patients positive for a *ROS1* rearrangement have a typical clinical profile, including young age at onset and nonsmoking history. *ROS1* fusions are associated with sensitivity to tyrosine kinase inhibitors that have "off-target" activity against ROS1; an example of this is crizotinib.[48]

ERCC1 and RRM1

Cisplatin-based chemotherapy is the standard of care for all patients with advanced stage NSCLC and is also used as adjuvant treatment for patients with completely resected stage II and III NSCLC.[1,49–51] Cisplatin impedes DNA replication by establishing DNA-platinum adducts. Breaks in the DNA strand occur when the DNA unwinds in anticipation of initiation of replication. ERCC1 belongs to the nucleotide excision repair (NER) family of proteins and is involved in the repair of these DNA strand breaks.[52] The ERCC1 protein works with its partner protein xeroderma pigmentosum complementation group F (XPF) in the final step of the NER pathway that recognizes and removes cisplatin-induced DNA adducts, allowing the tumor DNA replication to continue.[53] The NER pathway-mediated removal of platinum DNA reverses the tumoral DNA damage induced by cisplatin, thereby leading to cisplatin resistance (Fig. 47.1). High expression of ERCC1 in the tumor thus predicts for cisplatin resistance and serves as a predictive molecular determinant for the efficacy of this chemotherapy agent.[54]

The nature-envisioned purpose of ERCC1 is to effect DNA repair when DNA damage occurs after exposure to natural DNA-damaging entities, such as ionizing radiation and mutagenic compounds. A relatively preserved DNA repair mechanism, as suggested by high nuclear ERCC1 expression, therefore preserves genomic integrity. High tumoral levels of ERCC1 have therefore been associated with better outcomes in patients with early-stage disease who have had curative resection, presumably because of more indolent tumor behavior secondary to a relatively preserved genomic integrity. ERCC1 thus functions as a prognostic marker in patients with early-stage NSCLC.

RRM1 is the regulatory component of ribonucleotide reductase and is a nonredundant component of DNA synthesis.[55] Its primary function is to generate nucleotides that can be used for DNA synthesis and repair.[56] It is also the principal target of the commonly used cytotoxic agent, gemcitabine, and hence, high RRM1 levels predict for resistance to gemcitabine.[10,57] Analogous to ERCC1, RRM1 has been associated with different survival

outcomes in patients with NSCLC, with higher RRM1 levels predicting for a better prognosis and improved survival.[58] In preclinical trials, increased RRM1 expression was shown to be associated with decreased invasion and migration and with an overall more indolent behavior.[56] It is not entirely clear how RRM1 causes these effects, but it has been postulated that the effects are perhaps mediated through a direct correlation between RRM1 and expression of phosphatase and tensin homolog protein.[58] RRM1 therefore has both a predictive and prognostic function.[59,60]

The prognostic function of ERCC1 was first noted in a retrospective analysis of patients with NSCLC who had curative resection. ERCC1 was measured using reverse transcription (RT)-PCR, and its expression was normalized using 18SrRNA (a commonly used housekeeping gene) expression; therefore its levels were expressed as a unitless ratio. Using an ERCC1 value of 50 to dichotomize the cohort, researchers noted a significant difference in median survival for patients with ERCC1 expression of more than 50 in the tumor compared with patients with ERCC1 expression of less than 50 in the tumor (94.6 vs. 35.5 months; $p = 0.01$).[61] In multivariate analysis, high ERCC1 expression was found to be an independent predictor of better prognosis.

Olaussen et al.[62] further analyzed the prognostic value of ERCC1 in specimens obtained from the International Adjuvant Lung Trial (IALT). In the IALT study, patients with curatively resected NSCLC had been randomly assigned to receive adjuvant chemotherapy or no further therapy, as was the standard of care at that time. In the overall study population, adjuvant chemotherapy had improved 5-year survival by 4.1% ($p < 0.03$). Olaussen et al.[62] used IHC to analyze the tumor samples in that study for expression of ERCC1 (in addition to other markers) using an antibody that was then believed to stain for ERCC1 (murine antibody from clone 8F1; Neomarkers Inc, Fremont, CA, USA). Among patients with ERCC1-negative tumors, the 5-year overall survival rate was significantly longer for patients who received chemotherapy (47% vs. 39%; $p = 0.002$). However, among patients with ERCC1-positive tumors, overall survival did not differ between patients who received adjuvant chemotherapy and patients who did not. Of note, among patients who did not receive adjuvant chemotherapy, overall survival was significantly better for patients with ERCC1-positive tumors than for patients with ERCC1-negative tumors (adjusted HR for death, 0.66; 95% CI, 0.49–0.90; $p = 0.009$). This finding suggests an intrinsic prognostic function for ERCC1.

Given these results, the authors conducted a comprehensive analysis to compare various methods to measure ERCC1, as well as several antibodies used to measure ERCC1 by IHC.[63] They obtained 494 tumor specimens from two independent phase III trials (the National Cancer Institute of Canada Clinical Trials Group JBR.10 and the Cancer and Leukemia Group B 9633 trial from the Lung Adjuvant Cisplatin Evaluation Biology project). The researchers also repeated the staining of all 589 specimens in the original set of samples from the IALT study. They mapped the epitope recognized by 16 commercially available ERCC1 antibodies and investigated the capacity of the different ERCC1 isoforms to repair platinum-induced DNA damage. The investigators noted that ERCC1 was positive in 77% of the samples in the current study compared with 44% of the samples in the IALT study. Additionally, ERCC1 was no longer a predictive biomarker of the efficacy of chemotherapy ($p = 0.53$ for interaction). The 8F1 antibody used in the current study was different from that used in the initial analysis, and they concluded that there was a shift in the activity of the 8F1 antibody. Unfortunately the 8F1 antibody used in the IALT study had been totally consumed and was therefore not available for comparison.

Another significant finding was that each of the 16 antibodies tested could detect all of the four known isoforms of ERCC1. Because the epitopes are common in these four isoforms (201, 202, 203, and 204), none of the currently available antibodies could distinguish between them. For the purposes of RT-PCR, separate primers can be made for ERCC1 isomers 201 and 203;

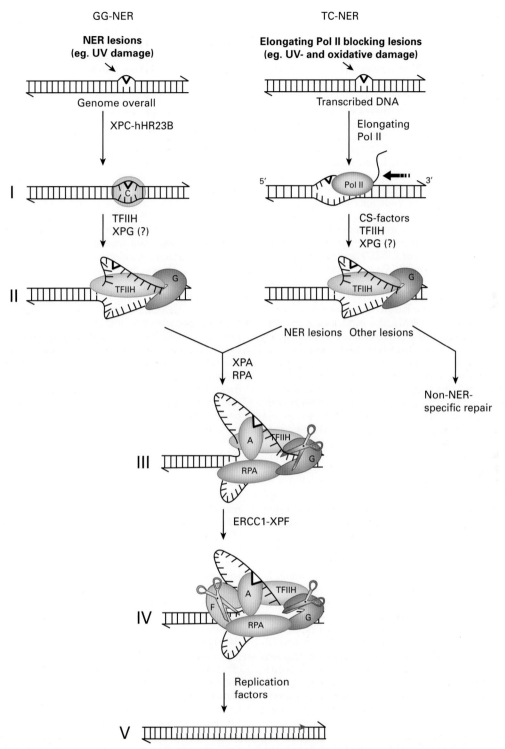

Fig. 47.1. Molecular model for the incision stage of nucleotide excision repair (NER). In global genome NER (GG-NER), XPC-hHR23B senses DNA helix-distorting nuclear excision repair lesions, leading to conformational alterations of the DNA, whereas in transcription-coupled repair (TC-NER), lesions are detected by the elongating RNA Pol II. In GG-NER, XPC-hHR23B at lesion attracts TFIIH (and possibly XPG). In both GG-NER and TC-NER, TFIIH creates a 10- to 20-nucleotide opened DNA complex around the lesion by virtue of its helicases XPB and XPD; this step requires ATP. XPA and RPA stabilize the 10- to 20-nucleotide opening and position other factors. XPA binds to the damaged nucleotides, RPA to the undamaged DNA strand. XPG stabilizes the fully opened complex. XPG, positioned by TFIIH and RPA, makes the 3′ incision. ERCC1-XPF, positioned by RPA and XPA, makes the second incision 5′ of the lesion. Dual incision is followed by gap-filling DNA synthesis and ligation. Drawn contacts between molecules reflect reported protein–protein interactions. *(Reprinted with permission from de Laat WL, Jaspers NG, Hoeijmakers JH. Molecular mechanism of nucleotide excision repair. Genes Dev. 1999;13(7):768–785.)*

however, because of substantial homology, primers cannot be separately made against 202 and 204. Thus, these two polymorphisms were measured in unison and there was no detectable difference in ERCC1-positive or ERCC1-negative samples in terms of overall or progression-free survival. However, in cell line experiments only the ERCC1 202 polymorphism seemed to predict for resistance to cisplatin; thus, this polymorphism may be the functional one. The authors concluded that measuring the clinically relevant functional ERCC1 202 polymorphism may be the better predictor of benefit for cisplatin in patients with NSCLC. Measuring the specific ERCC1 202 polymorphism will, however, be challenging because the high percentage of sequence homology among the four protein isoforms makes the generation of an ERCC1 202-specific antibody technically difficult. Making ERCC1 202-specific primers is onerous for the same reason.[63] However, the ERCC1 202 polymorphism may be detectable by sequencing at the DNA level, which would convert this nondiscrete biomarker into a discrete one.

To study the association between ERCC1 and RRM1, Zheng et al.[12] estimated the expression of ERCC1 and RRM1 at the protein level by AQUA and at the RNA level by RT-PCR and correlated the findings with survival. RRM1 expression was directly correlated with ERCC1 expression. Furthermore, patients who had tumors with high expression of RRM1 also had superior survival compared with patients who had tumors with low expression of RRM1 (disease-free survival, more than 120 vs. 54.5 months; HR, 0.46; $p = 0.004$; and overall survival, more than 120 vs. 60.2 months; HR, 0.61; $p = 0.02$). Other investigators also showed that patients who had tumors with high expression of both biomarkers had superior overall survival compared with patients who had tumors with low expression of either one of the biomarkers or both.[12]

The Southwest Oncology Group conducted a trial to assess the feasibility of selecting treatment based on in situ tumor levels of ERCC1 and RRM1 in a cooperative group setting.[64] Patients with stage I lung cancer were enrolled. ERCC1 and RRM1 expression were determined at the protein level with use of AQUA (range of expression, 1–255), and the level was classified as high or low based on previously established cutoff values of 65.0 for ERCC1 and 40.0 for RRM1. The treatment regimen consisted of cisplatin and gemcitabine (80 mg/m^2 on day 1 and 1 g/m^2 on days 1 and 8) for patients who had tumors with a low level of ERCC1 or RRM1 or both. Patients who had tumors with a high level of ERCC1 or RRM1 were followed up with observation, which is essentially the standard of care. In the protocol, feasibility was defined as the assignment of treatment within 12 weeks after surgery in at least 75% of the enrolled patients. Eighty-five patients were accrued between March 2009 and April 2011. ERCC1 and RRM1 levels were successfully determined in 83 patients, and 72 patients (87%) were successfully assigned appropriate therapy within the 12-week time frame. Of the 83 patients, 64 (77%) were assigned to chemotherapy and 19 (23%) to observation. ERCC1 levels ranged from 4.3 to 211.2 (median, 44.7), and RRM1 levels ranged from 2.5 to 234.4 (median, 39.3). The authors therefore concluded that assignment of chemotherapy was feasible in a multi-institutional cooperative group setting.

In the advanced stage NSCLC setting, Rosell et al.[59] analyzed samples from 100 patients to evaluate the association between expression of ERCC1 and RRM1 and survival. Patients in the study were treated with either gemcitabine and cisplatin; gemcitabine, cisplatin, and vinorelbine; or gemcitabine and vinorelbine followed by vinorelbine and ifosfamide. ERCC1 and RRM1 expression at the mRNA level was determined by RT-PCR in FFPE samples that had been obtained bronchoscopically. Again, a strong correlation between the expression of ERCC1 and RRM1 was noted ($p < 0.001$). Among patients treated with gemcitabine and cisplatin, the median survival was significantly longer for patients who had tumors with low RRM1 mRNA expression than for patients who had tumors with high RRM1 mRNA expression

(13.7 vs. 3.6 months; $p = 0.009$). In addition, the median survival was significantly longer for patients who had tumors with low expression of RRM1 and ERCC1 than among patients who had high levels of both genes ($p = 0.016$). These results essentially corroborated the earlier findings by the same group in a smaller cohort of patients in which ERCC1 mRNA expression was significantly associated with response to cisplatin and gemcitabine in patients with advanced stage NSCLC.[65]

The Genomic International Lung Trial (GILT) was the first prospective randomized trial designed to show clinical benefit of customizing chemotherapy.[66] In this phase III trial, 444 patients with previously untreated advanced NSCLC were randomly assigned in a 1:2 ratio to either a control arm of docetaxel and cisplatin or a genotypic arm in which treatment was assigned based on the level of ERCC1 mRNA expression in the tumor, as measured by RT-PCR. In the genotypic arm, patients received docetaxel and cisplatin if their tumors expressed ERCC1 mRNA levels lower than the median or received docetaxel and gemcitabine if the tumors expressed ERCC1 mRNA levels higher than the median. The study reached its primary end point of response, with a significantly better response rate in the genotypic arm than in the control arm (51.2% vs. 39.3%; $p = 0.02$). In multivariate analysis, low ERCC1 expression was an independent predictor of tumor response to cisplatin. The study was not powered to show survival differences, but neither progression-free survival nor overall survival was significantly different between the control and genotypic arms; the median progression-free survival was 6.1 months for the genotypic arm compared with 5.2 months for the control arm (HR, 0.9; $p = 0.30$), and the median overall survival was 9.9 months compared with 9.8 months for the genotypic and control arms, respectively (HR, 0.9; $p = 0.59$). Within the genotypic arm, relatively similar response rates were noted for patients with ERCC1-negative tumors treated with docetaxel and cisplatin (53%) and patients with ERCC1-positive tumors treated with docetaxel and gemcitabine (47%), with a median progression-free survival of 6.7 and 4.7 months, respectively, and a median overall survival of 10.3 and 9.4 months, respectively. In retrospect, given that expression of ERCC1 and RRM1 correlates with each other, a fact that was not known to the investigators at the time GILT was designed, cisplatin and gemcitabine would have been optimal treatment for patients who had tumors with low ERCC1 expression, and docetaxel with vinorelbine (rather than gemcitabine) would possibly be more desirable for patients who had tumors with high ERCC1 expression (because the presence of high ERCC1 expression suggests concomitant high expression of RRM1 and high RRM1 expression predicts for resistance to gemcitabine). The reason for the strong correlation between high ERCC1 and RRM1 expression is not clear but it is postulated that a steady supply of nucleotides, which are generated by RRM1, is necessary for efficient repair, which is carried out by ERCC1.

In an attempt to accelerate the application of this research to clinical practice, a prospective phase II trial, Molecular Analysis-Directed Individualized Therapy (MADe IT), assigned combination chemotherapy according to expression of ERCC1 and RRM1 (as measured by RT-PCR), with a primary end point of feasibility.[67] Patients who had tumors with low ERCC1 expression were treated with carboplatin, and patients who had tumors with low RRM1 expression were treated with gemcitabine; patients who had tumors with high expression of either marker were treated with docetaxel. Therefore, based on the expression of ERCC1 and RRM1, patients could be assigned to one of four treatment groups: gemcitabine and carboplatin (low expression of both RRM1 and ERCC); gemcitabine and docetaxel (low RRM1 expression and high ERCC1 expression); docetaxel and carboplatin (high RRM1 expression and low ERCC1 expression); or docetaxel and vinorelbine (high expression of both RRM1 and ERCC1). The response rate was 44%, with an overall survival of 13.3 months and a progression-free survival of 6.6 months (Fig. 47.2).[67]

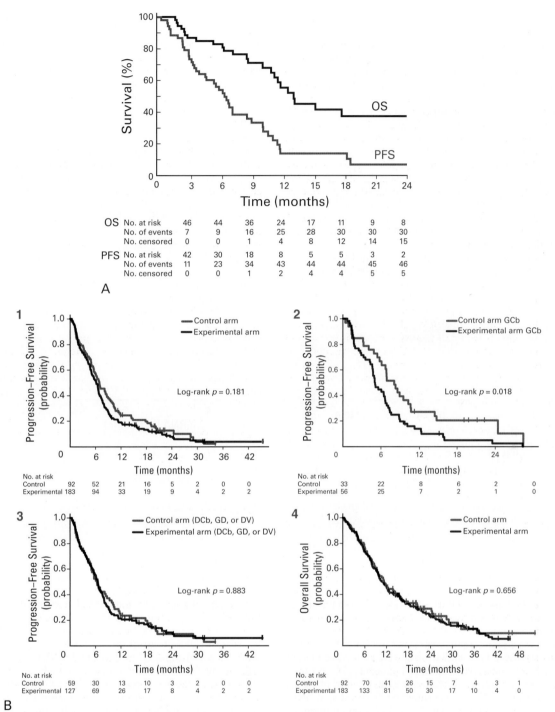

Fig. 47.2. (A) Overall survival (OS) and progression-free survival (PFS) for 53 patients with advanced nonsmall cell lung cancer treated with chemotherapy based on expression of the ribonucleotide reductase subunit 1 (*RRM1*) and excision repair cross-complementing group 1 (*ERCC1*) genes. ERCC1 and RRM1 were measured by reverse transcription polymerase chain reaction in this trial.[34] (B) Comparison of survival according to ERCC1 and RRM1 expression. ERCC1 and RRM1 in situ protein levels were used for dichotomization, with in situ protein expression measured with use of the automated quantitative analysis (AQUA) technique. (1) Progression-free survival. (2) Comparison of progression-free survival between the experimental and control arms for patients with low expression of both ERCC1 and RRM1 levels who received identical therapy (gemcitabine and carboplatin [GCb]). (3) Comparison of progression-free survival between the experimental and control arms for patients with high expression of RRM1 and low expression of ERCC1; low expression of RRM1 and high expression of ERCC1; and high expression of both RRM1 and ERCC1; patients in the experimental arm received either docetaxel and carboplatin (DCb), gemcitabine and docetaxel (GD), or docetaxel and vinorelbine (DV), and patients in the control arm received GCb. (4) Overall survival.

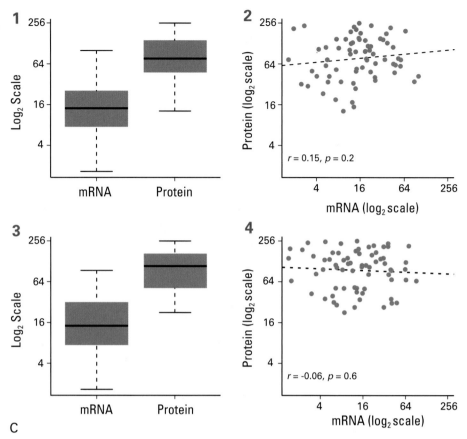

Fig. 47.2. con'd (C) No correlations were found in the expression of ERCC1 (1 and 2) and RRM1 (3 and 4). *(A. Reprinted with permission from Simon G, Sharma A, Li X, et al. Feasibility and efficacy of molecular analysis-directed individualized therapy in advanced non-small-cell lung cancer. J Clin Oncol. 2007;25(19):2741–2746; B. and C. Modified with permission from Bepler G, Williams C, Schell MJ, et al. Randomized international phase III trial of ERCC1 and RRM1 expression-based chemotherapy versus gemcitabine/carboplatin in advanced non-small-cell lung cancer. J Clin Oncol. 2013;31(19):2404–2412.)*

To further analyze the effect of treatment customization, three other trials were conducted in the same institution using similar eligibility criteria; however, all patients were treated with a similar regimen and the results were compared with the findings of the phase II MADe IT trial. The data were allowed to mature before these comparisons were made. Encouraged by the promising results of these studies,[68] a prospective randomized phase III trial (phase III MADe IT trial) was launched. In this trial, 275 eligible patients were randomly assigned in a 2:1 ratio to the experimental arm or the control arm. In the control arm, treatment was with gemcitabine and carboplatin. In the experimental arm, treatment was given according to ERCC1 and RRM1 expression as in the phase II trial. Progression-free survival was the primary end point and the trial was powered to show a 32% improvement in progression-free survival at 6 months.[69] In both arms, a median of four cycles of chemotherapy were given. There were no significant differences between the experimental and control arms in terms of progression-free survival (6.1 vs. 6.9 months) or overall survival (11.0 vs. 11.3 months). Of interest, a subset analysis demonstrated that, among patients who had tumors with low levels of both ERCC1 and RRM1 expression and received the same treatment (carboplatin and gemcitabine), progression-free survival was significantly better in the control arm than in the experimental arm (8.1 vs. 5.0 months; $p = 0.02$; Fig. 47.2B). The reason for

this finding is not clear. A key difference between the phase II and phase III trials was that ERCC1 and RRM1 expression was measured at the mRNA level by RT-PCR in the phase II trial, whereas, for dichotomization purposes, it was measured at the protein level using AQUA and the 8F1 antibody. Hence, the estimations of ERCC1 may have not been entirely accurate. Indeed, no correlation between ERCC1 mRNA and protein levels ($r = -0.06$) was noted in this trial. There were also no correlations between RRM1 mRNA levels and in situ protein levels measured by AQUA; this finding was thought to be due to different fixation and processing techniques used in these investigations.

Significant batch effects were also noted; that is, ERCC1 and RRM1 expression levels were higher or lower in batches. The expression levels also tended to vary according to when and where the tests were performed (personal communication, Michael Schell). Hence, it is quite likely that the fallacies in measurement may have led to the differences in efficacy with carboplatin and gemcitabine in the experimental arm and the control arm. It should be noted that these studies were done before the Centers for Medicare and Medicaid Services mandate that all molecular testing of tissue on which clinical decisions are made must be performed in Clinical Laboratory Improvement Amendments–certified laboratories.[69] Thus, the clinical uses of markers such as ERCC1 and RRM1 remain to be elucidated; however, exploring

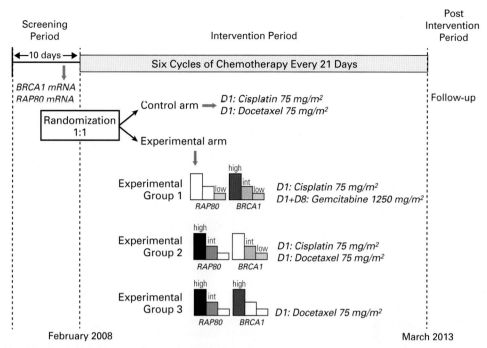

Fig. 47.3. Study design and intervention period for the Spanish Lung Cancer Group phase III randomized trial. During the 10-day screening period, BRCA1 and RAP80 mRNA expression was analyzed, and if the analysis was successful, patients were randomly assigned in a 1:1 ratio to either the control or experimental arm. The screening and intervention periods were similar for the Chinese phase II randomized trial, but patients were randomized in a 1:3 ratio to either the control or one of three experimental arms.

specific isoforms may provide further opportunities for additional investigation.

BRCA1

BRCA1 belongs to the mismatch repair pathway of genes and is typically instrumental in repairing single-strand breaks. It also functions as a differential regulator of chemotherapy-induced apoptosis.[70] In preclinical models, BRCA1 has been shown to be a sensitizer to apoptosis induced by antimicrotubulin agents, such as taxanes and vinca alkaloids, and also abrogates the apoptosis induced by a range of DNA-damaging agents, including cisplatin and etoposide.[71] BRCA1 mRNA expression has been shown to correlate with ERCC1 mRNA expression, and low expression of BRCA1 has been shown to predict for a more favorable outcome in patients with resected NSCLC who have received adjuvant cisplatin and gemcitabine.[72,73]

In a feasibility study, the Spanish Customized Adjuvant Trial and the Spanish Lung Cancer Group (SLCG) customized adjuvant chemotherapy based on BRCA1 mRNA levels in 84 patients with completely resected NSCLC.[74] Docetaxel was used to treat tumors with high levels of BRCA; docetaxel and cisplatin were used to treat tumors with intermediate levels; and cisplatin and gemcitabine were used to treat tumors with low levels. The median survival had not been reached for patients with high or intermediate BRCA1 levels at the time of the report and was 25.6 months for patients with low levels ($p = 0.04$). Interim analyses showed that single-agent docetaxel was not inferior to cisplatin and docetaxel in terms of survival for patients with high BRCA1 levels. Based on these results, the SLCG designed a phase III open multicenter randomized study of customized adjuvant chemotherapy, based on BRCA1 mRNA levels, for completely resected early-stage (II–IIIA) NSCLC. In this study, patients were randomly assigned to the control or experimental arms in a 1:3 ratio. In the control arm, patients received docetaxel plus cisplatin, and in the experimental arms, patients who had tumors

with higher BRCA1 transcriptional levels were treated with single-agent docetaxel and patients who had tumors with intermediate and low BRCA1 expression received cisplatin-based doublets. Postoperative radiotherapy was mandatory for patients with N2 disease. According to the preliminary results of the study,[75] differences in the safety profile of the treatment schedules were noted, with customized treatment requiring fewer dose reductions; the efficacy results had not been reported by the time of publication. Therefore, high BRCA1 levels predict resistance to cisplatin and possibly sensitivity to docetaxel.

In the SLCG phase II customized chemotherapy trial, BRCA1 and RAP80 expression had a combined effect on outcome for patients with advanced NSCLC. Based on this finding, the SLCG conducted a randomized phase III trial to compare nonselected cisplatin-based chemotherapy with therapy customized according to BRCA1 and RAP80 levels (the BREC study).[76] A parallel randomized phase II trial was carried out in China under the auspices of the SLCG (Fig. 47.3). Patients were randomly assigned to the control or experimental arm in a 1:1 ratio in the SLCG trial and in a 1:3 ratio in the Chinese trial. The primary end point was progression-free survival. The results of the two studies indicated a poor predictive capacity of RAP80 for customization. Indeed, the prespecified interim analysis showed a detrimental effect in the experimental arm (HR for disease progression, 1.35; $p = 0.03$) and, based on these results, the study was prematurely closed. However, a significant interaction between performance status and treatment arm was found; in the experimental arm, a favorable, although nonsignificant, effect was found for patients with a performance status of 0, whereas there was a negative effect for patients with performance status of 1, including a significantly increased risk of death. Despite previous findings showing a predictive capacity for RAP80, the results of the BREC study indicate that other molecular factors may also influence the BRCA1-RAP80 predictive model.[76,77] For instance, a preclinical model published in 2012 showed that BRCA1 protein, p53 binding protein 1 (53BP1), and RAD51 may assemble at double-strand breaks in RAP80-depleted cells, whereas RAP80 and 53BP1, but not RAD51, may assemble at double-strand breaks in BRCA1-depleted cells.[78] Therefore, the results of the BREC study may provide the groundwork for research to define better predictive models for chemotherapy outcomes. The benefit obtained from biomarker-directed treatment in patients with a performance status of 0, while not significant, may pave the way for further investigation in this subgroup of patients.

Class β-Tubulin

Increased expression of class III β-tubulin has been shown to correlate with resistance to antimicrotubule agents such as taxanes and vinorelbine in patients with advanced NSCLC.[79] However, interest in β-tubulin faded after the findings of a retrospective analysis of data from the JBR.10 trial were reported. The JBR.10 trial compared adjuvant cisplatin and vinorelbine with observation alone after curative-intent surgical resection of stage IB–II NSCLC. β-tubulin expression measured by semiquantitative IHC demonstrated that high expression of β-tubulin was associated with poorer recurrence-free and overall survival among patients treated with surgery alone, but not among patients treated with adjuvant chemotherapy.[80] Further study of β-tubulin as a predictor of taxane sensitivity has been halted.

Thymidylate Synthase

Thymidylate synthase is essential for purine synthesis required for DNA replication. 5-Fluorouracil is a prototypic drug known to inhibit thymidylate synthase. However, thymidylate synthase has also been proposed as a target for pemetrexed, which has become a cornerstone drug for patients with nonsquamous NSCLC. Levels of thymidylate synthase have been high in small cell lung carcinoma; among NSCLCs, thymidylate synthase expression has been higher in squamous cell carcinoma than in adenocarcinomas.[81] Preclinical studies suggest that low expression of thymidylate synthase, dihydrofolate reductase, glycinamide ribonucleotide formyl transferase, and *MRP4* gene expression correlate with response to pemetrexed.[82] In animal studies, overexpression of thymidylate synthase correlated with decreased sensitivity to pemetrexed.[83] Taken together, these data suggest that high expression of thymidylate synthase predicts resistance to pemetrexed.

High levels of thymidylate synthase in squamous cell lung cancer provide an explanation for the decreased activity of pemetrexed in patients with this histologic subtype of NSCLC. A randomized phase III trial compared pemetrexed with docetaxel in the second-line treatment of patients with advanced stage NSCLC. Overall, there was no difference in efficacy between pemetrexed and docetaxel. Pemetrexed, however, was significantly less toxic than docetaxel.[84] Among patients with nonsquamous carcinoma, pemetrexed led to better overall survival than docetaxel (9.3 vs. 8.0 months), whereas docetaxel appeared to yield better overall survival for patients with squamous cell carcinoma (7.4 vs. 6.2 months).

This differential benefit of chemotherapy according to histology was also evident in a phase III trial comparing cisplatin and gemcitabine (863 patients) with cisplatin and pemetrexed (862 patients) in advanced NSCLC, with a prespecified subset analysis based on histology.[85] Although there was noninferiority for the pemetrexed-containing regimen compared with the gemcitabine-containing regimen in an unselected cohort of patients (median survival, 10.3 vs. 10.3 months; HR, 0.94; 95% CI, 0.84–1.05), overall survival was significantly superior for pemetrexed compared with gemcitabine among 847 patients with adenocarcinoma (12.6 vs. 10.9 months) and 153 patients with large cell carcinoma (10.4 vs. 6.7 months). For 473

patients with squamous cell carcinoma, however, the reverse was true, with gemcitabine providing additional benefit (10.8 vs. 9.4 months).

Similarly, in a randomized double-blind study of 663 patients with stage IIIB or IV disease who did not have disease progression after four cycles of platinum-based chemotherapy, the authors postulated a differential expression of thymidylate synthase between squamous and nonsquamous histology as a possible mechanism for the histology-specific benefit for pemetrexed. In this study, patients were assigned to receive pemetrexed (500 mg/m², day 1) or best supportive care until disease progression.[86] Although maintenance therapy with pemetrexed was of benefit for the entire cohort of patients (overall survival, 13.4 vs. 10.6 months; HR, 0.79, p = 0.012) compared with best supportive care, the overall survival was significantly better for patients with nonsquamous histology (15.3 vs. 10.3 months; HR, 0.70; p = 0.002).

Given the findings of these studies, investigators have attempted to tailor chemotherapy based on ERCC1 and thymidylate synthase in the International Tailored Chemotherapy Adjuvant Trial. This ongoing phase III multicenter randomized trial is comparing adjuvant pharmacogenomic-driven chemotherapy with standard adjuvant chemotherapy for patients with completely resected stage II to stage IIIA NSCLC. ERCC1 and thymidylate synthase are assessed by quantitative RT-PCR on FFPE tumor specimens in a central laboratory. The primary end point is overall survival; secondary end points include disease-free survival, toxicity profile of the treatment regimen in relation to ERCC1, and thymidylate synthase mRNA quantification versus protein quantification. The total anticipated patient accrual is 700. Patients in each genomic category will be randomly assigned to receive either a standard chemotherapy selected by the investigator (cisplatin and vinorelbine, cisplatin and docetaxel, or cisplatin and gemcitabine) or an experimental treatment chosen according to the following algorithm: high expression of ERCC1 and thymidylate synthase: single-agent paclitaxel; high expression of ERCC1 and low level of thymidylate synthase: single-agent pemetrexed; low ERCC1 expression and high level of thymidylate synthase: cisplatin and gemcitabine; and low expression of ERCC1 and thymidylate synthase: cisplatin and pemetrexed. Four cycles of the selected chemotherapy will be administered in both the standard and experimental arms. Enrollment on this trial was ongoing at the time of publication.

Gene Expression Profiling

With the advent of high-throughput technologies, investigators have attempted to develop oligonucleotide array–based gene signatures that can be used as both a prognostic and predictive tool. Although multiple genes can be analyzed at one time with gene expression microarrays, the technique itself is complex and necessitates specialized techniques and complex bioinformatics. This complexity has precluded its wider application in community centers. Several private and for-profit entities have offered to analyze samples and provide the results on a fee-for-service basis.

Among the first gene expression signatures to be studied was a multivariate model that included p53, KRAS, and HRAS, which was used to determine prognosis in stage I resected NSCLC.[87] Chen et al.[88] reported on a five-gene signature that may provide prognostic value for patients with NSCLC. These authors first identified a 16-gene panel, utilizing oligonucleotide microarrays, which correlated with survival. From this panel of 16 genes, five genes (*DUSP6, MMD, STAT1, ERBB3,* and *LCK*) were selected for further studies by RT-PCR and decision-tree analysis. This gene profile dichotomized patients into two groups: high risk (59 patients) and low risk (42 patients). For patients in the high-risk group, the median overall survival was significantly shorter than for patients in the low-risk group (20 vs. 40 months; $p < 0.001$). The median progression-free survival was also significantly shorter in the high-risk group (13 vs. 29 months; $p = 0.002$).

Several other chemotherapy predictive or prognostic gene signatures have also been developed and are moving toward validation.[89–95] Gene-expression profile signatures are now used in clinical practice for breast cancer,[96–99] but have not been used widely in clinical practice, most likely because of the complexity of the technology itself and cost. In addition, the lack of clear understanding of the genes that constitute the panel raises questions about its validity and lack of validation in large data sets consisting of hundreds of patients.

HOST-RELATED FACTORS

In theory, specific chemotherapy regimens may be selected or avoided based on genetic factors within the host. These germline genetic factors typically predict for the risk of toxicity rather than efficacy. Single-nucleotide polymorphisms (SNPs) and substitutions of a single base in a DNA sequence account for approximately 90% of genetic variation in humans. SNPs are estimated to occur as frequently as every 100 to 300 bases, and, by definition, must be present in at least 1% of the population. SNPs are found in both coding and noncoding sequences and may alter DNA transcription rates, RNA splicing, translation efficiency, and protein function.

UGT1A1*28

Chemotherapy metabolism and detoxification are influenced by a large number of SNPs. As a key example, polymorphisms in the uridine diphosphate glucuronosyltransferase 1A1 (UGT1A1) gene have a substantial effect on gastrointestinal and myelosuppressive toxicity in patients treated with irinotecan. Gilbert syndrome has often been diagnosed in patients with the UGT1A1 gene, and people with this syndrome have a predominantly unconjugated hyperbilirubinemia that is asymptomatic.[100–103]

Irinotecan is activated to SN-38, which then exerts antitumor activity.[104] SN-38 is then detoxified to the pharmacologically inactive SN-38 glucuronide (SN-38G). UGT1A1 is the principal enzyme responsible for the glucuronidation of SN-38. The in vitro glucuronidation of SN-38 is strongly correlated with the UGT1A1 gene promoter polymorphism UGT1A1*28, which contains an additional TA repeat in the TATA sequence of the UGT1A1 promoter; i.e., the sequence is (TA)7TAA instead of (TA)6TAA.[104] Among patients with the (TA)7TAA sequence, the rate of SN-38 glucuronidation has been reported to be significantly slower than among patients with the normal allele ($p = 0.001$) and the rates of grade 4 toxicities, especially diarrhea and myelosuppression, have been significantly higher. These results suggest that screening for UGT1A1*28 polymorphism may identify patients with lower SN-38 glucuronidation rates and greater susceptibility to irinotecan-induced gastrointestinal and bone marrow toxicity.[103,105] Use of the UGT1A1 polymorphism to predict for toxicity to irinotecan is approved by the United States Food and Drug Administration (FDA) for use in clinical practice.

CYP3A

Polymorphic variants in cytochrome P450 (CYP) proteins are also recognized as determinants of chemotherapy activity and toxicity. This large and diverse family of enzymes catalyzes the metabolism of xenobiotics, including many anticancer agents.[106] CYP3A members are the most abundant type of CYP in the small intestine and liver, with substantial interindividual and interracial variation in expression attributed to SNPs.[107,108] CYP3A expression affects the pharmacokinetic disposition of multiple drugs

and may have an impact on the metabolism of environmental procarcinogens, thus influencing an individual's predisposition toward cancer. The role of SNPs in drug metabolism and disposition is complex, and efforts to define their utility for personalized medicine are ongoing.[109,110] Interindividual differences in host DNA repair capacity may also affect the response to chemotherapy. Multiple SNPs have been identified in genes involved in nucleotide excision repair, double-strand DNA break repair, nucleotide synthesis, and other DNA repair processes.[111,112] Decreased DNA repair capacity resulting from SNPs appears to contribute to lung cancer risk, particularly in patients who are young, female, and light smokers or nonsmokers.[113]

Although such host-related differences are typically considered on an individual patient basis, in a broader sense, genotyping studies may help to explain differences in patients' outcomes based on ethnic or racial background (i.e., population-related pharmacogenomics). For example, variations in taxane metabolism between Japanese and white populations have been reported and purported to account for differences in outcomes of taxane-based chemotherapy.[114] To address this question, joint studies between Japanese and United States investigators have been designed to identify population-related differences in drug pharmacogenomics using a so-called common-arm approach.[115] In such studies, separate phase III trials evaluating paclitaxel and carboplatin for advanced-stage NSCLC incorporated similar study criteria for patient eligibility and treatment. In a preliminary report, differences in allelic distribution for genes involved in paclitaxel disposition or DNA repair were found between patients in Japan and the United States. Genotype-associated correlations with clinical outcomes were observed for progression-free survival with CYP3A4*1B and for response with ERCC2 K751Q. This research strategy may assist in determining whether the significant differences in efficacy and toxicity that have been reported in these two populations are attributable to population-related genetic variance.[115]

CONCLUSION

Sensitizing EGFR mutations and the ALK fusion oncogene are now recognized as predictive biomarkers in lung cancer. KRAS mutational status is predictive of lack of therapeutic efficacy with EGFR tyrosine kinase inhibitors. MET and ROS1 genomic alterations are more rare driver mutations that, when detected, may enable more precision treatment for patients with lung cancer. Conversely, the use of molecular biomarkers such as ERCC1, RRM1, BRCA1, thymidylate synthase, and others remains investigational. The pharmacogenomic research community must come to an agreement on optimal ways of measuring these biomarkers. Because these biomarkers are discrete—measured at the DNA level with a clear and unambiguous answer (positive or negative)—they are most likely to have wide clinical application. With regard to host-related factors, one biomarker is FDA-approved for use in clinical practice: estimation of the UGT1A1 polymorphism to predict for toxicity to irinotecan. However, this biomarker also has not found wide application because of the limited use of irinotecan to treat lung cancer in the United States. Asymptomatic predominantly unconjugated hyperbilirubinemia is a hallmark of Gilbert syndrome, which in turn is caused by the UGT1A1*28 polymorphism. Thus, in the clinical setting, hyperbilirubinemia according to routinely performed metabolic or liver panels would provide a clue to the possibility of increased toxicity with irinotecan and may prompt formal testing for the UGT1A1*28 polymorphism.

The field of lung cancer pharmacogenomics has advanced exponentially since the early 2000s and yet is essentially still in its initial stages. The pace of development is expected to continue over the coming years, and research has highlighted several important lessons that will serve us well going forward.

KEY REFERENCES

1. National Comprehensive Cancer Network (NCCN). Clinical practice guidelines in oncology: Non-small cell lung cancer. Version 2.2017; October 26, 2016. http://www.nccn.org.

6. Aggarwal C, Somaiah N, Simon GR. Biomarkers with predictive and prognostic function in non-small cell lung cancer: ready for prime time? *J Natl Compr Canc Netw*. 2010;8(7):822–832.

12. Zheng Z, Chen T, Li X, et al. DNA synthesis and repair genes RRM1 and ERCC1 in lung cancer. *N Engl J Med*. 2007;356(8):800–808.

15. The Clinical Lung Cancer Genome Project (CLCGP). Network Genomic Medicine. A genomics-based classification of human lung tumors. *Sci Transl Med*. 2013;5(209):209ra153.

18. Johnson BE, Janne PA. Epidermal growth factor receptor mutations in patients with non-small cell lung cancer. *Cancer Res*. 2005;65:7525–7529.

26. Mok TS, Wu YL, Thongprasert S, et al. Gefitinib or carboplatin-paclitaxel in pulmonary adenocarcinoma. *N Engl J Med*. 2009;361(10):947–957.

34. Kwak EL, Bang YJ, Camidge DR, et al. Anaplastic lymphoma kinase inhibition in non-small-cell lung cancer. *N Engl J Med*. 2010;363:1693–1703.

37. Solomon BJ, Mok T, Kim DW, et al. First-line crizotinib versus chemotherapy in ALK-positive lung cancer. *N Engl J Med*. 2014;371:2167–2177.

40. Eberhard DA, Johnson BE, Amler LC, et al. Mutations in the epidermal growth factor receptor and in KRAS are predictive and prognostic indicators in patients with non-small-cell lung cancer treated with chemotherapy alone and in combination with erlotinib. *J Clin Oncol*. 2005;23:5900–5909.

44. Slebos RJ, Kibbelaar RE, Dalesio O, et al. K-ras oncogene activation as a prognostic marker in adenocarcinoma of the lung. *N Engl J Med*. 1990;323:561–565.

45. Sholl LM, Aisner DL, Varella-Garcia M, et al. Multi-institutional oncogenic driver mutation analysis in lung adenocarcinoma: the Lung Cancer Mutation Consortium Experience. *J Thorac Oncol*. 2015;10:768–777.

49. Sandler A, Gray R, Perry MC, et al. Paclitaxel-carboplatin alone or with bevacizumab for non-small-cell lung cancer. *N Engl J Med*. 2006;355(24):2542–2550.

50. Wakelee HA, Schiller JH, Gandara DR. Current status of adjuvant chemotherapy for stage IB non-small-cell lung cancer: implications for the New Intergroup Trial. *Clin Lung Cancer*. 2006;8(1):18–21.

66. Cobo M, Isla D, Massuti B, Montes A, et al. Customizing cisplatin based on quantitative excision repair cross-complementing 1 mRNA expression: a phase III trial in non-small-cell lung cancer. *J Clin Oncol*. 2007;25(19):2747–2754.

69. Bepler G, Williams C, Schell MJ, et al. Randomized international phase III trial of ERCC1 and RRM1 expression-based chemotherapy versus gemcitabine/carboplatin in advanced non-small-cell lung cancer. *J Clin Oncol*. 2013;31(19):2404–2412.

85. Scagliotti GV, Parikh P, von Pawel J, et al. Phase III study comparing cisplatin plus gemcitabine with cisplatin plus pemetrexed in chemotherapy-naive patients with advanced-stage non-small-cell lung cancer. *J Clin Oncol*. 2008;26(21):3543–3551.

88. Chen HY, Yu SL, Chen CH, et al. A five-gene signature and clinical outcome in non-small-cell lung cancer. *N Engl J Med*. 2007;356(1):11–20.

111. Kiyohara C, Yoshimasu K. Genetic polymorphisms in the nucleotide excision repair pathway and lung cancer risk: a meta-analysis. *Int J Med Sci*. 2007;4(2):59–71.

115. Gandara DR, Kawaguchi T, Crowley J, et al. Japanese-US common-arm analysis of paclitaxel plus carboplatin in advanced non-small-cell lung cancer: a model for assessing population-related pharmacogenomics. *J Clin Oncol*. 2009;27(21):3540–3546.

See Expertconsult.com for full list of references.

48 New Targets for Therapy in Lung Cancer

Aaron S. Mansfield, Grace K. Dy, Mjung-Ju Ahn, and Alex A. Adjei

SUMMARY OF KEY POINTS

- Treatment of lung cancer is rapidly evolving. Large cell carcinomas as a group have therapeutically relevant driver mutations in nearly 40% of cases.
- Despite the recent failures of some agents, in 2015 the US Food and Drug Administration issued seven approvals of agents for the treatment of lung cancer.
- Many additional promising agents that target several aberrant signaling pathways are under development.
- A large proportion of genomic alterations are not considered directly druggable targets, such as mutant p53 or amplified SOX2; this obstacle may be surmounted by identifying synthetically lethal changes amenable to drug therapy.
- Targeted therapy requires simultaneous development of the targeted agent along with biomarker assay platforms for patient selection to optimize therapeutic benefit.
- To avoid misinterpretation of clinical trial data, thorough understanding of drug activity and characterization of pharmacologic activity, particularly of small-molecule inhibitors, is necessary, particularly when an anticipated clinical benefit is not found.

Major advances in the therapy of cancer have occurred since the beginning of the new millennium. These advances were spurred by increased knowledge of the biologic hallmarks of cancer coupled with breakthroughs in genomic and pharmaceutical technologies. In the field of lung cancer, researchers discovered the oncogenic role of so-called druggable proteins arising from somatic mutations in the epidermal growth factor receptor (*EGFR*) gene and chromosomal rearrangements in the anaplastic lymphoma kinase (*ALK*) gene. These findings led to therapies resulting in substantially higher response rates and survival in patients with lung cancer being treated with EGFR and ALK inhibitors, respectively, compared with conventional chemotherapy.[1-3] Recognizing the integral role played by the tumor microenvironment in the initiation and maintenance of the malignant phenotype has also resulted in the development of antiangiogenesis agents with clinical relevance in various malignancies, such as the use of the monoclonal antibody bevacizumab in the nonsquamous subtype of nonsmall cell lung cancer (NSCLC).[4] Modulation of immune checkpoints is another highly promising approach. In this chapter, we review promising therapeutic drug targets for the treatment of NSCLC as of 2016.

Although the relevance of each target and its role in each signaling pathway is presented in a linear fashion to facilitate discussion, individual targets do not function in isolation because cells possess a complex architecture of signaling networks that are highly interconnected. Moreover, negative feedback loops and concurrent activation of multiple substrates involved in a number of important pathways can lead to paradoxical effects depending on the cellular context. Thus, the presence of a drug inhibitor can result in pathway activation that leads to cell survival or proliferation rather than cell death, resulting in ineffective therapies. This is a challenge in the therapy of malignancies such as lung cancer, which tend to harbor multiple molecular aberrations. Additionally, targeted therapies may also affect signaling networks within nonmalignant cells and modulate antitumor immunity or the tumor microenvironment.[5]

KEY SIGNAL TRANSDUCTION PATHWAYS

The two major signaling cascades that are triggered upon activation of growth factor receptors are the RAS/RAF/MAPK and the PI3K/AKT/mTOR pathways. Multiple relevant targets for drug therapy in NSCLC can be illustrated as they transduce signals through these two interconnected pathways (Fig. 48.1).

The RAS/RAF/MAPK pathway plays a major role in the signaling cascades of various growth factor receptors, such as EGFR, human epidermal growth factor receptor type 2 (HER2), fibroblast growth factor receptor (FGFR), and others. Upon activation of receptor kinase signaling, recruitment of adaptor proteins (e.g., Grb2, Shc, and others) triggers key downstream steps involving RAS activation. After this event, the serine/threonine kinase RAF (a member of the MAPK kinase or MAPKKK group of protein kinases), represented by the members ARAF, BRAF, and CRAF, phosphorylates two distinct serine residues on the MAPKs (also known as MEK) MEK1 and MEK2. MEK1/2 subsequently phosphorylates both serine/threonine and tyrosine residues in the final p44 and p42 MAPK (also known as ERK1/2) in the cascade, which then phosphorylates downstream substrates, resulting in proliferation and survival.[6,7]

Similarly, lipid phosphorylation via phosphoinositide 3-kinase (PI3K) signaling regulates various cellular functions such as proliferation, survival, metabolism, and metastasis. This pathway is normally regulated by receptor tyrosine kinases (RTKs), particularly signals generated by insulin and insulin-like growth factor 1 (IGF-1) receptors (IGF-1Rs).[8] The PI3K pathway is also frequently involved in the development and maintenance of the malignant phenotype arising from oncogenically driven RTK activation of the pathway. The class I PI3Ks are primarily involved in the generation of phospholipid messengers in response to RTK activation.[9] Termination of PI3K signaling in turn is mediated by phosphatases such as the tumor suppressor phosphatase and tensin homolog (PTEN) on chromosome 10.[10]

Phospholipid messengers generated upon PI3K activation bind to phosphoinositide-dependent kinase 1 (PDK1) and, downstream to it, protein kinase B (AKT) and other effector proteins through specific pleckstrin homology or other lipid-binding domains. PDK1 is the principal kinase responsible for phosphorylation and activation of the serine/threonine kinase AKT. AKT itself is also phosphorylated by downstream substrates, an example of nonlinear interactions that exist in signaling pathways. Activated AKT phosphorylates various substrates that mediate diverse functions, such as degradation of the Forkhead (FOXO) transcription factors and inhibition of BAD and BAX, resulting in reduced apoptosis and cell survival. AKT also activates mammalian target of rapamycin (mTOR) by direct phosphorylation as well as by phosphorylating the tumor suppressor tuberin (also known as TSC2), thus inhibiting the repressor function of the tuberin–hamartin (also known as TSC1) complex on mTOR.[11,12] mTOR kinase, a highly conserved serine/threonine kinase,

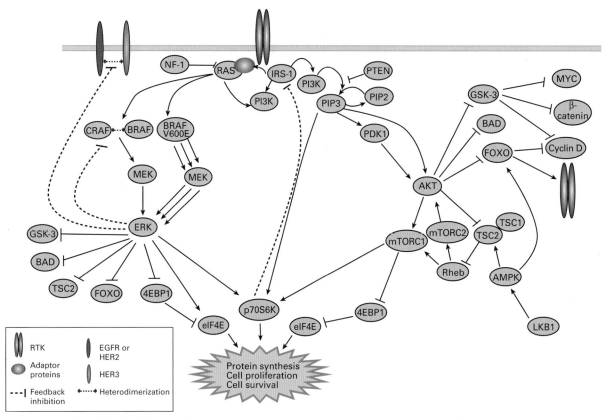

Fig. 48.1. Simplified signaling output mediated through relevant drug targets in nonsmall cell lung cancer.

subsequently regulates cellular metabolism and protein synthesis through downstream effectors such as p70S6K and 4EBP1. MEK/ERK signaling also activates mTOR by inactivating TSC2 upon phosphorylation by ERK1/2, one of the several links between the RAS/RAF/MAPK and PI3K/AKT/mTOR pathways.[13]

THERAPEUTIC TARGETS

This chapter provides a review of the frequency of genomic alterations found in relevant selected targets for two major histologic subtypes of NSCLC, squamous cell carcinoma and adenocarcinoma (Table 48.1). Large cell carcinomas as a group have therapeutically relevant driver mutations in nearly 40% of cases. The distribution of these mutations has been described and mirrors the classification of squamous and nonsquamous subtypes of NSCLC as defined by immunohistochemistry (IHC),[14] and thus is not categorized separately. Many drugs are in clinical use or in development for each corresponding drug target.

Receptor Tyrosine Kinases

Human Epidermal Growth Factor Receptor Type 2

HER2 (also known as ERBB2) belongs to the same family of HER RTKs as EGFR.[15] In contrast to EGFR, HER2 does not interact with any ligand directly but serves as the preferred dimerization partner of EGFR and other ErbB family members, such as HER3 and HER4, to trigger autophosphorylation and downstream signaling through both the MAPK and PI3K pathways described earlier.[16] HER2 gene amplification (defined as HER2/CEP17 ratio per cell of 2 or greater, and absolute HER2 signals in more than 4; or more than 15 copies in more than 10% of cells using fluorescence in situ hybridization [FISH] assay) is found in approximately 1% to 3% of lung cancers.[17,18] HER2 exon 20

insertions are found in approximately 3% of adenocarcinomas.[19] HER2 amplification is correlated with histologic subtype and tumor grade, such that high-level amplification appears to be concentrated in the subgroup of high-grade adenocarcinomas.[17] Intratumor heterogeneity in the level of HER2 amplification also appears frequently.[17] This latter feature may partly account for the negative results of clinical trials conducted a decade ago using trastuzumab in combination with chemotherapy for patients with NSCLC. In addition to patients with tumor heterogeneity, these studies included patients with potentially low-to-absent HER2 amplification (e.g., inclusion of patients with 2+ HER2 protein expression as determined by IHC).[20–22]

Afatinib, an oral pan-HER inhibitor, has been used as monotherapy in genotypically selected solid tumors (lung cancers excluded) with either EGFR or HER2 amplification but showed limited activity, with an objective response rate of 5%.[23] Lapatinib, an oral dual EGFR/HER2 inhibitor, demonstrated limited activity as monotherapy in a molecularly unselected population of NSCLC tumors. Of interest is that one of two patients with HER2 amplification (determined retrospectively) had a partial response, although this result was not confirmed.[24] Dacomitinib is another oral pan-HER inhibitor with demonstrated in vitro activity in selected HER2-amplified cell lines resistant to trastuzumab and lapatinib,[25,26] which resulted in a 12% response rate in patients with HER2 exon 20 insertions, but no responses in patients with HER2 amplification.[27]

HER2 amplification is also implicated in acquired resistance to therapy with EGFR tyrosine kinase inhibitors (TKIs) in laboratory models and in the clinical setting.[18,28] HER2 amplification is found in 12% to 13% of cases of acquired resistance to EGFR-TKIs wherein it is mutually exclusive with the EGFR T790M mutation among tumors with acquired EGFR-TKI resistance. In contrast, no HER2 exon 20 mutations were identified in patients who developed resistance to the irreversible EGFR-TKI

TABLE 48.1 Genetic Abnormalities in Squamous Cell Carcinoma and Adenocarcinoma of Lung[a]

Genetic Abnormality	Gene Location	Frequency (%)	
		Squamous Cell Carcinoma	Adenocarcinoma
HER2 overexpression	17q11.2–q12, 17q21	3–5	5–9
*HER2 amplification	17q11.2–q12, 17q21		
EGFR-TKI naïve		<1	1–4
Acquired EGFR-TKI resistance		—[b]	12–13
*FGFR1 amplification	8p12	22	1–3
PIK3CA amplification	3q26.3	33	6
c-MET amplification	7q31.1	3–21	3–21
HER2 mutation	17q11.2–q12, 17q21	1	2
*HER3 mutation	12q13	1	1
c-MET mutation	7q31.1	1	2
*FGFR2 mutation	10q26.13	3	1–2
*FGFR3 mutation	4p16.3	3	<1
DDR2 mutation	1q23.3	4	1
KRAS mutation	12p12.1	6	21
*NRAS mutation	1p13.2	—	<1
*BRAF mutation	7q34	<1–2	3–5
*MAP2K1 mutation	15q21	—	<1
*PIK3CA mutation	3q26.3	3–9	2–3
PTEN mutation	10q23.3	10	2
PTEN loss	10q23.3	8–20	8–20
AKT1 mutation	14q32.32	1	Very rare
LKB1 mutation	19p13.3	5	23
*LKB1/KRAS dual mutations	19p13.3/12p12.1	—	5–10
*PIK3CA/KRAS dual mutations	3q26.3/12p12.1	—	<1
*NRG1 fusion	8p12	—	<4[c]
*ROS1 fusion	6q22	0–1	1–3
*RET fusion	10q11.2	<1	1–2
*FGFR fusion	(FGFR1) 8p12 (FGFR2) 10q26.13 (FGFR3) 4p16.3	<1–2	<1
*BRAF fusion	7q34	—	3[c]

[a]Table adapted with permission from the American Association for Cancer: Perez-Moreno P, et al. Squamous cell carcinoma of the lung: molecular subtypes and therapeutic opportunities. *Clin Cancer Res.* 2012;18(9):2443–2451. Genetic abnormalities with an asterisk (*) pertain to data updated or not found in the original table.
[b]Denotes that no data have been published to date.
[c]Prevalence in never-smokers.
EGFR-TKI, epidermal growth factor receptor-tyrosine kinase inhibitor; *HER2,* human epidermal growth factor receptor type 2.

afatinib.[29] *HER2* amplification is also a putative mechanism of acquired resistance to ALK inhibitors in EML4–ALK-translocated lung cancer cells in vitro, although clinical studies have not confirmed this possibility to date.[30]

In comparison, mutations in *HER2* occur in 2% to 4% of NSCLC tumors, largely in high-grade and moderately to poorly differentiated adenocarcinomas.[19,31–33] More than 95% of the mutations described to date are small insertions in exon 20, mostly represented by an in-frame insertion of 12 base pairs that causes duplication of the amino acids YVMA.[31] Functional studies of this insertion mutation show that it confers greater transforming and antiapoptotic potential, in addition to its stronger catalytic activity, compared with wild-type *HER2*.[34] It can also trigger EGFR activation in the absence of cognate ligands and EGFR kinase activity.[34] *HER2* mutations appear to occur in greater proportions among women and never-smokers and are generally mutually exclusive with *EGFR* and Kirsten rat sarcoma (*KRAS*) mutations as well as *HER2* amplification, with rare exceptions.[35–37] An activating *HER2* V659E mutation sensitive to lapatinib was described in a specimen of lung adenocarcinoma from a patient with Li-Fraumeni syndrome.[38] It is anticipated that secondary *HER2* mutations, such as L755S, T862A, and the gatekeeper T798M mutation, can arise as a mechanism of acquired drug resistance similar to what is seen in *HER2*-amplified breast cancers after chronic therapy with lapatinib.[39,40]

Afatinib has been reported to induce tumor response or disease stabilization when used as monotherapy in *HER2*-mutant lung adenocarcinomas.[36] Similarly, trastuzumab-based combinations have induced partial responses.[36,37,41] Although lapatinib demonstrated preclinical activity against cells expressing the *HER2* insertion mutation,[34] tumor response has not been documented with monotherapy in the very limited number of patients reported on thus far.[36] Clinical activity has been documented, however, when lapatinib is used in combination with either chemotherapy or trastuzumab-based regimens in patients with NSCLC who have either a *HER2* exon 20 insertion or the *HER2* V659E mutation.[38,41] As per above, dacomitinib resulted in a 12% response rate in patients with *HER2* exon 20 insertions.[27] *HER2* exon 20 mutations, especially HER2YVMA, appear to be a promising target in lung cancer but needs to be validated.

Human Epidermal Growth Factor Receptor Type 3

HER3 (also known as ERBB3) is another representative of the four-member group in the HER RTK family. HER3 is generally considered to have functionally weaker kinase activity compared with EGFR.[42,43] Heterodimerization with other HER members, such as with HER2 upon binding of the ligand neuregulin, triggers autophosphorylation and recruitment of downstream signaling molecules. *HER3* mutations have been reported in approximately 1% of lung adenocarcinomas and 1% of squamous cell lung cancers.[44] Most of the *HER3* mutations identified to date are clustered in the extracellular domain (ECD), although some are mapped to the kinase domain.[44] The functional characteristics of most specific mutants described in NSCLC are yet to be verified; however, several *HER3* mutations in either the ECD or kinase domain have been shown to promote oncogenesis in a ligand-independent manner, although this effect required the presence of kinase-active HER2. Recently, an activating *HER3* V855A mutation that is homologous to *EGFR* L858R was identified in a patient with chemotherapy resistant NSCLC.[45] This mutation was transforming in murine and human cell line studies in the presence of wild-type *HER2*. Various small-molecule inhibitors and monoclonal antibodies against HER2 and HER3, as well as PI3K inhibitors, have demonstrated variable effectiveness depending on the specific *HER3* mutation.[44]

The recurrent fusion gene CD74-NRG1 found in mucinous lung adenocarcinomas of never-smokers appears to correlate with increased HER3 phosphorylation in tumor tissue.[46] This chimeric transcript results in the expression of the EGF-like domain in tumor tissue that is otherwise negative for neuregulin. Functional characterization of this fusion protein in vitro showed activation of the PI3K-AKT pathway.[46] Indeed, HER3 plays an integral role in activation of the PI3K survival pathway upon its heterodimerization with EGFR or HER2 in malignant cell lines.[47] EGFR-TKI-sensitive NSCLC cancer cell lines rely on HER3 signaling to activate the PI3K/AKT pathway.[48]

HER3 signaling is also implicated in acquired resistance to EGFR-TKIs. Persistent HER3-activated PI3K signaling is uncoupled from EGFR and is mediated instead through its interaction with MET, which is amplified in this setting.[49] Another mechanism that can sustain HER3-activated PI3K signaling is disruption of negative feedback networks. ERK signaling leads to feedback phosphorylation of the conserved T669 residue within the juxtamembrane domain of EGFR, HER2, and HER4, and this prevents transphosphorylation of HER3 (Fig. 48.1).[50] The loss of this dominant negative feedback suppression of HER3 by intact MEK/ERK signaling is thought to account for the increased AKT phosphorylation found with MEK inhibitors in EGFR- and HER2-driven malignant tumors.[50]

Blockade of HER3 signaling, through monoclonal antibody therapies or antisense oligonucleotides, improves the antitumor activity of EGFR and HER2 TKIs in preclinical models, including cell lines with acquired resistance to EGFR-TKIs.[51–53] Another proposed approach for reducing HER3-mediated activation to enhance EGFR-TKI activity involves modulation of circulating neuregulin ligands via inhibition of ADAM17, a membrane-associated metalloprotease that cleaves and releases HER ligands from cells to enable receptor binding.[54] Afatinib and dacomitinib are both oral irreversible pan-HER TKIs that have produced marked tumor regression in xenograft models that contained EGFR mutations, including the T790M mutation, which is associated with acquired resistance to EGFR-TKIs.[55,56] However, subsequent modeling showed that cytotoxicity against T790M can be accomplished only at clinically unachievable concentrations, thus accounting for the limited efficacy seen for this patient subset in the clinic.[57] Nonetheless, these agents can block HER2 heterodimerization with EGFR or HER3,[58] thus explaining the potential to overcome acquired resistance mediated by HER3. In a randomized phase II study comparing dacomitinib and erlotinib, dacomitinib demonstrated significantly improved progression-free survival in KRAS wild-type NSCLC with or without EGFR mutation.[59] A phase III study comparing first-line dacomitinib with gefitinib for patients who have NSCLC with EGFR-activating mutations was ongoing at the time of publication. Another phase III study comparing second- or third-line dacomitinib and erlotinib in patients with KRAS wild-type NSCLC has completed enrollment at the time of the publication of this chapter (ClinicalTrials.gov identifier: NCT01360554). A phase III clinical trial recently demonstrated statistically significant but modest improvements in progression-free and overall survival with afatinib compared with erlotinib in patients receiving second-line therapy for squamous cell NSCLC;[60] however, enthusiasm for these results has been muted by the advances seen with immunotherapy for this patient population. Various monoclonal antibodies against HER3 are being investigated in clinical trials, combining them with other inhibitors of the EGFR or HER2 pathway.

Hepatocyte Growth Factor Receptor

Binding of the ligand hepatocyte growth factor (HGF, also known as scatter factor), a paracrine factor secreted by stromal cells, to its cognate receptor MET facilitates receptor phosphorylation, leading to the activation of downstream signaling through the MAPK and PI3K pathways, which promote epithelial-to-mesenchymal transition (EMT), invasion, and metastasis.[61] Ubiquitin-mediated receptor degradation is regulated at the Cbl E3-ligase RTK binding domain, similar to what has been described for EGFR and HER2.[62] Mechanisms of aberrant activation of MET described in NSCLC include receptor overexpression (with or without HGF), c-MET gene amplification, or exon 14 skipping abnormalities. Levels of MET expression as high as 60% have been reported in various studies of NSCLC.[63] Both the EGFR and c-MET genes are located on chromosome 7, and an increased copy number of the c-MET gene as determined by FISH is associated with an increased copy number of the EGFR gene and confers a worse prognosis.[64] Coamplification of c-MET and EGFR is also described in up to 8.5% of NSCLCs not previously treated with EGFR-TKIs.[65] Amplification of c-MET also occurs infrequently with an incidence of 3% to 7% among patients not treated with EGFR-TKIs, but this incidence increases to 10% to 22% among patients with acquired resistance to EGFR-TKIs.[49,66] Exon 14 skipping mutations occur in about 3% of patients with NSCLC.[67] Patients with sarcomatoid pulmonary carcinomas are enriched for MET exon 14 skipping mutations, and one study identified that 22% of patients with this relatively rare form of lung cancer have this mutation.[68] MET can be transactivated through a variety of protein interactions and can heterodimerize with other RTKs, such as EGFR, HER2, HER3, and ret proto-oncogene (RET), in cells with c-MET amplification, representing an escape or bypass mechanism mediating resistance to inhibitors of these RTK-activated signaling pathways.[49,69,70] In a preclinical model, MET activation through paracrine secretion of HGF also served as a mechanism for resistance to second-generation selective ALK inhibitors such as ceritinib (LDK378), but not to the MET/ALK inhibitor crizotinib.[71]

Somatic intronic mutations of c-MET that lead to an alternatively spliced transcript, encoding a deletion of the exon-14 juxtamembrane domain spanning the amino acids 964 through 1010, result in loss of the Cbl binding site at Y1003.[62] This skipping mutation in exon 14 yields a functional MET protein with decreased ubiquitination and consequently sustained activation of the MAPK pathway through altered receptor downregulation.[62] This mutation variant appears to be mutually exclusive with mutations of other genes involved in the MAPK pathway (e.g., EGFR, RAS, and RAF).[62] Additional mutations have been described in both the ECD and juxtamembrane domains, some of which have transforming potential.[63,72,73] No reports have indicated nonsynonymous mutations in the kinase domain to date. Of note is that most of these other mutations reported are in fact germline.[74] The germline mutation N375S, which occurred at the highest frequency, appears to be associated with smoking and squamous histology. The MET-N375S mutation seems to confer resistance to the small-molecule MET kinase inhibitor SU11274.[74]

Various approaches for inhibiting the MET pathway have been tested or are in clinical development. These strategies include anti-HGF and anti-MET monoclonal antibodies, or small-molecule MET kinase inhibitors. The MET/ALK/ROS1 inhibitor crizotinib was reported anecdotally to induce a rapid and durable response in a patient with de novo c-MET amplification without ALK rearrangement.[75] Models of resistance to MET inhibitors predict the emergence of either secondary mutations or activation of EGFR signaling through increased expression of transforming growth factor-α.[76] A randomized phase III study in previously treated patients with NSCLC of erlotinib with or without tivantinib, initially thought to be a selective nonadenosine triphosphate (non-ATP) competitive MET inhibitor, was halted because of an increased incidence of interstitial lung disease; regardless, there was no improvement in overall survival.[77] Similarly, a separate phase III clinical trial conducted throughout Europe and the United States failed to show an overall survival benefit of erlotinib and tivantinib compared with erlotinib and placebo.[78] Nonetheless, preclinical data generated from two different groups suggest that although tivantinib can mitigate HGF-dependent MET activation, this is not its major mechanism of action.[79,80] Tivantinib (in contrast to crizotinib) did not inhibit MET autophosphorylation at doses that induced apoptosis. Instead, it exhibited cytotoxicity regardless of activation status of the MET pathway or the presence or absence of a functional MET kinase. In fact, growth inhibition and cytotoxicity reported with tivantinib may be mainly due to its effect on microtubule dynamics,[81] which is not found with other MET inhibitors.[79,80]

Onartuzumab (MetMAb), a monoclonal antibody that binds to the ECD of MET to prevent ligand binding, was evaluated in a randomized phase III study in combination with erlotinib as compared with placebo plus erlotinib in patients with NSCLC and MET-positive status as determined by IHC. The rationale for the study was based on promising results for progression-free survival (2.9 vs. 1.5 months; hazard ratio [HR], 0.53; $p = 0.04$) and overall survival (12.6 vs. 3.8 months; HR, 0.37; $p = 0.002$) noted in patients with MET-positive NSCLC who received the onartuzumab plus erlotinib combination compared with the placebo plus erlotinib treatment in the preceding randomized phase II study.[82] In contrast, patients with MET-negative NSCLC who received the combination had worse progression-free survival (1.4 vs. 2.7 months; HR, 1.82; $p = 0.05$) and overall survival (8.1 vs. 15.3 months; HR, 1.78; $p = 0.16$) compared with patients who received placebo plus erlotinib.[82] Unfortunately, the phase III clinical trial was stopped early due to futility as the experimental arm did not improve overall survival (OS), progression free survival (PFS), or overall response rate (ORR) compared with erlotinib alone.[83]

Whereas targeting MET based on protein expression has had challenges, *MET* amplification and *MET* exon 14 skipping mutations are emerging as promising targets. The interim analysis of a small study demonstrated that 4 of 12 patients with intermediate (2.2–5) or high (>5) ratios of MET to CEP7 responded to crizotinib.[84] An even more impressive response rate was observed in an interim analysis of a trial of the safety and efficacy of crizotinib for patients with *MET* exon 14 skipping mutations where 10 of 15 patients had confirmed or unconfirmed partial responses.[85] One case report showed that a patient with a *MET* exon 14 skipping mutation who demonstrated a response to crizotonib acquired a mutation in the *MET* kinase domain, D1228N, at the time of progression.[86] Responses have also been observed in patients with *MET* exon 14 skipping mutations treated with cabozantinib.[87] Other MET inhibitors in development include AMG337 and capmatinib (INC280). These ongoing trials will help clarify which MET abnormalities are potentially targetable in NSCLC, but *MET* exon 14 skipping mutations and amplification seem to be better predictors of response than MET expression by IHC at this time.

Fibroblast Growth Factor Receptor

The fibroblast growth factor receptor (FGFR) signaling module plays an important role in various cellular processes, such as vascular and skeletal development during embryogenesis, as well as regulation of angiogenesis and wound healing in adults. The FGF family of ligands, with more than 20 members, is sequestered to the extracellular matrix by heparin sulfate proteoglycans. Five FGFRs exist, of which *FGFRs* 1–4 are highly conserved and contain the classic tyrosine kinase motifs in their split kinase domain.[88] Moreover, *FGFRs* 1–3 are subject to alternate splicing, which results in variants with tissue-specific expression and varying ligand affinity. Dimerization of the ternary complex consisting of FGF, FGFR, and heparin sulfate proteoglycan activates downstream signaling, which ultimately leads to pathway activation of the RAS/MAPK and PI3K/AKT signaling cascades.[88]

Various mechanisms of oncogenic FGFR signaling have been described in NSCLC. Focal amplification of *FGFR1* is reportedly found in 22% of squamous-type NSCLCs.[89] *FGFR1* amplification appears to result in ligand-independent signaling and confers sensitivity to treatment using small molecule FGFR-TKIs.[89] Somatic gain-of-function mutations in *FGFR2* and *FGFR3*, a subset of which have transforming ability, have also been described in up to 6% of squamous NSCLCs.[90] These mutations are commonly coincident with mutations in *TP53* and *PIK3CA* and are mostly sensitive to inhibition by FGFR-TKIs.[90] Mutations in

FGFR2 or *FGFR3* can occur in either the kinase domain, causing constitutive activation, or in the ECD, which results in constitutive dimerization.[90] Cell models (i.e., fibroblasts) expressing the ECD mutations and exposed to a low concentration of multikinase inhibitors with anti-FGFR activity exhibited enhanced growth. This growth-promoting phenomenon was not seen with higher drug concentrations or with the use of selective FGFR inhibitors.[90]

Various chromosomal rearrangements involving *FGFR1–3* result in fusion products that also exhibit ligand-independent oligomerization capability, activation of the MAPK pathway, and sensitivity to FGFR-TKIs. Several of these reported in NSCLC include BAG4–FGFR1, FGFR2–CIT, FGFR2–KIAA1967, and FGFR3–TACC3. The FGFR3–TACC3 fusion, found in approximately 2% of squamous cell NSCLCs and rarely in adenocarcinoma, is the most frequently reported to date.[91–94] Other potential fusion partners that mediate oligomerization in other tumor types include BICC1, CCDC6, BAIAP2L1, CASP7, and OFD1.[94]

Similar to other TKIs, an anticipated mechanism of acquired resistance to FGFR inhibitors is the emergence of secondary mutations, such as the V555M alteration in *FGFR3*.[95] Oncogenic switch or constitutive activation of other pathways leading to activation of the MAPK or PI3K pathway, such as through MET,[96] may also underlie acquired or intrinsic resistance to FGFR inhibition, thus providing a rationale for investigations on combination therapy. Likewise, oncogenic switch to FGFR signaling has been suggested to mediate resistance to EGFR-TKIs,[97,98] as well as to HER2, MET, and angiogenesis inhibitors.[96,99–101]

Because of the high degree of homology between the vascular endothelial growth factor receptor 2 (VEGFR2) and FGFR tyrosine kinase domains, various oral multikinase inhibitors that are approved by the US Food and Drug Administration (FDA) or in clinical development (e.g., sorafenib, pazopanib, axitinib, regorafenib, ponatinib, cediranib, nintedanib) are able to inhibit FGFR1 in nanomolar concentrations. Several of these agents, such as dovitinib and brivanib, were in fact developed to have relatively greater selectivity for FGFR kinase than for VEGFR2. Nonetheless, hypertension is a common toxic effect of these agents, which suggests that inhibition of the VEGF pathway remains a major effect of these agents.[102–104] More selective FGFR inhibitors in early phase clinical testing include AZD4547 and BGJ398. On-target adverse effects, such as hyperphosphatemia and retinal detachment, have been reported.[105,106]

The results of the Lung Cancer Master Protocol, which includes the FGFR inhibitor AZD4547 in patients with squamous cell carcinoma of the lung, are eagerly awaited (NCT02154490).

c-Ros Oncogene 1

c-Ros oncogene 1 (ROS1) is a proto-oncogene that encodes an RTK closely related to ALK. Notably, ROS1 is expressed only transiently in the lung during murine development and is not found in healthy adult human lung tissue.[107,108] Its ligand has yet to be identified. A phosphoproteomic analysis of TK signaling demonstrated that ROS1 ranked among the top 10 RTKs activated in NSCLC.[109] Further analysis demonstrated that constitutive activation of ROS1 arose from the presence of SLC34A2–ROS1 fusion in an NSCLC cell line. Multiple other fusion partners have since been reported in NSCLC, such as CD74–, TPM3–, SDC4–, EZR–, LRIG3–, KDELR2–, CCDC6–, and FIG–ROS1.[110] The transforming potential of many of these fusions has been well established. Although localization to the Golgi apparatus of the FIG–ROS1 fusion appears to be crucial for its transforming ability, no discernible pattern of distribution has been found for the other variants.[110] ALK inhibitors have demonstrated preclinical and clinical activity against ROS1-rearranged NSCLCs.[111] This is not surprising given the close homology between ALK and ROS1. However, unlike FGFR, ALK, and RET fusions, in which the mechanism of constitutive kinase activation is attributed to the dimerization domain of the partner protein, the mechanism of activation of most ROS1 fusion proteins remains unclear because most partner proteins lack the dimerization domains.

In an unselected population of patients with NSCLC, the frequency of ROS1 rearrangement is 0.9% to 1.7%, with most cases found in adenocarcinomas.[110] This prevalence can increase to approximately 6% of EGFR/KRAS/ALK wild-type lung adenocarcinomas in East Asian never-smokers.[111,112] For patients who have lung cancer with ROS1 rearrangement, the objective response rate to pemetrexed appears to be higher and the median progression-free survival longer than in lung cancer patients without the ROS1 or ALK rearrangement.[112] One mechanism of acquired resistance to crizotinib is the acquisition of a secondary mutation in the ROS1 kinase domain that interfered with drug binding in a patient with CD74–ROS1 rearrangement.[113] Cabozantinib is one agent that may overcome resistance mutations in this setting.[114] Aside from crizotinib, other oral agents with anticipated or demonstrated activity against oncogenic ROS1 fusions as well as crizotinib-resistant ALK translocations in NSCLC include the selective ALK inhibitors ceritinib (LDK398), lorlatinib, the dual ALK/EGFR inhibitor brigatinib, and the ROS1/ALK/NTRK inhibitor entrectinib. Crizotinib is a more potent inhibitor than ceritinib. The expansion cohort of a phase I clinical trial with 50 patients with ROS1 mutations treated with crizotinib demonstrated a response rate of 72% with a median duration of 17.6 months.[115] A separate retrospective study of off-label use crizotinib for ROS1-rearranged NSCLC similarly reported an overall response rate of 80% with a median PFS of 9.1 months.[116] Crizotinib has since been approved by the US FDA for the treatment of ROS-1 rearranged NSCLC.

Rearranged During Transfection–RET

The primary mechanism of RET activation in NSCLC occurs through chromosomal rearrangements. Various oncogenic RET fusions have been described by separate investigators since the first publication in late 2011.[117] Fusion partners reported include KIF5B, CCDC6, TRIM33, and NCOA4, all of which contain coiled–coil domains that have oligomerization potential to induce constitutive TK activation.[118] Functional studies indicate that these RET fusions have oncogenic potential.[119]

RET rearrangements, similar to ROS1 and ALK, are observed primarily in lung adenocarcinomas from never-smokers and are also associated with poorly differentiated tumors.[120] Although the overall prevalence is only 1% to 2% in adenocarcinomas, the prevalence can be as high as 16% among never-smokers with nonsquamous histology negative for driver mutations in other oncogenes (EGFR, KRAS, NRAS, BRAF, HER2, PIK3CA, MEK1, AKT, ALK, and ROS1).[121] Vandetanib and cabozantinib are small-molecule inhibitors of multiple kinases, including VEGFR2 and RET, that are currently approved for treatment of metastatic medullary thyroid cancer. Other FDA-approved agents that demonstrate in vitro inhibition of RET include axitinib, sunitinib, regorafenib, sorafenib, and ponatinib (which exhibits the highest potency). Preliminary findings from a phase II study of cabozantinib in patients with NSCLC and RET rearrangements demonstrated objective tumor responses in two of three patients treated.[121] Clinical activity has also been reported with vandetanib.[122] Alectinib also has potent antitumor activity against RET rearrangements, including those with gatekeeper mutations (V804L and V804M).[123] In fact, in one report two of four patients responded to alectinib after failure of other RET inhibitors.[124] Mechanisms of acquired resistance are yet to be

established in the clinical setting. Preclinical modeling predicted the emergence of the gatekeeper V804L/M mutation, which is resistant to vandetanib but remained sensitive to ponatinib.[125,126]

Discoidin Domain Receptors

The members of the discoidin domain family of receptors, DDR1 and DDR2, are unusual RTKs that have as their ligand different types of collagen rather than a typical growth factor.[127] Both DDRs are activated by fibrillar collagens, but only DDR1 can be activated by nonfibrillar collagen.[127] DDR1 is mainly expressed in epithelial cells, whereas DDR2 is found in mesenchymal cells.[127] Novel somatic mutations in lung cancer of both DDR1 and DDR2 were first described in 2005.[128] Mutations are found in both the kinase domain and other regions. Functional characterization of DDR2 mutations, identified in approximately 3% to 4% of squamous cell lung cancers,[129] later established their oncogenic potential.[130]

DDR2-transformed cells appear to require the coordinated activity of both DDR2 and the Src family of kinases for maximal proliferation, which explains their exquisite sensitivity to dasatinib, a dual Src and DDR2 inhibitor, compared with either a DDR2- or Src kinase-specific inhibitor as a single agent.[130] Of the commercially available kinase inhibitors, dasatinib has the most potent activity against DDR2 (Kd value 5.4 nM) compared with other kinase inhibitors such as ponatinib (9 nM), imatinib (71 nM), nilotinib (35–55 nM), sorafenib (55 nM), and pazopanib (474 nM).[130–132] Clinical responses to dasatinib among patients with DDR2 mutation have been reported.[130,133] However, its therapeutic index is narrow because of its multiple off-target effects, particularly pleural effusion, and thus DDR2-selective agents are needed.

Tyrosine-Protein Kinase Receptor UFO (AXL) and Proto-Oncogene Tyrosine-Protein Kinase (MER)

The primary ligand for AXL and MER, both members of the TAM (representing the three members: Tyro-3, Axl, and Mer) receptor family of RTKs, is the vitamin K–dependent ligand growth arrest-specific protein 6 (Gas6).[134,135] Ligand binding induces dimerization that results in stimulation of proliferative and antiapoptotic signaling through the MAPK/ERK and PI3K/AKT pathways.[134,135] AXL is ubiquitously expressed, whereas MER is expressed in hematopoietic-derived cells, epithelium, and reproductive tissues.[135] Both are involved in regulation of the actin cytoskeleton and tumor cell migration and invasion. They exhibit transforming potential and have complementary roles in promoting tumor cell survival and resistance to chemotherapy in NSCLC.[134] Conversely, either knockdown or pharmacologic inhibition of AXL or MER using sulfasalazine reduces growth, suppresses invasiveness, and restores sensitivity to various cytotoxic agents.[134,136]

Overexpression of AXL and MER is reported in 93% and 50% to 69% of NSCLCs, respectively.[134,135] The Gas6 ligand is also frequently expressed in NSCLC, thus providing continuous signaling through autocrine and/or paracrine mechanisms. Overexpression of AXL, which can be upregulated during activation of EMT, appears to mediate resistance to targeted therapies as well as to EGFR and HER2 TKIs.[137,138] Inhibition of AXL restores sensitivity to EGFR-TKI therapy. A potentially oncogenic AXL fusion product that carries the tyrosine kinase domain and dimerization units (AXL–MBIP) was identified by transcriptome analysis of lung adenocarcinomas.[92] Taken together, these findings highlight the therapeutic potential of targeting AXL and MER. A caveat in drug development against these targets is that both proteins have an essential function in limiting inflammation. Increased inflammation seen in knockout mice lacking both receptors paradoxically fosters a tumor-promoting microenvironment in colitis-associated colon cancer.[139]

Tropomysin Receptor Kinase

The genes *NTRK1–3* encode the tropomysin receptor kinase (Trk) proteins Trk A, B, and C, respectively. The Trk receptors are transmembrane proteins critical for the development of both the central and peripheral nervous systems. Rearrangements of *NTRK* genes are the most common oncogenic mutations of these genes that result in constitutive activation of fusion proteins. *NTRK* gene rearrangements have been discovered in NSCLC and other malignancies such as colorectal cancer, papillary thyroid carcinoma, glioblastoma, and human secretory breast cancer. One patient with a soft-tissue sarcoma that harbored a LMNA–NTRK1 rearrangement had a dramatic response to the TRK inhibitor LOXO-101.[140] Similarly, a patient with metastatic colorectal cancer with a LMNA–NTRK1 rearrangement experienced a partial response to the pan-TRK inhibitor entrectinib.[141] In NSCLC, MPRIP–NTRK1 and CD74–NTRK1 rearrangments were the first to be reported and were found to be oncogenic.[142] This same study suggested that *NTRK1* gene rearrangements are present in 3% to 4% of patients without other known oncogenic alterations, but this may represent fewer than 1% of all patients with NSCLC. Regardless, the responses observed in other malignancies to the TRK inhibitors in development are similarly encouraging for NSCLC.

Nonreceptor Targets
RAS

The RAS superfamily of guanosine triphosphatases (GTPases) consists of three highly related proteins: KRAS, HRAS, and NRAS. These proteins interface with a large number of effectors, including RAF and PI3K. Although they share similar properties, each isoform may have preferential signaling. For example, KRAS is more potent than HRAS in RAF activation, and the opposite is true for PI3K activation.[143,144] Mutations in NSCLC resulting in constitutive activation of RAS proteins occur predominantly at codons 12, 13, and 61 of KRAS, particularly in smoking-related adenocarcinomas, of which approximately 30% harbor these mutations. Mutant *KRAS* alleles are also often amplified at higher levels in NSCLC compared with the wild-type allele, similar to observations seen with EGFR and suggesting that the preferential amplification of the mutant copy of the gene has functional significance.[145,146]

RAC1b, an isoform of the RAC1 GTPase that includes one additional exon, is found to be preferentially upregulated in lung cancer via splice–site mutations.[147] RAC1b appears to promote KRAS-induced lung tumorigenesis, and its expression appears to be associated with sensitivity to MEK inhibition.[148] Inactivating mutations in the tumor suppressor gene *NF1* are found in approximately 7% of lung adenocarcinomas.[145] Because *NF1* suppresses the activity of GTPase-activating proteins that stimulate the catalytic activity of RAS, its inactivation mimics a hyperactivated RAS phenotype even in the absence of *RAS* mutations.

Intact signaling through the PI3K pathway, specifically the binding of RAS to PI3K, is also required for tumorigenesis in mouse models of *KRAS*-driven lung tumors.[149] Other mouse models indicate that nuclear factor-κB and cell-cycle targets such as PLK1 and cyclin-dependent kinase (CDK) signaling, particularly CDK4 are essential for proliferation of *KRAS*-mutant lung adenocarcinoma, with lethal effects seen upon pharmacologic inhibition of these implicated pathways.[150–154] Additional observations also indicated that inhibition of proteasome function and of transcription factor pathways impaired the growth and increased the apoptosis of KRAS-mutant NSCLC.[153,155] Of

interest is that GATA2 dependency is also found in other similar oncogenically driven NSCLC tumors, such as those mediated by *EGFR*, *NRAS*, *NF1*, and EML4–ALK.[155]

Data based on *KRAS*-knockdown experiments showed variable effects on cell viability among *KRAS*-mutant cell lines, with some *KRAS*-mutant cell lines appearing not to be dependent on this pathway.[156,157] The same *KRAS*-knockdown experiments showed dependency on RAS signaling in various *KRAS* wild-type cell lines.[156] Based on this finding, a *KRAS*-dependency gene expression signature was developed that was more predictive of sensitivity or resistance to targeted therapies, such as MEK inhibitors, than was *KRAS* mutation status itself.[156] Presence of the *KRAS*-dependency gene expression signature in *KRAS*-mutant cell lines is associated with a well-differentiated tumor phenotype, whereas induction of EMT results in *KRAS* independence.[157] A potentially druggable target protein identified from integrated global transcriptome, proteome, and phosphoproteome analysis of a panel of NSCLC cell lines using this *KRAS*-dependency stratification is lymphocyte-specific tyrosine kinase (LCK).[158] Indeed, *KRAS*-dependent cell lines were sensitive to LCK inhibition, whereas *KRAS*-independent cell lines were not. MET inhibition also selectively impaired the growth of *KRAS*-dependent cell lines, as predicted based on this stratification.[158]

NRAS mutations are present in less than 1% of lung cancers and have been described predominantly in adenocarcinomas.[159] These mutations appear to be more common in current or former smokers. The nucleotide transversion mutations typically associated with smoking appear to be found less frequently in *NRAS*-mutant NSCLC (13%) than in *KRAS*-mutant NSCLC (66%).[159] In vitro studies showed that, similar to *KRAS* mutants, many of the NRAS-mutant cell lines were sensitive to MEK inhibition alone. In one MEK-resistant cell line that displayed high levels of IGF-1R, combination treatment with an IGF-1R and MEK inhibitor showed a greater antiproliferative effect compared with either drug used alone. These results parallel those seen with this combination in *KRAS*-mutant NSCLC, which exhibits increased dependence on IGF-1R signaling compared with *KRAS* wild-type cells.[160]

No direct RAS inhibitors have been successfully developed in the clinic as yet. Strategies explored have mainly sought to prevent plasma membrane localization of RAS, such as with the use of farnesyl transferase inhibitors, with disappointing results.[161] More recently, disruption of the interaction with phosphodiesterase δ, which facilitates plasma membrane localization, has been proposed as a novel approach.[162] Biochemical screening identified the derivative deltarasin, which inhibited RAS signaling and suppressed proliferation of *KRAS*-mutant pancreatic cancer cell lines in vitro and in vivo.[162] Inhibition of the mTOR pathway as monotherapy demonstrates only modest activity in *KRAS*-mutant NSCLC.[163] MEK inhibitors represented a promising approach for *KRAS*-mutant NSCLC. In a randomized second-line study of *KRAS*-mutant NSCLC, the combination of docetaxel with selumetinib (a MEK inhibitor) improved progression-free survival compared with placebo plus docetaxel (5.3 months vs. 2.1 months; HR, 0.58), with objective responses seen only in the selumetinib group (37% vs. 0%).[164] Adverse events were increased in the selumetinib group, such as febrile neutropenia (18% vs. 0%) and asthenia (9% vs. 0%). Recently it was reported in a press release that the SELECT-1 phase III clinical trial that randomized 510 patients to selumetinib or placebo in combination with docetaxel failed to improve progression-free survival.[165]

v-Raf Murine Sarcoma Viral Oncogene Homolog B–BRAF

Mutations in the RAF family most commonly occur in *BRAF*, whereas mutations in *CRAF* and *ARAF* are rare, found in less than 1% of human cancers.[166,167] Among patients with NSCLC, *BRAF* mutations are found in both squamous and nonsquamous histologies and tend to occur in smokers.[168,169] These mutations appear to promote constitutive BRAF–CRAF dimerization, resulting in RAS-independent activation of the MEK/ERK cascade.[170] Dimerization appears to be needed for downstream signaling for either wild-type or mutant BRAF, except for those characterized by high catalytic activity, such as the V600E and G469A mutations, wherein dimerization is not required for biologic function.[171] Oncogenic alterations in BRAF may also arise from chimeric fusion proteins. The SND1–BRAF fusion transcript has been described in 3% of lung adenocarcinomas among never-smokers. A few of these fusion transcripts are present concurrently in specimens with either EGFR or HER2 mutations.[172]

The constitutively activated V600E mutation represents nearly 50% to 60% of the BRAF mutations found in NSCLC. It is associated with micropapillary features, female gender, and poor prognosis.[168,169] In contrast to RTK-activated cells, which show feedback downregulation of RAF/MEK signaling upon ERK activation (Fig. 48.1), this physiologic feedback inhibition is missing in V600E BRAF-mutant tumors and is accompanied by high levels of MEK kinase activity.[173,174] The efficacy of MEK inhibitors in BRAF V600E mutants is attributed to this dependency on MEK activity for proliferation and survival. Non-V600E mutations, such as G469A, T599_V600insT, and V600_K601delinsE, demonstrate increased kinase activity relative to wild-type BRAF.[175] However, other non-V600E mutations are known to be kinase-impaired or inactivating (e.g., D594, G466, G496del, and Y472). Nonetheless, ERK activation can still be achieved through heterodimerization with CRAF,[176] thus predicting resistance to selective BRAF inhibitors (BRAFi). These kinase-impaired BRAF mutations, which have weak oncogenic potential,[176] appear to be sensitive to dasatinib.[177]

Tumor responses have been reported among patients with BRAF V600E-mutant NSCLC treated with vemurafenib and dabrafenib.[178–180] A recently published phase II clinical trial demonstrated a 63.2% overall response rate in patients with BRAF V600E mutations receiving dabrafenib and trametinib in the second line.[181] Despite the clinical success of BRAFi, resistance may develop due to the emergence of KRAS mutations.[180] Other anticipated mechanisms of acquired resistance to BRAFi, based on models of melanoma, include emergence of activating somatic mutations in NRAS or MAP2K1/MAP2K2, bypass signaling (e.g., other RTK-mediated pathways such as FGFR), BRAF amplification, or alternative BRAF splice isoforms.[182–184] MAPK-independent mechanisms also occur, with the PI3K pathway frequently implicated.[185] In contrast to the experience with various TKIs, secondary mutations in the target oncoprotein itself (i.e., BRAF or CRAF) are yet to be described in clinical samples, although several CRAF mutations generated from random mutagenesis experiments have been identified that can promote CRAF dimerization and confer resistance to RAF inhibitors.[186] The selective advantage from the relief of RAF autoinhibition due to the presence of RAF inhibitors (RAFi) may also paradoxically foster drug dependence for growth.[187,188]

Mitogen Activated Protein Kinase Kinase–MEK

A somatic activating mutation in the nonkinase region of the kinase in exon 2 of MEK1/2 (MAP2K1/MAP2K2), a dual-specificity serine/threonine and tyrosine kinase, has been reported in approximately 1% of lung adenocarcinomas and renders the cells sensitive to MEK inhibitors.[189] This G to T transversion mutation is known to be related to smoking and is found in specimens from former smokers. Because MEK1/2 activation represents the penultimate step of signaling in the canonical MAPK pathway, its inhibition has potential activity against tumors dependent on MAPK signaling, regardless of MEK mutation status. However, despite high basal ERK phosphorylation in EGFR mutant cells, these cells are uniformly resistant to MEK inhibition because of

the feedback mechanism discussed earlier.[173,174,190] In addition, MEK inhibition induces positive feedback of PI3K/AKT signaling as well in EGFR- and HER2-driven cancers through an increase in HER3 activation.[50]

MEKi demonstrate heterogeneous effects in KRAS-mutant tumors, which are in part attributed to the presence of activated parallel pathways such as PI3K/AKT/mTOR in KRAS-driven tumors.[191] Thus, synergistic effects have been documented with the combination of MEKi and PI3K inhibitors (PI3Ki),[192] although clinical development is challenging because of the serious toxicities encountered with combination therapy.[193] Results of a preclinical study suggest that an intermittent dosing regimen is effective and may be successful in mitigating toxicity with PI3Ki and MEKi combinations.[194] The effects of MEK inhibition in KRAS-mutant cancer cell lines also tend to be cytostatic, and xenograft models typically show reduction in tumor growth but not tumor regression with MEK inhibition alone.[195,196] These preclinical features predict the clinical experience thus far with MEK inhibitors used as monotherapy; that is, objective tumor responses are rarely seen.[197,198] In one pooled shRNA drug-screening approach to identify synthetically lethal combinations with MEKi in KRAS-mutant cancer cells independent of sensitivity to MEK/PI3K inhibition, the antiapoptotic member of the BH3 family of proteins BCL-XL was identified as a promising target.[195] MEK inhibition increases levels of the proapoptotic protein BIM, which, however, is bound and inhibited by antiapoptotic proteins such as BCL-XL. Indeed, the combination of MEKi and inhibitors of BCL-XL (BCL-XLi) caused marked tumor regression in vivo in KRAS-mutant xenografts and in a genetically engineered mouse model of KRAS-driven lung cancer.[195] Nonetheless, this strategy was not universally effective. KRAS-mutant cells exhibiting EMT demonstrated less sensitivity to this combination. Moreover, acquired resistance ultimately emerges.[195]

Phosphoinositide 3-Kinase

Class I PI3Ks are heterodimeric proteins composed of a regulatory and a catalytic p110 subunit that has four isoforms: α, β, δ, and γ. Tissue distribution and function vary according to the isoform, with cell proliferation and growth principally regulated by p110α. Amplification or activating mutations in PIK3CA, which encodes the p110α catalytic subunit, have both been described in NSCLC. Amplification of PIK3CA and mutation of PIK3CA appear to be mutually exclusive.[199] Somatic gain-of-function mutations in PIK3CA can be found in up to 9% of squamous NSCLCs.[200] These mutations most commonly occur either in the helical domain encoded by exon 9 (E542K, E545K), and therefore interfere with binding of the p85α regulatory subunit, or in the kinase domain encoded by exon 20 (H1047R, H1047L). Somatic mutations in the gene encoding p85α, PIK3R1, occur in approximately 40% of endometrial carcinomas and in approximately 1% of NSCLCs.[201,202] Although several mutants described in endometrial cancer have increased AKT signaling, others show no appreciable biologic effect. The functional consequences of PIK3R1 mutations in NSCLC are still unknown.

Loss of PTEN, the negative regulator of PI3K, results in a hyperactivated AKT phenotype.[203] Mechanisms implicated in the loss of PTEN include epigenetic silencing (e.g., promoter methylation), posttranslational modification, increased degradation, and mutations or homozygous deletions.[204] Genetic changes in PI3K (amplification or mutation) and mutation of PTEN appear to be more common in squamous cell carcinomas than in adenocarcinoma (9.8% vs. 1.6%, respectively), particularly within the Asian population.[205] Although both activating PIK3CA mutations and inactivating PTEN mutations augment AKT signaling in experimental systems, they do not appear to be functionally redundant in vivo because they can be found concurrently, such as in endometrial cancers.[206] Indeed, in contrast to the *PTEN* null setting, cell lines with *PIK3CA* mutations have variable degrees of AKT phosphorylation and often show diminished AKT signaling.[206]

Despite experimental preclinical data suggesting that these mutants can be exquisitely sensitive to PI3K or AKT inhibitors, clinical experience to date suggests that the mutation status alone is not a good predictive marker for tumor response because most patients with tumors harboring either a *PIK3CA* mutation or *PTEN* loss appear to have stable disease rather than objective response when treated with these agents.[207,208] Resistance to PI3K inhibitors is unlikely to arise from mutations at the gatekeeper residue alone, as indicated by modeling experiments showing that the mutated kinase has severely reduced catalytic activity and thus cannot be viable.[209] In a large phase II trial that screened over 1200 patients for *PI3K* mutations, the 12-week progression-free survival rates in response to buparlisib (BKM120) were 23.3% and 20.0% in squamous (*n* = 30) and nonsquamous groups (*n* = 33), respectively. Since the prespecified rate of 50% was not met by either group, this trial was halted.[210] Some PI3K inhibitors still in development include the PI3Kα inhibitors BYL719 and taselisib, and the dual PI3K/mTOR inhibitors SF1126 and PQR309.

Concurrent mutations in genes of the MAPK signaling pathway are common in lung adenocarcinomas with *PIK3CA* mutations.[211] Coexisting mutations that activate MAPK signaling render cells resilient to the effects of inhibiting a single pathway because of built-in redundancy from integration of both pathways to a final common effector, such as 4EBP1 phosphorylation.[196] Combined inhibition of ERK and AKT signaling is thus necessary to suppress tumor growth in such conditions. However, parallel pathway inhibition, although potentially efficacious, may cause greater clinical toxicity as a tradeoff.[212]

Protein Kinase B–AKT

The AKT family of kinases includes three isoforms—AKT1, AKT2, and AKT3—which belong to the protein kinase B family of serine/threonine kinases. Each isoform shows relative specificity, albeit considerable overlap, in its regulation of cellular processes and tissue distribution. These activities include antiapoptosis and cell survival for the ubiquitously expressed *AKT1*; maintenance of glucose homeostasis for *AKT2* in insulin-responsive tissues including liver, adipose tissue, and skeletal muscle; and brain development for *AKT3*.[213,214] The oncogenic E17K mutation in exon 4 of the pleckstrin homology domain of *AKT1* is uncommon in NSCLC, occurs primarily in the subset with squamous histology, and is generally mutually exclusive with the presence of *PIK3CA* mutations.[215,216] This mutation is associated with increased membrane localization, which results in elevated autophosphorylation of AKT1, increased levels of cyclin D1, and reduced sensitivity to an allosteric Akt kinase inhibitor.[216,217] In contrast, amplification of either *AKT1* or *AKT2* has been reported collectively in 7% of lung cancers but coamplification of these genes has not been found.[200,213] Although the reported cases involved small cell and large cell carcinomas as well, most cases appear to involve squamous histology rather than adenocarcinoma.[200,213]

The PI3K/AKT/mTOR signaling pathway is subject to feedback regulation similar to that of other pathways. Moreover, AKT activates multiple processes besides mTOR. Indeed, inhibition of AKT results in greater than a threefold increase in RTKs, such as HER3, RET, FGFR, and IGF-1R, across several cell lines, supporting the view that activation of AKT causes feedback inhibition of RTK expression.[218] This feedback regulation/inhibition of RTK expression effect appears to be independent of mTOR activity. Induction of HER3 phosphorylation appears to be the most prominent effect of AKT inhibition, particularly in HER2-driven tumors. These findings may provide an explanation for the

modest objective responses seen to date with these agents even in patients with an activated PI3K pathway signature.[219,220]

Mammalian Target of Rapamycin

mTOR interacts with a number of proteins to form two distinct complexes: mTOR complex 1 (mTORC1) and mTOR complex 2 (mTORC2).[221] mTORC2 is characterized by its association with the rapamycin-insensitive Rictor, and the interaction between Rictor and mTOR is mutually exclusive with that of Raptor, the binding partner in mTORC1. Physiologic activation of PI3K/AKT/mTOR signaling results in feedback downregulation of the pathway, with loss of expression of insulin receptor substrate-1 (IRS-1) (Fig. 48.1), which is the major substrate of IGF-1R and insulin receptors. The indolent behavior of several tumor types with an activated mTOR pathway has been ascribed to this negative feedback loop.[222] Inhibition of mTORC1 by rapamycin and its analogs paradoxically increases AKT activity through induction of IGF-1 signaling via inhibition of p70S6K-mediated IRS-1 downregulation.[223]

Unlike mTORC1, which is inhibited by rapamycin and its analogs, mTORC2 is generally insensitive to rapamycin, although prolonged treatment in several models can block mTORC2 assembly to cause its degradation.[221] Because mTORC2 plays an important role in AKT activation, this differential effect of rapamycin on the mTOR complexes also explains the phenomenon of feedback activation that probably underlies the modest responses seen in the clinic with rapalogues. This phenomenon also provided the impetus for the development of small-molecule inhibitors that can inhibit the catalytic activity of both mTORC1 and mTORC2 to avoid or mitigate the feedback AKT activation. In addition, a consequence of mTOR inhibition is feedback activation of RTKs as well as activation of ERK signaling through loss of p70S6K-mediated inhibition of PI3K.[218,222] These findings provide further evidence supporting the development of dual PI3K/mTOR inhibitors as well as the combination of MAPK and PI3K/AKT/mTOR pathway inhibitors described previously.

LKB1/STK11 is a serine/threonine kinase whose major phosphorylation target, AMP-activated protein kinase (AMPK), upon activation regulates various targets, including the TSC2 gene product tuberin, resulting in mTOR suppression.[224] LKB1/STK11 also phosphorylates related AMPK subfamily members (e.g., BRSK, MARK, NUAK), which have additional functions including regulation of cell polarity and cytoskeletal organization.[225] *LKB1/STK11* is the second most commonly mutated tumor suppressor after *p53* found in NSCLCs, particularly in adenocarcinomas, accounting for 20% to 30% of cases in the Western hemisphere.[145,205] Most *LKB1* mutations in lung tumors result in the generation of truncated and inactive LKB1 proteins.[226,227] *LKB1*-deficient cells exhibit aberrant upregulation of mTOR signaling with an attenuated AKT activation phenotype (similar to TSC2-deficient models) because of the previously mentioned negative feedback phenomenon in PI3K/AKT/mTOR signaling.[224,228] However, *LKB1*-deficient cells are paradoxically hypersensitive to apoptosis, relative to wild-type cells, during conditions of low-nutrient energy stress (e.g., glucose deprivation) or exposure to AMPK agonists (e.g., AICAR) because of an inability to restore metabolic homeostasis.[229] *LKB1*-deficient cells also exhibit alterations in dTTP metabolism and are sensitized to DNA damage and disruption of intracellular dTTP synthesis compared with *LKB1* wild-type cells; this finding suggests that deoxythymidylate kinase is a putative synthetic lethal target.[230]

Inactivating mutations of *LKB1* appear to be more frequent in patients with a history of smoking, and the higher frequency of these mutations among white compared with Asian populations is thought to be due in part to the higher prevalence of smokers in the West.[231] *LKB1* mutations often occur concurrently with *KRAS* mutations (up to 20% of *KRAS* mutants) or *BRAF* mutations (up to 25% of *BRAF* mutants, particularly non-V600 types).[231,232] Expression of the glucose transporter GLUT1 is elevated in *LKB1* mutant tumors, which results in increased glycolysis and the clinical observation of increased avidity on fluoro-deoxyglucose-positron emission tomography scanning.[233]

In a meta-analysis of published data on individual and coincident mutations in NSCLC, *LKB1/KRAS* double mutants were found in approximately 5% of adenocarcinomas in the western world and thus represent a distinct subset of NSCLC with epidemiologic and therapeutic relevance.[205] The degree of activation of the MAPK pathway in the *LKB1/KRAS* double mutants in vivo appeared to be decreased compared with *KRAS* mutants with wild-type *LKB1* status, and signaling was shown to occur primarily through the AKT, FAK, and SRC pathways.[233,234] That the signaling circuitry is shunted away from MAPK in *KRAS* and *BRAF* mutants when *LKB1* is inactivated explains why preclinical models of *LKB1/KRAS* double mutants were resistant to the combination of docetaxel and the MEK inhibitor selumetinib, which otherwise showed synergism in *KRAS* mutants with wild-type *LKB1*. It has been reported that dual *LKB1/KRAS* mutants exhibited a vigorous apoptotic response to phenformin, a mitochondrial inhibitor as an analog of metformin, regardless of the presence of other additional unique mutations (e.g., P53 loss or *PIK3CA* mutation).[235] However, efficacy is not sustained beyond 4 weeks, which suggests that the emergence of resistance and/or cellular adaptation will render monotherapy ineffective.

Heat Shock Protein 90

Heat shock protein 90 (HSP90) is one of the most abundant cellular proteins even under nonstress conditions, and at baseline it constitutes 1% to 2% of the total cellular protein content. HSP90 is named after its characteristic upregulation in response to temperature stress (to 4% to 6% of the total cellular protein content) as well as its molecular weight of about 90 kd.[236,237] This housekeeping protein is an evolutionarily conserved, specialized molecular chaperone with an intrinsic ATPase activity that, along with the assistance of various cochaperones such as the kinase-specific cochaperone Cdc37, ensures the proper folding of nascent polypeptides and the proper assembly of multimeric proteins to prevent aggregation of immature proteins.[238] HSP90 stabilizes and activates more than 200 client proteins, which fall into three main categories: protein kinases (including various mutant oncoproteins discussed previously), steroid hormone receptors, and proteins not involved in signal transduction, such as the transcription factor hypoxia-inducible factor-1alpha.[237,239] Research suggests some functional selectivity of HSP90 toward regulating most tyrosine kinases and tyrosine-like kinases, in contrast to other protein kinase families wherein nonclient proteins may be found in higher proportions.[240] In addition, members of the PI3K/AKT pathway are subject to regulation by HSP90 throughout the pathway, in contrast to the MAPK pathway (i.e., ERK is not a client protein).[240] Conversely, HSP90 itself is subject to post-translational modification from client protein kinases such as BRAF and WEE1; this phenomenon is thought to represent a positive feedback loop ensuring chaperone function.[241]

HSP90 is often overexpressed in cancer cells;[242] their reliance on this protein stems from the fact that mutant oncoproteins are often less stable and that additional cellular stresses are often incurred to maintain the malignant phenotype.[236] Inhibition of HSP90 can preferentially affect the mutant oncoproteins compared with their wild-type forms, such as EGFR, HER2, and BRAF, particularly since in some cases, the wild-type form (such as EGFR) may not be a client protein itself and is resistant to degradation induced by the HSP90 inhibitor.[243-245] This

differential protein stability and reliance on HSP90 function of mutant oncoproteins in NSCLC provides a rationale for investigating the role of HSP90 inhibition in this disease, particularly in combination approaches to overcome or prevent the oncogenic switch that is often seen as a mechanism of acquired resistance to kinase inhibitors used in the clinic. Moreover, inhibition of HSP90 has activity against tumor cells with gatekeeper or multiple other secondary mutations mediating acquired resistance to various kinase inhibitors.[246] HSP90 inhibitor monotherapy, such as with AUY992 or retaspimycin, has shown clinical activity in patients with ALK gene rearrangement, including patients with acquired resistance to crizotinib.[246,247]

Intrinsic resistance to HSP90 inhibitors may occur when specific mutant oncoproteins are innately not sensitive to these agents.[243] Various tumor suppressors are also subject to HSP90 regulation, and their inhibition may adversely spur the proliferation of clones harboring low-penetrant tumor suppressors.[248] WEE1 phosphorylation of HSP90 positively affects HSP90 function, but negatively affects binding of HSP90 inhibitors.[249] Pharmacologic inhibition of WEE1 sensitizes cancer cells to HSP90 inhibitors and thus provides a rationale for this combination. One mechanism of acquired resistance to HSP90 inhibition may arise through feedback activation of the heat shock transcription factor HSF1, a predictable response to currently available HSP90 inhibitors, which results in the induction of other heat shock proteins such as HSP70, HSP27, and HSP90 itself.[250] Lastly, an in vitro model showed that acquired resistance may arise by mutations that increase ATPase activity of HSP90.[251]

HSP90 as a drug target had eluded successful clinical development, largely because of issues regarding drug formulation, toxicities, and modest clinical responses seen with early-generation compounds, such as geldanamycin and its derivatives (17AAG/tanespimycin, 17-DMAG/alvespimycin).[252] The hepatotoxic effects were thought to be related to the nucleophilic reactions arising from the quinone component in the geldanamycin chemotype.[253] Next-generation compounds such as ganetespib, with different structural backbones, were thus developed. A randomized phase II study of docetaxel with or without ganetespib in patients with advanced lung adenocarcinoma showed improved overall survival among patients who received the drug combination, regardless of *EGFR* or *KRAS* mutation status. The incidence of febrile neutropenia was higher in the combination group, but no treatment-related deaths were seen.[254] The phase III trial of this combination in the treatment of patients with adenocarcinoma of the lung in the second line was terminated early for futility.[255]

Cyclin-Dependent Kinase

Cyclin-dependent kinases (CDKs) are serine/threonine kinases that, along with their associated cyclins, mediate cell cycle progression and transcription events. According to the classic model, CDK4 or CDK6 and D-type cyclins regulate events in the early G1 phase of the cycle; CDK2–cyclin E triggers the S phase; CDK2 or CDK1–cyclin A regulates the completion of the S phase; and CDK1–cyclin B is responsible for mitosis.[256-258] Although recurrent mutations of CDKs are rare, gene amplification or protein overexpression of the cyclin partners such as cyclin D1 is frequently encountered in various malignancies, including lung cancer.[259] In turn, the tumor suppressor that negatively regulates the cyclin D1–CDK4 complex, *p16INK4*, is often inactivated in lung cancer, most commonly by homozygous deletion, followed by promoter-region methylation, and rarely by point mutations.[260,261] Cyclin D-dependent kinases (CDK4 and CDK6) phosphorylate retinoblastoma, thereby inhibiting its growth-repressive effects that occur during its hypophosphorylated state.[262] Thus, cells with endogenous expression of functional p16 or mutant reti-noblastoma are thought to be mechanistically insensitive to CDK4/6 inhibitors.

Although early-generation pan-CDK inhibitors failed in clinical development because of toxicity, dramatic clinical results and a favorable toxicity profile have been reported in breast cancer using the small-molecule CDK4/6 inhibitor palbociclib (PD0332991), was approved by the US FDA in combination with letrozole for first-line treatment of estrogen receptor positive, HER2-negative advanced breast cancer.[263] These results have renewed interest in this class of agents. As discussed earlier, CDK signaling, particularly of CDK4, appears to be essential for proliferation of *KRAS*-mutant lung adenocarcinoma.[154] Inhibition of CDK4/6 also appears to be synergistic with trastuzumab in *HER2*-amplified breast cancer cell lines, suggesting the potential for similar activity in NSCLC cells with activated HER2 signaling.[264] A single-arm phase II study of palbociclib in patients with previously treated NSCLC with wild-type retinoblastoma and inactive p16 was closed to accrual after no responses were observed in 16 evaluable patients.[265] The Lung Cancer Master Protocol for patients with squamous cell carcinoma of the lung includes an arm with palbociclib.

CONCLUSION

Advances in our understanding of lung cancer biology and improvements in technology, especially genomic studies, have led to the identification of recurrent functional oncogenic events that represent potential targets for therapy. A large proportion of these genomic alterations are not considered directly druggable targets, such as mutant p53 or amplified SOX2. Nonetheless, this obstacle may be surmounted by identifying synthetically lethal changes amenable to drug therapy. Understanding of both forward signaling and feedback loops in physiologic as well as aberrant activation of oncogenic pathways facilitates the development of novel compounds and aids in the choice of drug combinations for clinical development. A multi-pronged approach entails the incorporation of immunotherapeutic and epigenetic approaches in future studies. Moreover, although tumor responses to certain targeted therapies in NSCLC can be dramatic, clinical benefit is always limited by the emergence of drug resistance, which commonly occurs through either secondary mutations in the drug target or activation of bypass alternative pathways. Other models of resistance, such as the counterintuitive phenomenon of tumor regression upon drug cessation because of acquired drug dependence for continued proliferation, provide a rationale for testing intermittent treatment strategies rather than the conventional approach of continuous dosing. The intermittent approach may also be necessary to mitigate toxicities incurred in the clinical setting, such as with PI3Ki and MEKi combinations, particularly when preclinical studies support this approach.

Targeted therapy requires simultaneous development of the targeted agent along with biomarker assay platforms for patient selection to optimize therapeutic benefit. Pertinent issues regarding standardization of assays and rigorous validation of biomarkers should be considered. Moreover, intratumor heterogeneity can contribute to suboptimal treatment outcomes even in the selected population. Coincident mutations also abrogate the therapeutic efficacy of monotherapy approaches, and these tumor subsets should be considered separately in prospective studies, although this approach inevitably introduces complexity and logistic challenges to the design and analysis of therapeutic trials. A thorough understanding of the spectrum of drug activity and characterization of pharmacologic activity, particularly of small-molecule inhibitors, is necessary to avoid misinterpretation of clinical trial data, particularly when an anticipated clinical benefit is not found.

KEY REFERENCES

3. Shaw AT, Kim DW, Nakagawa K, et al. Crizotinib versus chemotherapy in advanced ALK-positive lung cancer. *N Engl J Med.* 2013;368:2385–2394.
19. Kris MG, Johnson BE, Berry LD, et al. Using multiplexed assays of oncogenic drivers in lung cancers to select targeted drugs. *JAMA.* 2014;311:1998–2006.
77. Yoshioka H, Azuma K, Yamamoto N, et al. A randomized, double-blind, placebo-controlled, phase III trial of erlotinib with or without a c-Met inhibitor tivantinib (ARQ 197) in Asian patients with previously treated stage IIIB/IV nonsquamous nonsmall-cell lung cancer harboring wild-type epidermal growth factor receptor (ATTENTION study). *Ann Oncol.* 2015;26:2066–2072.
78. Scagliotti G, von Pawel J, Novello S, et al. Phase III multinational, randomized, double-blind, placebo-controlled study of tivantinib (ARQ 197) plus erlotinib versus erlotinib alone in previously treated patients with locally advanced or metastatic nonsquamous nonsmall-cell lung cancer. *J Clin Oncol.* 2015;33:2667–2674.
85. Drilon A, Camidge DR, Ou SH, et al. Efficacy and safety of crizotinib in patients (pts) with advanced MET exon 14-altered nonsmall cell lung cancer (NSCLC). *J Clin Oncol.* 2016:34.
103. Johnson PJ, Qin S, Park JW, et al. Brivanib versus sorafenib as first-line therapy in patients with unresectable, advanced hepatocellular carcinoma: results from the randomized phase III BRISK-FL study. *J Clin Oncol.* 2013;31:3517–3524.
109. Rikova K, Guo A, Zeng Q, et al. Global survey of phosphotyrosine signaling identifies oncogenic kinases in lung cancer. *Cell.* 2007;131:1190–1203.
111. Bergethon K, Shaw AT, Ou SH, et al. ROS1 rearrangements define a unique molecular class of lung cancers. *J Clin Oncol.* 2012;30:863–870.
119. Takeuchi K, Soda M, Togashi Y, et al. RET, ROS1 and ALK fusions in lung cancer. *Nat Med.* 2012;18:378–381.

See Expertconsult.com for full list of references.

49 Management of Toxicities of Targeted Therapies

James Chih-Hsin Yang, Chia-Chi (Josh) Lin, and Chia-Yu Chu

SUMMARY OF KEY POINTS

- Epidermal growth factor receptor (EGFR), anaplastic lymphoma kinase (ALK), BRAF, C-ros oncogene 1 (ROS1), ret proto-oncogene (RET) tyrosine kinase inhibitors (TKIs), several antiangiogenesis agents, and antiprogram death 1 (anti-PD1) immunotherapy are effective targeted treatments for lung cancer patients. Each class of agents has class side effects. In addition, each drug may have its own unique side effects.

- Dermatologic and gastrointestinal side effects are frequently encountered side effects of targeted therapy. These side effects are manageable and preventable.

- Interstitial lung diseases are a unique side effect occasionally encountered in lung cancer patients treated with TKIs or anti-PD1 monoclonal antibodies. Although these pulmonary side effects are rare, they may become fatal if left unnoticed. Patients should be informed about the symptoms of these side effects and seek medical care immediately if in doubt. Early intervention including discontinuation of medication and steroid administration is important to reverse the interstitial lung disease process.

- Physicians should be aware of other infrequent but important side effects such as QTc prolongation associated with some TKIs; hypertension, thromboembolic, or hemorrhage side effects associated with antiangiogenesis agents; autoimmune colitis, hepatitis, thyroiditis, or adrenitis associated with anti-PD1 therapy; and skin tumor associated with treatment with B-raf inhibitors.

- Different incidence of side effects between Asian and non-Asian populations may be due to intrinsic genomic differences or extrinsic differences in clinical practice.

Several classes of targeted agents are effective for the treatment of nonsmall cell lung cancer (NSCLC). EGFR TKIs such as gefitinib, erlotinib, and afatinib are very effective for the treatment of NSCLC in patients with EGFR activating mutations.[1] Novel EGFR TKIs such as osimertinib and rociletinib are efficacious in EGFR-mutant NSCLC patients with acquired EGFR T790M mutation.[1,2] EGFR monoclonal antibodies such as necitumumab enhance chemotherapy drug activity in patients with NSCLC (squamous and nonsquamous).[2] ALK inhibitors such as crizotinib, ceritinib (LDK378), alectinib (RO5424802 [CH5424802], AF802), and AP26113 are highly effective treatments for patients with ALK fusion oncoproteins. The most common of these proteins is echinoderm microtubule-associated protein-like 4-ALK, which is detected by ALK immunohistochemical staining or break-apart fluorescence in situ hybridization.[3] V-raf murine sarcoma viral oncogene homolog B (BRAF) inhibitors, such as dabrafenib or vemurafenib, are being tested in patients with BRAF V600E mutation.[4] ROS1 inhibitors such as crizotinib are highly active in patients with ROS1 rearrangements.[5] Foretinib (XL880) may also effectively inhibit ROS1 in patients with NSCLC.[6] These targeted therapies were designed to manage patients with tumors with specific driver mutations, and their side effects often can be predicted by the physiologic pathways that are inhibited. For example, the side effects of EGFR TKIs are diarrhea, skin toxicity, paronychia, hair changes, and mucositis. Rare side effects such as keratitis, nausea, and vomiting can also be linked to the physiologic function of the EGF–EGFR pathway. ALK, ROS1, and ret proto-oncogene (RET) inhibitors produce fewer but unpredictable side effects because less is known about the role of these genes in normal physiology.

Other classes of targeted agents inhibit general pathways that are involved in cancer development and growth. Antiangiogenic agents used in combination with chemotherapy have broad activity in various cancers, including lung cancer. Bevacizumab, a monoclonal antibody that targets vasculoendothelial growth factor (VEGF), improved response and survival in patients with lung adenocarcinoma treated with chemotherapy.[7] Small molecule inhibitors such as vandetanib or nintedanib also have demonstrated anticancer activity in clinical trials.[8] These agents usually cause side effects related to the vascular growth process, such as bleeding and thrombosis, and side effects related to disruption of VEGF pathways such as hypertension, proteinuria, and renal dysfunction.

Heat-shock proteins (HSPs) are chaperones that protect fragile proteins, especially oncoproteins, from disintegration. Inhibition of HSPs may lead to oncoprotein degradation and cancer cell death. HSP90 inhibitors are very effective in cancers such as NSCLC with ALK fusion proteins.[9] Because HSP90 is universally needed in normal physiologic function the consequences of HSP90 inhibition are less clear.

Another class of targeted therapy that has already proven effective in controlling NSCLC is immunotherapy that disrupts the immune checkpoint program death 1 (PD1) on T lymphocytes and its ligands (PD-L1 and PD-L2) on tumor cells. Monoclonal antibodies that target any of these surface proteins can be highly effective in lung cancers harboring PD-L1.[10] The blockage of this checkpoint is more specific on tumor cells than on normal cells. Therefore, these agents may produce fewer immunologic side effects than monoclonal antibodies that target upstream checkpoints such as ipilimumab, which blocks cytotoxic T lymphocyte antigen 4.[10]

Hepatocyte growth factor (HGF) and cMET inhibitors may have a role in inhibiting the growth of NSCLC cells. cMET amplification was noted in up to 20% of individuals with EGFR mutations in whom resistance to EGFR TKIs developed.[11] Monoclonal antibodies that target the ligand (HGF) or the receptor (cMET), as well as small molecule cMET kinase inhibitors, are under active development. The class side effects of HGF and cMET pathway inhibition are not very clear.[12]

Insulin-like growth factor (IGF) and its receptor (IGFR) belong to the insulin receptor family. Overactivity of the insulin signaling pathway has been implicated in tumor progression in several tumor types. Use of the IGFR1 inhibitor figitumumab with chemotherapy has increased response rates in patients with NSCLC.[13] Hyperglycemia and insulin resistance are typical side effects of IGF and IGFR pathway inhibitors.[14]

Phosphatidylinositol 3-kinase, AKT, mitogen-activated and extracellular signal-regulated kinase (MEK), extracellular signal-regulated kinase (ERK), and mammalian target of rapamycin are the central control molecules for cellular proliferation and apoptosis. Inhibitors of these proteins may lead to tumor control in some people with cancer. Unfortunately, substantial side effects have been reported.[15]

Some side effects from targeted therapy are related to the general molecular structures.[16] For example, infusion reactions, such as chills, fever, hypotension, or even rare anaphylactic reactions, are found with many antibody biologic agents. These side effects often can be alleviated or prevented by pretreatment with a corticosteroid. A unique side effect of many small molecule TKIs is interstitial lung disease, also called interstitial lung fibrosis.[17] Furthermore, similar to many other noncancer drugs or biologics, anticancer agents may have side effects that are not related to known pharmacologic or toxicologic properties. Therefore prescribing oncologists should be familiar with the side effect profiles of each targeted therapy.

DERMATOLOGIC SIDE EFFECTS

EGFR TKIs and Monoclonal Antibodies

Dermatologic side effects develop in a considerable number of patients treated with EGFR TKIs or monoclonal antibodies that target EGFR. A papulopustular (acneiform) eruption is the most frequent side effect; xerosis, eczema, telangiectasia, hyperpigmentation, hair changes, and paronychia may also occur.[18–20] Skin adverse events that result from treatment with EGFR TKIs may affect 45% to 100% of patients, and some of these side effects may be dose dependent.[20] By studying the development of resistance to the reversible EGFR TKIs erlotinib and gefitinib, researchers have learned about the molecular mechanisms underlying the signaling pathways involving EGFR. Novel molecularly targeted therapies have been developed to overcome EGFR T790M resistance. Afatinib is an irreversible ErbB family blocker, and its side effect profile is similar to other EGFR inhibitors, with skin toxicity (and diarrhea) being the most frequently reported adverse events.[21,22] Dacomitinib is another irreversible inhibitor of EGFR and human epidermal growth factor receptor-1 (HER1), HER2, and HER4. The monoclonal antibodies cetuximab and panitumumab also may produce skin toxicities because of their inhibition effect on EGFR.[23]

The common adverse effects of treatment with EGFR inhibitors are papulopustular (acneiform) rash, pruritus, and dry skin; nail, hair, and mucosal changes occur less frequently (Table 49.1).[23] Papulopustular (acneiform) rash associated with anti-EGFR therapy occurs in 43% to 94% of patients, with an incidence of approximately 73% in a 2011 meta-analysis.[24,25] The rash resembles acne vulgaris, but it is characterized by predominantly papular or pustular eruption, is not associated with comedones, and is pathologically and etiologically distinct from acne vulgaris (Fig. 49.1). Commonly affected areas are the face (nose, cheeks, nasolabial folds, chin, and forehead), V-areas of the upper chest and back, and, less frequently, the scalp, arms, legs, abdomen, and buttocks (Fig. 49.2). The palms, soles, and mucosa usually are spared. In general, the papulopustular rash manifests within 1 week to 3 weeks of starting an EGFR inhibitor, often commencing between days 7 and 14 and peaking by weeks 3 to 6.[23] The reaction is reversible, usually with complete resolution within 4 weeks of withdrawal from treatment, but the rash may reappear or worsen once treatment is resumed. Spontaneous improvement with resolution or stabilization of the rash occurs with continued treatment.

The incidence of papulopustular (acneiform) rash was highest among patients with metastatic colorectal cancer treated with cetuximab and in patients with lung cancer treated with afatinib.[21,24,25] The incidences of various cutaneous side effects of anti-EGFR treatments in various studies are hard to compare because the genetic background, clinical condition, treatment schedule, and patient characteristics differ in each trial (Table 49.1).[25] Patients with substantial cutaneous side effects are likely to benefit the most from treatment with EGFR inhibitors. Results from a 2013 systematic review and meta-analysis of 33 eligible trials showed that the presence of skin rash predicted the response to EGFR TKIs and the prognosis for patients with NSCLC.[26]

Among patients taking EGFR TKIs or monoclonal antibodies, 4% to 69% have dry skin with diffuse fine scaling after the onset of papulopustular rash.[21,23,25] Painful paronychial inflammation of the fingers and toes is seen in 6% to 47% of patients after 1 month to 4 months of anti-EGFR treatment.[25] This inflammation is often described as a periungual granulation type of paronychia or pyogenic granuloma-like changes, presenting as

TABLE 49.1 Spectrum of Dermatologic Adverse Effects Associated With Epidermal Growth Factor Receptor Inhibitors

Adverse Effect	Description	Frequency[21,23] (%)	Timing During Treatment
Papulopustular (acneiform) rash	Erythematous papular, follicular, or pustular lesions, which may be associated with mild pruritus Commonly affected areas: face (nose, cheeks, nasolabial folds, chin, forehead), V areas of the upper chest and back; less frequently, on the scalp, arms, legs, abdomen, and buttocks	60–94	Onset: between days 7 & 14 Peak: between weeks 3 & 5
Pruritus	Generalized itching sensation	16–60	Onset: between weeks 2 & 4 Peak: between weeks 3 & 6
Dry skin (xerosis)	Diffuse fine scaling on the whole body, especially the extensor areas	4–38	Onset: after appearance of rash
Paronychia	Painful periungual granulation lesions or friable pyogenic granuloma-like changes, associated with erythema, swelling, and fissuring of lateral nail folds or distal finger tufts	6–12	Onset: 2–4 months after start of treatment
Hair changes	Curlier, finer, and more brittle hair on scalp and extremities; extensive growth and curling of eyelashes and eyebrows	Unknown	Onset: as early as 7–10 weeks to many months after the start of treatment
Hypersensitivity reaction	Flushing, urticaria, and anaphylaxis	2–3	Onset: 1st day of initial dose
Mucositis	Mild to moderate mucositis, stomatitis, aphthous ulcers	2–36	Onset: during treatment, not related to dose or schedule

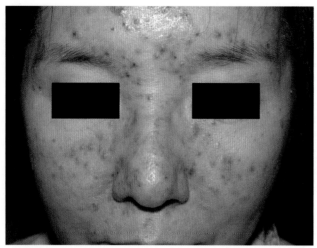

Fig. 49.1. Papulopustular (acneiform) rash associated with antiepidermal growth factor receptor therapy occurs in 60% to 94% of patients. Commonly affected regions are sun-exposed areas of the face such as the nose, cheeks, nasolabial folds, chin, and forehead.

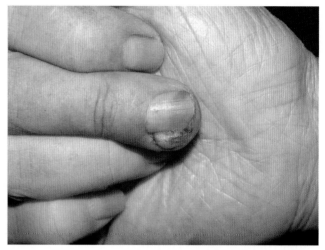

Fig. 49.3. Paronychia related to treatment with an epidermal growth factor receptor inhibitor often presents as painful periungual granulation lesions associated with erythema, tenderness, swelling, and fissuring of lateral nail folds or distal finger tufts.

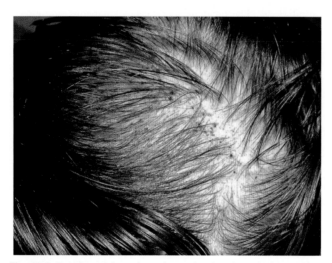

Fig. 49.2. Papulopustular rash on the scalp related to treatment with cetuximab.

erythema, tenderness, swelling, and fissuring of lateral nail folds or distal finger tufts (Fig. 49.3).

In patients who take anti-EGFR medications for several months, hair abnormalities may develop, such as curlier, finer, and more brittle hair on the scalp and extremities or slowed growth of beard hair. Androgenetic alopecia-like frontal alopecia has been noted (Fig. 49.4A). Extensive growth of the eyelashes and eyebrows has also been seen in some patients after many months of anti-EGFR therapy (Fig. 49.4B). Patients who report symptoms of eye irritation should be seen by an ophthalmologist because of the risk of trichiasis.[23]

Skin side effects related to EGFR inhibition are generally mild or moderate in severity. However, even mild events may increase the risk of secondary infections, and patients must cope with chronic discomfort, itching, and the disagreeable appearance of the rash. The rash predominantly affects visible areas of the body, which can cause distress, anxiety, negative self-image, and low self-esteem in some patients. Furthermore, high-grade (grade 3 or higher) skin reactions may lead to morbidity, treatment interruption, or dose modifications.[23] Dermatologic side effects may also affect compliance with treatment.[21] Survey results from 110

oncologists who administered EGFR inhibitor therapy indicated that 76% had interrupted therapy because of rash, whereas 32% had discontinued EGFR inhibitor therapy because of rash.[27] Dermatologic reactions also affect a patient's quality of life.[23]

The mechanism underlying the skin toxicities associated with EGFR inhibition is not fully understood, but it is thought to be related to the disruption of physiologic EGFR-mediated signaling processes in the epidermis, especially the basal keratinocytes.[20,21] Inhibition of EGFR-mediated signaling pathways affects keratinocytes in several ways, for example, inducing growth arrest and apoptosis, decreasing cell migration, increasing cell attachment and differentiation, and stimulating inflammation, which result in distinct cutaneous conditions.[20,21] An EGFR-independent pathway, known as c-Jun NH2-terminal kinase activation, may also be related to keratinocyte damage induced by EGFR TKIs.[28]

Several factors have been associated with an increased tendency for the development of rash. Among patients treated with erlotinib, rash is most likely to develop in nonsmokers, individuals with fair skin, and patients older than 70 years.[21] Men younger than 70 years of age are at an increased risk for the development of a rash with cetuximab therapy.[29] When exploring pharmacogenomic and clinical correlations, researchers found that variability in germline polymorphisms in EGFR was a determinant of cutaneous side effects in erlotinib-treated patients.[30]

Symptomatic and preventive treatments are usually helpful for patients. Strategies include use of topical moisturizers or corticosteroids, administration of systemic steroidal medications or antihistamine drugs to palliate pruritus and inflammation, and dose delay or reduction in the case of severe reactions. Although several guidelines for managing cutaneous side effects have been published, they are based mainly on anecdotal evidence and clinical experience.[20,31]

Patients initiating EGFR TKI or monoclonal antibody therapy should take precautions to protect their skin, such as using alcohol-free skin products and minimizing sun exposure by wearing protective clothing, a hat, and sunscreen with a sun protection factor greater than 30 and ultraviolet A and B protection. Some management strategies based on expert opinion have been proposed for the dermatologic side effects associated with anti-EGFR therapies (Tables 49.2–49.5).[21] For papulopustular (acneiform) rash, topical and oral corticosteroids or antibiotics can be used (Fig. 49.5 and Table 49.2). Patients in whom pruritus develops may benefit from topical, oral, or systemic

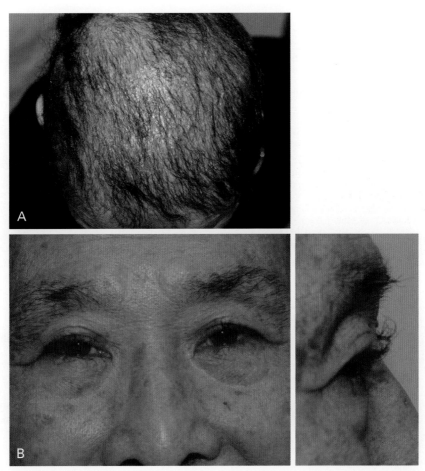

Fig. 49.4. (A) Hair abnormalities, such as curlier and brittle hair on the scalp, have been found in patients receiving dacomitinib for several months. Androgenetic alopecia-like frontal alopecia has also been reported. (B) Extensive growth of both eyelashes and eyebrows has occurred in some patients taking erlotinib for more than 6 months.

TABLE 49.2 Management of Papulopustular (Acneiform) Rash Associated With Epidermal Growth Factor Receptor (EGFR) Inhibitors

Severity of Side Effect[a]	EGFR Inhibitor Dose	Treatment
Grade 1: macular or papular eruption or erythema without associated symptoms	Continue at current dose	Topical corticosteroid[b] OR tacrolimus ointment, twice daily OR topical antibiotic[b] twice daily
Grade 2: macular or papular eruption or erythema with pruritus or other associated symptoms; localized desquamation or other lesions covering <50% of the body surface area	Continue at current dose	Oral antibiotic[c] for 6 weeks Stop topical antibiotic, if being used Topical corticosteroids[b] OR tacrolimus ointment twice daily
Grade 3 or higher: Severe, generalized erythroderma or macular, papular, or vesicular eruption; desquamation covering ≥50% of the body surface area Generalized exfoliative, ulcerative, or bullous dermatitis	Interrupt treatment; resume at reduced dose when effect is rated grade 2 or lower	Oral antibiotic[c] for 6 weeks Refer to dermatologist If infection is suspected (yellow crusts, purulent discharge, or painful skin or nares): change to a broad-spectrum oral antibiotic with gram-negative coverage Consider skin swab for bacterial culture

[a]Grade according to the National Cancer Institute-Common Terminology Criteria for Adverse Events.
[b]Topical corticosteroids may include (moderate or low strength) triamcinolone acetonide 0.025%, desonide 0.05%, alclometasone 0.05%, fluticasone propionate 0.05%, or hydrocortisone acetate 2.5%. Topical antibiotics include clindamycin 1-2%, erythromycin 1-2%, metronidazole 1%, or fusidic acid 2%.
[c]Oral antibiotics include doxycycline 100 mg twice daily, minocycline 100 mg twice daily, or oxytetracycline 500 mg twice daily.
(Adapted with permission from Lacouture ME, Schadendorf D, Chu CY, et al. Dermatologic adverse events associated with afatinib: an oral ErbB family blocker. Expert Rev Anticancer Ther. 2013;13(6):721–728.)

agents (Table 49.3). Topical corticosteroids, ammonium lactate, and moisturizing creams are recommended for xerosis (Table 49.4). For paronychia, topical antibiotics or antiseptics and silver nitrate applications can be beneficial (Fig. 49.6 and Table 49.5). Patients with an intolerable grade 2 skin reaction and

patients with a severe skin reaction (grade 3 or higher) should be referred to a dermatologist with experience managing patients taking EGFR inhibitors. These patients may also benefit from dose modification (Fig. 49.7). Temporary interruption of EGFR inhibitors may relieve severe skin symptoms but should not last

TABLE 49.3 Management of Pruritus Associated With Epidermal Growth Factor Receptor (EGFR) Inhibitors

Severity of Side Effect[a]	EGFR Inhibitor Dose	Treatment
Grade 1: mild or localized	Continue at current dose	Moderate-strength topical corticosteroid twice daily OR topical antipruritic (pramoxine 1% or doxepin 5% cream) once daily
Grade 2: intense or widespread	Continue at current dose	Moderate-strength topical corticosteroid twice daily OR topical antipruritic (pramoxine 1% or doxepin 5% cream) once daily AND oral antihistamine[b]
Grade 3 or higher: intense or widespread and interfering with activities of daily living	Interrupt treatment; resume at reduced dose when effect is rated grade 2 or lower	Oral antihistamine[b] AND GABA agonist[c] OR aprepitant OR doxepin[d] Refer to dermatologist

[a]Grade according to the National Cancer Institute-Common Terminology Criteria for Adverse Events.
[b]Oral antihistamines include levocetirizine 5 mg once daily, desloratadine 5 mg once daily, diphenhydramine 25 mg to 50 mg three times daily, or fexofenadine 60 mg two or three times daily.
[c]Gamma-aminobutyric acid (GABA) agonists include gabapentin 300 mg every 8 hours, or pregabalin 50 mg to 75 mg every 8 hours. The dose of either drug should be adjusted for patients with renal impairment.
[d]Aprepitant: 125 mg on day 1 and 80 mg on days 2 and 3; doxepin 25 mg to 50 mg every 8 hours.
(Adapted with permission from Lacouture ME, Schadendorf D, Chu CY, et al. Dermatologic adverse events associated with afatinib: an oral ErbB family blocker. Expert Rev Anticancer Ther. 2013;13(6):721–728.)

TABLE 49.4 Management of Xerosis Associated With Epidermal Growth Factor Receptor (EGFR) Inhibitors

Severity of Side Effect[a]	EGFR Inhibitor Dose	Treatment
Grade 1–2: Asymptomatic	Continue at current dose	Over-the-counter moisturizing cream or ointment to face and body twice daily
Symptomatic, not interfering with activities of daily living		Over-the-counter moisturizing cream or ointment, ceramide-dominant cream, or corneotherapy to face and body twice daily
Grade 3: interfering with activities of daily living	Interrupt treatment; resume at reduced dose when effect is rated grade 2 or lower	Over-the-counter moisturizing cream or ointment, ceramide-dominant cream, or corneotherapy to face and body twice daily AND ammonium lactate 12% cream, urea 10% cream, OR salicylic acid 6% cream to body twice daily[b] AND topical steroid[c] to eczematous areas twice daily

[a]Grade according to the National Cancer Institute-Common Terminology Criteria for Adverse Events.
[b]Avoid ammonium lactate, urea, or salicylic acid creams on erythematous, open skin areas, or fissure wounds.
[c]Topical corticosteroids may include (moderate or low strength) triamcinolone acetonide 0.025%, desonide 0.05%, alclometasone 0.05%, fluticasone propionate 0.05%, or hydrocortisone acetate 2.5%.
(Adapted with permission from Lacouture ME, Schadendorf D, Chu CY, et al. Dermatologic adverse events associated with afatinib: an oral ErbB family blocker. Expert Rev Anticancer Ther. 2013;13(6):721–728.)

TABLE 49.5 Management of Paronychia Associated With Epidermal Growth Factor Receptor (EGFR) Inhibitors

Severity of Side Effect[a]	EGFR Inhibitor Dose	Treatment
Grade 1: nail fold edema or erythema; disruption of cuticle	Continue at current dose	Topical antibiotic[b] AND vinegar soaks[c] AND topical ultrapotent corticosteroid
Grade 2: nail fold edema or erythema with pain, associated with discharge or nail plate separation, limiting instrumental activities of daily living; localized intervention indicated; oral intervention indicated	Continue at current dose	Topical antibiotic[b] AND vinegar soaks[c] AND topical silver nitrate weekly AND topical ultrapotent corticosteroid[d]
Grade 3 or higher: limiting self-care activities of daily living; surgical intervention or intravenous antibiotics indicated	Interrupt treatment; resume at reduced dose when effect is rated grade 2 or lower	Topical antibiotic[b] AND vinegar soaks[c] AND topical silver nitrate weekly; consider nail avulsion AND systemic antibiotic[e] Refer to dermatologist

[a]Grade according to the National Cancer Institute-Common Terminology Criteria for Adverse Events.
[b]Topical antibiotics include clindamycin 1%, erythromycin 1%, tetracycline 1%, or chloramphenicol 1%.
[c]Fingers or toes should be soaked for 15 minutes each day in a 1:1 solution of white vinegar and water.
[d]Topical ultrapotent corticosteroids include clobetasol propionate 0.05%, diflorasone diacetate 0.05%, or betamethasone dipropionate 0.25%.
[e]Systemic antibiotics include tetracycline, doxycycline, minocycline, or cephalexin.
(Adapted with permission from Lacouture ME, Schadendorf D, Chu CY, et al. Dermatologic adverse events associated with afatinib: an oral ErbB family blocker. Expert Rev Anticancer Ther. 2013;13(6):721–728.)

for more than 28 days. Anti-EGFR treatment should be permanently discontinued if dermatologic side effects remain at or above grade 3 despite dermatologic interventions and treatment interruption for 28 days. EGFR TKIs may be reintroduced at a lower dose for patients with a severe skin reaction (grade 3 or higher) that improves (grade 2 or lower) within 28 days of treatment interruption.[21]

Antiangiogenic Agents

Sorafenib, a multikinase inhibitor that targets rapidly accelerated fibrosarcoma (RAF) kinase, VEGF receptors (VEGFR-1 to VEGFR-3), platelet-derived growth factor-alpha, platelet-derived growth factor-beta, c-Kit, and RET, has been approved for use in various malignancies.[32] Hand–foot skin reaction is the

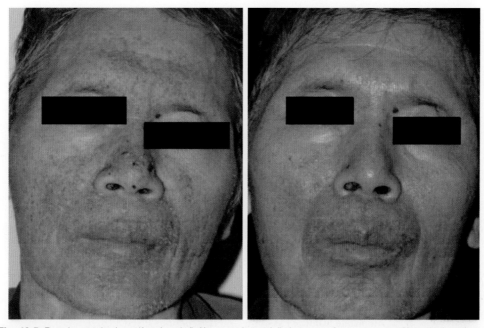

Fig. 49.5. Papulopustular (acneiform) rash (left) may substantially improve after treatment with topical cortico-steroids for 2 weeks (right).

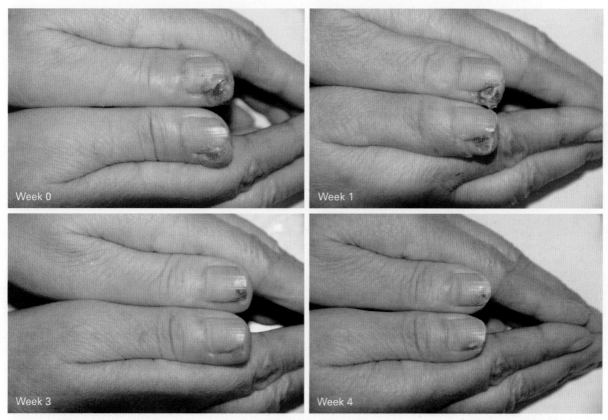

Week 0

Week 1

Week 3

Week 4

Fig. 49.6. Paronychia with granulation tissues improves after weekly applications of silver nitrate for 4 weeks.

major toxicity of sorafenib treatment requiring clinical management and dose modifications. This reaction is characterized by well-defined, tender palmoplantar hyperkeratotic or blistering lesions, especially in areas of trauma or friction (Fig. 49.8). When sorafenib is used alone, the development of hand–foot skin reaction is associated with dose.[32] However, patients treated with the combination of bevacizumab and sorafenib are at an increased risk of hand–foot skin reaction, suggesting that the pathophysiology may involve VEGF inhibition.[32] Other skin eruptions related to sorafenib therapy include facial or scalp erythema and dysesthesia, alopecia, splinter hemorrhage, keratoacanthoma, leukocytoclastic vasculitis, and epidermal inclusion cysts.

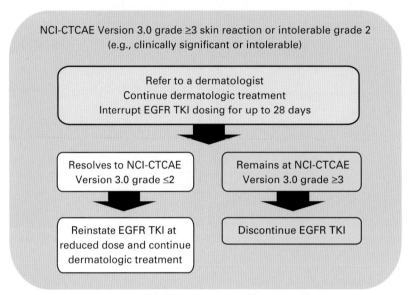

Fig. 49.7. Dose-modification strategy for patients with grade 3 or higher or intolerable grade 2 dermatologic side effects related to treatment with an epidermal growth factor receptor (EGFR) tyrosine kinase inhibitor (TKI). *(Adapted with permission from Lacouture ME, Schadendorf D, Chu CY, et al. Dermatologic adverse events associated with afatinib: an oral ErbB family blocker.* Expert Rev Anticancer Ther. *2013;13(6): 721–728.)* NCI-CTCAE, *National Cancer Institute-Common Terminology Criteria for Adverse Events.*

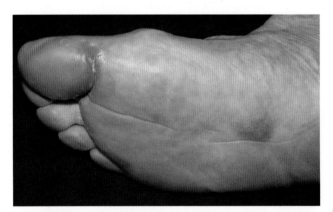

Fig. 49.8. Hand–foot skin reaction associated with sorafenib therapy is characterized by well-defined, tender palmoplantar hyperkeratotic or blistering lesions, especially in areas of trauma or friction.

Although skin rash (type unspecified) has been reported for some patients after infusion of bevacizumab, it is not a common toxicity of bevacizumab.

GASTROINTESTINAL SIDE EFFECTS OF EGFR INHIBITORS

Diarrhea is a common side effect during the first cycle of treatment with oral EGFR TKIs. The time of onset can vary widely. Diarrheal episodes are usually moderate and are generally well controlled with dose reduction and administration of loperamide.

Mechanism of Diarrhea

The pathophysiology of EGFR TKI-induced diarrhea remains unclear. Diarrhea is related to wild-type EGFR inhibition. Diarrhea is a common side effect for first-generation EGFR TKIs (e.g., gefitinib and erlotinib, which can inhibit wild-type and activating mutation of EGFR) and irreversible, second-generation EGFR TKIs (e.g., afatinib and dacomitinib, which inhibit wild-type, activating mutation, and probably T790M-resistant mutations). Diarrhea is less common in third-generation EGFR TKIs (e.g., osimertinib and rociletinib), which only inhibit wild-type EGFR at high concentrations.[22,33,34] Diarrhea induced by EGFR TKIs is thought to result from excess chloride secretion, causing a secretory form of diarrhea.[35] Little information is available about the histopathology of diarrhea induced by EGFR TKIs. In a phase I trial, microscopic analysis of tissue treated with neratinib (an irreversible EGFR TKI) showed mild duodenal mucosal gland dilatation and degeneration, as well as mild edema and slight villus atrophy in the small intestine.[36]

Incidence and Effect of Diarrhea

In the phase III trials of gefitinib (Iressa Survival Evaluation in Lung Cancer [ISEL] and Iressa Pan-Asia Study [IPASS]), the incidence of diarrhea of all grades was higher with gefitinib (27% to 46.6%) than with placebo (9%) or paclitaxel and carboplatin (21.7%). The incidence of high-grade (grades 3 to 5) diarrhea was greater with gefitinib (3% to 3.8%) than with placebo (1%) or paclitaxel and carboplatin (1.4%).[37,38]

In the phase III trials of erlotinib, the incidence of diarrhea of all grades was 57% in the European Randomized Trial of Tarceva versus Chemotherapy (EURTAC), in which erlotinib was used as first-line treatment, 19% in the Sequential Tarceva in Unresectable NSCLC (SATURN) trial of maintenance therapy with erlotinib, and 55% in the BR.21 trial in which erlotinib was used as second- or third-line treatment.[39–41] The incidence of high-grade diarrhea in patients receiving erlotinib was 5% in EURTAC, 2% in the SATURN trial, and 6% in the BR.21 trial. In the BR.21 trial, 5% of the erlotinib group required dose reductions because of diarrhea.[41] The incidence and severity of diarrhea were slightly lower in the SATURN trial than in the other studies, possibly because of the better performance status of SATURN trial patients or improved awareness and management of erlotinib-related adverse events by investigators.

Diarrhea is the most common adverse event related to treatment with afatinib. In the phase III trials of afatinib (LUX-Lung 3), the incidence of diarrhea of all grades was substantially higher with afatinib than with chemotherapy (95.2% vs. 15.3%).[42,43] The incidence of high-grade diarrhea was also much higher with afatinib than with chemotherapy (14.4% vs. 0%). Diarrhea led to treatment discontinuation in 1.3% of patients receiving afatinib. The incidence of grade 3 or grade 4 diarrhea was lower in an afatinib phase II study (7%) and another phase III study (5%).[44] The lower incidence of severe diarrhea may be a result of better management and prevention in the few centers that participated in these clinical trials. In the randomized phase II trial of dacomitinib, the incidence of all-grade diarrhea was higher with dacomitinib than with erlotinib (73.1% vs. 47.9%).[45] The incidence of high-grade diarrhea was higher with dacomitinib than with erlotinib (11.8% vs. 4.3%). Grade 2 diarrhea led to treatment discontinuation for one (1.1%) of 94 patients receiving dacomitinib. In the randomized phase II trial of afatinib versus gefitinib (LUX-Lung 7), all-grade diarrhea occurred more frequently in afatinib (90% vs. 61%). Grade 3 diarrhea was also more common with afatinib treatment (11.9% vs. 1.3%). Drug-related adverse events leading to discontinuation occurred in 6.3% and 6.3% of patients, respectively. However, the most common reason to discontinue afatinib was diarrhea in five patients (3.1%), whereas gefitinib increased alanine transaminase in five patients (3.1%).[45a]

Consequences and Management of Diarrhea

Severe diarrhea may result in fluid and electrolyte losses that lead to dehydration, electrolyte imbalances, and renal insufficiency.[22] Patients should be advised to take loperamide, 2 mg to 4 mg, after the first incidence of watery diarrhea. Two milligrams of loperamide can be taken every 4 hours to a maximum of 20 mg/day until diarrhea improves to grade 1. Patients with high-grade diarrhea or grade 2 diarrhea for more than 48 hours should temporarily discontinue the EGFR TKI therapy. Patients should consume enough water and electrolytes to prevent dehydration and renal damage. Because diarrhea is a common side effect of many cancer treatment regimens, guidelines for its management are well established.[46] Patients should be advised to discuss any symptoms of diarrhea with their health-care team immediately to facilitate early and effective management and prevent dose reductions or treatment discontinuation. Patients with frequent diarrhea should consume a light diet without dairy products. Dose reduction of EGFR TKIs should be considered for severe or recurrent diarrhea that affects the patients' quality of life.

PULMONARY SIDE EFFECTS: INTERSTITIAL LUNG DISEASE

Acute interstitial lung disease is an adverse event seen with all EGFR TKIs: gefitinib, erlotinib, afatinib, and osimertinib. More than one-third of reported cases are fatal. Patients with preexisting lung disease are at an increased risk.[47]

Mechanism of Interstitial Lung Disease

The development of EGFR TKI-induced interstitial lung disease is most likely related to decreased alveolar regeneration, a process normally regulated by EGFR, in a population with a high prevalence of preexisting pulmonary disease. Patients typically present with acute onset of dyspnea, cough, and pyrexia. In a series of Japanese patients, chest computed tomography images showed diffuse ground-glass opacities and evaluation of tissue samples indicated that there was diffuse alveolar damage with hyaline membrane formation.[48]

Incidence of Interstitial Lung Disease

Interstitial lung disease usually develops within 3 weeks to 7 weeks after the start of gefitinib therapy, and one-third of cases are fatal. The US Food and Drug Administration reported a 1% incidence of interstitial lung disease among 50,000 patients who received gefitinib worldwide.[49] In the ISEL trial, the frequency of interstitial lung disease events was similar in the two treatment groups (1%).[37] In IPASS, interstitial lung disease events occurred in 16 (2.6%) of 607 patients treated with gefitinib, three of whom died, and in eight (1.4%) of 589 patients treated with paclitaxel and carboplatin, one of whom died.[38] The incidence of interstitial lung disease has been reported to be higher in Japan (2%) than in the United States (0.3%).[49] In a review of data from more than 1900 Japanese patients with NSCLC treated with gefitinib over a 4-month period (3.5%) cases of interstitial lung disease were reported, of which 44% were fatal. Other than Japanese ethnicity, risk factors for the development of interstitial lung disease include male gender, a history of smoking, and a presence of interstitial pneumonia (odds ratios, 3.1, 4.79, and 2.89, respectively).[50] In addition, interstitial lung disease develops in 6.6% of men with a history of smoking. Approximately 90% of patients in whom gefitinib-induced interstitial lung disease develops have received prior radiotherapy or chemotherapy.[48]

Interstitial lung disease occurs in 1.1% of patients receiving erlotinib.[51] The onset of symptoms may range from 5 days to more than 9 months (median, 39 days) after initiating erlotinib therapy. The incidence of pneumonitis or pulmonary infiltrates of all grades was 1% when erlotinib was used as first-line treatment in EURTAC and 3% when it was used as a second- or third-line treatment in the BR.21 trial.[39,41] The incidence of grade 3 to grade 5 interstitial lung disease was 1% in EURTAC and less than 1% in the BR.21 trial. Serious interstitial lung disease, including fatal cases, can occur with erlotinib treatment. In the SATURN trial, the most frequently reported serious adverse event was pneumonia: seven (2%) cases were reported in the erlotinib arm, compared with four (less than 1%) in the placebo arm.[40] In the BR.21 trial, one of 485 patients in the erlotinib arm and one of 242 patients in the placebo arm died from pneumonitis.[41] Risk factors for the development of interstitial lung disease with erlotinib were similar to the risk factors identified in trials of gefitinib.

In a phase II study of afatinib that included 129 patients with EGFR mutations, four patients discontinued afatinib because of possible interstitial lung disease.[43] In the phase III randomized study, possible interstitial lung disease developed in three of 230 patients with lung adenocarcinoma positive for EGFR mutation who received frontline afatinib.[42]

Management of Interstitial Lung Disease

In most interstitial lung disease case series reports, the authors indicate that drug discontinuation, supportive therapy with mechanical ventilation, and high-dose corticosteroids are the only useful interventions and that up to 40% of cases are fatal.[48,50] Resuming EGFR TKIs after resolution of symptoms has been associated with recurrence of interstitial lung disease. EGFR TKIs should be withheld for acute onset of new or progressive unexplained pulmonary symptoms, such as dyspnea, cough, and fever. EGFR TKIs should be permanently discontinued if interstitial lung disease is diagnosed.[49,51] The best strategy for preventing severe interstitial lung disease seems to be early diagnosis and EGFR TKI discontinuation. Frequent chest radiography for a few weeks after initiating EGFR TKIs and patient education for early signs of interstitial lung disease are important steps to prevent complications in populations with a high prevalence of EGFR TKI-induced interstitial lung disease.[52]

BEVACIZUMAB AND RAMUCIRUMAB SIDE EFFECTS

Bevacizumab causes a wide range of class-related adverse effects. A noteworthy concern with this class of agents is the potential for vessel injury and bleeding, which has been seen in patients with squamous cell lung cancer.[53] Bevacizumab is contraindicated for patients with a history of hemoptysis, brain metastasis, or a bleeding diathesis, but in appropriately selected patients, the rate of life-threatening pulmonary hemorrhage is less than 2%.[7]

The safety of operating on patients treated with bevacizumab continues to be a major concern because of the risk of bleeding and poor wound healing. In a pooled analysis of two large clinical trials in patients with colon cancer, individuals who needed surgery while being treated with bevacizumab had a higher frequency of serious wound healing complications than individuals treated with placebo (13% vs. 3.4%).[54] In light of these data and because of the long half-life of bevacizumab, elective surgery should be delayed for at least 4 weeks from the last dose of antibody, and treatment should be not resumed for at least 4 weeks after surgery.[55]

Other toxicities characteristic of antiangiogenic drugs include hypertension and proteinuria. A majority of patients receiving bevacizumab require antihypertensive therapy, particularly patients receiving higher doses and more prolonged treatment.[7,56] The mechanism of bevacizumab-related hypertension is still unclear but may relate in part to decreased endothelial nitric oxide production.[57] Physicians should carefully monitor the blood pressure of all patients on bevacizumab and intervene with antihypertensives when appropriate. In some studies, reversible posterior leukoencephalopathy developed during bevacizumab treatment in patients with poorly controlled hypertension.[58-60] Bevacizumab has also been associated with congestive heart failure, probably secondary to hypertension.[61] Proteinuria often develops during bevacizumab treatment, but it is usually an asymptomatic finding and rarely associated with nephrotic syndrome.[62]

Arterial thromboembolic events (i.e., stroke or myocardial infarction) are serious concerns with antiangiogenic agents.[63] The authors of a meta-analysis reported that the incidence of arterial thromboembolic events was 3.8% in patients receiving bevacizumab-containing regimens compared with 1.7% in the control group.[63] To reduce the risk of arterial thromboembolic events, clinicians should carefully evaluate a patient's risk factors (e.g., age older than 65 years, clotting diathesis, a history of arterial thromboembolic events) before initiating treatment.

Gastrointestinal perforation, a potentially life-threatening complication of bevacizumab, has been reported in up to 11% of patients with ovarian cancer, perhaps related to the presence of peritoneal carcinomatosis and to prior abdominal surgery.[64] Colonic perforation is rare during bevacizumab treatment for colon cancer, but it occurs most frequently in patients with intact primary colonic tumors, peritoneal carcinomatosis, peptic ulcer disease, chemotherapy-associated colitis, diverticulitis, or a history of abdominal radiotherapy. The rate of colonic perforation is less than 1% in patients with breast or lung cancer who receive the antibody.[55,64] Gut perforation is an infrequent side effect of bevacizumab in patients with lung cancer. However, special caution should be taken for patients with lung cancer and peritoneal metastasis who are receiving bevacizumab.

Ramucirumab is a fully human immunoglobulin G1 monoclonal antibody that specifically binds to VEGFR-2. A randomized phase III trial of docetaxel plus ramucirumab versus docetaxel plus placebo as the second-line therapy in patients with NSCLC was reported. Incidence of febrile neutropenia was higher in patients treated with ramucirumab than in controls (grade 3: 10% vs. 6%; grade 4: 6% vs. 4%). Patients in the ramucirumab group had more bleeding events of any grade (29% vs. 15%), although rates of grade 3 or worse events were the same. Incidence of epistaxis of any grade was significantly higher in the ramucirumab group than in the control group, but few grade 3 or worse events occurred. Of note, this trial enrolled patients with both squamous cell and nonsquamous cell carcinoma excluding major blood vessel involvement and intratumor cavitation. Hypertension occurred more frequently in the ramucirumab group than in the control group, with one grade 4 hypertension event occurring in the ramucirumab group.[65]

ANAPLASTIC LYMPHOMA KINASE INHIBITOR SIDE EFFECTS

The most common adverse reactions to crizotinib, an ALK and MET inhibitor, are vision disorders, nausea, diarrhea, vomiting, edema, and constipation, which occur in 25% of patients or more.[66,67]

Given the role of ALK in the development of the visual system and gut, it is tempting to speculate that several of the common adverse effects result from direct anti-ALK effects on the native protein. Peripheral edema may be a notable exception, as this adverse effect also has been reported with MET inhibition.[68] Other ALK-specific inhibitors (e.g., AP26113, ASP3026, alectinib, ceritinib) are not associated with peripheral edema.[69] The visual disturbances associated with crizotinib include brief light trails, flashes, or image persistence occurring at the edges of the visual field, and these effects usually begin within days after treatment has started. The disturbances occur most commonly with changes in lighting. Studies in rats have demonstrated that crizotinib causes reductions in the rate of retinal dark adaptation but not the ability to achieve full dark adaptation, offering a partial explanation for these clinical findings. Severe side effects associated with crizotinib are rare. Drug holidays followed by rechallenge at a lower dose have allowed ongoing treatment in some cases of severe neutropenia or transaminitis, but permanent drug discontinuation is occasionally required.[70]

Crizotinib-induced hepatotoxicity has occurred with fatal outcomes. Biweekly monitoring of transaminases for the first 2 months of treatment is recommended. Severe, including fatal, treatment-related pneumonitis has occurred. Patients should be monitored for pulmonary symptoms indicative of pneumonitis. In patients with a history of or predisposition for QTc prolongation, or for patients who are taking medications known to prolong the QT interval, clinicians should consider periodic monitoring with electrocardiography and determination of serum electrolyte levels.[70]

Given reports that rapid-onset hypogonadism occurs in the majority of men taking crizotinib, serum testosterone levels should be routinely checked and replaced as appropriate during therapy.[71,72] Case reports of crizotinib-induced asymptomatic profound bradycardia and renal cysts were published between 2011 and 2013, the clinical significance of which remains uncertain.[70,73,74]

HEAT-SHOCK PROTEIN 90 INHIBITOR SIDE EFFECTS

HSP90 inhibitors (e.g., ganetespib [STA-9090], retaspimycin [IPI-504], luminespib [AUY922]) are currently being tested in patients with certain molecular subtypes of NSCLC, such as ALK fusion.[75,76] The side effect profile of the *N*-terminal-binding radicicol and geldanamycin analogs (e.g., retaspimycin) differs from that of the next-generation synthetic resorcinol-containing chemo-type agents (e.g., AUY922) because of structural differences.[77] For example, reversible visual disturbance has been reported in patients receiving AUY922 but not retaspimycin.[78]

BRAF INHIBITOR SIDE EFFECTS

BRAF inhibitors (e.g., vemurafenib, dabrafenib) have been approved in BRAF-mutated malignant melanoma and are currently being tested in clinical trials for BRAF-mutated NSCLC.[4,79,80] BRAF mutations occur in 1% to 2% of lung adenocarcinoma cases.[81–83] Cutaneous squamous cell carcinoma is a class side effect of BRAF inhibitors. Febrile reaction is unique to dabrafenib.

Skin tumors, especially keratoacanthoma and cutaneous squamous cell carcinoma, have developed in a high percentage of patients in clinical trials of vemurafenib or dabrafenib.[84] Experience from clinical trials of melanoma has shown that the most common grade 2 or higher toxicities were cutaneous squamous cell carcinoma or keratoacanthoma (5% to 11%), fatigue (8%), and pyrexia (3% to 6%). Palmoplantar hyperkeratoses and actinic keratoses were also common but mild. Phototoxicity was rare (3%).[85] Studies have shown that different RAF inhibitors activate the ERK pathway in cells with wild-type BRAF via a mechanism involving dimerization of BRAF and RAF proto-oncogene serine/threonine-protein kinase (CRAF) and transactivation of the inhibitor-free promoter in a RAS–guanosine triphosphate-dependent manner.[84] These findings provide the most likely explanation for the development of skin tumors during RAF inhibitor treatment. Cutaneous toxicities such as rash, hyperkeratosis, cutaneous squamous cell carcinoma, and keratoacanthoma occur with both vemurafenib and dabrafenib, but have been reported to occur to a lesser degree with dabrafenib. Of note, cutaneous squamous cell carcinoma has occurred in 19% of patients with vemurafenib and in only 5% of patients with dabrafenib.[85]

In a 2013 systematic dermatologic study of 42 patients, 100% of patients treated with vemurafenib presented with at least one adverse skin reaction.[86] The most common cutaneous side effects were verrucous papillomas (79%) and hand–foot skin reaction (60%). Other common cutaneous toxic effects were a diffuse hyperkeratotic perifollicular rash (55%), photosensitivity (52%), and alopecia (45%). Keratoacanthoma and cutaneous squamous cell carcinoma occurred in 14% and 26% of the patients, respectively.[86]

Several surgical approaches are available to manage keratotic growths. For small and superficial lesions, destructive modalities such as curettage and electrodessication or cryosurgery may be sufficient.[87] Mohs micrographic surgery may be needed for larger lesions. When surgical treatment is either impractical or undesirable, other strategies such as topical 5-fluorouracil may be used.[87] Reduction of vemurafenib or dabrafenib dose is another potential management strategy. Bexarotene and other systemic retinoids may be helpful for vemurafenib-associated cutaneous squamous cell carcinoma and keratoacanthoma.[87] Use of a MEK inhibitor in combination with vemurafenib or dabrafenib may block paradoxical mitogen-activated protein kinase signaling downstream of CRAF in keratinocytes.[86,87]

In the pivotal trial of vemurafenib in melanoma, cutaneous squamous cell carcinoma occurred in 40 (12%) of 336 patients treated with vemurafenib and in 1 (<1%) of 282 patients treated with chemotherapy.[88] In the pivotal trial of dabrafenib in melanoma, cutaneous squamous cell carcinoma and keratoacanthoma occurred in 14 (7%) of 187 patients treated with dabrafenib and in none of the patients treated with chemotherapy.[89] Across clinical trials of dabrafenib (586 patients), the incidence is between 6%

and 10%.[89–91] The median time to the first cutaneous squamous cell carcinoma was 9 weeks (range, 1 week to 53 weeks). Among patients in whom a cutaneous squamous cell carcinoma developed, at least one additional cutaneous squamous cell carcinoma developed in approximately 33% with continued dabrafenib. The median time between diagnosis of the first and second cutaneous squamous cell carcinoma was 6 weeks.[89–91]

Serious febrile drug reactions have occurred only with dabrafenib. In a melanoma trial, serious febrile drug reactions—defined as serious cases of fever or fever of any severity accompanied by hypotension, rigors or chills, dehydration, or renal failure in the absence of another identifiable cause (e.g., infection)—occurred in 7 (3.7%) of 187 patients treated with dabrafenib and in none of the patients treated with dacarbazine. The incidence of fever (serious and nonserious) was 28% in patients treated with dabrafenib and 10% in patients treated with dacarbazine.[89] In patients treated with dabrafenib, the median time to initial onset of fever (any severity) was 11 days (range, 1 day to 202 days) and the median duration of fever was 3 days (range, 1 day to 129 days).[89]

MEK INHIBITOR SIDE EFFECTS

MEK inhibitors (e.g., refametinib, selumetinib, trametinib, cobimetinib) have been tested in clinical trials for the treatment of NSCLC.[92] The most common adverse effects of MEK inhibitors (e.g., trametinib) are rash, diarrhea, peripheral edema, fatigue, and dermatitis acneiform.[93] MEK inhibitors also have unique cardiac and ophthalmologic side effects.[94]

Central serous retinopathy can occur during treatment with trametinib. In a melanoma trial, ophthalmologic examinations including retinal evaluation were performed at baseline and at regular intervals during treatment; central serous retinopathy developed in one patient (less than 1%) who received trametinib; however, no cases of central serous retinopathy were identified in chemotherapy-treated patients. In addition, no cases of retinal vein occlusion had been reported at the time of analysis.[94] Ophthalmologic evaluation should be performed any time a patient reports visual disturbances, and the results should be compared with baseline, if those data are available. If central serous retinopathy is diagnosed, trametinib should be withheld. If repeat ophthalmologic evaluation indicates resolution of the central serous retinopathy within 3 weeks, the patient may resume trametinib at a reduced dose.

PD1 AND PD-L1 MONOCLONAL ANTIBODY SIDE EFFECTS

NSCLC is now known to be an immunologically targetable cancer. Anti-PD1 antibodies (e.g., nivolumab, pembrolizumab [MK-3475]) and anti-PD-L1 antibodies (e.g., atezolizumab [MPDL3280A], durvalumab [MEDI4736]) have shown effectiveness in treating NSCLC.[95,96]

In a phase I trial, 296 patients were treated with nivolumab at 1 mg/kg to 10 mg/kg.[96] Treatment-related adverse events occurred in 70% of patients. As many as 14% of patients had grade 3 or grade 4 treatment-related adverse events, the most common of which was fatigue. Immune-related adverse events of all grades, including rash (12%), pruritus (9%), diarrhea (11%), transaminitis (3% or less), thyroid abnormalities (3% or less), and infusion-related reaction (3% or less), occurred in 41% of patients. Grade 3 or grade 4 immune-related adverse events occurred in 6% of patients, which mainly included diarrhea, rash, transaminitis, and thyroid abnormalities. Pneumonitis (any grade) developed in nine patients (3%); grade 3 or grade 4 pneumonitis developed in three (1%). Three patients died of pneumonitis.

Among 135 patients with melanoma who were treated with pembrolizumab (MK-3475), 2 mg/kg or 10 mg/kg, in a phase

I trial, adverse events occurred in 72% of patients.[97] As many as 9% of patients had grade 3 to grade 5 treatment-related adverse events, most commonly fatigue. Immune-related adverse events of any grade occurred in 15.9% of patients; these events included rash (4.5%), influenza (3.0%), pruritus (2.2% or less), eczema (2.2% or less), vitiligo (2.2% or less), and hypothyroidism (2.2% or less). Grade 3 or grade 4 immune-related adverse events occurred in 5.3% of patients, mainly thyroid abnormalities. Grade 1 or grade 2 pneumonitis developed in four patients (3%). Of note, no cases of pneumonitis were reported in the clinical trials of the anti-PD-L1 antibodies BMS-936559 and MPDL3280A.[98]

ETHNIC DIFFERENCES IN SIDE EFFECTS OF TARGETED THERAPY

Differences in drug-related side effects by patient ethnicity are a source of concern.[52] Several factors contribute to the different experience patients have in drug-related efficacy and toxicities. Extrinsic factors included medical practice pattern, patients' access to health care, dietary patterns, and living environment, among others. Intrinsic factors include body size, body composition, and, most importantly, genetic differences related to drug absorption, distribution, metabolism, and excretion. For most drugs, interpatient variability is usually higher than interethnic variability.

Interstitial lung disease is an important example of the effect of ethnicity on adverse event frequency. The frequency of treatment-induced interstitial lung disease reported in Japanese studies is 3.5% to 5.8% for patients managed with gefitinib or erlotinib; mortality from interstitial lung disease is 1.6% to 3.6%.[50,52] An independent review committee reported that in a postmarketing surveillance study of 3488 Japanese patients, interstitial lung disease occurred in 4.5% of erlotinib-treated individuals, of whom 55 (1.6%) died.[99] Interstitial lung disease developed in 42 of 1080 Taiwanese patients treated with gefitinib, and the condition was considered to be gefitinib related in 25 (2.3%) of them.[100] However, the frequency of interstitial lung disease among patients treated with EGFR TKIs outside Asia is around 1%.[49,51] It is unclear what factors contribute to this striking disparity. In the ISEL study, the frequencies of gefitinib-related side effects were not formally compared between the group of Asian patients and the overall study population, but there were no apparent differences in most side effects, including diarrhea or skin rash. A higher percentage of severe grade 3 and grade 4 pneumonia was seen among the 235 (6.4%) Asian patients compared with 891 (1.7%) non-Asian patients.[101]

In the LUX-Lung 3 study of afatinib compared with pemetrexed and cisplatin in patients with EGFR mutation, the frequency of grade 3 diarrhea was higher in Japanese patients (20%) than in white patients (11%). This result could be due to the low dosages of loperamide typically used in Japan or to the smaller body size of Japanese patients using the same 40-mg dose of afatinib.[42]

Preliminary data show that crizotinib concentration is higher in Asian patients than in other patients taking the same dosage. However, there were no differences in crizotinib-related side effects by ethnicity in phase II studies.[102]

Cytochrome P450 polymorphisms are distributed unequally among ethnic groups and may contribute to differences in the frequency of drug-related side effects. For example, tivantinib (ARQ197), a cMET inhibitor, is metabolized by 2C19, which has extensive-metabolizer and poor-metabolizer forms. Patients with the poor-metabolizer 2C19 polymorphism may have excessive hematologic toxicity if given the same dose of tivantinib as an individual with the extensive-metabolizer polymorphism (360 mg, twice daily). The 2C19 poor-metabolizer polymorphism is rare among white individuals but is present in 20% of Asian individuals. Therefore it is necessary to test for 2C19 polymorphisms in Asian patients to determine appropriate dosing.[103]

CONCLUSION

Targeted therapies are effective treatment options for patients with advanced lung cancer. Given rapid advances in molecular classification of lung cancers, targeted therapies have demonstrated increasingly good anticancer activity. The side effects of targeted therapy are different from the effects of chemotherapy. Most, if not all, side effects are manageable, preventable, and treatable. Early identification of the side effects followed by appropriate treatment is important to maximize the benefit of targeted therapy for patients with lung cancer.

KEY REFERENCES

1. Lee CK, Brown C, Gralla RJ, et al. Impact of EGFR inhibitor in non-small cell lung cancer on progression-free and overall survival: a meta-analysis. *J Natl Cancer Inst.* 2013;105(9):595–605.
20. Lacouture ME. Mechanisms of cutaneous toxicities to EGFR inhibitors. *Nat Rev Cancer.* 2006;6(10):803–812.
21. Lacouture ME, Schadendorf D, Chu CY, et al. Dermatologic adverse events associated with afatinib: an oral ErbB family blocker. *Expert Rev Anticancer Ther.* 2013;13(6):721–728.
22. Yang JC, Reguart N, Barinoff J, et al. Diarrhea associated with afatinib: an oral ErbB family blocker. *Expert Rev Anticancer Ther.* 2013;13(6):729–736.
29. Lacouture ME, Anadkat MJ, Bensadoun RJ, et al. Clinical practice guidelines for the prevention and treatment of EGFR inhibitor-associated dermatologic toxicities. *Support Care Cancer.* 2011;19(8):1079–1095.
38. Mok TS, Wu YL, Thongprasert S, et al. Gefitinib or carboplatin-paclitaxel in pulmonary adenocarcinoma. *N Engl J Med.* 2009;361(10):947–957.
42. Sequist LV, Yang JC, Yamamoto N, et al. Phase III study of afatinib or cisplatin plus pemetrexed in patients with metastatic lung adenocarcinoma with EGFR mutations. *J Clin Oncol.* 2013;31(27): 3327–3334.
50. Ando M, Okamoto I, Yamamoto N, et al. Predictive factors for interstitial lung disease, antitumor response, and survival in non-small-cell lung cancer patients treated with gefitinib. *J Clin Oncol.* 2006;24(16):2549–2556.
86. Boussemart L, Routier E, Mateus C, et al. Prospective study of cutaneous side-effects associated with the BRAF inhibitor vemurafenib: a study of 42 patients. *Ann Oncol.* 2013;24(6):1691–1697.
99. Nakagawa K, Kudoh S, Ohe Y, et al. Postmarketing surveillance study of erlotinib in Japanese patients with non-small-cell lung cancer (NSCLC): an interim analysis of 3488 patients (POLARSTAR). *J Thorac Oncol.* 2012;7(8):1296–1303.

See Expertconsult.com for full list of references.

50 Immunotherapy and Lung Cancer

Leena Gandhi, Johan F. Vansteenkiste, and Frances A. Shepherd

SUMMARY OF KEY POINTS

- Immunotherapy has entered a new era in lung cancer and is rapidly changing the standard of care.
- Vaccines as monotherapies have shown marginal efficacy in certain settings.
- Program death-1 (PD1) and PD1 ligand (PDL1) inhibitors have showed marked and durable responses for a broad subset of lung cancer patients with overall survival rates that far exceed what has been seen with chemotherapy. In addition, the overall toxicity rate is lower than what has been seen with chemotherapy.
- PDL1 is a potential but imperfect biomarker of response in nonsmall cell lung cancer.
- Combination therapies (with other immunomodulators, vaccines, chemotherapy, and radiation) are actively being explored to extend the benefit of PD1 inhibition to more patients.

Lung cancer is the leading cause of cancer-related death, and 85% of patients with this condition are diagnosed with nonsmall cell lung cancer (NSCLC). Modest improvements in cure rates have been observed among patients with early and locally advanced disease; nevertheless, the majority of patients die as a result of a metastatic progression of the cancer.[1] Patients with advanced-stage NSCLC have a median overall survival (OS) of 10 months and a 1-year survival rate of about 40% when treated with modern platinum-doublet chemotherapy, although this time frame has somewhat been extended to a median OS of 13.9 months with maintenance pemetrexed following cisplatin–pemetrexed in nonsquamous lung carcinoma.[2] Tumors with specific oncogenic drivers are particularly sensitive to specific tyrosine kinase inhibitors that represent significant improvements over chemotherapy for these subgroups. Such therapy is approved for tumors with activating epidermal growth factor receptor (EGFR) mutation, anaplastic lymphoma kinase translocation, or c-ros oncogene (ROS) translocation, and several other oncogenic drivers have targeted therapies in development. However, there are still large populations of NSCLC without any targeted therapy available to them.

Immunotherapy using programmed death receptor (PD1) or PD1 ligand (PDL1) inhibitors has already changed the outcomes for advanced NSCLC patients, in some cases more than doubling survival times, and the survival improvements that are possible with combination therapy are still to be determined. As in many tumor types, the rapid advent of immunotherapy-based regimens built on a backbone of PD1 or PDL1 inhibition is rapidly changing our standards of care. Many trials of PD1/PDL1 inhibitors are ongoing in patients in different stages of lung cancer, in combination with vaccines, chemotherapy, radiation, targeted therapy, and with novel immunotherapeutics, suggesting that more change is yet to come.

IMMUNOLOGIC DYSFUNCTION IN PATIENTS WITH LUNG CANCER

The principle of immunosurveillance, that is, the ability of the immune system to recognize malignant cells as foreign and, possibly, to eliminate them, has long been accepted, but the many potential mechanisms of tumor evasion from immune surveillance are now beginning to be targeted with therapeutic agents.[3]

Normal immunosurveillance starts with uptake of tumor antigens by antigen-presenting cells (APCs), particularly dendritic cells (Fig. 50.1). The antigens are internalized, processed into small peptide sequences, and displayed on the extracellular surface of the APC in the presence of the class I and class II major histocompatibility complex (MHC). The dendritic cell with antigenic peptides on its surface circulates to the draining lymph nodes and matures, leading to interaction with naive T lymphocytes.[4]

This interaction results in activation of the CD4+ T-helper lymphocytes—with liberation of several cytokines, for example, interleukin-2 (IL-2; Th1 cells), IL-12 (dendritic cells), and interferon gamma (Th1 cells)—and subsequent activation of CD8+ T cells into cytotoxic T lymphocytes.[5] For this T-cell activation to occur, there must be an interaction between the specific T-cell receptor on naive T cells and the antigen presented by the APC on an MHC molecule. A required costimulatory event is the interaction between the B7 molecules (B7-1 [CD80], B7-2 [CD86]) on the APCs and CD28 on the T cells (Fig. 50.2).[6] Finally, activated cytotoxic T lymphocytes will recognize tumor cells (TCs) that display the complementary peptide–MHC class 1 complex on their cell surface and induce apoptotic cell death.[3,7]

To prevent excessive reactions with autoimmunity and damage to normal host tissue, modulation of activated CD8+ cells is required. Activated CD8+ T cells also express cytotoxic T lymphocyte-associated antigen-4 (CTLA-4) on their surface. Binding of CTLA-4 with CD80 or CD86 on APCs provides an inhibitory signal and limits further T-cell activation. This mechanism against autoimmunity also may be responsible for the tolerance of tumor antigens.[8] Although PD1 was identified on exhausted T cells in 1992, it was after the discovery of the PDL1 ligand (B7-H1) on lymphoid and nonlymphoid tissues that the role of PDL1:PD1-mediated downregulation of immune activation in peripheral tissues was clarified.[9,10] Interaction of PD1 with its ligand results in downregulation of T-cell mediated cell killing, altered cytokine production, and ultimately apoptosis.[10–14] PDL1 is expressed in various normal tissues in response to inflammatory cytokine signaling to maintain self-tolerance. This same mechanism can be co-opted by TCs to avoid an acquired immune response to tumor-associated antigens.[15,16]

Overall, lung cancer and other tumors can induce major immunologic dysfunction through a variety of mechanisms. Downregulation of antigens and decrease of expression of MHC class I molecules and costimulatory molecules lead to failure of T-cell recognition and activation. Inhibitory cytokines such as indoleamine 2,3-dioxygenase and transforming growth factor-beta (TGF-β) impede the maturation of dendritic cells and promote the development of T-regulatory cells and myeloid-derived suppressor cells, which have a powerful immunosuppressive action. Inhibition of T-cell activation by the CTLA-4 interaction

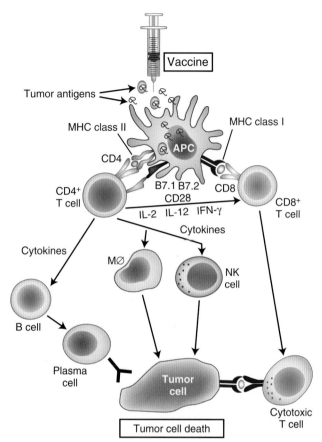

Fig. 50.1. Schema of the steps involved in tumor immunology and vaccination. *APC,* antigen-presenting cell; *IFN,* interferon; *IL,* interleukin; *MHC,* major histocompatibility complex; *MØ,* macrophage; *NK cell,* natural killer cell. *(Reprinted with permission from Mellstedt H, Vansteenkiste J, Thatcher N. Vaccines for the treatment of non-small cell lung cancer: investigational approaches and clinical experience.* Lung Cancer. *2011;73:11–17.)*

with B7 and PDL1–PD1 interactions to suppress effector T-cell function can contribute centrally and locally to immune suppression. Lastly, the failure to activate apoptotic mechanisms in response to the effect of cytotoxic T lymphocytes may render the lung cancer cells insensitive to immune control.[17]

SUPPORTING EVIDENCE FOR THE USE OF IMMUNOTHERAPY FOR LUNG CANCER

Although lung cancer historically was not considered to be an immunogenic malignancy, there is evidence suggesting that there may be important immune responses in patients with lung cancer. The LACE-Bio group, in a study of 1600 patients with resected early-stage NSCLC, found that marked infiltration of the tumor by lymphocytes was associated with significantly longer disease-free survival and OS (hazard ratio [HR], 0.57 [*p* = 0.0002] and 0.56 [*p* = 0.0003], respectively).[18] Other studies also have shown that increased stromal infiltration of CD4+/CD8+ T cells is independently associated with better prognosis in cases of early-stage NSCLC.[19,20] By contrast, high expression of tumor-infiltrating T-regulatory cells— that is, reduced antitumor immunity—has been associated with recurrence of disease.[21,22] Patients with advanced-stage NSCLC, in whom tumors have higher numbers of macrophages and CD8+ T cells compared with the surrounding stroma, have better survival rates.[23] The overexpression of PDL1 by TCs in NSCLC has been demonstrated in several retrospective studies, which have reported rates of 27% to 58%. Several of these studies report an increased

inflammatory infiltrate associated with PDL1 overexpression.[24–29] The expression of PDL1 by TCs may also be mediated by the activation of specific oncogenes associated with NSCLC including EGFR.[24,30–32] Smoking status has also been correlated with elevated PDL1 expression.[32] However, the association between OS and PDL1 expression remains controversial with reports of both an associated improvement and decrease in OS.[24–27] PDL1 overexpression and associated activation of the PD1 pathway thus appear to be broadly exploited by TCs in NSCLC as a means to evade T-cell-mediated antitumor activity. These findings support the strategy to use or manipulate the immune system to generate antitumor effects to improve the outcomes for patients with lung cancer.

The approaches toward therapeutic modulation of immune responses fall into two primary categories. The first, "active" immunotherapy includes modes of stimulating the immune response, such as ILs, interferons, or antigen-specific immunotherapy. Historically, and even in some recent large phase III trials, "active" immunomodulatory agents that stimulate immune response have been associated with disappointing results in lung cancer. Historical examples include trials investigating bacillus Calmette-Guérin,[33] levamisole,[34] or interferons and ILs.[35] More recent examples include trials investigating PF-3512676 (ProMune), an agonist of the toll-like receptor 9 that enhances maturation of dendritic cells,[36,37] and talactoferrin alpha, an oral recombinant human lactoferrin, acting by dendritic cell recruitment and activation in the gut-associated lymphoid tissue.[38]

Therapeutic cancer vaccination is a mode of antigen-specific "active" immunotherapy in which the immune system is primed to produce antigen-specific antibodies, CD4+ T-helper cells, and CD8+ cytotoxic T lymphocytes against relevant tumor-associated antigens. This has been an active area of research in lung cancer, but one that has had largely marginal benefits seen as monotherapies to date, which are reviewed in the following sections.

The second approach, "passive immunotherapy," involves blocking inhibitory signals that suppress immune responses against cancer. Examples of the latter include monoclonal antibodies that modulate T-cell activity by inhibiting CTLA-4, PD1, or PDL1, also known as immune checkpoint inhibitors. It is this latter category of therapy, specifically PD1 and PDL1 antibodies, that has galvanized the field of immunotherapy in lung cancer by demonstrating marked clinical benefit in subsets of patients and this, therefore, will constitute the majority of the discussion here.

VACCINES

Antigen-specific immunotherapeutic agents always have two major components. The first component consists of immunogenic tumor-associated antigens, which can be DNA, RNA, peptides, recombinant proteins, gangliosides, or whole TCs. However, the presence of tumor-associated antigens alone is insufficient for a therapeutic cancer vaccine as the immune system already has failed to control the cells expressing these antigens; otherwise, the tumor would not have grown to a clinical level. Therefore, a strong adjuvant is added to potentiate the immune response.[39] This immunoadjuvant can be a phospholipid or aluminum formulation, a viral vector, a dendritic cell, or a liposome preparation. There are many vaccination strategies and compounds in development. Most have been evaluated either in the adjuvant setting or following first-line chemotherapy in the advanced setting to determine whether they can stave off progression of disease. We will review some of the agents that are still in clinical development and the change in direction now being taken with the success of immune checkpoint inhibitors.

Melanoma-Associated Antigen-A3 Vaccine

Melanoma-associated antigen (MAGE)-A3 is expressed almost exclusively on TCs and is not expressed in normal tissue, except in male germ line cells; however, such cells do not present the antigen as they lack MHC molecules.[40] The function of MAGE-A3 is unknown, but its expression has been associated with worse prognosis in cases of lung cancer.[41] Expression has been documented in 35% of early-stage NSCLC.[42]

The vaccine contains a recombinant fusion protein (MAGE-A3 and protein D of *Haemophilus influenzae*) in combination with an immune response-enhancing adjuvant (AS02B in the phase II study and AS15 in the phase III study).[43]

For NSCLC, the proof-of-concept study was a double-blind, placebo-controlled randomized phase II trial.[44] Patients with completely resected MAGE-A3-positive stage IB to stage II NSCLC were randomly assigned to receive MAGE-A3 vaccine (122 patients) or placebo (60 patients). No adjuvant chemotherapy was given, as this therapy was not recommended at the time of the study. The disease-free interval was the primary end point of the study and, at a median of 70 months after resection, there was a nonsignificant trend in favor of MAGE-A3 (HR for disease-free interval, 0.75; 95% confidence interval [CI], 0.46–1.23; p = 0.254). A potential gene signature, which was found to be predictive of the clinical activity of the MAGE-A3 vaccine in a trial involving patients with metastatic melanoma,[45] was further validated in a separate study in early-stage NSCLC.[46] The disease-free interval was better for actively treated patients with NSCLC and a positive gene signature compared with patients who received placebo (HR, 0.42; 95% CI, 0.17–1.03; p = 0.06); among patients with a negative gene signature, no benefit was found (HR, 1.17; 95% CI, 0.59–2.31; p = 0.65).

On the basis of these data, a large double-blind, randomized placebo-controlled phase III trial (MAGE-A3 as Adjuvant NSCLC Immunotherapy Trial [MAGRIT]) was conducted from 2007 to 2012 and reported in 2016.[47] Patients with MAGE-A3 overexpression (4210 of 13,489 originally screened) who had completely resected stage IB to stage IIIA NSCLC and adjuvant chemotherapy as clinically indicated were randomly assigned (in a 2:1 ratio) to receive MAGE-A3 vaccine or placebo. There was no difference in disease-free survival between the two groups: median 60.5 months in the vaccinated group and 58.0 months in the placebo group (HR, 0.97; 95% CI, 0.80–1.18; p = 0.76). In the absence of any treatment effect, no gene signature predictive of response could be evaluated or validated. Further development of the MAGE-A3 vaccine in NSCLC has been stopped.

Mucinous Glycoprotein-1 Vaccines

Tecemotide (L-BLP25)

Mucinous glycoprotein-1 (MUC1) is a highly glycosylated transmembrane protein that is present in normal tissue only at the apical surface of the epithelial cell.[48] Its exact function remains unclear, but MUC1 may promote cell growth and survival.[49] In cancer cells, MUC1 is overexpressed with loss of polarity of expression and is underglycosylated or aberrantly glycosylated, which results in unmasking of its peptide epitopes, thus identifying a potential target for immunotherapy.[50]

Tecemotide (L-BLP25) is a peptide vaccine based on a 25-amino-acid sequence from the MUC1 protein in a liposomal delivery system (consisting of cholesterol, dimyristoyl phosphatidylglycerol, and dipalmitoyl phosphatidylcholine), which facilitates uptake by APCs, and monophosphoryl lipid A, which is added to enhance immune stimulation.[51]

In an open-label phase II randomized study, 171 patients with stage IIIB to stage IV NSCLC who had a response or stable disease after first-line therapy were randomly assigned to best supportive care plus tecemotide (88 patients) or best supportive care alone (83 patients).[52] The median OS was not significantly different in patients who were treated with tecemotide, compared with those treated with best supportive care alone (13.0 months; HR, 0.739; 95% CI, 0.509–1.073; p = 0.112). In a post hoc analysis by stage, tecemotide did not provide benefit to patients with stage IV disease but it did provide some benefit to patients with stage IIIB disease who were treated with chemoradiation therapy (HR, 0.524; 95% CI, 0.261–1.052; p = 0.069).

A phase III, double-blind study was conducted in stage III patients and confirmed these findings,[53] showing no significant survival benefit in those treated with vaccine (829 patients; median OS, 25.6 months; 95% CI, 22.5–29.2) compared with those treated with placebo (410 patients; median OS, 22.3 months; 95% CI, 19.6–25.5 months; adjusted HR for modified intention-to-treat population, 0.88; 95% CI, 0.75–1.03; p = 0.123). Again, in the subgroup of patients who received concurrent chemotherapy plus radiation (as opposed to sequential) prior to vaccination, there was a statistically significant benefit. The OS in the vaccinated group was 30.8 months (95% CI, 25.6–36.8) compared with 20.6 months (95% CI, 17.4–23.9) for those who received placebo (adjusted HR, 0.78; 95% CI, 0.64–0.95; p = 0.016). A follow-up report with longer follow-up confirmed these findings and suggested that high levels of serum MUC1 and antinuclear antibodies (ANA), correlated with a possible survival benefit (interaction p = 0.0085 and 0.0022) for tecemotide.[54] Further development of this vaccine as a monotherapy has been stopped.

TG4010 Vaccine

The TG4010 vaccine also targets MUC1 as well as IL-2. It uses a viral vector—attenuated Ankara virus—that has been genetically modified to express the full MUC1 protein and IL-2 and exogenous IL-2 used as an immunoadjuvant to try to overcome the T-cell suppression caused by the cancer-associated MUC1 mucin.[55] This vaccine was tested in a slightly different setting, given not as "adjuvant" therapy after chemotherapy, but in combination therapy in the metastatic setting.

In an open-label phase II randomized study, 148 untreated patients with MUC1-expressing stage IIIB to stage IV NSCLC were randomly assigned to receive up to six cycles of cisplatin and gemcitabine with or without TG4010. The 6-month rate of progression-free survival (PFS) was not statistically different between the two arms (43% vs. 35%; p = 0.13), but higher response rate was seen in the experimental arm (43% vs. 27%; p = 0.03). In a subgroup analysis, the level of activated natural killer (NK) cells acted as a possible predictive factor. In patients with normal levels of NK cells, the PFS rate at 6 months was 58%, compared with 38% for placebo (p = 0.04), and OS was significantly better (18 vs. 11.3 months; p = 0.02).[56] Side effects related to TG4010 were mild and most commonly included injection-site reactions, fever, and abdominal pain.

A phase IIb randomized, double-blind, placebo-controlled trial to evaluate first-line chemotherapy with or without TG4010 for patients with MUC1-positive (at least 50% expression on TCs) stage IV NSCLC was reported in 2016.[57] In this trial, patients received four to six cycles of a platinum-based doublet chemotherapy (bevacizumab allowed) and TG4010 or placebo until disease progression or treatment discontinuation for any reason. The primary end point was PFS to validate the predictive value of the previously identified TrPAL biomarker (CD16, CD56, and CD69 triple-positive activated lymphocytes) as a marker of benefit. From 2012 to 2014, 22 patients were randomized to TG4010 and chemotherapy and 111 to placebo. The median PFS in the vaccinated group was 5.9 months versus 5.1 months in the placebo group (HR, 0.74; 95% CI, 0.55–0.98; one-sided p = 0.019). The primary end point was met because in patients with the TrPAL biomarker less than the upper limit of normal, the HR for PFS was less than 1 (HR, 0.75; 95% CI, 0.54–10.3), although notably the

CI crosses 1. The phase III portion of the study is continuing with OS as the primary end point.

Belagenpumatucel-L

Belagenpumatucel-L is an allogeneic whole-tumor-cell vaccine derived from four irradiated NSCLC cell lines (two adenocarcinomas, one squamous cell carcinoma, and one large cell carcinoma) that have been transfected with a plasmid containing a TGF-β2 antisense transgene, which downregulates TGF-β2. Elevated levels of TGF-β2 are known to be linked to immunosuppression in patients with cancer, and TGF-β2 levels are inversely correlated with prognosis in patients with NSCLC.[58]

Whole-tumor-cell vaccines can expose the host immune system to a wide range of tumor antigens. Although autologous TCs generally are thought to provide the panel of antigens most representative of the tumor in an individual patient, their practical use is limited by the complex production process. The G-VAX vaccine initially was associated with promising findings in a phase II study involving 83 patients with NSCLC, but further development was abandoned because of logistic problems.[59]

Belagenpumatucel-L was investigated in a phase II single-arm dose-range study involving 75 patients with NSCLC of various stages that suggested improved survival among advanced-stage patients treated at high dose.[58] This vaccine was further studied in the phase III randomized STOP trial.[60] Patients with stage IIIA (T3 N2), stage IIIB, and stage IV disease, without progression after first-line chemotherapy, were randomly assigned to treatment with intradermal belagenpumatucel-L (270 patients) or placebo (262 patients), once monthly for 18 months and then once at 21 months and 24 months. There was no difference in survival for the vaccinated group (median OS, 20.3 months), compared with the placebo group (17.8 months; HR, 0.94; p = 0.594). There were also no differences in PFS. However, a prespecified Cox regression analysis demonstrated that time from chemotherapy (<12 weeks) and the receipt of radiation were associated with benefit, suggesting that there still may be a role for this vaccine in certain settings.[60]

Epidermal Growth Factor Vaccine

Given the prevalence of EGFR overexpression in NSCLC and the importance of EGFR signaling in multiple subtypes of NSCLC, an EGF vaccine (CimaVax) was developed in Cuba with recombinant human EGF coupled to a carrier protein (P64K *Neisseria meningitidis* protein) and emulsified in Montanide ISA-51.[61] A randomized phase III trial conducted in Cuba in 405 NSCLC patients with stage IIIB/IV disease who had completed first-line chemotherapy demonstrated a nonsignificant improvement in median survival for the vaccinated group (10.83 months, 95% CI, 8.85–12.71 months) versus the control group (8.86 months, 95% CI, 6.69–11.03 months).[62] When a weighted log rank was used, given the late separation of curves, the survival difference became significant. High baseline EGF levels were associated with poorer survival overall, but for those with high baseline EGFR, vaccination was associated with improved survival (HR, 0.41; 95% CI, 0.25–0.67; p = 0.0001); however, the CIs for median survival in each arm were very wide. A new international randomized trial, comparing best supportive care alone with best supportive care plus this vaccine after conventional first-line treatment for advanced NSCLC, was started in 2011 and is still ongoing (ClinicalTrials.gov identifier: NCT01444118).

Racotumomab

This compound, formerly known as 1E10, is an anti-idiotype ganglioside vaccine. Gangliosides are involved in cell–cell recognition, cell matrix adhesion, and cell differentiation and are expressed on the surface of TCs. The compound targets Neu-glycosylated sialic acid-containing ganglioside (NeuGc-GM3), a variant of the normal Neu-acetylated sialic acid ganglioside, which is identified almost exclusively in transformed cells, making NeuGc-GM3 an attractive target for immunotherapy.[63,64]

Racotumomab was evaluated in a prospective, randomized, open-label study in Cuba in 176 patients with stage III/IV NSCLC with objective response or stable disease after standard first-line treatment.[65] The intent to treat median OS was 8.2 months versus 6.8 months in the placebo arm (HR, 0.63; 95% CI, 0.46–0.87; p = 0.004), but the OS in both arms were notably low. Fewer than 30% of patients were evaluated for immune response. A confirmatory randomized phase III multinational trial is still ongoing (ClinicalTrials.gov identifier: NCT01460472).

Overall, strategies using vaccine in early- or later-stage lung cancer have proved disappointing, with marginal improvements in survival in select circumstances that require validation. However, one explanation for the lack of effectiveness of vaccines is the possibility that local immune suppression around the tumor prevents the mounting of a sufficient immune response to actually shrink tumors and halt growth. The advent of checkpoint inhibition may alter the potential for vaccines through combination strategies as described in the following section.

IMMUNE CHECKPOINT INHIBITORS: AGENTS AND CLINICAL DEVELOPMENT

Far more promising than the "active immunotherapy" agents studied to date is the recent experience with "passive immunotherapy," such as monoclonal antibodies that modulate T-cell activity by inhibiting CTLA-4, PD1, or PDL1 (immune checkpoint inhibitors).

CTLA-4 is an immunomodulatory molecule that acts as a negative regulator in the early phase of T-cell-mediated immune responses. With CTLA-4, immune activation takes place when there is binding between the antigen presented on the dendritic cell and the T-cell receptor in the presence of costimulatory binding of B7 and CD28, whereas inhibition takes place when coexistent B7 binding is with CTLA-4 (see Fig. 50.2 left panel). Anti-CTLA-4 antibodies prevent interaction between CTLA-4 and its ligands, resulting in relief of the inhibitory signal provided by CTLA-4 and consequent enhancement of activation and proliferation of tumor-specific T cells.[66,67]

In the later phase, immune effector functions take place when there is binding between an antigen presented on tumor tissue and the T-cell receptor. The normal role of PD1 and its ligands is to limit the activity of T cells in peripheral tissues at the time of an inflammatory response to limit autoimmunity.[68] In the context of antitumor activity of CD8+ lymphocytes, however, this same blockade does not allow efficient TC kill (see Fig. 50.2 right panel). Anti-PD1 and anti-PDL1 antibodies reverse this inhibition, and thus they restore antitumor immune effector functions.[69]

Checkpoint Inhibitors
Anti-CTLA-4 Antibodies

Ipilimumab. Ipilimumab is a humanized immunoglobulin G1 (IgG1) anti-CTLA-4 monoclonal antibody, which is an effective and approved agent for the treatment of melanoma but has had no clear single-agent activity in NSCLC or SCLC.[70,71] In a phase II trial in both NSCLC and SCLC, patients received six cycles of carboplatin–paclitaxel chemotherapy plus placebo or plus ipilimumab in two different sequences: either concurrent (four cycles of chemotherapy plus ipilimumab followed by two cycles plus placebo) or phased ipilimumab (two cycles of chemotherapy plus placebo followed by four cycles plus ipilimumab). For eligible patients, ipilimumab or placebo was administered every 12 weeks as maintenance therapy after chemotherapy and the

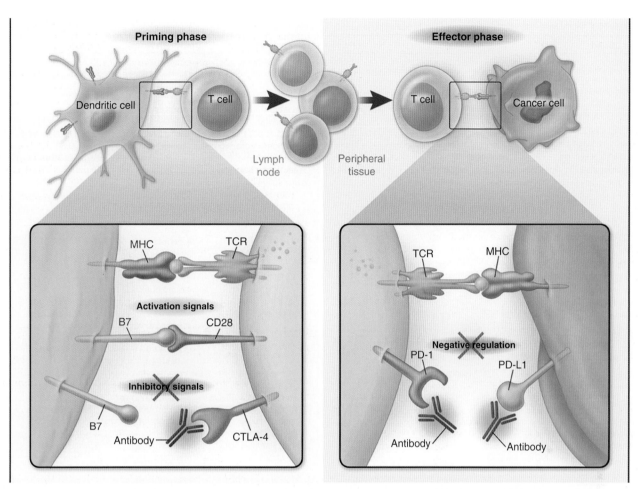

Fig. 50.2. Blockade of PD-1 or CTLA-4 signaling in tumor immunotherapy. T cells recognize antigens presented by the major histocompatibility complex (MHC) on the surface of cancer cells through their T-cell receptor (TCR). This first signal is not enough to turn on a T-cell response, and a second signal delivered by the B7 costimulatory molecules B7-1 (or CD80) and B7-2 (or CD86) is required. Cytotoxic T-lymphocyte–associated antigen 4 (CTLA-4) is up-regulated shortly after T-cell activation and initiates negative regulation signaling on T cells during ligation with the B7 costimulatory molecules expressed by antigen-presenting cells. When these molecules bind to CD28, they provide activation signals; when they bind to CTLA-4, they provide inhibitory signals. The interaction between CTLA-4 and the costimulatory molecules happens primarily in the priming phase of a T-cell response within lymph nodes. Programmed death 1 (PD-1) inhibitory receptor is expressed by T cells during long-term antigen exposure and results in negative regulation on T cells during ligation with PD-L1 and PD-L2, which are primarily expressed within inflamed tissues and the tumor microenvironment. The PD-1 interaction happens in the effector phase of a T-cell response in peripheral tissues. Its blockade with antibodies to PD-1 or PD-L1 results in the preferential activation of T cells with specificity for the cancer. *(Reprinted with permission from Ribas A.,* N Eng J Med. *2012;366:2517–2519.)*

primary end point was immune-related PFS (irPFS) as defined by Wolchok and colleagues.[72] In the NSCLC study, the irPFS was significantly better for patients treated with phased ipilimumab than for controls (HR, 0.72; $p = 0.05$), but it was not significantly better for patients treated with concurrent ipilimumab than it was for controls (HR, 0.81; $p = 0.13$, but in the small squamous cell subgroup, HR was 0.55).[70] Median irPFS rates were 5.7 months, 5.5 months, and 4.6 months for the phased ipilimumab, concurrent ipilimumab, and control groups, respectively. There was no significant difference in OS, and the rates of grade 3 and grade 4 immune-related adverse events were high (15%, 20%, and 6%, respectively).

The results of the SCLC study were similar.[73] Phased ipilimumab improved irPFS compared with the control (HR, 0.64; $p = 0.03$) but concurrent ipilimumab did not (HR, 0.75; $p = 0.11$). The median irPFS rates for the phased ipilimumab, concurrent ipilimumab, and control groups were 6.4 months, 5.7 months, and 5.3 months, respectively. There was no significant improvement in OS (HR, 0.75; $p = 0.13$). The overall rates of grade 3 and grade 4 immune-related adverse events were 17%, 21%, and 9%, respectively.

On the basis of these results, two phase III trials using phased ipilimumab were initiated with OS as the primary end point: one in squamous cell carcinoma and one in SCLC. Both studies showed absolutely no OS benefit or PFS benefit with increased rates of toxicities for the ipilimumab arm (squamous study [unpublished] and SCLC study).[73] In the squamous cell study, among 388 patients treated with blinded therapy with chemotherapy plus ipilimumab, the median OS was 13.4 months compared with 12.4 months in 361 patients treated with chemotherapy plus placebo (HR, 0.91; 95% CI, 0.77–1.07; $p = 0.25$; results not published but are presented on ClinicalTrials.gov [NCT01285609]). In the SCLC study, median OS was 11 months for the ipilimumab-containing arm and 10.9 months for the placebo plus chemotherapy arm (HR, 0.94; 95% CI, 0.81–1.09; $p = 0.38$).[73]

Anti-PD1 and Anti-PDL1 Antibodies

Several monoclonal antibodies are in various stages of research. We focus here on the antibodies currently approved for treatment of NSCLC, including nivolumab, pembrolizumab, and atezolizumab. Other agents, such as durvalumab and avelumab,

TABLE 50.1 First-Line Randomized Studies of Checkpoint Inhibition

Compound	Trial	Design	No. of Patients	Study Population	Treatment Arms	Primary End Point
Nivolumab[74]	Phase III CheckMate 026 NCT02041533	Randomized vs. first-line platinum-based chemotherapy	541	Treatment-naive metastatic NSCLC	Nivolumab vs. platinum-based chemotherapy	PFS in prespecified subset of those with ≥5% PDL1 expression
Pembrolizumab[75]	Phase III (KEYNOTE-024)	Randomized vs. first-line platinum-based chemotherapy	305 (randomized population)	Treatment-naive metastatic NSCLC with ≥50% PDL1 tumoral expression	Pembrolizumab vs. platinum-based chemotherapy	PFS: 10.3 months vs. 6.0 months for chemotherapy (HR, 0.50; 95% CI, 0.37–0.68; $p < 0.001$)
Pembrolizumab[76]	Phase III (KEYNOTE-042) NCT02220894	Randomized open-label	1240	Treatment-naive metastatic NSCLC with ≥1% PDL1 positivity	Pembrolizumab vs. platinum-based chemotherapy	OS
Atezolizumab[77]	Phase III: Several ongoing studies IMpower110 NCT02409342 (others ongoing as well)	Randomized open-label	570	Treatment-naive metastatic NSCLC	Atezolizumab vs. platinum + pemetrexed (nonsquamous) or platinum + gemcitabine (squamous)	PFS and OS
Nivolumab/ ipilimumab	Phase III CheckMate 227 NCT02477826	Randomized open-label	2220	Treatment-naive metastatic NSCLC	Nivolumab vs. nivolumab/ ipilimumab vs. platinum-based chemotherapy ± nivolumab	OS and PFS of the monotherapy vs. chemotherapy or combination vs. chemotherapy
Durvalumab/ tremelimumab	Phase III (MYSTIC) NCT02453282	Randomized open-label	810	Treatment-naive metastatic NSCLC in subgroups (PDL1 positive and PDL1 negative)	Durvalumab vs. durvalumab/ tremelimumab vs. platinum-based chemotherapy	PFS and OS of the combination vs. platinum-based chemotherapy
Durvalumab/ tremelimumab	Phase III (NEPTUNE) NCT02542293	Randomized open-label	800	Treatment-naive metastatic NSCLC in stratified subgroups (PDL1 positive and PDL1 negative)	Durvalumab/ tremelimumab vs. standard of care platinum-based chemotherapy	OS

CI, confidence interval; *HR,* hazard ratio; *NSCLC,* nonsmall cell lung cancer; *OS,* overall survival; *PDL1,* PD1 ligand 1; *PFS,* progression-free survival.

are also in clinical development in lung cancer, although the focus for these agents has been on combination studies, which are still in the early stage and ongoing at this time and so are beyond the scope of this chapter. Table 50.1 outlines some of the major completed and ongoing studies evaluating checkpoint inhibitors as an alternative to standard therapy. Table 50.2 outlines major trials completed and ongoing combining checkpoint inhibitors with standard chemotherapy.

Initial Phase I Studies

Nivolumab (BMS-936558, MDX-1106/ONO-4538, OPDIVO)

Nivolumab is a fully human IgG4 antibody targeting PD1. The proof-of-principle study was a phase I dose-escalation study involving 296 patients with refractory solid tumors who received intravenous nivolumab at a dosage of 1 mg/kg, 3 mg/kg, or 10 mg/kg every 2 weeks for 8 weeks.[80] Response was evaluated according to Response Evaluation Criteria in Solid Tumors (RECIST), and patients with nonprogressive disease or clinically stable disease (even with progression according to RECIST) could continue for as many as 12 8-week cycles or until disease progression or complete response occurred. The cumulative response rate was 18% (14 of 76) among patients with NSCLC. Responses were durable and lasted for more than a year in many cases. Clinical response was related to expression of PDL1 in tumor biopsy specimens (as determined using the 28-8 antibody on a DAKO platform),

which were available for only a small subset of 42 patients. The rate of grade 3 or grade 4 treatment-related adverse events was 14%, and there were three drug-related deaths from pneumonitis. Longer follow-up data demonstrated a median OS of 9.6 months for pretreated patients, with 1- and 2-year survival rates of 42% and 14%, respectively.[81]

Pembrolizumab (MK-3475, Keytruda)

Pembrolizumab is a fully humanized IgG4 antibody targeting PD1 that was also initially tested in lung cancer as part of a broader phase I study in multiple tumor types (KEYNOTE-001). Initial lung cancer data in 495 patients established a role for PDL1 as a predictive biomarker of response.[82] Patients treated at different doses and dosing schedules were pooled for the biomarker analysis but divided into a training and validation cohort to establish a cutoff for tumor PDL1 expression that was predictive of response to pembrolizumab. Tumor PDL1 expression was evaluated in a contemporaneous biopsy specimen (as opposed to nivolumab studies) using a distinct, proprietary IHC assay and PDL1 antibody (clone 22C3, Merck), also on a DAKO platform.

Overall, the study demonstrated a relative risk (RR) of 19.4% and a median duration of response of 12.5 months. In the overall study population, the median PFS was 3.7 months and the median OS was 12.0 months. A cutoff for tumor PDL1 positivity of 50% or greater was selected as a cutoff for predictive value based on receiver-operating-characteristic curve analysis of the

TABLE 50.2 First-Line Randomized Studies of Checkpoint Inhibition Plus Chemotherapy

Compound	Trial	Design	No. of Patients	Study Population	Treatment Arms	Primary End Point
Nivolumab (Rizvi et al. 2016)[78]	Phase I, CheckMate 012 NCT01454102	Open-label combination of nivolumab with platinum-based chemotherapy	56	Treatment-naive metastatic NSCLC	A. Nivolumab + cisplatin/gemcitabine B. Nivolumab + cisplatin/pemetrexed C. Nivolumab (10 mg/kg) + carboplatin/paclitaxel D. Nivolumab (5 mg/kg) + carboplatin + paclitaxel	**Safety RR** A. 33%; B. 47%; C. 47%; D. 43% **24-week PFR** A. 51%; B. 71%; C. 38%; D. 51% **2-year OS** A. 25%; B. 33%; C. 27%; D. 62%
Nivolumab	Phase III, CheckMate 227 NCT02477826	Randomized first-line platinum-based chemotherapy ± nivolumab vs. nivolumab alone vs. nivolumab + ipilimumab	2220	Treatment-naive metastatic NSCLC	Platinum-based chemotherapy ± nivolumab OR nivolumab/ipilimumab OR nivolumab alone	PFS and OS of nivolumab and nivolumab/ipilimumab vs. chemotherapy alone
Pembrolizumab (Langer et al. 2016)[79]	Phase II (KEYNOTE-021) NCT02039674	Open-label, randomized phase II pembrolizumab ± cisplatin/pemetrexed	123	Treatment-naive metastatic nonsquamous NSCLC	Cisplatin + pemetrexed ± pembrolizumab	RR: 55% RR in combination vs. 29% with chemotherapy alone PFS: 13 months vs. 8.9 months (HR, 0.53; 95% CI, 0.31–0.91; p = 0.0102)
Pembrolizumab	Phase III (Merck 189, NCT02578680 and Merck 407, NCT02775435)	Randomized first-line platinum-based chemotherapy ± pembrolizumab	570 (189) and 560 (405)	Treatment-naive metastatic NSCLC	Pembrolizumab vs. platinum–pemetrexed in nonsquamous NSCLC (189) or platinum–nab-paclitaxel in squamous NSCLC (405)	PFS
Atezolizumab	Phase III Several ongoing studies IMpower110 NCT02409342 (others ongoing as well)	Randomized open-label	570	Treatment-naive metastatic NSCLC	Platinum + pemetrexed (nonsquamous) or platinum + gemcitabine (squamous) ± atezolizumab	PFS and OS

CI, confidence interval; *HR,* hazard ratio; *NSCLC,* nonsmall cell lung cancer; *OS,* overall survival time; *PFR,* progression-free rate; *PFS,* progression-free survival; *RR,* response rate.

training cohort. Patients with tumor PDL1 expression levels above this threshold exhibited an RR of 45.2% in the validation cohort. The median PFS of patients above this threshold was 6.3 months and the median OS was not yet reached at the time of the publication; there was a clear separation of PFS and OS curves for the 50% or more subset compared with 1% to 49% or less than 1% curves (which tracked together). Treatment-related grade 3 to grade 5 adverse events occurred in 10% of patients with one death from pneumonitis.

Atezolizumab (MPDL3280A, Tecentriq)

Atezolizumab is a humanized IgG1 monoclonal antibody targeting PDL1. There may be benefits to targeting PDL1 rather than PD1 as this spares interruption of PDL2–PD1 interactions and therefore theoretically may have fewer side effects. In a phase I expansion study, pretreated patients with NSCLC were treated at doses of 1 mg/kg, 10 mg/kg, 15 mg/kg, or 20 mg/kg.[83] An objective response was noted in 12 (23%) of 53 evaluable patients with NSCLC. There were additional delayed responses after RECIST-determined progressive disease. Treatment-related grade 3 or grade 4 adverse events were reported in 11% of patients, with no patient having grade 3 or higher pneumonitis and only 1% of patients having diarrhea. Responses were

evaluated in the context of PDL1 expression (based on an assay using the Sp142 antibody on a VENTANA platform) on TCs and immune cells (ICs). There was a statistically significant improvement in response rate with higher PDL1 expression (p = 0.015) on ICs, but not with tumoral PDL1 expression (p = 0.920).[84] A T-helper type 1 like gene signature was also associated with response.

Second-Line Randomized Studies Establishing PD1/PDL1 Inhibition as a Standard of Care

Nivolumab (MDX-1108, OPDIVO)

Two separate phase III studies were conducted in patients with either nonsquamous (CheckMate 057) or squamous (CheckMate 017) advanced NSCLC after progression on initial chemotherapy.[85,86] The CheckMate 017 study randomized 272 squamous NSCLC patients to nivolumab versus docetaxel and met its primary end point of demonstrating improved OS with nivolumab (median 9.2 months) compared with docetaxel (median 6.0 months; HR, 0.59; 95% CI, 0.44–0.79; p < 0.001). The median PFS was higher in the nivolumab group (3.5 months vs. 2.8 months; HR, 0.62; 95% CI, 0.47–0.81; p < 0.001) as well as the objective response rate (ORR; 20%

vs. 9%; p = 0.008). No significant association between tumor PDL1 status and OS, PFS, or ORR was noted in patients treated with nivolumab with an ORR of 19% in those with 10% or more tumor PDL1 expression compared with 16% in those with 10% or less expression. However, a trend toward improved OS and PFS was noted when comparing high and low PDL1 expressing tumors.[59]

The CheckMate 057 study randomized 582 patients with nonsquamous NSCLC to receive either nivolumab or standard docetaxel in a similar trial design.[85] A similar improved OS of 12.2 months with nivolumab versus 9.4 months with docetaxel was seen. However, the benefit was not apparent early on in the study (<3 months into treatment), during which time nivolumab performed slightly worse than docetaxel, with a resulting lower median PFS (2.3 months vs. 4.2 months). Both the 1-year PFS (19% vs. 8%) and ORR (19% vs. 12%, p = 0.02) were superior with nivolumab. Unlike the squamous cell carcinoma study, this study showed a clear relationship between increasing PDL1 expression and improved outcome with an HR of 0.40 (95% CI, 0.26–0.59) for those with over 10% expression but an HR of 1.00 (95% CI, 0.76–1.31; p < 0.001) for those with less than 10% PDL1 expression.

Both studies examined tumor PDL1 expression with an IHC assay using a rabbit antihuman PDL1 antibody (clone 28-8, Epitomics) on a DAKO platform and used prespecified cutoffs for PDL1 positivity of over 1%, over 5%, and over 10%.[85,86] These thresholds for PDL1 positivity were derived from the initial phase I study of nivolumab and were subsequently evaluated in a phase II study of 117 advanced NSCLC patients (CheckMate 063), which demonstrated an ORR of 14% (7/51) among PDL1 positivity less than 5% of tumors and 24% (6/25) among PDL1 positivity in 5% or more tumors.[80,87]

Notably, based on the results from CheckMate 017, the Food and Drug Administration (FDA) granted approval to nivolumab in March 2015 for second-line treatment of squamous cell carcinoma, irrespective of PDL1 status. In October 2015, after the results of CheckMate 057 were published, the FDA expanded approval of nivolumab to include all NSCLCs. This updated approval also included new approval of the "complementary" PDL1 28-8 DAKO diagnostic test to "help physicians determine which patients may benefit most from treatment." However, there was no mandated PDL1 testing for any group, which led to rapid uptake of nivolumab as a standard second-line therapy.

Pembrolizumab

The KEYNOTE-010 study randomized 1034 advanced NSCLC patients to receive either second-line docetaxel or pembrolizumab at 2 mg/kg or 10 mg/kg.[88] This study enrolled patients with a minimum tumor PDL1 expression of 1% on an archival or contemporaneous biopsy (similar to nivolumab studies) using the Merck proprietary antibody. A significant improvement in OS was observed for pembrolizumab (2 mg/kg) over docetaxel (10.4 months vs. 8.5 months; HR, 0.71; 95% CI, 0.58–0.88; p = 0.0008) and pembrolizumab (10 mg/kg) over docetaxel (12.7 months vs. 8.5 months; HR, 0.61; 95% CI, 0.49–0.75; p < 0.0001). This effect was amplified among patients with tumor PDL1 expression of 50% or more in both pembrolizumab (2 mg/kg) to docetaxel (14.9 months vs. 8.2 months; HR, 0.54; 95% CI, 0.38–0.77; p = 0.0002) and pembrolizumab (10 mg/kg) to docetaxel (17.3 months vs. 8.2 months; HR, 0.50; 95% CI, 0.36–0.70; p < 0.0001) groups. Similarly, radiographic responses occurred at a higher rate among patients with 50% or more PDL1 expression treated with pembrolizumab at 2 mg/kg (30% vs. 18%) or 10 mg/kg (29% vs. 18%) but not docetaxel (8% vs. 9%).

Initially, the accelerated FDA approval of pembrolizumab as second-line therapy in NSCLC was based on KEYNOTE-001

and limited to the subset of patients with over 50% PDL1 expression as determined by the DAKO 22C3 PDL1 companion diagnostic assay.[82] Following the KEYNOTE-010 publication, approval was expanded to include all patients with at least 1% PDL1 expression (which has a prevalence of 66% based on that publication).[88] Notably, the incidence of treatment-related grade 3 to grade 5 adverse events was higher in this study (13% to 16%) than in the phase I study, although still significantly less than with docetaxel (35%).

Atezolizumab

The POPLAR trial was a randomized phase II trial of atezolizumab versus docetaxel in previously treated NSCLC patients, which also looked at outcomes relative to both TC expression of PDL1 and IC expression of PDL1.[89] Expression that was less than 1% was called TC0 or IC0, expression between 1% and 4% was called TC1 or IC1, expression between 5% and 49% was called TC2 or IC2, and expression over 50% was called TC3 or IC3. Expression was evaluated using the Sp142 VENTANA assay. OS was greater with atezolizumab (12.6 months; 95% CI, 9.7–16.4 months) compared with docetaxel (9.7 months; 95% CI, 8.6–12.0 months) with an HR of 0.73 (95% CI, 0.53–0.99; p = 0.04). Increasing improvement in OS was seen with increasing PDL1 expression in either the TC or IC compartment. At the highest level of expression, TC3 or IC3 (which were mostly non-overlapping), the HR was 0.49 (95% CI, 0.22–1.07; p = 0.068). However, without PDL1 expression, the HR crossed 1 (1.04; 95% CI, 0.62–1.75; p = 0.871).

The OAK trial was a randomized phase III trial of similar design to POPLAR that was published in 2016.[90] Notably this trial showed an improvement in OS for atezolizumab versus docetaxel in all groups, including those with IC0 or TC0. OS with atezolizumab was 13.8 months (95% CI, 11.8–15.7 months) versus 9.6 months with docetaxel (95% CI, 8.6–11.2 months) with an HR of 0.73 (95% CI, 0.62–0.87; p = 0.0003) similar to the POPLAR trial. In addition, the HR in the TC0 or IC0 group was similar (HR, 0.75; 95% CI, 0.59–0.96; p = 0.0102), although the HR for the TC3 or IC3 group was still better than the other subgroups (HR, 0.41; 95% CI, 0.27–0.64). This was the only group to show a PFS benefit as well. Between the POPLAR study and the OAK study, the vendor for the PDL1 assay changed, but the assay remained the same. However, it is notable that the percentage of IC0 and TC0 patients was discrepantly high in this study (45%) compared with 32% in the POPLAR study and rates close to 30% in other studies with other agents. Therefore it is unclear whether the beneficial effect seen in this subgroup was truly indicative of benefit in true PDL1 "negative" patients. However, these findings led to the FDA approval of atezolizumab in the second-line treatment of NSCLC patients, regardless of PDL1 status in December 2016.

In addition to showing improved outcomes, all of these drugs showed far lower toxicity rates than docetaxel although serious immune-related adverse events were seen with all drugs and it is not clear whether atezolizumab, a PDL1 inhibitor, has a lower toxicity rate than the PD1 inhibitors nivolumab and pembrolizumab.

First-Line PD1 Inhibition
Pembrolizumab

There are two first-line studies of pembrolizumab compared with standard first-line therapy: KEYNOTE-042, which enrolled patients regardless of PDL1 status, and KEYNOTE-024, which enrolled only those with PDL1 expression of over 50% by the 22C3 antibody DAKO assay. KEYNOTE-024 was reported in 2016 and showed a clearly superior PFS with pembrolizumab, compared with platinum-based therapy (HR, 0.5; 95% CI, 0.0.37–0.68; p < 0.001).[75] The median OS for the pembrolizumab subgroup has not been reached but the OS at 6 months was superior for the pembrolizumab arm (HR, 0.60; 95% CI, 0.41–0.89; p = 0.0005). Treatment-related grade 3 to grade 5 adverse events in the pembrolizumab subgroup were lower than with platinum-based therapy (26.6% vs. 53.3%), although arguably, this rate is higher than some earlier studies had shown. These findings have led to a rapid change in the standard of care for this subgroup of patients with the FDA approval coming shortly on the heels of the publication and presentation (October 24, 2016). As a by-product of this study, the standard of care has also changed in terms of testing for PDL1. Although two of the three approved drugs in second-line therapy have unrestricted approvals (no PDL1 threshold required) and results from studies of all three approved drugs suggest that there is a likely benefit among all patients (even though pembrolizumab was not tested in patients with no PDL1 expression), results at low-level PDL1 expression suggest identical outcomes to those with no expression from the phase I KEYNOTE-001 study.[82] However, in the absence of data in patients with less than 50% PDL1 expression, the FDA approval in a subset of patients will likely spark more widespread testing for PDL1 at diagnosis of metastatic disease.

Nivolumab

The CheckMate-026 study randomized untreated patients to receive nivolumab monotherapy versus first-line therapy with a platinum doublet (investigator's choice).[74] A prespecified analysis of tumors with over 5% PDL1 expression using the DAKO 28-8 assay showed no benefit in terms of PFS to nivolumab over chemotherapy. In fact, there was no benefit at any level of expression, including in those with over 50% expression. However, there were issues of imbalances that may have played a role including increased numbers of patients with high PDL1 expression randomized to the control arm and a greater number of women on the chemotherapy arm. These results were quite surprising given the very positive results of the KEYNOTE-024 study. Until now, the two drugs have been considered very similar in terms of efficacy and safety. The results from the ongoing KEYNOTE-042 study,[76] which is closer in patient population to the CheckMate 026 study, are eagerly awaited to better understand the appropriate group to receive first-line PD1 inhibitors.

Atezolizumab

The comparison of first-line atezolizumab with platinum-based chemotherapy is also ongoing (see Table 50.1).[91] Results from a cohort of a nonrandomized monotherapy study (BIRCH) that have been presented but not published suggest increasing response rates to atezolizumab in either the first- or second-line setting among those with higher levels of PDL1 expression.[77]

PDL1 Expression and Association With Response. The dependence on PDL1 expression for increased efficacy for all of these drugs has been hotly debated and is confounded by the use of different assays, different PD1 level cutoffs, and different biopsy requirements in studies of these different agents. In addition, heterogeneity of expression within the tumor is an important confounding factor as there is frequent geographic variation of expression.[92] An international effort at "harmonization" is ongoing through the IASLC, and a first publication reporting on the performance of four different antibodies on a set of 39 NSCLC specimens showed good concordance between three of the four antibodies:[93] the VENTANA Sp142 assay was an outlier (lower sensitivity). It is not clear whether this lower sensitivity may be a

factor in the high rate of PDL1 negatives seen in the OAK study. IC staining was more variable between all of the antibodies. A second study tested three of the same antibodies—the VENTANA Sp263 (used with durvalumab), DAKO 22C3 (pembrolizumab), and DAKO 28-8 (nivolumab)—in 500 NSCLC samples obtained commercially and showed an agreement of over 90% between the three antibodies.[94] Overall, all antibodies show some improvement in response to increasing PDL1 expression, but PDL1 IHC remains an imperfect biomarker, not only because of the aforementioned issues, but also because its predictive value is limited (at best, >50% expression predicts for about a 50% benefit with pembrolizumab, but for most of these, there can be benefit rates of 5% to 15% in those with negative expression as well). Alternative predictive biomarkers are an area of very active investigation. For instance, nonsynonymous mutation burden has been demonstrated to be a predictive biomarker for pembrolizumab benefit.[95] Although it does not necessarily perform better than PDL1 IHC, a quantitative measurement of mutation burden would not be subject to the same assay and geographic variation. Other measures, such as mass spectrometry, RNA sequencing, and neoantigen burden (and specific neoantigens), as well as cytokine or other immune signatures, continue to be areas of study.

COMBINATION STRATEGIES

A myriad of combination studies has been launched in the wake of the initial findings of activity of PD1/PDL1 inhibitors to improve upon the chances for durable response among the close to 80% of patients who do not respond to monotherapy. These strategies include combinations with other immune-oncology agents that either act to stimulate T-cell activation (OX40, 41BB, or GITR agonists) or block other inhibitors of T-cell activation (Lag3, Tim3, CTLA-4; reviewed by Mahoney et al.[96] Strategies to boost neoantigen production to stimulate an immune response or expression of genes associated with immune response with the use of histone deacetylase inhibitors or other epigenetic modifiers are active areas of study. Studies using blocking antibodies for inhibitory signals to NK cell activity (anti-KIR and others) as well as modified IL-15L ligand–receptor complexes are currently in clinical development in lung cancer.[97] Many other areas are being explored broadly in solid tumors including chimeric antigen receptor T cell or NK cell adoptive cell therapies that have shown great promise in hematologic malignancies.

In addition, combinations with chemotherapy (see Table 50.2) or radiation with the idea that cytotoxicity will expose more neoantigens and stimulate an immune response or using radiation's role in causing local inflammation to boost systemic immune responses are actively ongoing. Targeted therapy combinations are also actively being explored. Finally, the effectiveness of PD1 inhibition has reinvigorated the vaccine field given the potential of these drugs to block local immune suppression that can limit the effectiveness of vaccines. Multiple vaccine-PD1/PDL1 combination studies are currently in development or ongoing and will provoke a reevaluation of multiple vaccines that have ceased development.

The combination strategy that is furthest in development is the combination of CTLA-4 inhibition with PD1 or PDL1 inhibition. This strategy (using nivolumab, a PD1 inhibition, combined with ipilimumab, a CTLA-4 inhibitor) is already an approved combination for melanoma treatment, with notably superior activity to nivolumab alone in those whose tumors have low or no PDL1 expression.[98] In lung cancer, initial cohorts of a combination study (CheckMate 012) using doses similar to those used for melanoma (nivolumab [3 mg/kg] + ipilimumab [1 mg/kg] or nivolumab [1 mg/kg] + ipilimumab [3 mg/kg] every 3 weeks) showed unacceptable toxicity with 51% experiencing (25 of 49 patients) grade 3 to grade 4 toxicity.[99] The study was modified to evaluate much lower and infrequent doses of ipilimumab (1 mg/kg every 6 or 12 weeks) in combination with standard-dose nivolumab (3 mg/kg every 2 weeks). These cohorts were better tolerated, with grade 3 to grade 4 treatment-related adverse effect rates of 32% (every 12-week cohort) or 28% (every 6-week cohort). The ORR in the every 6-week and 12-week cohorts was 47%,[52] which is substantially higher than the 18% to 20% RR seen with monotherapy. Unexpectedly, response rates were higher with increasing PDL1 expression, with a 92% RR in those with over 50% expression, although the sample size was very small (13 patients). By contrast, a phase I study combining durvalumab with tremelimumab demonstrated the lowest grade 3–4 toxicity (17%) in a combination of 20 mg/kg durvalumab plus 1 mg tremelimumab every 4 weeks, which was chosen as the phase II dose.[100] In a group of 26 patients with over 24 weeks of follow-up treated with durvalumab (10–20 mg/kg) plus tremelimumab (1 mg/kg), the response rate was 23% and did not appear to be dependent on PDL1 status.

CONCLUSION

Modulation of the immune system as a treatment modality for lung cancer has entered a new era with the success of PD1/PDL1 inhibition in generating marked and durable response rates. Because of this success, the path forward for other immunotherapies such as vaccines, adoptive cell therapy, and other immunomodulators has been invigorated as well with the opportunity for synergistic combination. There is still much to learn about how we can best identify the right patients who will get durable benefit from monotherapy with PD1/PDL1 inhibitors (only about 20% of patients) and who will require alternative means to "activate" the immunogenicity of the tumor to generate a long-term response. In addition, the best way to optimize combination therapy with existing cytotoxic and targeted therapies remains poorly understood and will require carefully nuanced sequencing studies and robust biomarker evaluation to understand the best path forward. However, we have come a long way from platinum-doublet therapy for all patients in a very short time, so given the potential for combination therapies we can hopefully look forward to significant further improvement ahead.

KEY REFERENCES

9. Ishida Y, Agata Y, Shibahara K, Honjo T. Induced expression of PD-1, a novel member of the immunoglobulin gene superfamily, upon programmed cell death. *EMBO J.* 1992;11(11):3887–3895.

10. Freeman GJ, Long AJ, Iwai Y, et al. Engagement of the PD-1 immunoinhibitory receptor by a novel B7 family member leads to negative regulation of lymphocyte activation. *J Exp Med.* 2000;2;192(7):1027–1034.

11. Jin HT, Ahmed R, Okazaki T. Role of PD-1 in regulating T-cell immunity. *Curr Top Microbiol Immunol.* 2011;350:17–37.

12. Nishimura H, Honjo T. PD-1: an inhibitory immunoreceptor involved in peripheral tolerance. *Trends Immunol.* 2001;22(5):265–268.

13. Blank C, Gajewski TF, Mackensen A. Interaction of PD-L1 on tumor cells with PD-1 on tumor-specific T cells as a mechanism of immune evasion: implications for tumor immunotherapy. *Cancer Immunol Immunother.* 2005;54(4):307–314.

14. Butte MJ, Keir ME, Phamduy TB, Sharpe AH, Freeman GJ. Programmed death-1 ligand 1 interacts specifically with the B7-1 costimulatory molecule to inhibit T cell responses. *Immunity.* 2007;27(1):111–122.

15. Dong H, Strome SE, Salomao DR, et al. Tumor-associated B7-H1 promotes T-cell apoptosis: a potential mechanism of immune evasion. *Nat Med.* 2002;8:793–800.

16. Taube JM, Klein A, Brahmer JR, et al. Association of PD-1, PD-1 ligands, and other features of the tumor immune microenvironment with response to anti-PD-1 therapy. *Clin Cancer Res.* 2014;20(19):5064–5074.

24. Yang CY, Lin MW, Chang YL, Wu CT, Yang PC. Programmed cell death-ligand 1 expression in surgically resected stage I pulmonary adenocarcinoma and its correlation with driver mutations and clinical outcomes. *Eur J Cancer.* 2014;50(7):1361–1369.

25. Chen YB, Mu CY, Huang JA. Clinical significance of programmed death-1 ligand-1 expression in patients with non-small cell lung cancer: a 5-year-follow-up study. *Tumori.* 2012;98(6):751–755.

26. Chen YY, Wang LB, Zhu HL, et al. Relationship between programmed death-ligand 1 and clinicopathological characteristics in non-small cell lung cancer patients. *Chin Med Sci J.* 2013;28(3):147–151.

27. Mu CY, Huang JA, Chen Y, Chen C, Zhang XG. High expression of PD-L1 in lung cancer may contribute to poor prognosis and tumor cells immune escape through suppressing tumor infiltrating dendritic cells maturation. *Med Oncol.* 2011;28(3):682–688.

28. Boland JM, Kwon ED, Harrington SM, et al. Tumor B7-H1 and B7-H3 expression in squamous cell carcinoma of the lung. *Clin Lung Cancer.* 2013;14(2):157–163.

29. Konishi J, Yamazaki K, Azuma M, Kinoshita I, Dosaka-Akita H, Nishimura M. B7-H1 expression on non-small cell lung cancer cells and its relationship with tumor-infiltrating lymphocytes and their PD-1 expression. *Clin Cancer Res.* 2004;10(15):5094–5100.

30. Akbay EA, Koyama S, Carretero J, et al. Activation of the PD-1 pathway contributes to immune escape in EGFR-driven lung tumors. *Cancer Discov.* 2013;3(12):1355–1363.

31. Calles A, Liao X, Sholl LM, et al. Expression of PD-1 and its ligands, PD-L1 and PD-L2, in smokers and never smokers with KRAS-mutant lung cancer. *J Thorac Oncol.* 2015;10(12):1726–1735.

32. D'Incecco A, Andreozzi M, Ludovini V, et al. PD-1 and PD-L1 expression in molecularly selected non-small-cell lung cancer patients. *Br J Cancer.* 2015;112(1):95–102.

55. Trevor KT, Hersh EM, Brailey J, Balloul JM, Acres B. Transduction of human dendritic cells with a recombinant modified vaccinia Ankara virus encoding MUC1 and IL-2. *Cancer Immunol Immunother.* 2001;50(8):397–407.

60. Giaccone G, Bazhenova LA, Nemunaitis J, et al. A phase III study of belagenpumatucel-L, an allogeneic tumour cell vaccine, as maintenance therapy for non-small cell lung cancer. *Eur J Cancer.* 2015;51(16):2321–2329.

61. Rodriguez PC, Neninger E, García B, et al. Safety, immunogenicity and preliminary efficacy of multiple-site vaccination with an epidermal growth factor (EGF) based cancer vaccine in advanced non small cell lung cancer (NSCLC) patients. *J Immune Based Ther Vaccines.* 2011;9:7.

62. Rodriguez PC, Popa X, Martínez O, et al. A phase III clinical trial of the epidermal growth factor vaccine CIMAvax-EGF as switch maintenance therapy in advanced non-small cell lung cancer patients. *Clin Cancer Res.* 2016;22(15):3782–3790.

64. Vázquez AM, Hernández AM, Macías A, et al. Racotumomab: an anti-idiotype vaccine related to N-glycolyl-containing gangliosides—preclinical and clinical data. *Front Oncol.* 2012;23(2):150.

65. Alfonso S, Valdés-Zayas A, Santiesteban ER, et al. A randomized, multicenter, placebo-controlled clinical trial of racotumomab-alum vaccine as switch maintenance therapy in advanced non-small cell lung cancer patients. *Clin Cancer Res.* 2014;20(14):3660–3671.

76. De Lima Lopes G, Wu YL, Sadowski S, et al. P2.43: pembrolizumab vs platinum-based chemotherapy for PD-L1+ NSCLC: phase 3, randomized, open-label KEYNOTE-042 (NCT02220894): track: immunotherapy. *J Thorac Oncol.* 2016;11(10S):S244–S245.

82. Garon EB, Rizvi NA, Hui R, et al. KEYNOTE-001 investigators. *N Engl J Med.* 2015;372(21):2018–2028.

84. Herbst RS, Soria JC, Kowanetz M, et al. Predictive correlates of response to the anti-PD-L1 antibody MPDL3280A in cancer patients. *Nature.* 2014;515(7528):563–567.

85. Borghaei H, Paz-Ares L, Horn L, et al. Nivolumab versus docetaxel in advanced nonsquamous non-small-cell lung cancer. *N Engl J Med.* 2015;373(17):1627–1639.

86. Brahmer J, Reckamp KL, Baas P, et al. Nivolumab versus docetaxel in advanced squamous-cell non-small-cell lung cancer. *N Engl J Med.* 2015;373(2):123–135.

87. Rizvi NA, Mazières J, Planchard D, et al. Activity and safety of nivolumab, an anti-PD-1 immune checkpoint inhibitor, for patients with advanced, refractory squamous non-small-cell lung cancer (CheckMate 063): a phase 2, single-arm trial. *Lancet Oncol.* 2015;16(3):257–265.

88. Herbst RS, Baas P, Kim DW, et al. Pembrolizumab versus docetaxel for previously treated, PD-L1-positive, advanced non-small-cell lung cancer (KEYNOTE-010): a randomised controlled trial. *Lancet.* 2016;387(10027):1540–1550.

89. Fehrenbacher L, Spira A, Ballinger M, et al. Atezolizumab versus docetaxel for patients with previously treated non-small-cell lung cancer (POPLAR): a multicentre, open-label, phase 2 randomised controlled trial. *Lancet.* 2016;387(10030):1837–1846.

90. Rittmeyer A, Barlesi F, Waterkamp D, et al. Atezolizumab versus docetaxel in patients with previously treated non-small-cell lung cancer (OAK): a phase 3, open-label, multicentre randomised controlled trial. *Lancet.* 2017;389(10066):255–265.

91. Herbst RS, De Marinis F, Jassem J, et al. PS01.56: IMpower110: Phase III Trial comparing 1L atezolizumab with chemotherapy in PD-L1-selected chemotherapy-naive NSCLC patients: Topic: Medical Oncology. *J Thorac Oncol.* 2016;11(11S):S304–S305.

92. McLaughlin J, Han G, Schalper KA, et al. Quantitative assessment of the heterogeneity of PD-L1 expression in non-small-cell lung cancer. *JAMA Oncol.* 2016;2(1):46–54.

93. Hirsch FR, McElhinny A, Stanforth D, et al. PD-L1 immunohistochemistry assays for lung cancer: results from phase 1 of the "Blueprint PD-L1 IHC Assay Comparison Project." *J Thorac Oncol.* 2017;12(2):208–222.

94. Ratcliffe MJ, Sharpe A, Midha A, Barker C, Scorer P, Walker J. A comparative study of PD-L1 diagnostic assays and the classification of patients as PD-L1 positive and PD-L1 negative. In: *Proceedings of the 107th Annual Meeting of the American Association for Cancer Research, New Orleans, LA, April 16–20, 2016.* Philadelphia, PA: AACR; 2016. [Abstr LB-094].

95. Rizvi NA, Hellmann MD, Snyder A, et al. Cancer immunology. Mutational landscape determines sensitivity to PD-1 blockade in non-small cell lung cancer. *Science.* 2015;348(6230):124–128.

96. Mahoney KM, Rennert PD, Freeman GJ. Combination cancer immunotherapy and new immunomodulatory targets. *Nat Rev Drug Discov.* 2015;14(8):561–584.

97. Liu B, Kong L, Han K, et al. A novel fusion of ALT-803 (interleukin (IL)-15 superagonist) with an antibody demonstrates antigen-specific antitumor responses. *J Biol Chem.* 2016;291(46):23869–23881.

98. Larkin J, Chiarion-Sileni V, Gonzalez R, et al. Combined nivolumab and ipilimumab or monotherapy in untreated melanoma. *N Engl J Med.* 2015;373(1):23–34.

99. Hellmann MD, Rizvi NA, Goldman JW, et al. Nivolumab plus ipilimumab as first-line treatment for advanced non-small-cell lung cancer (CheckMate 012): results of an open-label, phase 1, multicohort study. *Lancet Oncol.* 2017;18(1):31–41.

100. Antonia S, Goldberg SB, Balmanoukian A, et al. Safety and antitumour activity of durvalumab plus tremelimumab in non-small cell lung cancer: a multicentre, phase 1b study. *Lancet Oncol.* 2016;17(3):299–308.

See Expertconsult.com for full list of references.

51 Adjuvant and Neoadjuvant Chemotherapy for Early-Stage Nonsmall Cell Lung Cancer

Giorgio V. Scagliotti and Everett E. Vokes

SUMMARY OF KEY POINTS

- Surgery remains the most effective curative approach for early-stage (IA–IIB) NSCLC. Selected cases with clinical stage IIIA disease equally benefit from radical resection.

- Stereotactic radiotherapy may be an alternative for selected medically inoperable patients.

- Long-term survival after surgical resection is stage-related, with the likelihood of recurrence increasing with advancing cancer stage (of course this is what staging is all about).

- Two comprehensive systematic reviews and meta-analyses, recently updated, showed a significant benefit of adding chemotherapy after surgery, with an absolute increase in survival of 4% at 5 years. The other meta-analysis in which surgery plus radiotherapy and chemotherapy was compared with surgery and radiotherapy showed indeed a significant benefit, representing an absolute improvement in survival of 4% at 5 years.

- The role of adjuvant radiotherapy for patients with N2 disease remains unclear, and an ongoing study is addressing the issue.

- The role of molecular targeted therapies currently remains generally unproven; studies investigating bevacizumab and epidermal growth factor receptor inhibitors in an imprecisely defined patient population did not show meaningful benefit.

- There is no clear role for molecular prognostic and predictive biomarkers or molecular signatures to assist in treatment selection.

Lung cancer is the most common fatal malignant disease among men and women worldwide.[1,2] Approximately 90% of lung cancers are tobacco-related. Primary prevention of lung cancer through smoking cessation is the first goal in reducing the incidence of lung cancer. However, tobacco consumption is increasing worldwide and the risk of lung cancer is higher for former smokers than for never-smokers; in the United States, more than 50% of lung cancers occur in former smokers.[3] Consequently, lung cancer will continue to be a relevant health problem for the foreseeable future.

More than 80% of all newly diagnosed cases of lung cancer are nonsmall cell lung cancer (NSCLC). Surgery is the main curative therapeutic approach for early-stage NSCLC (stages IA to IIB), but early-stage NSCLC is only a minority (20% to 25%) of all cases. Some groups of patients with stage III disease also benefit from pulmonary resection, usually in combination with other treatment modalities.

Long-term survival after surgical resection is stage-related, with the likelihood of recurrence increasing with advancing cancer stage. One-third of patients with stage IA will relapse and die of the disease within 5 years. Relapse occurs after resection in more than 50% of patients with stage II NSCLC.[4] The majority of these relapses are distant metastases, with a 10% risk of a local recurrence after complete resection. The brain is the most common site of metastatic recurrence, followed closely by bone, ipsilateral and contralateral lung, the liver, and adrenal glands. Histology influences the pattern of recurrence; local recurrence is more common in patients with squamous cell carcinoma and distant metastases are more likely in patients with adenocarcinoma (Table 51.1).[5–8] More than 80% of recurrences occur within 2 years after radical surgery. A 2010 investigation of the timing of local and distant failures showed that among 975 patients with stage I or II disease, recurrent disease developed in 250 patients: 43 at local sites, 110 at distant sites, and 97 at both local and distant sites.[9] The median times to local and distant failure were 13.9 months and 12.5 months, respectively (range, 1 to 79 months for both types of failure). In most patients who had both local and distant recurrence, the failure occurred at both sites simultaneously. This finding is important because only time to first failure has been reported in many trials, and additional sites of failure have not been subsequently analyzed. These results support the integration of local treatment modalities with systemic therapies.

Micrometastatic dissemination of cancer cells at levels that are undetectable with currently available imaging techniques seems to affect the prognosis of patients with clinical early-stage NSCLC. It has been shown consistently that positron emission tomography (PET), which is now routinely included in the staging workup for NSCLC, detects metastatic disease in 11% to 14% of cases otherwise cleared for resection using conventional screening methods and also better detects unsuspected disease in the mediastinal and hilar nodes.[10–12] Despite improved detection with PET, micrometastases are missed. In small retrospective studies, researchers have attempted to detect micrometastatic lymph node disease with immunohistochemistry (IHC) and real-time polymerase chain reaction to identify cytokeratins and carcinoembryonic antigens.[13–16] Patients with positive findings in otherwise morphologically normal lymph nodes were almost invariably more likely to have adverse outcomes than patients without occult micrometastatic disease. Quantification of free circulating DNA has been proposed as a potential additional diagnostic tool for use in patients with resected or persisting neoplastic disease.[17]

As screening techniques are incorporated into preventive and primary care models, it is hoped that the pattern of lung cancer diagnoses can be shifted from stage IV to earlier stages, leading to further interest in the use of systemic adjuvant therapies. This stage migration will be important for decreasing the mortality of lung cancer; however, as we increase the number of patients detected with stage I disease, we must also be able to have some noninvasive molecular or imaging modalities that will help to identify patients with stage I disease who may benefit from additional local and systemic treatments after a complete resection to improve long-term survival.

TABLE 51.1 Rates and Patterns of Relapse Following Radical Resection for Nonsmall Cell Lung Cancer

Author (Year)	Stage	No. of Patients	Pattern of Relapse (%)	
			Local–Regional Only	Distant Only
Martini et al. (1980)[5]	T1–2 N1 (S)	93	16	31
	T1–2 N1 (A)	114	8	54
	T2–3 N2 (S)	46	13	52
	T2–3 N2 (A)	103	17	61
Feld et al. (1984)[6]	T1 N0	162	9	17
	T2 N0	196	11	30
	T1 N1	32	9	22
Pairolero et al. (1984)[7]	T1 N0	170	6	15
	T2 N0	158	6	23
	T1 N1	18	28	39
Thomas et al. (1990)[8]	T1 N0 (S)	226	5	7
	T1 N0 (NS)	346	9	17

A, adenocarcinoma; *NS,* nonsquamous cell carcinoma; *S,* squamous cell carcinoma.

RATIONALE FOR ADJUVANT THERAPY

The use of adjuvant (postoperative) therapy for the treatment of various solid tumors is well established and is based on theoretical models and clinical observations. After complete resection, a patient's tumor load should be nonexistent or minimal. Any residual neoplastic cells present in micrometastatic deposits should contain few clones resistant to chemotherapy or radiotherapy. Experimental and clinical data support the Gompertzian model of tumor growth and regression in most human solid cancers: when a tumor is present microscopically but is clinically undetectable, its growth rate should be at its highest. Therefore, although the numerical reduction of malignant cells induced by cytotoxic chemotherapy is small, the fractional cell kill from an effective dose of chemotherapy should be high.

The decision to use adjuvant therapy involves balancing the need to treat a large number of patients who may be cured by surgery alone against the need for additional systemic therapy to eradicate remaining cancer cells in only a subset of these patients. Thus, if survival is increased for 10% of patients, the other 90% are exposed unnecessarily, either because they did not need the adjuvant treatment or because adjuvant therapy was ineffective in eradicating residual disease. Because no tools exist that determine prospectively who will benefit from adjuvant therapy, it is very important to select a tolerable regimen and limit the length of treatment (Fig. 51.1). In addition, careful pathologic staging enables better prediction of prognosis, facilitates patient selection, and permits comparison of treatment outcomes among trials.

The most appropriate treatment or regimen for the adjuvant setting has not been established. At a minimum, the chosen agent or agents should have proven activity in advanced disease and should be generally well tolerated.[18] Thus, in the case of cytotoxic chemotherapy, a platinum-based doublet regimen should be selected, initiated sufficiently early after radical surgery, and administered for at least three or four cycles.[19]

ROLE OF ADJUVANT RADIOTHERAPY

Before effective chemotherapy regimens were established, postoperative thoracic radiotherapy was the preferred adjuvant treatment. Although radiotherapy may improve local–regional control, it is unlikely to reduce systemic recurrence. Use of radiotherapy has been evaluated in many retrospective and prospective studies. Data from nine of these studies (2128 patients) were included in the Postoperative Radiation Therapy (PORT) meta-analysis. The authors of this meta-analysis concluded that postoperative radiotherapy had a significant detrimental effect on survival, especially for patients with stage I and II disease.[20] These results were

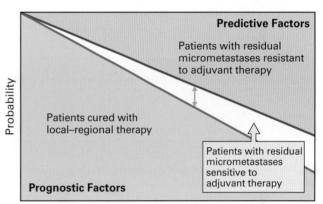

Fig. 51.1. Benefit of adjuvant chemotherapy in an unselected patient population and the role of potential prognostic and predictive factors in the adjuvant setting.

confirmed by a Cochrane systematic review and meta-analysis in 2000 and substantially updated in 2005, which demonstrated that postoperative radiotherapy may have a significant adverse effect on survival (hazard ratio [HR], 1.18).[21] The 18% relative increase in the risk of death is equivalent to an absolute detriment of 6% at 2 years (95% CI, 2% to 9%), reducing overall survival (OS) from 58% to 52%. Exploratory subgroup analyses indicate that this detrimental effect was most pronounced for patients with stage I or II disease. For patients with stage III N2 disease, there was no clear evidence of an adverse effect or potential benefit. This outcome is plausible because increased frequency of local–regional failure is associated with the bulky disease often seen in stage III NSCLC.

In most of the studies included in the PORT meta-analysis, patients were treated with older radiotherapy technology (e.g., cobalt 60) and outdated dosimetry, which are less effective than current treatment approaches, and the higher mortality rate in the radiotherapy groups can be attributed in part to an excess of deaths related to intercurrent disease. In a retrospective review, it was reported that use of new technologies and improved dosimetry for postoperative radiotherapy does not excessively increase the risk of death related to intercurrent disease.[22] Another shortcoming of the PORT meta-analysis is that it failed to include sufficient data on mediastinal lymph node dissection, and, additionally, the surgical procedure varied substantially across studies and centers.

Using data from the United States Surveillance, Epidemiology and End Results (SEER) database, researchers evaluated the

TABLE 51.2 Main Baseline and Treatment Characteristics of Patients Enrolled in Major Trials of Adjuvant Chemotherapy

	ALPI/EORTC[36]	IALT[37]	BLT[38]	ANITA[39]	NCIC-JBR.10[40]	CALGB 9633[43]
Regimen	Cisplatin, vindesine, and mitomycin (3 cycles)	Cisplatin and vindesine, vinblastine, vinorelbine, or etoposide (3–4 cycles)	Cisplatin and vindesine; cisplatin and vinorelbine; cisplatin, vinblastine, and mitomycin; or cisplatin, mitomycin, and ifosfamide (3 cycles)	Cisplatin and vinorelbine (4 cycles)	Cisplatin and vinorelbine (4 cycles)	Carboplatin and paclitaxel (4 cycles)
Sequential radiotherapy allowed	Yes	Yes	Yes	Yes	No	No
No. of patients enrolled/planned	1209/1300	1867/3300	381/500	840/800	482/450	344/384[b]
Median age (y)	61	59	61	59	61	61
Male:female ratio	86:14	81:19	65:35	85:14	66:34	65:35
Stage (%)						
I	39	37	29	36[a]	46	100[a] (all IB)
II	31	24	37	24	54	
IIIA	29	39	27	39	0	
Histology (%)						
Squamous	51	47	48	59	37	35
Nonsquamous	45	46	52	40	65	65
Rate of pneumonectomy (%)	26	35	NR	38	25	11

[a]Stage IB disease.

[b]The original sample size was 500 patients and was subsequently emended. The study was closed early based on the recommendation of the Data Safety Monitoring Board.

ALPI/EORTC, Adjuvant Lung Project Italy/European Organisation for Research and Treatment of Cancer; *ANITA*, Adjuvant Navelbine International Trial Association; *BLT*, Big Lung Trial; *CALGB*, Cancer and Leukemia Group B; *IALT*, International Adjuvant Lung Cancer Trial; *NCIC*, National Cancer Institute of Canada.

relation between survival and postoperative radiotherapy.[23] Factors with a negative effect on OS were older age, T3 or T4 tumor stage, N2 node stage, male gender, fewer lymph nodes sampled, and a greater number of involved lymph nodes. In this study, the use of postoperative radiotherapy was associated with increased survival for patients with N2 disease, but not for patients with N1 or N0 disease.

The role of radiotherapy for patients with N2 disease remains unclear, as no definitive conclusions can be drawn from the available literature. The Lung Adjuvant Radiation Therapy trial in Europe, still ongoing, includes patients with N2 NSCLC who have had surgery, with or without adjuvant chemotherapy.[24] Patients are randomly assigned to postoperative radiotherapy (54 Gy) or no radiotherapy, and it is hoped that results from this trial will define the role of adjuvant radiotherapy for patients with N2 NSCLC.

EARLY STUDIES OF ADJUVANT CHEMOTHERAPY

In the 1960s and 1970s, alkylating agents and nonspecific immunotherapies (e.g., levamisole and bacillus Calmette–Guerin vaccine) universally failed, and detrimental effects of these agents were occasionally reported.[25] These drugs are now known to have very limited or no activity in advanced NSCLC. Subsequently, the use of cisplatin-based chemotherapy was extensively tested in all stages of resectable NSCLC.[26–32] In all but one of these early studies, adjuvant therapy failed to show clinical benefit. Common flaws in the design of these trials were overestimation of the potential benefit of adjuvant chemotherapy, imbalance in relevant patient and treatment characteristics (for instance, the rate of incomplete mediastinal lymph node dissection), and unrealistic patient accrual goals. In addition, in most of the trials, chemotherapy dose delivery (total dose and dose intensity) was often inadequate, with only 50% of patients, on average, receiving the intended course of treatment. Given the toxicity of these regimens in the absence of good antiemetic supportive care and the lack of proven survival benefit from adjuvant therapy, physicians were reluctant to offer participation in adjuvant trials to their patients.

Nevertheless, the authors of a large meta-analysis, which included these trials, reported a 13% reduction in the risk of death with adjuvant cisplatin-based chemotherapy, a result of borderline significance ($p = 0.08$).[33] There was a 6% reduction in the risk of death among patients who received postoperative radiotherapy and cisplatin-based chemotherapy compared with patients who received postoperative radiotherapy only ($p = 0.46$). In contrast, adjuvant chemotherapy with alkylating agents was shown to be significantly detrimental (HR, 1.15; $p = 0.005$).

These findings failed to have an effect on clinical practice because they were of only borderline significance and were based on several flawed studies. In addition, the heterogeneity of surgical procedures and the difference in the staging modalities limited the applicability of the results. Nevertheless, the findings strongly supported a potential role for adjuvant chemotherapy and the need for a large, well-designed confirmatory trial.

LARGE-SCALE STUDIES ON PLATINUM-BASED ADJUVANT CHEMOTHERAPY

Given the evidence of a marginal benefit of adjuvant systemic treatment, several randomized studies were conducted to evaluate the role of modern, platinum-based regimens in all stages of resectable NSCLC (Table 51.2). Some of the trials were initiated prior to the publication of the PORT meta-analysis and thus included postoperative radiotherapy.

The first of these studies to be reported was an Eastern Cooperative Oncology Group (ECOG) trial, which compared the efficacy of four cycles of adjuvant cisplatin and etoposide plus concomitant thoracic radiotherapy (total dose of 50 Gy) with postoperative radiotherapy alone for 488 patients with stage II and IIIA disease.[34] There was no significant difference between the two treatment arms in terms of median time to progression. The median survival was 38 months for the concurrent chemoradiation therapy arm and 39 months for radiotherapy alone arm

TABLE 51.3 Five-Year Survival Rates Overall and by Disease Stage in Landmark Studies of Adjuvant Chemotherapy

Study	Overall	Stage I	Stage II	Stage III
	Hazard Ratio for 5-Year Survival (95% CI)			
ALPI/EORTC[36]	0.96 (0.81–1.13) p = 0.59	0.97 (0.71–1.33)	0.80 (0.60–1.06)	1.06 (0.82–1.38)
IALT[37]	0.86 (0.76–0.98) p < 0.03	0.95 (0.74–1.23)	0.93 (0.72–1.20)	0.79 (0.66–0.95)
BLT[38]	1.02 (0.77–1.35) p = 0.90	NT	NT	NT
ANITA[39]	0.80 (0.66–0.96) p = 0.017	1.14 (0.83–1.57)	0.67 0.47–0.94)	0.60 (0.44–0.82)
NCIC JBR.10[40]	0.69 (0.52–0.91) p = 0.04	0.94	0.59 (0.42–0.85)	NI
CALGB 9633[43a]		0.62 (0.41–0.95) p = 0.028	NI	NI

[a]Early data, collected after a median follow-up of 34 months.
ALPI/EORTC, Adjuvant Lung Project Italy/European Organisation for Research and Treatment of Cancer; *ANITA*, Adjuvant Navelbine International Trial Association; *BLT*, Big Lung Trial; *CALGB*, Cancer and Leukemia Group B; *IALT*, International Adjuvant Lung Cancer Trial; *NCIC*, National Cancer Institute of Canada; *NI*, not included; *NT*, not tested.

(HR, 0.93; 95% CI, 0.74–1.18). The lack of efficacy may have been due to the toxicity of radiation with concomitant administration of cytotoxic agents; this effect was more striking in patients with stage II disease. In a biologic correlative study of 197 tumors from this trial, neither p53 protein expression nor Kirsten rat sarcoma viral oncogene homolog (*KRAS*) mutation showed any relation to outcome.[35]

In a joint effort, the Adjuvant Lung Project Italy (ALPI) and the European Organisation for Research and Treatment of Cancer (EORTC) enrolled 1209 patients with completely resected stage I, II, or IIIA NSCLC between 1994 and 1999.[36] Patients were randomly assigned to either three cycles of chemotherapy with mitomycin, vindesine, and cisplatin (MVP) or to observation. Sixty-nine percent of patients completed the three cycles of MVP, with half of those patients needing dose reductions. Radiotherapy was administered sequentially according to the policy at each center, and 43% of patients received postoperative radiotherapy. There was no significant difference in OS between the two groups (HR for death, 0.96). The median OS was 55 months in the chemotherapy arm and 48 months in the observation arm (HR, 0.96; 95% CI, 0.81–1.13; p = 0.59). Subset analysis by stage showed that 5-year survival was better for patients with stage II disease than for patients with stage I or III disease (Table 51.3). Even though the HR for patients with stage II NSCLC was not significant, it is notable that, in this subset of patients, there was a 10% survival advantage at 5 years for patients who received chemotherapy. No significant association was found between *p53* or *Ki67* expression, and disease stage or tumor histology. The relation of *KRAS* mutation status to survival was analyzed using specimens from adenocarcinomas and large-cell carcinomas; mutations were found in 22% of 117 samples, with no relation to survival.

The International Adjuvant Lung Cancer Trial (IALT) was the first large trial to demonstrate a significant benefit of adjuvant chemotherapy. A total of 1867 patients with completely resected NSCLC were randomly assigned to cisplatin plus a second drug (vindesine, vinblastine, vinorelbine, or etoposide) or to observation.[37] Approximately 10% had stage IA disease, 27% had stage IB, 24% had stage II, and 39% had stage III. In the chemotherapy arm, 74% of patients received at least 240 mg/m² of cisplatin and 27% of patients received postoperative radiotherapy. Grade 3 or 4 toxicity was reported for 23% of patients (0.8% of toxicity-related deaths). Survival was significantly longer in the chemotherapy arm (HR, 0.86; 95% CI, 0.76–0.98; p < 0.03): 5-year survival in the chemotherapy and observation arms were 44.5% and 40.4%, respectively. The median survival was 50.8 months and 44.4 months, respectively, and the median disease-free survival was 40.2 months and 30.5 months (Table 51.3).

In the Big Lung Trial (BLT), 381 patients with resected stage I–III NSCLC were randomly assigned to three cycles of postoperative chemotherapy (cisplatin and vindesine; cisplatin, mitomycin, and ifosfamide; cisplatin, mitomycin, and vinblastine; or

cisplatin and vinorelbine) or to surgery alone.[38] Sixty-four percent of patients received all three courses of chemotherapy, and 40% of them needed dose reductions. Postoperative radiotherapy was used for only 14% of patients. No significant differences in survival were noted between the two groups. However, this trial was underpowered, had a short follow-up (29 months), and a 15% rate of incomplete resection.

In the Adjuvant Navelbine International Trial Association (ANITA) trial, 840 patients with resected stage IB–IIIA NSCLC were randomly assigned to cisplatin (100 mg/m²) every 4 weeks and vinorelbine (30 mg/m²) weekly or to observation; 301 patients (36%) had stage IB disease, 203 (24%) had stage II disease, and 325 (39%) had stage IIIA disease.[39] After a median follow-up of 76 months, the median survival was 65.7 months in the chemotherapy group and 43.7 months in the observation group. Overall, chemotherapy significantly reduced the risk of death (HR, 0.80; 95% CI, 0.66–0.96; p = 0.017) and conferred a survival advantage of 8.6% at 5 years, which was maintained at 7 years (8.4%). The 5-year survival rate was better for patients with stage III disease than for patients with stage I or II disease (Table 51.3). Grade 3 or 4 neutropenia was documented for 85% of patients, febrile neutropenia for 9%, and severe infection for 11%. The most common nonhematologic adverse effects were asthenia (28%), nausea and vomiting (27%), and anorexia (15%). As in many of the other studies of adjuvant chemotherapy already described, postoperative radiotherapy was administered according to the policy of individual centers. Radiotherapy was beneficial for patients with N2 disease and harmful for patients with N1 disease when combined with chemotherapy.

The role of adjuvant chemotherapy in the treatment of stage I and II NSCLC was investigated in the National Cancer Institute of Canada Clinical Trials Group JBR.10 trial, which was powered to detect a 10% improvement in 3-year survival.[40] Four hundred and eighty-two patients with resected stage IB and II NSCLC (excluding T3 N0) were enrolled and randomly assigned to receive four cycles of cisplatin (50 mg/m²) on days 1 and 8 every 4 weeks and vinorelbine (25 mg/m²) weekly for 16 weeks or to observation. Patients did not receive postoperative radiotherapy, and they were stratified by node status (N0 or N1) and *KRAS* mutation status. OS was significantly longer in the chemotherapy arm (94 vs. 73 months; HR, 0.69; 95% CI, 0.52–0.91; p = 0.04), as was recurrence-free survival (not reached vs. 47 months; HR, 0.60; p < 0.001). The 5-year survival rate was 69% in the chemotherapy arm and 54% in the observation arm (p = 0.03), with an absolute gain of 15% at 5 years. In the subset analysis by stage, patients with stage II disease had a greater survival benefit at 5 years (difference of 20% between study arms, p = 0.004) than patients with stage I disease (7% difference between study arms; not significant) (Table 51.3). Fifty-eight percent of the 231 patients who received chemotherapy received three cycles of cisplatin and vinorelbine. Nineteen percent of patients were hospitalized for problems related to chemotherapy toxicity. In an updated analysis of this study with a median follow-up of 9.3 years, adjuvant chemotherapy continued to produce a significant survival benefit ($p = 0.04$), with an absolute improvement of 11% in 5-year survival (67% in the chemotherapy arm vs. 56% in the observation arm) (Table 51.4). The benefit was particularly pronounced for patients with stage II disease (median survival, 6.8 vs. 3.6 years), and there was no survival benefit for patients with stage IB disease (median survival, 11.0 vs. 9.8 years). However, within the population with stage IB disease, tumor size was predictive of chemotherapy effect, with chemotherapy of benefit for patients with tumors 4 cm or larger (HR, 0.66) compared with patients with smaller tumors (HR, 1.73). The 5-year survival for patients with tumors 4 cm or larger was 79% for patients in the chemotherapy arm compared with 59% for patients in the observation arm. *KRAS* mutation was not associated with a differential effect of chemotherapy.[41]

Similarly, long-term data from the IALT trial were reported at a median follow-up of 7.5 years and the OS advantage was no longer significant ($p = 0.1$) (Table 51.4).[42] This late loss of survival benefit appears to be due to an excess of noncancer-related deaths in the chemotherapy arm.

Unfortunately, JBR.10 and ANITA, two of the positive studies, used chemotherapy doses and schedules that are not routinely used in current clinical practice. The most common dose of cisplatin currently used is 75 mg/m^2 on day 1; cisplatin on days 1 and 8 (as in the JBR-10 trial) is unusual and weekly vinorelbine for 16 weeks is associated with high toxicity and a challenge to safely administer in the adjuvant setting. These trials provide the necessary clinical evidence for adjuvant chemotherapy and may justify the use of other cisplatin-based doublets with similar activity for stage IV NSCLC at the same doses and schedules.

The Cancer and Leukemia Group B (CALGB) 9633 trial was unique in limiting enrollment to patients with resected stage IB disease and is the only large trial to have used a carboplatin-based regimen. The study was powered to detect a 13% improvement in OS at 5 years.[43] In this study, 344 patients were randomly assigned to receive carboplatin (AUC 6) and paclitaxel (200 mg/m^2) every 3 weeks for a total of four cycles, and the trial was closed early (90% of patients recruited) when an interim analysis showed a 12% absolute improvement in OS at 4 years (71% vs. 59%; HR, 0.62; $p = 0.028$). Chemotherapy delivery was excellent, with nearly 85% of patients receiving four cycles of chemotherapy. Toxicity in this group of patients was minimal, with 36% of patients having grade 3 or grade 4 myelosuppression and no treatment-related deaths.

Following initial closure and early reporting, the final analysis of the results of this trial could not confirm a significant favorable outcome. After an extended follow-up (74 months), there was only a nonsignificant trend toward improvement in survival (59% vs. 57%; $p = 0.125$) (Table 51.4).[44] It should be noted that the small sample size did not allow for adequate power to detect small differences in survival. The 3-year failure-free survival (66% vs. 57%) and the 3-year OS (79% vs. 70%; $p = 0.045$) continued to favor the chemotherapy group.

A pooled analysis of data from JBR.10 and CALGB 9633 was done to evaluate survival according to tumor size. The authors

found that the effect of chemotherapy seemed to increase with tumor size.[45] Thus, current entry criteria for adjuvant chemotherapy trials in North America specify a tumor size of 4 cm or larger. The impact of adjuvant chemotherapy use and tumor size on outcomes in stage I has been reviewed from 2003 to 2006 in the National Cancer Database in the United States. The results of the study indicate an increased use over time of adjuvant chemotherapy although it continues to frequently not be used. The analysis also supports the guidelines indicating adjuvant chemotherapy for stage I NSCLC tumors larger than 4 cm with a positive survival impact for patients whose tumors ranged from 3.0 to 8.5 cm.[46]

Overall three studies showed a positive impact of adjuvant chemotherapy in resectable NSCLC, with a survival benefit ranging from 4.1% (IALT) to 15% (JBR.10).[36,39,40] A few factors may help to explain the difference in survival among the landmark adjuvant studies (Table 51.3). First, the sample size differed substantially among the studies (from less than 500 patients to 3300 according to the planned sample sizes) to assess the same expected therapeutic effect in the same patient population. Effectively, the only two studies designed to detect a reasonable survival advantage were the ALPI and IALT trials, which, not surprisingly, demonstrated a relatively similar survival benefit: 3% and 4.1%, respectively.

Second, most of the landmark adjuvant studies do not include information about the proportion of patients who had systematic lymph node dissection or lymph node sampling. This detail is important, as one randomized clinical study showed that systematic lymph node dissection significantly influenced survival for every stage of resectable NSCLC.[47] Third, patients with lung cancer frequently have comorbidities, including chronic obstructive pulmonary disease and cardiovascular diseases, which can affect survival substantially.[48,49] Lastly, an unbalance in the proportion of patients who quit smoking after radical surgery may potentially account for survival differences, as was shown in two retrospective studies.[50,51] A common feature of most of these landmark studies, with the exclusion of the CALGB 9633, is the less than optimal compliance with adjuvant regimens. Because of treatment delays and dose reductions, the delivery of three cycles of adjuvant chemotherapy ranged from 58% to 74% in studies of cisplatin-based chemotherapy.[36–40,43] Reasons for low rates of treatment compliance may be related to the time needed to fully recover from the surgical procedure for lung cancer (which is longer than the time to recover from breast cancer surgery, for example). The rate of pneumonectomy in some of these studies far exceeded the rate in consecutive surgical series; pneumonectomy was done in 26% of patients in ALPI, in 35% of patients in IALT, and in 41% of patients in ANITA, and a subset analysis of the tolerability of chemotherapy in these subgroups has not been performed. Of note, in breast cancer, the survival benefit of adjuvant therapy has been more striking in patients who receive more than 85% of the intended total dose of chemotherapy.[52]

The impact of platinum-based adjuvant chemotherapy on survival has also been specifically evaluated in Asian patients with stage I–IIIA NSCLC. Among 2231 patients in the Taiwan cancer registry who had resection in 2004 to 2007, the mortality rate was lower for patients treated with chemotherapy for both stage II and IIIA disease. Multivariate analysis demonstrated that platinum-based adjuvant chemotherapy was an independent prognostic factor for OS for patients with stage II disease ($p = 0.024$), including both men and women and patients older than 70 years of age.[53]

Quality of Life and Adjuvant Cisplatin-Based Chemotherapy

The impact of adjuvant chemotherapy on quality-of-life outcomes has also been investigated. This specific outcome was evaluated in the JBR.10 trial through the EORTC quality-of-life

TABLE 51.4 Impact of Adjuvant Chemotherapy on Overall Survival in Studies With Prolonged Follow-Up

Study	Follow-Up (Y)	Hazard Ratio for Overall Survival (95% CI)
NCIC JBR.10[41]	9.3	0.78 (0.61–0.99) $p = 0.04$
IALT[42]	7.5	0.91 (0.81–1.02) $p = 0.1$
CALGB 9633[44]	6.2	0.83 (0.64–1.08) $p = 0.125$

CALGB, Cancer and Leukemia Group B; *IALT*, International Adjuvant Lung Cancer Trial; *NCIC*, National Cancer Institute of Canada.

questionnaire C30 and a trial-specific checklist at baseline and at weeks 5 and 9 for patients who received chemotherapy and for all patients at regular follow-up visits.[40] The impact of initial surgery on quality of life was similar for the two treatment arms (chemotherapy and observation), whereas the quality of life during chemotherapy was only modestly affected, (in particular, for fatigue, nausea, and vomiting), but without associated changes in global quality of life. These symptoms improved considerably at 3 months of follow-up, with more permanent side effects being limited to sensory neuropathy and chemotherapy-associated hearing loss. Thus, negative effects on quality of life appear to be modest and fairly short-lived. Investigators further followed up on these findings by assessing quality-adjusted time without symptoms or toxicity and reported that adjuvant chemotherapy was preferred for relapse and toxicity and had an overall better quality-adjusted time in the range of 5 to 6 additional months.[54,55]

STUDIES OF ADJUVANT TREATMENT WITH ORAL UFT

UFT, an oral fluoropyrimidine combining uracil and tegafur, has been extensively studied in Japan as adjuvant treatment as a single-agent or in combination with intravenous cytotoxic agents. In the largest trial of postoperative UFT therapy in resected NSCLC, by Kato et al.,[56] 979 patients with completely resected stage I adenocarcinoma were randomly assigned to either oral UFT (250 mg/m^2) for 2 years or to observation. OS favored the UFT arm (HR, 0.71; 95% CI, 0.52–0.98; p = 0.04) and the 5-year survival was 88% in the UFT arm compared with 85% in the observation arm. Subset analyses showed that the benefit was greatest for the subgroup of 263 patients who had T2 N0 disease (HR, 0.48; 95% CI, 0.29–0.81; p = 0.005) but not for the 716 patients who had T1 N0 disease (HR, 0.97; 95% CI, 0.64–1.46; p = 0.87). Compliance was limited to 74% at 12 months and 61% at 24 months. One questionable point in this trial is the absence of any advantage in disease-free survival for the patients in the UFT arm, and this finding clearly contrasts with the results of the positive studies of cisplatin-based adjuvant therapy (IALT, JBR.10, and ANITA), in which improvement in OS for patients receiving adjuvant chemotherapy was invariably associated with disease-free survival that was similar or of greater magnitude.

The results of other published studies of adjuvant UFT in smaller patient cohorts were completely or partially inconsistent with the data found in the study by Kato et al.,[56] and confirmatory data for white patients are lacking.[57–59] Additionally, questions regarding a specific genetic sensitivity to UFT in Japanese patients remain unanswered.

EFFICACY OF ADJUVANT CHEMOTHERAPY ACCORDING TO SYSTEMATIC REVIEWS, META-ANALYSES, AND CANCER REGISTRY DATA

Several systematic reviews and meta-analyses have confirmed the value of adjuvant cisplatin- or UFT-based chemotherapy for resected NSCLC (Table 51.5).[60–65] All of these reviews have consistently shown a benefit from adjuvant chemotherapy, with HRs ranging from 0.72 for adjuvant UFT to 0.89 for cisplatin-based chemotherapy.

Four of these meta-analyses are based on individual patient data rather than published study reports. In a meta-analysis comparing the outcomes for 2003 patients (in six studies) treated with adjuvant oral UFT as a single agent or in combination with other cytotoxic agents, UFT significantly improved OS (HR, 0.74; 95% CI, 0.61–0.88), corresponding to a 4.6% benefit at 5 years (p = 0.001) and 7% at 7 years (p = 0.001).[63]

A further analysis of randomized trials of UFT specifically evaluated the effect of the drug on stage I (T1a and T1b) disease in 1269 patients.[66] Among the 670 patients with T1a disease, the 5-year survival rate was 85% for patients who had surgery only and 87% for patients who received adjuvant UFT. Among the 599 patients with T1b disease, the 5-year survival rate was 82% for patients who had surgery only and 88% for patients who received adjuvant UFT (p = 0.011).

The Lung Adjuvant Cisplatin Evaluation (LACE) is a pooled analysis of data from 4584 patients in five randomized clinical trials of adjuvant therapy (ALPI, ANITA, BLT, IALT, and JBR.10).[64] The analysis demonstrated a significantly positive effect of chemotherapy in terms of OS (HR, 0.89; 95% CI, 0.82–0.96) and disease-free survival (HR, 0.84; 95% CI, 0.78–0.90), with a relative reduction in the risk of death of 11% (HR, 0.89; 95% CI, 0.82–0.96). For patients with stage II–III NSCLC, the gain in OS was 5.3% at 5 years (48.8% vs. 43.3%; HR, 0.83; 95% CI, 0.83–0.95). A small, insignificant survival gain was also evident for patients with stage IB disease (HR, 0.92; 95% CI, 0.78–1.10), and a detrimental effect was found for patients with stage IA disease (HR, 1.41; 95% CI, 0.96–2.1). The most active regimen seems to be cisplatin and vinorelbine, mainly because of the greater number of patients treated (1888 patients; HR, 0.80) and higher total doses of cisplatin administered in combination with that drug (320 to 400 mg/m^2).

Two comprehensive systematic reviews and meta-analyses were published in 2010[65,67] and recently updated.[68] One of these meta-analyses was based on 34 trials (8447 patients) in which surgery plus chemotherapy was compared with surgery alone. The data showed a significant benefit of adding chemotherapy after surgery, with an absolute increase in survival of

TABLE 51.5 Systematic Reviews and Meta-Analyses or Individual Patient Data Meta-Analyses of Trials Evaluating Cisplatin-Based or UFT-Based Adjuvant Treatment

Author	Adjuvant Treatment	Number of Studies (Patients)	Hazard Ratio (95% CI) for Overall Survival
Hotta et al.[59]	Cisplatin-based chemotherapy	8 (3786)	0.89 (0.81–0.97)
	Single-agent UFT	5 (1751)	0.79 (0.67–0.96)
Sedrakyan et al.[60]	Cisplatin-based chemotherapy	12	0.89 (0.82–0.96)
	Single-agent UFT	7 (total = 7200)	0.83 (0.73–0.95)
Bria et al.[61]	Cisplatin-based chemotherapy	12 (6494)	0.93 (0.89–0.95)[a]
Hamada et al.[62b]	UFT (single agent or combined with chemotherapy)	6 (2003)	0.74 (0.61–0.88)
Pignon et al. (LACE Collaborative Group)[63b]	Cisplatin-based chemotherapy	5 (4584)	0.89 (0.82–0.96)
NSCLC Meta-analyses Collaborative Group[64b]	Cisplatin-based chemotherapy	17 (4406)	0.90 (0.82–0.98)
	Single-agent UFT	16 (3848)	0.80 (0.71–0.90)

[a]Expressed as risk ratio.
[b]Individual patient data meta-analyses.
LACE, Lung Adjuvant Cisplatin Evaluation; *NSCLC*, nonsmall cell lung cancer; *UFT*, an oral fluoropyrimidine combining uracil and tegafur.

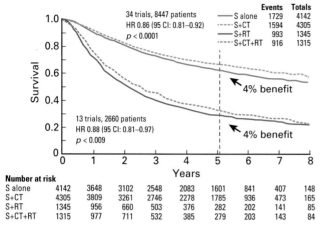

Fig. 51.2. Two meta-analyses of individual patient data comparing surgery alone (S) with surgery followed by chemotherapy (CT), with or without postoperative radiotherapy (RT), for operable nonsmall cell lung cancer. *HR*, hazard ratio. *(Modified with permission from NSCLC Meta-analyses Collaborative Group; Arriagada R, Auperin A, Burdett S, et al. Adjuvant chemotherapy, with or without postoperative radiotherapy, in operable non-small-cell lung cancer: two meta-analyses of individual patient data. Lancet. 2010;375(9722):1267–1277.)*

4% (95% CI, 3% to 6%) at 5 years (from 60% to 64%) (Fig. 51.2).[65] The other meta-analysis was based on 13 trials (2660 patients) in which surgery plus radiotherapy and chemotherapy was compared with surgery and radiotherapy. Again, adding chemotherapy was of significant benefit, representing an absolute improvement in survival of 4% (95% CI, 1% to 8%) at 5 years (from 29% to 33%) (Fig. 51.2).[67] In both meta-analyses, it was noted that there was little variation in effect according to the type of chemotherapy, other trial characteristics, or patient subgroup.

Douillard et al.[69] specifically evaluated cisplatin and vinorelbine compared with other regimens in four trials (IALT, BLT, JBR.10, and ANITA). Survival associated with cisplatin and vinorelbine was superior to that associated with other regimens, with improvement at 5 years of 8.9%.

Additional analyses support the safety and efficacy of adjuvant chemotherapy in standard clinical practice. Booth et al.[70] evaluated outcomes for patients with surgically resected NSCLC registered in the Ontario Cancer Registry and compared outcomes for patients treated in 2001–2003 with outcomes for a second cohort treated in 2004–2006. The proportion of patients receiving adjuvant chemotherapy increased from 7% to 31%, and postoperative admissions remained stable at 36% and 37%, respectively, within 6 months after surgery. Of note, there was a 33% reduction in the proportion of patients admitted to the hospital for subsequent metastatic disease and there was substantial improvement in the 4-year survival among patients who had surgical resection, increasing from 52.5% for the initial cohort to 56.1% for the second cohort. This analysis supports the use of adjuvant chemotherapy, with evidence of a survival benefit in clinical practice.

Overall, adjuvant chemotherapy has been shown, to a limited extent, to significantly increase survival rates, particularly for patients with stage II and early stage III disease, whereas its effect on stage I disease is not yet clearly established, specifically, for tumors of 4 cm or less.[71,72]

Miksad et al.[73] further evaluated the statistical evidence for a positive effect of adjuvant chemotherapy in a bayesian analysis. Using this approach, the probability of a 4% survival benefit was found to increase from 33% before IALT to 64% after IALT, and after sequential updating of the analysis with data from JBR.10

and ANITA, the probability increased to 82%. IALT produced the largest decrease in variance (61%) and decreased the chance of a survival decrement to 0%. However, sensitivity analyses did not support a survival benefit after IALT, and only the sequential updating substantiated a more than 90% probability of a 6% survival benefit and a 50% probability of a 12% benefit for patients with resected stage II and III NSCLC.

To date, no specific prognostic or predictive biomarkers have been identified that could assist in routine selection of patients for chemotherapy, including *KRAS* mutation, which was evaluated as a prognostic or predictive biomarker in four trials.[74]

ADJUVANT CHEMOTHERAPY FOR OLDER PATIENTS

More than 50% of lung cancers are diagnosed in patients older than 65 years, and approximately 30% of lung cancers are diagnosed in patients older than 70 years of age.[75] The favorable data on efficacy of adjuvant chemotherapy have been largely derived in younger patient cohorts, and separate data supporting its use in an older population would assist physicians in better advising such patients on the utility of adjuvant chemotherapy.

It is well known that older patients tolerate chemotherapy poorly because of comorbidities, mainly respiratory and cardiovascular diseases that are more prevalent in this population, and organ failure, especially declining renal function, which alters drug pharmacodynamics. Moreover, after a demanding surgery such as lobectomy or pneumonectomy, the risk of chemotherapy-induced toxicity is increased because of associated comorbidities in an older population. Higher toxicity or reduced compliance may diminish the potential survival benefit obtained with adjuvant chemotherapy.

A retrospective analysis was designed to evaluate the influence of age on survival, chemotherapy compliance, and toxicity in the JBR.10 trial.[76] Data for 155 patients 65 years or older and 327 younger patients were analyzed. Adenocarcinoma histology and better performance status were more common among the younger patients. The older patients received significantly fewer doses of chemotherapy ($p = 0.0004$ for vinorelbine, and $p = 0.001$ for cisplatin), with no significant difference in toxicities. Among the older patients, OS was significantly better with chemotherapy than with observation (HR, 0.61; $p = 0.04$), but survival was significantly shorter for the 23 patients older than 75 years compared with the patients 66 to 75 years old. These data suggest that, in clinical practice, older fit patients should not be denied adjuvant platinum-based chemotherapy.

Similarly, a pooled analysis was undertaken to assess patients older than 70 years in five large trials of cisplatin-based chemotherapy that were included in the LACE analysis.[77] Specifically, patients were divided into three groups according to age: younger than 65 years, 65 to 69 years old, and older than 70 years. Survival HRs for the three groups were 0.86, 1.01, and 0.9 respectively. More older patients died from noncancer-related causes. Similarly, older patients received lower total doses of cisplatin and fewer chemotherapy cycles.

A population-based study in Canada involving data from the Ontario Cancer Registry compared the uptake of adjuvant chemotherapy among patients 70 years or older with that among younger patients.[78] When data for 2001–2003 were compared with data for 2004–2006 (when adjuvant chemotherapy was introduced into practice), the 4-year survival rate for older patients increased significantly. In essence, more patients, including older ones, were offered adjuvant chemotherapy in the second time period (16.2% vs. 3.3%).

The impact of adjuvant chemotherapy for stage I NSCLC elderly patients with tumors >4 cm was investigated in the SEER Medicare database from 1992 to 2009. Overall, 84% of the patients were treated with resection alone, 9% received platinum-based adjuvant chemotherapy, and 7% underwent PORT with or without adjuvant chemotherapy. Platinum-based chemotherapy was associated with improved survival but also with an increased amount of serious adverse events especially in terms of hematologic toxicity.[79]

A study from South Korea investigated the quality of life for patients younger or older than 65 who were treated with postoperative chemotherapy and found no significant difference between the age groups in terms of quality of life.[80] Thus, based on the available data, it appears that adjuvant chemotherapy can be offered to older patients who have good performance status and good end-organ function, although age-specific prospective data have not been generated to date.

NEW CHEMOTHERAPY REGIMENS AND TARGETED THERAPY

In recent years, much has been learned about the activity of new chemotherapy regimens in stage IV disease that is relevant to adjuvant trials. In 2002, the ECOG 1594 trial directly compared four commonly used platinum-based doublets, and no difference was found among them in terms of response or survival.[81] In another trial, cisplatin and gemcitabine was compared with cisplatin and pemetrexed, and both regimens were shown to be of equal activity in the entire patient cohort.[82] However, a predefined subset analysis according to tumor histology showed that patients who had tumors with nonsquamous cell histology benefited significantly from the pemetrexed-based regimen, whereas patients who had tumors with squamous cell histology had longer survival when treated with gemcitabine. These results have influenced the choice of treatment for stage IV disease and can similarly be applied to both standard practice and investigational trial design in the adjuvant setting.

Few specific data for adjuvant chemotherapy with cisplatin and docetaxel or cisplatin and pemetrexed exist. However, some preliminary clinical experience has been published. For example, a chart review of 54 patients treated with adjuvant cisplatin and docetaxel (75 mg/m^2 for each drug in 3-week intervals) demonstrated that 85% of patients received all four planned cycles, usually at full dose.[83] The data suggested good dose delivery and patient convenience for this regimen. In a randomized phase II trial, 132 patients with completely resected NSCLC (10% stage IA, 38% stage IB, and 47% stage IIB) were randomly assigned to four cycles of cisplatin and either vinorelbine or pemetrexed, and having drug delivery and efficacy are end points. The feasibility of administering the combinations was 95.5% for cisplatin and pemetrexed and 75.4% for cisplatin and vinorelbine.[84] The pemetrexed based-regimen had significantly fewer hematologic grade 3 or 4 side effects ($p < 0.001$), whereas the rates of nonhematologic toxicities were similar.

Researchers have tried to enhance the efficacy of adjuvant chemotherapy by combining it with targeted therapy, including vascular endothelial growth factor (*VEGF*) inhibitors and epidermal growth factor receptor (*EGFR*) tyrosine kinase inhibitors (TKIs). *VEGF* is the most potent and specific angiogenic factor that has been identified, with a well-defined role in normal and pathologic angiogenesis. A correlation has been noted between the degree of tumor vascularization and the level of *VEGF* mRNA expression, and in virtually all specimens examined, *VEGF* mRNA is expressed in tumor cells but not in endothelial cells, whereas mRNAs for the two *VEGF* receptors, Flt-1 and KDR, are upregulated in endothelial cells associated with the tumor.[85] *VEGF* is also a strong prognostic indicator in NSCLC and is associated with early postoperative relapse and decreased survival.[86]

ECOG 4599 demonstrated that adding the antiangiogenic bevacizumab to carboplatin and paclitaxel for advanced NSCLC increased median survival time (12 vs. 10 months).[87] Therefore, the question of adding bevacizumab to chemotherapy in the

adjuvant setting is of great current interest. In general, bevacizumab is administered only to patients who have tumors with nonsquamous cell histology, given the increased risk of pulmonary hemorrhage reported in early trials for patients with squamous cell carcinoma. However, in the adjuvant setting, because there is no remaining macroscopic disease, the bleeding risk is eliminated and bevacizumab may be added to a doublet regimen of choice, usually cisplatin and pemetrexed for adenocarcinoma and large cell carcinoma and cisplatin combined with paclitaxel, docetaxel, or gemcitabine for patients with squamous cell histology. ECOG 1505 was a phase III study that evaluated the addition of bevacizumab to adjuvant chemotherapy in patients with resected stage IB, II, or IIIA NSCLC (ClinicalTrials.gov identifier: NCT00324805) having OS as the primary end point. Chemotherapy was investigator-selected and included cisplatin/ vinorelbine, cisplatin/docetaxel, cisplatin/gemcitabine, and cisplatin/pemetrexed. From July 2007 to September 2013, 1501 patients were enrolled and at the median follow-up time of 41 months the IDMC recommended releasing the trial results due to futility. The HR for disease-free survival was 0.98 (95% CI, 0.84–1.14) and for OS was 0.99 (95% CI, 0.81–1.21).[88] In subset analysis none of the four specific chemotherapy regimens was shown to be superior to control or another regimen.

In advanced NSCLC, *EGFR* TKIs such as gefitinib, erlotinib, and afatinib have been shown to increase progression-free survival for patients with sensitizing *EGFR* mutations when administered as a single agent in the first-line setting and in unselected patients in the second or third line (erlotinib only). Other targets with activity in NSCLC have been identified, in particular the echinoderm microtubule-associated protein-like 4 (*EML4*)-anaplastic lymphoma kinase (*ALK*) fusion gene and C-ros oncogene 1, receptor tyrosine kinase (*ROS1*) rearrangements. To date, the role of these targeted agents as adjuvant therapy has not been investigated. The clinical experience with *EGFR* TKIs in this setting is very limited, and most trials to date have not required that patients have molecular testing for a drug-specific molecular predictive factor. It has been shown that patients with sensitizing mutations appear to derive more benefit from adjuvant chemotherapy and that chemotherapy may reduce the frequency of *EGFR* mutations, suggesting a preferred response of those subclones to chemotherapy.[89,90]

A Japanese phase III study planned to randomly assign patients with completely resected NSCLC (stage IB–IIIA) to receive either adjuvant gefitinib at 250 mg/day or placebo 4 to 6 weeks following surgery, for 2 years, until recurrence or trial withdrawal. However, recruitment was stopped after 38 patients had been randomly assigned, because interstitial lung disease–type events were being increasingly reported in Japan in the advanced disease setting. Safety data for 38 recruited patients (18 who received gefitinib and 20 who received placebo) showed no unexpected adverse drug reactions, with the most common being grade 1 or gastrointestinal and skin disorders in 12 and 16 patients receiving gefitinib, respectively, and in 5 and 6 patients receiving placebo, respectively. Grade 3 or 4 adverse events occurred in 4 patients receiving gefitinib and in 1 patient receiving placebo. Interstitial lung disease–type events were reported in 1 patient receiving gefitinib (concomitantly with other interstitial lung disease–inducing drugs) who died and in 2 patients receiving placebo. Adverse events associated with surgical complications were reported in 6 patients receiving gefitinib and in 4 patients receiving placebo.[91]

In the same patient population, another phase III trial from the National Cancer Institute of Canada (JBR.19) compared gefitinib and placebo after four courses of cisplatin-based chemotherapy, but the trial was prematurely closed after accrual of only 503 patients as a consequence of the negative outcome of other phase III studies, such as Southwest Oncology Group (SWOG) S0023 (gefitinib compared with placebo for patients with nonprogressive stage IIIB disease after concurrent chemoradiation therapy and maintenance docetaxel) and the Iressa Survival Evaluation in Lung Cancer trial (second-line gefitinib compared with placebo).[92–94] Data from JBR.19 showed no advantage for the addition of maintenance gefitinib after adjuvant chemotherapy.[92] Few patients in this trial had documented *EGFR* mutations, and they also did not seem to derive benefit from gefitinib.

The Randomized Double-Blind Trial in Adjuvant NSCLC With Tarceva (RADIANT) trial compared adjuvant erlotinib with placebo after adjuvant platinum-based chemotherapy in patients with stage IB–IIIA NSCLC positive for *EGFR* expression according to IHC and/or fluorescence in situ hybridization [FISH]. The primary end point was disease-free survival (DFS); key secondary end points were OS and DFS and OS in patients whose tumors had *EGFR*-activating mutations (EGFRm-positive). A total of 973 patients were randomly assigned and there was no statistically significant difference in DFS (median, 50.5 months for erlotinib and 48.2 months for placebo; HR, 0.90; 95% CI, 0.74–1.10; $p = 0.324$). Among the 161 patients (16.5%) in the EGFRm-positive subgroup, DFS favored erlotinib (median, 46.4 vs. 28.5 months; HR, 0.61; 95% CI, 0.38–0.98; $p = 0.039$), but this was not statistically significant because of the hierarchical testing procedure and no effect on survival was demonstrated. The most common grade 3 adverse events in patients treated with erlotinib were rash (22.3%) and diarrhea (6.2%).[95] Potential limitations of the study are the relative unselected patient population, as FISH is positive in a large proportion of patients and a less sensitive biomarker than mutation testing, and thus, the role of FISH in early-stage disease is unproven. The onset of resistant secondary mutations or other resistance mechanisms may be another concern, as these mutations and resistance mechanisms have been noted frequently in stage IV disease.

Analysis of data from a surgical database of 167 patients with completely resected stage I–III NSCLC harboring sensitizing mutations and treated with adjuvant TKIs showed a 2-year survival of 89% compared with 72% for nontreated patients.[96] The findings support evaluation in prospective studies.

In another study, 36 patients with surgically resected stage IA–IIIA NSCLC harboring activating *EGFR* mutations were treated with 150 mg/day of erlotinib for 2 years after completion of any standard adjuvant chemotherapy and/or radiotherapy. After a median follow-up of 2.5 years, the 2-year disease-free survival was 94% (95% CI, 80% to 99%), suggesting an improvement over the historically expected rate of 70%.[97]

A definitive trial evaluating erlotinib and crizotinib in patients selected according to molecular testing was close to starting in the United States at the time of publication. This trial, Adjuvant Lung Cancer Enrichment Marker Identification and Sequencing Trial (ALCHEMIST), will initially focus on patients with tumors with *EGFR* mutations and *EML-ALK* fusions, but it is designed to allow for inclusion of additional targets, as active agents for them are identified.

Another recent randomized trial evaluated the efficacy of an anti-MAGE-A3 cancer immunotherapeutic as adjuvant therapy. Patients with completely resected stage IB–IIIA MAGE-positive NSCLC were randomly assigned to either receive intramuscular injections of recombinant MAGE-A3 with an added immunostimulant or placebo in a 2–1 randomization design. A total of 13,849 patients were screened for MAGE-A3 expression, and 4210 had a MAGE-positive tumor; 2312 of these patients met all eligibility criteria and were randomly assigned to treatment. Median DFS was 60.5 months for the MAGE group and 57.9 months for placebo (not significant). Thus, further development of this approach has been halted. It should be noted, however, that high interest currently exists to further study immune stimulatory approaches. These are now focused on inhibitors of the PD-1 mechanism.[93,98]

NEOADJUVANT CHEMOTHERAPY

Neoadjuvant (preoperative) chemotherapy offers potential advantages over postoperative chemotherapy, including greater therapeutic compliance and the ability to treat micrometastatic disease, to analyze the treatment-related effect on the primary tumor, and to select patients with responsive disease; patients with disease progression during chemotherapy will most likely not benefit from surgery.

Platinum-based doublets confer response rates in the preoperative setting that exceed rates achieved in advanced NSCLC,[99–102] and consequently, tumor downstaging may potentially lead to a higher percentage of radical resections. Disadvantages of neoadjuvant chemotherapy include the delay of surgery, less accurate staging (the pathologic staging is confounded by the induction treatment), and, potentially, increased surgical morbidity and mortality after chemotherapy, with a decrease in the quality of life.

In the 1990s, two small, randomized phase III trials, mainly designed for patients with stage III (N2) NSCLC, were terminated early based on interim analyses that showed significant improvements in OS for the combined approach of perioperative chemotherapy plus surgery compared with surgery alone.[103,104] However, results from these early trials may have been biased by imbalances between treatment groups in important prognostic factors. A large, randomized study by Depierre et al.[105] showed an 11-month improvement in survival with neoadjuvant chemotherapy compared with surgery alone for patients with stage I–IIIA disease (median, 37 vs. 26 months, $p = 0.15$).[105] The difference in OS between the treatment arms increased to 10.4% at 3 years, favoring neoadjuvant chemotherapy, with a significant reduction in the rate of disease-free survival ($p = 0.033$). In a subset analysis, the benefit of chemotherapy was confined to patients with N0 and N1 disease, with a relative risk of death of 0.68 ($p = 0.027$).

All of the aforementioned studies were conducted with doublet or triplet combinations that are not currently used. The feasibility and safety of neoadjuvant chemotherapy with carboplatin and paclitaxel for early-stage NSCLC were prospectively established in the Bimodality Lung Oncology Team trial.[106] This phase II trial enrolled two sequential cohorts of patients with clinical stage IB, II, and IIIA disease. Clinical staging was defined by CT imaging, and mediastinoscopy was required for all patients. Patients with mediastinoscopy-proven N2 disease or superior sulcus tumors were excluded from the trial. Patients were treated with paclitaxel and carboplatin before and after surgery; patients in cohort 1 received two cycles before surgery and three cycles after surgery, and patients in cohort 2 received three cycles before surgery and four cycles after surgery. For all the patients in both cohorts, the radiographic response rate was 51%, the complete resection rate was 86%, and the pathologic complete response rate was 5%. Three-year and 5-year survival rates were 61% and 45%, respectively, which are comparable to the rates in historical series. There were no significant differences in patient characteristics or outcome between the two cohorts. A detailed analysis showed a lack of correlation between radiographic and pathologic responses, with 50% of patients who were found to have equivalent or more extensive disease at surgery having a major response to chemotherapy. Two patients died postoperatively. Ninety-six percent of patients received the planned preoperative chemotherapy, and 45% received postoperative chemotherapy. A subsequent phase III study, SWOG S9900, compared the same induction chemotherapy for three cycles followed by surgery with surgery alone for patients with clinical stage IB, II, and IIIA NSCLC (excluding superior sulcus and N2 disease).[107] Mediastinoscopy was performed when a mediastinal lymph node was bigger than 1 cm, and the original statistical plan called for 600 patients in order to detect a 33% increase in median survival or a 10% increase in 5-year survival. This trial closed prematurely in June 2004 when new evidence demonstrated the superiority of adjuvant chemotherapy over surgery alone, making the accrual to the control arm of the study flawed. At the time of study closure, 336 of the planned 600 eligible patients had been enrolled. Neoadjuvant chemotherapy was well tolerated, with 79% of patients receiving all three cycles. Objective response was documented in 41%, and 7% had progressive disease. Seven patients in the chemotherapy arm died postoperatively, compared with four patients in the surgery alone arm. With a median follow-up of 53 months, the median survival was 75 months for the chemotherapy arm compared with 46 months for the surgery alone arm; the 5-year survival rates were 50% and 43%, respectively. Although the use of chemotherapy was associated with a 19% reduction in the risk of death (HR, 0.81), this difference did not achieve significance ($p = 0.19$). Progression-free survival trended in favor of perioperative chemotherapy (median, 33 vs. 21 months, $p = 0.07$).

The Neoadjuvant Taxol Carboplatin Hope (NATCH) trial compared surgery alone to either chemotherapy followed by surgery or surgery followed by chemotherapy.[108] A total of 624 patients with stage I (greater than 2 cm), II, and T3 N1 disease according to the sixth edition of the TNM staging classification for lung cancer were randomly assigned to the three arms. The primary end point of the study was DFS. In the preoperative arm, 97% of patients started the planned chemotherapy, and the radiographic response rate was 53.3%. In the adjuvant arm, 66.2% started the planned chemotherapy. Surgery was performed in 94% of patients; surgical procedures and postoperative mortality were similar across the three arms. There was a trend toward longer DFS for patients in the preoperative arm compared with patients in the surgery alone arm (5-year DFS, 38.3% vs. 34.1%; HR for progression or death, 0.92; $p = 0.176$). The 5-year DFS rate was 36.6% in the adjuvant arm (HR for comparison with surgery alone arm, 0.96; $p = 0.74$). Overall, this study failed to show significant differences in DFS with the addition of preoperative or adjuvant chemotherapy to surgery. In this trial, in which the treatment allocation was made before surgery, more patients were able to receive preoperative than adjuvant treatment.

Another phase III trial promoted by the Medical Research Council (MRC), with the participation of European cooperative groups (MRC LU22, NVALT 2, EORTC 08012), randomly assigned 519 patients with early-stage NSCLC to receive either surgery (261 patients) or three cycles of platinum-based chemotherapy followed by surgery (258 patients).[109] Before randomization, clinicians chose the chemotherapy that would be given from a list of six standard regimens. The primary outcome measure was OS, which was analyzed on an intent-to-treat basis. Most of the patients (61%) had clinical stage I disease; 31% had stage II disease, and 7% had stage III disease. Seventy-five percent of patients received all three cycles of chemotherapy. The overall response rate was 49% (95% CI, 43% to 55%) and disease was downstaged in 31% (range, 25% to 37%) of patients. The rate of postoperative complications was not higher in the combined-modality arm and no impairment of quality of life was noted. However, there was no evidence of a benefit in terms of OS (HR, 1.02; 95% CI, 0.80–1.31; $p = 0.86$).

In another pan-European phase III study, Chemotherapy for Early Stages Trial (ChEST), patients with chemotherapy- and radiotherapy-naïve NSCLC (stage IB, II, or IIIA) were randomly assigned to either treatment with three cycles of gemcitabine (1250 mg/m^2 on days 1 and 8, every 3 weeks) plus cisplatin (75 mg/m^2 on days 1 or 2, every 3 weeks) followed by surgery, or to surgery alone.[110] Randomization was stratified by center and disease stage (IB/IIA vs. IIB/IIIA). The primary end point was 3-year progression-free survival. The study was closed prematurely after the random assignment of 270 patients, 129 to combined therapy and 141 to surgery alone. Slightly more patients in the surgery alone arm had stage IB–IIA disease (55.3% vs. 48.8%). The chemotherapy response rate was 35.4%. The combined modality was

associated with significantly better progression-free survival (HR, 0.70; $p = 0.003$) and OS (HR, 0.63; $p = 0.02$). Preoperative chemotherapy had a significant impact on outcomes in the stage IIB–IIIA subgroup (3-year progression-free rate, 36.1% vs. 55.4%; $p = 0.002$). These findings are not consistent with the results of S9900, which found no difference in treatment effect by stage,[107] and the results of the trial by Depierre et al.,[105] in which the benefit of chemotherapy was greater for patients with earlier stages of disease. The NATCH trial, however, demonstrated greater benefit of chemotherapy among patients with clinical stage II (T3 N1) disease.[108]

A systematic review and meta-analysis not based on individual patient data was reported in 2006 by Burdett et al.[111] and updated to include results from the MRC trial.[109] The original meta-analysis included data from seven randomized trials published between 1990 and 2005 (988 patients globally). Neoadjuvant chemotherapy improved survival (HR, 0.82; 95% CI, 0.69–0.97), equivalent to an absolute benefit of 6% at 5 years. The update documented a shift of the HR to 0.87 (95% CI, 0.76–1.01), with loss of the significance of the improvement in outcome. In 2014, the NSCLC Meta-analysis Collaborative Group performed a systematic review and individual participant data meta-analysis to establish the effect of preoperative chemotherapy for patients with resectable NSCLC.[112] Analyses of 15 randomized controlled trials (2385 patients) showed a significant benefit of neoadjuvant chemotherapy on survival (HR, 0.87; 95% CI, 0.78–0.96; $p = 0.007$), a 13% reduction in the relative risk of death (Fig. 51.3). This finding is remarkably similar to the results of the LACE Collaborative Group, which further updated the data in the meta-analysis with the results of the phase III studies NATCH and ChEST. Consisting of nearly 2200 total patients from 10 trials, the combined analysis produced a HR favoring neoadjuvant chemotherapy and surgery of 0.89 (95% CI, 0.81–0.98; $p = 0.02$) (unpublished data). The combined HR from these meta-analyses suggests that the estimated benefit from neoadjuvant chemotherapy is similar in magnitude to that expected with adjuvant chemotherapy.

A French multi-institutional trial first compared in an open-label, randomized trial with a 2 × 2 factorial design preoperative versus postoperative chemotherapy, then two chemotherapy regimens (gemcitabine-cisplatin versus paclitaxel-carboplatin). The preoperative group received two preoperative cycles followed by two additional preoperative cycles, while the postoperative group underwent two preoperative cycles followed by two postoperative cycles, the third and fourth cycles being given only to responders in both cases. A total of 528 patients were randomized and the 3-year OS did not differ between the two groups (67.4% and 67.7%, respectively; HR, 1.01 [0.79–1.30], $p = 0.92$), nor did 3-year DFS, response rates, toxicity, or postoperative mortality. Chemotherapy compliance was significantly higher in the preoperative group.[113]

In summary, perioperative chemotherapy is a feasible and ethical approach for patients with stage II–IIIA NSCLC, and modern chemotherapy regimens produce a benefit in the neoadjuvant setting similar to the benefit in the adjuvant setting although the supportive database is smaller. Tumor response occurs in 40% to 50% of patients, with treatment compliance that is generally better than that for adjuvant chemotherapy. However, the tumor is downstaged in fewer than 20% of cases and the rate of complete response is low.

BIOMARKERS TO INDIVIDUALIZE ADJUVANT CHEMOTHERAPY

Current research efforts aim to identify subsets of patients who will derive the greatest benefit from adjuvant chemotherapy by using gene expression profiling and pharmacogenomic approaches.

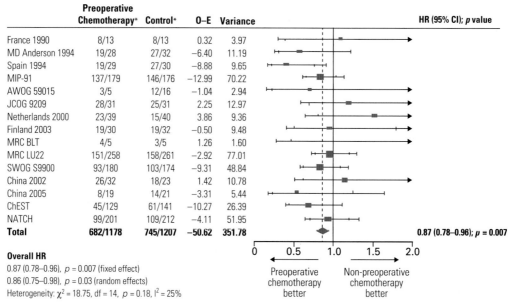

	Preoperative Chemotherapy*	Control*	O–E	Variance	HR (95% CI); p value
France 1990	8/13	8/13	0.32	3.97	
MD Anderson 1994	19/28	27/32	−6.40	11.19	
Spain 1994	19/29	27/30	−8.88	9.65	
MIP-91	137/179	146/176	−12.99	70.22	
AWOG 59015	3/5	12/16	−1.04	2.94	
JCOG 9209	28/31	25/31	2.25	12.97	
Netherlands 2000	23/39	15/40	3.86	9.36	
Finland 2003	19/30	19/32	−0.50	9.48	
MRC BLT	4/5	3/5	1.26	1.60	
MRC LU22	151/258	158/261	−2.92	77.01	
SWOG S9900	93/180	103/174	−9.31	48.84	
China 2002	26/32	18/23	1.42	10.78	
China 2005	8/19	14/21	−3.31	5.44	
ChEST	45/129	61/141	−10.27	26.39	
NATCH	99/201	109/212	−4.11	51.95	
Total	**682/1178**	**745/1207**	**−50.62**	**351.78**	**0.87 (0.78–0.96); p = 0.007**

Overall HR
0.87 (0.78–0.96), $p = 0.007$ (fixed effect)
0.86 (0.75–0.98), $p = 0.03$ (random effects)
Heterogeneity: $\chi^2 = 18.75$, df = 14, $p = 0.18$, $I^2 = 25\%$

Fig. 51.3. Effect of neoadjuvant (preoperative) chemotherapy on survival. Each square denotes the hazard ratio (HR) for that trial comparison, with the horizontal lines showing the 95% and 99% CIs. The size of the square is directly proportional to the amount of information contributed by the trial. The blue diamond gives the pooled HR from the fixed-effect model; the center of this diamond denotes the HR and the extremities the 95% CI. *BLT*, Big Lung Trial; *ChEST*, Chemotherapy for Early Stages Trial; *CI*, confidence interval; *df*, degrees of freedom; *JCOG*, Japanese Cancer Oncology Group; *MIP*, mitomycin, ifosfamide, cisplatin; *MRC*, Medical Research Council; *NATCH*, Neoadjuvant/Adjuvant Trial of Chemotherapy; *O–E*, observed minus expected; *SWOG*, South West Oncology Group.*Number of events/number entered. (*Reprinted from NSCLC Meta-analysis Collaborative Group. Preoperative chemotherapy for non-small cell lung cancer: a systematic review and meta-analysis of individual participant data. Lancet. 2014;383:1561–1571.*)

Microarray technologies allow researchers to explore the prognostic significance of thousands of markers using high-throughput and computational approaches. To date, more than 30 studies in lung cancer have been reported, showing that gene expression signature may stratify patients with early-stage NSCLC into different groups based on prognosis or survival.[114] Although most of these signatures have been validated in one or more independent patient cohorts, overlap of gene sets in the microarray datasets has been minimal. Thus, there is a strong possibility that sample collection methods, processing protocols, single-institution patient cohorts, small sample sizes, and peculiarities of the different microarray platforms are contributing substantially to the results. To address these issues, a multi-institutional collaborative study was conducted to generate gene expression profiles from a large number of samples with a priori determined clinical features, useful to evaluate proposed prognostic models for potential clinical implementation. A large series of lung adenocarcinomas was tested to determine whether microarray measurements of gene expression, either alone or combined with basic clinical covariates (stage of disease, age, and gender of the patient), can be used to predict OS. The risk scores produced correlated strongly with actual outcomes, especially when clinical and molecular information were combined to build prognostic models for early-stage lung cancer.[115]

A 14-gene expression assay based on quantitative polymerase chain reaction (PCR) that used formalin-fixed paraffin-embedded tissue samples and differentiated patients with heterogeneous statistical prognoses was developed in a cohort of 361 patients with resected nonsquamous NSCLC. The assay was validated in two different cohorts: 433 patients with resected stage I nonsquamous NSCLC and 1006 patients with resected stage I–III nonsquamous NSCLC from several leading Chinese cancer centers.[116] The signature segregated patients according to risk (low, intermediate,

and high), with 5-year survival rates of 71.4%, 58.3%, and 49.2%, respectively ($p = 0.0003$). Multivariate analysis in both cohorts indicated that no standard clinical risk factors could account for or provide the prognostic information derived from tumor gene expression. These data suggest that quantitative-PCR-based assays could reliably identify patients with early-stage nonsquamous NSCLC at high risk for mortality after surgical resection.

A DNA methylation microarray that analyzes 450,000 CpG sites was used to investigate tumoral DNA obtained from 444 patients with NSCLC that included 237 stage I tumors. The prognostic DNA methylation markers were validated in an independent cohort of 143 patients with stage I NSCLC. Unsupervised clustering of the 10,000 most variable DNA methylation sites in the discovery cohort identified patients with high-risk stage I NSCLC who had shorter relapse-free survival (RFS; HR [HR], 2.35; 95% CI, 1.29–4.28; $p = 0.004$). The study in the validation cohort of the significant methylated sites from the discovery cohort found that hypermethylation of five genes was significantly associated with shorter RFS in stage I NSCLC: *HIST1H4F*, *PCDHGB6*, *NPBWR1*, *ALX1*, and *HOXA9*. A signature based on the number of hypermethylated events distinguished patients with high- and low-risk stage I NSCLC (HR, 3.24; 95% CI, 1.61–6.54; $p = 0.001$).[117]

Although these types of molecular tools may add prognostic information beyond stage in early NSCLC or may serve as a stratification tool for future adjuvant studies, they are not routinely used in clinical practice.

Another approach that has been evaluated as a method for selecting patients for adjuvant chemotherapy is to identify a predictive molecular determinant for cisplatin. Cisplatin inhibits replication by binding to DNA and forming platinum–DNA adducts, causing strand breaks when the DNA helices unwind in preparation for replication. The nuclear excision repair (NER)

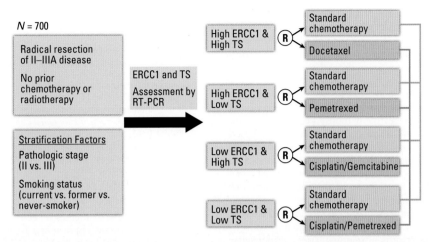

Fig. 51.4. The International Tailored Chemotherapy Adjuvant Trial, an ongoing phase III multicenter randomized trial comparing adjuvant pharmacogenomic-driven chemotherapy with standard adjuvant chemotherapy for completely resected stage II–IIIA nonsmall cell lung cancer. *ERCC1*, excision repair cross–complementation group 1; *RT-PCR*, real-time polymerase chain reaction; *TS*, thymidylate synthase.

family of genes is involved in repair of these DNA strand breaks.[118] The excision repair cross–complementation group 1 (ERCC1) enzyme is one of the proteins involved in the final step of the NER pathway that recognizes and removes cisplatin-induced DNA adducts. ERCC1 is also important in the repair of interstrand cross-links in DNA and in recombination processes. The removal of platinum-DNA adducts by the proteins of the NER pathway reverses the tumoral DNA damage induced by cisplatin, leading to cisplatin resistance. High tumoral *ERCC1* expression, therefore, was predicted to be associated with cisplatin resistance and hence serve as a predictive molecular determinant for this chemotherapy agent.

Exploratory studies in advanced disease confirmed this hypothesis,[119,120] but a later phase III trial failed to prove the superiority of this approach.[121] *ERCC1* expression may be investigated either at the protein level, with use of IHC, or at the mRNA level, with use of quantitative PCR. Initial data from the IALT Biology study appeared to confirm ERCC1 as assessed by IHC as a positive prognostic factor and negative predictive factor for benefit from chemotherapy in a sample of 761 tumor specimens obtained before administration of chemotherapy.[122] Thus, patients with tumors that overexpressed *ERCC1* had longer survival than patients with tumors that did not, but the addition of chemotherapy was of no additional benefit. Among patients with no ERCC1 protein detected in the tumor, the median survival was 14 months longer for patients who received chemotherapy than for patients who did not receive chemotherapy. Among patients with *ERCC1*-positive tumors, there were no differences in survival with or without chemotherapy. This observation prompted the initiation of a phase II study that enrolled 150 patients with completely resected nonsquamous cell stage II or IIIA (non-N2) tumors. Patients in the control arm (n = 74) were treated with four standard-dose courses of cisplatin plus pemetrexed (CP). In the customized treatment arm (n = 76), patients with activated *EGFR* mutations received erlotinib 150 mg for 1 year; *ERCC1*-negative patients received four CP courses, whereas *ERCC1*-positive patients underwent follow-up. The trial sought to demonstrate the feasibility of customized adjuvant chemotherapy based on timely biomarker analysis within a 2-month postsurgery delay.

The primary end point of the study was met but the subsequent phase III study was cancelled because the unreliability of the ERCC1 immunohistochemical read-outs became evident.[123] In fact in a further analysis of a larger number of samples, original results about the predictive role of ERCC1 IHC were not confirmed,[124] likely due to the fact that currently available monoclonal antibodies could not distinguish among the four ERCC1 protein isoforms, whereas only one isoform produced a protein that had full capacities for nucleotide excision repair and cisplatin resistance.[116,125] Thus, ERCC1 testing is not currently used in routine practice. Other genomic markers being investigated in ongoing randomized clinical trials in early disease to tailor adjuvant treatment include *BRCA1*, another gene involved in both homologous recombination repair and nonhomologous end joining,[125] and thymidylate synthase, a putative marker for pemetrexed sensitivity.[126]

In a Spanish multicenter study, completely resected stage II–III NSCLC patients were randomized to receive standard adjuvant chemotherapy or, in the experimental arm, three different treatment options based on the level of tumor *BRCA1* expression. The study failed to show a significant benefit from treatment customization, but a longer follow-up time is needed to conclude definitively in favor of a completely negative study. The study does not support the hypothesis of cisplatin-resistance in high *BRCA1* tumors, and cisplatin-based CT remains the standard of care.

Another phase III trial, the International Tailored Chemotherapy Adjuvant Trial, compared adjuvant pharmacogenomic-driven chemotherapy versus standard adjuvant chemotherapy in completely resected stage II–IIIA NSCLC by evaluating *ERCC1* and thymidylate synthase expression (Fig. 51.4) The trial has fully completed the accrual in 2014 and final results are eagerly awaited.

CONCLUSION

Randomized studies testing the efficacy of current standard adjuvant chemotherapy regimens have demonstrated a positive impact on DFS and OS. A precise quantitative estimate of the survival gain is not known, but meta-analysis suggests it is approximately 5% at 5 years. The findings of two randomized clinical trials conducted with selected patient populations support the use of adjuvant treatment after complete resection of stage IB–II NSCLC, and two other, larger, randomized clinical trials (one marginally positive and one marginally negative) support the use of adjuvant treatment after complete resection of all stages of NSCLC. A new meta-analysis that includes the most recent generation of these positive and negative randomized clinical studies will substantially contribute to determining the role of adjuvant chemotherapy.

There is a need, however, for reliable predictive and prognostic factors that stratify patients who do or do not need adjuvant therapy in order to avoid the exposure of most patients to unnecessary treatments. In the near future, genomic (or pharmacogenomic) and proteomic assays may drive the identification of patients who are ideal candidates for adjuvant therapy.

Neoadjuvant chemotherapy may be better suited than adjuvant therapy for evaluating novel agents, as the effect of the drug on the target can be assessed by pretreatment biopsy (at diagnosis) and after chemotherapy (at surgery). However, targeted agents matched to specific mutations may need to be administered for long periods of time, which is better accomplished in the adjuvant setting, where a curative resection option is not jeopardized in patients who fail to respond preoperatively. The duration of the administration of novel agents postoperatively, for example, in patients who have an initial response, will need careful evaluation in randomized trials. It is hoped that better patient selection and better matching of individual patients to a specific treatment regimen based on molecular profiling can lead to more effective treatment.

Smoking cessation and early detection of lung cancer remain of high importance. It is hoped that newer radiographic methodologies will allow for better characterization and even earlier detection of malignancies to decrease the number of diagnostic procedures performed to remove small lesions that are not malignant. In the long run, improved molecular technologies are likely to also allow for earlier detection by nonradiographic methods.

KEY REFERENCES

9. Boyd JA, Hubbs JL, Kim DW, et al. Timing of local and distant failure in resected lung cancer: implications for reported rates of local failure. *J Thorac Oncol*. 2010;5(2):211–214.
21. PORT Meta-analysis Trialists Group. Postoperative radiotherapy for non-small cell lung cancer. *Cochrane Database Syst Rev*. 2000;(2): CD002142.
33. Non-small Cell Lung Cancer Collaborative Group. Chemotherapy in non-small cell lung cancer: a meta-analysis using updated data on individual patients from 52 randomised clinical trials. *BMJ*. 1995;311(7010):899–909.
63. Hamada C, Tanaka F, Ohta M, et al. Meta-analysis of postoperative adjuvant chemotherapy with tegafur-uracil in non-small-cell lung cancer. *J Clin Oncol*. 2005;23(22):4999–5006.
64. Pignon JP, Tribodet H, Scagliotti GV, LACE Collaborative Group. Lung adjuvant cisplatin evaluation: a pooled analysis by the LACE Collaborative Group. *J Clin Oncol*. 2008;26(21):3552–3559.
65. NSCLC Meta-analyses Collaborative Group, Arriagada R, Auperin A, et al. Adjuvant chemotherapy, with or without postoperative radiotherapy, in operable non-small-cell lung cancer: two meta-analyses of individual patient data. *Lancet*. 2010;375(9722):1267–1277.
68. Burdett S1, Pignon JP, Tierney J, et al. Adjuvant chemotherapy for resected early-stage non-small cell lung cancer. *Cochrane Database Syst Rev*. 2015;(3): CD011430.
77. Fruh M, Rolland E, Pignon JP, et al. Pooled analysis of the effect of age on adjuvant cisplatin-based chemotherapy for completely resected non-small-cell lung cancer. *J Clin Oncol*. 2008;26(21): 3573–3581.
95. Kelly K, Altorki NK, Eberhardt WE, et al. Adjuvant Erlotinib Versus Placebo in Patients With Stage IB–IIIA Non-Small-Cell Lung Cancer (RADIANT): a Randomized, double-blind, phase III Trial. *J Clin Oncol*. 2015;33:4007–4014.
116. Kratz JR, He J, Van Den Eeden SK, et al. A practical molecular assay to predict survival in resected non-squamous, non-small-cell lung cancer: development and international validation studies. *Lancet*. 2012;379(9818):823–832.
122. Olaussen KA, Dunant A, Fouret P, et al. DNA repair by ERCC1 in non-small-cell lung cancer and cisplatin-based adjuvant chemotherapy. *N Engl J Med*. 2006;355(10):983–991.
124. Friboulet L, Olaussen KA, Pignon JP, et al. ERCC1 isoform expression and DNA repair in non-small-cell lung cancer. *N Engl J Med*. 2013;368(12):1101–1110.

See Expertconsult.com for full list of references.

52 Treatment of Extensive-Stage Small Cell Lung Cancer

Mamta Parikh, Karen Kelly, Primo N. Lara, Jr., and Egbert F. Smit

SUMMARY OF KEY POINTS

- Performance status is universally recognized as an independent prognostic factor and typically correlates with the extent of tumor burden.
- As first-line therapy, platinum agent plus etoposide or irinotecan remains the standard of care for the treatment of small cell lung cancer (SCLC).
- The ideal number of chemotherapy cycles for SCLC has not been defined; however, four to six cycles are considered the standard based on results from randomized trials.
- Despite an initially high response rate to frontline platinum-based chemotherapy, extensive-stage SCLC will universally relapse, often within 3 to 6 months.
- Alternative chemotherapy strategies have focused on modifying the dosage and schedules of established regimens.
- Dose-dense regimens have shown mixed results.
- Most trials employing a dose-intensification strategy did not show a survival advantage over standard therapy for patients with extensive-stage SCLC, and higher doses were typically associated with greater toxicity.
- Patients who receive no further therapy have a median survival of less than 3 months.
- Patients who have previously received platinum-based therapy are grouped into two general categories reflecting the platinum-sensitivity status of their disease: platinum sensitive and platinum refractory.
- Topotecan is approved as second-line treatment for patients with platinum-sensitive, relapsed disease based on symptom control. An oral formulation of topotecan was also developed for patients' convenience.
- Despite progress in the understanding of genomic alterations and signaling pathways in SCLC, clinical experiments with tyrosine kinase inhibitors, other small-molecule inhibitors, and antiangiogenic agents have been disappointing Other therapeutic areas of interest more recently evaluated include epigenetic modifiers, inhibitors of DNA repair and the cell cycle, immunocheckpoint inhibitors and inhibitors of the Notch pathway.

The chemosensitivity of small cell lung cancer (SCLC) was first identified 50 years ago with the recognition that methyl-bis-β-chloroethyl amine hydrochloride could cause tumor regression in more than 50% of patients.[1] Since then, numerous antineoplastic agents have been shown to produce objective response rates of at least 20% in previously untreated patients. Older active agents included nitrogen mustard, doxorubicin, methotrexate, ifosfamide, etoposide, teniposide, vincristine, vindesine, nitrosureas, and cisplatin and its analog carboplatin.[2] In the 1990s, six new agents were discovered to have activity against SCLC in untreated patients, including paclitaxel, docetaxel, topotecan, irinotecan, vinorelbine,

and gemcitabine.[3–11] In this century, two additional cytotoxic agents were evaluated: pemetrexed, a multitargeted antifolate agent evaluated as monotherapy in the relapse setting, and amrubicin, a topoisomerase II inhibitor that has produced impressive responses as first-line therapy.[12,13] This chapter discusses first-line and second-line therapy for patients with extensive-stage SCLC.

FIRST-LINE CHEMOTHERAPY

Combination Chemotherapy

Given the large number of active agents in SCLC, the evaluation of combination regimens quickly ensued. In the 1970s, randomized trials demonstrated the superiority of combination chemotherapy over single-agent therapy.[14] Furthermore, studies showed that simultaneous administration of multiple agents was more efficacious than the sequential administration of the same agents.[15,16] Cyclophosphamide-based regimens were commonly used to treat SCLC, including cyclophosphamide, doxorubicin, and vincristine (CAV); cyclophosphamide, doxorubicin, and etoposide (CDE); and cyclophosphamide, etoposide, and vincristine (CEV).

After the introduction of cisplatin, randomized trials with a regimen of cisplatin and etoposide showed that this combination was as effective as CAV and less toxic.[17,18] A meta-analysis of 36 trials demonstrated that regimens containing cisplatin and/or etoposide offered a significant survival advantage to patients with SCLC.[19] Thus cisplatin and etoposide became the preferred regimen for the treatment of extensive-stage SCLC, yielding overall response rates of 65% to 85%, complete response rates of 10% to 20%, and a median survival of 8 months to 10 months.[16–18] For patients with limited-stage SCLC, cisplatin and etoposide plus twice-daily thoracic radiotherapy was also considered the treatment of choice, producing an 87% overall response rate, a 56% complete response rate, a median survival of 23 months, and a 5-year survival rate of 44%.[20] Carboplatin is frequently substituted for cisplatin because of its more favorable toxicity profile. One small randomized trial comparing cisplatin and etoposide with carboplatin and etoposide in patients with limited- and extensive-stage disease showed similar efficacy, but the carboplatin-based combination was significantly less toxic.[21] A meta-analysis of individual data from 633 patients who participated in four clinical trials did not demonstrate any difference in efficacy between cisplatin- and carboplatin-based regimens, with a median survival of 9.6 months and 9.4 months, respectively.[22] Significant differences in toxicity were found; more neutropenia, anemia, and thrombocytopenia occurred with carboplatin-based regimens, whereas more nausea, vomiting, neurotoxicity, and renal toxicity developed with cisplatin-based regimens.

Years elapsed before the discovery of newer cytotoxic agents such as the topoisomerase II inhibitors, taxanes, gemcitabine, and vinorelbine, which were shown to have antitumor activity in SCLC. Many studies have summarized the results from novel combinations that were evaluated in phase III trials (Table 52.1).[23–55] Enthusiasm for the combination of cisplatin and irinotecan (PI) arose when Japanese researchers halted their phase III trial prematurely after an interim analysis showed a survival benefit for PI over cisplatin and etoposide.[23] One hundred and fifty-four patients were randomly assigned to receive either four

TABLE 52.1 Randomized Trials Comparing First-Line Combination Chemotherapy Regimens for Small Cell Lung Cancer

Author (y)	Regimen	No. of Patients	Overall Response Rate (%)	Progression-Free Survival (mo)	Median Survival (mo)	1-Year Survival Rate (%)
Noda et al.[23] (2002)	PI	77	84.4[a]	6.9[b]	12.8[c]	58.4
	PE	77	67.5	4.8	9.4	37.7
Lara, Jr. et al.[24] (2009)	PI	324	60	5.8	9.9	41
	PE	327	57	5.2	9.1	34
Hanna et al.[25] (2006)	PI	221	48	4.1	9.3	35
	PE	110	44	4.6	10.2	35
Zatloukal et al.[26] (2010)	PI	202	39	5.4	10.2	42
	PE	203	47	6.2	9.7	39
Kim et al.[27] (2013)	PI	173	62[d]	6.5	10.9	NR
	PE	189	48	5.8	10.3	NR
Hermes et al.[28] (2008)	IC	105	NR	NR	8.5	37[b]
	EC	104	NR	NR	7.1	19
Schmittel et al.[29] (2011)	IC	106	54	6.0	10.0	37
	EC	110	52	6.0	9.0	30
Eckardt et al.[31] (2006)	PT	389	63	6.0[b]	9.8	31
	PE	395	69	6.2	10.0	31
Fink et al.[32] (2012)	PT	357	56[e]	6.9[e]	10.3	40
	PE	346	46	6.1	9.4	36
de Jong et al.[33] (2007)	CDE	102	60	4.9	6.8	24
	CT	101	61	5.2	6.7	26
Socinski et al.[35] (2009)	PemC	364	31	3.8	8.1	NR
	EC	369	52[f]	5.4[g]	10.6[g]	NR
Kotani et al.[36] (2012)	AP	142	78	5.1	15.3	NR
	IP	142	72	5.7	18.3	NR
Mavroudis et al.[37] (2001)	PET	62	50	11.0[b]	9.5	38
	PE	71	48	9.0	10.5	37
Reck et al.[38] (2003)	CET CEV	301	72	8.1[h]	12.7	48
		307	69	7.5	11.7	51
Niell et al.[39] (2005)	PET	293	75	6.0	10.6	38
	PE	294	68	5.9	9.9	37
Pujol et al.[40] (2001)	PCDE PE	117	76[b]	7.2[i]	10.0	40[j]
		109	61	6.3	9.3	29

[a]$p = 0.02$.
[b]$p = 0.003$.
[c]$p = 0.0004$.
[d]$p = 0.0064$.
[e]$p = 0.01$.
[f]$p < 0.001$.
[g]$p < 0.01$.
[h]$p = 0.033$.
[i]$p < 0.0001$.
[j]$p = 0.0067$.

AP, amrubicin and cisplatin; CDE, cyclophosphamide, doxorubicin, and etoposide; CET, carboplatin, etoposide, and paclitaxel; CEV, carboplatin, etoposide, and vincristine; CT, carboplatin and paclitaxel; EC, etoposide and carboplatin; IC, irinotecan and carboplatin; IP, irinotecan and cisplatin; NR, not reported; PCDE, cyclophosphamide, carboplatin, doxorubicin, and epirubicin; PE, cisplatin and etoposide; PemC, pemetrexed and carboplatin; PET, cisplatin, etoposide, and paclitaxel; PI, cisplatin and irinotecan; PT, cisplatin and topotecan.

cycles of etoposide (100 mg/m^2) on days 1, 2, and 3 with cisplatin (80 mg/m^2) on day 1 every 3 weeks or four cycles of irinotecan (60 mg/m^2) on days 1, 8, and 15, and cisplatin (60 mg/m^2) on day 1. Patients treated with PI had a significantly better overall response rate (84.4% vs. 67.5%; $p = 0.02$), median survival (12.8 months vs. 9.4 months), and 1-year survival rate (58.4% vs. 37.7%; $p = 0.002$) than patients treated with cisplatin and etoposide. The PI combination was associated with a higher rate of grade 3 or grade 4 diarrhea ($p = 0.01$), whereas cisplatin and etoposide were associated with a higher rate of myelosuppression ($p = 0.0001$). The Southwest Oncology Group (SWOG) conducted a confirmatory trial using the identical study design but found no survival benefit for PI.[24] In this large trial of 651 patients, all efficacy parameters were very similar except for a trend toward improved progression-free survival time for PI (5.7 months vs. 5.2 months for cisplatin and etoposide; $p = 0.07$). Grade 3 or grade 4 neutropenia and thrombocytopenia were higher in the cisplatin and etoposide arm, whereas grade 3 or grade 4 nausea/vomiting and diarrhea were higher in the PI arm. A phase III superiority trial comparing a novel dose and schedule of the PI regimen (irinotecan [65 mg/m^2] with cisplatin [30 mg/m^2] given on days 1 and 8) with standard cisplatin and etoposide produced similar survival in both arms.[25] In Europe, a different schedule of PI (irinotecan [65 mg/m^2] on days 1 and 8 with cisplatin [80 mg/m^2] on day 1) was assessed in comparison with standard cisplatin and etoposide.[26] The data showed that the PI regimen was noninferior to cisplatin and etoposide, as hypothesized. The median overall survival rates were 10.2 months and 9.7 months, respectively, with a hazard ratio (HR) of 0.81 (95% confidence interval [CI], 0.61–1.01; $p = 0.06$). Overall response rates were 39% for PI and 47% for cisplatin and etoposide, and time to progression was 5.4 months and 6.2 months, respectively. The number of grade 3 or grade 4 adverse events was similar between the arms, but more patients in the PI arm had gastrointestinal toxicity and more patients in the cisplatin and etoposide arm had neutropenia. In 2013, Korean investigators reported the results from a phase III trial comparing PI with cisplatin and etoposide.[27] Irinotecan was administered on days 1 and 8 with cisplatin on day 1, and cisplatin and etoposide were given in the standard fashion. The trial, however, did not demonstrate the superiority of PI (HR, 0.88; 95% CI, 0.73–1.05; $p = 0.12$). The median overall survival was 10.9 months for PI and 10.3 months for cisplatin and etoposide. The overall response rate was significantly higher for PI (62.3% vs. 48.2%; $p = 0.0064$), but progression-free survival was not significantly different (6.5 months vs. 5.8 months, respectively). The frequency of anemia, nausea, and diarrhea was greater with PI.

Irinotecan has also been evaluated in combination with carboplatin. The IRIS study demonstrated superior survival for irinotecan plus carboplatin compared with oral etoposide plus carboplatin; however, overall survival in both study arms was low, at less than 9 months.[28] Drug dosages and schedules were unconventional and lower than other published regimens, with irinotecan (175 mg/m^2) and carboplatin (area under the curve [AUC] 4) administered on day 1, and etoposide (120 mg/m^2) orally on days 1–5 with carboplatin (AUC 4) on day 1. Another trial, conducted in Germany, randomly assigned 216 patients to receive either irinotecan (50 mg/m^2) on days 1, 8, and 15 with carboplatin (AUC 5) or intravenous (IV) etoposide (140 mg/m^2) on days 1–3 with carboplatin (AUC 5).[29] The irinotecan regimen was not found to be superior to the etoposide regimen in terms of overall survival (HR, 1.34; 95% CI, 0.97–1.85; $p = 0.072$). The median survival was 10 months and 9 months, respectively. The overall response rate and progression-free survival were similar for both treatment arms.

A meta-analysis of seven randomized trials including 2027 patients that compared irinotecan plus a platinum agent with etoposide plus a platinum agent showed a survival advantage for irinotecan regimens (HR, 0.81; 95% CI, 0.71–0.93; $p = 0.003$).[30] No significant differences in progression-free survival or overall response rate were noted. Irinotecan regimens produced significantly less hematologic toxicity but more gastrointestinal toxicity than etoposide regimens. Overall, the data suggest that combinations of irinotecan or etoposide plus a platinum compound are reasonable options as first-line therapy for patients with extensive-stage SCLC.

Topotecan, a drug with activity for disease relapse, was evaluated in the frontline setting. Two large phase III trials with oral or IV topotecan plus cisplatin did not show a survival advantage over standard cisplatin and etoposide. Efficacy parameters were similar between the regimens, with median survival times of 9 months to 10 months.[31,32] The IV topotecan regimen did produce a significantly higher overall response rate (56% vs. 46%; $p = 0.01$) and prolonged progression-free survival (7 months vs. 6 months; $p = 0.004$), but was associated with more hematologic toxicity.

Several other novel platinum combinations have been studied. One trial comparing paclitaxel plus carboplatin with CDE showed no benefit of the doublet over the standard regimen, but survival was modest in both arms, at less than 7 months.[33] A phase III trial of the combination of pemetrexed and carboplatin unexpectedly showed inferior efficacy to standard treatment. In a previous randomized phase II study of pemetrexed plus cisplatin or carboplatin, the carboplatin arm produced a median survival of 10.4 months and was well tolerated.[34] A phase III study, the Global Analysis of Pemetrexed in SCLC Extensive Stage, was designed to show noninferiority of pemetrexed (500 mg/m^2) and carboplatin (AUC 5) compared with etoposide and carboplatin. With 733 patients randomly assigned to treatment, the study was terminated prematurely when the predefined futility end point for progression-free survival showed inferiority of the experimental arm.[35] In the final analysis, overall survival was inferior (HR, 1.56; 95% CI, 1.27–1.92; $p < 0.01$). The median overall survival was 8.1 months for pemetrexed and carboplatin and 10.6 months for etoposide and carboplatin. The median progression-free survival was 3.8 months for pemetrexed and carboplatin and 5.4 months for etoposide and carboplatin ($p < 0.01$), and the

overall response rate also favored the etoposide and carboplatin combination (52% vs. 31%; $p < 0.001$). Significant neutropenia and more febrile neutropenia were seen in the etoposide arm. By contrast, death during therapy or within 30 days was higher for the pemetrexed arm than for the etoposide arm (16% vs. 10%; $p = 0.032$), and the rate of toxicity-related death was higher (1.4% vs. 0%; $p = 0.028$).

Another novel cytotoxic agent with promising early results that failed to show a survival advantage in the phase III setting was amrubicin. A phase III randomized study showed that amrubicin plus cisplatin was inferior to PI.[36] Two hundred and eighty-four patients were randomly assigned to receive either amrubicin (35 mg/m^2 to 40 mg/m^2) on days 1–3 and cisplatin (60 mg/m^2) every 3 weeks or cisplatin (60 mg/m^2) on day 1 and irinotecan (60 mg/m^2) on days 1, 8, and 15 every 4 weeks. The median overall survival for amrubicin plus cisplatin was 15 months, compared with 18.3 months for PI (HR, 1.33; 95% CI, 1.01–1.74; $p = 0.681$), and this result exceeded the noninferiority margin. The progression-free survival was 5.1 months for amrubicin plus cisplatin and 5.7 months for PI with an overall response rate of 78% and 72%, respectively. An increased incidence of grade 4 neutropenia (79% vs. 23%) and febrile neutropenia (32% vs. 11%) was found in the amrubicin plus cisplatin arm.

The favorable toxicity profiles of most of the newer agents led investigators to explore the possibility of integrating them into an active doublet (see Table 52.1). Three randomized trials evaluating the addition of paclitaxel to cisplatin and etoposide or carboplatin and etoposide did not produce a survival benefit over traditional doublets and were associated with increased toxicity.[37–39] French investigators evaluated a four-drug regimen in which they added cyclophosphamide and 4′-epidoxorubicin to cisplatin and etoposide (PCDE). A significant improvement in the complete response rate (13% vs. 21%; $p = 0.02$) and overall survival (9.3 months vs. 10.5 months; $p = 0.0067$) was noted for PCDE.[40] However, PCDE was associated with a significantly higher hematologic toxicity rate, with 22% of patients having a documented infection, compared with 8% in the cisplatin and etoposide arm ($p = 0.0038$). Toxicity-related death rates were similar, at 9% for PCDE and 5.5% for cisplatin and etoposide. Since the early 1990s, there have been no major breakthroughs with newer chemotherapy agents in the first-line setting. A platinum agent plus etoposide or irinotecan remains the standard of care for the treatment of SCLC.

Alternative Chemotherapy Strategies

Alternative chemotherapy strategies have focused on modifying the dosage and schedules of established regimens, including dose intensification, alternating non–cross-resistant chemotherapy, and prolonged treatment durations. However, with the discovery of molecularly targeted agents, investigators have largely abandoned the pursuit of optimizing current chemotherapy regimens.

Dose Intensification

Dose intensity is defined as the dose per meter squared per week. Dose intensification can be accomplished by increasing the dose administered or by shortening the interval between doses (dose density). Results from preclinical tumor models suggested that one of the simplest ways to overcome drug resistance was dose escalation.[41] In the late 1970s, Cohen et al.[42] randomly assigned patients to receive either standard dosages of cyclophosphamide, methotrexate, and lomustine or a higher dose of cyclophosphamide and lomustine plus a standard dose of methotrexate. Patients treated in the high-dose arm had a higher overall response rate that led to prolonged survival, and a subset of these patients were long-term survivors. These data resulted in a series of seven randomized trials comparing high-dose and conventional-dose chemotherapy in patients with limited-stage and extensive-stage SCLC.[43–49] Most of these trials were conducted in the 1980s and did not show a clinical benefit. The Spanish Lung Cancer Group reexamined this question in 2004.[49] They compared high-dose epirubicin (100 mg/m^2) plus cisplatin (100 mg/m^2) administered on day 1 with standard cisplatin and etoposide (cisplatin [100 mg/m^2] on day 1 and etoposide [100 mg/m^2] on days 1–3) in 402 patients with SCLC. Efficacy results were similar between the arms. A study of patients with limited-stage disease published in 1989 showed a superior 2-year survival rate of 43% when the dose of cisplatin and cyclophosphamide was increased by 20% in the first cycle of a PCDE regimen, compared with a 2-year survival rate of 23% for standard PCDE.[50]

Dose-dense regimens have shown mixed results. One such combination was an intense weekly regimen of cisplatin (25 mg/m^2) for 9 consecutive weeks, vincristine (1 mg/m^2) on even weeks for 9 weeks, and doxorubicin (40 mg/m^2) and etoposide (80 mg/m^2) on days 1–3 on odd weeks for 9 weeks (CODE). This was the first regimen to be associated with an impressive 2-year survival rate of 30% among 48 patients with extensive-stage SCLC.[51] The investigators were able to administer close to the intended full doses of all four agents, thereby increasing the dose intensity by twofold. The National Cancer Institute of Canada–Cancer Treatment Group (NCIC–CTG) in collaboration with SWOG conducted a phase III trial comparing the CODE regimen and conventional alternating CAV/cisplatin and etoposide for patients with extensive-stage SCLC.[52] Response rates were higher in the CODE arm, but no differences were found in progression-free or overall survival. Although rates of neutropenia and fever were similar, toxicity-related deaths occurred in 9 of 110 patients receiving CODE, compared with one of 109 patients receiving CAV/cisplatin and etoposide ($p = 0.42$). Given the high toxicity-related death rate and similar efficacy, CODE was not recommended. Japanese investigators subsequently demonstrated that adding granulocyte colony-stimulating factor (G-CSF) to CODE increased the mean total dose intensity received, reduced neutropenia and febrile neutropenia, and significantly prolonged survival (59 weeks vs. 32 weeks; $p = 0.0004$).[53] This led to a phase III trial of CODE plus G-CSF compared with CAV/cisplatin and etoposide.[54] The response rate was significantly higher for CODE, but there was no survival advantage. The toxicity-related death rate with CODE plus G-CSF was low, with only four reported deaths.

European investigators evaluated the dose-dense strategy with or without colony stimulation in seven phase III trials published between 1993 and 2002.[55–61] Two trials showed a survival advantage for the dose-dense arm, and the other trials reported similar outcomes between the standard and experimental arms. The trial by Steward et al.[58] showed a significant prolongation in survival with dose intensification of vincristine, ifosfamide, carboplatin, and etoposide (ICE) chemotherapy compared with standard dosing of this regimen. The median survival time was 443 days in the dose-dense arm and 351 days in the standard arm ($p = 0.0014$), with 2-year survival rates of 33% and 18%, respectively. There was no difference in response rate, despite the 26% increase in dose intensity in the experimental arm. The British Medical Research Council randomly assigned 403 patients to receive doxorubicin, cyclophosphamide, and etoposide in two or three weekly schedules.[59] In this trial, a 34% escalation in dose density was achieved. Although the response rates in the two arms were similar, a significant improvement was found in the complete response rate in the dose-dense arm (40% vs. 28%; $p = 0.02$) that translated into a 2-year survival benefit (13% vs. 8%; $p = 0.04$). Subgroup analysis showed that the survival advantage among patients with extensive disease was as large as that for patients with limited disease.

A possible explanation for the failure of the previous trials is that the dose intensity was insufficient to produce a survival benefit. To definitively answer the question about dose intensification, studies were conducted using stem cell rescue, which would allow for a 200% to 300% dose escalation of chemotherapy. Multiple small studies have shown this approach to be feasible. The original studies focused on patients who had a response with conventional cytotoxic therapy and then received high-dose consolidation with stem cell rescue. A randomized trial testing this late-intensification strategy was reported by Humblet et al.[62] in 1987. One hundred and one patients received standard induction chemotherapy, and 45 patients with chemotherapy sensitivity were randomly assigned to receive either one additional cycle with high-dose cyclophosphamide, carmustine, and etoposide or conventional doses of the same drugs. In this highly selected group of patients, the median overall survival was 68 weeks for the high-dose arm compared with 55 weeks for the conventional therapy ($p = 0.13$).

Because of its improved safety and feasibility, peripheral blood stem cell transplantation has largely replaced autologous marrow transplants. Japanese investigators reported promising results from a phase II study of high-dose ICE with autologous peripheral blood stem cell transplantation in 18 patients with limited-stage SCLC after concurrent, hyperfractionated chemoradiation therapy.[63] The complete response rate was 61% and the median survival time was 36.4 months. One toxicity-related death was reported. At the time of publication, a randomized trial based on these results was ongoing. Three randomized trials using high-dose ICE chemotherapy with peripheral blood rescue as first-line treatment for SCLC have also been reported.[64–66] The largest trial included 318 patients with predominantly limited-stage SCLC and compared six cycles of a dose-dense ICE regimen every 14 days, with G-CSF–mobilized whole-blood hematopoietic progenitors, with six cycles of the standard 28-day ICE regimen.[64] Despite doubling of the median dose intensity with the dose-dense regimen (182% vs. 88%, respectively), the median survival time and the 2-year survival rate were comparable (14.4 months and 22% vs. 13.9 months and 19%, respectively). By contrast, an identical study by Buchholz et al.[65] was halted after 70 patients were enrolled. They reported a favorable median survival of 30.3 months ($p = 0.001$), a 2-year survival rate of 55%, and a time to progression of 15 months ($p = 0.0001$) for the dose-intense arm compared with a median survival of 18.5 months, a 2-year survival rate of 39%, and a time to progression of 11 months for the standard-dose arm in this small, single-institution study. The European Group for Blood and Marrow Transplant conducted a similar study.[66] The study was closed after 140 of the planned 340 patients were enrolled because of poor accrual. The median dose intensity for the high-dose arm was 293%, but this dose did not yield a survival benefit; the median survival time was 18.1 months and the 3-year survival rate was 18% for the high-dose arm, compared with 14.4 months and 19%, respectively, for the standard ICE arm. None of the subgroups benefited from high-dose ICE.

Overall, most trials using a dose-intensification strategy did not show a survival advantage over standard therapy for patients with extensive-stage SCLC, and the higher doses were typically associated with greater toxicity. This approach should be abandoned in patients with extensive disease. In limited-stage SCLC, the optimal drug doses remain unclear, with several studies suggesting a possible benefit. Continued evaluation of dose intensity in the curative setting is reasonable.

Alternating Non–Cross-Resistant Chemotherapy Regimens

To achieve maximal antitumor effects using multiple active agents, they should be administered simultaneously at their optimal single-agent dose. However, because drug toxicities often overlap, strict adherence to this approach is often not possible in the clinical setting. In the 1980s, Goldie et al.[67] suggested that alternating two non–cross-resistant chemotherapy regimens of relatively comparable efficacy could minimize the development of drug resistance while avoiding excessive host toxicity. This strategy was particularly appealing for SCLC because both CAV and cisplatin and etoposide are highly active against SCLC and contain agents from divergent drug classes. Three randomized phase III trials were performed to evaluate CAV and CAV alternating with cisplatin and etoposide.[16,17,68] Studies from the United States and Japan showed similar efficacy between the study arms, whereas the NCIC–CTG reported superior efficacy for the alternating regimen, with overall response rates of 80% and 63%, respectively ($p < 0.002$), and survival times of 9.6 months and 8.0 months ($p = 0.03$). Investigators at the NCIC–CTG went on to test this approach in patients with limited-stage SCLC.[69] Patients were randomly assigned between two induction regimens, either alternating CAV/cisplatin and etoposide or sequential therapy with three cycles of CAV followed by three cycles of cisplatin and etoposide. Chemotherapy was followed by radiotherapy in patients with a disease response. The therapeutic outcomes in the study groups were not significantly different. SWOG conducted a similar study and found no advantage for the alternating CAV/cisplatin and etoposide regimen over the etoposide, vincristine, doxorubicin, and cyclophosphamide regimen in patients with limited-stage disease.[70]

The European Organization for Research and Treatment of Cancer reported a trial testing two relatively non–cross-resistant regimens: CDE and vincristine, carboplatin, ifosfamide, and mesna.[71] Patients with extensive-stage SCLC were randomly assigned to receive either a maximum of five courses of CDE or an alternating regimen consisting of CDE in cycles 1, 3, and 5 and vincristine, carboplatin, ifosfamide, and mesna in cycles 2 and 4. The trial accrued only 148 of the 360 planned patients. The median survival time was 7.6 months in the standard arm and 8.7 months in the alternating arm ($p = 0.243$).

Although no survival benefit for the alternating drug hypothesis was demonstrated, the emergence of newer active agents for the treatment of SCLC justified revisiting this strategy. The North Central Cancer Treatment Group conducted a trial of etoposide and cisplatin alternating with topotecan and paclitaxel.[72] The overall response rate was 77%, including four complete responses among 44 evaluable patients. The median survival was 10.5 months, with 1- and 2-year survival rates of 37% and 12%, respectively. This alternating regimen was associated with a high rate of grade 3 and grade 4 neutropenia (95%) despite the use of filgrastim in cycles 2, 4, and 6. The Hellenic Oncology Research Group treated 36 previously untreated patients with extensive-stage SCLC with cisplatin and etoposide alternating with topotecan.[73] The overall response rate was 64%, and 14% of patients had a complete response. Grade 3 and grade 4 neutropenia occurred in 39% of patients during the cycles of cisplatin and etoposide and in 55% after the topotecan treatment. These limited data incorporating newer chemotherapy agents into an alternating strategy were disappointing. Taken together, alternating newer and/or older cytotoxic agents to overcome drug resistance is an unsuccessful strategy and should not be pursued.

Treatment Duration and Maintenance Therapy

The ideal number of chemotherapy cycles for SCLC has not been defined; however, four to six cycles is considered the standard based on the results from the randomized trials described previously. Clinical trials specifically designed to investigate the role of prolonged treatment using a consolidation or maintenance approach have been performed. Three of 14 trials produced positive results.[74–76] All three trials were initiated in 1982.

In two trials of patients with limited-stage SCLC, two cycles to four cycles of consolidation therapy with cisplatin and etoposide were given to patients who had a response after induction CAV with or without thoracic radiotherapy.[74,75] The remaining trial randomly assigned patients with nonprogressing limited or extensive-stage disease to four additional cycles of CEV or observation.[76] Although this trial showed that four cycles of CEV were inferior, a second randomization to salvage chemotherapy compared with palliative care given at the time of disease progression demonstrated that the subset of patients who received eight cycles of CEV with or without salvage therapy did not live longer than patients who received four cycles of CEV and salvage therapy at the time of relapse. The role of consolidation and/or maintenance therapy with topotecan was evaluated by the Eastern Cooperative Oncology Group (ECOG).[77] Two hundred and twenty-three patients with nonprogressing, extensive-stage SCLC were randomly assigned to receive either four cycles of topotecan or observation. Progression-free survival from the date of randomization was significantly better with topotecan than with observation alone (3.6 months vs. 2.3 months; $p < 0.001$), but overall survival from randomization was not significantly different between the arms (8.9 months vs. 9.3 months; $p = 0.43$). A meta-analysis of 14 randomized trials of maintenance chemotherapy involving 1806 patients was published in 2013.[78] Maintenance chemotherapy failed to increase survival when compared with observation alone, with an odds ratio for 1-year mortality of 0.88 (95% CI, 0.66–1.19; $p = 0.414$). Maintenance treatment did, however, significantly prolong progression-free survival for patients with extensive-stage disease (HR, 0.72; 95% CI, 0.58–0.89; $p = 0.003$). This benefit was limited to patients who had switch maintenance therapy. Overall, chemotherapy after four to six cycles of a combination regimen is not warranted. Patients should be followed closely for signs and symptoms of relapse. Clinical trials evaluating maintenance regimens with molecularly targeted agents were ongoing at the time of publication.

In summary, a platinum-based doublet with etoposide or irinotecan remains the standard of care for patients with SCLC. Although extensive research has not altered the standard of care for SCLC in many years, an analysis of the Surveillance, Epidemiology, and End Results database showed a modest but significant improvement in survival with current therapies.[79] In 1973, the 2-year survival rate for extensive-stage SCLC was 1.5%, compared with 4.6% in 2000, whereas the 5-year survival rate for limited-stage SCLC increased from 4.9% to 10% during a similar period (Fig. 52.1). Moreover, the recent genomic characterization of SCLC provides optimism that novel, efficacious agents are forthcoming.

FIRST-LINE CHEMOTHERAPY FOR OLDER PATIENTS

According to the Surveillance, Epidemiology, and End Results database, 42% of patients with SCLC were aged 70 years or older at diagnosis.[80] Similar age distributions are seen worldwide.[81,82] Furthermore, the 5-year survival rate for SCLC was significantly worse for older patients than for younger patients ($p < 0.0001$) and had not changed over the 15 years studied.[80] For the period between 1998 and 2003, 5-year survival rates were 6.5% for patients younger than 70 years of age, 3.4% for patients aged 70 to 79 years, and 2.4% for patients aged 80 years or older.

Retrospective reviews to identify prognostic factors in SCLC have shown variable results with regard to age. The largest experience comes from SWOG.[83] An analysis of 2580 patients enrolled in six SWOG studies, of whom approximately 10% were older, showed that patients over the age of 70 years had a significant risk of death, with a HR of 1.5 ($p \leq 0.0001$) for limited-stage disease and a HR of 1.3 ($p = 0.006$) for extensive-stage disease. By contrast, a smaller study from 1991 reviewed 614 patients with limited- and extensive-stage disease from the University of Toronto

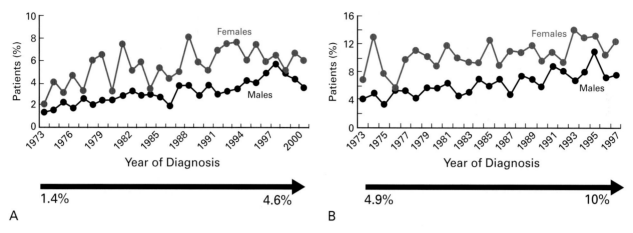

Fig. 52.1. All-cause survival trends in (A) extensive-stage small cell lung cancer (SCLC) from 1973 to 2000 and (B) limited-stage SCLC from 1973 to 1997. *(Modified with permission from Govindan R, Page N, Morgensztern D, et al. Changing epidemiology of small-cell lung cancer in the United States over the last 30 years: analysis of the Surveillance, Epidemiologic, and End Results database.* J Clin Oncol. 2006;24(28):4539–4544.)

clinical trial database and showed that age over 70 years was not a significant predictor of a poorer outcome.[84] A meta-analysis published by Pignon et al.[83] in 1992 examined 2140 patients with limited-stage disease from 13 randomized trials that were designed to determine the role of thoracic radiotherapy combined with chemotherapy compared with chemotherapy alone. The relative risk of death in patients older than 70 years of age receiving combination therapy was 1.07, higher than that of older patients receiving chemotherapy alone. Since this meta-analysis, a review of two NCIC–CTG trials, BR.3 and BR.6, involving 618 patients with limited-stage SCLC who received the same chemotherapy regimen, showed no difference in survival between patients aged younger and older than 70 years.[84] In the United States Intergroup study comparing once-daily and twice-daily radiotherapy for limited-stage SCLC, survival of younger patients was better than that for patients older than 70 years of age, with borderline significance ($p = 0.051$).[85]

Advanced age has been perceived as a strong rationale for the use of less aggressive therapies or no therapy, for fear of increasing toxicity. The literature is conflicting on this topic. Some retrospective reviews have reported that older age is associated with an increased risk of chemotherapy-related morbidity and mortality, whereas other studies have shown that despite toxicity and dose reductions, older patients receive a survival benefit with chemotherapy and/or radiotherapy compared with no treatment.[86–93] A review by the Royal Marsden Hospital investigated the survival outcomes of 322 older patients (aged 70 years or older) with SCLC treated with chemotherapy from 1982 to 2003.[94] Patients treated between 1995 and 2003 had a median survival of 43 weeks and a 1-year survival rate of 37%, compared with 25 weeks and 14%, respectively, for patients treated between 1982 and 1994 ($p < 0.001$). Patients who received a platinum combination had significantly better survival ($p < 0.001$) than patients who received single agents or another combination. No survival difference was found between a cisplatin and a carboplatin regimen. In a 2005 analysis of 54 older patients with limited-stage disease who participated in the North Central Cancer Treatment Group phase III trial of cisplatin and etoposide plus twice-daily or once-daily thoracic radiotherapy, survival was not different from that of their younger counterparts despite higher toxicity.[95] These results corroborate the United States Intergroup findings. More data are needed from phase III trials regarding age-specific outcomes.

To formally address the question of dose tolerability among older patients with SCLC, Ardizzoni et al.[96] randomly assigned

patients aged 70 years or older either to four cycles of cisplatin (25 mg/m²) on days 1–2 with etoposide (60 mg/m²) IV on days 1–3 every 3 weeks (the attenuated-dose regimen; 28 patients) or to cisplatin (40 mg/m²) on days 1–2 plus etoposide (100 mg/m²) IV on days 1–3 with prophylactic G-CSF (the full-dose regimen; 67 patients). Patients treated with the attenuated-dose regimen had a poorer outcome. The response rate was 39% in the attenuated-dose arm and 68% in the full-dose arm, with 1-year survival rates of 18% and 39%, respectively. No grade 3 or grade 4 myelotoxicity was reported in the attenuated-dose group, but 10% was noted in the full-dose group. There was one toxicity-related death in the full-dose arm. The median number of cycles was four in both groups; 75% of patients in the attenuated-dose group and 72% in the full-dose group completed all planned cycles. Japanese investigators conducted a phase III trial to test whether nearly full doses of carboplatin and etoposide were superior to their standard regimen for older patients, which consisted of a split dose of cisplatin and etoposide. Older was defined as an age of 70 years or more with an ECOG performance status of 0 to 2. Patients younger than 70 years of age with a performance status of 3 were also allowed to participate.[97] A total of 220 patients with extensive-stage SCLC were entered in the study, with 110 patients receiving carboplatin (AUC 5) on day 1 and etoposide (80 mg/m² IV) on days 1–3 every 3–4 weeks for four cycles, and 109 patients receiving cisplatin (25 mg/m²) on days 1–3 with etoposide (80 mg/m² IV) on days 1–3 every 3–4 weeks for four cycles. G-CSF was recommended in both treatment arms. As many as 92% of the patients met the criteria for older status, and 8% were poor risk. Objective response rates were identical in both treatment arms (73%). The median survival for the carboplatin and etoposide arm was 10.6 months and the 1-year survival rate was 41%, as compared with 9.9 months and 35%, respectively, for the split-dose cisplatin and etoposide arm. The rate of grade 3 or grade 4 neutropenia was high in both arms (95% for the carboplatin and etoposide arm and 90% for the split-dose cisplatin and etoposide arm). A significant difference in the rate of grade 3 or 4 thrombocytopenia was noted (56% for carboplatin and etoposide and 16% for split-dose cisplatin and etoposide; $p = 0.01$). There were four treatment-related deaths, three in the carboplatin and etoposide arm and one in the split-dose cisplatin and etoposide arm. The authors concluded that either regimen was a reasonable treatment option.

The optimal chemotherapy regimen for older patients with SCLC is not known. We have learned that chronologic age should not be the sole determinant of treatment decisions. Physiologic age determined by comorbidities and performance status provides a clearer framework for guiding treatment decisions. Among patients aged 70 years or older, categories such as fit elderly (performance status of 0 or 1) and frail (performance status of 2–4) are emerging as beneficial terms in both the clinical and research settings. Despite the limited data, we are encouraged that a survival benefit can be achieved in a subset of older patients with acceptable toxicity. As the older population continues to increase, it is crucial that we develop evidence-based treatment plans. Additional clinical research in this population is needed.

FIRST-LINE CHEMOTHERAPY FOR PATIENTS WITH POOR PERFORMANCE STATUS

Performance status is universally recognized as an independent prognostic factor and typically correlates with the extent of tumor burden. Several retrospective studies of large databases have confirmed that shorter survival times among patients with SCLC are associated with poor performance status.[98–100] Despite poor survival, patients with a performance status of 2 have routinely been eligible for clinical trials because our experience has taught us that patients whose poor performance status is attributed to tumor burden can respond to treatment with meaningful symptom palliation, improved performance status, and prolonged survival. However, the number of patients with poor performance status enrolling in clinical trials is low, and outcome data specific to performance status are not available.

Clinical trials specifically including patients with poor performance status are few and were conducted more than 20 years ago. Two trials evaluated the oral formulation of etoposide because it was presumed to be efficacious but less toxic. The first study randomly assigned previously untreated patients with a performance status of 2–4 to either oral etoposide (50 mg twice a day) for 10 days (171 patients) or standard chemotherapy with cisplatin and etoposide or CAV (168 patients).[101] The primary end point was palliation of symptoms at 3 months. The data safety and monitoring board stopped the trial early because of an inferior survival rate with oral etoposide. Survival was 130 days in the oral etoposide arm and 183 days in the standard arm ($p = 0.03$). Palliation rates were similar in both arms (41% vs. 46%, respectively). Grade 2 or greater hematologic toxicity was low in both arms (21% vs. 26%, respectively). The second trial, conducted by the London Lung Cancer Group, enrolled patients younger than 75 years of age with a performance status of 2 or 3 or patients equal to or older than 75 years of age with any performance status to receive 100 mg etoposide orally for 5 days (75 patients) or CAV alternating with cisplatin and etoposide (80 patients).[102] The authors hypothesized that oral etoposide would produce a similar survival rate but with improved quality of life. This study, too, was stopped prematurely because of a significantly inferior survival rate in the oral etoposide arm. The median survival was 4.8 months, with a 1-year survival rate of 9.8% for oral etoposide, compared with 5.9 months and 19.3%, respectively, for CAV/cisplatin and etoposide ($p < 0.05$). Grade 3 and grade 4 toxicities were infrequent and similar between the treatment groups, except that more nausea and vomiting were reported in the CAV/cisplatin and etoposide arm. In another study, the Medical Research Council Lung Cancer Working Party randomly assigned 310 patients with poor performance status either to a four-drug regimen of etoposide, cyclophosphamide, methotrexate, and vincristine (control arm) or to a less intense two-drug regimen of etoposide and vincristine.[103] No differences were found in symptom palliation, response rates, or survival times between the groups; however, more early deaths occurred with the four-drug regimen. Grade 2 or greater hematologic toxicity and mucositis were also worse with the four-drug regimen.

Despite the lack of data, experts generally agree that if a poor performance status is due to the disease itself, patients should be offered standard platinum-based chemotherapy with close monitoring because they have a reasonable chance of symptom palliation and prolonged survival.

SECOND-LINE CHEMOTHERAPY

Despite an initially high response rate to frontline platinum-based chemotherapy, extensive-stage SCLC will universally relapse, often within 3 to 6 months. The precise mechanisms of drug resistance that result in disease progression have not been well defined, but are likely to be multifactorial.[104] Relapse generally heralds a poor outcome. Patients who receive no further therapy have a median survival of less than 3 months.[105] Traditionally, patients who have previously received platinum-based therapy are grouped into two general categories reflecting the platinum-sensitivity status of their disease.[106] These categories include platinum sensitive, referring to relapse 90 days or more after the last dose of platinum; and platinum refractory, referring to relapse within 90 days of the last treatment. A third category, platinum resistant, has sometimes been assigned to patients whose disease progressed during platinum-based therapy; these patients are typically grouped together with the platinum-refractory category. The practice of categorizing disease according to platinum sensitivity arose from seminal observations in a small, single-arm phase II trial of salvage teniposide published in 1988.[107] In that experience involving 50 patients, the response to second-line teniposide appeared to be associated with a previous response to platinum-based therapy and with the length of time between the last line of therapy and the initiation of teniposide. Since then, clinical trials in the second-line setting have routinely stratified patients according to the platinum sensitivity of their disease, resulting in higher sample sizes and increased resource use. More recent data from SWOG among patients treated in a series of phase II trials in the second-line setting and beyond strongly suggest that platinum-sensitivity status may no longer be relevant in the modern era. In a pooled analysis of 329 patients with platinum-treated SCLC enrolled in three SWOG phase II trials, 151 patients had platinum-sensitive disease and 178 had platinum-refractory disease.[108] In this analysis, Cox proportional hazards models adjusted for baseline prognostic factors showed that only an elevated serum lactate dehydrogenase level (HR, 2.04; $p < 0.001$), male gender (HR, 1.36; $p = 0.04$), performance status of 1 (HR, 1.25; $p = 0.02$), and weight loss of at least 5% (HR, 1.53; $p = 0.01$) were independently associated with overall survival. Platinum-sensitivity status was not associated with either progression-free survival (HR, 1.11; $p = 0.49$) or overall survival (HR, 1.25; $p = 0.14$). However, these data must be prospectively validated before clinical use.

As a historic footnote, it is notable that before the establishment of cisplatin and etoposide as the frontline regimen for extensive-stage SCLC, systemic therapy consisted mostly of other multiagent chemotherapy regimens, most commonly CAV. During that era, cisplatin plus etoposide was a typical treatment choice for SCLC that had failed to respond to CAV. In a phase III SWOG trial, 103 patients with disease relapse who were categorized as having good or poor risk were randomly assigned either to cisplatin and etoposide or to a four-drug regimen (carmustine, thiotepa, vincristine, and cyclophosphamide). For good-risk patients, the median survival was 35 weeks with cisplatin and etoposide and 10 weeks with the four-drug regimen. Poor-risk patients in both treatment arms had an unfavorable response rate (9%) and a short median survival (10 to 12 weeks). In addition, CAV had no clear benefit for patients whose disease had failed to respond to cisplatin and etoposide.[16,17,107] Subsequently, several phase III trials of newer approaches have evaluated the role of these systemic therapies in the pretreated setting (Table 52.2).

TABLE 52.2 Phase III Trials of Second-Line Chemotherapy Regimens for Small Cell Lung Cancer

Author (y)	Regimen	No. of Patients	Overall Response Rate (%)	Median Survival	1-Year Survival Rate (%)
von Pawel et al.[109] (1999)	Topotecan CAV	107	24.3	25 wk	14.2
		104	18.3	18.3 wk	14.4
O'Brien et al.[110] (2006)	Topotecan	71	NR	25.5 wk[a]	NR
	Best supportive care	70	7	13.9 wk	NR
Eckardt et al.[111] (2003)	Topotecan (IV)	151	21.9	35 wk	29
	Topotecan (PO)	153	18.3	33 wk	33
Jotte et al.[112] (2011)	Topotecan (IV)	424	31	7.5 mo	28
	Amrubicin	213	17	7.8 mo	25

[a]$p < 0.05$.
CAV, cyclophosphamide, doxorubicin, and vincristine; *IV*, intravenous; *NR*, not reported; *PO*, oral.

The topoisomerase-1 inhibitor topotecan became available in the late 1990s and was found in early phase trials to have efficacy in previously treated SCLC. In a small phase III trial of 211 patients who had disease relapse more than 60 days after completion of induction therapy, topotecan (1.5 mg/m^2/day on days 1–5 every 21 days) was found to be comparable in efficacy with conventional CAV.[113] This trial had a primary end point of objective response, with a secondary end point of overall survival. At the final analysis, the overall response rates and median survival were not significantly different between the treatment arms (24.3% vs. 18.3% and 25 weeks vs. 24.7 weeks, respectively). In other words, topotecan failed to demonstrate a clear efficacy advantage over CAV. However, symptoms such as dyspnea, fatigue, anorexia, and hoarseness appeared to have been significantly improved with topotecan, despite a higher rate of grade 3 or grade 4 anemia and thrombocytopenia in that arm. The United States Food and Drug Administration (FDA) approved topotecan as second-line treatment for patients with platinum-sensitive, relapsed disease based on symptom control. An oral formulation of topotecan was later developed for patients' convenience. To evaluate the efficacy of this formulation, 141 patients with disease relapse were randomly assigned to receive either oral topotecan (2.3 mg/m^2/day for 5 days) plus best supportive care or best supportive care alone every 21 days.[109] Oral topotecan was superior to best supportive care, with a median survival time of 25.9 weeks, compared with 13.9 weeks for best supportive care ($p = 0.01$). A survival advantage was recognized in patients who had disease relapse both less than 60 days and more than 60 days from the end of their previous therapy. The most common toxicities with oral topotecan were hematologic events. Grade 3 and grade 4 neutropenia occurred in 61%, thrombocytopenia in 38%, and anemia in 25% of patients. Subsequently, oral topotecan was compared with IV topotecan in patients with platinum-sensitive disease that relapsed more than 90 days after chemotherapy.[110] One hundred and fifty-three patients received oral topotecan (2.3 mg/m^2/day on days 1–5 every 21 days), and 151 patients received standard doses of IV topotecan (1.5 mg/m^2/day on days 1–5 every 21 days). The response rate, median survival, and 1-year survival for the oral agent were 18.3%, 33 weeks, and 33%, respectively, compared with 21.9%, 35 weeks, and 29%, respectively, for IV administration. The incidence of grade 4 neutropenia was 47% with oral topotecan and 64% with the IV formulation. Quality of life appeared comparable between the arms. The FDA subsequently approved oral topotecan for the treatment of both sensitive and resistant/refractory SCLC.

The early years of the 21st century saw a renewed interest in the role of anthracyclines in relapsed SCLC. Specifically, amrubicin was developed principally in Japan, and this agent is currently approved for commercial use in Japan for treating SCLC. Two phase II Japanese trials were initially completed. One trial enrolled 60 patients with relapsed SCLC, 16 of whom had relapse within 60 days of platinum-based therapy (refractory) and 44 who had relapse after 60 days (sensitive). Patients received amrubicin (40 mg/m^2) for 3 days every 3 weeks.[112] A median of four cycles were delivered. Overall response rates were 50% (95% CI, 25% to 75%) and 52% (95% CI, 37% to 58%) for the refractory and sensitive cohorts, respectively. Overall median survival was 10.3 months and 11.6 months in the refractory and sensitive groups, respectively. Amrubicin resulted in high rates of myelotoxicity, with grade 3 or grade 4 neutropenia occurring in 83%. However, the rate of febrile neutropenia was only 5%, and no toxicity-related deaths were reported. In another phase II trial, 34 Japanese patients with relapsed SCLC (10 refractory, 24 sensitive) received amrubicin (45 mg/m^2) for 3 days every 3 weeks.[114] A median of four cycles were administered. Response rates were 60% (95% CI, 23% to 97%) for patients with refractory disease and 53% (95% CI, 35% to 70%) for patients with sensitive disease. The median survival was 6.8 months for patients with refractory disease and 10.4 months for patients with sensitive disease. Again, rates of myelosuppression were high, with grade 3 or grade 4 neutropenia reported for more than 70% of patients. At the higher amrubicin dose, however, the rate of febrile neutropenia was 35%, with one toxicity-related death from pneumonia.

In a randomized phase II trial from Japan, 60 patients were assigned to receive either amrubicin (40 mg/m^2 on days 1–3) or topotecan (1 mg/m^2 IV on days 1–5) every 3 weeks.[115] Overall response rates were 38% (95% CI, 20% to 56%) for amrubicin and 13% (95% CI, 1% to 25%) for topotecan. Among patients with so-called sensitive relapse, the response rates were 53% and 21% for the amrubicin and topotecan arms, respectively. Among patients with so-called refractory relapse, 17% responded to amrubicin compared with 0% for topotecan. The median progression-free survival was 3.5 months for patients in the amrubicin arm and 2.2 months for patients in the topotecan arm.

In the United States, a randomized phase II study was performed to evaluate the response rate of amrubicin compared with topotecan in patients with so-called sensitive-relapse disease.[116] Seventy-six patients were randomly assigned in a 2:1 fashion to receive the same dose of amrubicin (50 patients) or topotecan (26 patients) at 1.5 mg/m^2 IV on days 1–5 every 3 weeks. Treatment with amrubicin was associated with a higher response rate (44% vs. 15%; $p = 0.021$). The median progression-free survival and overall survival were 4.5 months and 9.2 months, respectively, with amrubicin, and 3.3 months and 7.6 months, respectively, with topotecan. Grade 3 or higher neutropenia and thrombocytopenia appeared to be more frequent in the topotecan group (78% and 61% vs. 61% and 39%, respectively). No evidence of anthracycline-induced cardiotoxicity was reported. In a phase II North American trial of amrubicin in patients with refractory or resistant disease progressing within 90 days,[117] 75 patients received amrubicin at 40 mg/m^2 on days 1–3 every 3 weeks. An overall response rate of 21.3% was reported, with an acceptable safety profile. Notably, no patient had early cardiotoxicity.

Lastly, a large global phase III trial was conducted to compare amrubicin and topotecan.[118] In this study, 637 patients were randomly assigned 2:1 to receive either amrubicin (40 mg/m^2 IV) on days 1–3 (424 patients) or topotecan (1.5 mg/m^2 IV) on days 1–5 (213 patients). The primary end point was overall survival. Patients with refractory relapse represented approximately 45% of the group. Grade 3 or higher adverse events (all $p < 0.05$) in the respective amrubicin and topotecan groups included neutropenia (41% vs. 53%), thrombocytopenia (21% vs. 54%), anemia (16% vs. 30%), infections (16% vs. 10%), and febrile neutropenia (10% vs. 4%). Transfusion rates were 32% in the amrubicin arm and 53% in the topotecan arm ($p < 0.01$). Despite a higher response rate in the amrubicin arm (31% vs. 17%; $p = 0.0002$), no difference was found in overall survival (HR, 0.88; $p = 0.17$). The median survival was 7.5 months and 7.8 months for the amrubicin and topotecan arms, respectively. This pivotal trial thus failed to show a survival benefit for amrubicin, precluding its commercial approval outside of Japan.

Using the same regimen as that in the frontline setting as salvage therapy can also be an option for selected patients. Two small case series totaling 18 patients have reported outcomes on 10 patients who had disease relapse more than 10 months after the end of previous therapy. In this database, durable responses were seen after treatment with the original regimen.[119,120] Thus considering salvage treatment with the original regimen is reasonable, particularly for patients with a long relapse-free interval.

Other agents commonly used in the salvage setting (second line and beyond), often as single agents, are taxanes (docetaxel and paclitaxel), gemcitabine, vinorelbine, ifosfamide, and other topoisomerase inhibitors (irinotecan and oral etoposide).[121] In general, clinical trials of these chemotherapeutic agents have yielded modest clinical benefits in this pretreated population, with response rates ranging from 10% to 20% and median survival of 2 months to 5 months. As expected, rates of response to subsequent therapies tend to be lower for patients with platinum-refractory disease, whereas the likelihood of response is better for patients with platinum-sensitive disease.

In summary, the topoisomerase inhibitor topotecan (whether delivered IV or orally) represents a reasonable standard of care for patients with relapsed SCLC. In Japan, amrubicin is also approved for SCLC therapy. However, efficacy for either of these agents is fairly modest and must be weighed against their known toxicities, particularly myelosuppression. Given the generally poor outcome of patients with relapsed or refractory SCLC, participation in clinical trials with novel approaches represents the principal standard of care.

NEW DRUGS

Improvements in clinical outcome after treatment of patients with extensive-stage SCLC will necessitate more effective systemic treatments. Drug development for extensive-stage SCLC has, however, been slow during the past 20 years. In contrast to treatments for nonsmall cell lung cancer, neither cytotoxic agents with novel mechanisms of action nor targeted agents have entered the clinical arena for SCLC.

Cytotoxic agents that have generated some interest in the past decade include belotecan, a novel camptothecin analog, and picoplatin, a platinum analog. Belotecan has been studied in patients with both untreated and pretreated extensive-stage SCLC. In untreated patients, a single-arm phase II study showed an overall response rate of 54%, a 4.6-month time to progression, and a 10.4-month median overall survival. As with other topoisomerase I inhibitors, myelosuppression was the main toxic effect, with grade 3 or grade 4 neutropenia occurring in more than 70% of patients.[122] Subsequently, the combination of belotecan and cisplatin was investigated in two phase II studies, which found an overall response rate of greater than 70% and a median overall

survival of more than 10 months.[123,124] At the time of publication, this doublet was undergoing phase III testing in untreated patients. In pretreated patients, the efficacy of belotecan seems to be no different from that of currently available topoisomerase I inhibitors. Three phase II studies demonstrated an overall response rate ranging from 14% to 24%, a median progression-free survival of 1.6 months to 3.7 months, and a median overall survival of 4.0 months to 13.9 months.[125–127] Of note, all three studies were performed in Asian populations, in whom this class of drugs seems to have more efficacy in SCLC. Taken together, the results obtained with belotecan suggest that this drug will not constitute a major step forward in the treatment of SCLC.

In vitro studies identified picoplatin (ZD0473) as a platinum analog capable of circumventing resistance to both cisplatin and carboplatin. After single-agent phase II studies in which no compelling results were obtained, a randomized phase III study was launched in which 401 patients with SCLC relapse (within 6 months of completing first-line therapy) were randomly assigned in a 2:1 fashion compared with best supportive care. No difference was found in overall survival between the treatment arms.[128]

Despite progress in our understanding of genomic alterations and signaling pathways in SCLC,[129–132] clinical experiments with tyrosine kinase inhibitors, other small-molecule inhibitors, and antiangiogenic agents have been disappointing (Table 52.3). Other therapeutic areas of interest more recently evaluated include epigenetic modifiers and inhibitors of DNA repair and the cell cycle. In a phase II study, romidepsin (a histone deacetylase inhibitor) did not show a meaningful benefit in relapsed extensive-stage disease SCLC (ED-SCLC).[133] Another phase II study of the histone deacetylase inhibitor panobinostat was stopped prematurely as patients did not meet Response Evaluation Criteria in Solid Tumors criteria for partial response.[134] Veliparib, a poly(ADP-ribose) polymerase inhibitor implicated in the DNA damage repair pathway, was recently studied in a small phase I dose-escalation study in combination with cisplatin and etoposide in newly diagnosed ED-SCLC.[135] Of the seven evaluable patients, 14.3% had a complete response, 57.1% had a partial response, and 28.6% had stable disease. As such, veliparib continues to be under investigation, including in one study of the combination of temozolomide, another DNA damaging agent, and veliparib. Inhibition of aurora A kinase, which regulates cell cycle transit from G_2 to cytokinesis, has shown promising preclinical activity and thus a phase I/II trial of alisertib was conducted in a variety of tumor types.[136] One arm enrolled 60 patients with relapsed or refractory SCLC; objective partial responses of 21% (95% CI, 10% to 35%) were seen in this trial. A follow-up phase II trial combining alisertib with paclitaxel in patients with platinum-refractory ED-SCLC has completed accrual.

Investigators hope that novel immune-modulating agents may alter the therapeutic landscape of SCLC. Mounting evidence suggests that these agents may work in concert with classic cytotoxic chemotherapy and, more importantly, with radiotherapy. Although phase III trials examining the role of tumor vaccines, mainly performed in the maintenance setting of responding patients, have been uniformly negative, results of early studies with immune checkpoint modulators have been encouraging.

Ipilimumab, a monoclonal antibody that blocks cytotoxic T-lymphocyte antigen-4, has been studied in a randomized phase II study including 130 patients with extensive-stage SCLC not previously treated with chemotherapy.[156] A total of 135 patients were treated with carboplatin and paclitaxel or the same regimen plus two schedules of ipilimumab. Although no differences were found in progression-free survival or overall survival, the so-called phased schedule of ipilimumab (i.e., administered after two courses of carboplatin and paclitaxel without ipilimumab) resulted in a higher immune-related progression-free survival and numerically increased overall survival (12.9 vs. 9.9 months). Concurrent ipilimumab and carboplatin and paclitaxel provided no benefit even

TABLE 52.3 Selected Targets and Agents Studied for Small Cell Lung Cancer

Target	Agent	Phase	Result	Comment
VEGF-A	Bevacizumab[137]	III	Negative	In combination with cisplatin + etoposide Statistically significant improvement in PFS but not OS
VEGFR-I–III	Cediranib[138]	II	Negative	
VEGFR, PDGFR, Raf-1	Sorafenib[139], thalidomide[140]	II, III	Negative	
VEGFR, PDGFR, Flt-3, RET, Kit	Sunitinib[141]	II, III	Negative	
VEGF-A, B	Aflibercept[142]	II	Negative	
	NGR-hTNF[143]	II	Negative	
VEGF, EGFR	Vandetanib[144]	II	Negative	
cKit	Imatinib[145]	II	Negative	cKit expression required
Src	Dasatinib,[146] saracatinib[147]	II	Negative	
mTOR	Everolimus,[148] temsirolimus[149]	II	Negative	
EGFR	Gefitinib[150]	II	Negative	Responses in EGFR MT patients
BCl-2	Oblimersen,[151] navitoclax,[152] obatoclax,[153] AT101[154]	I/II	Negative	
RAS	R115777[155]	II	Negative	
Aurora A kinase	Alisertib[136]	I/II	21% PR	Relapsed/refractory disease
HDAC	Romidepsin,[133] panobinostat[134]	II	Negative	
PARP	Veliparib[135]	I	Acceptable safety profile	In combination with cisplatin + etoposide in newly diagnosed ED-SCLC

BCl-2, B-cell CLL/lymphoma 2; *ED-SCLC*, extensive-stage disease small cell lung cancer; *EGFR*, epidermal growth factor receptor; *Flt-3*, Fms-like tyrosine kinase 3; *HDAC*, histone deacetylase; *MT*, mutated; *mTOR*, mammalian target of rapamycin; *NGR-hTNF*, CNGRC-human Tumor Necrosis Factor-alfa fusion protein; *OS*, overall survival; *PARP*, poly(ADP) ribose polymerase; *PDGFR*, platelet-derived growth factor receptor; *PFS*, progression-free survival; *PR*, partial response; *RAS*, rat sarcoma gene; *RET*, rearranged during transfection proto-oncogene; *VEGF*, vascular endothelial growth factor; *VEGFR*, VEGF receptor.

in numerical terms for progression-free survival or overall survival. Near doubling of the incidence of grade 3 or grade 4 adverse events was observed when ipilimumab-containing regimens were compared with standard chemotherapy. These findings prompted a phase III clinical trial evaluating the combination with standard platinum and etoposide.[157] In total, 1132 patients with newly diagnosed ED-SCLC were enrolled to randomized, blinded arms, with one arm treated with etoposide and platinum with placebo, and the other arm with etoposide and platinum and ipilimumab. As in the phase II study, ipilimumab or placebo was administered in a phased schedule. Unfortunately, the trial demonstrated no difference in median progression-free survival or overall survival between the arms. Patients treated with the combination of platinum, etoposide, and ipilimumab were found again to have a higher incidence of treatment-related diarrhea, colitis, and rash and more treatment-related deaths. Thus the combination of standard chemotherapy with ipilimumab did not result in improved efficacy in ED-SCLC but did result in added toxicity.

Ipilimumab was also recently studied in combination with a programmed cell death protein 1 (PD1) inhibiting antibody, nivolumab, in the CheckMate 032 trial. This phase I/II trial enrolled patients with limited and extensive-stage SCLC who had progressed after platinum-based chemotherapy.[158] Of the 216 patients enrolled, 98 were treated with nivolumab (3 mg/kg IV) every 2 weeks, with the remainder of patients enrolled into initial treatment with nivolumab (1 mg/kg IV) and ipilimumab (1 mg/kg IV) every 3 weeks. Patients who received the latter regimen could then undergo dose escalation such that 61 patients received nivolumab (1 mg/kg) and ipilimumab (3 mg/kg IV) every 3 weeks, and 54 received nivolumab (3 mg/kg) and ipilimumab (1 mg/kg) every 3 weeks, whereas three patients remained at the initial dose. All arms showed potential benefit, though treatment with nivolumab alone resulted in a modest 10% objective response rate. Although the study was not designed to detect efficacy differences between arms, the combination of nivolumab and ipilimumab did result in higher objective response rates (23% for nivolumab [1 mg/kg] + ipilimumab [3 mg/kg] and 19% for nivolumab [3 mg/kg] + ipilimumab [1 mg/kg], respectively).

However, patients treated with the combination discontinued therapy due to treatment-related adverse effects, and there were more grade 3 and grade 4 adverse effects with combination treatment, most commonly lipase elevation and diarrhea.

In addition to the aforementioned data with nivolumab, PD1 inhibition in ED-SCLC was also investigated in the KEYNOTE-028 trial.[159] This phase Ib trial has screened a cohort of 135 patients with ED-SCLC who had progressed on platinum-based chemotherapy, with 27% of patients subsequently testing positive for greater or equal to 1% PD1 ligand expression. Ultimately, 17 patients with ED-SCLC were treated with pembrolizumab (10 mg/kg IV) every 2 weeks. Of these patients, 25% had a partial response to treatment, with durable responses at greater than 16 weeks. There was also a high rate of drug-related adverse events; although there was only one patient with a greater than or equal to grade 3 drug-related adverse event, 53% of drug-related adverse events were reported. As of this publication, final results of this trial have not been reported. As such, while immune checkpoint inhibition remains of interest, to date modest efficacy findings have been tempered by significant toxicity.

A new target, DLL3, part of the Notch signaling pathway, has been identified due to its high expression in SCLC cells. DLL3 is thought to play a key role in the function and survival of tumor-initiating cells. An antibody–drug conjugate, rovalpituzumab tesirine, has been designed to bind DLL3. In a phase Ia/Ib trial, patients with SCLC who had progressed after first- or second-line therapy were treated with rovalpituzumab tesirine.[160] Although the trial was small and reported a modest partial response of 34% with 31% of patients achieving disease stability, duration of response was more than 178 days with no cases of disease progression. Moreover, although DLL3 status was not required for treatment, patients did require sufficient tumor sample for testing. About 67% of patients had tumor DLL3 expression greater than or equal to 50%; these patients tended to have better responses and an overall survival of 5.8 months. It is hoped that this novel targeted agent will demonstrate efficacy upon further investigation, and a phase II study is currently underway.

CONCLUSION

The optimal first-line treatment for good performance score ED-SCLC, regardless of age, is a platinum doublet with either etoposide or irinotecan. Although poor performance status (ECOG PS 2–4) patients are less able to tolerate platinum doublets, because the disease itself attributes most to the deterioration of performance status, a platinum-based regimen at standard doses should be offered with close monitoring. For second-line treatment, the standard of care consists of the topoisomerase I inhibitor topotecan, and in Japan, damrubicin. Because the therapeutic results of second-line treatments remain poor, enrollment of relapsed ED-SCLC in clinical trials with novel agents is also an acceptable standard of care. No new agents with clinically relevant activity have been identified during the last two decades in ED-SCLC, underscoring the unmet need in this area.

KEY REFERENCES

16. Roth BJ, Johnson DH, Einhorn LH, et al. Randomized study of cyclophosphamide, doxorubicin, and vincristine versus etoposide and cisplatin versus alternation of these two regimens in extensive small cell lung cancer: a phase III trial of the Southeastern Cancer Study Group. *J Clin Oncol.* 1992;10(2):282–291.
20. Turrisi 3rd AT, Kim K, Blum R, et al. Twice-daily compared with once-daily thoracic radiotherapy in limited small-cell lung cancer treated concurrently with cisplatin and etoposide. *N Engl J Med.* 1999;340(4):265–271.
22. Rossi A, Di Maio M, Chiodini P, et al. Carboplatin- or cisplatin-based chemotherapy in first-line treatment of small-cell lung cancer: the COCIS meta-analysis of individual patient data. *J Clin Oncol.* 2012;30(14):1692–1698.
23. Noda K, Nishiwaki Y, Kawahara M, et al. Irinotecan plus cisplatin compared with etoposide plus cisplatin for extensive small-cell lung cancer. *N Engl J Med.* 2002;346(2):85–91.
24. Lara Jr PN, Natale R, Crowley J, et al. Phase III trial of irinotecan/cisplatin compared with etoposide/cisplatin in extensive stage small cell lung cancer: clinical and pharmacogenomics results from SWOG S0124. *J Clin Oncol.* 2009;27(15):2530–2535.
26. Zatloukal P, Cardenal F, Szczesna A, et al. A multicenter international randomized phase III study comparing cisplatin in combination with irinotecan or etoposide in previously untreated small-cell lung cancer patients with extensive disease. *Ann Oncol.* 2010;21(9):1810–1816.
28. Hermes A, Bergman B, Bremnes R, et al. Irinotecan plus carboplatin versus oral etoposide plus carboplatin in extensive small-cell lung cancer: a randomized phase III trial. *J Clin Oncol.* 2008;26(26):4261–4267.
29. Schmittel A, Sebastian M, Fischer von Weikersthal L, et al. A German multi-center, randomized phase III trial comparing irinotecan-carboplatin with etoposide-carboplatin as first-line therapy for extensive-disease small-cell lung cancer. *Ann Oncol.* 2011;22(8):1798–1804.
32. Fink TH, Huber RM, Heigener DF, et al. Topotecan/cisplatin compared with cisplatin/etoposide as first-line treatment for patients with extensive disease small-cell lung cancer: final results of a randomized phase III trial. *J Thorac Oncol.* 2012;7(9):1432–1439.
79. Govindan R, Page N, Morgensztern D, et al. Changing epidemiology of small-cell lung cancer in the United States over the last 30 years: analysis of the Surveillance, Epidemiologic, and End Results database. *J Clin Oncol.* 2006;24(28):4539–4544.
97. Okamoto H, Watanabe K, Kunikane H, et al. Randomised phase III trial of carboplatin plus etoposide vs. split doses of cisplatin plus etoposide in elderly or poor-risk patients with extensive disease small-cell lung cancer: JCOG 9702. *Br J Cancer.* 2007;97(2):162–169.
105. Owonikoko TK, Behera M, Chen Z, et al. A systematic analysis of efficacy of second-line chemotherapy in sensitive and refractory small-cell lung cancer. *J Thorac Oncol.* 2012;7(5):866–872.
110. O'Brien ME, Ciuleanu TE, Tsekov H, et al. Phase III trial comparing supportive care alone with supportive care with oral topotecan in patients with relapsed small-cell lung cancer. *J Clin Oncol.* 2006;24(34):5441–5447.
120. Giaccone G, Ferrati P, Donadlo M, Testore F, Calciati A. Reinduction chemotherapy in small cell lung cancer. *Eur J Cancer Clin Oncol.* 1987;23(11):1697–1699.
130. Pfeifer M, Fernandez-Cuesta L, Sos ML, et al. Integrative genome analyses identify key somatic driver mutations of small-cell lung cancer. *Nat Gen.* 2012;44(10):1104–1110.
139. Gitliz BJ, Moon J, Glisson BS, et al. Sorafenib in platinum-treated patients with extensive stage small cell lung cancer: a Southwest Oncology Group (SWOG 0435) phase II trial. *J Thorac Oncol.* 2010;5:1835–1840.
142. Allen JW, Moon J, Redman M, et al. Southwest Oncology Group S0802: a randomized, phase II trial of weekly topotecan with or without ziv-aflibercept in patients with platinum-treated small-cell lung cancer. *J Clin Oncol.* 2014;23:2463–2470.
143. Cavina R, Gregorc V, Novello S, et al. NGR-hTNF and doxorubicin in relapsed small-cell lung cancer. *J Clin Oncol.* 2012:suppl. [Abstract 7085].
144. Arnold AM, Seymour L, Smylie M, et al. Phase II study of vandetanib or placebo in small-cell lung cancer patients after complete or partial response to induction chemotherapy with or without radiation therapy: National Cancer Institute of Canada Clinical Trials Group Study BR.20. *J Clin Oncol.* 2007;25:4278–4284.
159. Ott PA, Fernandez MEE, Hiret S, et al. Pembrolizumab (MK-3475) in patients (pts) with extensive-stage small cell lung cancer (SCLC): Preliminary safety and efficacy results from KEYNOTE-028. *J Clin Oncol.* 2015;33:suppl (Abstract 7502).

See Expertconsult.com for full list of references.

53

Malignant Mesothelioma

Paul Baas, Raffit Hassan, Anna K. Nowak, and David Rice

SUMMARY OF KEY POINTS

- Development of malignant mesothelioma is usually associated with asbestos exposure.
- The most common genetic alterations in mesothelioma are deletion of *CDKN2A/ARF*, inactivation of *NF2*, and mutation or deletion in *BAP1*.
- The eighth edition of the American Joint Commission on Cancer/Union for International Cancer Control staging manual has altered the T and N components for staging from the previous edition.
- Clinical, imaging, and serum biomarkers can contribute to prognostication in pleural mesothelioma.
- First-line palliative chemotherapy is cisplatin (or carboplatin) with pemetrexed; appropriate patients may benefit from the addition of bevacizumab.
- There is no standard second-line chemotherapy for pleural mesothelioma although reintroduction of a pemetrexed-containing regimen, or the use of vinorelbine or gemcitabine, would be considered reasonable.
- Optimal surgical management of malignant pleural mesothelioma remains controversial.
- Immunotherapies including mesothelin-targeted agents and immune checkpoint inhibitors have shown promising efficacy in mesothelioma but further research is required before these are adopted as standard therapy.

All mesothelioma tumors originate from the lining of the pleural cavity, the lung, the pericardium, and the abdominal cavity, including the tunica vaginalis. After transformation of the mesothelium or peritoneum, subtypes of mesothelioma can develop. Malignant mesothelioma (MM) occurs most frequently on one side of the thorax (Malignant Pleural Mesothelioma [MPM]—80%) with the remainder occurring in the abdomen as malignant peritoneal mesothelioma. Although the World Health Organization classification distinguishes three main histologic subtypes of mesothelioma, epithelioid (60%), sarcomatoid (10% to 15%), and biphasic (25% to 30%), there are different subtypes of the epithelioid histology. These subtypes include the papillary, pleomorphic, tubulopapillary, and small cell type. However, these subtypes are not standardly reported.[1]

The main cause of MPM is the exposure to asbestos fibers, which was first described by Wagner et al.[2] Other causes of mesothelioma are endemic erionite exposure in Turkey, ionizing radiation, and chronic inflammation in the pleura.[3,4] Unlike the case with lung cancer, cigarette smoking does not play a role in the development of MPM. MPM is one of the best-known occupational diseases and it is more likely to develop in men than in women (90% vs. 10%), primarily as a result of its association with mining and processing of asbestos fibers. Given the long latency period of 30 to 50 years, the prevalence of mesothelioma is expected to peak for the next decade. Regulations against handling and mining asbestos

in Western Europe and the United States were put in place in the 1990s. It is expected that the disease will be increasingly encountered in third-world countries because of the lack of legislation and increased export to these countries.

BIOLOGY OF MALIGNANT PLEURAL MESOTHELIOMA

Considerable progress has been made in understanding the molecular basis of mesothelioma, which has, in turn, led to an abundance of preclinical studies translating these discoveries to treatment.

Some people with mesothelioma have no history of asbestos exposure or prior radiotherapy.[4] In the case of peritoneal mesothelioma, many patients are teenagers or young adults. Good evidence now exists that at least in some people there may be a genetic basis for developing mesothelioma, which could lead to mesothelioma by itself or cause some individuals to be susceptible to asbestos carcinogenesis. Cyclin-dependent kinase inhibitor 2A/alternative reading frame (*CDKN2A/ARF*), neurofibromatosis type 2 (*NF2*), and BRCA1-associated protein 1 (*BAP1*) are the most frequently mutated tumor suppressor genes in mesothelioma.[5]

Cyclin-Dependent Kinase Inhibitor 2A/Alternative Reading Frame

CDKN2A/ARF is the most frequently inactivated tumor suppressor gene in malignant mesothelioma and encodes two important cell cycle regulatory proteins, p16 (*INK4A*) and, in an alternative reading frame, p14 (*ARF*).[6] p16, a cyclin-dependent kinase (CDK) inhibitor, blocks phosphorylation of retinoblastoma protein, and p14 (*ARF*) blocks murine double minute 2 (*MDM2*), thus resulting in a positive regulation of p53. Homozygous deletion of *CDKN2A/ARF* thus results in inactivation of two major tumor suppressing pathways, retinoblastoma protein and p53.[5]

CDKN2A deletion is found in about 70% of primary tumors and nearly all mesothelioma cell lines.[7]

Neurofibromatosis Type 2

The *NF2* gene encodes a tumor suppressor protein Merlin, a member of the band 4.1 family of cytoskeletal linker proteins. Inactivating *NF2* mutations are found in 35% to 40% of MPMs.[8] The mechanisms of Merlin-mediated tumor suppression are not well defined. Merlin mediates contact-dependent inhibition of cell proliferation in normal cells, primarily through inhibition of mammalian target of rapamycin (mTOR) in an AKT-independent manner. mTOR activity is aberrantly upregulated in the absence of Merlin, leading to increased cell proliferation.[5,9]

BAP1

Up to 60% of mesotheliomas have *BAP1* alterations, which include, among others, homozygous deletions of partial or entire *BAP1* and sequence-level mutations.[10] *BAP1* is located on chromosome 3p21.1, which is also deleted in several human malignancies.[11] Germline *BAP1* mutations were described in 2011 in mesothelioma families in which *BAP1* mutation carriers had an exceptionally high incidence of malignancies, including mesothelioma and uveal melanoma.[12] These malignancies did not develop in family members who did not carry germline *BAP1* mutations. *BAP1* is a nuclear protein that enhances BRCA1-mediated inhibition of breast cancer cell proliferation, acting as a tumor suppressor in the BRCA1 growth control pathway and regulating proliferation by deubiquitinating host cell factor.[1] *BAP1* influences a wide array of cellular functions, and its depletion induces significant changes in the expression of many genes that control various cellular pathways.[4,9]

DIAGNOSIS

Diagnosis of mesothelioma may be achieved by cytologic analysis of pleural effusions sampled by thoracentesis, blind pleural biopsy, computed tomography (CT)-directed fine-needle aspiration or core biopsy, and, increasingly more commonly, via pleuroscopy. However, in a considerable number of cases, evaluations of specimens obtained by these less invasive modalities are inconclusive, necessitating surgical biopsy. Video-assisted thoracoscopic surgery (VATS) is the preferred method for surgical diagnosis of MPM (Fig. 53.1). VATS allows large tissue samples to be obtained from multiple areas of the thoracic cavity, an important consideration, given the considerable tumor heterogeneity within individual mesothelioma tumors. Multiple separate biopsies by VATS increases the likelihood of accurately determining histologic subtype.[13] VATS can also be used to identify whether the tumor involves the visceral pleura as well as the parietal pleura, although this distinction is no longer required for staging with the updated American Joint Commission on Cancer (AJCC)/Union for International Cancer Control (UICC) eighth edition guidelines. VATS is otherwise of limited use for assessment of tumor or node stage. Although VATS is most easily performed in patients with a large effusive component, occasionally tumor burden is such that VATS is impossible due to fusion of the visceral and parietal pleurae and, in such instances, a small, 2-cm cutdown can usually allow access to the underlying pleural tumor under direct vision. A further merit of VATS is that it allows talc pleurodesis to be done at the time of tissue diagnosis, which often obviates the need for additional palliative procedures. Pleurodesis does not influence the ability to perform subsequent cytoreductive surgery (pleurectomy/decortication [PD] or extrapleural pneumonectomy [EPP]). Talc will cause fluorodeoxyglucose (FDG) activity in the pleural distribution and in mediastinal lymph nodes on positron emission tomography (PET) imaging. For this reason, initial staging with PET should be performed before talc pleurodesis.

Thoracotomy is to be avoided as a diagnostic method as it not only causes the patient unnecessary trauma but also hampers the performance of subsequent cytoreductive surgery due to disruption of tissue planes and risks iatrogenic tumor invasion of the chest wall.

STAGING

The AJCC/International Mesothelioma Interest Group staging system is based primarily on pathologic data and is, therefore, of limited use when applied to clinical staging of this disease.[14] Many of the factors that contribute to stage assignment, such as involvement of the pericardium, lung, and diaphragm; involvement of the endothoracic fascia; and lymph node metastases, for example, simply are not possible to determine accurately with current imaging technology. The staging system has recently undergone revision based on an international multicenter prospective data collection of detailed staging information and

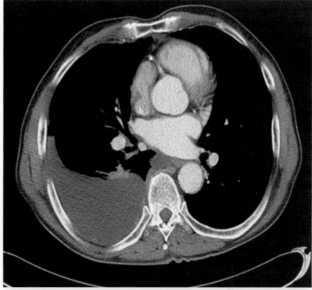

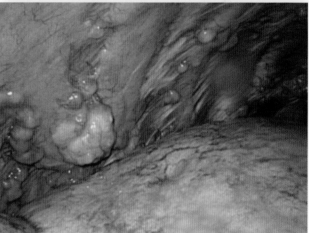

Fig. 53.1. (A) Computed tomography (CT) image of a male patient with a pleural effusion and minimal pleural thickening. (B) Image from video-assisted thorascopic surgery shows multiple nodules on chest wall at the level of the CT image. (B) The lung is partly collapsed and shows no involvement.

component descriptors (Table 53.1).[14a] The revision for the eighth edition AJCC/UICC staging system has made a number of important changes, including collapsing T1a and T1b into T1 and revising nodal staging such that any ipsilateral mediastinal involved lymph nodes are all included as N1 disease, whereas nodes previously categorized as N3 and reclassified as N2. PET is useful for identifying occult distant metastatic disease (present in up to 25% of cases), but it is inaccurate for determining T and N stage.[14b,14c,15]

Laparoscopy and Thoracoscopy

Extension of the tumor through the diaphragm into the peritoneal cavity or dissemination to the contralateral side can occur, which will influence the staging and treatment options. Rice et al.[16] reported on 109 patients who had routine laparoscopy before planned EPP and found nine (8.3%) patients with transdiaphragmatic extension of tumor and one (0.9%) with diffuse peritoneal carcinomatosis. Alvarez et al.[17] performed thoracoscopic examination of the contralateral side and found contralateral chest involvement in three (10%) of 30 patients from a selected group.

TABLE 53.1 IASLC Mesothelioma Staging Project: TNM Definitions*

Stage	Definition
Primary Tumor (T)	
TX	Primary tumor cannot be assessed
T0	No evidence of primary tumor
T1	Tumor imited to the ipsilateral parietal± visceral ± mediastinal± diaphragmatic pleura
T2	Tumorinvolving each of theipsi ateral pleural surfaces (parietal, mediastinal, diaphragmatic, and visceral pleura) with at least one of the following features: • involvement of diaphragmatic muscle • extension of tumor from visceral pleura into the underlying pulmonary parenchyma
T3	Describeslocally advanced but *potentially* resectable tumor. Tumor involving all of theipsilaterat pleuralsurfaces (parietal, mediastinal, diaphragmatic, and visceral pleura) with at least one of the following features : • involvement of the endothoracic fascia • extension into the mediastinal fat • solitary, completely resectabte focus of tumor extendinginto the soft tissues of the chest wall • nontransmurat involvement of the pericardium
T4	Describes locally advanced *technically* unresectable tumor. Tumor involving all of the ipsilateral pleural surfaces (parietal, mediastinal, diaphragmatic, and visceral pleura) with at least one of the following features: • diffuse extension or multifocal masses of tumor in the chest wall, with or without associated rib destruction • direct transdiaphragmatic extension of tumor to the peritoneum • direct extension of tumor to the contralaterat pleura • direct extension of tumor to mediastinal organs • direct extension of tumor into the spine • tumor extending through to the internal surface of the pericardium with or without a pericardial effusion, or tumor involving the myocardium
Regional Lymph Nodes (N)	
NX	Regional lymph nodes cannot be assessed
N0	No regional lymph node metastases
N1	Metastases in the ipsilateral bronchoputmonary, hilar, or mediastinal (including the internal mammary, peridiaphragmatic, pericardial fat pad, or intercostal lymph nodes) lymph nodes
N2	Metastases in the contralateral mediastinal, ipsilaterat, or contralateral supraclavicutar lymph nodes
Distant Metastasis (M)	
M0	No distant metastasis
MI	Distant metastasis present

IASLC MESOTHELIOMA STAGING PROJECT: STAGE GROUPING CHANGES

	N0		N1/N2	N1	N3	N2
Stage	Seventh Edition	Eighth Edition	Seventh Edition	Eighth Edition	Seventh Edition	Eighth Edition
TI	I (A, B)	IA	III		IV	IIIB
T2	II	IB	III		IV	IIIB
T3		IB	III	IIIA	IV	IIIB
T4	IV	IIIB	IV	IIIB	IV	IIIB
M1	IV	IV	IV	IV	IV	IV

*Modified from Rusch VW, Chansky K, Kindler HL, Nowak AK, Pass HI, Rice DC, et al. IASLC Staging and Prognostic Factors *Committee, advisory boards, and participating institutions.*The IASLC Mesothelioma Staging Project: Proposals for the M Descriptors and for Revision of the TNM Stage Groupings in the Forthcoming (Eighth) Edition of the TNM Classification for Mesothelioma. J Thorac Oncol. 2016;11(12): 2112-2119.*

Mediastinal Evaluation

Lymph node metastases occur in approximately 50% of patients with MPM undergoing multimodality therapy and portends a poor prognosis. Current imaging modalities are inaccurate for defining N stage, and, therefore, cervical mediastinoscopy has been advocated for pretreatment staging of MPM.[18] The sensitivity, specificity, and accuracy for cervical mediastinoscopy have been reported by two groups and vary from 60% to 80%, 71% to 100%, and 67% to 93%, respectively.[19,20]

Endobronchial ultrasound (EBUS)- and endoscopic ultrasound (EUS)-guided fine-needle aspiration of mediastinal lymph nodes have been highly effective for staging nonsmall cell lung cancer. Rice et al.[21] compared 50 consecutive patients with mesothelioma who had staging cervical mediastinoscopy with 38 patients who had staging EBUS. Sensitivity and negative-predictive value were 28% and 49%, respectively, for cervical mediastinoscopy, and 59% and 57%, respectively, for EBUS. Furthermore, 11 patients had EUS preoperatively, and metastases were found in the infradiaphragmatic nodes in five patients.

Tournoy et al.[22] performed EUS and fine-needle aspiration in 32 patients with presumed early-stage mesothelioma and identified N2 metastases in four patients (12.5%). In 17 patients who subsequently had extrapleural pneumonectomy, one false-negative result (4.7%) was found. Some centers now prefer to stage the mediastinum by combined EBUC and EUS before entering a patient into a multimodality trial.

BIOMARKERS

Biomarkers have the potential to play a key role in current oncology practice. They can be used in diagnosis (screening), measurement of response, and follow-up. The requisites that apply for biomarkers are technical reproducibility, validation, and clinical relevance. Diagnostic biomarkers can underpin screening programs and early detection in high-risk individuals, can help to direct diagnostic procedures, and can provide support for cytologic or histologic diagnoses. Biomarkers can be predictive for a response or can be prognostic. Predictive biomarkers can assist with treatment selection, in particular drug therapy. Biomarkers of response can accelerate drug development through surrogate end point and provide guidance during routine patient care. Prognostic biomarkers can give patients and clinicians valuable information, in addition to their use as stratification factors in clinical trials. Biomarkers can involve blood measurements (plasma or serum) or molecular genetics or can be based on imaging.

Diagnostic Biomarkers

The development of robust diagnostic serum biomarkers for mesothelioma is important, as exposure to the etiologic agent is often known. A population with heavy asbestos exposure would be rational participants in a screening program. The availability of a blood-based biomarker would facilitate early detection and treatment. The most important candidate diagnostic serum biomarkers are mesothelin (serum mesothelin-related protein), osteopontin, and fibulin-3. Elevated levels of mesothelin are highly specific, unless patients have concurrent renal failure, and add to the diagnostic certainty or direct additional investigations when a diagnosis of mesothelioma is suspected.[23,24] However, mesothelin lacks sensitivity at the time of diagnosis, thus limiting its use in screening.[25,26] Osteopontin does not perform as well as mesothelin.[27] In 2012, Pass et al.[28] reported on fibulin-3 as a blood and effusion biomarker. Plasma levels of fibulin-3 were significantly higher for patients with mesothelioma than in people exposed to asbestos without mesothelioma, with a sensitivity of 100% and specificity of 94% reported. Effusion levels of fibulin-3 were also significantly higher in effusions from mesothelioma than from other etiologies; nevertheless, these findings should be further validated before translation to practice. Carcinoembryogenic antigen is a well-known marker that will not be elevated in case of a MPM. It can be used for quick screening for other tumor types with pleural dissemination.

Prognostic Biomarkers

A number of simple prognostic biomarkers have been well established in the literature for MPM. At pathologic diagnosis, a diagnosis of sarcomatoid or nonepithelioid subtypes of mesothelioma is uniformly associated with poor prognosis.[29,30] The same large retrospective series, mostly based on collections of clinical trial data, has also validated readily available laboratory parameters, including low hemoglobin, thrombocytosis, high white blood cell count, and elevated serum lactate dehydrogenase level as poor prognostic indicators.[31] In 2010, Kao et al.[32] proposed and independently validated an elevated neutrophil-to-lymphocyte ratio as a poor prognostic indicator; however, the patient groups used were heterogeneous and relatively small, and others have been unable to confirm these findings. High serum vascular endothelial growth factor (VEGF) levels have been found to correlate with poor prognosis and advanced stage of disease.[33] A recent publication used a Classification and Regression Tree analysis to group patients into prognostic categories at diagnosis, deriving four prognostic groupings with median survivals ranging from 7.5 months (risk group 4) to 34 months (risk group 1) using readily available clinical indicators including weight loss, hemoglobin level, performance status, histology, and albumin level.[34]

Considering prognostic serum biomarkers more specific to mesothelioma, mesothelin levels at diagnosis may also be prognostic;[34] however, mesothelin levels appear to reflect tumor bulk, as the addition of tumor bulk metrics to the model eliminates the significance of serum mesothelin.[35] No strong evidence exists that serum osteopontin is useful in prognostication, although lower tissue expression of osteopontin may be associated with longer survival and plasma osteopontin as well as mesothelin were found to increase prognostic accuracy in combination with the EORTC and CALGB mesothlieoma prognostic indices.[36]

Many candidate tumor molecular and histologic prognostic markers have been reported (phosphatase and tensin homolog, VEGF expression, fibroblast growth factor 2, cyclooxygenase-2, platelet-derived growth factor, epidermal growth factor receptor, epithelial-to-mesenchymal transition, osteopontin, and c-MET expression); however, at the time of publication, none has been sufficiently validated to be entered into routine clinical use worldwide. The anticipation is that the extensive molecular profiling and characterization efforts proceeding worldwide will identify new molecular prognostic biomarkers that will translate to routine clinical practice in addition to providing potential molecular targets for therapy.

Prognostic Imaging Biomarkers

In addition to providing anatomic staging information regarding the sites of disease involvement, a substantial body of evidence indicates that the bulk of tumor as demonstrated on imaging and metabolic characteristics of tumor may be prognostic biomarkers. Tumor volume as measured by CT is a prognostic indicator, but it can be challenging to implement automated volumetric measurements due to the difficulty of distinguishing tumor from pleural fluid and atelectasis.[37,38] Quantitative parameters from FDG-PET may be simpler to implement reproducibly and with less manual input. FDG-PET has consistently shown prognostic value in MPM, although the appropriate metric for quantitative assessment remains the subject of debate. A higher maximum standardized uptake value (SUV) is a poor prognostic indicator.[39] However, the inclusion of volumetric parameters may also be important, with the concepts of total lesion glycolysis or total glycolytic volume incorporating both SUV and a measure of lesion volume and performing better than SUV alone in studies incorporating both measures.[40,41]

CHEMOTHERAPY

First-Line Chemotherapy

Combination cytotoxic chemotherapy remains the mainstay of palliative treatment of patients with MPM, with cisplatin and an antifolate being the most widely used and evidence-based first-line doublet. The authors of two studies reported that the combination of cisplatin and an antifolate produced a survival benefit over cisplatin alone, with a hazard ratio for overall survival of 0.77 and a median survival gain of 3 months.[42,43] Cisplatin and pemetrexed have become the standard of care and the backbone on which subsequent clinical trials in mesothelioma have been constructed.

The combination of cisplatin and either pemetrexed or raltitrexed was associated with better quality of life and symptom control than cisplatin alone, with improvements in pain, dyspnea, fatigue, and cough, as well as global quality of life.[42] The combination of cisplatin and raltitrexed improved dyspnea to a clinically meaningful extent compared with cisplatin alone, although other parameters remained stable.[43] However, selection of patients who are fit for treatment is important, as is supportive care and careful oversight of potential toxicities. Treatment with cisplatin and pemetrexed should be accompanied by supplementary folate and vitamin B12 starting 1 to 2 weeks before the first day of chemotherapy.

Recently, the addition of bevacizumab to cisplatin and pemetrexed has demonstrated further benefits in progression-free and overall survival. Bevacizumab was used in combination with cisplatin and pemetrexed, and with subsequent single agent bevacizumab continuing until disease progression after completion of up to 6 cycles of the combination therapy. This addition gave a hazard ratio for overall survival of 0.7, increasing the median survival from 16.1 to 18.8 months, with manageable toxicities.

The high cost of bevacizumab and modest benefits, as well as the lack of any predictive biomarker, has delayed widespread uptake into international routine clinical practice. However in selected patients without contraindications to anti-VEGF therapy this is an appropriate addition to standard chemotherapy.[44]

Response to first-line chemotherapy should be assessed with serial CT performed at baseline and then after every two or three cycles. FDG-PET to monitor response is not standard, but can supplement information from CT and may provide an indication of response or progression at an earlier time point than CT. Although changes in serum mesothelin levels may parallel tumor volume, the test has not been sufficiently validated in this context to replace or supplement imaging to monitor response.[45] The optimum number of cycles of platinum-based chemotherapy has not been demonstrated in clinical trials; however, four to six cycles of doublet chemotherapy is in keeping with the pivotal clinical trial data, allowing for cessation at four cycles if treatment is poorly tolerated. The spectrum of common cumulative toxicities includes fatigue, progressive anemia, and sensory peripheral neuropathy.

Timing of First-Line Chemotherapy

The timing of initiation of first-line palliative chemotherapy remains a matter of debate. A chemotherapy regimen used in one small randomized clinical trial was subsequently found to be inactive (mitomycin, vinblastine, and cisplatin or carboplatin) in a large, randomized study.[46,47] In this trial,[43] patients who were symptomatically stable were randomly assigned to receive either immediate chemotherapy or delayed treatment after the onset of symptoms. The investigators found a nonsignificant survival benefit for the immediate treatment arm. Nevertheless, in asymptomatic patients with minimal or nonmeasurable disease and epithelioid histology, for example, patients presenting with pleural effusion that has been effectively managed, it is reasonable to defer treatment if surgery is not planned.

Second-Line and Subsequent Chemotherapy

Patients often have a good performance status at progression after first-line chemotherapy and are fit for and desire further treatment. Although uncontrolled studies and anecdotal experience support the potential for second-line chemotherapy to elicit objective treatment responses, at the time of publication, no positive randomized controlled trial of any agent in the setting of uniform previous treatment with cisplatin and pemetrexed had been reported.

In the era before routine first-line treatment with a platinum agent and pemetrexed, authors of a well-conducted randomized clinical trial of second-line single-agent pemetrexed plus best supportive care compared with best supportive care alone in 243 patients reported partial response in 19% of patients receiving pemetrexed and 2% of patients receiving best supportive care alone. The disease control rate was 59% in the pemetrexed arm and 19% in the best supportive care arm, and progression-free survival favored the pemetrexed arm (median, 3.6 vs. 1.5 months) although there was no significant difference in overall survival (p = 0.7434).[46] Patients who had a response to their previous chemotherapy regimen were more likely to have a clinical benefit. Substantially more participants in the best supportive care arm (52% vs. 28%) received postdiscontinuation chemotherapy, which may have obscured any potential difference in overall survival.

Although these results are encouraging, this study does not give firm guidance in the post-pemetrexed setting. To attempt to address this question, patients from the pivotal trial of pemetrexed and cisplatin were evaluated for chemotherapy use after pemetrexed.[49] Eighty-four patients in the pemetrexed and cisplatin arm received subsequent chemotherapy, with 48 patients receiving single-agent treatment and 36 patients receiving combination chemotherapy. Regimens included gemcitabine, vinorelbine, anthracyclines, and platinum agents alone and gemcitabine-based combinations. Although the data available were not suitable to examine response or disease control rates, subsequent chemotherapy was significantly correlated with longer survival (p < 0.001), after adjustment for treatment group and prognostic factors. This finding may be explained by a benefit from second-line chemotherapy, but is also likely to be biased by the selection of fitter patients for subsequent treatment lines.

Support for reintroduction of pemetrexed-based chemotherapy for patients who had a previous response can be found in a number of uncontrolled clinical trials and case series (Table 53.2). In an observational study,[31] patients who had response or stable disease to previous pemetrexed-based therapy were further treated with pemetrexed either as a single agent (15 patients) or in combination with carboplatin or cisplatin (16 patients).[50] The overall response rate was 19%, and 52% of patients had progressive disease as their best response. The median progression-free survival was 3.8 months, median overall survival was 10.5 months, and the toxicity was manageable. Predictors of better outcomes included a longer interval between initial pemetrexed-based chemotherapy and additional treatment, previous objective response to therapy, and second-line rather than third-line treatment.

In a large retrospective assessment of patient outcomes with second-line therapy, 181 patients who had received second-line chemotherapy were identified from eight Italian centers.[51] Most (66%) of the patients had received prior pemetrexed-based treatment, of whom 42 patients received further pemetrexed-based therapy and 31 received platinum and pemetrexed. Again, good performance status and more than 12 months since first-line therapy predicted better outcomes after further treatment in all patients. Although the disease control rate was similar for patients who were retreated with pemetrexed alone or in combination with a platinum drug, progression-free survival and overall survival were better for patients retreated with a combination of a platinum agent and pemetrexed. Clear potential biases exist that limit interpretation of these data, in particular, that selection of single-agent chemotherapy over combination chemotherapy is likely to have been influenced by clinician perception of the tolerability of combination chemotherapy for individuals, with single-agent treatment more likely to have been recommended for patients who were less fit.

A number of other nonpemetrexed second-line regimens were used in this retrospective Italian series, either with or without platinum agents.[51] These regimens included combinations of cisplatin or carboplatin with gemcitabine or vinorelbine, as well as vinorelbine and gemcitabine alone or in combination. Overall, the disease control rate, progression-free survival, and overall survival were superior for patients who received repeat platinum-based treatment, however, we should interpret these data with the same potential for bias as just discussed.

The interpretation of these studies has substantial limitations, particularly in view of the heterogeneity of patient populations. In particular, in some studies not all patients had been previously treated with pemetrexed. Selection criteria and tumor measurement metrics were variable. Few studies included evaluation of symptom benefit, quality of life, or functional benefit as measured by lung function.

In recommendations for second-line therapy, it is appropriate to consider reintroduction of a pemetrexed-based regimen for patients who have had a response to first-line pemetrexed-based treatment, and who have had a long interval since previous treatment, with patients treated more than 12 months before reintroduction likely to have the most benefit. An appropriate regimen choice is pemetrexed with the alternative platinum drug or single-agent pemetrexed if the patient is unfit for combination therapy or has a contraindication to the platinum compounds.

TABLE 53.2 Selected Results of Repeat Induction Therapy or Other Regimens Studied in the Second-Line Setting

First-Line Treatment	Subsequent Treatment	No. of Patients	Objective Response Rate (%)	Disease Control Rate (%)	Progression-Free Survival (Mo)	Overall Survival (Mo)	Reference
Pemetrexed with or without platinum agent	Pemetrexed with or without platinum agent	31	19	48	3.8	10.5	Ceresoli et al.[50]
Pemetrexed with or without platinum agent	Gemcitabine and vinorelbine	30	10	43	2.8	10.9	Zucali et al.[a]
Pemetrexed and platinum agent	Pemetrexed with or without platinum agent	30	17	66	5.1	13.6	Bearz et al.[129]
None or 1 regimen	Gemcitabine and epirubicin	23	13 (high dose), 7 (low dose)	NR	4.2	5.7	Okuno et al.[130]
Various	Vinorelbine	63	16	68	NR	9.6	Stebbing et al.[131]
Pemetrexed and carboplatin	Gemcitabine and docetaxel plus G-CSF	37	19	62	7	16.2	Tourkantonis et al.[132]
Various (not pemetrexed)	Pemetrexed + BSC (vs. BSC)	123	19	59	3.6	8.4	Jassem et al.[48]
Various	Irinotecan, cisplatin, and mitomycin C	13	20	70	7.3	7.3	Fennell et al.[b]
Platinum and pemetrexed	BNC105P	30	3	46	1.5	8.2	Nowak et al.[c]
Platinum and pemetrexed	Sunitinib	53	12	77	3.5	6.1	Nowak et al.[d]
Various	Pembrolizumab	25	28	76	5.8	NR	Alley et al.[e]
Platinum and pemetrexed	Avelumab	53	9	58	4	NR	Hassan et al.[97]
Platinum and pemetrexed	Nivolumab	18	27	50	NR	NR	Quispel-Janssen et al.[f]

[a]Zucali PA, Ceresoli GL, Garassino I, et al. Gemcitabine and vinorelbine in pemetrexed-pretreated patients with malignant pleural mesothelioma. *Cancer*. 2008;112(7):1555–1561.

[b]Fennell DA, Steele JP, Shamash J, et al. Efficacy and safety of first- or second-line irinotecan, cisplatin, and mitomycin in mesothelioma. *Cancer*. 2007;109(1):93–99.

[c]Nowak AK, Brown C, Millward MJ, et al. A phase II clinical trial of the vascular disrupting agent BNC105P as second line chemotherapy for advanced malignant pleural mesothelioma. *Lung Cancer*. 2013;81(3):422–427.

[d]Nowak AK, Millward MJ, Creaney J, et al. A phase II study of intermittent sunitinib malate as second-line therapy in progressive malignant pleural mesothelioma. *J Thorac Oncol.*, 2012;7(9):1449–1456.

[e]Alley EW, Schellens JH, Santoro A, et al. Single-agent pembrolizumab for patients with malignant pleural mesothelioma (MPM). Denver: World Conference on Lung Cancer: 2015.

[f]Quispel-Janssen J, et al. Nivolumab in malignant pleural mesothelioma (NIVOMES): an interim analysis, in 3th International Conference of the International Mesothelioma Interest Group. Birmingham, UK: 2016.

BSC, best supportive care; *G-CSF*, granulocyte colony stimulating factor.

In patients for whom pemetrexed-based treatment is not recommended, such as patients with a shorter treatment-free interval, vinorelbine, either as a single agent or with gemcitabine, has an acceptable activity and toxicity profile. Treatment discussions should include careful consideration of patient preferences and disclosure regarding the limited data on functional and quality-of-life benefits.

A relative paucity of trials of second-line cytotoxic chemotherapy in malignant mesothelioma has been reported since 2009. Research efforts and enrollment into second-line trials have focused on identifying novel targeted agents that may have activity in mesothelioma and the prospect of molecular predictors of response to such agents. A realistic perception exists that the benefits of cytotoxic chemotherapy have reached a plateau, given the lack of development of new cytotoxic agents in favor of molecularly targeted agents, and there is likely to be limited benefit from further testing of existing cytotoxic agents in this setting. The current generation of clinical trials for second-line therapy in mesothelioma generates debate about an appropriate control arm. Placebo control is still considered appropriate for a phase III study, in the absence of data showing a survival benefit for second-line treatment after pemetrexed. Second-line trials should include testing of quality-of-life and functional parameters in order to draw robust conclusions about patient benefit in this population.

SURGERY

Surgery for MPM is indicated for diagnosis, staging of disease, palliation of symptoms (rarely), and cytoreduction.

Palliative Surgery

Patients with mesothelioma most commonly present with dyspnea, chest wall pain, cough, or constitutional symptoms such as fatigue, fever, and anorexia. Respiratory symptoms may be secondary to atelectasis, with ventilation reduction and shunting caused by the compressive effects of pleural effusion or tumor encasement. Symptoms may also be secondary to altered respiratory mechanics as a result of altered chest wall mechanics and impaired movement of the ribs and diaphragm. Surgical palliation for patients with these symptoms includes treatment of pleural effusion and lung collapse and amelioration of chest wall mechanics.

Pleural Drainage

Treatment of pleural effusion depends on the size of the effusion, the degree to which it is causing atelectasis, and the amount of underlying lung entrapment. Simple thoracentesis is rarely effective in providing long-term relief of pleural effusion; however, it is a reasonable initial procedure to help dyspnea, to obtain a diagnosis, and to evaluate the degree to which the lung will reexpand. In the absence of complete reexpansion, pleural symphysis is unlikely to occur with sclerotherapy (i.e., talc). In cases of effusion with lung entrapment, placement of an indwelling pleural catheter can be helpful. This simple outpatient procedure does not require complete lung reexpansion to be effective, and, although tumor progression along the catheter tract has been described, it appears to be an uncommon event.[52]

Palliative Pleurectomy

The aim of palliative pleurectomy is to free up an entrapped lung, allowing it to reexpand, to ameliorate the restrictive effect of chest wall tumor, and to reestablish pleural apposition and ultimately pleural symphysis. Palliative pleurectomy should be differentiated from cytoreductive PD, which is performed with the aim of achieving macroscopic complete resection of tumor in the hope of influencing time to recurrence and survival. Quality-of-life improvements after palliative pleurectomy have not been extensively documented, and no prospective comparisons between best supportive care and PD exist. Control of pleural effusion is good, with most reports citing success in 80% to 100% of cases.[53] Improvement in dyspnea and chest wall pain is generally less. Soysal et al.[54] retrospectively reviewed 100 consecutive pleurectomies performed for palliation of MPM. Pleural effusion was controlled in 52 (96%) of 54 patients who presented with symptomatic effusion, chest pain was relieved or improved in 85%, and cough and dyspnea improved in all patients. Most important, symptom relief was achieved for up to 6 months.

Although palliative pleurectomy can achieve excellent control of pleural effusion, it requires a thoracotomy, and the upfront morbidity of this procedure may negate some of its potential advantages, particularly with respect to pain control. VATS debulking has emerged as an alternative option. Waller et al.[55] first described use of VATS pleurectomy in 19 patients with malignant effusion and showed control of pleural effusion in 84% of patients at a median follow-up of 12 months; however, tumor seeding at port sites occurred in 5 (38%) of 13 patients with MPM. A phase III trial comparing VATS pleurectomy with talc pleurodesis (MESOVATS) indicated that the success of VATS pleurodesis was higher than that of talc pleurodesis, but no differences in overall survival were found.[56] The influence of histology on outcome following palliative pleurectomy was evaluated in 51 patients with MPM.[55] Significant improvement in dyspnea and pain score was achieved at 6 weeks and 3 months; however, prolonged benefit was found mainly for patients with epithelioid tumors and for patients without substantial weight loss. The median survival for patients with nonepithelioid tumors in this study was 4.4 months. The 30-day mortality was 8%, but increased to 14% by 6 weeks, calling into question the validity of palliative pleurectomy for patients with sarcomatoid and biphasic tumors.

Cytoreductive Surgery

The aim of cytoreductive surgery is to remove all macroscopic tumor from the hemithorax.[57,58] It is postulated, although unproven, that R0 or R1 cytoreduction prolongs survival for patients, particularly patients with epithelioid tumors and no lymph node metastases. The argument in favor of cytoreduction is supported by several observations. First, a large body of evidence from other disease sites shows a benefit to cytoreductive surgery in stage IV disease; the results of randomized trials support this procedure for advanced ovarian, colorectal, and renal cell cancers. Second, most long-term survivors of MPM have had surgery as a component of their therapy, whereas very few long-term survivors have been treated with nonoperative strategies. In

two studies, both published in 2010, the outcomes for patients with MPM in the Surveillance Epidemiology and End Results database were evaluated. In both studies, survival was longer for patients who had cancer-directed surgery compared with patients whose treatment did not include surgery (11 vs. 7 months).[59,60] Third, the median survival of patients in three phase III trials of chemotherapy was between 10 and 13 months,[42,43,46] whereas in three multicenter trimodality phase II studies that included cytoreductive surgery in the form of EPP, the median survival on an intent-to-treat basis was notably longer than 17 months.[61–63] Lastly, several retrospective studies appear to demonstrate longer survival for patients with mesothelioma who have undergone more complete cytoreduction compared with patients with larger tumor volumes after resection.[64] The two approaches to cytoreductive surgery for pleural mesothelioma are EPP and radical PD (or total pleurectomy).

Extrapleural Pneumonectomy

EPP involves the en bloc resection of the parietal and visceral pleura, lung, ipsilateral pericardium, and diaphragm (Fig. 53.2). The pericardium and diaphragm are usually reconstructed with prosthetic mesh, often polytetrafluoroethylene, although use of polyglycolic acid, polypropylene, and various biologic meshes has also been described. The procedure is extensive and has been associated with a high mortality rate, but in most large-volume centers perioperative mortality is below 8%. Postoperative morbidity is approximately 50% to 60% and most commonly includes supraventricular tachyarrhythmias (44% to 46%), which are easily treated, but also life-threatening events such as major hemorrhage (1%), cardiac herniation (1% to 2%), esophageal perforation (1% to 2%), bronchopleural fistula (1% to 2%), empyema (3% to 6%), acute respiratory distress syndrome (4% to 8%), and pneumonia (5% to 10%). Survival following EPP in the trimodality setting ranges from 10 to 28 months and is dependent on stage, histology, and whether survival is calculated from the date of surgery or from the date of diagnosis. Because the entire lung is removed with EPP, the at-risk area for local recurrence is limited to the inner aspect of the chest wall, the peridiaphragmatic area, and the ipsilateral mediastinum. Local recurrence rates with EPP alone range from 30% to 50%. For this reason, both adjuvant hemithoracic radiotherapy and intrapleural therapies, such as heated intrapleural chemotherapy (HIOC) and photodynamic therapy (described later), have been administered in an effort to reduce local recurrence.

Adjuvant radiotherapy has been a treatment component in several case series. In a phase II trial of adjuvant external-beam radiotherapy reported by Rusch et al.,[65] radiotherapy to the postpneumonectomy space to 50.4 Gy reduced the rate of local failure to 13%.[18] Sites of failure were predominantly in the posterior diaphragmatic sulcus, but authors of later reports suggested higher rates of local recurrences (approximately 30%) using standard anterior-posterior beam techniques.[65] Intensity-modulated radiotherapy (IMRT), which allows for better dose distribution and targeting of the postpneumonectomy space, has been applied in this setting. Unfortunately, systemic metastases remain a major problem. Distant metastases developed in many patients, most commonly in the contralateral lung or in the abdominal cavity. Caution should be maintained when using IMRT after pneumonectomy because of the potential for radiation toxicity to the remaining lung; in some reports, IMRT has been associated with fatal pneumonitis.[66] Lung toxicity can be minimized, however, by ensuring the volume of lung tissue receiving 20 Gy or more is less than 7% and the mean lung dose is less than 8.5 Gy.[19] Newer modalities, such as helical tomotherapy and intensity-modulated proton-beam therapy, show promise to provide good local control while minimizing toxicity to surrounding structures.

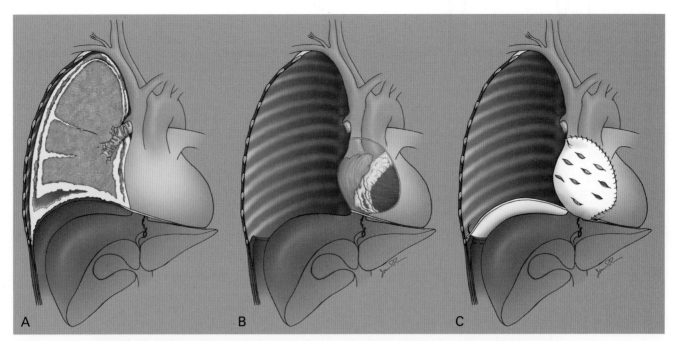

Fig. 53.2. Extrapleural pneumonectomy includes removal of all pleural lining, diaphragm, pericardium, and lung. (A) The yellow line indicates the spread of the mesothelioma over the pleural lining. (B) After removal of the lung and stripping of the parietal pleura, diaphragm, and pericardium, patches (white) (C) are placed to cover the abdominal structures and the heart. *(Reprinted with permission from David Rice, MD.)*

TABLE 53.3 Published Series of Extrapleural Pneumonectomy for Pleural Mesothelioma in Studies With at Least 70 Patients

Author	No. of Patients	Epithelial Subtype (%)	Stage III/IV (%)	Chemotherapy	Radiotherapy	Periop Mortality (%)	Median Survival (Mo)	Local Failure (%)	Distant Failure (%)
Sugarbaker et al.[67]	183	59	NR	Adjuvant	Hemithoracic	4	19	NR	NR
Edwards et al.[133]	105	74	85	Neoadjuvant	Hemithoracic	7	15	NR	NR
Flores et al.[134]	208	69	78	Neoadjuvant	Hemithoracic	5	14	NR	NR
Rice et al.[19]	100	67	87	None	Hemithoracic	8	10	13	54
Flores et al.[82]	385	69	75	Adjuvant	Not specified	7	12	33	66
Tilleman et al.[76]	96	55	81	HIOC (cisplatin)	None	4	13	17	62
Trousse et al.[135]	83	82	53	Neoadjuvant or adjuvant	Hemithoracic	5	15	NR	NR
Yan et al.[136]	70	83	NR	Not routinely	Hemithoracic	6	20	NR	NR

HIOC, heated intraoperative chemotherapy; *NR*, not reported; *Periop*, perioperative.

Survival following EPP is highly dependent on tumor stage, histology, and tumor volume (Table 53.3).[18,64,67] In a series of 183 patients with MPM treated at the Brigham and Women's Hospital, the median survival was 19 months overall and was 51 months for patients who had negative margins, epithelioid tumors, and negative nodes.[66] Analysis of 34 published reports showed an average survival of 18 months (range, 5 to 47 months).[68] The utility of EPP was questioned following publication of results of the Mesothelioma and Radical Surgery feasibility study, a small pilot study in 50 patients designed to test whether patients could be randomly assigned to receive either EPP or best supportive care following systemic platinum-based chemotherapy.[69] The trial was negative because it showed that it would not be feasible to randomize enough patients to reach the accrual goal of 670 patients, the number estimated to be required to have power to detect a survival difference. The results of this pilot study indicated that overall survival was worse in the EPP arm (14.4 vs. 19.5 months). The study has been criticized for several reasons, including high perioperative mortality (19%) in the EPP arm, small sample size,

failure to standardize chemotherapy regimens, crossover between treatment groups, lack of reporting of final histology, and survival analysis truncation at 18 months.[70,71]

Pleurectomy/Decortication

PD for cytoreduction of mesothelioma removes the involved visceral and/or parietal pleura with the aim of achieving macroscopic complete resection of tumor while preserving the underlying lung parenchyma. When structures such as the diaphragm or pericardium require resection, the procedure is termed extended PD (Fig. 53.2).[72] PD begins with complete extrapleural mobilization of the lung and involved parietal pleura to the level of the hilar structures, similar to that performed during the initial dissection for EPP. If the pleura/tumor is inseparable from the pericardium or diaphragm (as it often is), these structures are resected in a manner similar to that with EPP. Frequently, the pericardium does not require reconstruction because of the limited risk of cardiac torsion with the lung in situ. Once the lung

TABLE 53.4 Published Series of Pleurectomy/Decortication for Pleural Mesothelioma in Studies With at Least 40 Patients

Author	No. of Patients	Epithelial Subtype (%)	Stage III/IV (%)	Chemotherapy	Radiotherapy	Periop. Mortality (%)	Median Survival (Mo)	Local Failure (%)	Distant Failure (%)
Hilaris et al.[137]	41	68	NR	Adjuvant	Brachytherapy plus hemithoracic	0	21	71	54
Allen et al.[138]	56	50	NR	Adjuvant	Type not specified	5	9	NR	NR
Colaut et al.[139]	40	NR	23	Adjuvant	Local	3	11	86	0
Richards et al.[75]	44	55	39	HIOC (cisplatin)	None	11	13	57	43
Lucchi et al.[140]	49	80	82	Intrapleural IL-2 plus epidoxorubicin, adjuvant	Local	0	26	90	14
Flores et al.[134]	278	64	65	Adjuvant	Type not specified	4	16	65	35
Lang-Lazdunski et al.[141]	41	67	64	HIOC, adjuvant	Local	0	24	NR	NR
Nakas et al.[142]	67	78	100	None	None	3	13	44	18

HIOC, heated intraoperative chemotherapy; *IL-2*, interleukin-2; *NR*, not reported; *Periop*, perioperative.

and overlying pleura have been mobilized, an incision is made in the parietal pleura and taken through the tumor and visceral pleura down to the level of the lung parenchyma. Subpleural tumor deposits that remain adherent to the lung after visceral pleurectomy may be directly removed using sharp dissection or may be ablated using thermal energy. PD is generally associated with less risk than EPP, with perioperative mortality typically in the range of 0% to 5%. Reported complications include atrial arrhythmias (24% to 32%), prolonged air leaks (3% to 21%), pulmonary complications (9% to 11%), and empyema (2% to 8%).[72]

Because the lung is left in situ, PD offers a greater surface area for residual microscopic disease, as reflected in the higher rate of local recurrence compared with EPP, which is generally 1.5 to 2 times higher.[71] Because ipsilateral lung parenchyma remains in situ, the ability to deliver effective postoperative radiotherapy is compromised, which is not a limiting factor after EPP. Gupta et al.[73] reported on 123 patients who received hemithoracic radiotherapy (median, 43 Gy) following PD. Despite a preponderance of patients with early-stage disease (59%), the median survival was 14 months, and local recurrence developed in 56% of patients (Table 53.4).

Intrapleural Therapies

The relatively high local recurrence rate following cytoreductive surgery alone has prompted use of intrapleural therapies at the time of PD and EPP. These therapies have primarily involved intrapleural administration of platinum-based chemotherapy or intracavitary photodynamic therapy. Intrapleural therapies are attractive because they potentially treat the entire at-risk area of the hemithorax and lung. Topical administration of heated platinum agents has been shown to result in permeation of chemotherapy into tissue up to a depth of 5 mm. Most trials of intrapleural chemotherapy have been small phase I and II studies with limited numbers of patients, and the rate of local recurrence has ranged from 17% to 100%.[74] Earlier studies tended to rely on the instillation of the chemotherapeutic agent into the chest cavity via chest drains in the postoperative period, but later investigators employed HIOC, perfusing the cytotoxic agents in the chest at 42°C. Following a phase I/II study by Richards et al.[75] for patients with MPM who had PD and HIOC in which local failure occurred in 57%, Tilleman et al.[76] reported results of

heated cisplatin in 92 patients after EPP. Renal function was preserved by the concomitant administration of sodium thiosulfate and amifostine. Although recurrence within the ipsilateral chest was low (17%) and operative mortality was 4%, the median survival was 13 months. However, nearly half of the patients had stage III disease and 42% had nonepithelioid histology, which may have negatively influenced survival. A 1998 analysis from the same group compared patients with a good prognosis (epithelioid histology, low-volume disease, hemoglobin greater than 13g/dL, or female gender) who received HIOC with a similar group who did not and reported that the HIOC group had a longer interval to recurrence (27 vs. 13 months) and improved survival (35 vs. 23 months).[77]

Photodynamic therapy has been evaluated in a few phase I/II studies.[78–80] Local recurrence rates have varied between 15% and 76% and survival has ranged from 10 to 32 months. Treatment-related toxicity was an issue in some early studies, with reported deaths due to bronchial and esophageal fistulization.[79] A single, randomized study was performed by Pass et al.[81] to evaluate the effect of porfimer sodium after cytoreductive surgery. The study did not show any benefit of the addition of photodynamic therapy. In 2004, Friedberg et al.[80] reported promising results for 38 patients with MPM who had extended PD and intraoperative PDT. The median survival was 32 months, although local failure subsequently developed in 66% of patients and distant recurrence in 47%.

Choice of Extrapleural Pneumonectomy or Pleurectomy/Decortication

Controversy exists over the selection of the most appropriate surgical procedure (Fig. 53.3). A consensus statement from the International Mesothelioma Interest Group Congress in 2012 concluded that the goal of cytoreductive surgery should be the complete resection of all macroscopic tumor and that whether EPP or PD is applied to achieve this goal is of secondary importance and best left to the discretion of the surgeon based on patient and tumor characteristics.[71] Several comparison series have been published, but all have been retrospective in nature and thus subject to selection bias. The largest study to date was by Flores et al.,[82] who reported on 663 patients from three separate institutions. The overall median survival was 14 months and

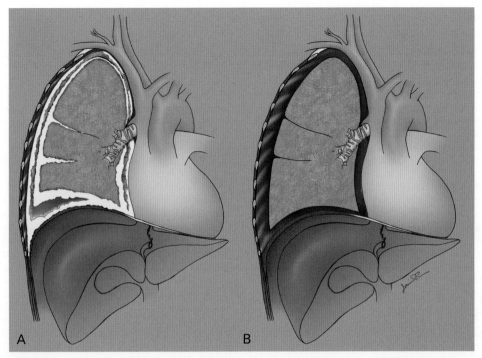

Fig. 53.3. Macroscopic complete resection is obtained when all macroscopic tumor (A) is resected, leaving the lung, diaphragm, and pericardium in situ (B). *(Reprinted with permission from David Rice, MD.)*

was significantly longer for the 278 patients who had PD than for the 385 patients who had EPP (16 vs. 12 months, $p < 0.001$). However, it should be recognized that significantly more patients in the PD group had early-stage tumors (35% vs. 25%, $p < 0.001$). In addition, the institutions involved in this study preferentially performed PD for patients with minimal visceral involvement and for patients with low tumor volume. This bias toward performing PD for patients with biologically more favorable tumors makes it difficult to draw firm conclusions from the data. Furthermore, a previous analysis from one of the institutions showed no difference in survival among 222 patients with EPP and 126 patients with PD.[83]

Another controversial topic relates to whether to offer EPP to patients with node metastases, which can occur in up to 50% of patients undergoing cytoreduction and which negatively influence survival. Investigators of a study published in 2007 compared outcomes for patients with node-positive disease who had EPP and PD and found no survival benefit for EPP over PD for patients with N2 disease.[57] However, accurately identifying N2 disease before EPP remains a problem. As already outlined, mediastinoscopy has poor sensitivity (approximately 30% to 40%) and, although EBUS and EUS may offer improved accuracy, a large number of positive nodes occur in locations where preoperative histologic sampling is not possible. Detailed intraoperative lymph node sampling following the initial extrapleural dissection in patients for whom EPP is planned affords the surgeon the ability to perform PD if node metastases are identified on evaluation of a frozen section specimen, thus sparing a patient likely to have a poor prognosis the risk of EPP.

In terms of postoperative quality of life, EPP is generally more deleterious than PD. In a 2012 study by Rena et al.,[84] quality of life for patients undergoing EPP or PD was measured using the validated Cancer Core Questionnaire from the European Organisation for Research and Treatment of Cancer. Patients who had EPP had significantly poorer functional scores at 6 and 12 months compared with patients who had PD and never approached a return to baseline. In terms of symptoms, pain scores increased and cough and dyspnea scores decreased, although to a lesser extent than for patients who had PD.

Controversy remains regarding the surgical management of MPM. In fit patients with epithelioid tumors and negative nodes, cytoreductive surgery as part of a multimodality regimen appears to improve survival compared with best supportive care or chemotherapy alone, although this result is unproven. Complete resection of all macroscopic disease is considered the goal of any therapeutic cytoreductive procedure, whether EPP or PD. EPP is associated with lower rates of local recurrence, particularly when combined with hemithoracic radiotherapy or HIOC, but it is also associated with higher perioperative morbidity and mortality than is PD. At the time of publication, no convincing evidence supports any major survival difference between the two procedures. Intrapleural therapies appear promising, particularly for patients with a good prognosis. Distant failure remains a substantial issue that limits long-term survival for patients who have undergone cytoreductive surgery, although in the future, it is possible that if micrometastatic disease can be successfully managed with improved chemotherapeutic or immunotherapeutic agents, the local control achievable with cytoreduction may translate into better survival.

IMMUNOTHERAPY FOR MESOTHELIOMA

Although mesothelioma is not considered particularly immunogenic, antitumor immune responses, including spontaneous tumor regressions in some patients with mesothelioma, have been reported. However, such spontaneous tumor regressions are rare, which suggests the presence of immune escape mechanisms. Mesothelioma is heavily infiltrated with many immune effector cells, and macrophages, natural killer cells, and T lymphocytes (both T-helper/inducer [CD4] and T-suppressor/cytotoxic [CD8] cells) constitute most of the inflammatory cells in malignant pleural effusions of patients with mesothelioma.[85]

Regulatory T Cells and Immunosuppressive Cytokines

Regulatory T cells are negative regulators of the immune system, which play an important role in maintaining peripheral tolerance. Hegmans et al.[85] demonstrated that mesothelioma tissue sections contained substantial amounts of regulatory T cells characterized by the Foxp3-positive, CD4-positive, CD25-positive immunophenotype. Authors of retrospective studies in a limited number of patients undergoing EPP indicate that the presence of high levels of CD8-positive tumor-infiltrating lymphocytes may be associated with better prognosis.[86] Preliminary evidence also suggests that blockade of regulatory T cells could enhance survival when combined with pemetrexed in established mesothelioma.[87]

Release of immunosuppressive cytokines is yet another mechanism employed by tumors to inhibit immune responses.[88] Transforming growth factor-β2 (TGF-β2) has been detected in the pleural fluid and malignant mesothelioma cell supernatants.[85] Although TGF-β blockade appeared promising in murine models of malignant mesothelioma, objective responses were not found in a phase II trial that evaluated GC1008, an anti-TGF-β monoclonal antibody.[89]

Immune Checkpoint Inhibition

Cytotoxic T lymphocyte-associated antigen 4 (CTLA-4) is a member of the CD28/B7 immunoglobulin superfamily of immune regulatory molecules. It shares its two ligands (B7-1 and B7-2) with its costimulatory counterpart CD28. CTLA-4 and CD28 and their ligands B7-1 (CD80) and B7-2 (CD86) are critically important for the initial activation of naive T cells and regulation of the clonal composition of the responding repertoire following migration of activated dendritic cells to lymphoid organs. The expression of CTLA-4 is upregulated following T-cell activation, and the pathway has been shown to play an important immunomodulatory role in cancer.

Preclinical data suggest synergy between CTLA-4 blockade and cytotoxic chemotherapy, possibly as the result of a variety of mechanisms, including induction of a long-lasting immunologic memory and inhibition of tumor cell repopulation.[90] In a murine mesothelioma model, the combination of gemcitabine and anti-CTLA-4 exerted a far greater antitumor effect than either agent alone, whereas a similar effect was lacking when CTLA-4 blockade was combined with cisplatin.[90] In a different murine mesothelioma model, anti-CTLA-4 monoclonal antibody administered between cycles of cisplatin led to inhibition of tumor cell repopulation and was associated with increased numbers of tumor infiltrating CD4 and CD8 T cells and upregulation of cytokines associated with cytotoxic T-cell function.[91] It is conceivable that the synergy of chemotherapy with CTLA-4 blockade is dependent on the type of cytotoxic agent, the schedule, and immunogenicity, all of which require further evaluation in clinical trials.

Tremelimumab, a monoclonal antibody to CTLA-4, was evaluated in a single-arm, phase II study of 29 patients with malignant mesothelioma who had progressive disease after a first-line platinum-based regimen.[92] Although the study did not reach its primary end point of demonstrating a 17% response rate, 2 (7%) patients had durable partial responses, one lasting 6 months and another lasting 18 months. In a further second-line single-arm study of dose-intensified tremelimumab, 14% partial responses were noted, with a median overall survival of 11.3 months.[92a]

Unfortunately a randomized phase IIb clinical trial of tremelimumab versus placebo did not reach its primary end point, with no evidence of benefit in overall survival or progression-free survival for patients with mesothelioma treated in the second-line setting.[93]

Encouraging early results have been presented for the program death 1 (PD1) targeting monoclonal antibodies, nivolumab and pembrolizumab in early-phase clinical trials. The results of the NivoMes trial in which 34 patients received nivolumab 3 mg/kg every 2 weeks with response evaluation at 6 weeks were recently presented.[94] PDL1 expression by immunohistochemistry was greater than 1% in 29% mostly in epithelial patients, but responses were seen irrespective of PDL1 expression. By 12 weeks, 50% of the patients had disease control, which decreased to 33% at 24 weeks, and median progression-free survival was 110 days. Pembrolizumab, 10 mg/kgm IV every 2 weeks, was delivered to 25 patients after failure of standard therapy as part of the KEYNOTE-28 trial.[95] Response rate was 20% with a median duration of 12 months, and at 6 months or later a clinical benefit rate of 40% was achieved. Progression-free survival was 5.4 months with a median overall survival of 18 months. An interim analysis of another Phase II trial of 35 patients treated at University of Chicago with pembrolizumab 200 mg IV every 21 days (median number of cyles, 9) noted a response rate of 21%, disease control rate of 80%, a median progression-free survival of 6.2 months, and an overall survival of of 11.9 months.[96] Again, PDL1 expression was independent of responses. However, in the largest clinical trial of an immune checkpoint inhibitor reported to date, the response rate was lower than reported with pembrolizumab and nivolumab. Fifty-three patients with heavily pretreated pleural or peritoneal mesothelioma received the anti-PDL1 antibody avelumab at a dose of 10 mg/kg every 2 weeks until disease progression or unacceptable toxicity. The overall response rate was 9.4% and the responses[97] were seen in patients with or without tumor PDL1 expression. Larger studies are needed to confirm efficacy of single agent immune checkpoint inhibitors in malignant mesothelioma. The current generation of clinical trials using immune checkpoint blockade are also exploring combinations of immunotherapies, immunotherapy with chemotherapy, and other PD1 and PDL1 blocking antibodies.

Dendritic Cell–Based Immunotherapy

Dendritic cells are potent antigen-presenting cells that originate from bone marrow precursor cells and are present in peripheral tissues, where they capture, process, and transport antigens to naive T cells in draining lymph nodes. When dendritic cells are immature, antigens are presented to T cells in the lymph node without costimulation, leading to either the deletion of T cells or the generation of inducible regulatory T cells. Immunogenic tumor-associated antigens are secreted or shed by tumor cells or released when tumor cells die and can be taken up by dendritic cells. Upon encountering an antigen, dendritic cells mature and express peptide-major histocompatibility complex (MHC) at the cell surface, as well as appropriate costimulatory molecules (Fig. 53.4). Mature dendritic cells migrate in large numbers to draining lymph nodes where they prime CD4-positive helper T cells and CD8-positive cytotoxic T lymphocytes, activate B cells, and initiate an adaptive immune response. Vaccination with ex vivo generated mature dendritic cells pulsed with tumor-associated antigens has successfully elicited therapeutic immunity in other solid tumors.

Ebstein et al.[98] demonstrated that dendritic cells from healthy donors pulsed with antigen preparations from apoptotic allogeneic mesothelioma cell lines were capable of inducing a class I restricted cytotoxic T-cell response against mesothelioma tumor cells.[98] Hegmans et al.[85] provided in vivo proof of the concept of antitumor immune responses generated by dendritic cell vaccination in mesothelioma and showed that mice who received tumor lysate-pulsed dendritic cells before tumor implantation had prolonged survival. Recently, preliminary results of an off-the-shelf allogenic tumor cell lysate from human mesothelioma cell lines (Pheralys) were reported.[99] Leucopheresis was performed to obtain an enriched monocyte fraction from which immature DC were generated, which were loaded with the allogenic lysate.

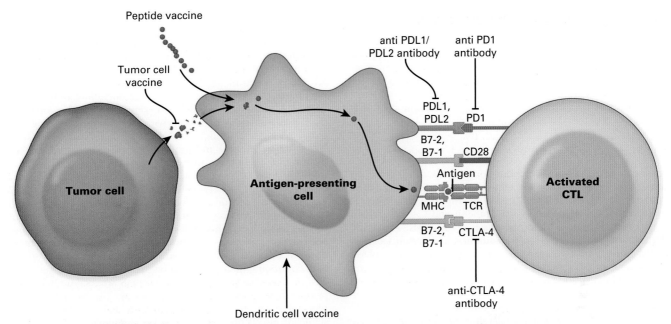

Fig. 53.4. Cellular processes involved in the immunomodulation of mesothelioma and potential targets for therapeutic intervention. The complex interaction between tumor cells and the immune system is presented in a simplified manner. Immunogenic tumor-associated antigens, which are shed by tumor cells or released when tumor cells die, are taken up by dendritic cells. Upon encountering an antigen, dendritic cells mature and express peptide-major histocompatibility complex (MHC) at the cell surface as well as appropriate costimulatory molecules, which lead to cytotoxic T-cell activation. Inhibitory processes from cytotoxic T lymphocyte-associated antigen 4 (CTLA-4), CD28, and program death 1 (PD1) regulate further activation of the immune system. Enhancing host immune system by antibody-mediated inhibition of T-cell coinhibitory receptors (e.g., CTLA-4, PD1) or their ligands (e.g., PDL1, PDL2) offers potential therapeutic opportunities in mesothelioma. Antigen-specific, tumor cell, and dendritic cell vaccines are other immunotherapeutic interventions that are being explored in mesothelioma. *TCR,* T cell receptor.

Immunotherapy with the allogenic tumor cell lysate was safe, and a randomized trial comparing DC therapy with Pheralys versus best supportive care as maintenance treatment after chemotherapy is planned.

Vaccination induced immunologic responses to keyhole limpet hemocyanin, and nine patients had increased CD3 and CD8 T cells expressing granzyme B after vaccination, suggesting lymphocyte activation by dendritic cell vaccination.[85,100] However, the measured humoral or cellular immunologic responses did not correlate with clinical responses. A phase I/II clinical trial ongoing at the time of publication is evaluating immune response to autologous RNA-modified dendritic cells engineered to express the WT1 protein for patients with malignant mesothelioma who have a good response to first-line chemotherapy (ClinicalTrials.gov identifier: NCT01291420). Based on indications from preliminary results (which included one patient with mesothelioma), this approach is feasible and capable of inducing immune responses.[101] The source of the tumor-associated antigens for dendritic cell loading, which requires care in identifying and characterizing antigenic epitopes, remains a critical issue that will determine the efficacy of dendritic cell–based vaccination in mesothelioma.[102]

Vaccination Using WT1

The transcription factor WT1 is overexpressed in malignant mesothelioma.[103] Although WT1 is a nuclear protein, it is processed and presented on the cell surface in the context of MHC molecules. In normal adult tissues, WT1 expression is restricted to low levels in nuclei of normal CD34 hematopoietic stem cells, myoepithelial progenitor cells, renal podocytes, and some cells in the testes and ovaries.[104]

Mesothelin-Targeted Therapies

Mesothelin is a tumor differentiation antigen that is present on normal mesothelial cells lining the pleura, peritoneum, and pericardium but is highly expressed in many solid tumors, including mesothelioma, ovarian and pancreatic cancer, and lung adenocarcinoma. In the case of mesothelioma, almost all epithelioid mesotheliomas express mesothelin, as does the epithelial component of biphasic tumors, but it is absent in sarcomatoid mesotheliomas. The mesothelin gene encodes a precursor protein of 71 kDa that is processed to a 31-kDa shed fragment megakaryocyte-potentiating factor and a 40-kDa fragment, mesothelin that is attached to the cell membrane by a glycosylphosphatidylinositol anchor. Both mesothelin and megakaryocyte-potentiating factor can be detected in serum and can be used as a biomarker of tumor detection or tumor response. The restricted expression of mesothelin on normal tissues makes it a good target for antibody- or cell-based immunotherapy.

Many mesothelin-targeted agents are being evaluated in clinical trials. These agents include an antimesothelin immunotoxin (SS1P), a chimeric antimesothelin antibody (MORAb-009, amatuximab), a mesothelin-targeted antibody drug conjugate (BAY94-9343), a mesothelin vaccine (CRS-207), and a chimeric antigen receptor (CAR)-based T-cell adoptive therapy.

SS1P

SS1P is a recombinant immunotoxin consisting of an antimesothelin variable fragment linked to a truncated Pseudomonas exotoxin A, PE38. After binding to mesothelin on the cell surface, SS1P is internalized and undergoes processing in the endocytic compartment of the cell and leads to inhibition of protein synthesis and, ultimately, cell death. In preclinical studies, SS1P showed significant antitumor activity against mesothelin-expressing tumor cells obtained from patients with mesothelioma.[105,106]

In 2013, a phase I trial was published on the use of SS1P for patients with recurrent MPM and showed promising and long-lasting responses.[107] Further studies will focus on the combination of this compound with chemotherapy.

Amatuximab (MORAb-009)

Amatuximab is a chimeric monoclonal antibody directed to mesothelin that kills mesothelin-expressing tumor cells by antibody-dependent cell-mediated cytotoxicity. In addition, it blocks the interaction between mesothelin and CA-125, which may potentially inhibit tumor metastasis.[108] In a phase I trial, the dose-limiting toxicities were transaminitis and serum sickness and the maximum tolerated dose was 200 mg/m^2.[109] In a phase II nonrandomized trial of chemonaive pleural mesothelioma patients, administration of amatuximab with pemetrexed and cisplatin resulted in overall survival of 14.8 months, which is better than historical controls with pemetrexed and cisplatin alone.[110] Analysis of the pharmacokinetic data showed that serum amatuximab trough concentrations above the population median of 38.2 µg/mL were associated with significant improvement of both progression-free as well as overall survival.[111] Pharmacodynamic modeling shows that administering amatuximab 5 mg/kg weekly will allow 80% of patients to achieve amatuximab trough concentrations above 38.2 µg/mL. Based on these data, a randomized phase II clinical trial of amatuximab plus pemetrexed and cisplatin versus pemetrexed and cisplatin for patients with newly diagnosed unresectable mesothelioma with a primary end point of overall survival has been initiated and is enrolling patients (Clinical trials.gov NCT02357147).

Antimesothelin Antibody Drug Conjugate (Anetumab Ravtansine)

Anetumab ravtansine (BAY94-9343) is a mesothelin-targeted antibody drug conjugate consisting of a humanized immunoglobulin G1 monoclonal antibody to mesothelin conjugated to DM4, a tubulin-binding drug. In preclinical studies, it has been extremely potent against mesothelin-positive cell lines and shows significant antitumor activity against mesothelin-expressing tumor xenografts.[112] In a phase I study, anetumab ravtansine was administered intravenously every 21 days (q3w) in 77 patients: 45 patients in 10 dose escalation cohorts from 0.15 to 7.5 mg/kg (21 mesothelioma, 9 pancreatic, 5 breast, 4 ovarian, 6 other), and 32 patients in two expansion cohorts (12 mesothelioma and 20 ovarian). A total of 38 patients were treated at maximum tolerated dose (MTD) in escalation and expansion cohorts (16 mesothelioma, 21 ovarian, 1 breast). The MTD of anetumab ravtansine given q 3 weeks was 6.5 mg/kg. The dose-limiting toxicity at the highest dose of 7.5 mg/kg was keratitis and neuropathy. The most common side effects included peripheral sensory neuropathy and corneal microdeposits. Out of 16 mesothelioma patients treated at the MTD, 5 (31%) patients had objective tumor responses and 7 (44%) patients had stable disease. However, in patients with pleural mesothelioma who received anetumab ravtansine as second-line therapy, 5 of 10 (50%) had objective partial responses and 4 (40%) had stable disease.[56] More important, the responses were durable with 3 patients having ongoing response at greater than 2 years.[113] Based on these results a randomized phase II registration clinical trial of anetumab ravtansine versus vinorelbine as second-line therapy for pleural mesothelioma, with a primary end point of progression-free survival, has been initiated (Clinical trials.gov NCT02610140).

Mesothelin Vaccine (CRS-207)

Mesothelin is an immunogenic protein and can elicit an antitumor immune response. CRS-207 is the only mesothelin vaccine in clinical trials at the time of publication. It consists of a live attenuated strain of the bacterium *Listeria monocytogenes* encoding human mesothelin. The safety and induction of antimesothelin immune response by CRS-207 were established in a phase I dose-escalation study of patients with mesothelin-expressing cancers.[114] A phase Ib study is evaluating the combination of CRS-207 with pemetrexed and cisplatin for patients with untreated pleural mesothelioma who are not candidates for surgical resection. On this study patients received two doses of intravenous CRS-207 given 2 weeks apart (prime vaccination), followed 2 weeks after the second dose of CRS-207 by pemetrexed and cisplatin administered on the standard dose and schedule for four to six cycles. If patients had stable disease or decreased tumor burden at completion of chemotherapy, they received two more doses of CRS-207 3 weeks apart as boost vaccination. Patients with continuing tumor response or stable disease could get CRS-207 as maintenance vaccination every 8 weeks. A total of 38 patients have been enrolled on this study. The most frequently reported adverse events related to CRS-207 consisted of transient side effects of fever, chills or rigor, and nausea. There were no additive or cumulative toxicities observed from combination treatment of CRS-207 and chemotherapy. Out of the 36 patients evaluable for tumor response, 1 (3%) had complete response, 20 (56%) had partial response, 13 (36%) had stable disease, and 2 (6%) had progressive disease as their best overall response and the median progression-free survival and overall survival were 7.6 (95% confidence interval [CI], 7.1–10.1) and 16.4 (95% CI, 11.0–20.6) months, respectively.[115]

Mesothelin-Directed CAR Therapy

The limited expression of mesothelin on normal tissues makes it a good candidate for CAR-directed T-cell therapies. Clinical trials of mesothelin-directed CAR T-cell agents are currently ongoing.[116] Results of initial clinical trials show that this approach is safe and some activity seen in patients with solid tumors.[117] More recently, preclinical studies have shown increased efficacy when antimesothelin CAR T cells are administered into the pleural cavity, and this approach is now being studied in patients.[118]

Oncolytic Viral Therapies

Oncolytic viruses are replicating microorganisms that have been selected or engineered to grow inside tumor cells.[119] Oncolytic viruses take advantage of tumor-specific mutations, signaling pathways, or antigens, allowing their selective replication in tumor cells leading to tumor cell lysis but sparing normal cells. For example, activation of viral transcription under a regulatory region of the gene that is preferentially transcribed in target tumors is commonly used to achieve tumor specificity. In addition to direct cytotoxicity, therapeutic virus-mediated destruction or damage of tumors can also lead to an antitumor immune response. Phagocytosis of apoptotic measles virus–infected mesothelioma cells induced spontaneous dendritic cell maturation, activation, and a significant amplification of mesothelin-specific CD8 T cells.[120]

A number of oncolytic viruses, which replicate preferentially within tumors, such as adenovirus, measles, retroviruses, Newcastle disease, herpes simplex viruses, and vesicular stomatitis viruses, have been examined for their cytotoxicity and efficacy in mesothelioma.[121]

One of the challenges with oncolytic viral therapy in mesothelioma is tumor penetration of the oncolytic viruses. Extracellular matrix and tumor-associated fibrous tissue hampers the spread of viruses released from infected tumors. Coexpression of enzymes that destroy extracellular matrix, such as heparanase, has been used successfully in preclinical studies to overcome the resistance from fibrous tissue, which prevents the penetration of oncolytic viruses.[122]

Gene Therapy

With the limited pattern of spread of mesothelioma, which is mostly restricted to the pleural cavity, and the ease of intrapleural delivery, local–regional administration of tumor selective adenoviruses and carrier cells, such as PA1STK cells, has been explored for therapeutic purposes.[123,124] In a phase I study of 21 patients with treatment-naive pleural mesothelioma, intrapleural delivery of Ad.HSVtk, a replication incompetent adenovirus with a transgene encoding herpes simplex virus thymidine kinase gene (HSVtk), was safe and well tolerated.[123] Tumor specificity in this study was achieved by the use of the HSVtk gene, whose protein product is an enzyme that converts ganciclovir into a highly cytotoxic phosphorylated form. Ad.HSVtk was administered into the pleural cavity following which patients received 2 weeks of ganciclovir intravenously. Anti-Ad humoral and cellular immune responses were generated, and posttreatment biopsies indicated presence of intratumoral transgene for patients who received a higher dose of Ad.HSVtk.

Clinical experience with Ad.HSVtk and preclinical data indicating that HSVtk generates a strong Th1-type antitumor immune response suggest that cell kill was primarily due to antitumor immune responses induced by Ad.HSV.tk/ganciclovir, rather than direct cytotoxicity.[125] Subsequently, several studies were conducted to enhance antitumor immune responses using adenoviral vector expressing human interferon (IFN)-β gene, which augments expression of the MHC class I antigens and induces apoptosis.[126] Although these trials demonstrated the safety of Ad.IFN-β and showed induction of antitumor humoral and cellular immune responses, the rapid rise in serum anti-Ad neutralizing antibody titers minimized target-cell transduction and IFN-β gene expression. Although these clinical studies have consistently demonstrated generation of antitumor immune responses, radiographic and clinical antitumor responses have been limited, possibly because of large tumor volumes and the presence of immunoinhibitory networks. At the time of publication, studies were underway to evaluate the combination of Ad.IFN-β gene transfer with chemotherapy and surgery based on preclinical data that have shown markedly enhanced antitumor efficacy of Ad.IFN-β when combined with chemotherapy or with debulking surgery.[127,128]

CONCLUSION

MPM continues to be a controversial and difficult to eradicate tumor. Consensus on the use of surgery and even the type of surgery has not been reached, yet there is a movement toward lung-sparing procedures in these patients. Cisplatin and pemetrexed together remains the standard of care with regard to cytotoxic therapy, but novel therapies are under investigation. There is abundant in vitro evidence for human immune reactivity against mesothelioma. However, such responses are often ineffectual in situ, as the tumor exerts locally immunosuppressive effects. Strategies being explored in mesothelioma to overcome this inhibition include local manipulation of immunoregulatory molecules in the tumor microenvironment (e.g., immune checkpoint inhibitors) and antigen-specific activation of the immune system (e.g., vaccines). A number

of investigational strategies focus on mesothelin, a tumor differentiation antigen that is present on normal mesothelial cells, but is highly expressed on mesothelioma.

KEY REFERENCES

2. Wagner JC, Sleggs CA, Marchand P. Diffuse pleural mesothelioma and asbestos exposure in the North Western Cape Province. *Br J Ind Med.* 1960;17:260–271.
11. Carbone M, Yang H, Pass HI, et al. BAP1 and cancer. *Nat Rev Cancer.* 2013;13(3):153–159.
12. Testa JR, Cheung M, Pei J, et al. Germline BAP1 mutations predispose to malignant mesothelioma. *Nat Genet.* 2011;43(10):1022–1025.
14. Rusch VW. A proposed new international TNM staging system for malignant pleural mesothelioma. From the International Mesothelioma Interest Group. *Chest.* 1995;108(4):1122–1128.
23. Robinson BW, Creaney J, Lake R, et al. Mesothelin-family proteins and diagnosis of mesothelioma. *Lancet.* 2003;362(9396):1612–1616.
28. Pass HI, Levin SM, Harbut MR, et al. Fibulin-3 as a blood and effusion biomarker for pleural mesothelioma. *N Engl J Med.* 2012;367(15):1417–1427.
40. Nowak AK, Francis RJ, Phillips MJ, et al. A novel prognostic model for malignant mesothelioma incorporating quantitative FDG-PET imaging with clinical parameters. *Clin Cancer Res.* 2010;16(8):2409–2417.
42. Vogelzang NJ, Rusthoven JJ, Symanowski J, et al. Phase III study of pemetrexed in combination with cisplatin versus cisplatin alone in patients with malignant pleural mesothelioma. *J Clin Oncol.* 2003;21(14):2636–2644.
44. Zalcman G, Mazieres J, Margery J, et al. Bevacizumab for newly diagnosed pleural mesothelioma in the Mesothelioma Avastin Cisplatin Pemetrexed Study (MAPS): a randomised, controlled, open-label, phase 3 trial. *Lancet.* 2016;387:1405–1414.
46. Muers MF, Stephens RJ, Fisher P, et al. Active symptom control with or without chemotherapy in the treatment of patients with malignant pleural mesothelioma (MS01): a multicentre randomised trial. *Lancet.* 2008;371(9625):1685–1694.
58. Sugarbaker DJ. Macroscopic complete resection: the goal of primary surgery in multimodality therapy for pleural mesothelioma. *J Thorac Oncol.* 2006;1(2):175–176.
62. Krug LM, Pass HI, Rusch VW, et al. Multicenter phase II trial of neo-adjuvant pemetrexed plus cisplatin followed by extrapleural pneumonectomy and radiation for malignant pleural mesothelioma. *J Clin Oncol.* 2009;27(18):3007–3013.
64. Pass HI, Kranda K, Temeck BK, Feuerstein I, Steinberg SM. Surgically debulked malignant pleural mesothelioma: results and prognostic factors. *Ann Surg Oncol.* 1997;4(3):215–222.
67. Sugarbaker DJ, Flores RM, Jaklitsch MT, et al. Resection margins, extrapleural nodal status, and cell type determine postoperative long-term survival in trimodality therapy of malignant pleural mesothelioma: results in 183 patients. *J Thorac Cardiovasc Surg.* 1999;117(1):54–63.
82. Flores RM, Pass HI, Seshan VE, et al. Extrapleural pneumonectomy versus pleurectomy/decortication in the surgical management of malignant pleural mesothelioma: results in 663 patients. *J Thorac Cardiovasc Surg.* 2008;135(3):620–626.
107. Hassan R, Miller AC, Sharon E, et al. Major cancer regressions in mesothelioma after treatment with an anti-mesothelin immunotoxin and immune suppression. *Sci Transl Med.* 2013;5(208):208ra147.
131. Stebbing J, Powles T, McPherson K, et al. The efficacy and safety of weekly vinorelbine in relapsed malignant pleural mesothelioma. *Lung Cancer.* 2009;63(1):94–97.

See Expertconsult.com for full list of references.

Mediastinal Tumors

Christopher Hazzard, Andrew Kaufman, and Raja Flores

SUMMARY OF KEY POINTS

- Knowledge of the anatomy of the mediastinum is critical to establishing the differential diagnosis and choosing the best diagnostic and therapeutic interventions.
- A wide variety of possible etiologies must be considered including solid and lymphatic malignancies, benign cysts, and benign neoplasms.
- Computed tomography (CT) and magnetic resonance imaging (MRI) are essential tools for the diagnosis and planning of surgical approach and choice of surgical technique.
- Thymoma and lymphoma are common anterior mediastinal masses in adults. Lymphoma and benign cysts are the most common middle mediastinal lesions. Neurogenic tumors are seen only in the posterior mediastinum.
- Vital visceral, vascular, and neurologic structures exist in the mediastinum, and precise surgical technique is paramount to avoid complications.
- Surgical resection of benign cysts should be reserved for bronchogenic or esophageal cysts; pericardial cysts do not warrant invasive tissue sampling or removal.
- Bronchogenic and esophageal cysts can acquire significant adhesions to surrounding structures, making minimally invasive resection challenging in some patients.
- Electrocautery should be used with caution near the spinal foramina to avoid central nervous system injury.
- Known complications from surgery include phrenic nerve injury and paralysis, chyle leak, bronchial or esophageal perforation, and bleeding.

The mediastinum is the region of the thorax between the pleural cavities, commonly described in three compartments: anterior, visceral or middle, and posterior. The anterior mediastinum contains the thymus, lymph nodes, connective tissue, and fat. The visceral mediastinum contains the heart and its vasculature within the pericardium, trachea and proximal bronchi, esophagus, thoracic duct, lymph nodes, and the vagus, phrenic, and recurrent laryngeal nerves. The posterior mediastinum contains the sympathetic chain and proximal intercostal arteries, veins, and nerves. The differential diagnosis for a mediastinal mass is influenced by its anatomic position (Table 54.1).[1]

Mediastinal masses are often asymptomatic and present as an incidental finding during workup, surveillance, or screening for an unrelated condition. Malignant disease is more likely to be symptomatic.[2] Symptoms resulting from local compression and invasion include superior vena cava syndrome, dyspnea, dysphagia, hoarseness, cardiac tamponade, and Horner syndrome. Systemic symptoms may occur because of endocrine tumor activity or fever, chills, and weight loss associated with malignancy (Table 54.2).[1] Certain syndromes have commonly associated tumors and symptoms, including myasthenia gravis and anterior mass with

thymoma or café-au-lait spots and posterior mass with von Recklinghausen neurofibromatosis.

The most common anterior mediastinal masses in adults are thymoma, germ cell tumor (GCT), lymphoma, and displaced thyroid. In the visceral compartment, the most common mass is lymphadenopathy associated with metastatic disease. Other visceral masses are usually congenital cysts. Most posterior masses are neurogenic tumors.[3]

CT can provide information about the size, density, and anatomic relationship of mediastinal masses. Intravenous contrast medium used with CT will usually assist in the definition of mediastinal masses. MRI of the mediastinum is hindered by cardiac and respiratory motion artifacts. MRI of mediastinal masses is normally reserved for assessing intraspinal involvement of paravertebral tumors.[4]

GERM CELL TUMORS

Extragonadal GCTs result from errors in cell migration during embryogenesis (Fig. 54.1). These tumors are most commonly found in the mediastinum, where they account for 15% of anterior mediastinal masses in adults.[5] Most mediastinal GCTs present in the second through fourth decade of life. Approximately 85% of mediastinal GCTs are benign and occur at similar rates in men and women;[6] however, 90% of malignant GCTs occur in men. With malignant GCTs, scrotal ultrasound is necessary to detect possible primary gonadal tumors. Histologically, there are three types of GCTs: benign teratoma, seminoma, and nonseminomatous GCT (NSGCT).[3]

Benign Teratoma

Benign teratomas are composed of multiple germ cell layers, and are also referred to as mature teratomas. These teratomas may contain any type of tissue, including teeth, hair, bone, cartilage, and occasionally higher order structures. Although many patients will be asymptomatic, benign teratomas have the capacity to compress, erode, rupture, and fistulize into surrounding structures.[7] Rarely, these benign tumors undergo malignant transformation.[8] Elevated serum levels of beta-human chorionic gonadotropin (beta-hCG) or alpha-fetoprotein (AFP) may indicate malignant GCT. Total surgical excision of benign teratoma is recommended. The treatment approach for benign teratomas can vary and has included median sternotomy and lateral thoracotomy. The preferred treatment, particularly with GCTs, is the hemiclamshell approach, which is a unilateral extension into the hemithorax. For large masses with bilateral extension, a clamshell incision (a combined upper median sternotomy and anterior thoracotomy) provides excellent exposure. Benign teratomas are often adjacently adherent, which can make dissection challenging, and total resection is not always possible. However, postsurgical prognosis is excellent, even with incomplete excision.[7] There is no indication for chemotherapy or radiotherapy.

Seminoma

Seminomas occur almost exclusively in men and usually present in the third to fourth decade of life. Seminomas often grow quite large before discovery, and metastatic disease is present in 60%

to 70% of cases.[9] The serum AFP level is normal in pure semi-noma and the beta-hCG level can be elevated in some patients. An elevated AFP level implies a nonseminomatous component, but workup and treatment should be the same as for NSGCTs; however, a CT-guided needle biopsy should be considered over surgical biopsy.[10,11] Because of the prevalence of systemic disease, treatment with radiotherapy alone is associated with significantly lower progression-free survival compared with that associated with bleomycin, etoposide, and cisplatin chemotherapy.[12] Even

TABLE 54.1 Differential Diagnosis of Mediastinal Mass by Compartment[1]

Anterior	Middle	Posterior
Thymoma	Lymphoma	Neurogenic tumor
Teratoma, seminoma	Pericardial cyst	Bronchogenic cyst
Lymphoma	Bronchogenic cyst	Enteric cyst
Carcinoma	Metastatic cyst	Xanthogranuloma
Parathyroid adenoma	Systemic granuloma	Diaphragmatic hernia
Intrathoracic goiter		Meningocele
Lipoma		Paravertebral abscess
Lymphangioma		
Aortic aneurysm		

TABLE 54.2 Systemic Symptoms of Mediastinal Tumors[1]

Syndrome	Tumor
Myasthenia gravis, red blood cell aplasia, hypogammaglobulinemia, Good syndrome, Whipple disease, megaesophagus, myocarditis	Thymoma
Multiple endocrine adenomatosis, Cushing syndrome	Carcinoid, thymoma
Hypertension	Pheochromocytoma, ganglioneuroma, chemodectoma
Diarrhea	Ganglioneuroma
Hypercalcemia	Parathyroid adenoma, lymphoma
Thyrotoxicosis	Intrathoracic goiter
Hypoglycemia	Mesothelioma, teratoma, fibrosarcoma, neurosarcoma
Osteoarthropathy	Neurofibroma, neurilemoma, mesothelioma
Vertebral abnormalities	Enteric cysts
Fever of unknown origin	Lymphoma
Alcohol-induced pain	Hodgkin lymphoma
Opsomyoclonus	Neuroblastoma

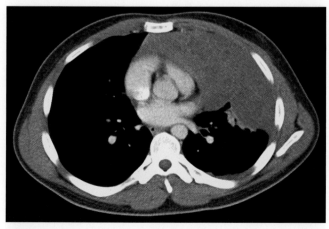

Fig. 54.1. Anterior mediastinal germ cell tumor with extension into the left hemithorax.

in the case of a residual mass, there is little, if any, role for surgical interventions.[9]

Nonseminomatous Germ Cell Tumor

NSGCTs can include embryonal carcinoma, yolk sac carcinoma, choriocarcinoma, or a mixed histology. Primary mediastinal NSGCT appears to be biologically distinct from testicular NSGCT and is associated with a poor prognosis.[13] Primary mediastinal NSGCTs grow rapidly and metastatic disease is found in 80% of patients.[14] Overall survival after multimodality treatment is 40% to 50%. Hematologic malignancies present with NSGCT in 6% of cases, most commonly in patients with acute megakaryoblastic leukemia, and myelodysplastic syndrome is the most common.[15] The serum AFP level is elevated in 80% of patients and the beta-hCG level is elevated in 30% to 35%. Substantial elevation of tumor marker levels can preclude biopsy.[12] However, if biopsy is performed, fine-needle aspiration can be ambiguous and is discouraged in favor of core-needle biopsy or anterior mediastinotomy.[16]

The standard treatment for NSGCT is four courses of bleomycin, etoposide, and cisplatin; ifosfamide has been recommended over bleomycin to avoid pulmonary complications prior to surgical resection.[12] Residual mass after chemotherapy should be surgically resected, regardless of the serum marker levels; the prognosis is poor for patients with unresectable residual masses. When active germ cell cancer is present in the surgical specimen, two additional courses of chemotherapy should be given. Patients who have no residual tumor should be followed closely with history and physical examination, determination of serum markers, and CT. Patients who have disease recurrence have a particularly poor prognosis, although a small number of patients may benefit from salvage chemotherapy.[13] A 20% survival rate following surgical resection for relapsed primary mediastinal NSGCT has also been reported.[17]

LYMPHOMA

Lymphomas represent a variety of hematologic neoplasms. Proper management of lymphoma depends on subtyping and staging. Approximately 15% of mediastinal masses are lymphomas, typically in the anterior or middle compartment (Fig. 54.2). About 90% of mediastinal lymphomas represent disseminated disease, and one-third are Hodgkin lymphomas. Most patients present with some combination of systemic B symptoms, and symptoms associated with local compression.[18] Positron emission tomography is frequently used to stage and monitor the progress of lymphoma.[19]

Hodgkin Lymphoma

Mediastinal involvement occurs in as many as two-thirds of Hodgkin lymphoma. Diagnosis typically requires tissue quantities only obtainable by surgical biopsy. Typically, video-assisted thoracoscopy (VATS) or anterior mediastinotomy will yield definitive samples; however, mediastinoscopy is not always sufficient.

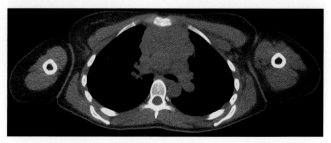

Fig. 54.2. Lymphoma in the anterior mediastinum.

CD15- and CD30-positive Reed-Sternberg cells, which are diagnostic for Hodgkin lymphoma, can be difficult to identify in a small biopsy.[18] Disease is staged according to the Ann Arbor Staging System;[20] early-stage Hodgkin lymphoma is treated with chemoradiation therapy and late-stage disease is treated with chemotherapy only.[21]

Non-Hodgkin Lymphoma

Large B-cell lymphoma and lymphoblastic lymphoma are the most common forms of non-Hodgkin lymphoma of the mediastinum. As in Hodgkin lymphoma, a sizable biopsy sample is often required for diagnosis. However, lymphoblastic lymphoma is usually first identified in bone marrow and peripheral blood; thus a mediastinal biopsy is not necessary. Lymphoblastic lymphoma is particularly aggressive, and treatment with chemotherapy and possible bone marrow transplant should not be delayed by staging procedures. Large B-cell lymphoma is treated with chemotherapy, and some centers also use radiotherapy for the treatment of B-cell lymphoma and lymphoblastic lymphoma.[18]

NEUROGENIC TUMORS

Approximately three-quarters of posterior mediastinal tumors are neurogenic (Fig. 54.3). These neurogenic tumors arise from the sympathetic chain or intercostal rami, and they most commonly take the forms of nerve sheath tumors (schwannoma and neurofibroma). Nearly all neurogenic tumors are benign, and approximately 30% of neurofibromas are associated with von Recklinghausen disease. Neurogenic tumors may erode osseous structures; this contributes to the development of an intraspinal (dumbbell) extension. MRI is essential if intraspinal involvement is suspected, as failure to recognize involvement can result in devastating spinal cord injury during attempted excision; resection of intraspinal tumor requires neurosurgical expertise. Simple nerve sheath tumors, whether benign or malignant, should be surgically resected, and a VATS approach is usually sufficient. Relative contraindications for complete resection include a mass greater than 6 cm and spinal artery involvement. Chemotherapy and radiotherapy may be used when complete resection is not possible.[4]

BENIGN CYSTIC MASSES

Bronchogenic Cysts

Bronchogenic cysts arise from errors in embryonic budding of the tracheobronchial tree (Fig. 54.4); they are the most

common mediastinal cysts and are frequently found behind the carina. The majority of bronchogenic cysts are discovered before the onset of symptoms, but most do eventually cause symptoms. Bronchogenic cysts can cause local compression and erosion and may become infected.[22] Resection of asymptomatic cysts can be controversial, but because of their potential to cause later complications and the favorable outcomes from early surgical intervention, VATS or mediastinoscopic resection is recommended.[22–24]

Esophageal Cysts

Esophageal cysts, also called esophageal duplications, arise in a similar manner as bronchogenic cysts. Like bronchogenic cysts, esophageal cysts can also cause local compression and may become infected. There is also risk of hemorrhage and rupture into the esophagus or airways. VATS excision is recommended, with care taken to minimize disruption of the esophageal muscularis.[22]

Pericardial Cysts

Pericardial cysts are mesothelium-derived and in close proximity to the pericardium. Pericardial cysts are typically benign and require no intervention. However, a growing pericardial cyst can cause hemodynamic compromise, and excision should be performed for symptomatic patients.[25] VATS is recommended, if feasible.

SUBSTERNAL GOITER

Goiters are enlargements of the thyroid and are deemed substernal when more than half of the gland extends inferior to the sternal notch (Fig. 54.5). Substernal goiters are the most common superior mediastinal tumors, usually found in the anterior mediastinum; however, 10% to 15% of substernal goiters are found in the posterior compartment.[26] The most common symptoms of substernal goiters are caused by local compression and include dyspnea, cough, and hoarseness. Approximately 25% of patients will be asymptomatic. A palpable thyroid is present in 88% of patients, and 16% of patients have hyperthyroidism.[27] Serum levels of thyroid-stimulating hormone, free T4, and total T3 can be useful in the diagnosis and detection of subclinical hyperthyroidism.[28] Spirometry can assess the extent of airway compression and may identify abnormalities in asymptomatic patients. CT is used to determine the extent and position of the goiter. Although malignancy is possible, needle biopsy is not indicated, as the malignant focus may be missed and its presence does not alter the operative indication.[29] Presence of substernal goiter is itself an indication for resection. Further enlargement worsens compression-associated symptoms and can complicate surgical

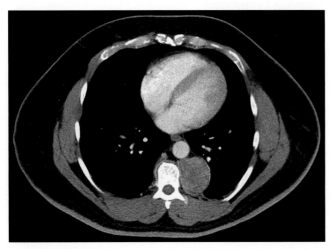

Fig. 54.3. Paravertebral mass typical of neurogenic tumors.

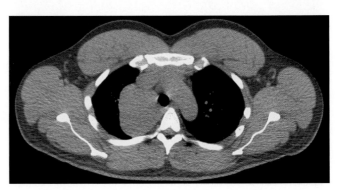

Fig. 54.4. Bronchogenic cyst in the visceral mediastinum.

treatment that would otherwise be associated with low post-operative morbidity.[27] Total thyroidectomy is recommended and can usually be accomplished by a collar incision. When the extent of thoracic involvement does not permit resection by a collar incision, possible approaches include manubrial split, sternotomy, and thoracotomy. Postoperative complications are infrequent and include hypoparathyroidism and recurrent laryngeal nerves paralysis.[29]

PARATHYROID ADENOMA

Primary hyperparathyroidism is most commonly a result of adenoma of the parathyroid glands (Fig. 54.6). Approximately 22% of parathyroid adenomas are found in a mediastinal parathyroid gland.[30] Resection of the tumor is curative in nearly every case.[31] The preferred surgical approach is minimally invasive and relies on precise preoperative localization. The mainstay of parathyroid adenoma localization is technetium-99m sestamibi scintigraphy; when combined with three-dimensional single-photon emission CT, the sensitivity and specificity are high.[32] Ultrasound is often used to complement other modalities. Localization has no diagnostic role and is used only for preoperative planning in biochemically proven cases. Most mediastinal parathyroid tumors can be resected transcervically, and videomediastinoscopy may be useful in difficult cases. VATS has also been used for the resection of parathyroid adenomas, but precise localization is particularly important with this approach. Intraoperative monitoring of the parathyroid hormone level is used to confirm systemic cure.[33]

LEIOMYOMA

Leiomyoma in the mediastinum usually arises from the esophagus or large vessels (Fig. 54.7). Primary mediastinal leiomyoma not associated with adjacent organs is exceedingly rare.[34] These lesions are firm and well circumscribed, and symptoms are typically due to local compression. Complete excision is the definitive treatment;[35] esophageal leiomyoma is treated using VATS enucleation.[36]

SURGICAL APPROACH

The appropriate surgical approach depends on the nature and position of the lesion within the mediastinum. A minimally invasive approach is often possible for uninvolved benign masses. More aggressive exposure is used for large and/or malignant tumors, for which complete resection is crucial and dissection is potentially challenging.

Access to small anterior midline tumors is commonly approached by a median sternotomy, with the patient in the supine position with the arms tucked to the side. In this position, the mediastinal vasculature, left and right hemithoraces, and lung hila are well exposed; however, exposure of the left lower lobe and posterior aspect of the lungs is poor. In some cases, a partial sternum-sparing approach will allow for sufficient exposure, such as a manubrial split for superior mediastinal mass. A collar incision may also provide sufficient access to the superior mediastinum if the mass can be accessed through the neck.

For large tumors extending into either of the hemithoraces, a hemiclamshell incision provides good exposure.[37] The patient should be placed in the supine position, with a longitudinal roll

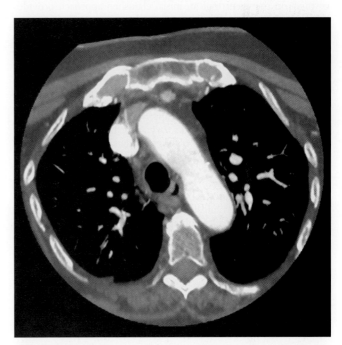
Fig. 54.6. Parathyroid adenoma in the superior anterior mediastinum.

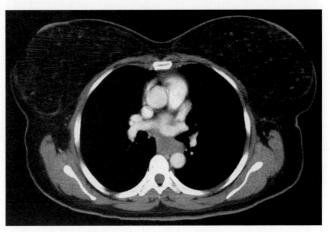
Fig. 54.7. Leiomyoma of the thoracic esophagus.

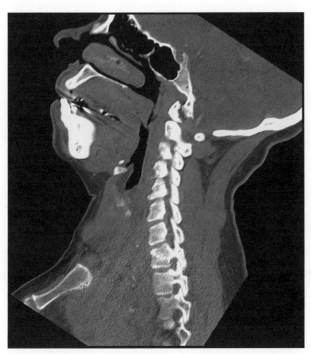
Fig. 54.5. Substernal goiter in the superior mediastinum.

elevating the thoracotomy side by 30 degrees and the arms tucked to the side. The ipsilateral lung may be collapsed to allow for anatomic resection of involved lobes, if necessary, and access to the posterolateral aspect of the tumor. If the tumor has substantial cervical extension, the upper sternotomy may be extended superiorly along the anterior border of the sternocleidomastoid.[38] This approach exposes the carotid and jugular vessels if vascular dissection is necessary. Rarely, resection of the subclavian vessels will be needed for a GCT. In these cases, a so-called trap door incision, created by extending the upper sternotomy along the superior margin of the clavicle, will allow for appropriate exposure. Excision of the medial third of the clavicle may also assist in exposure of the tumor.

A large tumor that extends into both right and left hemithoraces may be resected through a bilateral clamshell incision, with the patient in the supine position and the arms abducted or flexed over the forehead. A curvilinear incision should be made along the inframammary crease from the right to left anterior axillary lines for access to the fourth intercostal space; the mammary vessels are then ligated, and the sternum is divided transversally. Retraction is provided by two Finochietto retractors. An upper sternal split may be made in the event that an initial clamshell approach provides inadequate exposure of the superior mediastinum.

CONCLUSION

The mediastinum is dense with multiple organ systems, and the tumors thereof are equally varied. Appropriate management and surgical approach require careful assessment of each case. Indications for chemotherapy, radiotherapy, and surgical treatment of mediastinal GCTs vary according to the histologic subtypes. Surgical exposure of large mediastinal GCTs is often best approached by hemiclamshell or bilateral clamshell incision. Lymphoma of the mediastinum is usually a disseminated disease. Surgical biopsy provides sufficient tissue for diagnosis, but treatment is nonsurgical and based on the subtype and stage. Posterior masses are typically neurogenic tumors. MRI is essential for assessment of intraspinal involvement. Small uninvolved neurogenic tumors should be treated by VATS. Congenital cystic masses of the bronchial tree and esophagus should be resected by minimally invasive approach. Resection of pericardial cysts is reserved for symptomatic patients. A substernal goiter is an indication for total thyroidectomy. A collar incision is often sufficient, but more involved goiters can require a sternal split. Parathyroid adenomas causing primary hyperparathyroidism should be resected with a minimally invasive approach. Precise preoperative localization of parathyroid adenoma is crucial to successful resection. Leiomyomas are typically of the esophagus or large vessels and should be excised.

KEY REFERENCES

2. Davis Jr RD, Oldham Jr HN, Sabiston Jr DC. Primary cysts and neoplasms of the mediastinum: recent changes in clinical presentation, methods of diagnosis, management, and results. *Ann Thorac Surg*. 1987;44(3):229–237.
6. Mullen B, Richardson JD. Primary anterior mediastinal tumors in children and adults. *Ann Thorac Surg*. 1986;42(3):338 345.
12. Albany C, Einhorn LH. Extragonadal germ cell tumors: clinical presentation and management. *Curr Opin Oncol*. 2013;25(3):261–265.
14. McNamee CJ. Malignant primary anterior mediastinal tumors. In: Sugarbaker DJ, Bueno R, Krasna MJ, Mentzer SJ, Zellos L, eds. *Adult Chest Surgery*. New York, NY: McGraw-Hill; 2009:1154–1158.
16. Alam N, Flores R. Management of mediastinal tumors not of thymic origin. In: Pass HP, Carbone DP, Johnson DH, et al., eds. *Principles and Practice of Lung Cancer*. 4th ed. Philadelphia, PA: Wolters Kluwer Health/Lippincott Williams & Wilkins; 2010.
18. Smith S, van Besien K. Diagnosis and treatment of mediastinal lymphomas. In: Shields TW, Lociciero J, Reed CE, Feins RH, eds. *General Thoracic Surgery*. 7th ed. Vol. 2. Philadelphia, PA: Wolters Kluwer Health/Lippincott Williams & Wilkins; 2009:2379–2387.
22. Ferraro P, Martin J, Duranceau ACH. Foregut cysts of the mediastinum. In: Shields TW, Lociciero J, Reed CE, Feins RH, eds. *General Thoracic Surgery*. 7th ed. Vol. 2. Philadelphia, PA: Wolters Kluwer Health/ Lippincott Williams & Wilkins; 2009:2519–2538.
36. Vallböhmer D, Hölscher AH, Brabender J, Bollschweiler E, Gutschow C. Thoracoscopic enucleation of esophageal leiomyomas: a feasible and safe procedure. *Endoscopy*. 2007;39(12):1097–1099.
37. Bains MS, Ginsberg RJ, Jones 2nd WG, et al. The clamshell incision: an improved approach to bilateral pulmonary and mediastinal tumor. *Ann Thorac Surg*. 1994;58(1):30–32. discussion 33.

See Expertconsult.com for full list of references.

55 Neuroendocrine Tumors of the Lung Other Than Small Cell Lung Cancer

Krista Noonan, Jules Derks, Janessa Laskin, and Anne-Marie C. Dingemans

SUMMARY OF KEY POINTS

- Neuroendocrine cancers of the lung share some fundamental pathology features but span a broad range of clinical behaviors.
- The clinical behavior varies with the degree of differentiation: typical carcinoids are more indolent and localized, atypical carcinoids are intermediate and tend to spread systemically, and large cell neuroendocrine cancers are high grade and aggressive similar to small cell cancers.
- Unlike midgut carcinoids, bronchial carcinoids seldom present with carcinoid syndrome.
- Surgical resection is the preferred treatment for early-stage disease.
- Standard chemotherapy treatments for metastatic disease are platinum based but little phase III evidence exists to support a specific regimen.
- Clinical trials of molecularly targeted therapy are urgently needed.

Pulmonary neuroendocrine tumors represent a spectrum of tumors that develop from neuroendocrine cells of the bronchopulmonary (BP) epithelium. Although neuroendocrine tumors have similar morphologic and immunohistochemical (IHC) features, they span a broad clinical–pathologic spectrum and are characterized by differing biologic behavior. Typical carcinoids are low-grade, slow-growing malignancies that rarely metastasize; atypical carcinoids are intermediate-grade malignancies; and large cell neuroendocrine carcinoma (LCNEC) and small cell lung cancers (SCLCs) are high-grade carcinomas.[1]

BP carcinoid tumors are part of a heterogeneous group of neuroendocrine tumors arising from the Kulchitzky cells present in the bronchial mucosa and account for approximately 1% to 2% of all lung malignancies in adults. The incidence of BP carcinoid tumors in the United States has increased by approximately 6% per year over the past 30 years, with rates ranging from 0.2 to 2 per 100,000 individuals per year.[2–5]

LCNEC is an uncommon tumor of the lung with an incidence of approximately 3%, as reported in surgical case series.[6] LCNEC has only recently been described as a form of high-grade lung cancer that expresses neuroendocrine features. Because of the low incidence, evolving classification, and high degree of diagnostic difficulty, many aspects of LCNEC are still unknown.

CLASSIFICATION

Although neuroendocrine tumors of the lung exhibit divergent behavior, they share similar morphologic and biochemical characteristics, including an ability to secrete neuropeptides, and the presence of neuroendocrine granules. Of the pulmonary carcinoids, 80% to 90% are typical carcinoids, whereas 10% to 20% are atypical carcinoids.

Before the introduction of LCNEC, neuroendocrine tumors of the lung were subdivided into three classes: typical carcinoids, atypical carcinoids, and SCLC. In 1991, after reviewing a set of neuroendocrine tumors (typical and atypical carcinoids and SCLC), Travis et al.[7] found a group of tumors that deviated from the known classification in prognosis and morphology. They classified this new group as a high-grade neuroendocrine non small cell lung cancer (NSCLC) and placed it in between atypical carcinoid and SCLC.

In 1991, LCNEC was recognized in the World Health Organization (WHO) classification of lung tumors as a large cell carcinoma (LCC) based on its cytologic parallels (large cell size and abundant cytoplasm).[7] LCNEC is different from other LCCs because of its combination of neuroendocrine differentiation and morphology. Other LCC histologies can express neuroendocrine morphology, but not in combination with neuroendocrine differentiation.

Other regularly used terms referring to LCNEC are neuroendocrine carcinoma (NEC) grade 3, poorly differentiated NEC, and high-grade NSCLC; however, these terms are also used for SCLC and thus may include tumors with SCLC and/or LCNEC histology.

The most recent WHO/International Association for the Study of Lung Cancer classification of neuroendocrine lung tumors was established in 2004 by Travis et al.[8] (Table 55.1).[9]

DIAGNOSIS

Histology

Bronchopulmonary Carcinoids

A diagnosis of BP carcinoid can be challenging because of small biopsies, crush artifacts, and poor fixation of the specimens. BP carcinoids are composed of cells containing round to oval nuclei, a moderate amount of eosinophilic cytoplasm, finely granular chromatin, and indistinct or absent nucleoli. The cells tend to be uniform and can be arranged in a variety of patterns, including trabecular, palisading, spindle cell, glandular, follicular, rosette-like, sclerosing, clear cell, and papillary.[7,10] Rarely, BP carcinoids can show oncocytic or melanocytic features.[7,11,12] Stromal hyalinization, calcification, ossification, and amyloid deposition can also occasionally be seen.[13,14] Two features that distinguish atypical from typical carcinoids are the presence of necrosis and number of mitoses per square millimeter. Typical carcinoids must have no necrosis and fewer than 2 mitoses/2 mm^2 (10 high-power fields [HPFs]; Fig. 55.1). Atypical carcinoids should have either punctate necrosis or 2 mitoses to 10 mitoses/2 mm^2 (10 HPFs; Fig. 55.2),[15] and exhibit neuroendocrine differentiation, confirmed by more than 10% of positive cells for a neuroendocrine marker, such as chromogranin, synaptophysin, and/or neural cell adhesion molecule (NCAM; CD56).

TABLE 55.1 Criteria for Diagnosis of Neuroendocrine Tumors From the World Health Organization Guidelines[8,9]

Neuroendocrine Tumor	Criteria for Diagnosis
Typical carcinoid	Tumor with carcinoid morphology and <2 mitoses/2 mm^2 (10 HPFs), lacking necrosis, and ≥0.5 cm
Atypical carcinoid	Tumor with carcinoid morphology with 2–10 mitosis/2 mm^2 (10 HPFs) OR necrosis (often punctate)
Large cell neuroendocrine carcinoma	Tumor with a neuroendocrine morphology (organoid nesting, palisading, rosettes, trabeculae)
	High mitotic rate: ≥11/2 mm^2 (10 HPFs), median of 70/2 mm^2 (10 HPFs)
	Necrosis (often large zones)
	Cytologic features of a nonsmall cell carcinoma (NSCLC): large cell size, low nuclear-to-cytoplasmic ratio, vesicular, coarse or fine chromatin, and/or frequent nucleoli. (Some tumors have fine nuclear chromatin and lack nucleoli, but qualify as NSCLC because of large cell size and abundant cytoplasm.)
	Positive immunohistochemical staining for one or more neuroendocrine markers (other than neuron-specific enolase) and/or neuroendocrine granules by electron microscopy
Small cell carcinoma	Small size (generally less than the diameter of three small resting lymphocytes)
	Scant cytoplasm
	Nuclei: finely granular nuclear chromatin, absent or faint nucleoli
	High mitotic rate: ≥11/2 mm^2 (10 HPFs), median of 80/2 mm^2 (10 HPFs)
	Frequent necrosis often in large zones

HPFs, high-power fields.

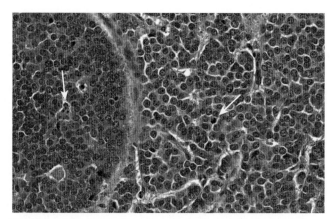

Fig. 55.2. Atypical carcinoid demonstrating increased mitoses *(right arrow)*, apoptotic bodies *(left arrow)*, and punctate necrosis seen within the nests and sheets of tumor cells. *(Courtesy Brenda Smith.)*

On slides stained with hematoxylin and eosin, these neuroendocrine growth patterns are recognized as organoid nesting, trabeculae, rosette-like structures, or palisading cells (Fig. 55.3). All LCNECs have a high proliferative rate, with more than 10 mitoses/mm^2 on HPF examination. Total HPF examination should include an area of 2 mm^2, preferably in the regions with the highest mitotic activity and viable cells. Besides high mitotic activity, areas of necrosis are frequently noted. By definition, all LCNECs express neuroendocrine differentiation, which is immunohistochemically confirmed when focal activity (more than 10% positive cells) is found with use of neuroendocrine markers (chromogranin, synaptophysin, or NCAM [CD56]) (Fig. 55.4). The presence of neuroendocrine granules on electron microscopy examination is also sufficient for diagnosis of LCNEC. The morphologic features of LCNEC resemble those of NSCLC, because the cells are large with abundant eosinophilic cytoplasm and a low nuclear-to-cytoplasmic ratio. The nuclei are round to oval shaped with granular chromatin (so-called salt and pepper). Nucleoli are also frequently seen (Fig. 55.3).

Cytology

It can often be challenging to make a diagnosis of atypical or typical carcinoid on cytologic examination, given the limited number of cells and the absence of tissue structure. BP carcinoids present as small, polyhedral-shaped cells with oval or round nuclei. The cells are arranged in a regular fashion, consisting of nests, sheets, ribbons, or spindle structures, separated by a fibrovascular stroma; however, a spindle-cell variant exists.[10,16–18] Necroses are only seen in atypical carcinoids,[15,19] which have 2 mitoses to 10 mitoses/10 HPFs. Typical carcinoids have less than 2 mitoses/10 HPFs. Nucleoli are common in atypical carcinoids and are occasionally seen in typical carcinoids; both typical and atypical carcinoids have finely granular chromatin.

Although cytologic smears are not suitable for establishing a diagnosis of LCNEC, cytologic examination can be useful during the initial evaluation of a tumor. On cytologic smears, the presentation of LCNEC is medium-to-large round or polygonal cells arranged in groups or as a single cell. The LCNEC cells can be arranged in rosette-like structures or peripheral palisading cells, and nuclear molding can be seen. In the background of the cytologic smears, necrosis and nuclear streaking are commonly seen. LCNEC cells have scant or moderate amounts of cytoplasm with a high nuclear-to-cytoplasmic ratio, which is dependent on the fixation material (air dried vs. alcohol

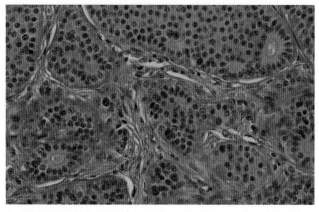

Fig. 55.1. Typical carcinoid shows an organoid nesting growth pattern and is composed of a homogeneous population of cells with finely granular cytoplasm chromatin and eosinophilic cytoplasm. No necrosis is seen, and if present, mitoses are rare. *(Courtesy Brenda Smith, British Columbia Cancer Agency, Vancouver, BC, Canada.)*

Large Cell Neuroendocrine Carcinoma

The diagnosis of LCNEC is also complex and often requires a large surgically resected lung biopsy specimen, mainly because small biopsy specimens are susceptible to crushing artifacts that may disturb the neuroendocrine morphology and cell size, two features that are critical for the diagnosis of LCNEC. To establish a LCNEC diagnosis, several histologic criteria have to be confirmed (Table 55.1). LCNECs express a neuroendocrine growth pattern (morphology) that is similar to that seen in low-grade neuroendocrine tumors (carcinoids).

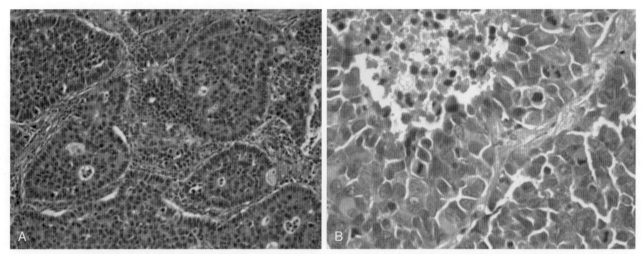

Fig. 55.3. (A) Large cell neuroendocrine carcinoma (hematoxylin and eosin, 100×). Nests of tumor cells with peripheral palisading and central necrotic foci and rosette-like structures. (B) High-magnification view (hematoxylin and eosin, 400×). Note large cells with abundant eosinophilic cytoplasm and round to oval nuclei with a fine granular (so-called salt-and-pepper) to more clumped chromatin with occasional nucleoli. Numerous mitotic figures and necrosis *(upper left corner)* are present. *(Courtesy Dr M. Béndek, Maastricht University Medical Centre, the Netherlands.)*

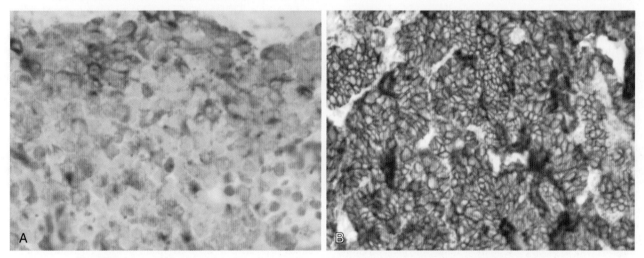

Fig. 55.4. Immunohistochemistry of a pulmonary large cell neuroendocrine carcinoma. (A) Granular cytoplasmic staining with chromogranin-A (100×); and (B) diffuse membrane positivity of CD56 (neural cell adhesion molecule, 100×) can be seen. *(Courtesy Dr M. Béndek, Maastricht University Medical Centre, the Netherlands.)*

fixated).[20] Most often, the nuclear shape is round or oval, and nuclear mitoses are frequently found. Nuclear pleomorphism and nucleoli are occasionally present.

Differential Diagnosis

Histology

Diagnosing LCNEC is a highly complex process and was addressed in interobserver studies on resected pulmonary neuroendocrine tumors. In a study performed by a panel of expert lung pathologists, a moderate interobserver variation with κ ranging from 0.35 to 0.81 was reported.[21–23] The most common overlapping diagnoses with LCNEC were SCLC, LCC, atypical carcinoid, basaloid carcinoma, and the poorly differentiated NSCLC tumors expressing a neuroendocrine phenotype.[6,21] Undoubtedly, these uncertainties are secondary to the morphologic and cytologic similarities of lung

tumors with LCNEC. In the interobserver studies of BP carcinoids, there was a variability of results, from substantial agreement (κ > 0.7) in one study[21] to fair to moderate (κ = 0.39–0.87) in another study by Lee et al.[24] The fact that there were only two pulmonary pathologists in the Lee et al.[24] study may have had an influence on the results.

Although differentiating pulmonary NEC from overlapping tumors can be a challenge, several criteria may help guide the diagnosis. The differentiation of atypical carcinoid from high-grade NEC can be achieved with the help of the mitosis count; on average, 2 mitoses to 10 mitoses/2 mm² are expressed in atypical carcinoid compared with more than 11 mitoses/2 mm² in high-grade NEC. Moreover, necrosis in atypical carcinoid predominantly consists of punctate foci, whereas necrosis is more prominent in LCNEC.[15]

A distinction between LCNEC and SCLC can be established only with the help of cytology-based criteria. Compared with

LCNEC, SCLC has a smaller cell size (less than the diameter of three lymphocytes), a higher nuclear:cytoplasmic ratio, and absent or faint nucleoli. Although it was demonstrated in several studies that LCNEC and SCLC had a considerably different mean cell size, the standard deviations did overlap. Therefore whether cell size is the most adequate criteria to differentiate LCNEC from SCLC should be questioned.[25–27] The mitosis count, which is useful in atypical carcinoid, is not helpful in differentiating LCNEC from SCLC.

Both SCLC and typical carcinoid cells may be similar in size and shape and may appear uniform. Variation in size may be a helpful distinguishing feature, from less than onefold (mild) in typical carcinoid to more than twofold to threefold in atypical carcinoid and high-grade neuroendocrine tumors.[28–30] In addition, SCLC cells are arranged in more cohesive groups and three-dimensional clusters, which are not present in bronchial carcinoids.[31–33] Ki-67 (MIB-1) staining may also be useful because SCLC will show a proliferation index of more than 50%, whereas carcinoids have a proliferation index of less than 20%.[34]

In addition to atypical carcinoid and SCLC, other forms of nonsmall carcinomas—such as the basaloid carcinoma—must be distinguished from LCNEC. The morphology of basaloid carcinoma is comparable to that of LCNEC; differentiation is possible with the help of IHC with neuroendocrine markers, which are negative in basaloid carcinomas.[8]

As for the basaloid carcinoma, poorly differentiated adenocarcinomas or squamous cell carcinomas can also be distinguished from LCNEC with the help of IHC markers, which are addressed later in the chapter.

Cytology

The value of cytology in the diagnosis of BP carcinoids has been examined in several studies. The main factor in distinguishing typical carcinoid from high-grade neuroendocrine neoplasms or other carcinomas is adequate evaluation of nuclear features. Typical carcinoids tend to have fine, evenly dispersed granular chromatin with inconspicuous or undetectable nucleoli; SCLC has coarsely granular chromatin and occasional chromatin clumping, and poorly differentiated carcinoma has more clumped chromatin in a vesicular nucleus.[29,35,36] The cytologic diagnosis of atypical carcinoid can be quite difficult, as it has features that may be found in typical carcinoid or SCLC. In atypical carcinoid, tumor cells tend to be larger than those noted in typical carcinoid or SCLC, and nuclear pleomorphism and atypia are also common. The finely granular chromatin is present, and mitoses range from 2 HPF to 10/10 HPFs.[37]

Compared with histology, misdiagnoses are even more common when LCNEC is diagnosed on cytology specimens. Preoperatively obtained cytologic smears from confirmed resected LCNEC have been reviewed in several studies.[20,38,39] In about 80% of smears, the cytology was initially diagnosed as NSCLC, SCLC, LCC with neuroendocrine features, poorly differentiated adenocarcinoma or squamous cell carcinoma, or combined SCLC. However, during the period between 1990 and the beginning of 2000, when the majority of the series in these studies were diagnosed, LCNEC was a new entity and pathologists may have been unaware of it. In 2005, a study was published in which 9 (90%) of 11 LCNEC cases ($N = 11$) were correctly diagnosed before surgery.[40]

Cytokeratin Markers. High-molecular-weight cytokeratin (CK) types 1, 5, 10, and 14 (antibody clone 34E1β2) are almost solely expressed in non-NECs such as basaloid carcinoma and poorly differentiated adenocarcinoma or squamous cell carcinoma. In tissue microarray panel studies, 3% to 17% of pure LCNEC[41] showed positive staining for clone 34E1β2.[26,40,42] Other commonly used high-molecular-weight CK types such as CK5/6,

CK7, and CK20 were positive in 2% to 13%, 57% to 77%, and 2% to 10% of LCNECs, respectively.[43,44] CK18 and CK19 were positive in 97% and 59%, respectively.[44,45] In combined LCNEC, expression of 34E1β2 has been noted in the adenocarcinoma/squamous cell carcinoma component.[40]

Markers for Differentiating Atypical From Typical Carcinoid. Counting mitoses may be challenging, especially if there is crush artifact or poor sample fixation. Ki-67 expression may be used as a surrogate to help differentiate between atypical and typical carcinoids. In a study by Warth et al.,[46] a low interobserver agreement was demonstrated when using mitotic count (median κ = 0.213) to distinguish between atypical and typical carcinoids, and the overall κ for Ki-67 was higher (0.746). Ki-67 expression is also prognostic; carcinoids with Ki-67 expression higher than 5% were associated with a worse overall survival.[37,47,48]

Markers for Differentiating Large Cell Neuroendocrine Carcinoma From Squamous Cell Carcinoma. In addition to high-molecular-weight CKs, markers such as desmocollin-3 and p63 may be useful in discriminating poorly differentiated squamous cell carcinomas from LCNEC. Desmocollin-3 was negative in 99% of all pure LCNECs and therefore appears to be a promising specific marker but requires further validation.[43] Expression of p63, a highly sensitive and specific marker for diagnosing squamous cell carcinomas, was detected in 0% to 18% of LCNECs. Therefore p63 may not be appropriate as a specific marker for poorly differentiated NSCLC when LCNEC is a possibility in the differential diagnosis.[26,43,49] When compared with p63, the nontransactivating isoform of the p63 gene, delta Np63 (p40), was found to be a more reliable marker for squamous differentiation. Expression of p40 was lower compared with p63 in LCNEC and therefore more accurate.[50] These results were confirmed in a study subtyping LCC with IHC; none of the confirmed LCNECs stained for p40.[51]

Markers for Differentiating Large Cell Neuroendocrine Carcinoma From Adenocarcinoma. Thyroid transcription factor-1 (TTF-1), a marker commonly used in defining the appropriate histotype of lung cancer and that is also sensitive and specific for lung adenocarcinoma, is expressed in about 50% of all resected lung LCNEC. The expression ranges of TTF-1 mainly depend on the antibody used. The more sensitive clone, SPT24, is positive in 23% to 77% of LCNECs,[43,44,52] and the 8G763 clone is positive in 23% to 48%.[42,43,53,54] Therefore TTF-1 is not useful in differentiating LCNEC from poorly differentiated NSCLC (adenocarcinoma).

A new marker named Napsin-A, specific to adenocarcinomas, was negative in 100% of LCNECs, but further validation of this marker is required.[43] In addition, collapsin response mediator protein (CRMP) is known to be involved in neurogenesis and was studied in a group of lung tumors. CRMP was expressed in 4 (100%) of 4 LCNECs and in 54 (100%) of 54 SCLCs. The expression of CRMP was negative in 0% of 22 adenocarcinomas and positive in 1 (8%) of 12 squamous cell carcinomas. The number of LCNECs studied was very small, but CRMP was shown to be a promising marker that also requires further validation.[55]

Markers for Differentiating Bronchopulmonary Carcinoid From Small Cell Lung Cancer. Ki-67 staining may be of value because SCLC shows a proliferation index of more than 50%, whereas carcinoids have a proliferation index of less than 20%.[34,56,57] K homology domain (KOC) protein and paired box gene 5 (PAX5) expressions have been evaluated in small samples.[58,59] The KOC protein was strongly positive in 90% of SCLCs and negative in 20 of 21 cases of typical and atypical carcinoids. PAX5 expression was present in 29 (78%) of 37 high-grade neuroendocrine tumors and 0 of 51 typical and atypical carcinoids. Validation in larger samples is required before such markers are used routinely for differentiation.

Markers for Differentiating Large Cell Neuroendocrine Carcinoma From Small Cell Lung Cancer. As of the time of publication, distinguishing LCNEC from SCLC by IHC is not feasible. Several markers have been proposed, but lack practical usefulness. Both CK7 and 18 are commonly expressed in LCNEC and were reported in several studies to have a considerably higher expression intensity in LCNEC compared with SCLC.[44,60] These results were similar in studies comparing the expression intensity of E-cadherin and β-catenin in LCNEC and SCLC, where both markers were shown to have considerably higher expression intensity in LCNEC.[44,60] Villin1, a promising marker located in the brush border of epithelial cells, was found to be expressed in 62% of LCNECs and 4% of SCLCs.[45,60] However, these results must be confirmed in larger studies. In a smaller study, IHC expression of neuronatin was examined in LCNEC and SCLC after an increased complementary DNA transcription of neuronatin in LCNEC was noted. Among the SCLC samples, 8% were positive for neuronatin with IHC staining compared with 43% among the LCNEC samples.[61] A neurogenesis-regulating gene (NeuroD) was also found to be differentially expressed between LCNEC and SCLC.[26] NeuroD was expressed in 53% of LCNECs and 13% of SCLCs. Therefore several markers may differentiate LCNEC from SCLC, but none of these is very specific or sensitive and further validation is required.

Markers for Differentiating Atypical and Typical Carcinoids From Large Cell Neuroendocrine Carcinoma. Separating atypical and typical carcinoids from LCNEC is possible with the Ki-67 index. The expression index in LCNEC is approximately 40% (range, 25% to 52%); for carcinoids, the expression index is reported to be below 20% (typical carcinoid, less than 2%; atypical carcinoid, less than 20%, typically ± 10%).[34,56,57,62] Consequently, Ki-67 may be useful in differentiating LCNEC from atypical and typical carcinoids, although the diagnosis has to be confirmed with a mitoses count.

Immunohistochemical on Cytology. IHC neuroendocrine markers such as chromogranin, synaptophysin, and NCAM were found to be positive in 28% to 31%, 64% to 75%, and 45% of cytologic smears, respectively.[20,63]

MOLECULAR BIOLOGY

Approximately 5% of BP carcinoids may occur as a result of the multiple neuroendocrine neoplasia type 1 gene (MEN1); 95% are sporadic tumors of uncertain etiology. Various techniques have been used to evaluate the molecular biology of BP carcinoids, including in vitro cell line studies, chromosomal evaluation, comparative genomic hybridization (CGH), polymerase chain reaction, and, most recently, whole genome sequencing. Swarts et al.[64] performed an extensive review of the molecular biology of neuroendocrine lung tumors, and Cakir and Grossman[65] examined the molecular pathogenesis of BP carcinoids. The molecular basis of LCNEC is also still unknown. SCLC and LCNEC are known as highly undifferentiated pulmonary tumors that express similar characteristics. However, according to WHO classification, LCNEC is categorized as a subtype of LCC. The molecular biology of LCNEC, determined by different techniques, has been addressed in several studies and the findings were compared with SCLC and LCC.

Loss of Heterozygosity

BP carcinoids may have loss of heterozygosity (LOH) on a variety of different chromosomes. LOH at 11q has been seen in 27% to 55.5% of typical carcinoids and 0% to 73% of atypical carcinoids.[66,67] LOH at 11q13, the locus of the MEN1 gene, was detected in 50% to 63.6% of atypical carcinoids and 22% to 73% of typical carcinoids.[66,68] In several other small studies, LOH was found on several chromosomes in bronchial carcinoids, including 3p14.2 (fragile histidine triad gene);[68,69] 5q;[67] 5q21 (adenomatous polyposis coil/mutated in colon cancer gene);[68] 9p;[67,70] 9p21 (p16);[68] 9q;[67] 13q;[67] 13q14.1–14.2 (retinoblastoma [Rb]);[68] 17p;[67] 17q13.1 (p53);[68,70] and X (microsatellite markers).[71]

In an evaluation of LOH with microsatellite markers at chromosomes 3p, 5q, 9p, 11q, and 13q, several similarities between SCLC and LCNEC were demonstrated.[68] These chromosomal findings were in accordance with the results from another study that compared LOH in LCC, LCNEC, and SCLC.[72] LOH was examined for chromosomes 3p, 5q, 9p, 10p, 10q, and 13q. Significant differences were noted between all three tumor types except for SCLC and LCNEC, emphasizing the close relation between these high-grade neuroendocrine tumors.

LOH has also been examined in combined SCLC and LCNEC tumors. Depending on the region being examined, combined tumors can express an SCLC or LCNEC phenotype. Investigators separately studied SCLC and LCNEC regions and found a high degree of similarity in the genetic profile. These findings suggest that there is a common origin of combined SCLC and LCNEC tumors.[71]

Chromosomal Aberrations

CGH and other genetic analyses to assess chromosomal aberrations in BP carcinoids,[73–79] high-grade pulmonary NECs,[80–85] or both have been examined in several studies.[85–88] Swarts et al.[64] performed a meta-analysis of these studies, which included typical carcinoids, 38 atypical carcinoids, 33 LCNECs, 48 SCLCs, and 11 unclassified high-grade neuroendocrine tumors. Chromosomal aberrations more than 10 Mb were much more frequent in LCNEC (average 13.7 aberrations per tumor) and SCLC (18.8 aberrations per tumor), as compared with atypical carcinoids (6.1 aberrations per tumor) and typical carcinoids (2.8 aberrations per tumor). The investigators assumed that smoking habit may explain the differences. The most frequent aberrations for bronchial carcinoids are −11q, +19P, −13q, +19q, +17q, −11p, −6q, +16p, +20p, and −3p. These aberrations differ from those present in the high-grade neuroendocrine tumors, with the exception of 3p and 13q losses.

Chromosomal aberration in LCNEC and SCLC has also been studied. Through CGH, loss of chromosomes 3p, 4, 5p, 6q, 8p, 9p, and 21q, and gain in 5p, 8q, 12p, and 22 was found in three patients with LCNEC. Similarities between chromosomal aberrations in LCNEC and SCLC included loss of 3p, 4q, 5q, and 13q and gain of 5p. Noticeable chromosomal aberrations between SCLC and LCNEC were found at chromosomal arms 3q (gain), 10q (loss), and 17p (loss) in favor of SCLC, and gain of 6p in favor of LCNEC.[82] Compared with atypical carcinoid, no similarities were detected.[86] In a study by Peng et al.,[85] several similarities between LCNEC and SCLC were found when the genetic profiles were analyzed with high-density bacterial artificial chromosome array. Frequently gained loci were located at 1q, 2q, 3q, 5p, 7q, 8q, 12q, and 18q; lost loci were located at 1p, 3p, 4q, 5q, 10q, 13q, 16q, 17p, and 22q. Considerably different chromosomal aberrations compared between all stages of SCLC and LCNEC were located at 2q (gain), 3p (loss), 4q (loss), and 6p (loss). Although it may appear that SCLC and LCNEC share a common genetic profile, the majority of similarities may not be very specific, because numerous chromosomal aberrations are commonly encountered in other forms of lung cancer, including pulmonary NEC.

Microarray Comparison

Anbazhagan et al.[89] performed hierarchical clustering of gene expression profiles of two carcinoids, two SCLCs, and two brain tumors. Although the carcinoids clustered together with the brain tumors, SCLC was more closely related to normal bronchial epithelial carcinoma. Swarts et al.[90] used gene expression profiling to explore pathways involved in lung carcinoid progression and found that in carcinoids with poor prognosis, a significantly higher number of downregulated genes were located at chromosome 11q (p = 0.00017). In addition, a number of upregulated genes were found to be involved in the mitotic spindle checkpoint, the chromosomal passenger complex, mitotic kinase CDC2 activity, and the BRCA/Fanconi anemia pathway. At the individual gene level, BIRC5 (survivin), BUB1, CD44, IL20RA, KLK12, and OTP were independent predictors of patient outcome. For BIRC5, the number of positive nuclei was also related to poor prognosis within the group of carcinoids. Aurora B kinase and BIRC5, major components of the chromosomal passenger complex, were particularly upregulated in high-grade carcinomas and may therefore be indicative of therapeutic targets for these tumors.[90]

When examining the clinical behavior of high-grade neuroendocrine tumors, classification based on genetic profiling may be more appropriate than histologic classification. Jones et al.[91] examined complementary DNA microarray data obtained from neuroendocrine lung tumors (8 LCNECs [2 combined with SCLC], 17 SCLCs [2 combined with LCNEC], and 13 LCCs). Surprisingly, neither SCLC nor LCNEC clustered as single entities in the way that LCCs did. In support of this molecular description of neuroendocrine lung tumors, Shibata et al.[92] found three high-grade neuroendocrine subclasses when data from comparative genome hybridization were hierarchically clustered (8 SCLC and 15 LCNEC). The three subclass branches were subdivided into groups named BR1, BR2, and BR3. Patients in the BR2 group had a significantly different survival compared with the BR1 and BR3 groups (p = 0.028). However, contrary to findings from Jones et al.,[91] almost all SCLCs clustered.[92]

Mutation Analysis

In a recent study by Sachithanandan et al.[93] of patients with MEN1, 5% had been diagnosed with BP carcinoids. MEN1 is an autosomal dominant disorder associated with mutations in the gene locus on 11q13. MEN1 gene activation is evident in 70% of patients with atypical carcinoid, 47% with typical carcinoid, 52% with LCNEC, and 41% with SCLC. A single mutation was found in a small study of MEN1 in LCNEC.[94]

Capodanno et al.[95] assessed 190 patients with bronchial neuroendocrine tumors (75 typical carcinoids, 23 atypical carcinoids, 17 LCNECs, and 75 SCLCs) and found that there was an increasing frequency of phosphatidylinositol 3-kinase (PI3K) mutations, with increased biologic aggressiveness of the bronchial neuroendocrine tumors, except in LCNECs. PIK3CA mutations were present in 13% of typical carcinoids, 39% of atypical carcinoids, 31% of SCLCs, and only 12% of LCNECs.[95]

Mutations in LCNEC that are commonly encountered in lung cancer have been examined in several studies (Table 55.2). Kirsten rat sarcoma viral oncogene homolog (KRAS) and epidermal growth factor receptor mutations are uncommon in LCNEC, although there have been published reports in cases of combined LCNEC and adenocarcinomas.[68,96,97] Aberrant expression of anaplastic lymphoma kinase (ALK) by IHC was demonstrated in a single case of LCNEC. No ALK rearrangement or mutation was noted in further analyses.[98] Two PIK3CA mutations have been found at c.3145 G>A and c.3140 A>G.[95] In 29% of resected LCNECs, a mutation in the neurotropic tyrosine receptor kinase gene family was demonstrated.[96]

TABLE 55.2 Overview of Mutations Analyzed in Pure and Combined Large Cell Neuroendocrine Carcinoma of the Lung[a]

Mutation	Type of LCNEC (Number of Samples With Mutation/Total Number of Samples)			
	Pure	With SCLC	With Squamous Cell Carcinoma	With Adenocarcinoma
ALK	0/106[b]	ND	ND	ND
BRAF	0/24	2/9	0/3	ND
EGFR	1/62	0/10	0/3	0/8
KRAS	2/83	1/10	ND	1/9
NRAS	0/34	0/6	ND	ND
PIK3CA	2/43	1/10	ND	ND
ROS1	ND	ND	ND	ND
HRAS	1/17	0/8	0/3	ND
MEN1	1/13	ND	ND	ND
TP53	32/61	3/10	ND	1/1
KEAP1	2/19	0/9	0/1	ND
NTRK	6/21	ND	ND	ND
NFE2L2	1/19	0/9	ND	ND
STK11	8/28	1/10	ND	ND
CDK4	0/28	0/10	0/3	ND
DDR2	0/1	0/2	0/1	ND
ERBB2	2/26	0/10	0/3	ND
FGFR2	1/24	0/10	0/1	ND
FGFR3	0/25	0/9	0/2	ND
C-Kit	0/83	ND	ND	ND
C-met	0/83	ND	ND	ND
PDGFR alpha	0/83	ND	ND	ND
PFGFR beta	0/83	ND	ND	ND

[a]Published data only.
[b]By immunohistochemical analysis.
LCNEC, large cell neuroendocrine carcinoma; ND, no data have been reported on this mutation in the specified type of lung carcinoma; SCLC, small cell lung cancer.

In a 2013 study, a large group of molecularly analyzed lung tumors was reported by the Clinical Lung Cancer Genome Project and Network Genomic Medicine.[99] A total of 261 lung tumors (31 LCCs) were included for unsupervised hierarchical clustering of gene expressions. Although the analyzed carcinoid tumors harbored no noteworthy mutations, a number of mutations were identified in pure LCNEC and the combination of SCLC and LCNEC (Table 55.2). Based on genetic modeling, the authors of the study were able to classify the majority of all LCCs as adenocarcinoma, squamous cell carcinoma, or SCLC. Thereby, the diagnosis of LCC as a separate entity was brought into question. Whole-exome (15 tumors) and transcriptome (10 tumors) sequencing of LCNEC showed overlapping mutations between LCNEC and SCLC (T53, RB1, and EP300). Several mutations typically found in adenocarcinomas or squamous cell carcinomas were detected in LCNEC, but these findings were not significant. Additional information about the whole-exome and transcriptome sequencing of LCNEC is expected to be published in the near future.[99]

Pathways

The p53 gene, which helps to maintain genomic stability, is mutated in approximately 4% of typical carcinoids, 29% of atypical carcinoids, 80% of LCNECs, and 75% of SCLCs.[68,70,100–104]

The p16/cyclin D1/Rb pathway is affected in 9% to 20% of typical carcinoids, 22% of atypical carcinoids, 62% of LCNECs, and 71% to 90% of SCLCs.[62,78,79,104–109] The Rb gene is a tumor suppressor with a critical role in cell cycle control through the regulation of the G_1 growth arrest. p16 is a cyclin-dependent kinase inhibitor that inhibits binding of cyclin-dependent kinases to cyclin D1 and prevents phosphorylation (inhibition) of Rb. Therefore downregulation of p16 and Rb may lead to uncontrolled cell growth. Loss of Rb expression was demonstrated in 47% to 91% of LCNECs. Loss of p16 expression and overexpression of cyclin D1 were found more frequently in LCNEC than in SCLC.[26,57,62,72,110]

The intrinsic apoptosis pathway, including Bcl2, Bcl2L1, and BAX genes, has been found in several studies to be inhibited in high-grade neuroendocrine tumors, moderately affected in atypical carcinoids, and almost intact in typical carcinoids.[111,112]

The expression of AKT and mammalian target of rapamycin (mTOR) as part of the PI3K/AKT/mTOR pathway in a group of neuroendocrine lung tumors has also been evaluated in several studies; however, there were contradicting results for AKT expression (19% to 82%) and mTOR expression (50% to 77%) in these tumors.[113,114] Righi et al.[115] described a pattern of mTOR intensity expression that decreased from low- to high-grade neuroendocrine tumors. The authors also noted that mTOR expression correlated with SSRT-2/3 expression and hypothesized that mTOR may be a possible regulator of SSRT expression.

CLINICAL CHARACTERISTICS

BP Carcinoids

As a result of endobronchial obstruction and tumor ulceration, approximately 58% of patients with BP carcinoids present with symptoms including cough (32%), hemoptysis (26%), and pneumonia (24%).[1,116–123]

Contrary to midgut carcinoids, BP carcinoids produce less serotonin and thus patients with BP carcinoids have a lower rate of carcinoid syndrome. Carcinoid syndrome, which occurs in 1% to 3% of BP carcinoid cases, may be atypical, with episodes of flushing accompanied by disorientation, tremor, periorbital edema, lacrimation, salivation, hypotension, tachycardia, diarrhea, dyspnea, asthma, and edema.[116,123] In addition, the risk of carcinoid crisis with BP carcinoids is so low that routine prophylaxis with octreotide prior to tumor manipulation is not typically recommended.

Approximately 1% to 2% of BP carcinoids are associated with ectopic adrenocorticotropic hormone production.[12] Even more rare is the production of growth hormone-releasing hormone from BP carcinoids causing acromegaly,[124,125] hypoglycemia,[126] and hypercalcemia.[127,128]

Large Cell Neuroendocrine Carcinoma

Because of the difficulty in diagnosing LCNEC on small biopsy specimens and cytology samples, most clinical data come from surgical series, which may bias the results (i.e., selection of younger patients with less comorbidity). Reported symptoms at initial presentation often include coughing, weight loss, hemoptysis, chest pain, and fever.[129–131] Classic paraneoplastic syndromes, such as Cushing syndrome seen in SCLC or the carcinoid syndrome rarely associated with lung carcinoids, are seldom diagnosed in LCNEC.[132,133]

The incidence of LCNEC is about 3% in reviewed case series of resected pulmonary malignancies.[6] In these LCNEC series, the average age of initial presentation was 64 years (range, 30 years to 88 years) with the majority of patients being male (mean, 80%; range, 54% to 89%) and former heavy smokers (89% to 100%; Table 55.3). Data from two studies have challenged that the incidence of LCNEC is substantially higher in men. In 100 cases of confirmed resected LCNEC, the female-to-male ratio was 5:9 (46%:54%).[134] In a study of clinical characteristics extracted from the Surveillance, Epidemiology, and End Results

database, the findings were similar, with a female-to-male ratio of approximately 5:9 (45%:55%).[135]

STAGING

No classification staging system currently exists that specifically addresses BP carcinoids or LCNEC; therefore the seventh edition of the tumor, node, and metastasis (TNM) staging for NSCLC is used for staging LCNEC.[136]

IMAGING

Computed Tomography

Computed tomography (CT) and magnetic resonance imaging are recommended for staging of BP carcinoids. Typical carcinoids are well-defined, spherical, or ovoid masses that may narrow or obstruct airways and may result in secondary atelectasis.[137] Although typical carcinoids tend to be centrally located, atypical carcinoids are usually peripherally located. Davila et al.[138] noted that 15% of BP carcinoids were located peripherally, with 10% in the mainstem bronchi and 75% in the lobar bronchi. Calcification may be present in 30% of BP carcinoids.[118]

Most typical carcinoids present as stage I tumors, with 87% of patients having no lymph node metastases. In one series, 10% of patients with typical carcinoids had N1 disease; 3% had N2; and no patients had N3 disease. By contrast, the presence of N0, N1, N2, and N3 disease in patients with atypical carcinoids was 43%, 29%, 14%, and 14%, respectively.[116]

Large Cell Neuroendocrine Carcinoma

Findings of LCNEC on CT are nonspecific and comparable to that of other solid pulmonary malignancies. LCNEC is predominantly situated in the periphery (67% to 97%) of the lungs but, like SCLC, can also be centrally located (3% to 33%).[129,130,139,140] In radiologic and surgical case series, LCNEC had a slight tendency to be situated in the upper lobes. The border of the tumor is usually lobulated, but can be spiculated. On CT evaluation, the average diameter of the primary tumor is approximately 40 mm (range, 7 mm to 100 mm).[129,130,139,140] Necrosis is commonly seen and can present as an inhomogeneous enhancement, especially in larger nodules.[129] Calcification has been reported in 7% to 21% of all primary LCNEC tumors, and it has been hypothesized that these are dystrophic calcifications that can arise in areas of necrosis.[130,139,141]

Positron Emission Tomography

Imaging studies in which the effectiveness of positron emission tomography (PET) is evaluated are scarce. ^{68}Ga-DOTATOC PET, which targets the somatostatin receptor, was evaluated in neuroendocrine tumors and had a specificity of 90% to 92%, a sensitivity of 81% to 97%, and an accuracy of 87% to 96%.[142,143] ^{11}C-5-hydroxytryptophan, a radiolabeled precursor of 5-hydroxytryptophan synthesis, may be more specific for bronchial carcinoids. In one study, ^{11}C-5-hydroxytryptophan scanning was compared with CT for the identification of tumor lesions; ^{11}C-5-hydroxytryptophan identified tumor lesions in 95% of patients and detected more lesions than CT and somatostatin receptor scintigraphy (SRS) in 58% of patients.[144] The available data suggest that LCNEC has a high uptake of fluorine ^{18}F-2-deoxy-D-glucose (FDG) with a mean standardized uptake value of 12.0 (range, 3.9 to 25.6),[139,145] comparable with results found in SCLC.[146] The use of FDG is controversial for the imaging of BP carcinoids as they usually have low metabolic activity and therefore tend to have less FDG uptake compared with LCNEC and SCLC.[147]

TABLE 55.3 Overview of Clinical Characteristics in Select Large Studies of Surgically Resected Large Cell Neuroendocrine Carcinomas

Characteristics	Takei et al.[6]	Rossi et al.[172]	Veronesi et al.[174]	Varlotto et al.[135]	Fournel et al.[131]	Tanaka et al.[173]	Sarkaria et al.[134]	Grand et al.[241]	Grand et al.[241]	Kinoshita et al.[233]	Asamura et al.[234]
Period	1982–1999	1990–2004	1988–2004	2001–2007	2000–2010	2001–2009	1992–2008	1980–2009	1980–2009	1995–2010	NA
Pathology review board, number of pathologists	3	3	1 at each center	No review	1	1	2	NA	NA	3	Central, 6
No. of centers	1	2	Multicenter	Multicenter	1	1	1	2	2	1	Multicenter
No. of pure LCNEC (%)	82 (94)	83	144	324	63	63	77 (77)	52	52	56 (69)	126 (89)
No. of combined LCNEC (%)	5 (6)	—	—	—	—	—	23 (23)	—	50	25 (31)	15 (11)
Men (%)	86	88	81	55	77	87	54	71	86	85	89
Mean age (y)	62	NR	63	67	64	67	64	60.5	61.4	70	66
Smokers (%)	98	96	94	NR	89	92	98	95	94	100	99
SURGERY (%)											
Segment/wedge resection	9	NR	10	22	6	13	9	13	6	0	NR
Lobectomy	70	NR	66	73	73	87	80	63	48	95	NR
Bilobectomy	7	NR	5	NR	1	0	0	4	6	0	NR
Pneumonectomy	14	NR	17	6	19	0	11	19	40	5	NR
Systematic node dissection (%)	Yes (69)	Yes	Yes (94)	NR	Yes	NR	NR	Yes	Yes	Yes	NR
R0 resection (%)	NR	NR	94	NR	100	100	90	96	86	NR	NR
LYMPH NODE STATUS (%)											
N0	49	75	NR	69	46	NR	65	52	58	NR	54
N1	20a	25a	NR	17	24	NR	15	19	22	NR	18
>N2	20a	25a	NR	12	30	NR	23	29	20	NR	26
STAGE (%)b											
I	47 (4)	66 (6)	51 (NR)	57 (NR)	35 (7)	45 (6)	44 (7)	38 (7)	40 (7)	59 (7)	45 (5)
II	15 (4)	20 (6)	20 (NR)	16 (NR)	25 (7)	26 (6)	27 (7)	25 (7)	28 (7)	21 (7)	16 (5)
III	34 (4)	14 (6)	28 (NR)	18 (NR)	40 (7)	19 (6)	25 (7)	33 (7)	26 (7)	19 (7)	32 (5)
IV	3 (4)	0 (6)	1 (NR)	0 (NR)	0 (7)	0 (6)	4 (7)	2 (7)	4 (7)	1 (7)	7 (5)
Adjuvant chemotherapy (%)	14	34	17	NR	Yes (% NR)	32	25	NR	NR	Yes (% NR)	NR
5-Year survival (%)	57	27.6	43	41c	49.2	44.9	NR	39	38	53.3	40.3
5-YEAR SURVIVAL BY STAGE (%)											
I	67	33	52	60c	NR	NR	53	NR	NR	NR	58
II	75	23	59	NR	NR	NR	61	NR	NR	NR	32
III	45	8	20	NR	NR	NR	24d	NR	NR	NR	NR
IV	0	—	—	—	NR	NR	24d	NR	NR	NR	NR
Median follow-up (mo)	NR	17	27	15	NR	32.3	34	73e	73e	60	60
Recurrence (%)	39	62	40	NR	NR	NR	38	NR	NR	NR	48

aRepresents total of N1 and N2 lymph node status combined.

bThe edition of the American Joint Committee on Cancer staging classification differed among the studies. The fourth edition was used by Takei et al.,[6] the fifth edition was used by Rossi et al.,[172] and Tanaka et al.,[173] and the seventh edition was used by Fournel et al.,[131] Sarkaria et al.,[134] Grand et al.,[241] and Kinoshita et al.;[233] the sixth edition was used by Asamura et al.,[234] the edition used was not noted in the studies by Veronesi et al.[174] and Varlotto et al.[135] (various classifications).

cCalculated for 4 years of survival.

dRepresents the total of stage III and IV tumors combined.

eReported as mean value.

LCNEC, large cell neuroendocrine carcinoma; NA, not available; NR, not reported.

Somatostatin Receptor Scintigraphy

Expression of somatostatin is frequently found in neuroendocrine tumors and is known for its regulation of hormones including glucagon, gastrin, insulin, and the growth hormone. Currently, five somatostatin subtype receptors (SSTRs) are known and classified as SSTR-1 through SSTR-5. In a surgical series, the different receptors were found to be present to varying degrees in typical carcinoid, atypical carcinoid, and LCNEC. With the exception of SSTR-5, there was a tendency toward decreased expression in well- to poorly differentiated NECs.[148,149]

Radiographic detection of SSTR in tumors is possible with indium-111 pentetreotide scintigraphy (octreotide scan). An octreotide scan detects radiolabeled octreotide, a synthetic analog of somatostatin, which binds with a high affinity to SSTR-2, SSTR-3, and SSTR-5 after intravenous injection.

Approximately 80% of bronchial neuroendocrine tumors can be imaged with octreotide scanning.[150] In a study by Rodrigues et al.,[151] results from two different radioligands—[111]In-DOTA-D: Phe(1)-Tyr(3)-octreotide and ^{111}In-DOTA-lanreotide—were compared and the overall sensitivity was 93% and 87%, respectively. The sensitivity of SRS to detect the primary malignancy instead of metastatic disease can vary. Granberg et al.[152] identified a sensitivity of approximately 80% for primary bronchial carcinoids and 60% for liver metastases; however, the main limitation of SRS is its specificity, as it detects positivity in many other tumors, granulomas, and autoimmune diseases. The role of SRS in preoperative staging is controversial, taking into account that extrathoracic metastatic disease is rare.[153]

Although SRS is commonly used for detection of BP carcinoids, studies of LCNEC are scarce. In a small study evaluating LCNEC preoperatively, 55% of primary lesions (10 of 18) showed activity on octreotide scan.[154] In another study, the use of technetium-99m ethylene diamine diacetic acid/hydrazinonicotinyl-Tyr³-octreotide (99mTc-TOC) scintigraphy was evaluated for the detection of LCNEC.[155] A high sensitivity

was found for primary lesions (100%) and supradiaphragmatic metastases (83%), whereas none of the infradiaphragmatic (adrenal glands) metastases was detected and only 11% of all skeletal metastases were detected. Table 55.4 provides a summary of the clinical, pathologic, and imaging findings in neuroendocrine cancers of the lung.

THERAPY

Surgery

Bronchopulmonary Carcinoids

The standard of care for BP carcinoids is surgical resection, with the approach dependent on location, size of tumor, and tissue type. For central, localized typical carcinoid, lung preservation resection, such as sleeve resection, wedge, or segmental resection, is preferred.[156] The optimal treatment of atypical carcinoid with or without lymph node metastases is controversial, and the use of conservative resection in these two scenarios has been called into question. Typically, a more extensive resection, such as lobectomy, bilobectomy, and pneumonectomy, is recommended.[121,138,157,158] The goal is en bloc resection with preservation of as much normal lung as possible. Surgical margins that are as narrow as 5 mm are considered adequate, as bronchial carcinoids do not tend to spread submucosally.

Because 5% to 20% of typical carcinoids and 30% to 70% of atypical carcinoids metastasize to lymph nodes, a complete mediastinal lymph node sampling or dissection is indicated.[159–161] If the mediastinal lymph nodes are positive, a full dissection is recommended, as this does not preclude the possibility of cure.

It is possible to attempt a bronchoscopic resection of an intraluminal typical carcinoid. A variety of bronchoscopic strategies have been utilized, including neodymium:yttrium aluminum garnet laser, with or without photodynamic therapy, an approach

TABLE 55.4 Comparison of Clinical, Pathologic, and Imaging Findings in Neuroendocrine Tumors of the Lung

	Typical Carcinoid	Atypical Carcinoid	Large Cell Neuroendocrine Carcinoma	Small Cell Lung Cancer
DEMOGRAPHICS				
Median age (y)	40–50	50–60	60–70	50–70
Associated with smoking	No	Yes	Yes	Yes
Male-to-female ratio	1:1	1:1/2:1	>2.5:1	>2.5:1
HISTOPATHOLOGIC FEATURES				
Mitoses per 10 HPFs	<2	2–10	>10 (median, 70)	>50 (median, 80)
Necrosis	No	Yes (punctate)	Yes (large zones)	Yes (large zones)
Nucleoli	Occasional	Common	Very common	Absent or inconspicuous
Nuclear-to-cytoplasmic ratio	Moderate	Moderate	Low	High
Nuclear chromatin	Finely granular	Finely granular	Usually vesicular, may be finely granular	Finely granular
Shape	Round, oval, spindled	Round, oval, spindled	Round, oval, polygonal	Round, oval, spindled
IMAGING				
Central-to-peripheral ratio	3:1	3:1	1:4	10–20:1
Calcification/ossification (%)	30	30	9	Up to 23
Stage (%)[117,136]				
I	87	43	18.2	2.6
II	10	29	6.6	1.5
III	3	14	24.1	26.8
IV	0	14	42	57.8
Unknown	NA	NA	9.1	11.4
Extrathoracic metastases[234]	3%	21%	35%	60–70%
Enhancement	High; central or rim	High; central or rim	High	High with necrosis
FDG uptake on PET	Low	Low	High	High
SRS uptake (%)	80	80	55	Primary: 95; metastasis: 45–60

FDG, ¹⁸F-2-deoxy-D-glucose; *HPFs,* high-power fields; *NA,* not available; *PET,* positron emission tomography; *SRS,* somatostatin receptor scintigraphy.

that has been shown in several small series to be feasible.[162] This strategy may be effective for patients who are deemed inoperable because of comorbidities, or for patients who refuse surgery. New radiation technologies such as stereotactic ablation radiotherapy may also be useful in this setting, but definitive evidence is lacking and surgery, when possible, remains the standard of care.

Large Cell Neuroendocrine Carcinoma

Surgical treatment of LCNEC may be indicated for stage I and II disease, similar to other NSCLC histologic types. However, surgical treatment is rarely an option, as approximately 45% of patients present with metastatic disease (Table 55.4).[135,163] In addition, evidence regarding surgical treatment for LCNEC is rare because no randomized trials have been conducted on the subject.

In a selection of studies, surgical case series of LCNEC were reported, spanning the period from 1982 to 2010 (Table 55.3). The majority of the studies included a pathologic review of all resected tissues. Lobectomy was the most frequently used surgical treatment modality (48% to 95% of patients with LCNEC), although several patients received a pneumonectomy or bilobectomy. Systematical node dissection was performed in most cases, and the reported resection status, R0, was 84% to 100%. The stage of disease was recorded according to pathologic TNM staging editions IV to VII. There was no lymph node involvement in 46% to 75% of patients, but metastasis after resection was reported in 0% to 7% of the cases studied. After resection, 14% to 34% of the patients were treated with adjuvant chemotherapy, although the majority of the postsurgical data were missing.

The reported 5-year survival of patients with resected LCNEC ranged from 28% to 57%, with an average overall survival rate of 43%; however, it should be considered that the vast majority of the patients had stage I to III disease. Five-year survival of patients ranged from 33% to 67% for those with stage I disease and 23% to 75% for those with stage II disease. However, any conclusion is limited by the use of different TNM staging systems, and the adoption of adjuvant chemotherapy varied considerably from one study to another. Recurrence of disease was reported in 40% to 62% of patients.

Adjuvant Treatment
Bronchopulmonary Carcinoids

No prospective trials have directly addressed the benefit of adjuvant therapy for patients with BP carcinoids, although several single-institution retrospective series have evaluated the use of adjuvant radiation and/or chemotherapy. However, these studies tend to be small and had apparently discordant results.[118,156,164–167] Carretta et al.[164] reviewed 44 patients treated with surgical resection, and one patient with clinical stage IIIA disease received neoadjuvant mitomycin-c, vinblastine, and cisplatin and had a partial response, but disease recurred 2 months postoperatively. Of the five patients with N1 disease who received postoperative radiotherapy, none of them had local recurrence.[164] In the study by Paladugu et al.,[168] seven patients with atypical carcinoid who had distant metastases were treated with surgery followed by chemotherapy and all were alive at follow-up (range, 23 months to 127 months). By contrast, Mills et al.[169] did not detect any difference in survival when they compared seven patients with atypical carcinoid treated with adjuvant chemotherapy and radiotherapy with six patients who had a surgical procedure only. Thus adjuvant therapy for completely resected typical or atypical carcinoid, with or without regional node involvement, remains controversial. Despite these limited data, the National Comprehensive Cancer Network suggests the use of chemotherapy with or without radiotherapy for resected stage II or III atypical carcinoid and for stage IIIb typical carcinoid. The North American Neuroendocrine Tumor Society guidelines indicate that there are insufficient data to recommend adjuvant therapy,[159] whereas the European Society for Medical Oncology clinical practice guidelines do not specifically address adjuvant therapy.[170]

Large Cell Neuroendocrine Carcinoma

Evidence regarding adjuvant chemotherapy and radiotherapy for resected LCNEC is limited. Several retrospective case series and one prospective study have been reported. In this chapter, only studies in which treatment for pure or mixed LCNEC were assessed are reviewed. Studies that include LCC with neuroendocrine morphology without neuroendocrine differentiation are not addressed.

In 2006, Iyoda et al.[171] conducted a single-arm, nonrandomized, unblinded prospective trial of patients with resected LCNEC who were treated with postoperative adjuvant cisplatin and etoposide (two cycles). Fifteen patients with resected LCNEC (13 with stage I disease and 4 with stage II or higher), including radical lymph node dissection, were included. The results of the prospective study were compared with the results from a retrospective cohort of 23 patients treated with resected LCNEC without adjuvant chemotherapy; clinical characteristics of the two series were comparable. The authors reported a difference in overall survival, however, with an advantage for the cohort that received adjuvant treatment. The 2-year and 5-year overall survival was 88.9% and 88.9%, respectively, in the treatment group compared with 65.2% and 47.4% in the control group, respectively.

Rossi et al.[172] examined a cohort of 83 patients with resected LCNEC, including 28 patients who received adjuvant chemotherapy. The chemotherapy consisted of SCLC regimens (13 patients) and NSCLC regimens (15 patients), including cisplatin and gemcitabine, carboplatin and paclitaxel, and cisplatin and vinorelbine. Multivariate regression analysis for survival showed that treatment with an NSCLC adjuvant chemotherapy regimen resulted in a relative risk of 15.52 compared with an SCLC regimen, favoring the SCLC regimen ($p = 0.0001$). Stage and tumor size had a relative risk of 2.31 ($p = 0.029$) and 2.15 ($p = 0.013$), respectively. The chemotherapy regimens were not analytically reported. The results were similar in the study by Tanaka et al.[173] of 63 patients with completely resected (R0) LCNEC. Twenty-three (37%) of 63 patients were treated with induction chemotherapy (3 patients) or adjuvant chemotherapy (20 patients). Regimens differed, although all contained a platinum agent (combinations of carboplatin or cisplatin with etoposide, paclitaxel, docetaxel, or vinorelbine). Multivariate analyses showed improved survival for patients treated with adjuvant chemotherapy (hazard ratio [HR], 0.323; $p = 0.037$). Pathologic stage (I vs. II/III) was not a predictor for survival (HR, 0.645; $p = 0.29$). The authors also reported possible chemotherapy resistance in patients with LCNEC who were positive for three neuroendocrine markers (NCAM+, chromogranin A+, and synaptophysin+). In this group of patients with triple-positive LCNEC, chemotherapy did not contribute to increased survival.

Sarkaria et al.[134] evaluated 100 patients with surgically resected LCNEC (and combined LCNEC). Twenty-four patients received induction chemotherapy with a response rate of 63% (15 with partial response, 8 with stable disease, and 1 with progressive disease); 22 (92%) of the 24 patients received a platinum-based chemotherapy regimen. A total of 25 patients received adjuvant chemotherapy, mostly consisting of platinum-based regimens (80%), and 60% received a platinum-based regimen combined with etoposide. Adjuvant radiotherapy was administered to 15 patients. Forty-two patients received both induction chemotherapy and adjuvant chemotherapy. In patients with completely resected IB–IIIA disease, treatment with platinum-based chemotherapy correlated with a nonsignificant trend in increased survival. Multivariate analysis for survival was significant for stage (HR for stage III/IV vs. stage I/II, 2.21; $p = 0.011$), gender, and pulmonary comorbidities. In a study by Veronesi et al.,[174] in which patients with resected LCNEC were evaluated in a retrospective and multicenter setting, 21 patients received induction chemotherapy; among the 15 patients evaluable for response, the response rate was 80% (1 complete response, 11 partial responses, 2 stable disease, and 1 progressive disease). In addition, several patients received radiotherapy postoperatively. Chemotherapy combined with surgery compared with surgery alone was not a significant predictor in the multivariate analysis for survival (HR, 0.6; $p = 0.274$). Stage of disease, age, and type of surgery were significant independent prognostic factors.

Iyoda et al.[175] found that recurrence of disease occurred less frequently among 30 patients who received platinum-based adjuvant chemotherapy compared with 42 patients who received nonplatinum-based adjuvant chemotherapy; disease recurred in 33% of patients who received platinum-based chemotherapy compared with 62% of patients who received nonplatinum-based treatment ($p = 0.017$). However, no information was reported about the type of node dissection, the status of surgical margins (R0, R1, and R2), the exact type of chemotherapy, and the median follow-up of patients.

Preliminary results of neoadjuvant therapy in potentially surgically resectable patients with LCNEC who had a preoperative octreotide scan have been reported in only one study. All patients with positive findings on the scan received the somatostatin analog octreotide, and several patients also received radiotherapy. The results of this study were promising: a significant survival difference ($p = 0.0007$) was found for patients treated with octreotide compared with nontreated patients. Limitations of the study included small sample size (total of 18 patients, 10 of whom were treated) and its retrospective nature.[154]

Currently, in two prospective studies, the efficacy of adjuvant chemotherapy for resected LCNEC is being evaluated. The UMIN000001319 trial is a Japanese single-arm, multicenter, nonblinded randomized phase II study in which the effect of four cycles of cisplatin and irinotecan in both LCNEC and limited-disease resected SCLC is being assessed. Preliminary results from this study showed an overall and recurrence-free survival rate at 3 years of 86% and 74%, respectively, for the LCNEC cohort. Patients were classified as having IA to IIIA disease, and 83% of patients completed chemotherapy.[176] The other prospective study, also from Japan (Trial identifier: UMIN000010298), is a two-arm, randomized double-blind phase III trial in progress that is comparing adjuvant cisplatin and irinotecan with cisplatin and etoposide for stage I–IIIA resected LCNEC.[177]

Therapy for Metastatic Disease

Although there are no definitive guidelines for the treatment of BP carcinoids, the European Neuroendocrine Tumor Society has suggested treatment options according to prognosis. Patients with a good prognosis, including asymptomatic patients with typical carcinoid and no growth within 6 months to 12 months, may be treated with active surveillance, locoregional therapy, or somatostatin analogs. Patients with a poor prognosis (atypical carcinoid or growth within 6 months to 12 months) may be treated with peptide-receptor radiotherapy or palliative chemotherapy, such as temozolomide, streptozotocin (streptozocin) plus interferon, or everolimus.

Palliative Chemotherapy

As BP carcinoids are relatively rare and include a spectrum of pathologic features, there is a lack of robust clinical trial evidence to guide treatment choices. In general, treatment recommendations stem from the experience of treating gastrointestinal carcinoids or extrapolating information from trials on SCLC.

Sun et al.[178] conducted a phase II/III trial in symptomatic carcinoids, randomly assigning patients to 5-fluorouracil (5-FU) and streptozocin or 5-FU and doxorubicin. Response rates were nearly identical at 16% and 15.9% in the two arms, respectively, but the median progression-free survival associated with 5-FU and streptozocin was superior (24.3 months vs. 15.7 months; $p = 0.0267$). At the time of progression, patients received dacarbazine, with a resulting response rate of 8.2%.[178]

In retrospective studies, cisplatin and etoposide have been assessed for the treatment of atypical carcinoid, and the objective response has ranged from 7% to 39%, with a median duration of response ranging from 4 months to 102 months.[177,179–184] Guigay et al.[185] performed a retrospective study in 37 patients with progressive atypical carcinoid, 34 of whom had liver or bone metastases. Patients were treated with either cisplatin and etoposide or 5-FU and streptozocin or other regimens combining 5-FU or doxorubicin. The overall response rate to first-line chemotherapy was 32%; 5-FU and streptozocin resulted in a partial response in six (35%) of 17 patients and stable disease in five (33%). Cisplatin and etoposide resulted in a partial response in three (25%) of 12 and stable disease in four (33%) of 12 in the whole population, and a partial response in two (22%) of nine and stable disease in three (33%) of nine in the population with metastases.

In a number of small studies, temozolomide was evaluated for the treatment of BP carcinoids.[186–188] In a study by Ekeblad et al.,[188] 13 patients with BP carcinoids (10 typical and 3 atypical carcinoids) were treated with temozolomide; four (31%) had a partial response and an additional four patients had stabilization of disease. Crona et al.[187] evaluated 31 patients (14 with typical carcinoid and 15 with atypical carcinoid) also treated with temozolomide and found that 14% of patients had a partial response, 52% had stable disease, and 33% had progressive disease.

Other agents that have resulted in tumor shrinkage include capecitabine and oxaliplatin; capecitabine and liposomal doxorubicin; and 5-FU, dacarbazine, and epirubicin.[189–192] In small studies and case reports of these agents, patient responses fall in the range of 20% to 30% and generally have a short duration. Given the small size of these studies and lack of prospective data, no specific recommendation for a specific chemotherapy regimen can be made and patient participation in a clinical trial should be strongly encouraged.

Liver Metastases-Directed Therapy

The liver is the predominant site of metastases. Hepatic resection may be considered in selected patients with BP carcinoids who have isolated, low-volume liver metastases. Although not curative in nature, this may provide palliation of symptoms secondary to paraneoplastic syndromes and may result in potentially prolonged survival.[193] If liver resection is not feasible, other liver-directed therapies may be performed, including hepatic artery embolization and chemoembolization, radiofrequency ablation, and cryoablation. Treatment of liver metastasis has been shown to be associated with a biochemical response as high as 96%[193] and to reduce carcinoid-related symptoms.[159,194]

Managing Hormonal Symptoms

Somatostatin receptor analogs such as octreotide control symptoms caused by secretion of biologically active peptides or amines in 60% of patients with BP carcinoids. Although partial response is rare (5% to 10%), stable disease occurs in 30% to 50% of patients.[190] Interferon-alpha (IFN-α) is another option, with symptomatic remission reported in 30% to 70% of patients.[195–202] Acromegaly secondary to paraneoplastic growth hormone-releasing hormone secretion is rare, but usually responds to somatostatin or surgical debulking. Cushing syndrome may be treated with ketoconazole, aminoglutethimide, metyrapone, or mifepristone.[159] Octreotide was compared with placebo and shown to have antiproliferative effects in midgut carcinoids with an increase in progression-free survival from 6 months to 14 months (HR, 0.34; $p < 0.0001$).[203] Whether these data can be extrapolated to foregut tumors is uncertain.

Palliative Radiotherapy

BP carcinoid tumors are relatively radiotherapy resistant, and radiotherapy may only be considered when surgery is not feasible or after an incomplete resection. It may also provide pain relief in the case of bone metastases.[182,204]

Peptide receptor radiotherapy uses either [90]yttrium, [111]indium, or [177]lutetium radionuclides linked to a somatostatin analog to allow for targeting of somatostatin receptor-expressing tumor cells. Studies have shown complete and partial response rates of 0% to 8% with [[11]In-DTPA[0]]octreotide;[205,206] 4% to 33% with ^{90}Y-DOTA[0]-Tyr[3]octreotate;[207–211] and 17% to 38% with [117]Lu DOTA[0]-Tyr3octreotate.[212–215] One of the agents, DOTA[0]-Tyr[3]octreotate, was evaluated in 16 patients with foregut carcinoids, of which nine were BP carcinoids. Of the nine patients with BP carcinoids, five had a partial response, one had a minor response (tumor size reduction between 25% and 50%), two had stable disease, and one had progressive disease. The median time to progression was 31 months.[216] Long-term side effects of radiopeptide treatment may include decreased renal function, pancytopenia, and myelodysplastic syndrome. This therapeutic strategy is being evaluated further in several ongoing randomized, prospective trials. While the results are awaited, the use of radiopeptides for the treatment of advanced bronchial carcinoids remains investigational. Ongoing trials include the randomized registration trial of [117]Lu-octreotate plus octreotide acetate injection (30 mg every 4 weeks), compared with high-dose octreotide acetate injection (60 mg every 4 weeks) in midgut carcinoids only.

Surgery

In patients with indolent-behaving BP carcinoids and limited metastatic disease, surgical intervention may be warranted. Not only has surgery been shown to palliate symptoms, but it also may provide a disease-free survival benefit and potential cure. Que et al.[217] demonstrated that resecting liver metastases in liver-only metastatic bronchial carcinoids could result in a so-called cure in 20% of the treated patients.

Interferon

IFN-α has been shown to have a tumor response rate of 12% in a pooled analysis of several studies;[218] it has also been studied in combination with somatostatin analogs. Compared with octreotide alone, the combination of octreotide and IFN-α improved progression-free survival (HR, 0.28; 95% confidence interval, 0.16–0.45).[219] However, objective response rates were equally low in a study comparing IFN-α (4%), lanreotide (4%), or lanreotide plus IFN-α (7%).[220]

Molecularly Targeted Therapy

A subgroup of 44 BP carcinoids was included in a randomized phase III trial (RADIANT-3) comparing octreotide acetate injection with or without everolimus in 429 patients with advanced carcinoid tumors. Thirty-three patients were randomly assigned to everolimus plus octreotide and 11 to placebo and octreotide. The median progression-free survival was increased in the group receiving everolimus (13.6 months vs. 5.6 months). However,

almost half of patients who received everolimus had grade 3 or grade 4 adverse events, including stomatitis, diarrhea, and thrombocytopenia.[221] RAMSETE is a phase II trial evaluating everolimus as monotherapy in advanced nonpancreatic neuroendocrine tumors (35% foregut). Of the 19 patients with foregut carcinoids, none had a complete response or partial response, 12 had stable disease, and 7 patients had progressive disease. The median progression-free survival was 189 days.[222]

In a small series of 17 typical carcinoids, 5 tumors were shown to be IHC positive for c-Kit, 9 for platelet-derived growth factor beta, 12 for platelet-derived growth factor receptor alpha, and 7 for epidermal growth factor receptor. This raised the question of whether the use of specific tyrosine kinase inhibitors targeting these pathways is of clinical utility.[184]

Antiangiogenic agents have been assessed in several small phase II trials in advanced neuroendocrine tumors; however, foregut or BP carcinoids were only included in three studies.[223–226] Yao et al.[223] evaluated bevacizumab and octreotide LAR in 22 patients (4 bronchial carcinoid) and reported an overall response rate of 18%; Kulke et al.[224] investigated sunitinib in 107 patients (14 foregut) and reported an overall response rate of 2.4% and disease stabilization in 82.9% of patients. The median time to disease progression was 10.2 months. Castellano et al.[225] evaluated sorafenib and bevacizumab in 44 patients (19 foregut carcinoids) and found an overall response rate of 10%; however, Chan et al.[226] found no objective responses in the group of patients with carcinoid tumors in a phase II trial who were treated with temozolomide and bevacizumab. Based on these data, no definite conclusions can be made on the efficacy of antiangiogenic agents for the treatment of bronchial carcinoids.

An ongoing phase III trial (RADIANT-4) is comparing everolimus with placebo for advanced neuroendocrine tumors of gastrointestinal or lung origin (ClinicalTrials.gov identifier: NCT01524783). Other ongoing trials include the LUNA study, a randomized three-arm trial of pasireotide compared with everolimus alone or in combination for patients with advanced neuroendocrine tumors of the lung or thymus (ClinicalTrials.gov identifier: NCT01563354). Both trials have progression-free survival as the primary end point.

Therapy for Metastatic Large Cell Neuroendocrine Carcinoma

There is minimal evidence supporting the use of systemic therapy for metastatic LCNEC. As previously mentioned, LCNEC is a rare disease and diagnosis is based on histology from larger surgical biopsy specimens. In metastatic lung cancer, surgical biopsies are scarce. In the majority of studies reporting on advanced LCNEC, the diagnosis is based on a small biopsy sample or resected LCNEC case series containing metastatic recurrence of disease after surgical resection.

At the time of publication, two small single-arm, prospective multicenter phase II studies have been conducted in metastatic LCNEC. Both studies evaluated an SCLC chemotherapy regimen; in a European study of 42 patients, the regimen was cisplatin and etoposide; in a Japanese study of 44 patients, the regimen was cisplatin and irinotecan.[227,228] All patients had stage IIIB or IV disease, were chemotherapy naïve, and had an Eastern Cooperative Oncology Group performance status of less than 2. A central pathology review was performed in more than 95% of the patients. The diagnosis was revised in 25% of the patients who received cisplatin and etoposide and 28% of the patients who received cisplatin and irinotecan. The majority of revised diagnoses were SCLC.

In the cisplatin and irinotecan study, patients with confirmed LCNEC had a response rate of 47%; no patients had a complete response, 14 had a partial response, 10 had stable disease, and

6 had progressive disease. The median progression-free survival time was 5.8 months (range, 3.8 months to 7.8 months), and median overall survival was 12.6 months (range, 9.3 months to 16.0 months). Compared with the 10 patients who were diagnosed with SCLC in this study, patients with LCNEC had a significantly shorter overall survival time (12.6 months vs. 17.3 months; $p = 0.047$), although median progression-free survival was similar. Thirty patients (65%) completed four cycles of chemotherapy. Second-line chemotherapy consisted mostly of amrubicin (a drug registered only in Japan), platinum-based chemotherapy, and docetaxel. The response rate of second-line chemotherapy was not reported.

In the study of cisplatin and etoposide, patients with confirmed LCNEC had a response rate of 34%: no patients had a complete response, 10 had a partial response, and 9 had stable disease, with progression-free survival of 5.0 months (range, 4.0 months to 7.9 months) and overall survival of 8.0 months (range, 3.7 months to 7.9 months). In the other histology group, which consisted of nine patients with SCLC, one with atypical carcinoid, and one with neuroendocrine-expressing NSCLC, the progression-free survival was 3.1 months (range, 2.8 months to 8.5 months) and overall survival was 7.0 months (range, 3.0 months to 9.0 months). There was no significant difference between patients with LCNEC and the other histology group ($p = 0.55$). The reported median follow-up was 37.2 months.

The published literature includes several retrospective studies in which NSCLC-based regimens are evaluated; however, only a limited number of cases are reported. Rossi et al.[172] reported on 15 patients with resected LCNEC who were treated with cisplatin and gemcitabine or carboplatin and paclitaxel and gemcitabine monotherapy at the time of disease recurrence. None of the patients who received NSCLC-based therapy had a response, but six patients who received an SCLC regimen had an objective response. Sun et al.[229] performed a study of 45 patients with LCNEC treated with regimens specifically for SCLC or NSCLC. The authors reported a response rate of 73% (8 of 11 patients) in the group treated with SCLC regimens compared with a rate of 50% (17 of 34 patients) in the group treated with NSCLC regimens ($p = 0.19$). Platinum-based regimens combined with etoposide or irinotecan yielded a response rate of 73% in the SCLC group and 100% in the NSCLC group. Platinum-based regimens containing gemcitabine resulted in a response in 41% of the patients. In another study, approximately five of seven patients had a response to a combination of a platinum agent and paclitaxel.[230]

Available information about second-line chemotherapy for the treatment of LCNEC is almost nonexistent. In one retrospective study, a response rate of 23% (3 of 13 patients) was documented for second-line amrubicin monotherapy.[231] A single-arm, nonblinded phase II study of bevacizumab and docetaxel for second-line chemotherapy after platinum-based chemotherapy has been initiated in Japan (Trial identifier: UMIN000011713).

Molecularly Targeted Therapies

Targeted therapies have yet to be fully investigated for the treatment of LCNEC. In addition, the role of octreotide analogs has not been investigated in LCNEC.

There has only been one study in which SSTR-targeted therapies have been described, and prolonged overall survival was reported in patients with SSTR-positive metastatic disease.[232]

In a multicenter open-label, single-arm phase II study in Germany that was ongoing at the time of publication, the mTOR inhibitor everolimus is combined with paclitaxel and carboplatin for the treatment of advanced LCNEC. Recruitment is ongoing, and results have not been presented as yet.

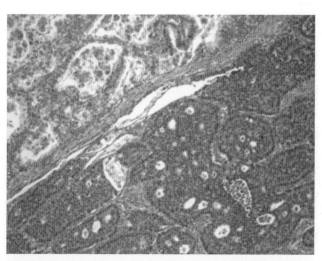

Fig. 55.5. Low-magnification view of a pulmonary large cell neuroendocrine carcinoma *(lower right corner)* combined with adenocarcinoma *(upper left corner*; hematoxylin and eosin, 40×). *(Courtesy Dr M. Béndek, Maastricht University Medical Centre, the Netherlands.)*

COMBINED LCNEC

LCNEC can be expressed as a pure form of the disease, but it can also be expressed in combination with other solid tumors. LCNEC is commonly seen in combination with an adenocarcinoma or squamous cell carcinoma component (Fig. 55.5). Other rare forms are combinations of LCNEC and giant cell carcinoma or spindle cell carcinoma. The exact incidence of combined LCNEC is unknown, but it has been reported to be between 6% and 31% in large series of surgically resected LCNEC (Table 55.3).[6,134,233,234] At the present time, combined tumors with an LCNEC component should be classified as combined LCNEC and treated as LCNEC, with the exception of LCNEC combined with SCLC, which should be classified as a combined SCLC and treated as SCLC.

PROGNOSIS

Bronchopulmonary Carcinoids

Patients with typical carcinoids have an excellent prognosis after surgical resection, with 5-year survival rates of 87% to 100% and 10-year survival rates of 82% to 87%. Typical carcinoids tend to be indolent tumors, with only 7% metastasizing after adequate resection. The prognostic effect of lymph node positivity is controversial. In some studies, no negative impact of node involvement was found, although other studies have shown a negative impact.[119,216,235,236] The only accepted negative prognostic feature is incomplete resection.

Atypical carcinoids have lower 5-year survival rates, ranging from 30% to 95%, depending on the series; corresponding 10-year survival rates are 35% to 56%. Atypical carcinoids have a higher propensity to metastasize (16% and 23% in two large series) and to recur locally (3% and 23% in the same two series).[237] In contrast to typical carcinoids, lymph node metastases in atypical carcinoids have a clear negative effect on prognosis.[238] In a series from the Mayo Clinic, 19 (83%) of 23 patients with typical carcinoids and lymph node metastases remained alive and disease free; however, four (17%) had distant recurrence, two of whom died.[239] Conversely, only four of 11 patients with atypical carcinoids and lymph node involvement were alive without recurrence, and six of seven in whom distant metastases developed died. More recently, evaluation of potential prognostic biomarkers was performed by quantitative real-time polymerase chain reaction. Low mRNA expression levels of CD44 and orthopedia homeobox and high levels of ret proto-oncogene (RET) were strongly associated with a low 20-year survival in patients with carcinoids. A direct link between gene expression and protein levels was confirmed for CD44 and orthopedia homeobox, but not for RET.[144,240]

Large Cell Neuroendocrine Carcinoma

Asamura et al.[234] reported that the survival curve for LCNEC is superimposable to that for SCLC. Depending on the series, 5-year survival rates ranged from 33% to 62% for stage I, 18% to 75% for stage II, 8% to 45% for stage III, and 0% for stage IV.[171,172,174,234]

CONCLUSION

Bronchial neuroendocrine tumors are a class of tumors arising from the neuroendocrine cells of the BP epithelium. The behavior of bronchial neuroendocrine tumors varies with their degree of differentiation: typical carcinoids have a more indolent behavior, rarely metastasizing; atypical carcinoids that are intermediate grade have an increased tendency to spread systemically; and LCNECs are high grade, with an aggressive phenotype similar to that in SCLC. Surgical resection of localized disease remains the standard of care for bronchial neuroendocrine tumors. For metastatic carcinoids, no current standard of care exists and participation in clinical trials should be considered for patients with these rare entities. Although metastatic LCNEC resembles SCLC in clinical behavior, the optimal chemotherapy regimen is not clear in this setting.

KEY REFERENCES

8. Travis WD, Brambilla E, Müller-Hermelink HK, Harris CC. *World Health Organization Classification of Tumours. Pathology & Genetics. Tumours of the Lung, Pleura, Thymus and Heart.* Lyon, France: IARC Press; 2004:19–25.
123. Filosso PL, Rena O, Donati G, et al. Bronchial carcinoid tumors: surgical management and long-term outcome. *J Thorac Cardiovasc Surg.* 2002;123(2):303–309.
149. Righi L, Volante M, Tavaglione V, et al. Somatostatin receptor tissue distribution in lung neuroendocrine tumours: a clinicopathologic and immunohistochemical study of 218 "clinically aggressive" cases. *Ann Oncol.* 2010;21(3):548–555.
157. Lucchi M, Melfi F, Ribechini A, et al. Sleeve and wedge parenchyma-sparing bronchial resections in low-grade neoplasms of the bronchial airway. *J Thorac Cardiovasc Surg.* 2007;134(2):373–377.
159. Phan AT, Oberg K, Choi J, et al. NANETS consensus guideline for the diagnosis and management of neuroendocrine tumors: well-differentiated neuroendocrine tumors of the thorax (includes lung and thymus). *Pancreas.* 2010;39(6):784–798.
178. Sun W, Lipsitz S, Catalano P, Mailliard JA, Haller DG. Eastern Cooperative Oncology Group. Phase II/III study of doxorubicin with fluorouracil compared with streptozocin with fluorouracil or dacarbazine in the treatment of advanced carcinoid tumors: Eastern Cooperative Oncology Group Study E1281. *J Clin Oncol.* 2005;23(22):4897–4904.
181. Fjallskog ML, Granberg DP, Welin SL, et al. Treatment with cisplatin and etoposide in patients with neuroendocrine tumors. *Cancer.* 2000;92(5):1101–1107.
221. Fazio N, Granberg D, Grossman A, et al. Everolimus plus octreotide long-acting repeatable in patients with advanced lung neuroendocrine tumors: analysis of the phase 3, randomized, placebo-controlled RADIANT-2 study. *Chest.* 2013;143(4):955–962.
229. Sun JM, Ahn MJ, Ahn JS, et al. Chemotherapy for pulmonary large cell neuroendocrine carcinoma: similar to that for small cell lung cancer or non-small cell lung cancer? *Lung Cancer.* 2012;77(2):365–370.

See Expertconsult.com for full list of references.

56 Thymic Tumors

Enrico Ruffini, Walter Weder, Pier Luigi Filosso, and Nicolas Girard

SUMMARY OF KEY POINTS

- Thymic tumors are rare malignancies and represent a wide array of tumors.
- Histologic classification distinguishes three separate entities: thymomas, thymic carcinomas, and neuroendocrine thymic tumors.
- Thymomas are characterized by variability in histologic appearance as well as in clinical behavior.
- Systemic paraneoplastic syndromes occur in almost 40% of patients, with myasthenia gravis being the most commonly reported.
- Patients with thymoma have an increased risk for the development of second malignancies and less than 40% of the patients will die from the original neoplastic disease, with the percentage being stage dependent.
- Several staging systems have been proposed, with the Masaoka staging system being more frequently used. A new tumor, node, metastasis (TNM) staging system will be implemented as the result of a global collaboration.
- Stage at presentation is the main prognostic factor.
- Surgery is the main treatment for thymic tumors, and radical resection is the goal.
- Other treatment modalities including radiotherapy and chemotherapy are used in the context of a multimodality approach.
- Thymic tumors are generally chemosensitive, with thymomas being more sensitive than thymic carcinomas. Exclusive chemotherapy is usually considered for patients medically or technically not qualified for surgical resection or in the presence of metastatic disease.

Thymic tumors are rare, although they are the most common tumors in the anterior mediastinal compartment. Despite their common term, thymic tumors represent a wide variety of tumors that, until recently, have been considered within one category. The most recent histologic classification, however, clearly distinguishes thymic tumors as three separate entities: thymomas, thymic carcinomas, and neuroendocrine thymic tumors (NETTs). In the past decade, the scientific community has been increasingly interested in thymic malignancies, resulting in the creation of many thymic tumors working groups and international thymic interest groups. As a consequence, dramatic advances have been made in our knowledge of the clinical and basic aspects of these rare diseases, providing important benefits for patients.

This chapter provides an overview of the most recent findings in the diagnosis, staging, histology, and management strategies of thymic tumors.

THYMOMA

Demographics and Clinical Presentation

Thymomas are rare neoplasms arising from the thymic epithelial cells. They are characterized by an extreme variability in histologic appearance, as well as in clinical behavior. The actual incidence of these diseases is unknown, but data from 2003 show an overall incidence in the United States of 0.15 cases/100,000 person-years.[1] Thymomas are the most common anterior mediastinal tumors in adults, accounting for about 50% of all mediastinal tumors. They can occur in all ages, but a peak in the incidence of thymomas associated with myasthenia gravis has been noted among individuals between the ages of 30 years and 40 years. A peak has also been noted among people (primarily women) aged between 60 years and 70 years who do not have myasthenia gravis.[2] Although in most series the gender distribution differs, the difference is not significant, and men and women are equally affected, especially when clinical series of more than 100 patients are considered.[3] Other malignant lesions (e.g., lymphoma, parathyroid and thyroid tumors, germ cell tumors, and mesenchymal and neurogenic neoplasms) as well as nonmalignant masses in the anterior mediastinum (e.g., aneurysms, granulomas, pericardial and esophageal cysts, and Morgagni hernias, as well as thymic hyperplasia) should be taken into account in the differential diagnosis. About 30% of patients with thymoma are asymptomatic. In these cases, the lesion is incidentally discovered, usually on chest radiographs. Among symptomatic patients, approximately 40% have local symptoms related to the intrathoracic mass, 30% have systemic symptoms, and the remaining have symptoms related to associated myasthenia gravis.[4] The most common local symptoms are chest pain, cough, and shortness of breath. In case of invasive neoplasms, common symptoms include superior vena cava (SVC) syndrome (Fig. 56.1), hemidiaphragm paralysis caused by phrenic nerve involvement (Fig. 56.2), and hoarseness due to recurrent laryngeal nerve infiltration. Pleural effusion and chest pain have also been noted in cases of pleural spread of the tumor.

Systemic paraneoplastic diseases occur in about 40% of patients with thymoma (Table 56.1).[4]

Myasthenia Gravis

Myasthenia gravis is, by far, the most commonly associated paraneoplastic disease in patients with thymoma. Thymoma has been found in 10% of patients with myasthenia gravis, and myasthenia gravis ultimately develops in 30% to 50% of patients with thymoma. Between 4% and 7% of patients with thymoma and myasthenia gravis have more than one paraneoplastic syndrome. Myasthenia gravis is very rarely associated with thymic carcinoma or type A or type AB thymoma, but, according to the World Health Organization (WHO) histologic classification, myasthenia gravis is significantly present in type B tumors and is usually found in early-stage disease.[5,6] Patients with thymoma and myasthenia gravis tend to be 10 to 15 years older than patients with myasthenia gravis who do not have thymoma, and slightly younger than patients with thymoma who do not have myasthenia gravis. Although the association between thymoma and myasthenia gravis is concurrent, it is not unusual to diagnose

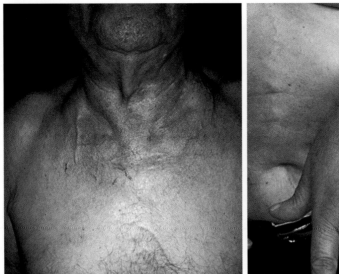
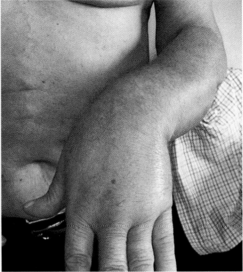

Fig. 56.1. Superior vena cava syndrome in a patient with advanced thymoma causing superior vena cava obstruction. The superficial chest venous network and the upper limb edema are evident.

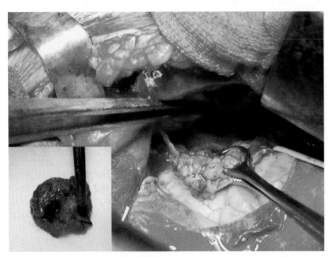

Fig. 56.2. Phrenic nerve involvement in an invasive thymic carcinoma.

thymoma up to a few years after myasthenia gravis. Kondo and Monden[7] reported that postoperative myasthenia gravis developed in about 1% of their patients who underwent complete thymoma resection. The authors concluded that resection of the thymus gland does not prevent myasthenia gravis from developing postoperatively.

Other Neurologic Syndromes

Neuromyotonia, isolated or in association with central nervous system involvement (Morvan syndrome), is frequently found in patients with thymoma.[8] Neuromyotonia is characterized by the presence of generalized muscle twitching and cramps, with electromyographic findings that are consistent with hyperexcitability of peripheral motor nerves (myokymic and neuromyotonic discharges). Other neurologic syndromes have been reported in association with thymic tumors.[9]

Hematologic Disorders

Pure red cell aplasia and hypogammaglobulinemia (Good syndrome) are the other two conditions more frequently associated with thymoma, occurring in 2% to 5% of cases.[10] Patients with

pure red cell anemia are usually older than patients with thymoma alone (mean age, 60 years), and the mean age is 50 years for patients with Good syndrome. Women are slightly more commonly affected than men.

Extrathymic Second Malignancies

According to the scientific literature, patients with thymoma have an increased risk for the development of second malignancies. Filosso et al.[11] reported that patients with thymoma have an approximately twofold higher risk for the development of a second cancer, compared with the normal population. An intrinsic immune abnormality, of which the tumor itself may be a marker, was suggested as a possible explanation. As noted by Welsh et al.,[12] these tumors are true second cancers rather than cancers related to possible postoperative treatment (e.g., radiotherapy) of thymoma.

Diagnostic Imaging Techniques

Imaging plays a central role in diagnosing and staging thymoma. The initial decision to either perform surgery or further investigate the tumor with tissue analysis is primarily based on the findings of computed tomography (CT), magnetic resonance imaging (MRI), and/or positron emission tomography (PET)/CT. The chosen imaging modality should allow the physician to determine the tumor size, local invasion, and the presence of distant spread of the disease. Based on the information, the physician decides if direct surgery is indicated or if preoperative (induction) therapy (stage III or IV disease) is needed. Follow-up imaging of treated patients is used to identify recurrence and resectable recurrent disease. Patients with completely resected recurrent disease have similar outcomes to those without recurrence.[13] Conventional chest radiography is usually the chosen imaging modality for the initial investigation of thymoma, followed by chest CT. It is important to differentiate between nonneoplastic thymic enlargement and thymoma. In young children, the thymus and the hyperplastic thymus can mimic a mediastinal mass. On CT images, thymic hyperplasia appears as a diffusely and symmetrically enlarged thymus with smooth borders and preservation of the normal thymic shape.[14] It may also alter the shape to a more nodal appearance, and it can even show an uptake of ^{18}F-2-deoxy-D-glucose (FDG).[15] Chemical-shift magnetic resonance (MR), with in-phase and out-of-phase gradient echo sequences, may be

TABLE 56.1	Paraneoplastic Syndromes Associated With Thymoma
Hematologic syndromes	Red cell aplasia
	Pancytopenia
	Multiple myeloma
	Megakaryocytopenia
	Hemolytic anemia
Neuromuscular disorders	Myasthenia gravis
	Lambert–Eaton syndrome
	Myotonic dystrophy
	Myositis
	Neuromyotonia (Morvan syndrome)
	Stiff-person syndrome
	Limbic encephalopathy
Collagen diseases and autoimmune disorders	Systemic lupus erythematosus
	Sjögren syndrome
	Rheumatoid arthritis
	Polymyositis
	Myocarditis
	Sarcoidosis
	Scleroderma
	Ulcerative colitis
Endocrine disorders	Addison disease
	Hashimoto thyroiditis
	Hyperparathyroidism
Immunodeficiency syndromes	Hyopogammaglobulinemia
	T-cell–deficiency syndrome
Dermatologic disorders	Pemphigus
	Alopecia areata
	Chronic mucocutaneous candidiasis
Renal diseases	Nephrotic syndrome
	Minimal change disease
Bone disorders	Hypertrophic osteoarthropathy
Malignant diseases	Carcinomas (lung, colon, stomach, breast, thyroid)
	Kaposi sarcoma
	Malignant lymphoma

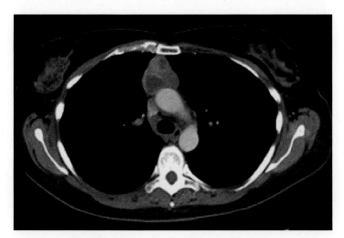

Fig. 56.3. Computed tomography of thymoma.

helpful for differentiation because it identifies the normal fatty infiltration that is unlikely in thymoma.[16,17]

CT with an intravenous contrast medium is the imaging modality of choice for evaluating thymoma and can help distinguish thymoma from other anterior mediastinal abnormalities (Fig. 56.3). Typically, on CT images, thymomas appear as spherical or ovoid, smooth, 5-cm to 10-cm anterior mediastinal masses. They have been described as ranging from a few millimeters to 34 cm in diameter. The tumor enhances homogeneously and may present with lobulated borders. In cases of hemorrhage or necrosis, it becomes heterogeneous or even cystic. The tumor can be partially or completely outlined by fat and may contain punctate,

coarse, or curvilinear calcifications.[18] Ipsilateral pleural nodules are suggestive of stage IVA (disseminated pleural) disease. CT has been thought to have a limited role in the detection of tumor invasiveness. Retrospective studies showed that partial or complete obliteration of fat planes around the tumor was not helpful in differentiating stage I thymoma from more advanced disease. Lobulated or irregular contours, cystic or necrotic regions within the tumor, and multifocal calcifications were more suggestive of invasive thymoma.[14,19]

Although the use of MR has decreased with the advances in multidetector CT and has been insufficiently studied for staging and follow-up, it still plays an important role in the investigation of the anterior mediastinal masses and in the staging of thymoma in patients with contraindication to CT. Thymoma presents with low to intermediate signal intensity on T1-weighted images and with high signal intensity on T2-weighted images.[20] Signal intensity is heterogeneous in tumors with necrosis, hemorrhage, or cystic change. Especially in patients with cystic masses, MR allows a distinction between congenital cyst and cystic thymoma, because fibrous septa and/or mural nodules are typically present in cystic thymoma but absent in a congenital cyst. These septa and nodules are often not evident on CT. Although CT is superior to MRI in the depiction of calcification within thymomas, MRI can occasionally reveal fibrous septa within the mass and can permit better evaluation of the tumor capsule. The presence of fibrous septa was shown to be associated with a less aggressive histologic classification.[21] In addition, the predominance of a necrotic or cystic component and heterogeneous enhancement were seen as signs of aggressiveness and were much more common with thymic cancer than with thymoma.[21]

Nuclear medicine plays a minor role in the routine evaluation of thymoma. Indium-111 octreotide shows uptake in thymoma and is used to identify patients who may respond to treatment with octreotide, which is considered to be the second or third choice of therapy when conventional chemotherapy fails.[22] The precise role of FDG-PET in the management of thymomas is unclear. One difficulty is that increased physiologic FDG uptake is common in a normal or hyperplastic thymus, especially in children and in adults younger than 40 years of age.[14]

Imaging During Follow-Up

The International Thymic Malignancies Interest Group (ITMIG) and the European Society for Medical Oncology (ESMO) Clinical Practice Guidelines suggest that, at a minimum, yearly chest CT should be performed for 5 years after surgical resection, and then alternating annually with chest radiography until year 11, followed by annual chest radiography alone, because late recurrences are common.[23,24] For patients with advanced-stage disease (stage III or IVA), thymic carcinoma, or for those who had incomplete tumor resection, chest CT every 6 months for 2 to 3 years is recommended. The ITMIG also suggests using MR to reduce the cumulative radiation dose. However, there is no study comparing the accuracy of CT with that of MR for identifying tumor recurrence.

Histologic Diagnosis

When the results of imaging techniques are equivocal for a diagnosis of a thymic tumor, cytohistologic diagnosis is required. In the past, it was suggested that, to obtain a definite diagnosis, every anterior mediastinal lesion should be subjected to biopsy before deciding on final treatment. In more recent years, however, refinements in imaging techniques have resulted in an improved diagnostic yield, and the need for a mediastinal biopsy has dramatically decreased. In a survey among European Society of Thoracic Surgeons (ESTS) members, 90% of the interviewed centers stated that they do not routinely look for a histologic confirmation of a suspected thymoma.[25] However, there is a general agreement that biopsy should be considered in the case of undefined CT findings that may suggest lymphoma, or in the case of unresectable tumors before induction chemotherapy or definitive chemoradiation therapy.[26–29]

Mediastinal Biopsy Techniques

Nonsurgical Biopsies. Nonsurgical biopsies include fine-needle aspiration biopsy and core-needle biopsy using transthoracic ultrasound or CT. Both techniques are performed with the patient under local anesthesia and light sedation and require patient compliance. Because of the broad spectrum of tissue types in the anterior mediastinum and the variety of cell morphologies even within the same lesion, the results of pathologic evaluation are extremely dependent on the area where aspiration is performed. In one report, the accuracy of evaluation of fine-needle biopsy samples was relatively poor in several areas, including differentiation between invasive and noninvasive thymoma, differentiation between thymoma and lymphoma, diagnosis of thymic hyperplasia, diagnosis of Castleman disease, subtyping of lymphoma, and differentiation among nonseminomatous germ cell tumor, carcinoma, and large cell lymphoma.[30] Percutaneous core-needle biopsy is suitable for large tumors located mostly in the anterior mediastinum. This procedure provides a larger volume of tissue than fine-needle aspiration does, and the architecture of the material sampled is preserved, allowing for more sophisticated laboratory analysis, such as electron microscopy, flow cytometry, immunocytochemistry, and measurement of surface tumor markers, all of which increase diagnostic specificity.[31] In a series of 70 patients who had percutaneous core cutting-needle biopsy for masses in the anterior mediastinum, adequate material was obtained in 89% of the patients, with an overall sensitivity of 92%.[32] Evaluation of a specimen obtained by CT-guided fine-needle aspiration established the diagnosis in 69% of cases, with a sensitivity and a specificity of 71% and 94%, respectively, and with fewer side effects than are associated with core-needle biopsy. However, this technique decreases the possibility of an adequate discrimination between thymic carcinoma and thymoma, which is crucial for the correct treatment of patients.[33] The advantages of the percutaneous image-guided fine-needle aspiration and core-needle biopsies are that they are minimally invasive, safe, and reproducible. They can be done in an outpatient setting, achieve good cosmetic results, and are cost-effective. The disadvantages are the low diagnostic accuracy and higher morbidity in small lesions, an unnecessary delay in diagnosis and therapy if not conclusive (thymoma and lymphoma), and the requirement for an expert investigator and an experienced cytopathologist. Accuracy of biopsies are also dependent on the use of immunocytochemical and histochemical markers, including cytokeratins (CKs) and p63 expression for normal and neoplastic epithelial cells and terminal deoxynucleotidyl transferase expression in immature T cells (usually observed in types AB, B1, B2, and B3 thymomas, and absent in carcinomas and type A thymomas).[28]

Surgical Biopsies

Surgical biopsies include anterior mediastinotomy (Chamberlain procedure), video-assisted thoracoscopic surgery (VATS), and mini-thoracotomy.[34] VATS permits excellent exposure of the entire mediastinum and allows precise dissection. This technique is a valuable tool, particularly in cases of masses with difficult access that require direct vision, such as tumors with proximity to neurovascular structures or to the vessels of the heart.[35] In addition to the possibility of allowing selective and large biopsies of mediastinal masses, VATS provides a better evaluation of the relationship to other thoracic organs as well as an evaluation of invasion of extracapsular spread.[36]

The sensitivity of the surgical techniques is far higher (more than 98%) than that of nonsurgical techniques, although the morbidity and the surgical stress should be taken into consideration in the choice of the technique.

The complication rate is generally low after histologic techniques on the mediastinum, and pneumothorax is the most common complication of nonsurgical techniques, occurring in 5% to 30% of the cases, depending on the location of the mass. Complications of surgical procedures are minimal. Seeding of the pleural space or the biopsy site has been a concern in the past, but there is no evidence to support that in the literature.[37]

Staging Systems

Before an official stage classification system for thymic malignancies has been defined by the Union Internationale Contre le Cancer and The American Joint Commission on Cancer,[38] several different systems (Masaoka, Masaoka–Koga, TNM Classification of Malignant Tumours [TNM], Groupe d'Etude des Tumeurs Thymique) are actually being used.[25] Historically, the proposed staging systems were designed on single-center experience of small series of patients who had surgery. In most cases these systems are empirically derived. Although several studies have provided some correlation with outcomes, the limited number of patients and infrequent validation in an independent set of patients generally provide little basis for choosing between one system and another.

Non-TNM Staging Systems

During the 1960s, thymoma was classified as invasive and non-invasive, and four histologic subtypes were recognized. The first staging system was proposed by Bergh et al. in 1978.[39] They designed a three-stage classification system based on 43 patients with thymoma who were treated from 1954 to 1975. Wilkins and Castleman[40] proposed a second staging system, based on minor changes to the system by Bergh et al. Masaoka et al.[41] first highlighted that the clinical course of thymoma is influenced by its local invasion, infiltration, and, finally, by distant spread with lymphogenous or hematogenous metastases. They also demonstrated the clinical importance of tumor local invasiveness as compared with lymphogenous or hematogenous metastasis, with a step-wise decrease in survival. A four-stage system was proposed in 1981, based on 93 patients (Box 56.1). Lastly, Koga et al.[42] proposed a revised Masaoka staging system in 1994 (see Box 56.1). The Masaoka–Koga staging system was clinically validated in a large series by Kondo et al.,[43,44] and it was recommended by the ITMIG in 2011. In 2012, Moran et al.[45] proposed a four-tiered staging system designed exclusively for thymomas. The major changes from the Masaoka system were the addition of stage 0 for encapsulated tumors (Masaoka stage I) and the shifting to a stage I, II, and IIIA,B from Masaoka stages II, III, and IVA,B, respectively. Moran et al.[45] considered stage 0 thymoma similar to an in situ malignancy or a premalignant neoplasm.

TNM-Based Staging Systems

In thymomas, the rate of lymphogenous and hematogenous metastases is about 2% and 1%, respectively. Local spread is the most common pattern of tumor invasion, and it may be precisely evaluated by the surgeon at the time of intervention. In this case, a staging system based on local invasion (such as Masaoka or Masaoka–Koga) seems to be suitable. However, thymic carcinomas and NETTs frequently present with lymphogenous (25%) and hematogenous metastases (12%). For these tumors, a TNM-based staging system is advisable. Several TNM-based staging systems for thymic tumors have been proposed in the past. Yamakawa and Masaoka[46] translated the Masaoka system into a new TNM-based system. In their new system, the T descriptor was the same as in the Masaoka system, and the anterior mediastinal lymph nodes around the thymus were considered the primary lymph nodes, and classified as N1. Tumors were classified as M0 or M1 according to the absence or presence of hematogenous spread. Tsuchiya et al.[48] proposed a TNM system specifically for thymic carcinoma. In their system, the N descriptor was the same as in the Yamakawa and Masaoka system, but tumors penetrating through the mediastinal pleura or pericardium were classified as T3, and the stage grouping allowed a much greater role for node involvement. In 2004, a TNM-based staging system for thymic tumors was proposed by the WHO, in which the T descriptor paralleled the stratification in the Masaoka system, and the N descriptor included involvement of anterior mediastinal nodes (N1), intrathoracic nodes other than anterior mediastinal ones (N2), and extrathoracic nodes (including scalene, supraclavicular, etc., N3; see Box 56.1). The stage grouping divided stage III (N1) from stage IV (N2). All TNM-based systems, however, lack validation. Staging became even more confusing when Weissferdt and Moran[47] proposed a three-stage TNM classification for thymic carcinoma in 2012. In this system, the major features are the classification of T1 as a tumor confined to the thymus and T3 as direct extension outside the chest, the limitation of node categories to intrathoracic, and the grouping of any T3, N1, or M1 tumors as stage III.

A new TNM-based system is expected in 2017, based on a collaborative effort between the ITMIG and the International Association for the Study of Lung Cancer (IASLC), through the analysis of survival in a retrospective international database of more than 10,000 cases (Table 56.2).[48] Given the major switch that the TNM system represents and the limited amount of fair level of evidence data to support our current treatment strategies (especially postoperative radiotherapy), the value of the TNM system to drive the therapeutic strategy has to be assessed. Meanwhile, the new TNM staging may even provide more help in formalizing resectability: T1–T3 level of invasion refers to structures amenable to surgical resection, whereas T4 level of invasion includes unresectable structures. A proposed nodal map is available from the ITMIG.[49] The proposed N descriptor in the staging system includes:

- the anterior region (N1), which involves the anterior mediastinal nodes (prevascular, para-aortic, ascending aorta, superior and inferior phrenic, and supradiaphragmatic) and the anterior cervical nodes (low anterior cervical); and
- the deep region (N2), which includes the middle mediastinal (internal mammary, upper and lower paratracheal, subaortic, subcarinal, and hilar) and the deep cervical (lower jugular and supraclavicular).

HISTOLOGY OF THYMIC TUMORS

Thymoma

Thymomas are epithelial tumors mixed with reactive lymphocytes. They are ultrastructurally characterized by desmosomes and tonofilaments and are primarily found in the anterosuperior mediastinum.[2] Atypical localization within the thyroid, the pericardium, the lung parenchyma, and hilum is documented, and they can even coat the pleura in a mesothelioma-like fashion.

Overall, thymomas are generally solid, lobulated, yellow-gray tumors. Eighty percent are encapsulated, and the remainder infiltrates the surrounding structures. Foci of necrosis and cystic degeneration, with eventual hemorrhage, are common, sometimes making a differential diagnosis against multilocular thymic cyst difficult.

The histologic classification of thymomas has been debated for more than 50 years. Lattes and Jonas[50] (in 1957) and Bernatz et al.[51]

(in 1961) proposed a classification based on the major morphologic pattern, including predominantly lymphocytic, predominantly epithelial, predominantly mixed, and predominantly spindle-cell-type thymoma. In 1978, Levine and Rosai[52] separated thymoma from a variety of other thymic neoplasms, such as thymic carcinoid, various lymphomas, and germ cell tumors. They divided thymomas into benign, or noninvasive, and malignant, or invasive, tumors. In 1985, Muller-Hermelink and Marino[53] proposed a system that used both topography and morphology. Their system included six subtypes: medullary, mixed, predominantly cortical, cortical, well-differentiated carcinoma, and thymic carcinoma. Lastly, in 1999, WHO reached a consensus on thymoma classification based on both morphology and the epithelial cell-to-lymphocyte ratio.[54] Six subtypes were identified: type A (spindle cell, medullary), type AB (mixed), type B1 (organoid), type B2 (cortical), type B3 (well-differentiated thymic carcinoma), and type C (thymic carcinoma).

Type A thymomas consist of cells with a spindle- or oval-shaped nucleus and a uniform bland cytology, reminiscent of cells in the atrophic adult thymus (Fig. 56.4). Rosette-like, storiform, or gland-like formations can be seen. Few intermingled lymphocytes are found. In nearly all cases, the epithelial tumor cells are positive for CK19, and in 50% of cases, they are positive for the B lymphocyte marker CD20. If staining for CK19 is negative, monophasic synovial sarcoma, or solitary fibrous tumor, must be ruled out. Reticulin stains are very useful in assessing the spindle cell, type A pattern. A well-recognized variant is called micronodular thymoma with lymphoid stroma, presenting epithelial micronoduli with intraepithelial CD1a-positive immature T cells and florid lymphoid follicular hyperplasia of the stroma. Myasthenia gravis occurs less frequently with type A thymomas, although secondary mucosa-associated lymphoid tissue (extranodal marginal zone B cell) lymphoma may develop.

Type B thymomas consist of round or polygonal epithelioid cells. They are further subdivided based on the proportional increase in epithelial cell content in relation to the reactive lymphocytes and the degree of cytologic atypia: from B1 (number of lymphocytes greater than number of epithelial cells) to B2 (number of lymphocytes epithelial cells equal) to B3 (number of lymphocytes less than number of epithelial cells). B1 thymomas are lymphocyte rich (organoid), containing only small nonatypical, CK19-positive epithelial cells. They resemble a normal functional thymus: cortical areas have CD1a-positive lymphocytes; edematous perivascular spaces include CD20-positive lymphocytes; and nodularity is vague. Unfortunately, positivity for epithelial CK19 and lymphocytic CD1a is physiologic in the cortex. Thus the differential diagnosis between normal thymus, thymoma, and lymphoblastic lymphoma may be very challenging, particularly with evaluation of a frozen section. In newborns and children less than 3 years of age, it will mostly be a true thymic hyperplasia, but in older children or adolescents, T-cell lymphoblastic lymphoma must be ruled out. Although thymomas in children are unusual, a few documented cases have occurred in children around puberty. Thymomas are p63 positive, but this marker may also be present in mediastinal B-cell lymphomas.

In type B2 thymomas (cortical), scattered plump tumor cells show vesicular nuclei with prominent nucleoli. Perivascular spaces eventually include palisading of lymphocytes, and Hassall bodies are rare. In type B3 thymomas (epithelial, atypical), proliferative invasive CK19-positive epithelium is associated with immature lymphocytes positive for CD99 and CD1a (Fig. 56.5). A diagnosis of combined thymoma is made if, for example, the components B2 and B3 both achieve 50% of tumor surface. Thymomas combining type A with type B features are designated as type AB (mixed) and they contain lymphocyte-rich and lymphocyte-poor areas. Rare thymomas include the metaplastic, the microscopic, and the sclerosing variant, and the so-called lipofibroadenoma.

BOX 56.1 Staging Systems for Thymic Tumors

NON-TNM SYSTEMS

MASAOKA STAGING SYSTEM

Stage	Description
I	Macroscopically encapsulated tumor without microscopic invasion of capsule
IIA	Macroscopic invasion into surrounding fatty tissue or mediastinal pleura
IIB	Microscopic invasion into capsule
III	Macroscopic invasion into nearby organs (i.e., pericardium, great vessels, or lung)
IVA	Pleural or pericardial dissemination
IVB	Lymphogenous or hematogenous metastasis

MASAOKA–KOGA STAGING SYSTEM

Tumor Stage	Description
I	Grossly and microscopically completely encapsulated tumor
IIA	Microscopic transcapsular invasion
IIB	Macroscopic invasion into thymic or surrounding fatty tissue, or grossly adherent but not breaking through mediastinal pleura or pericardium
III	Macroscopic invasion of nearby organs (pericardium, great vessels, or lung)
IVA	Pleural or pericardial dissemination
IVB	Lymphatic or hematogenous metastasis

WORLD HEALTH ORGANIZATION TNM-BASED STAGING SYSTEM

T Descriptor

T1	Macroscopically completely encapsulated and microscopically no capsular invasion
T2	Tumor invades pericapsular connective tissue
T3	Invasion into nearby organs (i.e., pericardium, great vessels, lung, pleura)
T4	Pleural or pericardial dissemination

N Descriptor

N0	No lymph node metastasis
N1	Metastasis to anterior mediastinal lymph nodes
N2	Metastasis to intrathoracic lymph nodes, except anterior mediastinal lymph nodes
N3	Metastasis to scalene or supraclavicular lymph nodes

M Descriptor

M0	No hematogenous metastasis
M1	Hematogenous metastasis

Stage Grouping

Stage	T	N	M
I	T1	N0	M0
II	T2	N0	M0
III	T1	N1	M0
	T2	N1	M0
	T3	N0–N1	M0
IV	T4	Any N	M0
	Any T	N2–N3	M0
	Any T	Any N	M1

TNM, tumor, node, metastasis.

TABLE 56.2 The Proposed Tumor, Node, Metastasis Staging (International Association for the Study of Lung Cancer Prognostic Factors Committee/International Thymic Malignancy Interest Group)[4,49]

Stage		Descriptors
TUMOR		
T1	T1a	Encapsulated or unencapsulated, with or without extension into the mediastinal fat
	T1b	Extension into the mediastinal pleura
T2		Direct invasion of the pericardium (partial or full thickness)
T3		Direct invasion of the lung, the brachiocephalic vein, the superior vena cava, the chest wall, the phrenic nerve, and/or hilar (extrapericardial) pulmonary vessels
T4		Direct invasion of the aorta, arch vessels, the main pulmonary artery, the myocardium, the trachea, or the esophagus
NODE		
N0		N0, no nodal involvement
N1		N1, anterior (perithymic) nodes (IASLC levels 1, 3a, 6, and/or supradiaphragmatic/inferior phrenics/pericardial)
N2		N2, deep intrathoracic or cervical nodes (IASLC levels 2, 4, 5, 7, 10, and/or internal mammary nodes)
METASTASIS		
M0		No metastatic pleural, pericardial, or distant sites
M1	M1a	Separate pleural or pericardial nodule(s)
	M1b	Pulmonary intraparenchymal nodule or distant organ metastasis

STAGE GROUPING		CORRESPONDING MASAOKA–KOGA STAGE
I	T1N0M0	I, IIA, IIB, III
II	T2N0M0	III
IIIA	T3N0M0	III
IIIB	T4N0M0	III
IVA	T any N0,1 M0,1a	IVA, IVB
IVB	T any N0-2 M0-1b	IVB

IASLC, International Association for the Study of Lung Cancer.

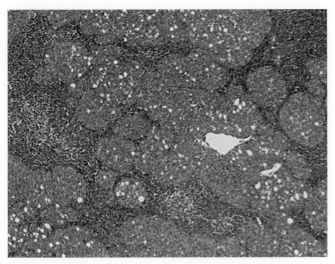

Fig. 56.4. Spindle cell type A thymoma with micronodular pattern.

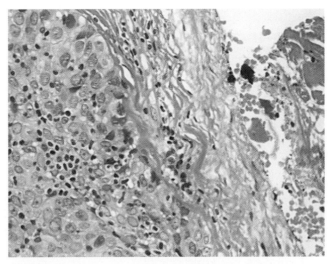

Fig. 56.5. Type B3 thymoma with atypical epithelial cells intermingled with sparse lymphocytes. Fine capsule with ink marking of the cauterized resection margin.

With the challenging criteria, it is evident that the opportunity for achieving interobserver agreement on histologic classification of thymomas is limited. The recent proposal of major and minor morphologic and immunohistochemical criteria to better individualize each thymic epithelial tumor entity aims at addressing those issues and has been integrated into the updated WHO classification.[6,55] As previously mentioned, immunohistochemistry may be valuable, and a list of useful markers is integrated into the WHO classification.

Diagnosis on evaluation of core biopsies may differ from the follow-up analysis of whole tumor sections. To overcome these problems, Suster and Moran, in 2008,[56] proposed a simplified classification into three subtypes: thymoma (well-differentiated tumors), atypical thymomas (intermediate differentiation), and thymic carcinomas (poorly differentiated tumors); others, maintaining the WHO classification, demonstrated that among the six subtypes, only three WHO categories were prognostically significant: types A, AB, and B1; types B2 and B3; and type C. Ultimately, thymoma subtyping on small biopsies is usually not needed for the therapeutically relevant distinction between lymphoma and solid tumor. In any case, diagnostic discrepancies between core-needle and resection specimen histology can be anticipated, given the frequent occurrence of histologic tumor heterogeneity that may be missed due to sampling error. Of note, histologic switch from lymphocytic lesions to more epithelial tumors has been reported, and may be related to tumor heterogeneity, as well as the effect of previous corticosteroid and chemotherapy treatment.[57,58]

Thymic Carcinoma

The 2004 WHO update maintained the range from type A to B3, but separated thymic carcinomas from thymomas with the rationale that thymomas are organotypic, unique tumors, because the combination of epithelial tumor cells with reactive lymphocytes may not be found in other organs (Table 56.3).[55] For this reason, the C category was abandoned. Thymic carcinomas display the common neoplastic morphologies found in other body sites, and they do not have the capacity to promote the maturation of intratumoral immature T cells. For thymic carcinomas, 11 histologic variants are recognized. The most common are squamous cell carcinomas, lymphoepithelioma-like carcinomas, and neuroendocrine tumors (considered as a separate entity in some series). As in other organs, the precise clinical relevance concerning therapy and prognosis is difficult to assess, and tumor heterogeneity is often found.

TABLE 56.3 World Health Organization Histologic Types of Thymic Tumors

Type of Thymic Tumor	Histologic Types
Thymoma	Type A (spindle cell; medullary)
	Type AB
	Type B1 (lymphocyte rich, lymphocytic, predominantly cortical, organoid)
	Type B2 (cortical)
	Type B3 (epithelial, atypical, squamoid; well-differentiated thymic carcinoma)
	Micronodular thymoma
	Metaplastic, sclerosing, microscopic thymoma
	Lipofibroadenoma
Thymic carcinoma	Squamous cell, epidermoid keratinizing
	Epidermoid nonkeratinizing
	Basaloid
	Lymphoepithelioma-like
	Mucoepidermoid
	Sarcomatoid
	Clear cell
	Mucoepidermoid
	Papillary
	Undifferentiated
	Combined
Neuroendocrine tumors	Well-differentiated neuroendocrine tumors or carcinomas, including typical and atypical carcinoids
	Poorly differentiated neuroendocrine carcinomas, including large and small cell neuroendocrine carcinoma

TABLE 56.4 International Thymic Malignancy Group Recommendations for Outcome Measures for Thymic Tumors

Outcome Measure	End Point	Patient Population
Overall survival	Death from any cause	All patients
Freedom from recurrence	Recurrence	Complete resection (R0), complete response after nonsurgical treatment
Time to progression	Disease progression	Incomplete resection (R1 or R2), stable disease, or progression of disease after nonsurgical treatment

Most patients with thymic carcinomas are symptomatic, reflecting the high stage III to stage IV at diagnosis. Autoimmune phenomena associated with thymoma, such as myasthenia gravis or pure red cell aplasia, are rarely found. Lymph node and distant metastases are common. Squamous cell carcinoma may be keratinizing or nonkeratinizing, and no thymopoiesis or autoimmunity is present. Immunohistochemistry is of some help for the differential diagnosis. In contrast to lung squamous cell carcinoma, staining for CD117 (c-Kit) may be positive in thymic squamous cell carcinomas, but less than 10% of patients have a CD117 mutation. Epstein-Barr virus may be found in lymphoepithelioma-like carcinomas and in nasopharyngeal carcinomas. Many thymic adenocarcinomas are CD5 positive, a lymphocyte marker considered to be rare in carcinomas, but negative for thyroid transcription factor 1 and thyroglobulin.

Neuroendocrine Thymic Tumor

The thymus exhibits the same spectrum of neuroendocrine tumors as the lung, although with different frequencies. In the lung, typical carcinoid and small cell lung carcinoma (SCLC) are the most common histotype, but in the thymus, the most frequent histotype is atypical carcinoid. According to the WHO 2004 classification (see Table 56.3), carcinoids are classified as well-differentiated neuroendocrine tumor/carcinoma and considered separate from the high-grade tumors, large cell neuroendocrine carcinoma, and SCLC. Thymic carcinoids are often locally invasive and metastasize distantly. Endocrine manifestations, other than Cushing syndrome, are infrequent. They can also be associated with multiple endocrine neoplasia (MEN) type 1 or 2a, and they are very rarely associated with myasthenia gravis. Morphologic variants include the spindle cell pattern, which can be confused with a type A thymoma if diagnosis is not corroborated by immunohistochemical results for neuroendocrine markers, such as synaptophysin. For diagnosis of primary thymic SCLC, a mediastinal metastasis of a lung neoplasm must be carefully ruled out. SCLC can be present in combination with squamous cell carcinoma or carcinoid.

OUTCOME MEASURES AND PROGNOSTIC FACTORS IN THYMIC TUMORS

Outcome Measures

The standard outcome measure for most clinical studies is overall survival. Although easily reproducible and comparable across different series, overall survival has some limitations in slow-growing malignancies like thymic tumors. Indeed, many patients with thymoma have a long life expectancy, and it is not unusual to have survival of 30 years or more. Overall, less than 40% of patients with thymoma die from the thymoma, and this percentage is also stage dependent (stage I, 3%; stage II, 30%; stage III, 58%; stage IV, 78%). In addition, unlike other more aggressive solid neoplasms, in which patients with a recurrence almost invariably die from that neoplasm, many patients with thymoma may live many years with a recurrence and may die from causes unrelated to thymoma. For these reasons, other outcome measures seem more appropriate in thymic tumors. Among other measures, some have been discussed and proposed in the literature. They include disease-related survival, disease-specific survival, cause-specific survival, cancer-specific survival, disease-free survival, freedom-from-recurrence, progression-free survival, and time to progression. All these survival measures considered a specific end point (death and different causes of death, recurrence after complete resection, disease progression after incomplete resection) and a specific patient population (all patients, complete resection [R0], and incomplete resection [R1 or R2]). In a 2011 report, the ITMIG addressed this important issue and came to the conclusion that the assessment of efficacy of any treatment in thymic malignancy is best measured when recurrence is considered as the end point.[23] Therefore the ITMIG recommends that, along with the calculation of overall survival, any study in which outcomes after treatment of thymic tumors are reported should indicate freedom from recurrence for any patient undergoing a treatment aimed at obtaining complete disease eradication, as indicated by a complete resection (R0) in surgically treated patients or complete radiographic response in nonsurgically treated patients (Table 56.4). For any patients in whom a residual disease is expected after treatment (partial radiographic response or incomplete resection [R1 or R2]), time to progression should be used.

Prognostic Factors

A prognostic factor can be defined as a variable that can be used to estimate the chance of recovery from a disease, or the chance of disease relapse. Prognostic factors are divided into tumor-related, host-related, and environmental-related factors.[59] The most important prognostic factor in all human cancers is the stage at presentation, which is the anatomic extent of the disease. By using a set of definitions indicating the anatomic tumor

TABLE 56.5 Prognostic Factors in Thymic Tumors[38]

Variable	Significance		
	Consistent Prognostic	Inconsistent	Consistent Nonprognostic
Stage (Masaoka)	X		
Complete resection	X		
Gender			X
Myasthenia gravis			X
Tumor size		X	
Age		X	

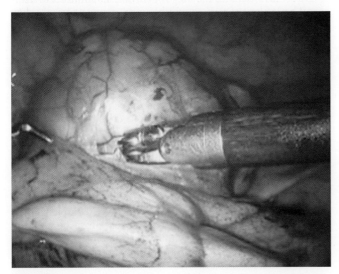

Fig. 56.6. Robotic-assisted thoracoscopic surgery for thymoma resection. Intraoperative view of a patient with Masaoka stage II thymoma (type AB according to the World Health Organization system), with a size of 5 × 5 × 3 cm.

spread, we can allocate each individual's tumor into a category that is associated with a different outcome. As a consequence, the inclusion of any nonanatomic variable into a stage classification (completeness of resection, histology, etc.) seems inappropriate, and the term "prognostic model" should be used instead. A number of studies investigating possible prognostic factors in thymic tumors have been published in the past decades. The authors of one review analyzed prognostic factors for thymic tumors in the literature.[60] When only studies using multivariate analysis were considered, a total of 29 studies reporting prognostic predictors for survival were identified, and 12 studies reporting prognostic predictors for recurrence were identified. Most prognostic predictors for survival were also predictors for recurrence. The only validated prognostic factors for both survival and recurrence were the stage at presentation (Masaoka or Masaoka–Koga staging systems) and the completeness of resection. As for the stage, the majority of studies did not find a significant difference between stage I and stage II, which were collapsed into a single stage in some cases. Gender and myasthenia gravis are consistently reported as not being significant predictors for either survival or recurrence. Histology, according to WHO classification, does not seem to be a validated prognostic factor, with the exception of thymic carcinoma. Other prognostic factors, including age, tumor size, and other parathymic syndromes, were inconsistently reported as significant prognostic factors (Table 56.5). The next step will be the integration of the different prognostic factors (tumor related, host related, and environmental related) into a prognostic model. This is a necessary step to get to a prediction of prognosis from a population basis to an individual basis.[61] Any

proposed prognostic model should be validated, either internally or externally, and it should be flexible enough to include any new factor as it emerges, and should also indicate the degree of uncertainty, especially when the prognostic index is applied to individual patients.

TREATMENT OF THYMOMA

Surgery

Surgical resection is the mainstay for the treatment of thymoma, with a reported operative mortality of 2% and a complication rate of approximately 20%.[62] Treatment of thymoma depends on the location and its stage.[63] Early-stage thymomas are eligible for complete surgical resection, with an excellent early and long-term outcome. Complete resection should always be the primary goal. Results depend on the localization and the size of the tumor. The ITMIG recommends en bloc resection, including complete thymectomy and resection of the surrounding mediastinal fat, because of the possibility of subtle macroscopically invisible invasion of the tumor.[64] Some studies recently reported good results in early-stage, nonmyasthenic thymomas, after thymomectomy only, and without thymectomy, although results after long-term follow-up are expected before drawing definite conclusions.[64] The 10-year survival rates after surgical resection of thymomas are 90%, 70%, 55%, and 35% for stages I, II, III, and IVA thymoma, respectively. The recurrence rate is 3%, 11%, 30%, and 43% in resected stage I, II, III, and IVA thymoma, respectively. The disease-free survival at 10 years is 94%, 88%, 56%, and 33% for stages I, II, III, and IVA, respectively.[65]

Extent of Resection

Significantly better survival rates have been noted in patients who underwent complete resection.[3] After complete resection, 10-year survival is expected at 80%, 78%, 75%, and 42% for stages I, II, III, and IVA, respectively. Of interest, long-term survival rates for patients with stage I and III are similar when complete resection is performed. In a large series Regnard et al.[3] have shown that complete resection was the only significant prognostic factor in multivariate analysis.

Surgical Approach

Most of the experts recommend a sternotomy as the optimal incision for thymoma, because it might not be possible to perform a complete thymectomy via thoracotomy.[66,67] The transcervical approach has also been used for this purpose.[24] Minimally invasive approaches, including VATS and robotic-assisted thoracoscopic surgery (RATS) for early-stage thymomas, have been reported and are gaining popularity in specialized centers.[68–73] In particular, RATS allows an excellent exposure and precision of resection in tumors of adequate size and location (Fig. 56.6).[74] An alternative approach that we use at our institution in Zurich is a hybrid approach, which includes RATS and anterolateral thoracotomy. In this approach, we use RATS to release the left innominate vein and part of the thymus from the side where there is less tumor extent and then we dissect and retrieve the tumor from the contralateral side through an anterolateral thoracotomy. ESMO guidelines suggest that minimally invasive surgery is an option for presumed stage I and possibly stage II tumors in the hands of appropriately trained thoracic surgeons, given its similar results to those of open approaches.[75,76] Recently, a subxiphoid approach has been proposed, using either VATS or a combined VATS/RATS assistance, with excellent results for early-stage thymoma. The technique has been associated with a lower postoperative pain and a better exposure of both phrenic nerves.[77]

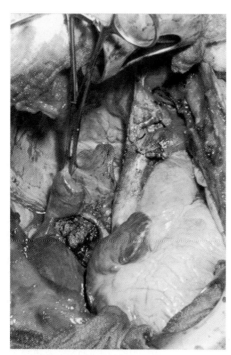

Fig. 56.7. Right-sided hemiclamshell incision for resection of thymoma.

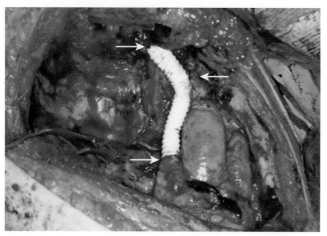

Fig. 56.8. Intraoperative view of a patient with Masaoka stage III disease who had resection of the superior vena cava, including part of the right and left innominate veins. Right upper lobectomy and partial resection of the pericardium were also done. Reconstruction was performed with a polytetrafluoroethylene-ringed graft between the atrio-caval junction and the right and left innominate veins (white arrows).

Surgical Management of Stage III Thymoma

Thymoma is classified as stage III, locally advanced stage, when it has invaded the surrounding structures, such as pericardium, great vessels (SVC, innominate veins, ascending aorta, and main pulmonary artery), lung parenchyma, phrenic nerves, and chest wall. Median sternotomy is the standard approach for all stage III thymomas. This approach provides an excellent exposure if the tumor invades the adjacent mediastinal and lung structures. A clamshell (bilateral anterolateral thoracotomy with transversal sternotomy) incision has also been proposed for large tumors extending in both pleural cavities.[78] Alternatively, a hemiclamshell incision, which allows excellent exposure of the mediastinum and the involved pleural space, is recommended (Fig. 56.7). This exposure starts with anterolateral thoracotomy through the

fourth or fifth intercostal space and is completed with partial median sternotomy.[79] This incision provides an excellent exposure of the brachiocephalic vessels and phrenic nerve, compared with standard sternotomy incision. As in early-stage thymoma, complete resection is mandatory for a good outcome in any stage III thymoma. The left brachiocephalic vein, SVC, right atrium, pericardium, lung, and diaphragm should be resected if necessary. Resection of one phrenic nerve, and resection and reconstruction of the ascending aorta and main pulmonary artery, may occasionally be indicated to achieve a complete resection. Invasion of the myocardium precludes the resection.[78]

Direct invasion into the lung is generally not difficult to manage. The infiltrated part should be en bloc resected depending on the respiratory function of the patient. Wedge resection, segmentectomy, or lobectomy can be performed based on the extent of invasion into the lung. Pneumonectomy or extrapleural pneumonectomy is rarely performed, but should be considered to achieve a complete resection if the patient has adequate physiologic reserve to tolerate this procedure. In patients with appropriate lung reserve, one phrenic nerve may be resected, but resection of both nerves should be avoided. Meanwhile, phrenic nerve preservation does not affect overall survival, but increases the risk of local recurrence.[80] If the phrenic nerve is resected, plication of the diaphragm should be considered.[81] The SVC and the brachiocephalic vein(s) can be resected and reconstructed, if a complete resection could be achieved.[82] Partial resection of the wall of the SVC, with direct repair or patch, can also be done. If more than 30% of the circumference is involved, complete resection and reconstruction are needed. In such a case, reconstruction of the SVC can be done with a polytetrafluoroethylene graft (Fig. 56.8). When there is intra-atrial involvement of the SVC, resection and reconstruction of the ascending aorta and main pulmonary artery require using cardiopulmonary bypass.[83] Routine removal of anterior mediastinal nodes and anterior cervical nodes is recommended,[75,84] particularly in thymic carcinomas. Systematic sampling of other intrathoracic sites is encouraged (i.e., paratracheal, aortopulmonary window, and subcarinal areas, depending on tumor location) in stage III/IV tumors. Systematic lymphadenectomy (N1 + N2) is strongly recommended in case of thymic carcinoma. Meanwhile, the new IASLC/ITMIG TNM staging system of thymic tumors leads to the recommendation that local–regional lymphadenectomy should be carried out during resection of all types of thymic tumors.[85]

Minimally Invasive Resection

Although open surgical approaches are generally accepted as the criterion standard for thymoma resection, the use of both VATS and RATS for thymoma resection has been reported.[68–73] The main concerns for a minimally invasive thymoma resection are complete resection and the size of the tumor. With advances in the instrumentation and techniques, VATS thymectomy is being performed more frequently at many institutions. VATS thymectomy for thymoma is indicated for encapsulated or early-stage tumors (Masaoka stage I–II); generally, there is no indication for using VATS or RATS resection in more advanced stages (Masaoka stage III–IV). Although thymomas larger than 5 cm are technically difficult to remove with VATS, Takeo et al.[71] reported that 15 of 35 thymomas were larger than 5 cm in diameter. These authors use a method that lifts the sternum and takes the tumor out using a subxiphoid incision. They recommend that VATS can be used safely for clinical Masaoka stages I and II. Ye et al.[69] evaluated short-term outcomes of 46 patients who underwent surgery for Masaoka stage I thymoma with VATS and RATS. They reported comparable results between these two technologies. In a retrospective study, Rückert et al.[73] compared thymectomy by VATS and RATS and reported significant improvement in the RATS group compared with the VATS group, which included

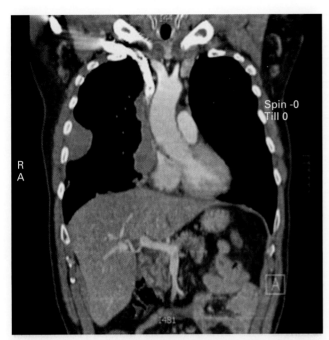

Fig. 56.9. Coronary view of a patient with Masaoka stage IVA disease. After induction chemotherapy, we performed right pleuropneumonectomy using a right-sided hemiclamshell incision. The patient had partial resection of the superior vena cava, pericardium, and diaphragm, as well as reconstruction with synthetic patches.

17 cases of thymoma. We reported on 20 thymoma cases that involved thymectomy with RATS; the median tumor size was 4 cm, and the median follow-up was 26 months with no local, but two pleural, recurrences.[70] For our studies, and for other studies, longer follow-up is needed to conclude that the results are oncologically sufficient.

Stage IVA Thymoma

Stage IVA thymoma is defined as intrapleural or intrapericardial dissemination of tumor cells without any distant metastasis (see Fig. 56.4). Surgical options in this stage, in addition to thymus and thymoma resection, are excision of pleural/pericardial implants, total pleurectomy, and pleuropneumonectomy.[86] Although it seems to be a very aggressive approach, pleuropneumonectomy has been shown to be feasible with good outcomes in these patients (5-year survival rates between 75% and 78% in selected series).[87] In one case, after induction chemotherapy, we performed a right pleuropneumonectomy using right-sided hemiclamshell incision (Fig. 56.9). The patient had partial SVC resection and reconstruction with a pericardium patch. We also performed pericardium and diaphragm resection and reconstruction with a synthetic patch. This patient (male) did not receive any adjuvant treatment, and he was alive, without recurrence, after 48 months of follow-up. Most patients may also require diaphragm and pericardium resection as performed in mesothelioma surgery.[88]

Radiotherapy

Thymic tumors have a tendency toward local recurrence and show moderate-to-high radiosensitivity profiles. This has always been considered a prerequisite for the adoption of radiotherapy in the whole treatment strategy. Unfortunately, the rarity of these tumors, and the lack of prospective, randomized trials, makes it difficult to draw evidence-based recommendations about the efficacy of radiotherapy in the different clinical settings. It may be

delivered before surgery or after surgery, either in patients not eligible for surgical intervention or for treatment of recurrent tumors. The standard radiotherapy technique in thymic tumors is three-dimensional (3-D) conformal radiotherapy, but in most centers, to reduce the exposure of thoracic structures, such as the heart, lung, and esophagus, intensity-modulated radiotherapy (IMRT) is gradually being substituted for 3-D conformal radiotherapy. There have been no dedicated studies comparing the outcomes (efficacy and toxicity) of 3-D conformal radiotherapy with IMRT in thymic neoplasms. In other thoracic tumors such as lung cancer, toxicity was lower for IMRT.[89] Four-dimensional (4-D) CT is an advance in technology that further improved target localization and, in the process, reduced the dose to normal structures. It allows for quantitative tumor motion evaluation during treatment planning and delivery. Motion management may be important, especially when the target includes structures in the lower portion of the thoracic cavity, closer to the diaphragm. By several methods, margins can be reduced and the dose to normal tissues decreased when the clinical volumes are large. This may often occur in adjuvant radiotherapy. Proton therapy has been adopted for treating invasive thymomas, especially when the anterior mediastinum is involved. The dosimetric advantages of proton therapy in such situations should be proven to offer better clinical outcomes. In several institutions, a combination of intensity-modulated proton therapy, 4-D imaging, and adaptive radiotherapy is under investigation, with the aim of maximizing the therapeutic index.[90] The delivered doses vary based on the clinical setting, ranging from 45 Gy as neoadjuvant therapy, to 45 to 55 Gy as postoperative therapy, to 60 to 66 Gy as exclusive treatment, with conventional fractionation (1.8 Gy/day to 2.0 Gy/day).[91]

Preoperative Radiotherapy

To improve resectability rates, preoperative radiotherapy has been used alone or in combination with chemotherapy (sequential or concurrent) in a neoadjuvant (induction) setting.[92–94] Unfortunately, with the exception of a few reports, most of the studies failed to show significantly better resectability rates and survival when compared with neoadjuvant chemotherapy alone.

Postoperative Radiotherapy

Postoperative radiotherapy is usually performed within 3 months after the surgical procedure, for a total dose of 50 to 54 Gy in 1.8-Gy to 2.0-Gy fractions. Indications for postoperative radiotherapy depend on the stage at surgery, complete or incomplete resection, and factors such as WHO histology, and possibly tumor size and presence of necrosis (Fig. 56.10).[75] In Masaoka stage I disease, adjuvant radiotherapy has no role. For stage II disease, the largest series so far found either no differences with or without radiotherapy or a detrimental effect.[43,95] However, it should be noted that a more recent series suggested an improved disease-free survival using postoperative radiotherapy for WHO type B2 or B3 thymoma and thymic carcinoma.[96–98] Adjuvant radiotherapy has a well-established role in the treatment of stage III disease in clinical practice, although the level of evidence is low. Several earlier studies demonstrated a decrease in the rate of recurrence (0% to 20%) after complete resection and postoperative radiotherapy, which was significantly lower than after surgery alone.[99] More recent studies have demonstrated the efficacy of postoperative radiotherapy for stage III to stage IV disease,[100,101] whereas other trials have failed to show any significant advantage.[51,102] A study of data on 626 invasive thymomas in the US Surveillance, Epidemiology and End Results (SEER) registry showed a similar cause-specific survival for postoperative radiotherapy and surgery alone (91% vs. 86%, $p = 0.12$).[103] Similar results were obtained in a 2009

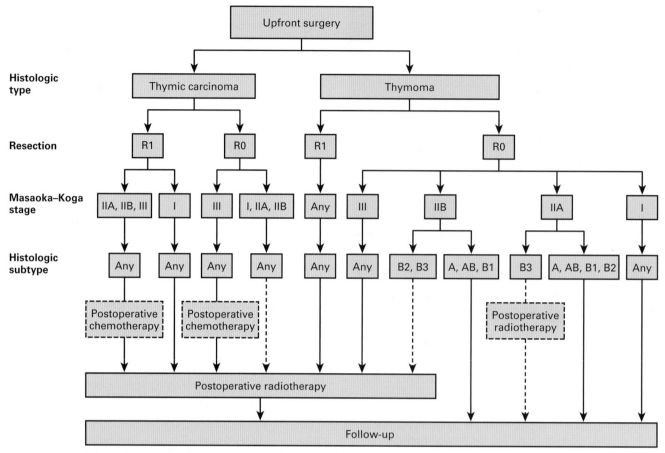

Fig. 56.10. Postoperative management of thymoma and thymic carcinomas: European Society for Medical Oncology clinical practice guidelines algorithm.[75]

meta-analysis incorporating stage II and III disease.[104] Among 592 patients from 13 different studies, no significant difference was found between surgery alone and surgery plus radiotherapy (odds ratio, 1.05; p = 0.63).

Ultimately, the global trend over the past years has been toward a less frequent use of postoperative radiotherapy in thymoma, and to keep it in reserve for high-risk cases.[75] This is based on recent reports from large databases,[103,105–109] as well as pooled analyses of retrospective studies,[104] indicating

- the absence of survival benefit after radiotherapy in stage I thymoma, or after R0/1 resection of stage II to stage III thymoma;[103,106,107]
- a similar rate of recurrence in patients who received postoperative radiotherapy or not after complete resection of thymoma;[104,110] and
- a recurrence-free survival and overall survival benefit with postoperative radiotherapy after resection of thymic carcinoma.[106,108,109]

Stage and completeness of resection are thus the most relevant criteria in the decision making, followed by histology. Those factors are the most significant predictors of survival; however, one must take into account that retrospective analyses are likely to be biased, because postoperative radiotherapy is most likely administered in patients with incomplete resection or high-grade tumors. Therefore the absence of survival differences may then suggest that postoperative radiotherapy reduced or overcame the risk of recurrence in those patients. Another point to consider is that recurrences of thymic epithelial tumors occur outside the mediastinum in more than 60% of cases.[111]

Therefore it appears that the evidence to support using postoperative radiotherapy for completely resected, invasive thymomas is lacking. Incorporating additional factors, including high-risk WHO histologic subtypes, large tumors (more than 8 cm), and close margins, may be taken into account when considering whether postoperative radiotherapy is indicated for an individual patient. Conversely, a higher level of evidence seems to support the use of adjuvant radiotherapy for patients who have an incomplete resection (R1 or R2). The ESMO Clinical Practice Guideline recently proposed a decision algorithm for postoperative radiotherapy, integrating those data (see Fig. 56.10).

Definitive Radiotherapy

Radical (so-called curative) radiotherapy is customarily used for patients who are not surgical candidates, or for patients who have inoperable disease after induction chemotherapy. For such patients, chemoradiation therapy is usually delivered in a sequential manner, to a total dose of 54 to 70 Gy. The response rate reaches 70%, with a 5-year survival projection of 70% to 80%. These results are similar to those reported after surgery with incomplete resection.[92,112]

Chemotherapy

As for other thoracic malignancies, chemotherapy regimens are selected in accordance with the intended use in patients with thymic neoplasms. This depends on the tumor size, signs of infiltration on imaging, stage, and histology. Thymic tumors are generally chemosensitive, although thymomas are more sensitive

TABLE 56.6 Polychemotherapy Regimens in Stage III to Stage IV Thymic Tumors in Small Series

Author (Year)	No. of Patients	Percentage of Complete Resection (R0)	Treatment		Polychemotherapy		Partial Response or Better (%)
			Induction	Postoperative	Regimen	Schedule	
Venuta et al. (1997)[112]	21	86	Chemotherapy	Chemoradiation therapy	Cisplatin 75 mg/m², day 1 Etoposide 120 mg/m², days 1, 3, and 5 Epirubicin 100 mg/m², day 1	Three 21-day cycles	100
Bretti et al. (2004)[116]	25	44	Chemotherapy	Radiotherapy	Cisplatin 50 mg/m², day 1 Doxorubicin 40 mg/m², day 1 Vincristine 0.6 mg/m², day 2 Cyclophosphamide 700 mg/m², day 4	Four 21-day cycles	72
Kim et al. (2004)[117]	22	76	Chemotherapy	Chemoradiation therapy	Cisplatin 30 mg/m², days 1, 2, and 3 Doxorubicin 20 mg/m², days 1, 2, and 3 Cyclophosphamide 500 mg/m², day 1 Prednisone 100 mg, days 1, 2, 3, 4, and 5	Three 21-day cycles	77
Lucchi et al. (2006)[118]	30	77	Chemotherapy	Chemoradiation therapy	Cisplatin 75 mg/m², day 1 Epirubicin 100 mg/m², day 1 Etoposide 120 mg/m², days 1, 3, and 5	Three 21-day cycles	73
Yokoi et al. (2007)[119]	17	22	Chemotherapy	Radiotherapy	Cisplatin 20 mg/m², days 1, 2, 3, and 4 Doxorubicin 40 mg/m², day 1 Methylprednisolone 1000 mg, days 1, 2, 3, and 4 Methylprednisolone 500 mg, days 5 and 6	Four 21-day cycles	92
Wright et al. (2008)[93]	10	80	Chemoradiation therapy	Chemotherapy	Cisplatin 33 mg/m², days 1, 2, and 3 Etoposide 100 mg/m², days 1, 2, and 3	Two 28-day cycles	40
Kunitoh et al. (2009)[120]	27	NG	Chemotherapy	None	Cisplatin 25 mg/m², days 1, 8, 15, 22, 29, 36, 43, 50, and 57 Vincristine 1 mg/m², days 1, 8, 36, and 50 Etoposide 80 mg/m², days 1, 2, 3, 15, 16, 17, 29, 10, 31, 43, 44, 45, 57, 58, and 59 Doxorubicin 40 mg/m², days 1, 2, 3, 15, 16, 17, 29, 10, 31, 43, 44, 45, 57, 58, and 59		59
Rea et al. (2011)[121]	38	81	Chemotherapy	Chemoradiation therapy	Cisplatin 50 mg/m², day 1 Doxorubicin 40 mg/m², day 1 Vincristine 0.6 mg/m², day 3 Cyclophosphamide 700 mg/m², day 4	Three 21-day cycles	68
Park et al. (2013)[122]	27	79	Chemotherapy	None	Cisplatin 75 mg/m², day 1 Docetaxel 75 mg/m², day 1	Three 21-day cycles	63

NG, Not given.

to chemotherapy than thymic carcinomas. As described earlier, the primary goal of treatment is the complete surgical resection (R0) of the thymic neoplasm. Chemotherapy strategies include chemotherapy used both as initial treatment and as treatment in case of recurrence. Chemotherapy as initial treatment can be further divided into chemotherapy with curative intent (primary or preoperative chemotherapy or postoperative chemotherapy) and chemotherapy with palliative intent.[75,110] Exclusive (palliative) chemotherapy is administrated in patients medically or technically not qualified for surgical procedures, or for patients with metastatic disease.

Primary (Induction, Preoperative) Chemotherapy

The major goal of induction chemotherapy is to downstage the tumor prior to surgery. Therefore, chemotherapy regimens have to be evaluated based on their ability to induce response (Table 56.6). In 2013, a Cochrane meta-analysis was performed to evaluate the role of induction therapy. Forty-nine relevant, randomized studies were identified, but none of them met the criteria necessary for a Cochrane analysis.[113] Therefore all published guidelines related to multimodal treatment of thymic neoplasm continue to be based on expert opinions. The majority

TABLE 56.7 Selected Chemotherapy Combination Regimens for Thymomas and Thymic Carcinomas

Regimen	Agents	Doses
ADOC	Adriamycin	40 mg/m²/3 weeks
	Cisplatin	50 mg/m²/3 weeks
	Vincristine	0.6 mg/m²/3 weeks
	Cyclophosphamide	700 mg/m²/3 weeks
CAP	Cisplatin	50 mg/m²/3 weeks
	Adriamycin	50 mg/m²/3 weeks
	Cyclophosphamide	500 mg/m²/3 weeks
PE	Cisplatin	60 mg/m²/3 weeks
	Etoposide	120 mg/m² × 3/3 weeks
VIP	Etoposide	75 mg/m² × 4 d/3 weeks
	Ifosfamide	1.2 g/m² × 4 d/3 weeks
	Cisplatin	20 mg/m² × 4 d/3 weeks
CODE	Cisplatin	25 mg/m²/1 week
	Vincristine	1 mg/m²/2 weeks
	Adriamycin	40 mg/m²/2 weeks
	Etoposide	80 mg/m² × 3/2 weeks
Carbo-Px	Carboplatin	AUC 5–6 mg/m²/3 weeks
	Paclitaxel	200–225 mg/m²/3 weeks
CAP–GEM	Capecitabine	650 mg/m² bid 14 days/3 weeks
	Gemcitabine	1000 mg/m² × 2 days/3 weeks

AUC, Area under the curve.

of reported primary chemotherapy regimens are part of multimodality treatments. This may include presurgical or additional postoperative radiotherapy with and without chemotherapy. Therefore, the rate of complete resections (R0) and the response rates after induction chemotherapy are often difficult to evaluate, because different regimens are used. On average, for patients with stage III to stage IV thymic neoplasm, induction therapy achieved a response rate of 71% (29% to 100%) and surgery resulted in a complete resection in 68% (22% to 86%). All regimens consisted of a combination of multiple drugs. The backbones of the induction therapies were cisplatin, anthracyclines, etoposide, and cyclophosphamide. A 2013 study showed that a combination of a taxane and cisplatin achieved response rates of 63% and 79% in complete resections (R0).[114] Overall, about 75% of patients with advanced thymic neoplasm who received multimodal therapy survived 5 years.[115] These induction chemotherapy regimens are associated with toxicities that have to be taken into account. Predominantly, the induction regimens resulted in hematologic toxicity. Patients treated with induction treatment with multiple-drug chemotherapy have to be medically fit enough to have a performance status after induction that allows major surgery. However, patients with thymic malignancies tend to be younger with less comorbidities compared with patients who have lung cancer. This means that even intense chemotherapy regimens with multiple drugs can be administered in this patient population.

Postoperative (Adjuvant) Chemotherapy

In the majority of the cases, postoperative therapy after resection of thymic tumors consists of radiotherapy or both radiotherapy and chemotherapy. In contrast to lung cancer, improved local control is the main focus of adjuvant therapy in thymic neoplasms. For this reason, chemotherapy alone is rarely used in an adjuvant setting. Authors of a Japanese retrospective study that included more than 1300 patients with thymoma found no improvement of survival in a subgroup of 473 patients with complete resection (R0) who were treated with induction therapy and postoperative chemotherapy, compared with patients treated with induction therapy only.[43,75]

Exclusive (Palliative) Chemotherapy

In cases when metastatic spread, or other reasons, prohibits local treatment with surgery or radiotherapy, exclusive chemotherapy with palliative intent is offered. Patients with relapse after curative-intent therapy are also treated with palliative chemotherapy. Monotherapies with cisplatin, ifosfamide, and paclitaxel were used in these patients.[123] Recently, amrubicin, a new anthracycline, was tested in nine patients with platinum-refractory disease, resulting in a 44% response rate.[124] In addition, for 13 patients who were pretreated with pemetrexed, the overall response rate was 17%.[125] The combination of steroids and octreotide was used for symptom and tumor control. Overall, patients treated with single-agent therapies achieved a response rate of 28%, and a median overall survival of about 2 years.[126]

The current standard is combination chemotherapy, based on cisplatin regimens (Table 56.7).[127–129] No randomized studies have been conducted, and which regimen should be considered standard remains unknown. Multiagent combination regimens and anthracycline-based regimens appear to have improved response rates compared with etoposide-based regimens. A combination of cisplatin, doxorubicin, and cyclophosphamide is preferred.[75]

Combined Radiotherapy and Chemotherapy

Radiotherapy is the mainstay of postoperative therapy, and is included in the majority of multimodal therapy concepts. The rationale for combining chemotherapy and radiotherapy (chemoradiation therapy) is to augment cytotoxicity against remaining tumor cells. In one study, chemoradiation therapy was used as induction therapy, resulting in a response rate comparable to chemotherapy alone.[93] Chemoradiation therapy can also be used in the postoperative setting if a large unresectable tumor volume remains in the thorax after resection (i.e., an R2 resection). In addition, chemoradiation therapy is the definitive treatment for patients who are not medically fit for surgery or who have a thymic neoplasm that is technically not resectable.[91] Twenty-three patients with unresectable thymoma were treated with a combination of cisplatin, doxorubicin, and cyclophosphamide, and thoracic radiation. A total of 5 complete and 11 partial responses to chemotherapy (overall response rate of 69.6%) were reported. The 5-year survival rate was 52.5%.[130]

Targeted Therapy

When it comes to targeted therapies, the differences between thymomas and thymic carcinomas become even more obvious at the molecular level. The expression of major histocompatibility molecules, autoimmune regulator, and the capacity to mature lymphocytes are different because both entities are differentially developed from their common epithelial progenitor cell. This results in different expression of target molecules, such as KIT mast/stem cell growth factor receptor, epidermal growth factor receptor, and insulin-like growth factor receptor-1.[131]

When analyzed by immunohistochemical methods, KIT is overexpressed in 2% of thymomas and in 79% of thymic carcinomas.[132] There are activating mutations in exons, 9, 11, 13, and 17 only in thymic carcinomas.[75,129,132,133] Imatinib is a small-molecule multikinase inhibitor that blocks KIT, Bcr-Abl, and platelet-derived growth factor receptor. Treatment with imatinib resulted in short disease stabilization in phase II studies.[134]

Angiogenesis is of special importance during the development of thymic neoplasm. Vascular endothelial growth factor-A levels were elevated in serum samples from patients with thymic carcinomas, and vascular endothelial growth factor-R1 and R2 were expressed in the malignant thymic tissue. Therefore

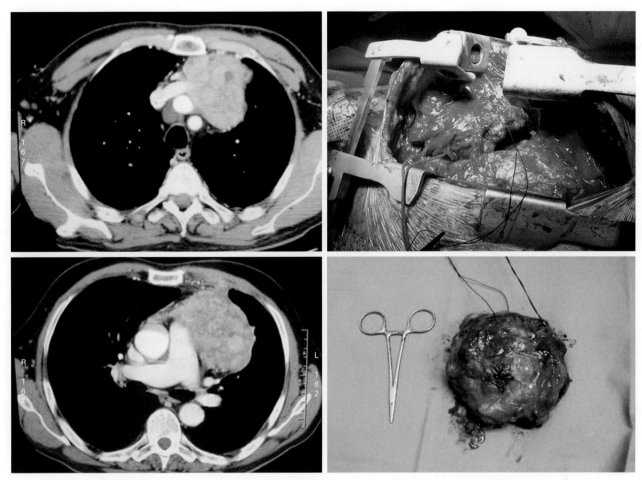

Fig. 56.11. Thymic carcinoma: computed tomography images, surgical access, and operative specimen.

angiogenesis appears treatable with small-molecule, multi-tyrosine kinase inhibitors, such as sunitinib.[135,136] A phase II trial recently demonstrated the efficacy of sunitinib in terms of response and disease control rate (DCR) in thymic epithelial tumors, including thymic carcinomas (objective response rate, 26%; DCR, 91%) and, to a lesser extent, thymomas (objective response rate, 6%; DCR, 81%).[109] Sunitinib may then represent an off-label option as a second-line treatment of thymic carcinomas, independently from KIT status.[137]

More recently, everolimus was evaluated in thymic epithelial tumors in a recently reported phase II trial reporting on a 22% response rate, as well as a 93% DCR. Everolimus may, therefore, represent an off-label option for refractory tumors.[136]

THYMIC CARCINOMA

Thymic carcinomas are rare tumors of the mediastinum, with a prevalence of one to three cases per 10 million people.[1] Among thymic tumors, 15% to 20% are thymic carcinoma. Until recently, thymic carcinoma has been considered a subtype of thymoma (type C thymoma). The 2004 WHO histologic classification clearly defines thymic carcinoma as a distinct tumor from thymoma. In contrast to thymomas, thymic carcinomas show a distinct histology (cytologic atypia, lack of an organotypic appearance, and resemblance to carcinomas occurring elsewhere in the body), have a more aggressive clinical behavior, and have a poorer prognosis. Population-based studies show an average 16% resection rate in patients with thymic carcinoma. The 5-year survival rate is 17% for patients who do not have surgery.[138]

Clinical Presentation and Diagnosis

Approximately 60% of patients with thymic carcinoma are symptomatic; approximately 40% have node metastases at the time of presentation and 10% have distant metastases. Symptoms include chest pain, dyspnea, cough, or sign of SVC compression. Associated paraneoplastic syndromes—represented by polymyositis or dermatomyositis or erythropoietin hypersecretion—are rare in thymic carcinoma.[2] Myasthenia gravis is rarely seen with thymic carcinoma, with a prevalence reported in the literature of 0% to 15%.[139] Imaging techniques most often reveal a poorly defined mediastinal mass showing radiographic signs of infiltration of the surrounding organs (loss of surrounding fat plane), sometimes with associated pleural effusion, pleural nodules, and lymph nodal enlargement, as evidence of advanced disease (Fig. 56.11). MRI may be of help to better define the direct vascular invasion. Some investigators have found FDG-PET to be useful in the differential diagnosis with thymomas and in detecting node or distant metastases.[140]

Histology

The 2004 WHO classification clearly separates thymic carcinomas from thymomas. This classification also recognizes 11 subtypes of thymic carcinoma, including NETTs, which are considered, by most authors, as a separate entity. The most frequent subtype thymic carcinoma is squamous cell carcinoma (40%), followed by lymphoepithelioma-like (15%).[141] According to some studies, the squamous cell type is associated with a better prognosis than other subtypes.[142] The differential diagnosis of thymic carcinoma from more aggressive subtypes of thymomas (type B3, well-differentiated thymic carcinoma) may be difficult, and large interobserver variability in the histologic allocation to these two groups has been reported. The ITMIG addressed this important issue with a dedicated consensus statement that tried to establish objective criteria for optimal differentiation among the histologic categories.[28]

Staging System

There is no general agreement about optimal staging of thymic carcinoma. The ITMIG recommends using the Masaoka and Masaoka–Koga staging systems, which are consistently applied in thymomas. Some authors, however, did not find a good survival stratification among Masaoka stages and have proposed modifications of the original Masaoka staging system, including the collapse of stages I and II and stages III and IV into a two-tiered system.[147] The high prevalence of node metastases in thymic carcinoma prompted some authors to suggest the use of a TNM-based system, as recommended by WHO.[47] A further staging classification that recognizes three-stage categories based on the extent of the regional involvement (stage I and II) and metastatic/distant disease (stage III) has been proposed.[144]

The new TNM-based system expected in 2017 will be most suitable for thymic carcinomas, given the integration of nodal and metastatic involvement, which are more frequent as compared with thymomas (see Table 56.2).[49,85]

Treatment

As in other thymic malignancies, surgery represents the cornerstone of therapy for thymic carcinoma. A complete resection should always be attempted, because it represents the single most important prognostic factor. The approach to treatment for most patients with thymic carcinoma involves using a median sternotomy access, which allows an excellent view of the anterior mediastinum and both pleural cavities. As in NETT, the surgeon should be ready to perform extended resection to neighboring structures, including mediastinal pleura, lung, pericardium, phrenic nerve (monolateral), and the SVC. When the tumor invades nonresectable intrathoracic structures (aorta, heart, bilateral phrenic nerves), residual tissue is left behind, and clips are placed to facilitate postoperative radiotherapy. Very often, in locally advanced tumors, a combined sternothoracic approach, using extended accesses (clamshell, hemiclamshell, sternothoracotomy), is performed to gain a view to the intrathoracic structures, which should be resected. Similar to the situation with NETT, when treating thymic carcinoma, there is little room for minimally invasive techniques (VATS and RATS). Resection of the tumor should be associated with a regional lymphadenectomy for staging.

The role of chemotherapy and radiotherapy as adjuncts to surgery is far less established in thymic carcinoma than it is in thymomas, due to the rarity of the condition. Most cases include in their population both thymomas and thymic carcinoma, and sometimes it is difficult to extrapolate the results for thymic carcinoma. As evidenced in an ESTS survey, most surgeons agree that thymic carcinoma should be approached in a multimodality setting.[25] When the tumor is considered nonresectable, induction (primary) chemotherapy may be indicated, followed by surgical resection. After resection, the role of adjuvant therapies (mostly radiotherapy) remains undefined. In a landmark Japanese series, including 92 patients with thymic carcinoma who had complete resection, survival was better after adjuvant chemotherapy than after no additional treatment, radiotherapy, or chemoradiation therapy.[43] Some series failed to find any survival advantage with the use of postoperative radiotherapy after resection of thymic

carcinoma,[144] but others found a marginal benefit.[145,146] A study based on a retrospective review of data in the ESTS database found that surgery followed by radiotherapy conferred a significant survival advantage over surgery alone.[139] The lack of prospective studies and the unavoidable selection bias of all the published retrospective studies somehow present a limitation. Therefore, a reasonable suggestion, based on the published literature, seems to recommend postoperative chemoradiation therapy after resection of thymic carcinoma—if there was no preoperative treatment—and radiotherapy only if primary chemotherapy was used (see Fig. 56.10).[75,147,148] For patients who are considered to be inoperable, chemotherapy and radiotherapy have produced response rates of 20% to 60%. The discovery of an overexpression of some molecular markers (such as KIT) in thymic carcinomas (up to 79% of the cases) stirred some enthusiasm for a possible biologic therapy.[149] Unfortunately, despite the high overexpression of KIT, only a small percentage of patients with thymic carcinoma have KIT mutations (9%), consisting of mutations observed in gastrointestinal stromal tumors or melanomas (V560del, L576P), or restricted to thymic carcinomas (H697Y, D820E).[75,147] Responses were reported with the use of KIT tyrosine kinase inhibitors imatinib, sunitinib, or sorafenib, mostly in single-case observations.[121] KIT sequencing (exons 9–17) is an option for refractory thymic carcinomas in the setting of potential access to such inhibitors, particularly in the context of clinical trials.[75]

Immunotherapy using the program death-1 checkpoint inhibitor pembrolizumab was recently assessed in refractory thymic carcinomas.[150] An ongoing phase II trial enrolled 30 patients, with a 24% response rate. Most of the responses were durable, an observation similar to that observed in nonsmall cell lung cancer in the second-line setting; the safety profile was characterized by some frequent and severe toxicities such as myositis, myocarditis, and pemphigus.

Survival and Prognostic Factors

In almost all cases, thymic carcinoma portends a poorer prognosis than do thymomas. Five-year survival rates vary from 30% to 85% according to most authors;[145,151] improved survival rates have been reported in later series. Based on results from the most recent studies, complete resection is associated with the best survival rates, although incomplete resection seems to confer a survival advantage over simple biopsy.[152] Therefore some authors advocate a debulking resection rather than no resection at all, in the case of nonresectable tumors.[139] Among different prognostic predictors, complete resection and early stages seem to be the most consistent factors among all the published series, and tumor size, associated paraneoplastic syndromes, and histologic subtypes are not uniformly reported to be significant in the largest series (Table 56.8).

NEUROENDOCRINE THYMIC TUMOR

NETTs represent around 2% of all neuroendocrine tumors and about 5% of all thymic malignancies.[156] Similar to their counterparts in other organs, they are often associated with endocrinopathies or other paraneoplastic syndromes. About 400 cases of NETT have been reported in the literature so far.

Clinical Presentation and Diagnosis

NETTs are more often seen in men, with a male-to-female ratio of 3:1. Mean age at presentation is 54 years, with a wide age range (16–97 years). Unlike thymomas, NETTs are usually symptomatic (70% of the cases).[157] The most frequent symptoms include cough, asthenia, chest pain, dyspnea, and, sometimes, SVC syndrome. On other occasions, patients present with signs and

TABLE 56.8 Comparison of Results in Published Series of Patients With Thymic Carcinoma

Author (Year)	No. of Patients	No. (%) of Complete Resections (R0)	5-Year Overall Survival (%)	Prognostic Predictors
Kondo et al. (2003)[43]	186	92 (71)	51	Complete resection, adjuvant therapy
Yano et al. (2008)[152]	30	7 (23)	48	Hematogenous metastasis, complete resection
Lee et al. (2009)[145]	60	14 (35)	39	Masaoka stage, surgical intervention, complete resection
Hosaka et al. (2010)[153]	21	14 (67)	61	Masaoka stage, histologic grade
Okereke et al. (2012)[154]	16	14 (88)	65	None
Weissferdt et al. (2012)[144]	65	21 (45)	66	Masaoka stage, tumor size, lymph node status
Okuma et al. (2013)[138]	40	—a	30	Response
Weksler et al. (2013)[151]	290	121 (89)	40	Gender, surgical intervention, Masaoka stage, histologic grade
Thomas de Montpréville et al. (2013)[155]	37	22 (60)	66 (3 years)	Masaoka stage, complete resection
Ruffini et al. (2014)[139]	229	140 (71)	61	Masaoka stage, complete resection, adjuvant radiotherapy

aStudy included advanced-stage disease only, and no surgery was performed (chemotherapy was given).

symptoms of associated endocrinopathies or of distant metastases. Twenty percent of patients have metastases at presentation, with a prevalence of extrathoracic metastases as high as 30%. CT and MRI both show a large, lobulated mass, with radiographic evidence of invasion of the surrounding organs. Less often, they present as a well-circumscribed, capsulated lesion with few signs of invasion. [18]FDG–PET/CT is of little diagnostic use in NETT. Among new diagnostic tools, promising results involving the use of ^{68}Ga-1,4,7,10-tetraazacyclododecane-N[I],N[II],N[III],N[IIII]-tetraacetic acid (D)-Phe1-thy3-octreotide (DOTATOC) PET/CT have been published.[158] The presence of receptors for somatostatin (subtype 2, sst2) suggests the use of specific scintigraphy (octreotide scan) using 111-indium-diethylenetriamine pentaacetic acid-D-phenylalanine-octreotide.[159] As with other neuroendocrine malignancies, NETTs are frequently associated with paraneoplastic syndromes (endocrinopathies), including adrenocorticotropic hormone secretion (Cushing syndrome), MEN type 1 (MEN-1 or Wermer syndrome, with tumors of the parathyroids, pancreatic islet cells, and pituitary gland), and growth hormone-releasing hormone hypersecretion with ectopic acromegaly. Other less frequent syndromes include prolactin secretion, MEN-2, peripheral neuropathy, and Lambert–Eaton syndrome. Unlike lung and gastrointestinal neuroendocrines, carcinoid syndrome is unusual. Lastly, the association with myasthenia gravis is also unusual, with only one case reported in the literature.[159]

Histologic Classification

According to the 2004 WHO classification, NETTs are considered a subtype of thymic carcinomas and separate from thymomas.[55] Several histologic subtypes of NETTs have been proposed. The two most used classifications are the WHO and the Armed Forces Institute of Pathology. Some authors still use the standard classification of NETTs as typical and atypical carcinoids, and large and small cell neuroendocrine carcinomas. The WHO classification categorizes NETT into well-differentiated neuroendocrine carcinomas (including typical and atypical carcinoids) and poorly differentiated neuroendocrine carcinomas (including small and large cell neuroendocrine carcinomas).[160] The Armed Forces Institute of Pathology classification divides NETT into well, moderately, and poorly differentiated forms, based on morphologic criteria and mitotic count.[161] The pivotal roles of the proliferation index (mitotic count) and the Ki-67 index have been recognized, and both indexes have been incorporated into the European Neuroendocrine Tumor Society grading classification. The European Neuroendocrine Tumor Society system includes three groups: G1 (<2 mitoses per 10 high-power fields [HPFs] and/or Ki-67 index of ≤2%); G2 (2–20 mitoses per 10 HPFs and/

or Ki-67 index of 3% to 20%); and G3 (>20 mitoses per 10 HPFs and Ki-67 index >20%.).[162] In 2010, the revised WHO classification of neuroendocrine tumors confirmed the importance of proliferative indexes and defined three groups of tumors according to the combination of morphologic features and of mitotic count and/or Ki-67 index: neuroendocrine tumor/neoplasm G1, neuroendocrine tumor/neoplasm G2, and neuroendocrine carcinomas.[163] The validity of this classification has been successfully tested in gastroenteropancreatic neuroendocrine tumors and, more recently, in NETTs.[164]

Staging System

There is no official staging system for NETTs. Customarily, most series used the Masaoka or Masaoka–Koga staging systems, which are currently used for other thymic malignancies. A TNM staging system for thymic tumors has been proposed by the WHO and has been used in some series, based on the finding that node or distant metastases are present in about 50% of NETTs at the time of diagnosis.[47] Recently, Gaur et al.,[167] using the SEER database, proposed a staging system based on the localized, regional, or distant extension of disease. According to this staging system, tumors that remain in situ or confined to the organ are regarded as localized. Tumors that locally invade or metastasize to regional lymph nodes are considered to be regional, and tumors that spread to distant organs are categorized as distant. The IASLC/ITMIG Staging Committee is working on the forthcoming eighth edition of the TNM staging manual of thoracic malignancies and will propose a common TNM staging system for all thymic tumors, including NETTs. This system is expected to be fully operative by 2017.

Treatment

Surgery remains the mainstay of therapy for NETTs. As in other thymic malignancies, the possibility of performing a complete resection (R0) is the most important prognostic factor. The efficacy of treatment of NETT has been evaluated in several published series (Table 56.9). The preferred surgical access is median sternotomy, which allows an optimal view of the anterior mediastinum and both pleural spaces. If the tumor invades the lung, it may be necessary to use a combined sternothoracotomic approach, with a hemiclamshell or clamshell incision (Fig. 56.12). Resection of the tumor should be associated with a regional lymphadenectomy for staging. Because of the frequent local extent of the tumor, minimally invasive techniques have no indications in NETTs. In case of associated MEN-1 syndrome with hyperparathyroidism, a concurrent thymectomy and cervical

TABLE 56.9 Comparison of Results in the Published Surgical Series (Since 1990) of More Than 10 Patients With Neuroendocrine Thymic Tumors

Author (Year)	No. of Patients	Mean Age (Years) (Range)	Associated Disease (No. of Patients)	No. (%) of Complete Resections	Histology (No. of Tumors)	Postoperative Treatment (No. of Patients)	Recurrence Rate (%)	Survival Rate (%) 5 Years	Survival Rate (%) 10 Years
Fukai et al. (1999)[165]	15	51 (19–73)	Cushing syndrome (2); myasthenia gravis (1)	13 (86.7)	Typical carcinoid (1); atypical carcinoid (9); SCNC (5)	Radiotherapy (5); chemotherapy (1); chemoradiation therapy (1)	67	33	7
Moran and Suster (2000)[157]	80	58 (16–100)	Cushing syndrome (4)	NA	Typical carcinoid (29); atypical carcinoid (36); SCNC (15)	NA	47	28[a]	10[a]
Tiffet et al. (2003)[166]	12	58 (35–78)	MEN-1 (2); Cushing syndrome (1)	9 (75)	Typical carcinoid (3); atypical carcinoid (6); LCNC (2); SCNC (1)	Radiotherapy (3); chemotherapy (1); chemoradiation therapy (1)	83	50	NA
Gaur et al. (2010)[167]	160	57	NA	NA	Typical carcinoid (75); atypical carcinoid (13); LCNC (16)	Radiotherapy (70)		50	20
Ahn et al. (2012)[168]	21	49 (20–72)	Cushing syndrome (3)	17 (81)	Atypical carcinoid (18); LCNC (3)	Radiotherapy (21)	38	[b]	
Cardillo et al. (2012)[169]	35	53	Cushing syndrome (11)	34 (97)	Typical carcinoid (17); atypical carcinoid (13); LCNC (5)	Radiotherapy (20)	26	84	61
Crona et al. (2013)[164]	28	46 (19–64)	Cushing syndrome (4); MEN-1 (6)	3 (14)	NA	Radiotherapy (18)		79	41

[a]Based on 50 patients.
[b]The mean overall survival was 42 months.
LCNC, large cell neuroendocrine carcinoma; *MEN-1*, multiple endocrine neoplasia, type 1; *NA*, not available; *SCNC*, small cell neuroendocrine carcinoma.

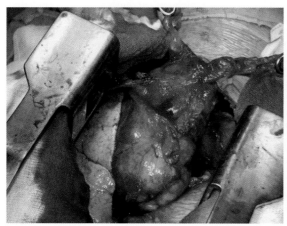
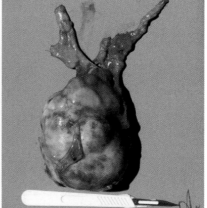

Fig. 56.12. Neuroendocrine thymic tumor: surgical access and operative specimen.

neck exploration should be considered to prevent recurrent disease from spreading to the supernumerary glands. Some authors suggest a routine prophylactic thymectomy in male patients with MEN-1 who are undergoing cervical neck exploration for hyperparathyroidism.

Resectability rates largely depend on the centers and their experience in major resection of intrathoracic structures. Sometimes, the surgeon is forced to leave residual tissue on nonresectable structures (e.g., heart, aorta, the phrenic nerves). Incomplete resection has been recommended by some authors for symptom relief (associated endocrinopathies) and to facilitate adjuvant treatments.

The role of chemotherapy and radiotherapy in NETT is far less established than in other thymic tumors. Preoperative (primary or induction) chemotherapy or radiotherapy has been suggested in the case of tumors that are not considered to be resectable at the time of diagnosis.[170] Radiotherapy has been investigated as a way to reduce recurrence and to improve long-term survival after surgery. Although postoperative radiotherapy is commonly used, a report based on data in the SEER database demonstrated that postoperative radiotherapy had a detrimental effect on long-term survival, although the authors pointed out a potential preselection bias in this group of patients.[167] Other series, however, have demonstrated a reduced risk of recurrence with postoperative radiotherapy.[159] Lastly, postoperative chemotherapy is associated with limited efficacy and a non-negligible toxicity. Cisplatin-based chemotherapy is currently used for patients with poorly differentiated tumors presenting with metastatic or nonresectable disease. Other authors reported good response rates using a combination of temozolomide and a platinum-based regimen. They suggest using temozolomide as first-line therapy for patients with well- or moderately differentiated NETT, because of fewer side effects.[156]

The expression of somatostatin receptors in NETT, and the antiproliferative activity of somatostatin, led some investigators to evaluate somatostatin analogs (octreotide and lanreotide) for the treatment of these tumors. Unfortunately, the results have not been promising so far, and their use cannot be recommended outside approved clinical trials. A promising new therapeutic strategy includes the use of radiolabeled (^{111}IN-DTPH 3) octreotide for radionuclide therapy.[171] The radionuclide could theoretically be replaced with a chemotherapeutic agent specific to NETT. The efficacy of this therapy, although theoretically appealing, is yet to be defined. Ultimately, everolimus represents an approved treatment for advanced, lung, and digestive nonfunctional NETTs, which may be used off-label in refractory thymic NETTs.[172]

Prognostic Factors, Recurrence, and Follow-Up

NETTs are more aggressive than neuroendocrine tumors in other organs. In addition, among thymic tumors, NETTs are associated with the lowest survival rate and the highest rate of local–regional, lymph node, and distant metastases. Five-year survival rates after treatment of NETT vary considerably, from as low as 28% to 84% (see Table 56.9). This variation may reflect the different accrual of the centers, as well as the evolving management strategies over the years. More recent series generally demonstrate better results than do historical ones.[137] A number of prognostic factors have been correlated with survival. The most important prognostic factors reported in almost all of the largest series include the stage (Masaoka, TNM, or system used by Gaur et al.[167]), the completeness of resection, and the degree of histologic differentiation. According to some series, the association of endocrinopathies (MEN-1 and Cushing syndrome) is also associated with a poorer survival. Less validated prognostic factors include tumor size (5-cm or 7-cm cutoff) and Ki-67 index.[169,173] As with other thymic tumors, recurrence is not uncommon in NETT. According to the ITMIG recommendations, recurrences may be divided into local, regional, or distant. Treatment of recurrence largely depends on its extent. Repeat resection may be considered for local or regional recurrence, with reported satisfactory long-term survival.[159,166] Systemic therapy should be considered for unresectable or distant recurrences. Because of the high risk of long-term recurrences, lifelong follow-up is mandatory in NETT; CT is the recommended imaging technique. In case of suspected recurrence, MRI or octreotide scan should be considered for the assessment of resectability.

RECURRENT THYMIC TUMORS

Although surgery remains the mainstay of treatment for all thymic tumors, relapse after surgery is not infrequent. Because of the relatively slow-growing nature of these tumors (with the notable exceptions of thymic carcinoma and NETT), and the fact that many patients with relapse may live a long time and die of another cause, the issue of treatment for recurrence of these tumors is of particular importance. Even after complete resection, recurrence rates are reported in the range of 10% to 30%, and up to 50% in more aggressive tumors.[174–176] The average time to recurrence is 5 years, although recurrences have been recorded up to 20 years after initial resection. Time to recurrence has been reported to be longer for stage I than stage II to stage IV disease (10 vs. 3 years). The recurrence rate largely depends on the stage, being negligible after resection of stage I thymomas (<4%) and progressively increasing from stage II to stage IVA (20% to 50%).[142] Recurrence

rates increase with histology from type A to B3 in thymoma (from 5% to 15%), and they also increase in thymic carcinoma (30% to 40%) and NETT (40%). Until recently, there has been confusion regarding the exact terminology in recurrent thymic tumors. The ITMIG addressed this issue and proposed using the term recurrence only after a complete resection (R0).[23] In addition, three patterns of recurrence were identified: local, in which recurrent disease appears in the anterior mediastinum or lower neck or is contiguous to the initial thymoma; regional, in which intrathoracic recurrent disease occurs in the pleura (visceral or parietal) or pericardium not contiguous with the thymus bed; and distant, in which recurrence is outside the thorax or lower neck or in the form of intrapulmonary nodules. Overall, the distribution pattern includes local recurrence in 30% to 35%, regional recurrence in 50% to 55%, and distant recurrence in 5% to 10% of patients.[177] An increased prevalence of distant recurrences has been reported in thymic carcinoma and NETT. The ITMIG analyzed 12 studies evaluating prognostic factors for recurrence; the single most important predictor of recurrence was the stage at presentation (almost all these studies used Masaoka or Masaoka–Koga stage).[61] Many studies did not find a significant difference between stage I and stage II disease (which were collapsed into one stage in some studies) and between stage III and stage IV disease. Completeness of resection, with safe surgical margins, is obviously a determinant for recurrence, and is part of the definition of recurrence. WHO histology (for thymic carcinoma), although prognostic for survival, was of less prognostic significance when recurrence was analyzed; furthermore, many authors tend to dichotomize the different WHO subgroups to achieve the so-called best results. Among other prognostic factors, only tumor size and invasion of great vessels were occasionally reported as prognostic for recurrence.

Diagnosis

Recurrence after resection of thymic tumors is diagnosed at follow-up, which raises the issue of the frequency and duration of follow-up for these tumors. There is a general agreement that, due to the possibility that disease will not recur until very late in the disease history, a life-long follow-up is mandatory for all thymic tumors.[139] As for the frequency of follow-up, some authors recommend yearly CT for the first 5 years, followed by alternating CT and chest radiography on a yearly schedule until year 11, and then chest radiography thereafter.[20] For high-risk thymomas (WHO stage B2 or B3), incomplete resections, and thymic carcinomas or NETTs, CT every 6 months is advisable for the first 3 years. MRI may be an attractive alternative, especially for young patients. PET/CT is not indicated for routine follow-up, and its use should be reserved for selected cases. Histologic confirmation of a suspicious recurrence is not routinely indicated, because treatment may be instituted in the presence of imaging evidence. There is a great amount of literature that investigates the role of postoperative (adjuvant) treatments (chemotherapy, radiotherapy, or chemoradiation therapy) in reducing recurrence rates after complete resection of thymic tumors. Adjuvant therapy (radiotherapy or chemoradiation therapy) is currently used for as many as 60% of patients with invasive (stage II–IV) thymic tumors, according to a survey by the ESTS.[25] This empirical attitude, however, seems to be mostly based on historical single series and retrospective series, lacking consistent validation. The authors of two studies questioned the usefulness of postoperative radiotherapy after complete resection of stage II to stage IV thymic tumors.[43,103] A 2009 meta-analysis confirmed the results of these two studies, indicating no evidence of a survival advantage associated with the use of postoperative radiotherapy after complete resection of thymic tumors (all stages).[104] Although many of these series focused their results on survival, similar results have also been obtained for recurrence.[26] Indeed, most thymomas relapse in the pleura, which is outside the radiation field of post-operative radiotherapy.[178] Using low-dose, whole hemithorax radiation to prevent pleural relapse has also been advocated by some authors.[179] In the absence of approved guidelines for the use of postoperative radiotherapy after complete resection of invasive thymomas, radiation therapy should be considered on an individual basis and further refined based on different covariates (tumor size, distance of free margins, WHO histology, invasion of great vessels).

Treatment

Treatment of recurrent thymic tumors after curative treatment is not standardized and depends on the extent of the relapse. The pattern of relapse has been found to be significantly different in thymoma and in thymic carcinoma. Thymic carcinoma has been associated with a higher rate of distant recurrence, earlier onset, and lower progression-free survival compared with thymomas.[180]

Surgical resection seems to be the optimal treatment for single, local, and easily resectable relapse and should be recommended. At the other end of the spectrum, surgery should not be considered for patients with bulky, local–regional unresectable recurrence or distant metastases. Instead, chemoradiation treatment may be offered (chemotherapy only for cases of distant relapse).[176] In patients with marginally resectable recurrent disease without distant metastases, surgery may be challenging, with the need for repeat sternotomy or extended surgical accesses and extended resection, or iterative surgery. In these cases, a multimodality approach using induction chemotherapy seems an attractive option, potentially increasing the resectability of residual tumor. The paucity of studies and patient series addressing this issue may partly explain the individualized approach that is being used at most centers. Overall, the resectability rate of recurrent thymic tumor ranges from 50% to 75%.[95,175,181,182] All series but one demonstrated improved survival,[183] if complete resection of recurrence was feasible (which occurs in about 65% of the cases), with survival rates comparable with those of the initial stages, ranging from 50% to 70% at 10 years for complete resections, compared with 0% to 20% for incomplete resections. In one series, published in 2012, surgical resection was associated with a better outcome in recurrent thymoma, but played a limited role for recurrent thymic carcinoma.[184] Chemotherapy seems to be a more effective treatment strategy. Iterative surgery is also indicated in case of subsequent resectable relapse. Surgery should be extensive and complete, particularly in case of pleural dissemination. The authors of two series reported excellent survival rates after aggressive surgery, including extrapleural pneumonectomy and the use of hyperthermic intrapleural chemotherapy, in the management of pleural recurrence of thymic malignancies.[178,185] Nonsurgical treatments of recurrence include chemotherapy or chemoradiation therapy, which have been associated with reasonable outcomes (5-year survival of 25% to 50%).[26,175,177]

RECOMMENDED MANAGEMENT OF THYMIC TUMORS

Several reviews on the management of thymic tumors are available in the literature.[2,26,147,186–188] In addition, the US National Cancer Institute developed guidelines that are available on its website (http://www.cancer.org/cancertopics/pdq/treatment/thymoma/healthprofessional) and that are periodically updated. Lastly, two volumes of *Thoracic Surgery Clinics* (February 2009 and February 2011) and a supplement of the *Journal of Thoracic Oncology* (July 2011) have focused on thymic tumors. ESMO Clinical Practice Guidelines dedicated to thymic tumors were in 2015. These resources provide an excellent overview of all the major aspects and topics related to thymic malignancies. The interested reader is strongly advised to refer to these sources.

Based on the published information, a treatment algorithm can be proposed according to the stage at presentation (Masaoka) and the type of thymic tumor (thymoma, thymic carcinoma, NETT, or recurrent tumor).

Thymoma

Upfront surgery should be done for stage I tumors. The use of any adjuvant therapy is not recommended. A complete resection is expected in all patients.

Stage II tumors should be treated as stage I tumors. A complete resection is expected in more than 90% of the patients. No adjuvant therapy is recommended after complete resection. Postoperative radiotherapy may be considered for incomplete resections and high-risk thymomas (type B2 or B3).

For stage III to stage IV tumors, the multidisciplinary team should make a decision about whether the tumor is resectable. For resectable tumors, upfront surgery is recommended, with the intent of a complete resection. Postoperative radiotherapy may be considered if there is concern about positive surgical margins, high-risk thymomas (type B2 or B3), thymic carcinoma, or NETT. For nonresectable tumors, primary chemotherapy is indicated. Surgery, with the intent of a complete resection, is performed for patients who have radiographic response.

Thymic Carcinomas and Neuroendocrine Thymic Tumor

Although the treatment strategies for thymic carcinoma and NETT are similar to those used for thymomas, the more aggressive behavior of thymic carcinoma and NETT very often requires a multidisciplinary approach, with the use of postoperative radiotherapy and/or chemotherapy, even in early stages, and the use of primary chemotherapy before surgery.

Recurrence

The extent of the recurrence should be carefully evaluated with use of imaging techniques. Histologic confirmation of recurrence is seldom required. In case of distant recurrence, definite chemotherapy is administered. In case of local or regional recurrence, the multidisciplinary team should decide if the recurrence is resectable. If it is, upfront surgery is indicated. Nonresectable recurrences should be treated with chemoradiation therapy.

THE GLOBAL EFFORTS

Thymic tumors are classified as an orphan disease because of their low prevalence. For this reason, robust scientific progress has been hampered, and advancements in management strategies have been slow. In addition, the lack of coordination among centers that have sufficient experience to provide consistent results has been a major obstacle. In an era of globalization and ease of communication, there is no excuse for the lack of cooperation that has occurred so far. To address this issue, several important thoracic societies have promoted the development of dedicated thymic groups.

A major step forward in the scientific advancement of thymic tumors has been the creation, in 2010, of the ITMIG (http://www.itmig.org), which was endorsed and supported by the most representative medical and surgical societies around the globe.[189] The mission of the ITMIG is to promote the advancement of clinical and basic science related to thymic malignancies. It provides infrastructure for international cooperation, maintains close collaboration with other related organizations, and facilitates the spread of knowledge about thymic neoplasms. The ITMIG works in close cooperation with thymic groups of international societies, including ESTS, the European Association of Cardio-Thoracic Surgeons, and the Japanese Association for Research of the Thymus. The ITMIG is a multidisciplinary organization, involving thoracic surgeons, radiation and medical oncologists, pathologists, pulmonologists, radiologists, and basic science researchers. It includes more than 500 members from all continents.

The ESTS (http://www.ests.org) started its thymic working group in 2010, and, since then, it has launched a retrospective thymic database that collects patient data among interested centers. In 2011, ESTS published the results of a survey of its members about the management of thymic malignancies.[25] Multiple articles about prognostic factors in thymic tumors and in thymic carcinomas have been published in the *European Journal of Cardio-Thoracic Surgery* and the *Journal of Thoracic Oncology*.[105,109,139,190] The ESTS also has a prospective database integrated into the official ESTS database platform (https://ests.dendrite.it/csp/ests/intellect/login.csp).

In France, the Réseau Tumeurs THYMiques et Cancer (RYTHMIC, http://www.rythmic.org), which is supported by the French National Cancer Institute, is a very active network. Its objective is to coordinate, at a national level, the diagnostic and therapeutic process in patients with thymic tumors. RYTHMIC initiatives include the creation of a national reference book for thymic tumors (Referentiel RYTHMIC), the organization of periodical regional and national thymic tumor boards, the establishment of a Web-based image and diagnostic archive, the development of a system for systematic double-checking histologic consultation, and the sponsorship of an annual educational meeting.[191]

The ultimate effort in thymic research is the institution, within the IASLC International Staging Committee (now the Staging & Prognostic Factors Committee; SPFC) of the SPFC Thymic domain, which is charged with developing a staging classification proposal for the *Eighth Staging Manual in Thoracic Oncology*, expected in 2017. The committee includes members from different countries, representing a variety of specialties (thoracic surgery, medical and radiation oncology, pathology, radiology). The committee is currently working at analyzing a collaborative database from the three main thymic organizations in the world (Japanese Association for Research of the Thymus, ITMIG, and ESTS). Overall, data on more than 8000 cases have been collated for analysis, representing the most important collaborative effort in the history of thymic research. The committee was asked to present a proposal for a consistent TNM-based staging classification for all thymic tumors (thymomas, thymic carcinomas, and NETTs).

CONCLUSION

A dramatic improvement in our knowledge of the diagnosis and management of thymic tumors has occurred in the last few years. This improvement has primarily resulted from an increased interest in these rare tumors at some dedicated centers, and, above all, from the creation of a worldwide international effort that succeeded in putting together large-volume, top-quality centers all over the world. The results of this amazing international cooperation will soon be available, resulting in a major improvement in the outcomes for a patient population that, until now, has had the same challenges as patients with an orphan disease.

Acknowledgments

The authors thank Thomas Frauenfelder (Department of Radiology, University Hospital Zürich, Switzerland), Alex Soltermann (Institute for Pathology, University Hospital Zürich, Switzerland), Ulf Petrausch (Department of Oncology, University Hospital Zürich, Switzerland), and Andrea Filippi (Department of Radiotherapy, University of Torino, Italy) for their support.

KEY REFERENCES

6. WHO histological classification of tumours of the thymus. In: Travis WB, Brambilla A, Burke AP, Marx A, Nicholson AG, eds. *World Health Organization Classification of Tumours. Pathology and Genetics of Tumours of the Lung, Pleura, Thymus and Heart*. Lyon, France: IARC Press; 2015.

23. Huang J, Detterbeck FC, Wang Z, et al. Standard outcome measures for thymic malignancies. *J Thorac Oncol*. 2011;6(7 Suppl 3):S1691–S1697.

28. Marx A, Ströbel P, Badve SS, et al. ITMIG consensus statement on the use of the WHO histological classification of thymoma and thymic carcinoma: refined definitions, histological criteria, and reporting. *J Thorac Oncol*. 2014;9:596–611.

44. Detterbeck FC, Nicholson AG, Kondo K, Van Schil P, Moran C. The Masaoka-Koga stage classification for thymic malignancies; clarification and definition terms. *J Thorac Oncol*. 2011;6:S1710–S1716.

49. Detterbeck FC, Stratton K, Giroux D, et al. The IASLC/ITMIG thymic epithelial tumors staging project: proposal for an evidence-based stage classification system for the forthcoming (8th) edition of the TNM classification of malignant tumors. *J Thorac Oncol*. 2014;9(suppl 2):S65–S72.

60. Detterbeck F, Youssef S, Ruffini E, Okumura M. A review of prognostic factors in thymic malignancies. *J Thorac Oncol*. 2011;6(7 Suppl 3):S1698–S1704.

62. Detterbeck FC, Parsons AM. Management of stage I and II thymoma. *Thorac Surg Clin*. 2011;21:59–67.

75. Girard N, Ruffini E, Marx A, Faivre-Finn C, Peters S. ESMO Guidelines Committee. Thymic epithelial tumours: ESMO Clinical Practice Guidelines for diagnosis, treatment and follow-up. *Ann Oncol*. 2015;26(suppl 5):v40–v55.

76. Hess NR, Sarkaria IS, Pennathur A, et al. Minimally invasive versus open thymectomy: a systematic review of surgical techniques, patient demographics, and perioperative outcomes. *Ann Cardiothorac Surg*. 2016;5(1):1–9.

78. Venuta F, Rendina EA, Klepetko W, Rocco G. Surgical management of stage III thymic tumors. *Thorac Surg Clin*. 2011;21(1):85–91.

91. Girard N, Mornex F. The role of radiotherapy in the management of thymic tumors. *Thorac Surg Clin*. 2011;21(1):99–105.

113. Wei ML, Kang D, Gu L, Qiu M, Zhengyin L, Mu Y. Chemotherapy for thymic carcinoma and advanced thymoma in adults. *Cochrane Database Syst Rev*. 2013;(8):CD008588.

149. Girard N. Chemotherapy and targeted agents for thymic malignancies. *Expert Rev Anticancer Ther*. 2012;12:685–695.

159. Ruffini E, Oliaro A, Novero D, Campisi P, Filosso PL. Neuroendocrine tumors of the thymus. *Thorac Surg Clin*. 2011;21(1):13–23.

177. Ruffini E, Filosso PL, Oliaro A. The role of surgery in recurrent thymic tumors. *Thorac Surg Clin*. 2009;19(1):121–131.

See Expertconsult.com for full list of references.

57   Lung Cancer Emergencies

Ken Y. Yoneda, Henri Colt, and Nicholas S. Stollenwerk

SUMMARY OF KEY POINTS

- The main oncologic emergencies most germane and specific to lung cancer are central airway obstruction, massive hemoptysis, and massive pleural effusion.

- Central airway obstruction due to lung cancer is traditionally classified as exophytic (intraluminal tumor), extrinsic (compression of the airway by tumor within or external to the wall of the airway), or mixed.

- Treatment of central airway obstruction generally correlates with the type of lesion: ablative modalities (e.g., laser, cryotherapy, argon plasma coagulation) for exophytic lesions; airway stenting for extrinsic compression; and combined therapies for mixed lesions.

- While treatment of central airway obstruction can improve survival, the major aim is the relief of symptoms.

- Massive hemoptysis may present in a dramatic fashion and with a rapidly fatal outcome. Rapid, efficient, and expert management and treatment are therefore of paramount importance.

- Patients with massive hemoptysis generally die of asphyxiation, not exsanguination, and although not all patients with massive hemoptysis require endotracheal intubation and mechanical ventilation, airway management with vigilant ongoing attention to airway assessment and management is a primary concern.

- Endovascular embolization (bronchial artery in 90% of cases) is the mainstay treatment of massive hemoptysis.

- Malignant pleural effusion is the most common cause of a massive pleural effusion.

- Point-of-care ultrasound is an important part of the evaluation and management of massive pleural effusions.

- Indwelling pleural catheters are an effective and safe method to help in the management of symptoms for patients with malignant pleural effusions.

The oncologic emergencies encountered by patients with lung cancer are not exclusive to lung cancer and, for the most part, may affect all cancer patients. Nevertheless, some circumstances and aspects of lung cancer emergencies are unique. Worldwide, lung cancer ranks first in cancer incidence and mortality,[1] but in the United States, it ranks third in incidence behind prostate and breast cancer.[2] Yet, among patients who present to the emergency department, more than three times as many have lung cancer as the next most common type, colorectal cancer. Not surprisingly, respiratory problems are the most common chief complaint for patients with lung cancer on presentation to the emergency department.[3,4] These patients also appear to be more acutely ill; more than five times as many patients with lung cancer die in the emergency department as compared with patients with colorectal cancer.[5] Although most lung cancer emergencies, such as pneumonia, respiratory failure, neutropenic sepsis, shock,

intracranial catastrophe, spinal cord compression, and pathologic fracture, also occur among patients with other cancers, three problems stand out as being most specific and germane to lung cancer, including central airway obstruction, massive hemoptysis, and massive pleural effusions. This chapter offers practical insights and perspectives into the etiology, evaluation, and management of these three complex, controversial, and dreaded complications of lung cancer.

CENTRAL AIRWAY OBSTRUCTION

For the purposes of this chapter, central airway obstruction is defined as obstruction of the trachea and main bronchi as well as of the lobar and segmental bronchi. Central airway obstruction is a complex and frequent sign of progressive disease in patients with lung cancer and in patients with malignancies that metastasize to the lungs and airways. Lung cancer-related central airway obstruction often requires emergent evaluation and treatment to prevent hospitalization and admission to the intensive care unit, to control progression of disease, to palliate and treat other life-threatening diseases, and to avoid immediate death.

Central airway obstruction is associated with many presenting signs and symptoms, a handful of diagnostic modalities used in its evaluation, a multitude of available interventional therapies, and, most importantly, a number of patient-related issues relevant to the diagnostic and therapeutic management of this emergency. In this chapter, we briefly address some of these issues as they relate to the oncologist, radiologist, cytopathologist, interventional pulmonologist, critical care specialist, thoracic surgeon, medical ethicist, and radiation oncologist operating as members of a multidisciplinary team for lung cancer management.

Types of Central Airway Obstruction Presenting as Emergencies

Traditionally, central airway obstruction is classified as exophytic (intraluminal), extrinsic (i.e., compression of the airway from tumor beyond or involving the airway wall), or mixed (Fig. 57.1). This classification is enhanced by specifying the location and extent of the airway abnormality; describing whether the obstruction is focal, multifocal, or diffuse; and indicating whether associated abnormalities are present, such as edema, bronchitis, airway necrosis, purulent secretions, obvious infection (which may be primary or secondary), bleeding, perforation or fistula, dehiscence, or airway distortion. It is also helpful to ascertain whether the abnormality is a primary or secondary disorder. For example, central airway obstruction may be a result of new, progressive, or recurrent disease, or it may be an iatrogenic complication after a procedure, such as airway intubation, mechanical ventilation, stent insertion, brachytherapy or laser resection, other bronchoscopic airway manipulation, external-beam radiotherapy, or thoracic surgical intervention.

Additional features that may be relevant in management decisions include whether the obstructing lesion is dynamic (alters the size of the airway during inspiration and expiration) or fixed (airway diameter remains unchanged during respiratory cycles), whether the lesion has associated malacia (softening of airway

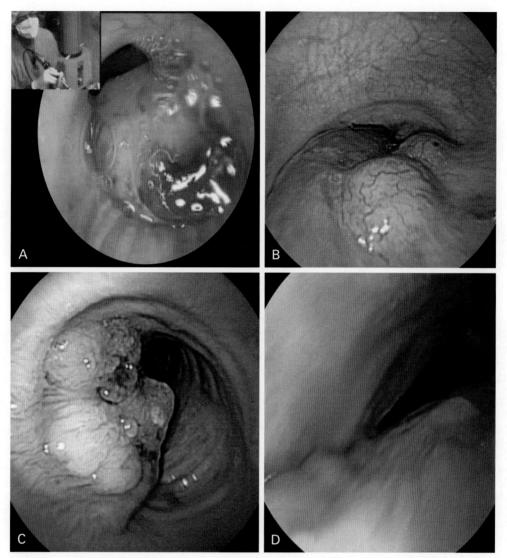

Fig. 57.1. Bronchoscopic images of four types of central airway obstruction prompting emergency intervention. (A) Exophytic lesion causing nearly total obstruction. Thermal ablation can be performed to restore airway patency. Note the external view of rigid bronchoscopy in the upper left-hand corner. (B) Nearly total tracheal obstruction by multilobulated hypervascular tumor involving the posterior membrane. Stent insertion will restore airway patency. Bronchoscopic tumor resection is not absolutely necessary. (C) Mixed obstruction (exophytic and extrinsic compression) by easily bleeding tumor involving the airway wall. Thermal ablation can be used to resect much of the intraluminal tumor. A stent will help maintain airway patency in the case of rapid tumor regrowth. (D) Nearly total airway closure from extrinsic compression by a mediastinal mass at the level of the carina and origin of the right main bronchus. Palliation is possible by airway stent insertion.

cartilage) or excessive dynamic airway collapse (exaggerated invagination of the posterior membrane), and the extent to which symptoms adversely affect the patient's functional status and quality of life. When the airway obstruction has caused an emergency, one must determine whether the emergency is immediately life-threatening. This last point has important implications for diagnosis, treatment, and ethical aspects of care.

Symptoms of Lung Cancer-Related Central Airway Obstruction

The symptoms of central airway obstruction associated with lung cancer are similar to those found in other instances of central airway obstruction and include dyspnea, cough, hemoptysis, hoarseness, and respiratory failure. These symptoms may be progressive or of sudden onset, and can easily be considered to be consistent with the patient's preexisting symptoms of the lung cancer itself. They can be signs of progressive although manageable disease or represent an immediate precursor or cause of death. Central airway obstruction should be suspected in all cases of new onset or increasing symptoms in any patient with known or suspected lung cancer and in patients who have recently undergone palliative or curative therapeutic interventions for their lung cancer. Of course, a patient's comorbidities may be contributing to or causing these nonspecific symptoms. The medical evaluation, therefore, must ascertain the presence, severity, and contributing roles of possible heart failure; esophageal extension; pleural disease; other malignancies extending to the lung, mediastinum, and airways; emphysema and chronic bronchitis; pneumonia; radiation-induced lung or airway injury; clinical depression; malnutrition; and failure to thrive.

Central airway obstruction can be suspected during an outpatient clinic visit, prompt the patient to make an emergency room

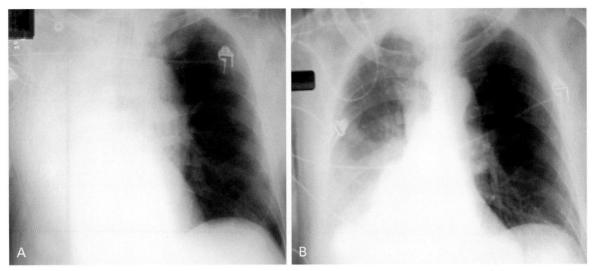

Fig. 57.2. Chest radiograph showing resolved right atelectasis after emergency intervention with flexible bronchoscopy in a patient with a known right lower-lobe tumor. In this case, respiratory insufficiency and radiographic abnormalities (ipsilateral mediastinal shift and atelectasis) were due to mucus plugging seen and removed at the time of emergent inspection bronchoscopy. (A) Shows complete collapse of the right lung. (B) After bronchoscopy.

visit, or be responsible for sudden deterioration requiring intubation, hospitalization, or both. Central airway obstruction often requires admission to the intensive care unit. On some occasions, the obstruction is discovered only after a patient has emergency intubation and is placed on mechanical ventilation. In other cases, symptoms of significant obstruction may warrant intubation, raising issues about life-sustaining treatment, appropriate use of medical resources, costs, and roles of palliative care and procedures. A third scenario may involve a patient with dyspnea or other complications who is denied admission to the intensive care unit and further diagnostic evaluation, either because the diagnosis of central airway obstruction is not considered or because the condition is diagnosed but may be considered irreversible. This last scenario raises issues of professionalism, competency, and resource allocation because levels and quality of care depend, in part, on physician expertise, team experience, institutional biases, finances, and societal philosophies regarding extent of care for patients with life-threatening illnesses. Good communication with the patient and with other health-care providers involved in the patient's care is essential, and a properly executed informed consent is a prerequisite to a thorough understanding of available therapeutic alternatives, including the potential consequences of choosing to accept or refuse minimally invasive surgical interventions.

The setting of emergency central airway obstruction is often complex and stressful for health-care providers, patients, and their families. Patients with malignant central airway obstruction may have a median survival as short as 3 months. One-year survival may be only 15%.[6] In general, the survival rate beyond 90 days in nonsurgical patients with lung cancer requiring admission to the intensive care unit is only 37%,[7,8] and in the case of associated acute respiratory failure, the prognosis is very poor.[9] Usually, respiratory failure in patients with lung cancer is caused by pneumonia, acute lung injury or acute respiratory distress syndrome, diffuse alveolar hemorrhage, airway bleeding, or venous thromboembolism, as well as central airway obstruction. Mortality increases with the number of failed organs, severity of comorbidities, and presence of airway obstruction. In one study, the hospital mortality rate was 83% for patients with lung cancer and central airway obstruction who were receiving mechanical ventilation, compared with 62% in patients without an obstructed airway.[10] In other studies, when respiratory failure was caused by airway obstruction, only 25% of patients were successfully

weaned from mechanical ventilation,[9] although some patients with malignant central airway obstruction benefited from interventional bronchoscopic procedures aimed at restoring airway patency.[11]

Diagnosis of Central Airway Obstruction

The diagnosis of central airway obstruction is made with a combination of clinical findings, radiographic imaging, and bronchoscopic techniques. Because they are noninvasive, chest radiography or computed tomography (CT) is usually performed first. In some life-threatening situations, flexible bronchoscopic inspection is performed to provide immediate information to assist in establishing indications for or against therapeutic interventions to restore airway patency, alleviate dyspnea, postpone or prevent the onset of respiratory failure requiring intubation, or palliate other symptoms (such as hemoptysis).

Clinical Findings

Findings related to central airway obstruction may include decreased breath sounds on chest auscultation, prolonged expiration, and unilateral wheezing. Patients may lose the ability to phonate in cases where an airway stent has migrated proximally to impinge on the vocal cords from below. Vocal cord paralysis may be suggested by cough, hoarseness, change in voice, or episodes of recurrent aspiration and may be related to a primary lung mass or enlarged mediastinal lymph node impinging on the recurrent laryngeal nerve. Hemoptysis may suggest central airway obstruction in patients with known lung cancer or cancers that are known to metastasize or otherwise spread into the airways (such as colon cancer, malignant melanoma, renal cell carcinoma, thyroid cancer, esophageal cancer, adenoid cystic carcinomas, sarcomas, and some lymphomas).

Chest Radiographs Often Aid in Diagnosis

Chest radiographs may show atelectasis, ipsilateral mediastinal shift, lobar consolidation, stent migration, or a mass impinging on the central airway (Fig. 57.2). CT is used to confirm the diagnosis and obtain more detailed information about the cause, extent, type, and morphology of the obstructing lesion. Associated findings include, among others, mediastinal widening, other lung or airway lesions, pleural disease, volume loss, atelectasis, and consolidation. Patients with a history of radiotherapy may have signs of fibrosis or radiation pneumonitis. CT may also provide information regarding the extent of peribronchial involvement and airway distortion, which may be underestimated by bronchoscopy alone. In some instances, ventilation–perfusion scans can be performed to ascertain whether functional lung exists beyond the level of the obstruction, but the results are not always precise and negative findings do not necessarily preclude successful reestablishment of airway patency and restored ventilation.

Flexible Bronchoscopic Examination

Flexible bronchoscopy provides information about the morphology, extent, etiology, and severity of the airway obstruction. It also provides information pertaining to associated airway abnormalities that may affect management decisions and indications for or against palliative or curative interventions to restore airway patency. In experienced hands, airway inspection is performed very quickly with minimal risk to the patient. Depending on the setting, bronchoscopy can be performed through the nares or the mouth (using a bite block), from behind the head of the patient or standing in front of and to the side of the patient, always in conjunction with supplemental oxygen and with or without sedation. For example, in a patient with impending respiratory failure, bronchoscopy can be performed with the patient receiving high-flow oxygen and/or through a continuous positive airway pressure mask, without sedation (to avoid risks of iatrogenic respiratory suppression), and with the patient in the seated position (to avoid aspiration or respiratory suppression related to the supine position).[12] Such a procedure done in the emergency department, hospital ward, or procedure suite may prompt an immediate referral to the operating room for a therapeutic bronchoscopic intervention. If absolutely necessary, the patient can be intubated temporarily with an endotracheal tube over the flexible bronchoscope, or, after appropriate sedation and airway management, intubation can be performed via laryngoscopy before transport to the operating room or interventional bronchoscopy suite.

Evaluation of Patients

Patients with a diagnosis of lung cancer–related central airway obstruction require a careful evaluation to obtain information that will guide management. Many decision points must be considered, some of which are disease related, whereas others are lesion related, patient related (e.g., clinical status and treatment preferences), and health-care team related (Table 57.1). To be certain that information is obtained to address each of these aspects of care, a four-step approach can be used that includes an initial evaluation, a review of procedural strategies, procedural techniques and expected/known results, and a long-term management plan (Table 57.2).[13,14] Many examples for dealing with cancer-related central airway obstruction can be found in the textbook *Bronchoscopy and Central Airway Disorders: A Patient-Centered Approach*.[15]

Treatment Modalities for Emergency Management of Lung Cancer–Related Central Airway Obstruction

The goals of therapy are to restore airway patency, improve symptoms, enhance quality of life, improve patients' functional status so they may undergo additional systemic or local–regional therapies, transfer hospitalized patients to a lower level of care (from the intensive care unit to the wards or from the wards to home), and increase survival. In recent years, a commonly used therapeutic palliative approach is the combination of endobronchial

TABLE 57.1 Examples of Factors That May Influence Management Decisions for Patients With Lung Cancer–Related Central Airway Obstruction in the Emergency Setting

Category	Description
Disease related	Severity and extent of comorbid conditions
	Extent of disease (organ failure, metastases)
	Prognosis without further systemic therapy
	Prognosis with additional systemic therapy
Lesion related	Extent of abnormalities
	Duration of central airway obstruction and symptoms of respiratory insufficiency
	Amenable to bronchoscopic removal or palliation
	Amenable to stent insertion
	Potential response to radiotherapy
Patient status and preference related	Functional status
	Expected survival in the absence of central airway obstruction
	Do-not-resuscitate status
	Response to informed consent
	Family support system
	Risk tolerance
	Desire to live: goals, expectations
Health-care team related	Team experience with bronchoscopic techniques
	Physician competence and experience
	Multidisciplinary team management
	Palliative care and medical ethics consultation availability
	Resource availability (intensive care unit beds, equipment, instruments)
	Proactive versus reactive behavioral profiles
	Realistic, nihilistic, or unrealistic desires and expectations
	Cost, health-care insurance, societal philosophies regarding resource allocation

TABLE 57.2 Four-Step Evaluation for Possible Intervention in Patients With Lung Cancer–Related Central Airway Obstruction

Initial Evaluation	Procedural Strategies
1. Physical examination, complementary tests, and functional status assessment	1. Indications, contraindications, and expected results
2. Patient's significant comorbidities	2. Operator and team experience and expertise
3. Patient's support system (including family)	3. Risk–benefits analysis and therapeutic alternatives
4. Patient's (and family's) preferences and expectations	4. Respect for persons

Procedural Techniques and Results	Long-Term Management Plan
1. Anesthesia and other perioperative care	1. Outcome assessment
2. Techniques and instrumentation	2. Follow-up tests, visits, and procedures
3. Anatomic dangers and other risks	3. Referrals to medical, surgical, or palliative/end-of-life subspecialty care
4. Results and procedure-related complications	4. Quality improvement and team evaluation of clinical encounter

debulking (using thermal, nonthermal, or mechanical techniques) with or without stent insertion, followed by external-beam radiotherapy and/or systemic therapy, if indicated or possible.

Bronchoscopic Laser Resection

Bronchoscopic laser resection, usually using the neodymium: yttrium aluminum garnet (Nd:YAG) laser, is a mainstay of emergency bronchoscopic intervention for patients with central airway obstruction. Laser can be used in conjunction with mechanical debulking and stent insertion, but requires that the health-care team have experience with laser technologies and, most importantly, knowledge of various laser–tissue interactions related to the use of low- and high-power densities. According to numerous studies, laser resection is an effective palliative procedure for central airway obstruction. Complications are uncommon in well-trained hands, but physicians should always consider the possibility of failure to control the airway, airway fires (especially with indwelling airway stents or endotracheal tubes), failure to control bleeding, and airway necrosis. In general, the depth of penetration of the Nd:YAG laser allows excellent coagulation of vessels that are several millimeters in diameter because this thermal ablative technique achieves substantial vasoconstriction and vaporization of tissues.[16]

Airway Stenting

Silicone airway stents are extremely valuable for emergency treatment of central airway obstruction. Not only can these stents be deployed, if necessary, without prior thermal ablative techniques, but they also ensure airway patency and give health-care providers time to address other issues relevant to a patient's care. Data from numerous studies confirm the efficacy of silicone stents to restore and maintain airway patency, although complications such as stent migration, kinking, obstruction by tumor or mucus, and even infection have been reported.[17] Silicone stents, however, require rigid bronchoscopy and general anesthesia. Models are available in all shapes and sizes, including stents that fit onto the carina or secondary bifurcations. By improving functional status, stent insertion allows the medical team to proceed with palliative chemotherapy or radiotherapy if indicated (Fig. 57.3).

Stent insertion becomes necessary when symptomatic airway stenosis is mixed, when stenosis is caused by extrinsic compression, or when a patient has had repeated removal of an intraluminal lesion at short intervals because of a fast-growing tumor. Stent selection has traditionally been based on an operator's previous experience with a particular stent and the local availability of various stents and other equipment. Stent retrievability is important among patients with malignancy for whom a temporary stent placement is expected; these include patients with malignant central airway obstruction who will undergo further surgical or systemic chemotherapy and/or radiotherapy (e.g., patients with thyroid cancer, primary lung cancer, and esophageal cancer impinging on or involving the airways).

In addition to the morphology and consistency of the tumor, the mechanical properties of the stent should be considered in selecting the appropriate stent. The expansile force (strength) and ability to withhold angulation (also known as buckling) vary among different types of stents. The studded-silicone-type stent has a high expansile force. In a distorted, curved airway, angulation properties are important because they determine whether a stent can conform to the acutely angulated airway and remain patent (Fig. 57.4).[18] Patients with indwelling airway stents benefit from having a stent medical-alert card, which informs emergency room physicians about stent type, size, location, and construction and provides instructions about emergency procedures in case of stent-related complications.[15]

External-Beam Radiotherapy

External-beam radiotherapy is a feasible, noninvasive therapeutic alternative, but when the patient has associated severe airway obstruction resulting in atelectasis, the response rate is 20% to 50% in studies involving more than 50 patients.[19] Smaller studies showed that bronchial obstruction can be relieved in

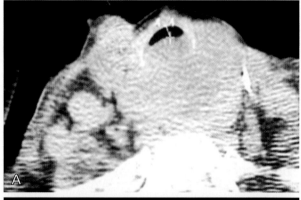

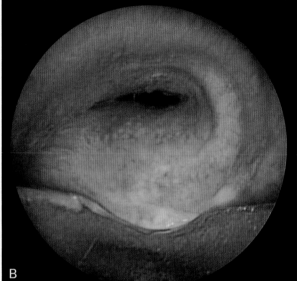

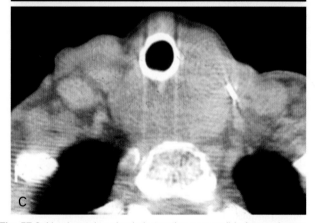

Fig. 57.3. Nearly total tracheal obstruction responsible for respiratory insufficiency required emergency intervention with rigid bronchoscopy and silicone stent insertion. (A) Computed tomography (CT) image demonstrates airway obstruction. (B) Central airway obstruction viewed at the time of emergency rigid bronchoscopy. (C) CT image shows restored airway patency after silicone stent insertion.

up to 74% of patients, resulting in complete or partial reexpansion of the collapsed lung. The time to initiation of treatment matters, because 71% of patients who had radiotherapy within 2 weeks after radiographic evidence of atelectasis had complete reexpansion of their lungs, compared with only 23% among patients having radiotherapy after 2 weeks.[20] The main limitation of external-beam radiotherapy is unwanted exposure

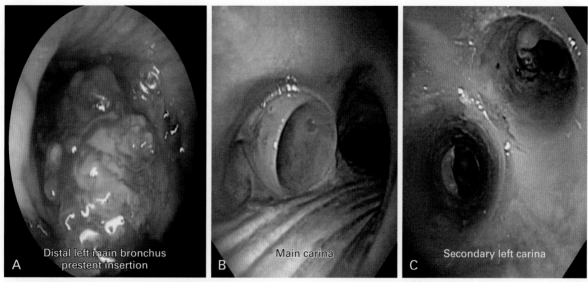

Fig. 57.4. Example of nearly total left bronchial obstruction. (A) Exophytic central airway obstruction from tumor extending from the origin of the left main bronchus to the entrance of the left upper-lobe and lower-lobe bronchi. (B) Proximal aspect of studded silicone Y stent in the left main bronchus extends slightly above the main carina. (C) More distally, the bifurcated silicone Y stent ensures patency of the left upper-lobe and left lower-lobe bronchi.

of the normal lung parenchyma, heart, spine, and esophagus. Improvements in imaging and treatment planning using three-dimensional conformational radiation and respiratory gating can precisely target radiation delivery and, by decreasing normal tissue margins included to account for uncertainties in position, can diminish the risk of clinically significant pneumonitis and esophagitis.[21] The restoration of airway patency usually improves a patient's functional status and performance score, accelerates the initiation of systemic therapy if indicated, and can improve survival.

Endobronchial Brachytherapy

Endobronchial brachytherapy has proven efficacy in patients with endoluminal tumor even when a substantial extrabronchial component is present. This treatment is based on the principle of the inverse square law, which states that dose rate decreases as a function of the inverse square of the distance to the source center, making it possible to achieve a high radiation dose in the center of the radiation source with a fast decrease toward the periphery. Endobronchial brachytherapy offers palliation, with rates of recanalization ranging from 60% to 90%. Symptomatic improvement is seen in 70% to 80% of well-selected patients. The variability in reported results is explained by patient selection, different treatment schemes, and the use of additional treatments. For palliation of symptoms of nonsmall cell lung cancer (NSCLC), however, a Cochrane meta-analysis concluded that endobronchial brachytherapy alone was less effective than external-beam radiotherapy.[22] Endobronchial brachytherapy is usually performed via flexible bronchoscopy. Treatment effects are delayed and complications include hemoptysis, which can be fatal in up to 21% of patients. Other complications include fistula formation, radiation bronchitis (10%), and bronchial stenosis. Squamous cell histology and, most importantly, treatment in the upper lobes are associated with the highest incidence of hemoptysis, probably because of the proximity of the great vessels. Radiation delivered anywhere in the vicinity of major vessels, however, probably increases bleeding risk, as does combined therapy such as laser resection plus endobronchial brachytherapy,

which together may augment the likelihood of tissue necrosis. Patients with poor performance status may also be at higher risk for periprocedural complications such as cough, bronchospasm, and pneumothorax caused by placement of the brachytherapy catheter.

Photodynamic Therapy

Photodynamic therapy can also be performed via flexible bronchoscopy and is approved for local–regional palliation for advanced NSCLC. This modality is most effective when the patient has more than 50% narrowing from mucosal disease.[23] The outcome of photodynamic therapy seems to be the best, however, when patients have a relatively good performance status.[24] In addition, this therapy is less than ideal in the emergency setting because the therapeutic effect is delayed for at least 48 hours and the associated risk of phototoxicity is approximately 20% at 4 weeks after the intervention. Photodynamic therapy may actually worsen airway obstruction during the initial posttreatment period because of sloughing of airway mucosa and retained tumor debris. Sloughed tissue can occlude the airway and cause complete obstruction, resulting in worsening symptoms and postobstructive pneumonia.[25] Similar to endobronchial brachytherapy, photodynamic therapy is contraindicated among patients at high risk for fatal massive hemoptysis. Hemorrhage has been reported for 0% to 2.3% of patients, but the risk may be higher when the disease involves major blood vessels.

Cryotherapy

Cryotherapy causes thrombosis and necrosis of tumor tissues. Although cryotherapy poses no risk of airway fire or perforation, it can cause cold-induced bronchospasm. Cryotherapy has been shown to be most effective when performed in combination with external-beam radiotherapy.[26] Similar to photodynamic therapy and endobronchial brachytherapy, cryotherapy has a delayed effect and initially may worsen airway obstruction, causing postobstructive pneumonia from sloughed necrotic tissue. Among patients with lung cancer and endoluminal obstruction, cryotherapy is reportedly effective in up to 75% of cases, but it is not a therapy of choice in the emergency setting or when extrinsic compression is present.

Argon Plasma Coagulation

Argon plasma coagulation and electrocautery allow removal of exophytic disease and provide superficial cauterization (3 mm to 6 mm), which may not be sufficient to stop large airway bleeding. Depth of penetration and distribution of heat-induced necrosis within tissues are not as predictable as they are with lasers because electrical current follows the path of least electrical resistance within different tissue types. Argon gas is heavy, inert, and much less soluble in the body than carbon dioxide. As gas is forced into the airway wall, perforation may occur, or gas may collect in a blood vessel and pass into the systemic circulation, causing life-threatening gas embolism.[27] Erosion from tumor also presents a risk to major vessels. Risks may be increased when treating highly vascularized lesions and in the proximity of large blood vessels.

Covered Self-Expanding Metal Stents

Self-expanding metal stents, also called hybrid stents, have been used to relieve airway obstruction and seal off fistulae to avoid symptoms of aspiration. Among patients receiving mechanical ventilation, self-expanding metal stents can be inserted via rigid bronchoscopy under general anesthesia or via flexible bronchoscopy under fluoroscopic guidance.[28] Some patients, however, are not suitable candidates for rigid bronchoscopy with a general anesthetic because of the severity of their illness and comorbidities or their unwillingness to have an operation. Fluoroscopy requires special facilities that may not be available in every intensive care unit. Self-expanding metal stents are more costly than silicone stents and can be difficult to remove.

Bronchoscopic Balloon Dilatation

Balloon dilatation is usually performed for airway strictures and is probably not ideal for cases of mixed obstruction from malignant disease. A balloon can be used to expand the airway lumen to facilitate the atraumatic passage of a rigid bronchoscope or endotracheal tube in cases where the operator has limited procedural experience. Mechanical resection of exophytic disease is possible using a specially designed resector balloon.[29]

Expected Outcomes of Emergency Bronchoscopic Management of Central Airway Obstruction

It is not the purview of this chapter to cite the results of bronchoscopic treatment of central airway obstruction. It is common sense, and many studies show, that restoring airway patency improves symptoms, quality of life, exercise capacity, and survival. Therefore, bronchoscopic treatments have universally become the standard of care and should be considered for all patients with a diagnosis of central airway obstruction related to lung cancer.

In some settings, referral to the appropriate specialist is necessary. When in doubt, it is better to ask the specialist to evaluate the patient than to assume that intervention is not technically possible, that the patient cannot tolerate or survive the procedure because of a poor functional status, or that the intervention will not improve quality of life or survival. To enhance the care of all patients with lung cancer, including patients who require emergency treatment for central airway obstruction, the benefits of consulting a multidisciplinary team cannot be overemphasized. Such a team can help make lung cancer management decisions, has ready access to airway specialists with experience and knowledge of minimally invasive interventional techniques, and is well trained in one or more therapeutic bronchoscopy procedures.

Because this section is dedicated to airway emergencies in patients with central airway obstruction, it is reasonable to comment on the subject of patients with respiratory failure due to central airway obstruction. In these cases, interventional bronchoscopic procedures such as mechanical debulking, thermal ablation, and stent insertion have more immediate results than external-beam radiotherapy,[30,31] help obviate the need for continued mechanical ventilation, provide time to initiate additional therapies, and prolong survival and quality of life.[32] In many instances, patients who seem close to death are able to live productive, comfortable lives after airway patency is restored.

The Society of Critical Care Medicine recommends admission to the intensive care unit for all patients with advanced cancer who have a reversible condition such as pulmonary embolism, cardiac tamponade, or airway obstruction.[33] Accompanying this recommendation is a prioritization scale identifying patients who will benefit most from admission to the intensive care unit (priority 1) and patients who will not benefit at all (priority 4). Patients with cancer complicated by airway obstruction are assigned priority 3, defined as unstable patients who are critically ill but have a reduced likelihood of recovery because of underlying disease or the nature of their acute illness. It is well recognized that emergency bronchoscopic intervention can be beneficial in many critically ill patients. In 2012, we reported the results of emergent therapeutic bronchoscopic intervention in 12 patients with NSCLC who had intubation and mechanical ventilation in the intensive care unit during a 6-year study period.[34] Airway patency was restored in 11 (92%) of 12 patients. Bronchoscopic intervention resulted in immediate extubation and discontinuation of mechanical ventilation in 9 (75%) of 12 patients. The overall median survival was 228 days (range, 6 days to 927 days). For 9 individuals who were extubated within 24 hours after intervention, the median survival was 313 days (range, 6 days to 927 days).

In another study, Jeon et al.[32] reported the results for 36 patients with respiratory failure and malignant central airway obstruction from various tumors. They noted that patients who had systemic therapy or radiotherapy in addition to bronchoscopic intervention survived longer than patients who had bronchoscopic palliation of central airway obstruction alone (median survival, 38.2 months vs. 6.2 months).[32] In a retrospective study from Holland, 14 patients with advanced disease from esophageal cancer (5 patients) or NSCLC (9 patients) had immediate symptomatic relief after bronchoscopic intervention. As a result, Dutch general practitioners responsible for terminal home care remarked that bronchoscopic intervention and airway stent insertion are worthwhile elements of a patient-focused treatment plan.[35]

MASSIVE HEMOPTYSIS

Hemoptysis is not a rare event, and it will occur at some point in approximately 20% of patients with lung cancer. Massive hemoptysis is far less common, but 3% of patients will have massive hemoptysis as their terminal event.[36] When hemoptysis is trivial in amount, it is usually straightforward to diagnose and treat; yet it may also foreshadow a more critical or fatal event. At times, hemoptysis has such a sudden onset and large volume that it prompts emergent hospitalization and treatment, yet is not considered massive by all definitions in the literature. At other times, it may arise or advance in such dramatic volume and fashion as to be truly shocking to both patient and clinician. With this unmistakable presentation, it is universally acknowledged as massive and is clearly recognizable as a critical life-threatening condition. However, no universally accepted term is used (major, massive, catastrophic, life-threatening, and severe have all been used) to describe these different scenarios, and even more elusive is a precise volume or clinically relevant definition. Perhaps most important is the physiologic effect of hemoptysis; for example, although 500 mL of blood loss is insufficient to cause exsanguination, it can lead to rapid asphyxiation and death. Rapid and efficient evaluation and treatment of hemoptysis are therefore of paramount importance. Mobilizing the resources to accomplish this task is a challenge, particularly in centers that may have limited experience and resources. Therefore, not surprisingly, the reported mortality rate is highly variable, ranging from 0% to 78%, depending on the definition, etiology, era, treatment center, study design, and, potentially, the treatment approach.[37–39]

For the purposes of this review, the term massive hemoptysis is used to encompass the various terms and definitions encountered in the medical literature, but the reader is encouraged to consider the broader context of potentially life-threatening hemoptysis. Data regarding massive hemoptysis specifically in the context of lung cancer are limited. Therefore much of the following discussion is derived from data regarding hemoptysis in general, but, wherever possible, the discussion is focused on lung cancer. Accumulating, albeit imperfect, evidence suggests the benefit of a multidisciplinary approach to the diagnosis and management of massive hemoptysis for patients with lung cancer.

Definition

The volume of expectorated blood that has been used to define massive hemoptysis varies from more than 100 mL to more than 1000 mL in 24 hours,[40,41] but is often considered to be greater than 600 mL. The volume of expectorated blood has long been recognized to correlate with disease severity and outcome, including mortality. In a retrospective, single-institution review of 887 patients with hemoptysis of greater than 200 mL in 24 hours, Corey and Hla[41] found that the mortality rate was 58% for patients with hemoptysis greater than 1000 mL in 24 hours, whereas the rate was 9% for patients with less than 1000 mL in 24 hours. However, the volume of expectorated blood is difficult for patients to quantify and is somewhat subjective. Furthermore, the expectorated volume may vastly underestimate the amount of blood remaining in the alveolar spaces and airways. For this reason, a chest x-ray may reflect more accurately the clinical significance of the bleeding. Perhaps more important than the precise volume of expectorated blood is its physiologic effect. It has been estimated that 400 mL of blood in the alveolar spaces is sufficient to impair oxygen transfer.[42] The same volume of blood can cause significant obstruction of the large airways, asphyxiation, and death. In addition, the rate of bleeding, underlying morbidity, and the patient's ability to maintain a patent airway all affect severity, independent of the absolute volume. Alternative definitions based more on the physiologic effects of airway obstruction and hemodynamic instability have been proposed.[43–45]

In a large series published in 2012, Fartoukh et al.[38] shed light on predicting the in-hospital mortality and severity of hemoptysis and hence clarified how we may consider, define, characterize, and manage this disorder. In their study, the volume of expectorated blood was an apparent predictor of mortality in a univariate analysis, but no longer remained an independent predictor of death after adjustment for other factors. Using data from a retrospective review of 1087 patients with hemoptysis admitted to the intensive care unit or step-down unit over 14 years at a single institution, they developed and validated a multiregression model for predicting in-hospital mortality. They devised a simple scoring system assigning points for chronic alcoholism (1 point), cancer (2 points), aspergillosis (2 points), pulmonary artery involvement (1 point), two or more chest x-ray quadrants (1 point), and initial mechanical ventilation (2 points). In-hospital mortality increased with increasing score, as follows: 0 = 1%, 1 = 2%, 2 = 6%, 3 = 16%, 4 = 34%, 5 = 58%, 6 = 79%, and 7 = 91%. These results suggest that rather than using a cutoff of expectorated volume for defining massive hemoptysis, a scoring system might better define hemoptysis and stratify patients according to the level of risk. Only with this type of objective and standardized definition can we begin to study how best to triage, manage, and treat these patients.

Etiology of Hemoptysis

Regarding massive hemoptysis in general, infectious etiologies (tuberculosis, bronchiectasis, mycetomas, and necrotizing pneumonia) predominate worldwide. Lung cancer is the cause in 3% to 10% of the cases that are severe enough to require bronchial artery embolization and in 17% of patients admitted to the intensive care unit.[37,38,46,47] Tuberculosis is the most common cause in specific areas of the world, yet is a rare cause in other areas.[48] Lung cancers, like most other cancers, are highly vascular and, particularly when endobronchial, may lead to massive hemoptysis. Patients with lung cancer may have chemotherapy-induced thrombocytopenia, comorbidities such as renal disease and/or liver disease, vascular disease requiring antiplatelet therapy, or thrombotic disorders requiring anticoagulation, and these factors compound the problem. Some of these conditions and medication effects can be mitigated, corrected, or reversed. Of special note are the antiangiogenesis factors and tyrosine kinase inhibitors (some of which also have significant angiogenesis inhibition) that can lead to massive hemoptysis.[49] The biologic effect of these medications cannot be reversed and lasts for weeks.

Massive hemoptysis in a patient with lung cancer should not be automatically assumed to be coming directly from the lung cancer lesion. As already discussed, patients often have comorbidities that may predispose them to various other etiologies of hemoptysis, including cancer-related hypercoagulability leading to pulmonary emboli, coagulopathy leading to alveolar hemorrhage, and immunosuppression leading to necrotizing pneumonia. The clinician must therefore thoroughly evaluate hemoptysis in patients with lung cancer without assuming that the lung cancer is the source of the hemoptysis. This evaluation is important in treatment considerations; for example, patients with diffuse alveolar hemorrhage and/or coagulopathy respond to specific treatments and are not likely to derive benefit from invasive therapeutic procedures such as endovascular embolization.

Vascular Source of Bleeding

In approximately 90% of cases of hemoptysis, the bronchial artery circulation is the source of bleeding. This circulation is of relatively low flow, representing only a small percentage of cardiac output. Consequently, the bleeding may be self-limited and minimal in quantity. However, the bleeding is at the same time driven by high systemic pressures that may flow directly into the airways, where no counter-pressure exists to provide tamponade against the bleeding. This so-called high-pressure–low-flow source of bleeding can rapidly overwhelm the patient's ability to keep the airways clear and avoid suffocation. Malignancy and chronic lung inflammation promote neovascularization, recruitment, hypertrophy, and proliferation of bronchial arteries. Chronic pleural inflammation promotes abnormalities in the circulation, which may originate from the mammary, subclavian, intercostal, thoracic, pericardial, phrenic, and thyrocervical arteries. These vessels may enter the lung through the pulmonary ligament or parietal or diaphragmatic pleura and represent another high-pressure–low-flow source, which has been reported in 3% to 25% of cases of hemoptysis.[39,46,47] Conversely, although the pulmonary artery circulation is driven by relatively low right ventricular pressures, a pulmonary artery bleed may represent a significant percentage of the cardiac output. This relatively low-pressure–high-flow circulation is responsible for only a minority

TABLE 57.3 Vascular Source of Hemoptysis

Source	Approximate Incidence (%)
Bronchial circulation	90
Other systemic circulation	3–25
Pulmonary vascular circulation	6

of cases of massive hemoptysis, but may be just as dramatic in presentation, such as with a ruptured Rasmussen artery in patients with tuberculosis. Remy et al.[50] detected a pulmonary vascular source of bleeding in 11 (6%) of 189 patients treated with transcatheter bronchial or pulmonary artery embolization for massive or repeated hemoptysis, and Wang et al.[51] recognized a pulmonary artery source in 2 of 30 patients. The authors of other large series have failed to report the pulmonary artery circulation as a significant source of hemoptysis. However, failure to consider the pulmonary circulation as a potential source of hemoptysis may explain why angiography fails to identify a definitive source of hemoptysis in approximately 11% of cases.[47,52] Of final note, the pulmonary venous circulation is also not well recognized as a potential source of massive hemoptysis. It has even lower pressures, equivalent to left atrial pressures, and represents a potential very-low-pressure–high-flow source of massive hemoptysis (Table 57.3).

Bronchial artery anatomy can be quite variable, and a thorough understanding and evaluation are necessary to determine the precise vascular origin of hemoptysis. The bronchial arteries originate from the descending aorta between T5 and T6 in 70% of people. Another 20% of people have ectopic branching arising from the subclavian, internal thoracic, pericardiacophrenic, innominate, thyrocervical trunk, and inferior phrenic arteries or abdominal aorta. In 10%, the bronchial arteries arise from other regions of the descending thoracic aorta and aortic arch.[53] Branching patterns of the bronchial arteries themselves are highly variable, with nine patterns described.[54] Multidetector CT provides an accurate road map for embolization by identifying the etiology and origin of the hemoptysis. It can depict the precise anatomy and nature of the bronchial and nonbronchial arteries involved, their course and size, and their relationship to the spinal artery.

Clinical Assessment, Initial Resuscitation, and Stabilization

Although assessment, resuscitation, and stabilization will be addressed separately from the approach to diagnosis, in reality all of these tasks are performed in parallel and are to a great degree integrated. As in most critical care situations, the initial clinical assessment, resuscitation, and stabilization of massive hemoptysis generally take precedence over complex or comprehensive diagnostic testing. Given that most patients die of asphyxiation rather than exsanguination, airway assessment and management are the priority. Initial hospital management should take place in the emergency room or the intensive care unit, with the most experienced personnel available rendering care. Whenever possible, these patients should be cared for at centers with the expertise and resources to optimally manage them. Transfer to tertiary centers may be advised.

Airway assessment is similar to that for any emergency patient, and the decision to perform endotracheal intubation and initiate mechanical ventilation rests on sound clinical judgment. If the patient has evidence of respiratory distress, one should not hesitate to secure an airway. However, not all patients with massive hemoptysis require endotracheal intubation. The aims of endotracheal intubation are to establish a secure airway, achieve adequate ventilation and oxygenation, and maintain airway clearance, which, in the nonintubated patient, are dependent on several

factors, including the flow, volume, and duration of hemoptysis; cough and airway clearance mechanics; and cardiopulmonary reserve. Prophylactic intubation is not usually warranted for a patient with massive hemoptysis who is not in distress. Nevertheless, one must pay careful attention to signs that a patient is failing to maintain airway clearance, such as tachycardia, tachypnea, hypertension, hypotension, and hypoxemia. A chest x-ray with two or more quadrants involved indicates a large volume of aspirated and incompletely cleared blood, suggesting that these patients are at an increased risk of death.[38] Early intubation may be warranted for these and other selected patients. Again, clinical judgment must be exercised, taking into consideration such factors as the patient's ability to tolerate transport, supine positioning, and sedation for angiography or other procedures.

Patients should be confined to bed rest and should be in a decubitus position with the bleeding lung down. When intubation is deemed necessary, a large-bore tube, size 8 or larger (to facilitate bronchoscopy and suctioning), should be inserted by the most experienced operator available. Bronchoscopic intubation is often preferred because it not only facilitates intubation, but may also be diagnostic and therapeutic. Furthermore, it allows selective intubation of the nonbleeding right or left lung when it is deemed necessary. Selective intubation of the left main bronchus can rapidly establish a secure airway as well as isolate and protect a nonbleeding left lung. Selective intubation of the right main bronchus is more problematic given the very proximal right upper-lobe takeoff. Placement of a balloon in the bleeding bronchus will cause tamponade and terminate hemoptysis, as well as further protect the nonbleeding lung. A double-lumen endotracheal tube can accomplish the same goals. Although placement of a double-lumen endotracheal tube has been advocated to isolate and protect the nonbleeding lung, its use is not without problems: misplacement occurs in about 50% of cases,[55] life-threatening trauma to the airway has been reported,[56] and the small diameters of the lumen make bronchoscopy and suctioning difficult.

Rigid, as opposed to flexible, bronchoscopy has been advocated as a means of securing an airway and simultaneously providing a platform to diagnose and control massive hemoptysis.[45,57] However, it is not readily available at all centers, and two large series on the management of massive hemoptysis suggested that flexible bronchoscopy (preferred as first-line therapy over rigid bronchoscopy) can be used safely, with a mortality rate of 0% to 4%.[37,52] Without head-to-head comparisons, the choice of rigid or flexible bronchoscopy remains largely based on individual experience, availability, and institutional practice.

Two large-bore intravenous catheters should be placed, and a central venous catheter should be considered. Appropriate aggressive volume resuscitation including blood and, when necessary, intravenous vasoactive medications should be administered. Chest x-ray, laboratory testing, and type and screening for blood should be performed. Disorders of coagulation should be corrected whenever possible.

As discussed earlier, the in-hospital mortality rate is 34% for patients with a score of 4 or more on the scoring system by Fartoukh et al.,[38] and admission to the intensive care unit should be strongly considered for these patients. Death from massive hemoptysis is difficult to predict, and even patients with a score of 3 or less may benefit from admission to the intensive care unit; clinical judgment must be exercised.

A thorough history and physical examination should be performed, with attention paid to the following: (1) the quantity, duration, and quality of hemoptysis; (2) the patient's lung cancer history including type, status, radiotherapy, surgical procedures, and antineoplastic drug therapy; (3) medication history; (4) underlying liver, kidney, and cardiopulmonary diseases; (5) signs and symptoms of respiratory distress; (6) signs and symptoms of other sites of bleeding; and (7) history of alcohol use.

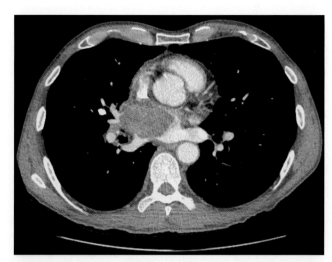

Fig. 57.5. Computed tomography of the chest shows invasion of a lung mass into the left pulmonary vein and right atrium, indicating multiple potential vascular sources of hemoptysis.

Approach to Diagnosis

The major diagnostic studies for massive hemoptysis are laboratory tests to evaluate for coagulopathy and other potential causes of hemoptysis (e.g., vasculitis and alveolar hemorrhage), chest x-ray, CT of the chest, and bronchoscopy. Laboratory testing is aimed at identifying correctible or treatable causes of hemoptysis, whereas the remaining diagnostic studies are aimed at rapid and efficient triage of patients for definitive invasive interventional treatment. Although a chest x-ray should be performed as an important prognostic indicator and may guide triage decisions,[38] chest x-rays are not helpful in approximately 50% of cases.[48]

In the critical setting of massive hemoptysis, localization of bleeding to a specific site or at least the relevant side is crucial in allowing the interventional radiologist to narrow his or her focus and to perform endovascular embolization in an efficient manner. CT images provide information on the site and potential causes of bleeding and may indicate the precise vascular origin and source (Fig. 57.5). Bronchoscopy more accurately identifies endobronchial lesions and provides a potentially temporizing and, on occasion, a definitive therapeutic option. A practical approach is to perform CT if the bleeding has been stabilized and to perform a diagnostic and potentially therapeutic bronchoscopic procedure on patients who are not stable enough for transport to CT because of uncontrolled bleeding. When necessary, these procedures can be performed sequentially.

Computed Tomography

In cases of severe and massive hemoptysis, CT identifies the side and specific site of bleeding in approximately 70% to 100% of patients and a specific cause in 60% to 100% of patients.[58,59] How well this information applies specifically to patients with lung cancer is unknown.

More recently, multidetector-row CT angiography has been used to identify bronchial and nonbronchial sources of bleeding as well as to depict the anatomy of the pathologic vessels. These results may help when planning endovascular embolization,[60] particularly for massive hemoptysis.[61] This road map may be extremely helpful because bronchial artery branching is highly variable and the origin and anatomy of the bronchial artery responsible for massive hemoptysis are not always easily identifiable.[62] Although the bronchial arteries usually arise from the aorta between T5 and T6, they may also arise from the lower thoracic aorta, subclavian arteries, brachiocephalic artery, internal mammary artery, costocervical trunk, pericardiacophrenic artery, thyrocervical trunk, or inferior phrenic artery. Multidetector-row CT may identify ectopic bronchial artery origins in more than 30% of cases of hemoptysis.[63,64] In a prospective study of multidetector-row CT for hemoptysis, this modality was diagnostic in 25 of 27 cases of massive, moderate, and/or recurrent hemoptysis.[60]

Bronchoscopy

For hemoptysis in general, CT identifies the side and specific site of bleeding in approximately 63% of patients.[65,66] The addition of bronchoscopy improves the yield to 93%,[48] and its routine use has long been advocated.[43,67] To what degree these studies can be extrapolated to massive hemoptysis in patients with lung cancer is unclear, and no clear consensus exists on the diagnostic role of bronchoscopy in this population. These studies do, nevertheless, provide insight and evidence that the two modalities are complementary. In cases of massive hemoptysis, bronchoscopy should certainly not supersede clinical evaluation, establishment of a secure airway, and hemodynamic stabilization. In the limited case series comparing flexible bronchoscopy and CT for massive hemoptysis, bronchoscopy and CT appeared equivalent in identifying the side or site of bleeding, and both methods had more than 70% yield. The two modalities may be complementary, but both are not always necessary. For identifying the specific cause of bleeding, CT appears to be far superior to bronchoscopy, but again the methods may be complementary.[58,59,68]

Treatment

Until the 1950s, the management of massive hemoptysis was mainly supportive and included rest, sedation, cough suppression, vitamin K supplementation, and systemic coagulants. For the most severe cases, emergency phrenic nerve crush, intentional induction of a pneumothorax and/or pneumoperitoneum, plombage (extrapleural introduction of inert substances), and/or thoracoplasty was used to collapse and induce tamponade in the hemorrhaging lung. Although pulmonary resection for traumatic pulmonary hemorrhage had been widely recognized, pulmonary resection for nontraumatic massive hemoptysis was not an accepted option until Ryan and Lineberry[69] in 1950, and Ross[70] in 1953, reported the first successful emergent surgical pneumonectomies for massive hemoptysis due to underlying lung disease (tuberculosis in both cases). By the late 1960s, conservative medical management of massive hemoptysis was increasingly recognized as having an unacceptably high mortality rate of 78% to 85%, compared with a rate of 0.9% to 19% after surgical intervention for patients who were considered operative candidates.[39,71,72] An aggressive surgical management approach was therefore advocated. However, up to 39% of the patients with massive hemoptysis were not considered operative candidates, and emergency surgical procedures carried a mortality rate of 37% to 43%.[39,73,74] Therefore by the late 1970s and early 1980s, coinciding with, and perhaps relating to, a decline in tuberculosis as the leading cause of hemoptysis in the United States, a number of centers advocated a return to more conservative management of even operable patients with massive hemoptysis. The mortality rate of this approach to major and massive hemoptysis was reported to be low, at 11% for operable patients who did not undergo an operation or endovascular embolization.[41] A paradigm shift to the modern era of hemoptysis management began with the first description of bronchial artery embolization by Remy et al.[75] in 1973, and by the late 1980s, its use was widespread.[41] Endovascular (including bronchial artery) embolization is now the standard first-line treatment for massive hemoptysis due to lung cancer, with surgical intervention reserved for selected refractory cases.[52] Although not useful in the acute setting of massive hemoptysis, radiotherapy may prevent recurrence of hemoptysis once the patient has been stabilized with conservative measures, such as bronchoscopic intervention and/or endovascular embolization.[76]

Bronchoscopy

Bronchoscopic intervention alone may be a definitive treatment, but in most cases of massive hemoptysis, bronchoscopy is used as a means of controlling airway bleeding until endovascular embolization or, rarely, a surgical procedure can be employed as the definitive treatment.[52] Occasionally, bronchoscopy can be used as a stopgap measure for controlling hemoptysis until an underlying coagulopathy or other reversible cause can be corrected. No consensus exists on the role of therapeutic bronchoscopy in the management of massive hemoptysis, and its use varies with local and regional practice and expertise. In two large case series, flexible bronchoscopy was routinely used in the management algorithm of massive hemoptysis with very low mortality rates of 0% and 4%, suggesting that it is an important intervention in the management of massive hemoptysis.[37,52] As discussed previously, when flexible bronchoscopy is used to guide endotracheal intubation, it may be reasonable and practical to proceed to a quick but thorough diagnostic and potentially therapeutic bronchoscopic intervention. Also, as mentioned earlier, when persistent bleeding renders a patient too unstable for transport for more definitive treatment, bronchoscopy may be considered the treatment of choice. When bronchoscopic intervention is undertaken, the bronchoscopist should be prepared for and have resources available for managing any complications that may occur.

Rigid bronchoscopy, or a combination of rigid and flexible bronchoscopy, has been advocated over flexible bronchoscopy alone, largely because it establishes a secure airway, allows selective isolation of the unaffected airway, and has greater suctioning capacity for maintaining airway clearance, while providing a platform for further endoscopic interventions.[47,57] However, no prospective studies have validated this approach as being superior, and the decision to use one over the other is largely based on individual experience and availability.

A variety of bronchoscopic means have been used to mitigate bleeding in patients with massive hemoptysis, all of which, with the exception of direct-pressure tamponade with the rigid bronchoscope, can be performed with either flexible or rigid bronchoscopy. The superiority of one method over another has not been studied in a systematic fashion; the choice is somewhat subjective and highly dependent on the operator's expertise and the available resources. Cold saline lavage is widely used and has been shown to be effective in controlling bleeding in massive hemoptysis due to lung cancer.[77,78] It is therefore considered a standard primary bronchoscopic treatment for massive hemoptysis.[79] Endobronchial instillation of topical vasoconstrictive agents such as epinephrine and norepinephrine has been recommended for the management of postbiopsy hemoptysis,[80,81] but in general this strategy is not very effective in massive hemoptysis because the drug is diluted and cleared by the active bleeding. Nevertheless, the combination of cold saline followed by epinephrine has been found to be effective in individual cases.[82] Potentially fatal arrhythmias have been reported with endobronchial instillation of epinephrine,[83] and norepinephrine has been offered as an alternative agent because of its reduced beta-adrenergic effect.[81] Concerns regarding the use of both epinephrine and norepinephrine have been raised, and experts in the field have called for the removal of vasoactive drugs for the management of airway bleeding.[84] However, phenylephrine may be a safe and acceptable alternative, given its pure alpha-adrenergic vasoconstrictive properties.

When endobronchial instillation of cold saline and vasoactive drugs fails to control bleeding, endobronchial balloon catheter tamponade can be used to temporize massive hemoptysis from lung cancer and can be performed without great difficulty by most bronchoscopists.[85] The balloon can be left in place until more definitive treatment and/or until transfer to a regional center with greater expertise in the management of hemoptysis. More advanced bronchoscopic techniques, such as endobronchial laser and argon plasma coagulation, are not widely available but have been reported to be effective in controlling massive hemoptysis when bleeding from an endobronchial tumor is visible and within reach of the bronchoscope.

Endobronchial application of the Nd:YAG laser for control of massive hemoptysis due to lung cancer was first reported by Edmondstone et al.[86] in 1983. Various types of lasers are available today, but Nd:YAG remains the most common laser used within the airway. Multiple case series have demonstrated its effectiveness in relieving airway obstruction and dyspnea due to endobronchial and endotracheal tumors, but few studies have addressed its effectiveness in controlling hemoptysis, particularly massive hemoptysis. Although it has been generally reported to be approximately 60% effective in controlling hemoptysis,[36,45,87] a substantially higher rate of 94% was reported in a case series published in 2007.[88] The effectiveness of the Nd:YAG laser in controlling massive hemoptysis is not clear, but its use for this purpose is common and continues to be advocated.[36,45,89]

In one study, endobronchial application of argon plasma coagulation was used to control hemoptysis in 56 of 56 patients (6 of whom had hemoptysis >200 mL/d) without recurrence during a mean follow-up of 97 days.[90] Like Nd:YAG laser therapy, argon plasma coagulation is a noncontact application, but it differs in that it delivers electrically conducted argon (plasma) that produces rapid coagulation at a lower depth of penetration than Nd:YAG. Like the Nd:YAG laser, its use for massive hemoptysis has not been well validated, but its use continues to be advocated.[36,45]

Endobronchial electrocautery has been used to control hemoptysis due to lung cancer,[91,92] but limited evidence is available for its use in massive hemoptysis. Its routine use therefore cannot be advocated.

Other advanced bronchoscopic procedures, including endobronchial instillation of tranexamic acid,[93] fibrinogen–thrombin,[94,95] airway stent tamponade,[96] and oxidized regenerated cellulose hemostatic plug,[82] have all been reported to be successful for at least temporarily terminating massive hemoptysis from lung cancer, but none has been well validated. In addition, airway placement of a silicone spigot and endobronchial instillation of *n*-butyl cyanoacrylate glue have been used to temporize massive hemoptysis in patients without lung cancer.[97,98] Routine use of these agents and devices cannot be recommended, and their use should be determined only on a case-by-case basis.

Probe cryotherapy and brachytherapy have been used to treat endobronchial tumor and hemoptysis.[99–104] However, their effects are not rapid enough to control massive hemoptysis, and their use cannot be recommended for this indication.[36] Spray cryotherapy has also been used to treat endobronchial tumor and hemoptysis,[105,106] and although its use in massive hemoptysis has not been reported, it offers a potentially novel means of controlling massive hemoptysis.

Endovascular Embolization

Angiographic signs that confirm a source of bleeding are as follows (Figs. 57.6–57.8):[107,108]

- hypertrophy or enlargement (diameter >3 mm)
- tortuous bronchial arteries
- parenchymal hypervascularity

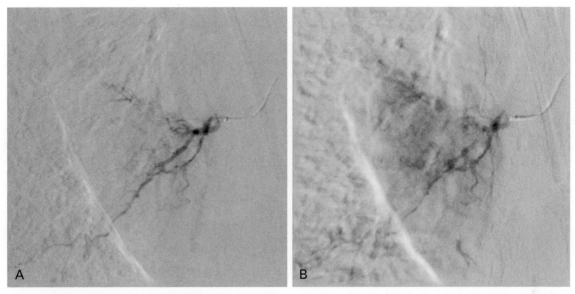

Fig. 57.6. Right bronchial arteriogram demonstrates (A) tortuous bronchial arteries and parenchymal hypervascularity; and (B) parenchymal staining.

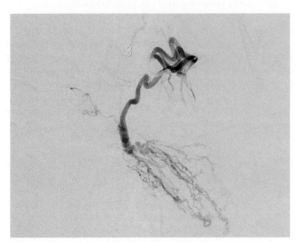

Fig. 57.7. Bronchial arteriogram shows hypertrophied, tortuous bronchial arteries with parenchymal hypervascularity.

- parenchymal staining
- bronchial artery aneurysms or pseudoaneurysm
- bronchial artery to pulmonary vein shunting
- bronchial artery to pulmonary artery shunting
- extravasation of contrast medium
- thrombus

Endovascular embolization is now the accepted first-line treatment for massive hemoptysis, and it is preferred to surgical resection because it is minimally invasive. Two large case series showed 0% and 4% mortality for severe or massive hemoptysis, and these results support a strategy of bronchial embolization as first-line treatment over surgical intervention.[37,52] Angiography identifies a definitive site of bleeding in approximately 90% of patients who undergo angiography for hemoptysis.[47,52] The findings of large case series suggest that endovascular embolization is successful in controlling bleeding in 81% to 98.5% of patients for whom a site of bleeding is identified.[47,52,109–111] Recurrent hemoptysis leading to death or requiring a surgical procedure or reembolization occurs in 10% to 25% of patients who require embolization for hemoptysis, and the highest failure rate is found for patients with cystic fibrosis and aspergilloma.[47,52,109,110] However, among all patients with hemoptysis who require bronchial artery embolization, individuals with cancer have the highest mortality rate, at up to 92%.[112]

Failure of embolization or recurrence after embolization may be due to incorrect technique, incomplete embolization, failure to visualize nonbronchial systemic vessels responsible for hemoptysis, development of new vessels, recanalization of embolized vessels, or failure to recognize a pulmonary artery or vein as the source of hemoptysis. Thorough mapping before the procedure is essential in avoiding incomplete exclusion of all branches involved. Embolization should be as peripheral as possible to prevent deep branches from receiving collateral flow from other systemic sources. Polyvinyl alcohol is probably the most commonly used embolic material. It consists of industrially manufactured, nonabsorbable particles between 150 μm and 700 μm in diameter,[47,113] although the use of material with a diameter greater than 325 μm has been recommended because this is the size of the largest bronchopulmonary anastomosis found in the human lung.[114]

Although serious complications from endovascular embolization are rare, minor complications are not. Spinal artery embolization with infarction is the most dreaded complication of bronchial artery embolization. This complication has been reported in 1% to 6% of cases and occurs because of unintended embolization of an anomalous spinal artery arising from a bronchial artery. With increased awareness and technical improvements over time, the incidence appears to be much lower and is now probably less than 1%.[47] Superselective bronchial artery embolization with a coaxial microcatheter system allows more stable cannulation distal to the spinal artery and has been reported to reduce spinal artery complications.[115] Minor complications of endovascular embolization include chest pain (24% to 91%) and dysphagia (0.7% to 18%).[47,116] Dysphagia may occur 2 days to 7 days after embolization and is likely due to compromise of small arterial branches supplying the esophagus.[117] Other rarer complications of endovascular embolization have been reported, such as myocardial infarction, possibly due to embolization via coronary-to-bronchial artery fistula; multiple systemic embolization; bronchial necrosis; and stroke (Table 57.4).[47,118,119]

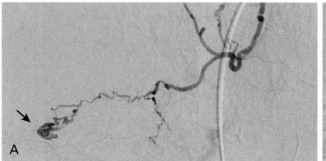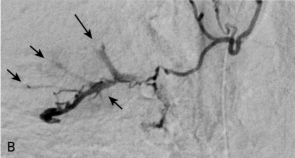

Fig. 57.8. Bronchial arteriogram shows (A) bronchial artery aneurysm/pseudoaneurysm *(arrow)*; and (B) shunting from the bronchial artery to the pulmonary artery or vein *(arrows)*.

TABLE 57.4 Complications of Endovascular Embolization

Complication	Incidence (%)
Chest pain	24–91
Dysphagia	0.7–18
Spinal artery embolization	<1–6
Myocardial infarction	<1
Stroke	<1
Multiple systemic embolization	<1
Bronchial necrosis	<1

Surgery

Although surgery plays a primary role in the prevention of recurrent hemoptysis in benign disorders such as aspergilloma, its role in lung cancer is limited, mainly because of the overall poor condition and prognosis of patients with lung cancer and hemoptysis. As an emergent procedure, it carries a high mortality rate, and it is rarely indicated for patients with lung cancer. Although emergent surgical intervention for massive hemoptysis has been widely quoted to cause death in approximately 40% of cases,[120] more recent data suggest hospital morbidity and mortality rates of approximately 27.5% and 11.5%, respectively.[121] Nevertheless, surgery remains warranted only for selected patients with lung cancer after conservative therapy, including endovascular embolization, has failed.

Outcomes

Hippocrates recognized hemoptysis as a herald to death. Even today, massive hemoptysis is a terrifying event for the lay person and is pathognomonic for death when depicted in movies and on television. Even the seasoned clinician is moved to a state of heightened awareness, knowing that despite efficient and appropriate diagnosis and treatment, death may be imminent. Only in the modern era has the short-term mortality rate been reduced to approximately 6.5% for severe hemoptysis of all etiologies.[52] Nevertheless, among all patients with hemoptysis, patients with lung cancer have among the highest in-hospital and 1-year mortality rates (up to 59% and 92%, respectively).[38,41,48,112] Treatment of patients with lung cancer and massive hemoptysis should therefore be considered largely palliative.

MASSIVE PLEURAL EFFUSIONS

A pleural effusion is considered large when it opacifies two-thirds or more of a hemithorax on chest x-ray. Massive pleural effusion is defined as complete or almost complete opacification of a hemithorax on chest x-ray.[122] Approximately 10% of patients with a pleural effusion have a massive effusion at the time of presentation. These patients are usually symptomatic and malignancy causes most of these cases, reported as 65% in two studies.[123,124]

Pleural Physiology

Pleural fluid arises from systemic pleural vessels in both the visceral and parietal pleura. Under normal physiologic conditions, fluid flows passively into the pleural space and exits via the parietal pleural lymphatics.[122] Pleural effusions occur because of an imbalance between pleural fluid flowing into and out of the pleural space. Most commonly, pleural fluid accumulates because of increased interstitial hydrostatic pressure in the lung, increased negative intrapleural pressure, increased pleural space oncotic pressure, and/or blockage of parietal pleural lymphatics.[125–127] Malignant effusion is believed to result directly from one or more of the following: pleural metastasis with increased pleural permeability, pleural metastasis with obstruction of pleural lymphatics, mediastinal lymph node involvement with decreased pleural lymphatic drainage, thoracic duct interruption, bronchial obstruction leading to increased negative pleural pressure, or pericardial disease.[122]

Massive pleural effusions lead to compressive atelectasis of the lung and a restrictive respiratory physiology in one of two settings: (1) increased intrapleural pressure with associated mediastinal shift away from the side of the pleural effusion, or (2) trapped lung physiology without a mediastinal shift or with a mediastinal shift toward the side of the effusion. Both underlying processes cause symptoms and impair respiratory physiology.[122,128,129]

Etiology and Pathogenesis

Pleural malignancies are usually metastatic, but primary pleural malignancies such as mesothelioma and lymphoma must also be considered. Lung carcinoma is the most common malignancy that metastasizes to the pleura, accounting for nearly 40% of all malignant pleural effusions.[130] Although breast cancer and lymphoma are the second and third most common causes, respectively, nearly all neoplasms have been reported to involve the pleura.[131,132] Mesothelioma should be considered in persons with an appropriate environmental exposure and geographic location; however, mesothelioma is not always associated with asbestos exposure.[133] In approximately 10% of patients, a primary site for malignancy is not identified.[130]

Pleural metastases occur via lymphatic spread, hematogenous spread, or direct invasion. Pleural tumors can then directly lead to pleural effusions, as detailed previously in the "Pleural Physiology" section.[134] Pleural effusions can also result indirectly from a tumor, a phenomenon referred to as a paramalignant effusion.

This cause of effusion can be associated with local inflammation and leaky capillaries, downstream lymphatic obstruction, or trapped lung physiology due to bronchial obstruction or lung parenchymal invasion by a tumor.[135]

Clinical Presentation

Malignant pleural effusions most commonly cause dyspnea, but patients may also present with cough and chest pain.[131] Because of the systemic effects of malignancy, the respiratory symptoms are generally accompanied by weight loss, malaise, and anorexia.[130] Although similar in presentation, massive pleural effusions should be expected to cause more severe symptoms because of more extensive pleural disease.

A massive pleural effusion often results in increased intrapleural pressure and a mediastinal shift away from the side of the pleural effusion. This massive volume and pressure can result in decreased chest wall compliance, compressive atelectasis of the ipsilateral lung, central airway compression, and hemodynamic effects related to the mediastinal shift.[136,137]

When a mediastinal shift is not evident or is toward the side of the effusion, one should suspect a trapped lung with fixation of the mediastinum, occlusion of the mainstem bronchus by a tumor, or extensive pleural involvement.[138] Whether the lung is trapped or not, the patient's symptoms will be similar because of decreased lung volume and compliance, as well as stimulation of chest wall and parenchymal lung receptors.

These two distinct underlying pathophysiologies of a massive pleural effusion (trapped lung or compressed lung) are important to understand and recognize. Therapeutic thoracentesis of a massive pleural effusion with a trapped lung will not satisfactorily address the underlying physiologic defect, will not completely relieve the patient's symptoms, and may lead to complications.[122,136]

Clinical examination is expected to be abnormal when a massive effusion is present. Ipsilateral breath sounds should be absent and dullness to percussion should be present on examination. Additional signs and symptoms including adenopathy, breast mass, neck mass, and cachexia support an associated diagnosis of malignancy.[131]

Initial Management

Guidelines for the management of malignant pleural effusion from the American Thoracic Society, British Thoracic Society, and European Respiratory Society separate diagnosis from treatment.[130,138,139] In our review, the initial treatment and diagnostic evaluation are deliberately presented simultaneously. A massive pleural effusion can be an emergency and, at minimum, it warrants an organized and efficient evaluation. In the clinical setting, management and diagnosis often occur simultaneously, or in whichever order is best for the patient's safety and management of symptoms.

Initial Presentation

Patients with a massive pleural effusion, whether it is malignant or nonmalignant, often present with dyspnea, cough, and chest pain. Nonmassive pleural effusions can also present with these symptoms, however, patients with massive pleural effusions tend to present with more severe symptoms and/or impaired cardiac or respiratory physiology.[122,128,129]

Guidelines from the American Thoracic Society, British Thoracic Society, and European Respiratory Society all recommend history, physical examination, and chest x-ray as the initial steps in evaluating a malignant pleural effusion.[138,139] These are sound recommendations; however, we believe that in the setting of massive pleural effusion, thoracic point-of-care ultrasonography

should be employed early. In skilled hands, lung ultrasound is more sensitive and specific for a pleural effusion than is chest x-ray.[140] Ultrasound of the lung and pleural space also has the advantage of distinguishing simple from complex effusions, as well as identifying pleural or lung masses suggestive of malignancy.[141] Algorithms have been developed for the evaluation of massive pleural effusion, with and without point-of-care ultrasonography (Fig. 57.9).

Point-of-care ultrasonography is a rapidly performed bedside examination that is focused and goal directed. It should have a defined purpose linked to improving the patient's outcome.[142] When point-of-care ultrasonography is performed in the critical care setting, it is also referred to as critical care ultrasonography. Both techniques have been widely adopted by many physicians in emergency medicine, pulmonary medicine, and critical care medicine.

Point-of-care ultrasonography is particularly helpful in the evaluation of dyspnea, hemodynamic instability, and undifferentiated shock.[143–145] In the setting of suspected massive pleural effusion, point-of-care ultrasonography also allows the physician to assess for cardiovascular compromise and to evaluate for alternative causes among patients presenting with dyspnea, cough, and chest pain.[146,147] Although this chapter focuses on massive pleural effusions, it is important to recognize that patients with malignancy and pleural effusion are at risk of pulmonary embolism, pneumothorax, postobstructive pneumonia, congestive heart failure, acute kidney injury, and hepatic dysfunction.

Ultrasound is not available in all clinical settings; however, the use of point-of-care ultrasonography in the emergency room is becoming the standard of care,[148] and many clinics now have access to portable ultrasound machines, making the implementation of bedside ultrasound for the initial evaluation of massive effusion a realistic consideration. The value of chest x-ray should not, however, be minimized. Chest x-ray is often available for review at the time of the physician's initial assessment. Furthermore, the clinical environment may not allow the use of point-of-care ultrasonography. Chest x-ray can improve the clinical assessment by confirming the presence and size of a suspected effusion, identifying an associated lung mass or airspace disease, ruling out a large pneumothorax, and helping to detect a mediastinal shift (Fig. 57.10).[137] Chest x-ray and ultrasound are complementary in the evaluation of possible massive pleural effusions. When available, lung and pleural ultrasound should not be delayed in favor of a chest x-ray, and in the appropriate clinical setting, point-of-care ultrasonography should be integrated into the initial physical examination and history.

Initial Therapeutic Intervention

The initial intervention for a massive pleural effusion is aspiration of pleural fluid to alleviate symptoms (Fig. 57.9). Thoracentesis should be performed under ultrasound guidance, unless ultrasound is not available and the aspiration is an emergency. The complication rate for thoracentesis performed under ultrasound guidance is very low (0% to 2.5%) when performed by skilled groups of physicians.[149–151] This rate is notably less than the commonly quoted complication rate of more than 10% for thoracentesis performed in the preultrasound era.[152,153] In addition to locating a safe site for pleural puncture, ultrasound is helpful for assessing a complicated pleural space.[154] This information helps the clinician avoid potential complications and optimize both diagnostic yield and safety.

The amount of fluid to remove and the method of removal depend on the patient and the clinical situation. For most patients, thoracentesis is the preferred method. It is recommended that pleural pressure be monitored during fluid drainage.

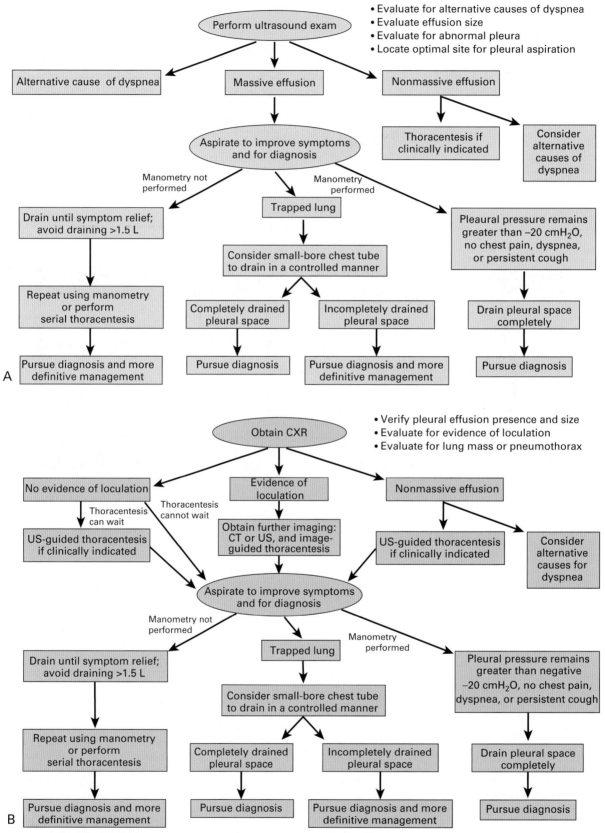

Fig. 57.9. Management algorithms for massive pleural effusion in two scenarios: (A) using point-of-care ultrasonography; and (B) without the availability of point-of-care ultrasonography. *CT*, computed tomography; *CXR*, chest x-ray; *US*, ultrasonography.

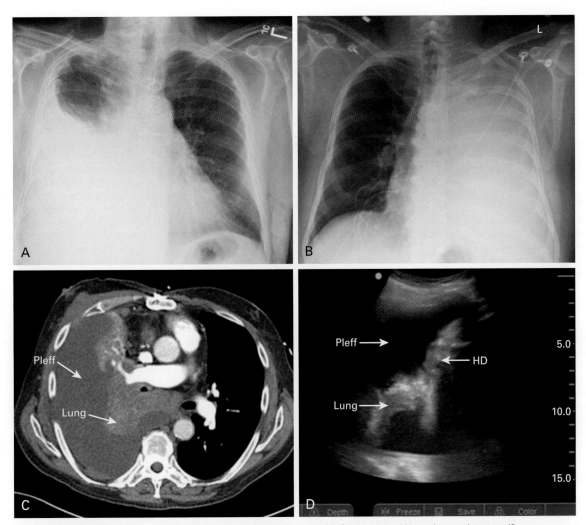

Fig. 57.10. Comparative images of massive pleural effusions. (A) Chest x-ray with nearly complete opacification of the right hemithorax. (B) Chest x-ray with complete opacification of the left hemithorax. The trachea is deviated to the right, consistent with a massive effusion. (C) Computed tomography of the chest of the same patient as in image A. Pleural effusion (Pleff), lung atelectasis, and mediastinal shift can be seen. (D) Thoracic ultrasonography of the same patient as in image A. Pleural effusion, lung atelectasis, and an abnormal right hemidiaphragm (HD) are visualized. Note the thickened diaphragm rather than the expected thin hyperechoic line. This finding is consistent with pleural metastasis.

Pleural manometry has many advantages for patients with massive pleural effusion. It can diagnose trapped lung, which will help in future management.[155] In addition, pleural manometry helps indicate when to stop fluid removal. Pleural pressure of less than -20 cmH$_2$O is associated with discomfort and reexpansion pulmonary edema.[156]

Common teaching and many experts recommend drainage of no more than 1.5 L of fluid.[122,130,157] However, this one-size-fits-all approach is flawed, especially for very large or complicated pleural effusions. Reexpansion pulmonary edema has been shown to be rare, and large-volume thoracentesis is generally well tolerated. In a series of 185 patients undergoing large-volume thoracentesis (1 L to 6.5 L withdrawn), only one patient had clinical reexpansion pulmonary edema, and this patient had only 1.4 L of fluid withdrawn. Only 22% of patients had pleural closing pressure less than -20 cmH$_2$O after large-volume thoracentesis.[158] In his text, Light recommends stopping fluid drainage if cough or pain develops or, based on animal studies, when pleural pressure reaches less than -20 cmH$_2$O, because of the risk of reexpansion pulmonary edema; significant edema commonly develops if pleural pressure is less than -40 cmH$_2$O. Patients who had discomfort after thoracentesis were more likely to have a more negative closing pleural pressure and a larger total change in pleural pressure.[156]

We recommend that the pleural space be completely drained, when possible and safe, both for controlling symptoms and improving physiologic parameters. Limiting the volume of pleural fluid drained will decrease the effectiveness of this procedure. We recommend both manometry and monitoring of symptoms, including cough, chest tightness or pain, and vasovagal symptoms.[156] However, if pleural pressure is not monitored, then an approach to large effusions as outlined by the British Thoracic Society guidelines is reasonable. The pleural effusion should be drained in a controlled fashion, with initial drainage of no more than 1.5 L and any additional fluid drained 1.5 L at a time at 2-hour intervals. Symptoms should be monitored, and the procedure should be stopped if the patient reports chest discomfort, persistent cough, or vasovagal symptoms.[130]

Small-bore pleural catheters that can be placed using a modified Seldinger technique and under ultrasound guidance should also be considered for appropriate patients. The small bore of the catheter and modified Seldinger technique make the procedure not much more invasive than therapeutic thoracentesis. This approach has the advantages of removing the fluid slowly, or at a constant pressure (setting the pleural drain to no less than -20 cmH$_2$O). In addition, if fluid is accumulating quickly, this approach avoids the need for multiple repeat thoracenteses. The major disadvantage to this approach is the need for pleural tube management after placement, meaning that this procedure is generally not appropriate for patients returning home immediately after placement. In addition, physician familiarity and skill are required for performing this procedure.

Subsequent Management

After the initial assessment and intervention, a plan is needed for subsequent and long-term management. This is best accomplished after the patient has a diagnosis. As noted earlier, 65% of massive pleural effusions are malignant, and the type of malignancy should be identified.

Additional Chest Imaging

Chest CT aids in identifying pleural-based masses, pleural thickening, loculated effusions, lung masses, parenchymal lung disease, and mediastinal adenopathy.[159] More complicated diagnostic imaging, such as positron emission tomography and magnetic resonance imaging, can have a role in evaluating for chest wall involvement and distant metastasis. Magnetic resonance imaging is most helpful in evaluating mesothelioma and differentiating benign from malignant pleural masses; however, it should be reserved for the appropriate setting, whether for staging, treatment, or long-term management.[160–163]

Pleural Fluid Analysis

Pleural fluid is often analyzed for lactate dehydrogenase, total protein, cholesterol, glucose, pH, amylase, and nucleated cell count. The initial pleural fluid analysis should be focused.[122] Heffner et al.[164] showed that the analysis of pleural fluid for lactate dehydrogenase and cholesterol alone was comparable to Light's criteria and avoided the need for simultaneous serum laboratory testing. Malignant effusions are commonly bloody, but less than half are grossly bloody. Lymphocytes or monocytes often predominate, but this is a nonspecific finding.[165]

In addition to focused chemistries, determination of pleural fluid pH can be helpful in the setting of both inflammation and malignancy. Malignant effusions have a pH less than 7.3 about one-third of the time, and this finding appears to be associated with increased tumor mass in the pleural space.[166] In addition to helping make a diagnosis, pH measurement has been shown to aid in prognosis. Malignant effusions with a low pH and glucose concentration have been shown to have a higher initial diagnostic yield on cytologic evaluation, a worse survival rate, and worse response to pleurodesis than those effusions with normal glucose and pH.[166–168] However, this dictum is not universally accepted. Aelony et al.[169] showed that talc pleurodesis was effective in a case series of patients with pH less than 7.3. Their findings are supported by Heffner et al.'s[170] analysis showing that pleural pH did not have adequate predictive value to recommend against pleurodesis, either because of pleurodesis failure or predicted short survival.[171] Although biochemical analysis and cell count of the pleural fluid are helpful when evaluating the etiology and management of pleural disease, ultimately the most important predictor of survival is likely to be the patient's overall health. In a study performed by Burrows et al.,[172] Karnofsky performance status was the most important predictor of survival at the time of pleuroscopy.

Histologic Analysis

In the absence of a clear cause for a massive unilateral effusion, and given the high percentage of massive effusions associated with malignancy, a sample should be sent for cytologic analysis. Positive results of pleural fluid cytology can be used to identify a specific malignant cell type, to perform immunohistochemical analysis, to test for molecular markers, and to indicate advanced disease. Initially, a cytologic sample alone should be sent. Although the purported yield of cytology varies considerably, a commonly referenced study of 414 patients had a diagnostic yield of nearly 60%.[173] The addition of closed pleural biopsy increased the yield by only 7%. The volume of fluid sent also improves yield; 150 mL of pleural fluid has been recommended.[174]

No single tumor marker can identify malignancy. A panel of markers can help guide further diagnostic procedures. In the initial evaluation, the routine use of tumor markers is not recommended and does not warrant the increased cost.[175]

As noted, closed pleural biopsy provides only a small additive diagnostic yield and hence is not part of the routine initial evaluation of a massive pleural effusion. Closed pleural biopsy should be considered when the initial focused evaluation, including thoracentesis and fluid cytology, is negative. Alone, closed pleural biopsy has a diagnostic yield of only approximately 40% and is associated with serious complications, including vasovagal syncope, hemothorax, pneumothorax, empyema, and death. In medical centers where it is available, CT-guided pleural biopsy using a cutting needle offered a yield of nearly 80%.[176] Neither closed pleural biopsy nor CT-guided pleural biopsy is warranted at initial evaluation; however, both can be considered subsequently, depending on local expertise.

More Definitive Management

Medical Thoracoscopy and Video-Assisted Thoracoscopic Surgery

The decision to pursue video-assisted thoracoscopic surgery as opposed to medical thoracoscopy will depend on local availability and expertise with each procedure. As a diagnostic procedure, medical thoracoscopy has the advantage of not requiring general anesthesia. This approach allows a less invasive and less expensive procedure. The diagnostic yield of medical thoracoscopy (95%) is much better than that of pleural fluid cytology and closed pleural biopsy combined (74%).[177] As described earlier, the initial therapeutic management and diagnostic evaluation does not include thoracoscopy. If the expertise in medical thoracoscopy is available and the initial evaluation does not yield a diagnosis, thoracoscopy should be used early.[178]

Serial Thoracentesis

Reaccumulation of fluid is common, and repeated thoracentesis is associated with pleural adhesions, making future management difficult. For these reasons, observation with as-needed thoracentesis is generally reserved for patients with minimal symptoms who require thoracentesis less than once per month.

However, in patients with limited life expectancy, this option can be less invasive and should be considered.[130,172]

Pleurodesis and Indwelling Pleural Catheter

For patients who are expected to survive longer than 1 month and who have a Karnofsky performance greater than 30%, more definitive management must be considered.[172] The optimal method to use, however, is not clear. Pleurodesis using tetracycline, bleomycin, or talc is commonly used. Talc has been shown to be the most effective sclerosant, with evidence suggesting that thoracoscopic talc poudrage is preferred over talc slurry. The benefit of, and decision to pursue, thoracoscopic talc poudrage over talc slurry is debatable and beyond the scope of this discussion for the emergency management of massive pleural effusion.[179,180] Indwelling pleural catheters have both advantages and disadvantages when compared with talc pleurodesis. These catheters can be placed in an outpatient setting[181] and have been shown to improve quality of life and dyspnea scores compared with talc slurry.[182] However, a large study did not show a significant difference in dyspnea, quality of life, or survival. Indwelling pleural catheters did reduce hospitalization time, but caused more adverse events, including catheter malfunction and infection.[183] The decision to pursue talc pleurodesis instead of an indwelling pleural catheter should be made on an individualized basis. However, it is generally accepted that indwelling pleural catheters are the preferred therapy for loculated malignant effusions and trapped lung.

CONCLUSION

Central airway obstruction, massive hemoptysis, and massive pleural effusions are three lung emergencies that are the most specific to lung cancer. Rapid diagnosis, careful evaluation, and a well-coordinated and carefully implemented treatment plan will satisfactorily address the problems that arise in the care of most patients with central airway obstruction due to lung cancer. Effective management will give patients improved functional status, better exercise tolerance, enhanced quality of life, reduced need for prolonged high-level care during hospitalization, longer survival, and the ability to consider and more safely undergo additional systemic therapy if indicated. The physician's technical ability to palliate severe central airway obstruction can improve with experience as he or she takes on increasingly difficult and challenging cases. Of course, one must never perform procedures for the procedure's sake, and bronchoscopic intervention must be considered within a patient-focused philosophy of care. A careful risk–benefit analysis helps safeguard against unnecessary interventions, although some may argue that when the alternative is death, even the most potentially heroic palliative interventional procedures may be warranted. Such attempts must be carefully weighed against the benefits and reasonableness of supportive care. In case of doubt, it is extremely beneficial to discuss decisions with a palliative care specialist, medical ethicist, and other members of the lung cancer multidisciplinary team, including with an expert more experienced with airway management procedures. In addition, bronchoscopists should track the indications and outcomes of their procedures, including procedure-related complications and postprocedure survival. As for any medical or surgical procedure, treatment of central airway obstruction requires a system of accountability to ensure that patients undergoing these interventions are appropriately selected, cared for, and monitored.

Hemoptysis is not a rare event for patients with lung cancer, but it may arise or advance in such dramatic volume and fashion as to be shocking to both the patient and clinician. With this unmistakable presentation, hemoptysis is universally acknowledged as massive and is easily recognized as a critical life-threatening condition. However, no universally accepted definition of massive hemoptysis exists. Although the volume of expectorated blood has traditionally been used to define massive hemoptysis, a grading system incorporating the patient's underlying disease, physiologic state, chest x-ray findings, and vascular source of bleeding more accurately predicts mortality. Rapid and efficient evaluation and treatment are of paramount importance, yet mobilizing the

resources to accomplish these tasks is a challenge. A multidisciplinary approach focused on rapid evaluation, stabilization in the intensive care unit, and endovascular embolization is recommended. Bronchoscopy may play an important diagnostic and therapeutic role, whereas surgery is rarely indicated. Transfer of these patients to a tertiary care center with the experience, personnel, and resources required for a multidisciplinary approach to the management of massive hemoptysis should be considered.

Massive pleural effusion can be a life-threatening emergency and therefore necessitates an organized, efficient, and safe approach to treatment. Therapeutic management and diagnosis often occur simultaneously. However, it is important to recognize that the initial intervention for the relief of symptoms and improvement in respiratory physiology—while ensuring patient safety—takes precedence over diagnosis. Pleural aspiration remains the key intervention in the initial management of massive pleural effusions. We have outlined an approach that we believe is both thoughtful and efficient.

Massive pleural effusions are usually associated with malignancy. For this reason, there must be a high clinical suspicion of malignancy when evaluating and managing a massive pleural effusion.

We recommend that, whenever possible, ultrasound be integrated early into the evaluation algorithm and that pleural pressure be monitored and managed during pleural fluid drainage. This approach will help minimize complications and maximize pleural fluid drainage.

Long-term management will depend on the cause of effusion, local expertise, and the available therapeutic and diagnostic modalities.

KEY REFERENCES

11. Chhajed PN, Baty F, Pless M, et al. Outcome of treated advanced non-small cell lung cancer with and without central airway obstruction. *Chest.* 2006;130(6):1803–1807.
15. Colt HG, Murgu S, eds. *Bronchoscopy and Central Airway Disorders: a Patient-Centered Approach.* Philadelphia, PA: Elsevier Saunders; 2012.
16. Hoag JB. Use of medical lasers for airway disease. In: Ernst A, Herth FJF, eds. *Principles and Practice of Interventional Pulmonology.* New York, NY: Springer Science + Business Media; 2013:357–366.
34. Murgu S, Langer S, Colt H. Bronchoscopic intervention obviates the need for continued mechanical ventilation in patients with airway obstruction and respiratory failure from inoperable non-small-cell lung cancer. *Respiration.* 2012;84(1):55–61.
35. Vonk-Noordegraaf A, Postmus PE, Sutedja TG. Tracheobronchial stenting in the terminal care of cancer patients with central airways obstruction. *Chest.* 2001;120(6):1811–1814.
38. Fartoukh M, Khoshnood B, Parrot A, et al. Early prediction of in-hospital mortality of patients with hemoptysis: an approach to defining severe hemoptysis. *Respiration.* 2012;83(2):106–114.
51. Wang GR, Ensor JE, Gupta S, Hicks ME, Tam AL. Bronchial artery embolization for the management of hemoptysis in oncology patients: utility and prognostic factors. *J Vasc Interv Radiol.* 2009;20(6):722–729.
124. Jimenez D, Diaz G, Gil D, et al. Etiology and prognostic significance of massive pleural effusions. *Respir Med.* 2005;99(9):1183–1187.
158. Feller-Kopman D, Berkowitz D, Boiselle P, Ernst A. Large-volume thoracentesis and the risk of reexpansion pulmonary edema. *Ann Thorac Surg.* 2007;84(5):1656–1661.
182. Demmy TL, Gu L, Burkhalter JE, et al. Optimal management of malignant pleural effusions (results of CALGB 30102). *J Natl Compr Canc Netw.* 2012;10(8):975–982.

See Expertconsult.com for full list of references.

58 The Role of Palliative Care in Lung Cancer

Mellar Davis and Nathan Pennell

SUMMARY OF KEY POINTS

- The best palliative outcomes are obtained when palliative care is involved early in advanced lung cancer.
- Integration of palliative care early in the advanced cancer patient has important health utilization and economic outcomes besides patient-related outcomes.
- Supportive oncology and palliative care are not the same. Supportive oncology involves therapies to treat or minimize anticancer therapy toxicity.
- There is in general a misunderstanding of palliative care as hospice care. This misunderstanding is a barrier to referral.
- Patient-related outcome measures predict relevant outcomes such as survival, tolerance to chemotherapy, and performance status.
- Hope in advanced lung cancer can be maintained without the promise of therapies that are unlikely to alter the cause of cancer.
- There are multiple symptom and quality-of-life tools with lung cancer–specific items that can be used to assess pain, nonpain symptoms, and quality of life in lung cancer.
- Pain, fatigue, dyspnea, cough, and anorexia can be successfully treated using guidelines established for specific symptom management.

DEFINITION OF PALLIATIVE CARE

The World Health Organization (WHO) defines palliative care as the "holistic care of patients with advanced progressive illness. Managing pain and other symptoms, and providing psychosocial and spiritual support are paramount. The goal of palliative care is to achieve the best quality of life for patients and their families. Many aspects of palliative care also apply earlier in the course of illness, in conjunction with curative, disease-modifying or rehabilitating treatments."[1,2] This definition establishes three important points: (1) palliative care is patient-oriented rather than disease-oriented; (2) palliative care is interdisciplinary, using multiple medical and nonmedical specialties to achieve the best quality of life for the patient and family; and (3) palliative care is complementary to disease-related care.[3] However, this definition does not provide clinical guidelines for successfully implementing early integration of palliative care. Specific guidelines are necessary for defining when and how palliative care needs to be integrated into clinical pathways for successful implementation.[3]

Many palliative care programs have adopted multiple names, including supportive care, to facilitate early integration. According to National Council for Hospice and Specialist Palliative Care Services, supportive care helps the patient and family cope with cancer and treatment, from before diagnosis through the process of diagnosis, treatment, cure, continuing illness or death, and (family) bereavement. Supportive care helps patients maximize the benefits of cancer treatment and live as well as possible with the side effects of the disease and its treatment. Supportive care is of equal priority with diagnosis and treatment. Supportive care

originally focused on side effects from anticancer therapies, such as neutropenic fever and nausea, related to chemotherapy agents. Unlike palliative care, supportive care does not have a recognized subspecialty status. Like palliative care, supportive care is multidisciplinary. Many trials have used the term best supportive care, but this term is not defined in trial documents. In one review, best supportive care was largely limited to biomedical support, such as transfusions, antibiotics, and antiemetics, and did not include advance directives, communication, and psychosocial or spiritual care or support.[4]

End-of-life care has been largely associated with hospice care. In the United States, because of the hospice Medicare benefit, end-of-life care is assumed to be the 6 months, or less, prior to the patient's death.[5] Definitions of end-of-life care have broadened considerably regarding disease trajectory, when end-of-life care should be introduced, and the clinical conditions on which it focuses. As noted previously, there are multiple of terms and definitions for end-of-life care and palliative care. The fact that programs frequently use several descriptors leads to confusion.[6–8] The reason palliative care programs have adopted the term supportive care is largely due to the fact that physicians and patients find the term more acceptable than palliative care.[9]

The first inpatient palliative care unit in North America was established by Dr. Balfour Mount at the Royal Victoria Hospital, Montreal, Canada in 1975. The establishment of this unit was just 8 years after St. Christopher's Hospice was opened in London, England by Cicely Saunders.[10] The term "palliative" was adopted at that time to describe the function of the unit and the purpose of the program. The main reason for opening this inpatient palliative care unit within an acute care hospital was because of disturbing deficiencies in the care of patients with incurable illnesses.[10] Dr. Mount recognized the misalignment between the goals for treating incurable and terminal illnesses, and the main goals of the acute care hospital, which were to investigate, diagnose, cure, and prolong life. In contrast, the three main goals of cancer treatment were to cure, prolong life, and palliate. Prior to the establishment of the palliative care unit, most, if not all, effort and resources were being applied toward curing or prolonging life. The palliative needs of terminally ill patients and their families, including medical, emotional, and spiritual needs, were generally neglected in an acute care hospital.

PHILOSOPHICAL DIFFERENCES BETWEEN ONCOLOGY AND PALLIATIVE CARE

A shift to a scientific-based, disease-oriented medical model, which occurred in the latter half of the 19th century, resulted in major advances in health care. Louis Pasteur's germ theory led to Joseph Lister's management of surgical wounds and the remarkable reduction in postoperative mortality and morbidity due to infections. Florence Nightingale used statistics and collected mortality data to prove that sanitary conditions reduce mortality,[11–19] and the randomized clinical trial based on disease models and evidence-based therapeutics became the language of medicine. However, the adverse outcome of this shift was to objectify patients and identify them with their disease (e.g., cancer patients) and to depersonalize the healing process through reductionism. Quantification of outcomes became a priority when treating large populations.[11]

The curative and the disease-modifying models include the inherent assumptions that analytical, rational, and clinical encounters are the basis for scientific inquiry.[20] The object of analysis is the disease rather than the patient and their experience of illness. Symptoms are valued as clues to a diagnosis instead of a disease worthy of treatment. Cure is contingent on effective diagnosis and treatment. Treatment is largely empiric, uniformly applied, rather than person-centered, and based on stringently controlled trials of persons with similar disease states and measurable disease-related objective outcomes that are viewed as most important (survival, disease-free survival, or progression-free survival).[20] Laboratory and radiographic data are trusted more than the patient's self-report, and patient-related outcomes are of secondary importance to disease-related outcomes. In fact, most physicians are unfamiliar with patient-related outcomes and outcome measures.[21] Few oncologists routinely use patient-related outcome measures in practice and largely depend on laboratory and radiographic disease states to guide treatment and clinical decisions. The disease-oriented and curative model tends to ignore phenomena that cannot be scientifically explained.[20] Patients are perceived as component parts, and treatment is delivered by subspecialists. Physicians tend to think in terms of molecules, cells, organ systems, and genomes, particularly those with critical cancer-related (so-called addicted) pathways.[20,22,23] They place secondary importance on relational perspectives.[20] Oncology within the cancer center is largely hierarchical and physician centered. Multidisciplinary tumor boards are almost entirely comprised of physicians from various subspecialties and rarely involve nonmedical and noncancer medical specialties such as nursing, palliative care, social work, and rehabilitation services. Discussions within tumor boards are almost entirely centered on managing the disease; treatment recommendations are largely biomedical in nature and limited to radiotherapy, surgery, and chemotherapy, or a combination of antitumor therapies. Death in a curative model is seen as defeat. There are no so-called good deaths in oncology.[20] The most commonly heard excuses are that treatment failed, or, even worse, the patient failed the treatment, or nothing more can be done. The curative model fosters the involvement of palliative care in a transitional approach, in which palliative care is considered only when anticancer therapy is exhausted, rather than as simultaneous care. As a result, in the absence of palliative care support, physicians do what they have been trained to do; they give chemotherapy or targeted agents even in a terminally ill patient with little-to-no expected benefit.[24,25] Reviews published regarding management of nonsmall cell lung cancer (NSCLC) have sometimes explicitly used an either-or approach when comparing chemotherapy with palliative care.[26] In the curative model, palliative care is considered end-of-life care, and referral is made once treatment is no longer effective.[27,28]

In the palliative-care approach, treatment centers around the patient and family, with the goals of providing relief of pain and other symptoms, reducing psychosocial and spiritual stressors, restoring function, including social life and the role within the family, and improving quality of life. Palliative care supports patient values, concerns and personal choices. Treatment of pain and other symptoms is a legitimate outcome and goal of medicine. Diagnosis is not a predetermined goal, but is pursued if compatible with the patient's personal goals.[20,29] Treatment is individualized based on evidence from guidelines. Palliative care, like hospice, seeks neither to hasten nor delay death and sees death as a natural part of living.[20,30] The structure of palliative care services is nonhierarchical, with multiple medical and nonmedical specialists, including physicians, forming an interdisciplinary team that recognizes different roles and responsibilities. Encounters are usually lengthy. To achieve the most favorable outcome, palliative care is best practiced within multiple encounters over a prolonged period of time and is best used early in the course of illness, rather than as a crisis intervention or as a death management service at the end of life.[20,25,31–34]

There are three basic integrated palliative care models. The first involves the oncologist playing both roles in cancer care. This requires extensive time and expanded expertise, and, in general, it is impractical, because of time constraints and the need for secondary training. Oncologists should be skilled in basic palliative care. In areas where there is a lack of palliative care services, this is the default model.[35] The second approach is the so-called cafeteria model, in which the oncologist forms an interdisciplinary team by arranging multiple consultations with specialists in radiotherapy, surgery, palliative care, social work, psychology, and spiritual care. The oncologist makes up the hub of the wheel and multiple specialists serve as the spokes of the wheel. This approach is time-consuming and expensive for patients who have to make multiple visits to many consultants. A breakdown in communication is also more likely to occur, and knowing which specialist to contact for which symptom, stressor, family concern, or financial matter may be problematic for the patient.[35] The third model involves a simultaneous consult with a palliative care specialist and the oncologist, early in the course of cancer treatment. Communication and rapport can be established with both specialists, and the oncologist is free to focus on cancer management. This is a time-efficient practice that improves communication between two services.[35] In this model, the palliative care specialist may potentially act as a so-called treatment broker. As the patient and oncologist gain trust in the palliative care specialist, the patient may feel free to use the palliative care specialist as a sounding board to clarify preferences and goals of care.[24,36] Palliative care includes several components, and interdisciplinary palliative care teams have many distinct characteristics (see Boxes 58.1 and 58.2).

WHY PALLIATIVE CARE IS NEEDED EARLY IN THE MANAGEMENT OF ADVANCED LUNG CANCER

Symptoms

Individuals presenting with lung cancer are usually highly symptomatic. Most patients with advanced disease have at least four distressing symptoms.[37–41] Their average pain severity is 6 to 7, which is considered moderate, based on a numerical

---

BOX 58.1 Palliative Care Structure

1. Outpatient clinics
   - Early referral
2. Consultation services
   - Inpatient/outpatient
   - Crisis intervention
3. Inpatient units
   - Direct care
4. Association or affiliation with hospice services
5. Home palliative care services
6. Education
   - Fellowships
   - Grand Rounds and other teaching modalities
   - Provision for teaching internal medicine residents, oncology fellows, other fellows (gynecology, oncology, radiation, pain management)
7. Research
   - Quality-improvement projects
   - Prospective observational and interventional studies
   - Dedicated time, fellows, personnel, and resources
   - Integration into oncology as supportive care trials

BOX 58.2 Characteristics of Palliative Care Interdisciplinary Teams

1. Continuity: reconciliation of service lines
2. Assessment of symptoms: expert use of patient-related outcome measures
3. Treatment of cancer complications and associated symptoms (expertise in pharmacologic and nonpharmacologic management of symptoms)
4. Communication
   - Treatment goals and prognosis
   - Assess values and preferences and understanding regarding disease stage, course, outlook, and goals of care
   - End-of-life care and decisions, preference for site of care
   - Advance directives
5. Transition facilitation
   - Active cancer treatment plus palliative care to active palliative care
   - Active palliative care to hospice
6. Family care
   - Facilitate family meetings
   - Understand family systems
   - Management of family distress, dysfunction, and family grief
7. Psychosocial care
   - Management of distress, depression, demoralization
   - Management of anticipatory grief, complicated grief, and depression in grief
8. Spiritual care
   - Recognize existential suffering
   - Able to take a spiritual history
   - Understand diverse religious practices
9. Rehabilitation
   - Referral to pulmonary and nonpulmonary rehabilitation, physical therapy, and occupational therapy
10. Supportive care
    - Treatment of toxicity and complications related to anticancer therapy
11. Care of the actively dying
12. Bereavement
13. Research in supportive and palliative care interventions, service structures, and complex research designs

---

rating scale with 0 being no pain and 10 being severe pain.[42] The most frequently reported symptoms are anorexia, cough, dyspnea, fatigue, pain, and insomnia. Individuals with lung cancer experience a greater prevalence of depression and anxiety than individuals with other cancers and also have more frequent and prolonged fatigue compared with patients with other cancers.[43,44] Breathlessness occurs in 70% of patients, is associated with a substantially greater symptom burden, and can adversely influence the experience of caring for a loved one.[45] Symptom burden may, in fact, be greater than patients indicate. That is why it is important to use a standardized symptom questionnaire. Studies have shown that, when presented with a symptom checklist, patients report three to four times more symptoms than they volunteer.[46]

Even individuals with relatively early-stage lung cancer (stages I–IIIB) have substantial symptoms. When using the Lung Cancer Symptom Scale at disease presentation, patients reported an average of 11 symptoms, and, even when successfully treated, they reported an average of 6 to 7 symptoms still present a year after treatment.[39] As mentioned previously, individuals with early-stage lung cancer experience lack of energy, worry, dyspnea, cough, and insomnia. The Karnofsky performance status often remains impaired at 36 to 52 weeks after treatment, but symptom distress gradually declines by 1 year. Symptom distress is the primary reason for clinical encounters in the outpatient setting and the primary reason for unscheduled admissions.[47] Despite treatments for NSCLC, there is gradual deterioration in physical function, activities of daily living, and cognitive function and an increasing need for social support.[48]

Physicians frequently believe that tumor reduction is a surrogate for improved patient-related outcomes. However, based upon a systematic review of quality of life associated with standard chemotherapy for advanced NSCLC, there are no major changes in the global quality of life for patients on standard chemotherapy regimens.[49] There is only a modest correlation (0.35) between objective tumor size and symptoms. Improved patient-related outcomes with treatment last a much shorter time (3.8 months on average) than duration of objective tumor response (6.4 months). Objective tumor response and patient-related outcomes contribute unique, independent information. One cannot be substituted for the other.[50] Unfortunately, most oncologists are unfamiliar with standard symptom questionnaires, and most are not aware of clinically meaningful differences in patient-related outcome measures.[21] However, having patients complete quality-of-life and symptom questionnaires gives patients a sense of better continuity with their physician and the feeling that their treating oncologist has considered their daily activities and emotional state. Patients think that such questionnaires are helpful and not burdensome.[51] Longitudinal assessment of symptoms is also important because treatment reduces certain symptoms but increases others.[52]

At least 40% of outpatients with cancer are undertreated for pain, as measured by the Pain Management Index. This reflects inadequate analgesic choices based on pain severity, but does not reflect pain response. Despite the fact that greater than 60% of patients have substantial pain, there is no change in the Pain Management Index score with follow-up. Oncologists self-rate their ability to manage pain as high (7 to 10, with 10 being the best management), but rate their colleagues' ability to control pain lower (3 to 10). Oncologists perceive lack of assessment, time constraints, and patient reluctance to complain as barriers to pain management.[53] Most oncologists know the WHO analgesic stepladder and prescribe opioids around-the-clock for chronic pain. However, most (greater than 60%) fail to correctly answer questions regarding opioid management (dose, schedule, conversion and rotation ratios, and titration) when tested through clinical scenarios.[53] This has been documented in several studies.[54,55] Symptom burden increases in intensity and number of symptoms as cancer progresses and then plateaus in the last month of survival. Eighty percent have increasing fatigue, dyspnea, and anorexia, and most have chest pain in the last 3 months of life.[39] Left poorly managed, these individuals experience a painful death, and families experience complicated grief or depression in bereavement.[56] Integrating palliative care into outpatient oncology practice early in the course of cancer reduces symptom burden, improves quality of life, and provides the care and support patients and families want (see Box 58.3).[25,57]

Communication

Honest communication is important but can be marred when a patient and physician maintain false hope in anticancer therapy. Good communication includes discussions about alternative therapies, prognosis, the goals of therapy, advance directives, and end-of-life care. Giving bad news requires some special skills, and few oncologists have had that type of communication training. In the US Cancer Care Outcomes Research and Surveillance (Can CORS) study, only half of patients with advanced cancer had discussions about hospice care, and yet greater than 70% died within 6 months.[58] Of the more than 4000 physicians caring for Can CORS patients, most would not initiate discussions

BOX 58.3 Patients and Families Need and Want To

Be treated as individuals
Be heard
Be valued for their skills and knowledge
Exercise real choice about treatment and services
Receive detailed, high-quality information about the disease, disease trajectory, prognosis, and goals of care
Know options and alternatives, including access to support groups, self-help services, and complementary therapy
Know they will undergo interventions that they have been informed of and have agreed to
Have excellent face-to-face communication
Know that services are well coordinated and are of high quality
Know that physical symptoms will be assessed and managed to their satisfaction and within the physician's current expertise and knowledge
Have services available that can provide support and advice about financial concerns, including employment
Have access to spiritual care and be supported spiritually
Die in the place of choice
Be assured that the family will be supported throughout their illness and into bereavement

about prognosis, advance directives, resuscitation, and hospice care, even if death was expected within 6 months and despite national guidelines. Most physicians stated that they would postpone these discussions until the patient was highly symptomatic or failed disease-modifying therapy. Some will not conduct these discussions unless initiated by the family or patient.[59] Medical oncologists explain the disease course in 53% of consultations and discuss the absence of cure in 84%.[60] However after consultation, most patients with advanced lung cancer still believe there is some chance of cure with chemotherapy.[61] Even after being fully informed using decision aids, one-third of patients with incurable cancer feel that their cancer has some chance of being cured with chemotherapy.[62] Patients do want to be fully informed about the stage at diagnosis and the prognosis, but comprehension often lags behind.[62] Within consultations, oncologists address symptoms in 35% of patient encounters and discuss prognosis in 39%. Patients may perceive prognosis differently than incurability, which has no time line.[60] Even when prognosis is discussed, physicians tend to be overly optimistic.[63,64] Documentation of discussions about prognosis appears in less than 40% of medical charts.[65] However, documented discussions about prognosis are also associated with documented discussions about options regarding ongoing anticancer therapy (odds ratio 5.8), and documented do-not-resuscitate (DNR) orders (odds ratio, 2.2).[65] Individuals with advanced cancer who overestimate their prognosis or who are given an overly optimistic estimate of survival are more likely to choose therapies for which the burden outweighs the benefit, are less likely to discuss preferences with surrogates, and are less likely to obtain information that would improve the quality of end-of-life care.[58,66,67]

The picture may be a bit different from the patient's perspective. In a study involving 276 patients from four major medical centers, 40% of patients rated communication with their oncologist about the potential for cure of their lung cancer low, and 80% gave low ratings about communication regarding resuscitation, life-sustaining treatments, and preparation of advance directives. Over half of patients reported that communication with their oncologist was inadequate.[68] These findings may be related to a patient's perception and inability to comprehend the seriousness of the situation, which is only realized as cancer progresses.

A large number of patients choose palliative chemotherapy at the end-of-life, for little to no benefit, because it helps them maintain a sense of control. Adverse effects are less of a concern for patients who value quantity of life.[69] In this situation, alternatives are frequently not discussed.[70] There are few, if any, decision aids to help patients make choices when considering palliative chemotherapy.[71] Patients who have a priority of a longer life rather than better quality of life and who have had a previous response to anticancer treatment are likely to choose aggressive treatment.[72] Patients experience cognitive dissonance when oncologists attempt to discuss end-of-life care and palliative chemotherapy within the same visit. Few patients with advanced cancer have completed advance directives, and less than one-quarter of patients want to discuss advance directives with their oncologists.[73] Sixty percent of oncologists prefer not to discuss advance directives and end-of-life care, including resuscitation and hospice, until anticancer treatments are exhausted.[74]

A collusion of hope surrounding anticancer therapy is maintained by continuing aggressive anticancer therapies despite little or no benefit. Although once important, patients seem to disregard quality of life and give precedence to quantity of life in choosing salvage chemotherapy.[69] Physicians are inclined to continue anticancer therapy, despite lack of benefit, to maintain hope rather than provide supportive and palliative care.[69] Paradoxically, this occurs despite the fact that there is little survival benefit with chemotherapy given within 1 to 3 months of death. In fact, chemotherapy may shorten survival, and early palliative care and hospice care may prolong survival.[25,75]

As a result, the average time from the last chemotherapy to death is 50 to 60 days, and the time from the last targeted therapy to death is 40 to 50 days. Fourteen to eighteen percent of individuals receive chemotherapy or targeted therapy within 30 days of dying.[76,77] The most common targeted agents used at the end of life are erlotinib and bevacizumab. Patients with lung cancer had greater odds (2.6) of being on a targeted agent within the last 30 days of life than individuals with other advanced cancers.[76] In one study at a large cancer center, the median time from palliative care consult to death was 1.4 months (interquartile 0.5 to 4.2 months) but the median length of time from the first encounter with an oncologist to consultation about palliative care was 20 months (interquartile 6 to 45). Therefore, there were multiple missed opportunities to include palliative care as part of patient care earlier in the course of disease.[78] Half of patients with lung cancer are within 2 months of death before end-of-life care and hospice are mentioned.[58] The average stable performance score of patients with lung cancer, as measured by the Palliative Prognostic Index, a modification of the Karnofsky performance score, is 8 to 9 months. Once the Palliative Prognostic Index has dropped to 30 or less, the average survival is 0.38 months. At this stage, very few patients (less than 5%) will have improvement in their performance score.[31] Consulting palliative care services after the patient has become bedridden, or has a poor performance score, provides little time to manage symptoms and primarily requires crisis intervention. Offering additional anticancer therapy when a performance score improves is unlikely to occur and, if discussed with the patient, will lead to a false sense of hope and will delay advanced care planning and hospice referral. Even patients with technically treatable small cell lung cancer and an Eastern Cooperative Oncology Group performance score of 3 or 4 do poorly. Only 20% of them will finish the standard four cycles. With a performance score of 4, the median survival is 7 days, and, with a performance score of 3, it is 64 days.[79]

The end results of poor communication and a collusion of hope in anticancer therapy are aggressive care at the end of life, chemotherapy in the last 14 days of life, intensive care unit admissions in the last 30 days of life, and acute hospital-based care in the last 30 days of life. About half of patients with advanced lung cancer will have aggressive therapy at the end of life.[77,80,81] The detrimental effect of aggressive care at the end of life is not just economic. It also creates a greater risk of caregiver depression and complicated grief.[82] In retrospect, many patients and families regret their choices of aggressive therapy near the end of life.[69,72,83,84]

In general, patients feel that advance directives should be discussed earlier than physicians do,[85] and the majority of families wished palliative care had been involved earlier in the course of cancer treatment.[86] In one study, end-of-life care discussions took place a median of 33 days before death.[87] In hospitalized patients with advanced cancer, palliative consults usually occur late within the hospital stay, when death is imminent, after a substantial hospital stay, or after admission to an intensive care unit. Consultations often involve the transfer of care.[88]

Most patients in large cancer centers do have a DNR directive in place at the time of death. The average time of signing a DNR directive is less than 3 days before death, and one-third are signed by surrogates.[89] As few as 5% of individuals with advanced cancer who die in the hospital have signed outpatient DNR directives.[89]

BENEFITS OF EARLY INTEGRATION OF PALLIATIVE CARE INTO ONCOLOGY

Symptom Management, Prognostic Information, and Hope

One of the benefits of integrating palliative care into outpatient oncology is decreased symptom burden.[25,34,57] The use of symptom assessment questionnaires will uncover more bothersome symptoms, which can then be managed by the palliative care team.[46,90] Individuals referred to palliative care early in the course of treatment are more likely to perceive and retain accurate information about prognosis and are less likely to receive aggressive chemotherapy at the end of life.[91,92] Prognostic discussions do not dampen hope. They empower individuals by providing realistic expectations to help them make informed choices about their medical care.[62,93] Early palliative care is associated with longer intervals between the last chemotherapy and death and increased hospice enrollment more than 7 days before death (60% compared with 33%).[94] Individuals who have less than 30 days of exposure to palliative care are more likely to receive chemotherapy within 30 days of death.[92] Hope is more influenced by a caring relationship between patient and physician than by prognostic disclosure.[95] The great majority of caregivers feel that avoiding discussions about prognosis is an inappropriate way of maintaining hope.[96]

Communication, Quality of Life, and Patient-Related Outcomes

Palliative care programs use quality-of-life questionnaires that have been shown to improve communication.[97] Providing palliative care during anticancer therapy improves quality of life.[25,41] Patient-centered communication takes time and involves sensitivity. Physicians must be able to respond to emotive verbal and nonverbal cues. Oncologists respond to approximately 20% to 30% of emotional cues and are quite responsive to informational cues.[98,99] Within family meetings, physicians often do most of the talking (71%) compared with family members (29%).[97,100] One of the core competencies required of physicians completing a fellowship in palliative medicine is to be able to conduct a family meeting. Therefore, when compared with oncology trainees, palliative medicine specialists are more likely to be better equipped to effectively communicate within the family conference. Emotional and psychosocial issues assume greater importance at the end of life. Communication training, which is part of a palliative medicine fellowship, can improve physicians' attitudes and their responses to emotions, as well as the satisfaction of the

patients' families. Time constraints are a major issue for cancer specialists because cancer treatment and related issues need to be addressed.[101-103] Paradoxically, despite the intensive involvement oncologists have with their patients, patients prefer to have conversations and communications about end-of-life care with physicians other than their oncologist. They want their oncologist to remain "optimistic" and focused on treating their cancer.[73,104]

Rehabilitation

General rehabilitation, exercise with strength training, and aerobics and pulmonary rehabilitation are often neglected in the various phases of treating patients with lung cancer. Many individuals with lung cancer have chronic obstructive lung disease (COPD), and evidence indicates pulmonary rehabilitation in chronic lung disease improves quality of life, dyspnea, and fatigue and empowers patients to be involved in their own therapy.[105] Although moderate physical activity reduces fatigue and improves symptoms, function and quality of life three-fourths of patients with lung cancer in the United States do not meet physical activity guidelines, and 51% do not participate in moderate activities.[106-112] For some individuals with cancer who have undergone potentially curative therapy, physical exercise can actually reduce recurrences and all-cause mortality.[113-115] Physical exercise is safe and feasible and may even potentially benefit individuals with advanced incurable cancer.[116,117] There is an open trial that is investigating the benefits of 2 months of a physical exercise intervention on fatigue and quality of life in patients with unresectable lung cancer.[118] Rehabilitation and physical exercise are most often discussed in palliative care, interdisciplinary team meetings rather than in oncology tumor boards.[119] Therefore, patients who are seen by the palliative care team are more likely to be considered for pulmonary rehabilitation and exercise training.

Research and complementary therapies of integration of palliative care into cancer treatment have resulted in supportive and complementary therapeutic trials during standard chemotherapy. In one trial, patients using American ginseng had improved cancer-related fatigue, particularly during chemotherapy.[120] In another trial, patients using omega-3 fatty acids during chemotherapy for NSCLC experienced improved muscle mass compared with standard treatment.[121,122]

Health-Care Economics

Early integration of palliative care into cancer care not only reduces aggressive care at the end of life, but also has economic advantages, without adversely influencing survival.[5,25,123] Nearly 40% of Medicare dollars are spent in the last months of life.[124] Even when palliative care is used as crisis intervention, transfer of appropriate patients from inpatient acute care to inpatient palliative care reduces costs by 66%.[125] Palliative care inpatient consult teams reduce daily inpatient costs by US $239.[126] The authors of two randomized trials and a cohort study found that care provided in inpatient palliative care units reduced costs by 38% to 50% compared with care provided in regular hospital wards.[124,127,128] Likewise, using in-home palliative care teams reduces readmissions to the hospital and emergency department compared with standard outpatient cancer care. The average costs per day for in-home outpatient care was $95, which was substantially less than the usual care ($213).[129] Financial comparisons of acute care hospital services have been possible using the Centers for Medicare & Medicaid Services case mix index (CMI) and All Patient Refined-Diagnosis Related Group (APR-DRG) data. Based on CMI and APR-DRG data, Cleveland Clinic's Inpatient Palliative Medicine acute care unit's total mean charges per admission are $7800 lower than at peer institutions without palliative care inpatient units, despite an equivalent severity of illness, longer length of stay, and higher mortality. The lower charges are due primarily to lower laboratory and pharmaceutical charges.[130] A systematic review of costs and cost-effectiveness of palliative care has been published,[131] but the quality of the studies varied, studies used different methods, and some studies were small. Cohort studies were at risk of bias through potentially unobserved confounding variables. However, all palliative care service structures (inpatient, home, and outpatient palliative care) were found to have economic advantages, largely due to reduced health-care utilization (readmissions and referral to hospice) and direct-care cost savings. For example, earlier palliative care enrollment reduced acute care days.[131]

Survival

Early integration of palliative care into cancer care does not shorten survival, and may actually prolong survival.[5,25,35,84,132] Early palliative care also leads to earlier hospice transition, which has a short-term survival advantage for patients with lung cancer.[133] The survival advantage of palliative care needs to be confirmed by other studies because this information was based on a post hoc analysis in the Boston Study,[25] and there has been much speculation about the mechanism used to calculate the survival advantage. Quality of life and mood are associated with survival; reduced quality of life and depression are associated with shortened survival; and improved quality of life is associated with improved survival.[134-140] Interventions such as palliative care improve quality of life and reduce depression, and may have a biologic effect related to prolonged survival.[25] It is interesting to note that, in the Boston Study, mood was improved without increased use of antidepressants.[25] Survival benefits also may be related to reduced aggressive care at the end of life.[25,75] Lastly, greater social support fostered by the palliative care team and the integration of the family into the plan of care may improve survival.[141,142]

STUDIES DOCUMENTING BENEFITS TO INTEGRATING PALLIATIVE CARE INTO CANCER CARE

The feasibility of integrating palliative care into oncology has been demonstrated in multiple clinical trials. In general, patients participating in these trials have experienced improved symptoms, quality of life, patient satisfaction, less aggressive care at the end of life, and no decrease in survival. It is important to note that the greatest benefit occurred when palliative care was integrated early in the course of advanced cancer.[25,129,132,143-147]

Several studies involving different cancers have evaluated benefits to home nursing and symptom-support visits during chemotherapy and after treatment. Certain symptoms, including depression and dyspnea, improved. In addition, chemotherapy toxicity was lower than in the control group, patient satisfaction improved, and there were fewer emergency room visits and hospitalizations.[129,148,149]

The benefits of inpatient palliative care consultations are relatively small unless palliative care teams assume direct care of patients. Without the palliative care team's involvement in direct care, recommendations for medical management are carried out in less than a quarter of patients. Also, although mild improvements in anxiety and dyspnea were noted, compared with care given without palliative care consultation, there was no improvement in depression or pain.[145,147]

Acute inpatient palliative care units with an interdisciplinary palliative care team have some advantages. Individuals directly managed by a palliative care team in an inpatient unit have fewer intensive care admissions, longer median hospice stays, and a greater number of completed advance directives. There were no detrimental effects on survival.[144]

Benefits to early integration of palliative care into cancer care were found in two large studies. The Educate, Nurture,

Before Life Ends (ENABLE) study involved education, problem-solving, symptom management, advanced-care planning, and monthly telephone follow-up. A full palliative care interdisciplinary team was not involved in care. The primary outcomes of mood and quality of life improved. There were no changes in symptom intensity or health-care utilization. There was a trend toward better survival with the intervention (14 vs. 8.5 months) ($p = 0.14$).[132,143] The second trial, conducted by Temel et al[25] involved individuals with newly diagnosed advanced lung cancer. Patients were randomly assigned to either usual care or integrated palliative care. The interdisciplinary team saw patients as outpatients within 8 weeks of diagnosis. Individuals were repeatedly seen when they returned to the clinic, or at least monthly. Management was guided by the National Consensus Project for Quality Palliative Care. The primary criteria were mood and quality of life at 12 weeks, using patient-related outcome measures (Functional Assessment of Cancer Therapy-Lung and Hospital Anxiety and Depression Scale). Other criteria were aggressive care at the end of life and survival. The results were improved mood without an increase in antidepressant use, improved quality of life as demonstrated by a clinically meaningful change in the quality-of-life scale, earlier referral to hospice, and significant improvement in survival.[25] The study was not powered for survival. As a result of several prospective studies, multiple national and international organizations have recommended early integration of palliative care into cancer treatment.[150-153]

BARRIERS TO INTEGRATING PALLIATIVE CARE INTO CANCER CARE

The collusion of hope between patient and physician, associated with aggressive anticancer therapy, leads to a belief that survival benefit increases with each salvage therapy, and delays or prevents palliative care referrals.[69,154] If discussions about prognosis and end-of-life care are put off, or not introduced, until crisis episodes, it is likely that palliative care will not be used until needed for crisis intervention, or not at all. Continuing to offer therapies that are unlikely to offer benefit, and then attempting to introduce discussions regarding end-of-life care, can confuse patients. Under these circumstances, end-of-life care discussions are not likely to be well received, or may be put off by patients in favor of continuing anticancer therapy.[104,155] Continuing aggressive care may be perceived by patients as the only reasonable choice and may be framed in terms of wanting to live, implying a survival advantage to ongoing aggressive therapy. These patients will have a false "either or" dichotomy between cancer therapy and palliative care.[154] Physicians delay referral because they don't want to destroy the patient's hope by recommending a palliative care specialist.[37] There is a false impression that palliative care services are dependent on disease outcomes and prognosis, rather than symptom burden, regardless of stage or expected disease outcomes. To overcome these barriers, the term supportive care has been adopted because it is more acceptable to patients and physicians and does not imply end-of-life care.[35,156,157]

Palliative care is under resourced. Although most patients with advanced cancer have a substantial symptom burden, and nearly 40% die from cancer, only 1% of the National Institutes of Health budget is devoted to palliative care.[158] Although palliative care services are available in more than 90% of National Cancer Institute (NCI) designated facilities and more than 75% of community cancer centers, and despite the fact that the great majority (over 80%) of cancer specialists rate palliative care as important to cancer care, less than 20% of cancer programs are likely to devote resources toward integrating palliative care into cancer treatment.[159,160] The average number of full-time equivalent physicians per cancer program is only two, and they are largely overworked.[159,160]

Other reasons for late referrals to palliative care include inequitable access to services and lack of standardized criteria for referral. In addition, physicians often lack an understanding of the extent and availability of services.[161-163] They also lack education and information about palliative care.[59,164,165] These factors can lead to delayed referral or no referral. Although standardized symptom assessment and measured patient-related outcomes are key to understanding symptom burden and patients' needs, most oncologists do not routinely use symptom assessment tools and have had little palliative care experience during training.[158,165,166] Because most patients do not report the full extent of the symptoms they are experiencing, the oncologist will remain unaware of the needs of patients.[167]

A review of 12 textbooks published by multiple medical specialties found that hematology-oncology textbooks ranked 10th in the palliative care content.[168,169] There has been improvement over the decade since that review was written, but it is interesting that, among reviews in managing advanced lung cancer published in major journals, palliative care often is either not included or is added as the last paragraph; outcomes of therapy are usually described in terms of progression-free survival and overall survival.[170,171] Although there are exceptions,[172] these data seem to indicate that oncologists have little exposure to information on palliative care in the materials they are reading to remain current in their specialty.

Some palliative care services, such as hospice, will not follow-up on patients who are being treated with chemotherapy.[163] Integration of palliative care into cancer treatment may be difficult if palliative care specialists do not have an understanding of the natural history of cancer, treatment by stage and histology, common chemotherapy side effects, and new developments in anticancer therapies, including new targeted agents and their toxicity. As a result, palliative care specialists may refer patients to hospice programs prematurely, because they mistake treatment toxicities for progressive cancer. To overcome this barrier, palliative care specialists need to have a fundamental knowledge of oncology, a basic understanding of new developments, and close communication with the oncologists.

Public exposure to information on palliative care is minimal, but public exposure to information on cancer is usually high, because of major news stories about sensational new discoveries and individual reports of dramatic successes based on N-of-1 experiences.[160] Because public fundraising is largely motivated by cure rather than care (e.g., Race for the Cure campaigns),[173] funding care may be seen as less important than funding cure.

Health-care policy involving changing from pay for services to value-based reimbursement may be responsible for either improving or diminishing palliative care services.[174] Value-based reimbursement is based upon cost-effectiveness and requires quality indicators. Palliative care quality indicators are different from those of oncology, and consensus about quality indicators is not universal. Palliative care quality indicators related to cancer care are underdeveloped.[175] Based on value-based reimbursement determined by health-care policy, inpatient units with high mortality may be viewed as unfavorable. In addition, if direct costs alone, rather than direct costs plus indirect cost savings, are not taken into account within the administrative matrix, then inpatient palliative care units may be seen as losing propositions.[131] Compared with general inpatient wards, the type of patient admitted to palliative care units may have higher or lower costs; but deaths are certainly higher than in the general wards. Patients on palliative care inpatient units have greater symptom severity, more serious psychosocial problems, and higher complexity of care.[176,177] The All Patient Refined-Disease Related Index, although useful, may not adequately reflect the complexity of care, severity of illness, or risk of mortality seen on inpatient palliative care units.[178] Part of the art of demonstrating case mixed severity is to use the appropriate word codes for symptoms and diseases to demonstrate for administrators and policymakers the type of patient treated on inpatient palliative care wards.[178]

As palliative care expands to chronic nonmalignant illnesses and moves upstream to comanage cancer patients undergoing disease modifying therapy, there will be negative consequences based on availability of services. There is not enough funding, enough training programs, or enough time to train the number of palliative care specialists needed to meet the demand.[179] It is unlikely that the medical system can take another layer of specialized care for seriously ill patients on top of expensive and already complex health care.[179] Bundling payments will discourage the practice of multiple consultations. If palliative care specialists are able to assume all of the tasks of palliation, other specialists will begin to believe that basic symptom assessment, management and psychosocial care are not part of their responsibility.[179]

To address these barriers, programs in all medical specialties should include training in basic palliative care skills, with treatment centered on patient goals and values, and basic symptom assessment and management. Core competency would include symptom assessment using standardized instruments, basic management of pain and nonpain symptoms, and screening for distress and psychosocial and spiritual concerns. Oncologists should discuss prognosis, goals of care, suffering, and advance directives and assess the patient's understanding of these issues.[180-182] To give providers an opportunity to assess the value of palliative care in improving the quality of oncologic care, the American Society of Clinical Oncology, through a grant from the Agency for Healthcare Research and Quality, in collaboration with the American Academy of Hospice and Palliative Medicine, is developing and disseminating a primary palliative care curriculum based on best evidence. The aim is to enhance oncologists' understanding of basic palliative care, while palliative care specialists concentrate on more complex or refractory symptoms and problems.[179,183]

END-OF-LIFE CARE

As lung cancer and its symptoms progress, the preference for information also progresses. Although the preference for information regarding diagnosis, prognosis, and treatment options does not change, the preference for information about palliative care and end-of-life decisions (if not integrated early into cancer care) does change. Preferences may be for either more information or less information.[184] As a result, it is important that oncologists update patients on disease status and prognosis and ask patients if they want information about palliative care, advance directives, and end-of-life care.

There are no universal definitions of end-of-life care, regardless of whether it is any length of time or a disease state or the patient's preference. Unfortunately, the WHO definition of palliative care is used as a master definition for end-of-life care.[6] Although the term end-of-life care is commonly used, there is no consensus about the components of its definition. It tends to imply either a time frame of survival or boundaries between cure and care that can be detrimental to integrating palliative care into cancer care (if palliative care is used synonymously with end-of-life care).[6]

ASSESSING SYMPTOMS AND QUALITY OF LIFE IN LUNG CANCER

Symptom control remains one of the most important practices in cancer care, palliative care, and end-of-life care and should be done continuously throughout the course of cancer treatment and into survival.[185,186] System assessment is one of the major limitations to symptom management. Fatigue, dyspnea, pain, anorexia, and cachexia are the most common physical symptoms related to lung cancer.[187-191] As symptom burden increases, global health and survival decreases.[188,192] For patients with lung cancer, symptom burden, when measured by the number of symptoms and severity, inversely correlates with quality of life and prognosis.[193,194] Symptom burden increases up to the last 4 weeks of life and then plateaus.[194]

Over the last decade, more than 50 tools have been developed to measure quality of life in individuals with lung cancer.[192] Commonly used quality-of-life measurement tools include the Functional Assessment of Cancer Therapy-Lung (FACT-L) and its modification (NCCN-FACT-17), Lung Cancer Symptom Scale (LCSS), and the European Organization for Research and Treatment of Cancer Quality of Life Questionnaire-Lung Cancer (EORTC-LC-13).[38,195–197] The FACT-L and the EORTC-LC-13 are generic, quality-of-life instruments with specific items related to lung cancer symptoms attached as a disease-specific module.

The FACT-L consists of 41 self-assessment questions, of which 34 pertain to five domains. Combining the physical, functional, and lung cancer modules creates the Trial Outcome Index, a tool that is sensitive to change over time and has provided clinically meaningful, patient-related outcomes in clinical trials.[25] Symptoms (dyspnea, difficulty breathing, cough, chest tightness, appetite and weight loss, and cognitive function) are assessed using a categorical scale with a time frame of 1 week. A change of 2 points on the 7-item symptom scale is clinically significant.[196,198,199] The questionnaire is relatively insensitive to treatment-related symptoms.

The LCSS consists of two scales, one rated by physicians and one rated by patients. The patient questions include six symptoms and three summary questions that are marked on a visual analog scale (a 100-mm horizontal line). The mean of the six symptom items is the average symptom burden. Physician items involve six main lung cancer symptoms. A change of 10 mm in the patient's scale is clinically meaningful. The LCSS does not measure social or affect quality-of-life domains, which is a drawback.[200]

The EORTC-LC-13 is a 13-item, lung cancer symptom module that includes cough, hemoptysis, dyspnea (3 items), sore mouth or tongue, dysphagia, hair loss, tingling hands, tingling feet, pain (3 items), and pain medications. All questions are framed in a 4-point categoric scale and a 7-point numerical scale, with the time frame of 1 week. This quality-of-life scale is clinically valid and useful. It is also sensitive to treatment-related symptoms.[197]

There are problems with measuring quality of life. There can be intraobserver and interobserver errors, missing data, fatigued patients, particularly for long questionnaires, and attrition, which can favorably influence the outcomes, because patients who fail to complete questionnaires are usually sicker or have dropped out of the study. In the case of attrition, statistical adjustments need to be made to prevent bias.[201,202] Comparison across studies is difficult because of differences in patient mix. Visual analog scales are more difficult for patients to understand and complete.[203,204] A shift response may occur as patients recalibrate the severity of their symptoms or change their priorities and feelings about the relative importance of quality-of-life domains over time.[205–208] More severe symptoms will tend to lower the mean over time.[208–211] Lastly, the quality of dying cannot be measured by quality-of-life questionnaires.[212,213] What patients and their loved ones want at the end of life has been identified (see Box 58.4).

Patients should complete quality-of-life questionnaires during the initial consultation and whenever there is a reevaluation of cancer response during treatment. In between, a symptom scale may be helpful. The Edmonton Symptom Assessment System (ESAS) is a nine-question scale with an additional question for patient-specific symptoms not covered in the nine questions. It gauges symptom burden by the number and severity of symptoms using a numerical rating scale (0 = no symptoms, 10 = severe symptoms). Completion rate is high, and it can be completed daily in the inpatient setting.[214–216] The ESAS may be a good way to screen for distress.[217] Distress is a multifactor, unpleasant, emotional experience of a psychosocial and spiritual nature that may interfere with the ability to effectively cope with cancer. Pain

---

> **BOX 58.4** What Patients and Families Want at the End of Life
>
> Mental awareness
> Peace with God or a supreme being
> Legacy (being of some help to others)
> Ability to pray and/or meditate
> Ability to make funeral arrangements
> Absence of burden to others
> Feeling that one's life is complete
> Closure on relationships (being able to reconcile and say goodbye)

and fatigue are the major contributors to distress.[218,219] It is recommended that all patients with cancer be assessed for distress. It is most often recommended that a so-called 11-point distress thermometer be used to screen patients and that a triage system be used to manage patients with distress.[220,221]

MANAGING LUNG CANCER SYMPTOMS

Symptoms are present both at diagnosis and with recurrent cancer. Symptoms recur, or new symptoms develop, with relapse after definitive therapy, or with progression on maintenance therapy, and are usually associated with weight loss. At least half of individuals with lung cancer make emergency department visits for intolerable symptoms sometime during the course of their cancer.[222] Part of the reason for high emergency department utilization is that disease progression—not symptoms—is used frequently as an indicator of relapse. As mentioned earlier, symptom progression, on average, occurs before disease progression. An alternative to detection of relapse would be symptom monitoring, using self-assessed symptom forms that are completed by outpatients on a weekly basis. A categoric, self-assessment scale, which measures the severity of weight loss, fatigue, pain, cough, and breathlessness on a weekly basis, has been developed and used in a feasibility study.[223] Sensitivity, specificity, and positive predictive value of these sentinel symptoms and weight loss were 86%, 93%, and 86%, respectively. Relapses were detected 6 weeks earlier on average than would have occurred with planned imaging. Use of this assessment tool may reduce the number of imaging procedures (which usually have a low yield in asymptomatic individuals) and allow for earlier intervention before symptoms become severe and require emergency department visits or emergency inpatient admissions.

Fatigue

Fatigue is almost universally experienced by individuals with advanced cancer and is the main symptom that detrimentally influences quality of life.[224,225] Fatigue is a distressing persistent sense of tiredness or exhaustion that interferes with daily activities. Unlike normal physical fatigue, it occurs with normal activity and can occur without any physical activity. It is pervasive and lasts beyond the normal expected recovery time. Descriptors for fatigue, such as tiredness, induration, lack of vigor, and asthenia, may not exactly describe every patient's experience.[226] Fatigue can be screened through a numerical rating scale (0 = no fatigue, 10 = severe fatigue), with fatigue ratings greater than 4 being clinically significant.[227,228] People with cancer who have fatigue should be screened for depression. Cancer-related fatigue is not associated with anhedonia, hopelessness, or worthlessness.[229] Insomnia and pain should be treated. Patients with obstructive sleep apnea will also experience fatigue and may benefit from continuous positive airway pressure while sleeping.[230] Anemia, hypothyroidism, and hypogonadism will contribute to the severity of fatigue, and treatment for these conditions may improve fatigue. Comorbidities, such as heart failure and COPD, should be assessed and treatment maximized.

In one randomized double-blind trial, cancer-related fatigue was improved with corticosteroids.[231] However, the long-term use of corticosteroids is associated with side effects, including osteoporosis, myopathy, insomnia, thromboembolism, and psychotomimetic side effects. Dexamethasone (4 mg in the morning and at noon) was used in this trial. Doses should be tapered to the lowest effective dose, or discontinued if no response is observed after a 2-week trial period. In a second randomized, double-blind trial, American ginseng was effective in reducing cancer-related fatigue. The side effects were similar to those with placebo, and ginseng had few drug interactions.[120] Psychostimulants were reported to be effective in prospective, single-arm studies, but these positive results have not been duplicated in randomized trials.[232,233] Strength and endurance training may help to address fatigue and loss of physical function during chemotherapy, as such training has been shown to increase the 6-minute walk time, stair climbing, strength capacity, and, in patients with dyspnea, perception of shortness of breath during submaximal walking.[234]

Dyspnea

Dyspnea can be described as chest tightness, rapid shallow breathing, air hunger, and not getting enough air,[235] and each descriptor reflects a different pathophysiology. Chest tightness is associated with coronary artery disease. Rapid shallow breathing is the result of a mismatch between respiratory drive and lung capacity. Air hunger is associated with increasing retention of carbon dioxide. Not getting enough air is associated with hyperinflation. Most patients with cancer have dyspnea at the end of life.[236]

In advanced cancer, particularly lung cancer, there are usually a multitude of reasons for dyspnea. These reasons include loss of lung volume from treatment and tumor size, pleural effusions, cardiac tamponade, COPD, coronary artery disease, thromboembolism, pneumonia and wasting, anxiety and depression, and uncontrolled pain.[237] Wasting is associated with quantitative and qualitative changes in the diaphragm muscle, which leads to reduced tidal volume with exertion and inspiratory capacity.[238,239]

Dyspnea can be screened by the numerical scale within the Edmonton Symptom Assessment System.[240] The Cancer Dyspnea Scale and the Dyspnea Numeric Scale, which assess dyspnea interference with activities, may also be used.[241]

Depending on the underlying etiology, treatment for cancer-related dyspnea may include surgery, chemotherapy, radiotherapy, thoracentesis, pericardiocentesis, the use of drainage tubes, bronchoscopy with laser or stenting, brachytherapy, corticosteroids and antibiotics, and transfusions. Nonintervention approaches may also reduce dyspnea. Pulmonary rehabilitation and walking aids that activate accessory muscles can improve dyspnea.[242] Oxygen should be used for patients who are hypoxic (oxygen saturation of less than 90%). Blowing air across the face, by way of a room or handheld fan, may reduce dyspnea in those who have normal oxygen levels.[243–245] Noninvasive ventilation, using bilevel positive airway pressure, reduces dyspnea and avoids intubation.[246] It does not require sedation.

Morphine reduces dyspnea without causing hypercapnia. Initial dose is 2.5 mg to 5 mg every 4 hours, as needed. If patients are opioid tolerant, a 25% increase in the opioid dose may be helpful.[247–249] Nebulized opioids and furosemide should not be used as standard therapy, because of lack of evidence supporting their effectiveness.[250,251] Most individuals with chronic dyspnea also have episodes of worsening dyspnea, or air hunger, that should be treated with an opioid, as needed. Benzodiazepines and sedating phenothiazines have been used to treat dyspnea, but there is conflicting evidence. There are negative and positive trials with few high-quality randomized studies.[252–255] Both benzodiazepines and sedating phenothiazines may be added or substituted for opioids

if patients are intolerant of opioids or wish not to go on opioids. Lastly, for patients with refractory dyspnea, palliative sedation, using subcutaneous phenobarbital, or using parenteral haloperidol plus a benzodiazepine (e.g., midazolam or lorazepam), may be necessary to control dyspnea. Palliative sedation should be discussed with patients and families before instituting treatment. The patient should have a DNR order, and, if gastric tube feedings are in place, they should be removed.[256–258]

Cough

Symptomatic cough will occur in at least half of patients with lung cancer.[259] Patients with advanced lung disease have greater dependence on cough for mucus clearance than healthy individuals. In patients with lung cancer, the cough response is prompted by excessive noxious stimulation of afferent sensory fibers through the vagus. There also can be central sensitization of neurons governing the cough reflex.[260,261] Evaluation of cough should include whether the cough is productive or not, what triggers the cough, the timing of the episodes (daytime or nocturnal), the patient's medications, (e.g., angiotensin-converting enzyme inhibitors), and the underlying comorbidities. A cough scale can be used to gauge frequency and severity.[260–262] The Manchester Cough and Lung Cancer Scale uses 10 items to assess cough in lung cancer. It is presently being validated.[263] Chest radiographs and computed tomography (CT) images may demonstrate an obstructive bronchus, pleural or pericardial effusions, atelectasis, pneumonia, bronchopleural or bronchoesophageal fistula, lymphangitic carcinomatosis, superior vena cava obstruction, or treatment-related pneumonitis.[260–262]

Radiotherapy, laser therapy, brachytherapy, or stenting may relieve an obstructive bronchus. Thoracentesis, chest tube drainage plus pleurodesis, or placement of tunnelled indwelling pleural catheter can reduce cough and dyspnea associated with pleural effusions. Pericardiocentesis may be relieved with a cardiac tamponade. Simple hydration, humidification, and mucolytics may be helpful, particularly with mobilization of secretions. However, there are no well-conducted randomized trials that support the use of mucolytics in the management of cough.[264,265] There is also sparse evidence for chest wall vibration and manual clearance of secretions.[266] Flutter valve oscillation through a mouthpiece has been used.[267] Positive end-expiratory pressure, via face mask, for 45 minutes per day improves cough and dyspnea.[268,269]

Cough suppression is desirable when cough is no longer useful as a function or if cough produces pain or is fatiguing. Opioids commonly used as cough suppressants include codeine, dextromethorphan, and morphine. Dextromethorphan controls the intensity of cough better than codeine.[270] Sustained-release morphine reduces cough severity by 40%. There is no evidence of a dose–response relationship when using morphine, or of one opioid being superior for the treatment of cough.[271–274]

Proton-pump inhibitors can reduce cough caused by gastric reflux, and gabapentin has been shown to reduce cough stemming from central sensitization.[275] Prednisone (30 mg daily for 2 weeks) may reduce cough associated with bronchospasm, or pleural, pericardial, or diaphragmatic irritation caused by the tumor or treatment.[272] Baclofen may also work, if standard therapies have been ineffective. For patients who are imminently dying, treatment with a cholinergic inhibitor, such as glycopyrrolate, may reduce secretions and the so-called death rattle.[276] The recommended glycopyrrolate dose is 0.1 mg to 0.2 mg (IV or subcutaneous) every 6 to 8 hours. It is best given around-the-clock because it prevents, rather than treats, secretions. Glycopyrrolate is a quaternary scopolamine derivative that does not cross into the central nervous system, thus preventing anticholinergic-induced cognitive dysfunction or delirium.[277] Alternatives are inhaled ipratropium or scopolamine ophthalmic solution dropped onto the tongue.[278]

Cachexia and Anorexia

Cachexia is most often recognized as involuntary weight loss. Precachexia is defined as a weight loss of less than 5%, and cachexia is defined as weight loss greater than 5%. However, if the body mass index (BMI) is less than 20, then a greater than 2% body weight loss would be defined as cachexia. Symptoms associated with cachexia include sarcopenia, loss of fat mass, anorexia, fatigue, and elevated inflammatory cytokines and acute phase reactants.[279] Anorexia is a cluster of symptoms that includes bloating, early satiety, taste and smell changes, dysgeusia, and diurnal variations in food intake.[280]

Peripheral and central mechanisms generate cachexia and anorexia. Inflammatory cytokines upregulate the transcription factor NF kappa-B in muscle that in turn, upregulates myostatin, proteasomes, and prostaglandins. Satellite cell proliferation is inhibited and muscle synthesis, through MyoD and mTOR/Akt, is blocked. Mitochondrial function and calcium metabolism) are also adversely affected, leading to reduced oxidative phosphorylation. In addition, there is an increase in reactive oxygen species.[281,282] Anorexia results from increased neurotransmission of proopiomelanocortin-containing neurons within the arcuate nucleus of the hypothalamus. There is also a simultaneous reduction of neuropeptide Y signals. Neurotransmission through proopiomelanocortin neurons is increased through activation of serotonin receptors (5-HT2C) as well as throughout regulation of interleukin-1.[281,282]

Inflammatory cytokines (tumor necrosis factor-alpha, interleukin-1, and interleukin-6) increase production of C-reactive protein from the liver and muscle. Hypoalbuminemia develops from loss of the endothelial barrier and extravasation into interstitial spaces.[283] Elevated C-reactive protein is associated with progressive weight loss and is a poor prognostic indicator in lung cancer.[284] Both serum albumin and C-reactive protein are combined in the Glasgow Prognostic Score.[285–287] Pretreatment Glasgow prognostic score is a useful and important predictor of cancer-specific survival in patients with inoperable NSCLC. It is predictive of the most important aspects of platinum-related toxicity.

Assessment of cachexia is complex. Factors that have been used to follow the course of cachexia and sarcopenia include changes in weight, BMI, anthropometric measurements, bioelectrical impedance, dual-energy x-ray absorptiometry, and measurement of muscle area at the level of the L3 vertebral body. Using CT to measure muscle mass at the L3 vertebral body level has been validated. These measurements can be done routinely to follow the course of cancer.[288] Assessment of anorexia can be made through the Edmonton Symptom Assessment Score. The Functional Assessment of Anorexia Cachexia Therapy scale, which is a 12-item module attached to the Functional Assessment of Cancer Therapy quality-of-life tool, can also be used.[289,290] There are multiple other nutritional scales, but they do not separate starvation from cachexia. In a study evaluating use of the Mini Nutritional Assessment scale for individuals with lung cancer, the score on the scale correlated with laboratory parameters of inflammation and was independently associated with survival.[291]

The best method for treating cancer-related cachexia is to cure the cancer. If this is not possible, then the goals of therapy are to maintain muscle mass, nutritional intake, and function.[292] Because it is unlikely that a single drug will have a major impact on cancer cachexia and anorexia, treatment should be multimodal. Appetite stimulants include corticosteroids, progesterone, and olanzapine.[293] In a randomized trial, the combination of megestrol acetate and olanzapine was superior to megestrol acetate as a single agent, with substantial improvements in appetite, nausea, weight gain, and quality of life.[294] Cachexia has been treated with single-agent antioxidants, l-carnitine, omega-3 fatty acids, thalidomide, nonsteroidal antiinflammatory drugs (NSAIDs),

and megestrol acetate, with little to marginal benefit. Recent trials of drug combinations have proven to be more effective than single agents in increasing lean body mass, decreasing energy expenditures, and improving appetite.[295] Ghrelin analogs and selective androgen receptor modulators are presently in development.[296–299]

Pain

At least half of individuals with advanced cancer will have chronic pain.[300] There are well-described cancer pain syndromes. Approximately 75% of individuals with cancer have pain related to their cancer, and 25% have pain related to treatment or comorbid illnesses. Many individuals with cancer have cancer pain syndromes because of widespread metastases, and these syndromes have been well described.[301–304] Clinicians can mistake existential suffering for physical pain. Characteristically, somatic pain does not respond to treatment with opioids.[305,306]

To properly assess pain, clinicians need to know pain intensity, the point from where it radiates, temporal pattern, pain quality, and provocative and relieving factors. The cause, pathophysiology, and pain syndrome can be inferred from the history and confirmed by physical examination and radiographs.[306] Pain intensity is largely used when choosing analgesics and adjusting doses, but interference with activity and function are equally important. Pain intensity may change little, but function, mood, sleep, and vitality may improve with treatment.[307] Another area that needs to be assessed when considering treatment is the side effects associated with analgesics. Pain can be assessed on a numerical rating scale. Mild pain is less than 4 on an 11-point numerical rating scale; moderate pain is 5 to 7; and severe pain is greater than 7. A reduction of baseline pain severity between 30% and 50% is clinically significant.[308–310] The Brief Pain Inventory is a validated tool and can be used in the initial assessment.[311,312] Before prescribing opioids for moderate to severe pain, the patient's substance abuse history, family substance abuse history, and patient's history of depression, anxiety disorder, or personality disorder should be obtained.[306]

Classifying pain into somatic, visceral, or neuropathic is an oversimplification of clinical reality. There are features of neuropathic pain in patients who have visceral metastases, as demonstrated in animal models. Central sensitization can occur in all three subclasses of pain.[313–315]

For mild pain, acetaminophen or NSAIDs can be used as the analgesics of choice, but should not be used for patients with coagulopathy, or heart or kidney failure. NSAIDs are also not recommended for treating older individuals. Prophylaxis with proton-pump inhibitors should be considered.[316] There is evidence that the combination of NSAIDs and acetaminophen may improve analgesia.[317]

For moderate pain, tramadol, tapentadol, codeine, or low doses of a potent opioid, such as morphine, are reasonable choices.[318,319] Although it had been assumed that codeine is an analgesic—through conversion to morphine via the cytochrome CYP 2D6—newer evidence suggests that there is actually synergy between codeine and morphine. Therefore, codeine may have to be converted to morphine for analgesia.[320] If patients were originally treated with nonopioid analgesics, such as acetaminophen or NSAIDs, these drugs can be added or continued.

For severe pain, potent opioids such as oxycodone, morphine, hydromorphone, or fentanyl may be used as first-line analgesics.[321] Starting doses are as follows: morphine, 5 mg every 4 hours by mouth; oxycodone, 5 mg every 4 hours; hydromorphone, 1 mg every 4 hours; and transdermal fentanyl at 12 μg per hour. If pain is acute or unstable, transdermal fentanyl should not be used.[321–323] Sustained-release morphine (15 mg every 12 hours) or oxycodone (10 mg every 12 hours) may be used in place of immediate-release preparations. Most patients have breakthrough pain. A rescue dose of one-sixth of the total daily opioid dose should be provided every 1 to 2 hours.[324–327] Transient flares of pain may be related to activities (incident pain) or spontaneous. End-of-dose failure is considered suboptimal around-the-clock opioid dosing. If this occurs, the around-the-clock dose should be increased. There are considerable differences in dose requirements between patients who will require dose titration of no less than 25% and no more than 100% of the total daily dose. As an alternative, transmucosal, buccal, sublingual, or intranasal fentanyl have been approved for breakthrough pain. These preparations are expensive and should be reserved as second-line treatments for individuals whose breakthrough pain is unresponsive to oral, immediate-release opioids.[328–330]

Titration of potent opioids is required to control pain in most individuals. To reach steady-state levels, the dose of immediate-release opioids should not be changed more often than every 24 hours. The dose of sustained-release opioids should not be changed more often than every 48 hours, and the dose of transdermal fentanyl should not be changed more often than every 48 to 72 hours. If pain remains a problem, then the rescue dose can be titrated to response, and the around-the-clock dose adjusted once steady-state is reached.[306,331] Patients with severe liver disease should be treated with morphine or hydromorphone because these opioids are conjugated and glucuronidation is relatively spared.[332] For patients who are in renal failure, methadone or buprenorphine are the opioids of choice.[333–336] Because of its unique pharmacology, methadone should be used only by designated prescribers.[306]

Adjuvant analgesics can improve pain and reduce opioid requirements. Antiseizure drugs, predominantly gabapentinoids, tricyclic antidepressants, and selective norepinephrine serotonin reuptake inhibitors (duloxetine and venlafaxine), can improve neuropathic pain. Because tricyclic antidepressants have substantial side effects, secondary amine tricyclic antidepressants may be better tolerated.[337] When adjuvant analgesics are used, the number needed to treat to substantially reduce neuropathic pain in an individual patient ranges from three to five.[338–340] Corticosteroids reduce symptoms and pain from tumor-related compressive neuropathy, brain metastases, and bowel obstruction.[341–343] Bisphosphonates have been used for bone pain.[344,345] For patients in whom pain does not respond to a first-line opioid, or in whom dose-limiting toxicity develops (e.g., confusion, myoclonus, hallucinations, nightmares, or severe nausea), switching to or rotating with an alternative opioid will improve pain control and reduce side effects.[346–348] Because of noncross tolerance, doses that are 50% to 70% of the equianalgesic dose should be used and further dose adjustment should be made, based on clinical context, including potential drug interactions and organ function. Routine use of analgesic tables can be dangerous.[349,350] As an alternative, switching to spinal opioids may improve the opioid therapeutic index by reducing side effects. Spinal adjuvant analgesics include bupivacaine and clonidine.[351,352]

Side effects related to opioids can add symptom burden to patients or may be mistaken for progressive cancer. Constipation, if severe, not only produces nausea and vomiting, but can also resemble a bowel obstruction. Because there is no tolerance for constipation, stool softeners and laxatives should be started proactively when opioids are prescribed.[353,354] Opioid-induced constipation that is unresponsive to laxatives and enemas should be treated with methylnaltrexone.[355] Opioid-induced sedation may respond to a methylphenidate.[356] The anticholinergic side effects of opioids, (dry mouth, urinary retention, and nausea) may require targeted approaches to management. Antiemetics, such as metoclopramide, prochlorperazine, or ondansetron, may be used to manage nausea.[357] For most individuals, nausea is mild and tolerance develops over several days. Most opioids, except for buprenorphine, induce hypogonadotropic hypogonadism, which can result in altered mood, hot flashes, loss of libido and

sexual function, and, over a period of time, loss of muscle and bone.[358] When treatment with an opioid is started or doses are adjusted, there can be mild sedation and mild muddled thinking, which usually resolves over several days. Patients should be taking stable doses of opioids for approximately 2 weeks before they consider driving a car. Overt confusion and delirium induced by opioids require opioid rotation or change in route rather than antipsychotics. Nonpharmacologic modalities should be considered concurrently with analgesics. Mind-body approaches and integrative interventions can be helpful, both in improving pain and in reducing the opioid requirements.[306] Correction of impending fractures of long bones; kyphoplasty; and brachial, celiac, or hypogastric blocks can improve pain and improve opioid responses.[359]

LUNG CANCER AND THE INTENSIVE CARE UNIT

In selected individuals in the United States, intensive care unit survival and hospital survival can be excellent depending on the clinical situation. Intensive care unit survival and hospital survival are 72% and 60%, respectively, but hospital survival is substantially decreased if mechanical ventilation is required (62% compared with 47%). In cancer specialty hospitals, intensive care unit survival is reported to be 40%, and only 30% of patients survive mechanical ventilation. This may be related to differences in the patient population.[360–365] For patients who require intensive care and survive hospitalization, fewer than 30% survive for 6 months. Individuals with lung cancer and progressive cancer prior to intensive care admission, and patients with preexisting poor performance status or progressive organ dysfunction, or both, have very high mortality rates in intensive care.[362] For patients with advanced lung cancer, admission to the intensive care unit should be considered a sign that hospice care is warranted. End-of-life care discussions should take place. Patients with progressive cancer, poor performance status, or progressive organ failure should be discouraged from being admitted to the intensive care unit because the outlook is so dismal. Unfortunately for most individuals, discussions about resuscitation preferences and intensive care admissions usually do not take place before transfer to intensive care.

LUNG CANCER AND CARDIOPULMONARY RESUSCITATION

For patients with lung cancer, survival to discharge after cardiopulmonary arrest is 16%, and only 8.5% return home. Many do not recover neurologic function and require placement in extended care facilities or inpatient hospices. Survival is even worse if either vasopressors or mechanical ventilation, or both, are required postarrest.[366–368] Cancer is not an independent predictor of the success of resuscitation, but progressive cancer prior to arrest, along with the number and severity of comorbidities, are predictive of a low chance for survival. Rather than simply asking patients whether or not they want to be resuscitated, discussions should be based on goals of care, outlook, benefits, and detriments.

CONCLUSION

The advances in oncologic therapies for lung cancer have prolonged the short-term survival of patients with advanced lung cancer. Along with increased survival, patients experience multiple cancer symptoms and impaired quality of life as the disease course evolves. There is now a shift in cancer treatment that favors early integration of palliative care, based on clinical and patient-related outcomes. Delivery of effective palliative care will require financial resources for palliative care fellowships, outpatient and inpatient palliative care services, and medical and public education. It will also require changes in health-care policy that promote integration of palliative care into cancer treatment.[369]

KEY REFERENCES

9. Fadul N, Elsayem A, Palmer JL, et al. Supportive versus palliative care: what's in a name? A survey of medical oncologists and midlevel providers at a comprehensive cancer center. *Cancer.* 2009;115(9):2013–2021.
21. Meldahl ML, Acaster S, Hayes RP. Exploration of oncologists' attitudes toward and perceived value of patient-reported outcomes. *Qual Life Res.* 2013;22(4):725–731.
24. Earle CC. It takes a village. *J Clin Oncol.* 2012;30(4):353–354.
25. Temel JS, Greer JA, Muzikansky A, et al. Early palliative care for patients with metastatic non-small-cell lung cancer. *N Engl J Med.* 2010;363(8):733–742.
33. Von Roenn JH, Temel J. The integration of palliative care and oncology: the evidence. *Oncology (Williston Park).* 2011;25(13):1258–1265.
35. Bruera E, Hui D. Integrating supportive and palliative care in the trajectory of cancer: establishing goals and models of care. *J Clin Oncol.* 2010;28(25):4013–4017.
36. The AM, Hak T, Koeter G, van der Wal G. Collusion in doctor-patient communication about imminent death: an ethnographic study. *BMJ.* 2000;321(7273):1376–1381.
46. Homsi J, Walsh D, Rivera N, et al. Symptom evaluation in palliative medicine: patient report vs systematic assessment. *Support Care Cancer.* 2006;14(5):444–453.
61. Weeks JC, Catalano PJ, Cronin A, et al. Patients' expectations about effects of chemotherapy for advanced cancer. *N Engl J Med.* 2012;367(17):1616–1625.
69. de Haes H, Koedoot N. Patient centered decision making in palliative cancer treatment: a world of paradoxes. *Patient Educ Couns.* 2003;50(1):43–49.
80. Earle CC, Landrum MB, Souza JM, Neville BA, Weeks JC, Ayanian JZ. Aggressiveness of cancer care near the end of life: is it a quality-of-care issue? *J Clin Oncol.* 2008;26(23):3860–3866.
85. Johnston SC, Pfeifer MP, McNutt R. The discussion about advance directives. Patient and physician opinions regarding when and how it should be conducted. End of Life Study Group. *Arch Intern Med.* 1995;155(10):1025–1030.
91. Temel JS, Greer JA, Admane S, et al. Longitudinal perceptions of prognosis and goals of therapy in patients with metastatic non-small-cell lung cancer: results of a randomized study of early palliative care. *J Clin Oncol.* 2011;29(17):2319–2326.
94. Greer JA, Pirl WF, Jackson VA, et al. Effect of early palliative care on chemotherapy use and end-of-life care in patients with metastatic non-small-cell lung cancer. *J Clin Oncol.* 2012;30(4):394–400.
131. Smith S, Brick A, O'Hara S, Normand C. Evidence on the cost and cost-effectiveness of palliative care: a literature review. *Palliat Med.* 2014;28(2):130–150.
158. Abrahm JL. Integrating palliative care into comprehensive cancer care. *J Natl Compr Canc Netw.* 2012;10(10):1192–1198.

See Expertconsult.com for full list of references.

59 Clinical Trial Methodology in Lung Cancer: Study Design and End-Point Considerations

Sumithra J. Mandrekar, Mary W. Redman, and Lucinda J. Billingham

SUMMARY OF KEY POINTS

- Lung cancer is increasingly understood at the molecular level; N-of-1 trials are becoming more relevant with the use of biomarker assessment and targeted therapies.

- The failure of promising agents in randomized studies has prompted reconsideration of the standard dose-finding paradigm in early phase trials, with the recognition that improved drug development strategies for single agents and combination therapies are required.

- The choice of end points and trial design options in the phase II and phase III setting is driven by the purported mechanism of the action of the drug and the availability of a biomarker to "enrich" patient population leading to either (a) larger randomized phase II, phase II/III, or phase III trials (all-comers design with retrospective subgroup assessment), or (b) smaller (including nonrandomized) phase II trials in an enriched subpopulation targeting larger differences.

- Adaptive designs are becoming a reality with advances in mobile computing, electronic data capture, and integration of research records with electronic medical records.

- Master protocols incorporating a central infrastructure for screening and identification of patients who can be funneled into multiple subtrials testing targeted therapeutics have become an efficient way to conduct definitive trials in lung cancer.

- Newer approaches to clinical trial end points and design strategies that challenge the historical paradigm of drug development are critical to accelerate the drug development process so that the right therapies can be delivered to the right patients.

In oncology, the development of new therapeutics typically follows the phase I, phase II, and phase III drug development paradigm. In phase I, the primary goal is to understand the safety profile of a new treatment in a small group of patients before further investigation. In the phase II setting, the primary goal is to determine if there is an efficacy signal worthy of further investigation; a secondary objective is to gain a better understanding of the treatment's safety. Phase II trials may have a single arm or may be a randomized trial in a homogeneous study population, with the trial size varying from less than 100 patients to as many as 300 patients. If the drug is considered safe and has a promising efficacy signal, then a phase III trial is initiated. The primary goal of the phase III trial is to compare the new treatment with the standard of care to demonstrate a clinical benefit or, in some cases, cost-effectiveness. Phase III trials are usually large, comprising a few hundred to thousands of patients, and they are conducted in a homogeneus group of patients at multiple institutions.

As biomarker assessment and use of targeted therapies increase in cancer treatment, N-of-1 trials—studies in which an individual is the single subject of study—are becoming more relevant. Biomarker assessment is a critical aspect of targeted therapy because biomarkers can identify patients who are more likely to benefit from a particular treatment. The Biomarkers Definitions Working Group defined a tumor marker or a biomarker as "a characteristic that is objectively measured and evaluated as an indicator of normal biologic processes, pathogenic processes, or pharmacologic responses to a therapeutic intervention."[1] In oncology, the term biomarker refers to a broad range of measures derived from tumor tissues, whole blood, plasma, serum, bone marrow, or urine. In principle, the pathway from basic discovery of a biomarker to its use in clinical practice is similar to a traditional drug development process, but there are some basic differences, which will be described here.[2] An extensive guideline for reporting studies on tumor markers has been developed and published.[3]

Biomarker-based trials deviate from the standard paradigm for developing a treatment or regimen. In the context of biomarkers, a phase I study tests the methods of assessing marker alteration in normal and tumor tissue samples. Results from this study may help to determine the cut points for quantitative assessment and meaningful interpretation of test results. The feasibility of obtaining the specimens, as well as the reliability and reproducibility of the assay, needs to be established at this stage. A phase II study is typically a careful retrospective assessment of the marker to establish its clinical usefulness. In phase III trials, the marker is prospectively evaluated and validated in a large, multicenter population that provides adequate power to address issues of multiple testing.[2]

For a biomarker to be useful in clinical practice, its assay results should be accurate and reproducible (analytically valid) and its value should associate with the outcome of interest (clinically valid). Further, for a biomarker to be useful in clinical practice there must be a specific clinical question, proposed alteration in clinical management, and improved clinical outcomes (the so-called clinical utility).[4] An elaborate tumor marker utility grading system was developed that defined the data quality or level of evidence needed for grading the clinical utility of markers.[5] In brief, level I evidence, which is similar to a phase III drug trial, is considered definitive. Levels II to V represent varying degrees of hypothesis-generating investigations, similar to phase I or II drug trials.

The high failure rate of phase III trials in oncology, including lung cancer, may be attributable to several factors, including inaccurate predictions of efficacy based on the hypothesis-generating phase II trials; failure to identify an appropriate dose or schedule (the so-called optimal dose) in a phase I trial; or problems with the phase III trial design.[6] Assessing the safety profile and establishing the maximum tolerated dose remain the primary focus of phase I trials, including trials of targeted therapies and vaccines. However, it is becoming more common for phase I trials to assess preliminary efficacy signals and identify the subsets of patients most likely to benefit from the new treatment. Tumor size response metrics based on longitudinal tumor size models are promising new end points in phase II clinical oncology studies;[7,8] however, these metrics have not been validated yet for routine use in clinical trials. Response is being measured as progression-free survival instead of using the Response Evaluation Criteria in Solid Tumors (RECIST). Variants of progression-free survival, such as disease control rate at a predetermined time point, have been shown to be acceptable alternate end points for rapidly screening new agents in phase II trials in patients with extensive-stage small cell lung cancer and advanced-stage nonsmall cell lung cancer (NSCLC).[9–12] For phase III trials, overall survival, defined as the time from random assignment or registration to death from any cause, is still the standard criterion end point because it is a measure of direct clinical benefit to a patient. As an end point, overall survival is unambiguous and can unequivocally assess the benefit of a new treatment relative to the current standard of care. Although improving overall survival remains the ultimate goal of new cancer therapy, an intermediate end point such as disease-free survival in early-stage disease has been used in the phase III setting to evaluate the treatment effect of new oncologic products.[13,14] However, overall survival continues to be an appropriate end point in trials without an intermediate end point or validated surrogate end points, such as for phase III trials in extensive-stage small cell lung cancer and advanced-stage NSCLC.[9]

This chapter is organized into sections that focus on the end points and design considerations for cytotoxic agents and targeted therapies for early phase, dose-finding trials; phase II trials; and phase III trials. Where possible, examples of ongoing or completed lung cancer clinical trials are used to explain the concepts. The chapter ends with a brief summary and a discussion of future perspectives on clinical trial design in lung cancer research.

EARLY PHASE TRIALS

Historically, dose-finding trials in oncology have been designed to establish the maximum tolerated dose of a therapeutic regimen, with safety as the primary outcome. These trials, which are usually the first to test a new agent in humans, may include patients with multiple tumor types when no other treatment is available. A fundamental assumption of these designs is that toxicity and efficacy are directly related to dose, that is, the higher dose, the greater the risk of toxicity and greater the chance of efficacy.[15] Although this paradigm works for cytotoxic agents, it is not readily applicable for molecularly targeted therapies, vaccines, or immunotherapy. The postulated mechanisms of action for these agents are not straightforward because (a) the dose–efficacy curves are usually unknown and may follow a nonmonotone pattern such as a quadratic curve or an increasing curve with a plateau (Fig. 59.1), and (b) dose–toxicity relationships are expected to be minimal.

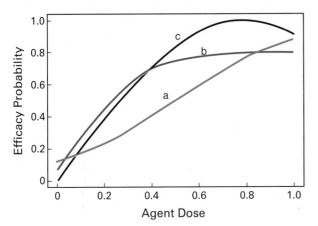

Fig. 59.1. Examples of dose–efficacy curves for molecularly targeted agents. *a,* Monotonic increasing; *b,* increasing with a plateau; *c,* unimodal.

With regard to targeted therapies, erlotinib, gefitinib, and bevacizumab have demonstrated clinical benefit in several cancers, including lung cancer, whereas others such as R115777 and ISIS 3521 have produced negative results.[16–18] Problems with the design of phase I studies provide plausible explanations for the lack of clinical activity seen with these drugs, despite understanding the pathway of action for such drugs. The phase I studies were designed primarily to assess maximum tolerated dose, and the patients enrolled in these studies were unselected (e.g., all-comers vs. patients whose tumors express a specific molecular target). Consider, for example, an immunotherapy administered to stimulate the patient's own immune system to fight the tumor. Overstimulation of the immune system could interfere with the drug's efficacy or prove harmful for the patient.[19]

Ideally, dose-finding studies for immunotherapies or targeted agents would include a secondary measure of efficacy to identify the biologically optimal dose or the minimum effective dose, instead of the maximum tolerated dose. However, barriers to measuring efficacy in early phase trials are the absence of validated assays or markers of efficacy, the time required to measure an efficacy outcome, and incomplete understanding of drug metabolism and its pathway. These limitations also preclude patient selection for phase I trials, although an enrichment strategy is being used more often—either during the dose-escalation or dose-expansion phase—to identify subsets of patients who are likely to benefit most from the treatment. Successful examples of using enrichment strategy in early phase trials include the development of vemurafenib to treat patients with melanoma positive for v-raf murine sarcoma viral oncogene homolog B (*BRAF*) mutation and crizotinib for patients with NSCLC-positive anaplastic lymphoma kinase (ALK) rearrangement.[20,21]

Phase I trial designs can be broadly categorized as either model based or rule based (also called algorithm based).[22] In the rule-based designs, small numbers of patients are treated starting at the lowest dose level. The decision to escalate, deescalate, or treat additional patients at the same dose level is based on a prespecified algorithm related to the occurrence of unacceptable dose-limiting toxicity. The trial is terminated once a dose level is reached that exceeds the acceptable toxicity threshold. The initial dose level often is derived from animal studies or trials conducted in a different setting. The interval between successive dose levels is usually based on a modified Fibonacci sequence.[15,23] Examples of rule-based designs commonly used in oncology studies include the traditional cohorts-of-three design and its variants, the accelerated titration design, and the two-stage design.[23]

The continual reassessment method introduced the concept of dose–toxicity models to guide the dose-finding process.[24,25] The dose–toxicity model represents the investigator's a priori belief in the likelihood of dose-limiting toxicity according to the delivered dose. The model is updated sequentially using cumulative patient toxicity data. Several modifications have been proposed to address the safety concerns associated with the original continual reassessment method, such as starting the trial at the lowest dose level, prohibiting skipping of dose levels during escalation, and requiring at least three patients at each dose level prior to escalation.[26–28] The trials with a model-based design using the continual reassessment method have demonstrated better operating characteristics than trials with rule-based designs in simulation settings. Specifically, a higher proportion of patients are treated at levels closer to the optimal dose level, and fewer patients are needed to complete the trial. A key characteristic of all these designs, model based or rule based, is that they use only toxicity to guide dose-escalation and do not incorporate a measure of efficacy in the dose-finding process.

Current statistical approaches extend the standard continual reassessment method in two directions to allow toxicity and efficacy outcomes to be modeled in a phase I trial. One example is the bivariate continual reassessment model, which uses a marginal logit dose–toxicity curve and a marginal logit dose–disease progression curve with a flexible bivariate distribution of toxicity and progression.[29] Other examples are the design proposed by Thall and Cook[30] that uses efficacy–toxicity trade-offs to guide dose finding;[30] the dose-finding scheme proposed by Yin et al.[31] using toxicity and efficacy odds ratios; and bivariate probit models for toxicity and efficacy proposed by Bekele and Shen,[32] and Dragalin and Fedorov.[33] Another statistical approach assumes that the observed clinical outcomes follow a sequential order: no dose-limiting toxicity and no efficacy, no dose-limiting toxicity but efficacy, or severe dose-limiting toxicity, which renders any efficacy irrelevant. In this case, the joint distribution of the binary toxicity and efficacy outcomes can be collapsed into an ordinal trinary (three-outcome) variable, which may be appropriate in the setting of vaccine trials and viral-reduction studies in patients with human immunodeficiency virus, among others.[34,35]

The design and end-point considerations are further complicated in the study of combination therapies. Ideally, the underlying biologic rationale for the combination would be known; for example, whether the efficacy of the two agents is additive, complementary, or synergistic. Understanding the interaction between the drugs may help investigators to anticipate whether the toxicity profiles of the agents are overlapping or additive. Typically, a set of predetermined dose-level combinations are explored based on either the maximum tolerated dose of one agent or other preclinical data demonstrating synergy. The dose of one agent under investigation is escalated, while the dose of the second agent remains constant until a tolerable combination dose level is achieved. Often it is unfeasible to explore all possible combination levels. Despite increased testing of combination treatments in oncology, few designs for dose escalation of two or more agents have been proposed.[36–39] Gandhi et al.[40] used a non-parametric, up-and-down, algorithmic-based sequential design to explore 12 dose combinations out of a possible 16 combinations. The maximum-tolerated-dose combinations were chosen based on the highest tolerated dose of each agent, achieving a targeted dose-limiting toxicity rate less than 33%. Two maximum-tolerated-dose combinations were identified using this design: 200 mg neratinib plus 25 mg temsirolimus and 160 mg neratinib plus 50 mg temsirolimus.[40]

The failure of promising agents in randomized studies has prompted reconsideration of the standard dose-finding paradigm, with the recognition that improved drug development strategies for single agents and combination therapies are required. Although the assumption of a monotonically increasing dose–toxicity curve is almost always appropriate from a biologic standpoint, a monotonically increasing relationship between dose and efficacy has been challenged by the recent development of molecularly targeted therapies, vaccines, and immunotherapies. Model-based designs are certainly not perfect or recommended for every dose-finding study, but they can be an attractive alternative to the traditional algorithm-based, up-and-down methods. However, the application of these designs to dose-finding studies in oncology has been limited for considerable scientific and pragmatic reasons.[22,41,42] The acceptance and use of these designs may be quicker and easier if they are developed in concert with a clinical paradigm.[40,43]

PHASE II TRIALS

The primary objective of a phase II trial is usually to determine whether there is sufficient evidence of efficacy to warrant further evaluation of a treatment (Fig. 59.2). Secondary goals of phase II trials are to establish which patients are most likely to benefit from this treatment and to evaluate toxicity in a larger study population. Phase II trials are often called screening trials, because they screen new agents or regimens for definitive evaluation in a phase III study. These trials usually include the minimum number of

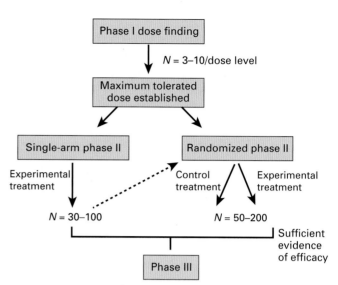

Fig. 59.2. Typical drug development pathway. *N*, total number of study participants.

patients necessary to achieve the study goals and are relatively short in duration so that the experimental treatment can continue to phase III testing. As with any phase of testing, the study goals dictate the specifics of design and end-point selection.

End-Point Considerations

Generally, different end points are used for phase II and III trials of the same treatment. For example, although overall survival is the criterion standard outcome for phase III studies, it is not time efficient to use it in phase II studies. For a phase II trial to be informative, the selected end point should be a surrogate for the phase III outcome of interest, and the magnitude of changes in the surrogate end point should relate directly to changes in the main end point.[44,45] Because clinically relevant outcomes depend on so many disease- and treatment-related variables, validation of a surrogate outcome is challenging.

As discussed earlier, commonly used end points for phase II trials in patients with advanced disease are response rate, progression-free survival, and disease control rate; for trials in patients with early-stage disease, disease-free survival is frequently used. The best outcome measure for a phase II study depends on the experimental agent's mechanism of action. For example, response rate was often used for cytotoxic treatments that were expected to affect survival by shrinking the tumor or reducing overall tumor burden. Since the early 2000s, trials of cytostatic agents, which are thought to prolong survival by shrinking the tumor or stabilizing tumor growth, have been designed to measure progression-free survival or disease control rate. In fact, there is evidence that stable disease predicts overall survival better than tumor response does, which is a reason for including measures of disease stability in chemotherapy trials.[11] The effect of agents that act on the immune system rather than directly on the tumor may not be adequately captured by the traditional measures defined by the RECIST; new criteria for immunotherapies have been developed.[46,47]

The choice of a summary statistic for time-to-event outcomes, such as progression-free or disease-free survival, should also be disease and treatment related. The median times summarize the point at which the event of interest has occurred in at least 50% of study participants. A landmark time can be used to summarize a single time point, for example, the percentage of patients who are progression free at 6 months. The hazard ratio, which is a summary measure of the relative benefit found in the treatment arm averaged over the entire study period, places equal value on differences between the study arms at every point. For treatments expected to have a delayed effect, such as immunotherapies, the average may not represent the treatment's efficacy; for these agents, a landmark time may be a better representation of the treatment effect. End points that may prove useful in the future are imaging-based measures or longitudinal biomarker measures.[48]

Randomized and Single-Arm Designs

Since the early 2000s, phase II trials have shifted from single-arm to randomized design. In a single-arm study, all participants receive the experimental treatment and study results are compared with historical data from patients receiving the standard of care. Studies with a single-arm design typically have 90% power and 5% one-sided type I error, with sample sizes ranging between 20 patients and 100 patients. The validity of this type of study depends on the availability of accurate historical data for the patient population. Biased historical data have been blamed for numerous failed phase III studies after a positive phase II study. In addition, single-arm biomarker studies cannot differentiate between a prognostic and predictive association with the clinical outcome.

Randomized phase II studies avoid the problem of bias in historical data by directly comparing patients who have been randomly assigned to receive an experimental treatment or the standard of care. Randomized studies are typically two to four times larger than single-arm phase II studies and have larger error rates (e.g., type I error of at least 10%).[49,50] A sufficiently powered, randomized phase II trial can differentiate between prognostic and predictive biomarkers.

Assessing Biomarker-Based Subgroups: Design Considerations

Information from phase II studies is often used to establish the patient population for a phase III study. Because therapies are being developed to target a specific biologic mechanism of the tumor or host, biomarker evaluation is an important consideration when designing a phase II study. Possible design choices are an all-comers design with secondary marker evaluation; a biomarker-stratified design with specific accrual targets within biomarker-defined subgroups; enrichment or targeted designs, which enroll only marker-positive patients; and multiple hypothesis designs, which specify both an overall population assessment and a subgroup assessment (Fig. 59.3).[51,52] Any of these designs may be used for the randomized phase II trial in an overall drug development strategy (Fig. 59.2).

In an all-comers design with secondary marker evaluation, the marker can be evaluated either at registration or at the end of the study. When the marker is evaluated at registration, the random assignment can be stratified to ensure balance of the marker between the treatment arms. Secondary evaluation is a reasonable approach when multiple biomarkers are to be assessed and little is known about the markers. However, depending on the prevalence of a marker, studies using this approach may be unpowered. For example, if the prevalence of the marker is 10%, in a two-armed study of 100 patients with 1:1 randomization, there would be only about five patients per arm for subgroup evaluation.

In a study with a biomarker-stratified design, specific accrual targets are established per stratum, based on stratum-specific objectives. All patients are assessed for marker status at registration, and this design ensures adequate power to detect effects within biomarker subgroups.[53] However, accrual for each stratum could differ substantially based on the marker prevalence, making this design impractical. In all cases, it is important to keep

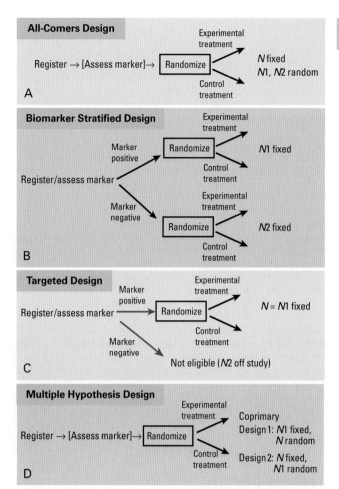

Fig. 59.3. Phase II designs incorporating potential biomarkers. (A) All comers; (B) biomarker stratified design; (C) targeted design; (D) multiple hypothesis design. *N*, total number of study participants; *N1*, patients with marker-positive tumors; *N2*, patients with marker-negative tumors.

in mind that the apparent differences in effect estimates across subgroups could be due to random variation alone.

In studies with an enrichment or targeted design, only individuals with the biomarker are enrolled and studied. Although this approach may be the most efficient design to screen a biomarker–drug combination, this design provides no information about how the therapy performs in the population with marker-negative tumors.[53]

A multiple hypothesis design specifies coprimary objectives for evaluating the treatment within a biomarker-defined subgroup and the overall study population, splitting the study-wide type I error between the two objectives. Determining the target sample size is a key distinction between an all-comers design and a multiple hypothesis design. If the multiple hypothesis study is designed to have a specific number of patients with marker-positive tumors (N1), then the total sample size is the number of patients (N) needed to accrue N1 patients. Alternatively, if the study is designed around the entire study population (N), then the percentage of the study population that has marker-positive tumors determines N1. In this design, marker status can be either evaluated at registration or during the study.

Any of these strategies for establishing biomarker-based subgroups may be used in a single-arm trial by simply assigning all registered patients to the experimental therapy. However, except for studies of patients with rare tumors and small biomarker subsets, a randomized phase II design is typically used, so that the prognostic value of the biomarker can be evaluated in the control arm. For example, in studies evaluating ALK inhibitors, it appears that patients who have tumors with the echinoderm microtubule-associated protein like 4 (EML4)–ALK fusion may also derive greater benefit from pemetrexed plus an ALK inhibitor than do patients who have tumors negative for the fusion.[21]

Adaptive Designs

In its 2010 draft guidance, the US Food and Drug Administration defines an adaptive design clinical study as a study with a prospectively planned opportunity for modification of one or more of the study design features based on analysis of (usually interim) data from participants in the study.[54] Examples of adaptations are modification of the randomization ratio between treatment arms, the study population, the treatment arms, and target treatment effect. A noteworthy example of an adaptive design study is the Biomarker-Integrated Approaches of Targeted Therapy for Lung Cancer Elimination phase II program, in which the randomization ratio is altered within biomarker-defined subgroups based on interim estimates of treatment efficacy within the treatment arm–subgroup combinations; the goal of the trial is to identify biomarker–drug combinations for further study.[55]

The usefulness of adaptive randomization is the subject of debate.[56] Parmar et al.[57] have described an approach to expedite drug development by allowing investigators to drop and add treatment arms to an ongoing study. It is important to note that a group sequential design, which is a design using interim monitoring with prespecified rules for early stopping due to either efficacy or futility, is not an adaptive design because the design features are not modified based on analysis of study data.

PHASE II/III AND PHASE III TRIALS

Traditional Designs

The primary objective of a phase III trial is to gather sufficient evidence of the benefits of a new treatment to potentially change clinical practice. Any design that achieves this objective is permissible, but phase III trials typically are large randomized controlled trials in which the new treatment is compared directly with the current standard treatment in a robust, unbiased manner. Generally, the comparison is made in terms of superiority of efficacy, with the result that progressively better treatments become the standard of care. However, designs that test for noninferiority are becoming more common and will be discussed in greater detail.

The choice of a primary outcome measure for comparing treatments in phase III oncology trials is related to the type of cancer, stage of disease, and type of intervention. In advanced lung cancer, survival time is generally considered to be the most clinically relevant measure of benefit to patients and hence it is the most commonly chosen primary outcome measure. Survival time is defined as the time from random assignment to a treatment arm to death. Patients who are still alive at the time of analysis are included in the comparison with a survival time that is censored at the date last known to be alive. Analysis of such data requires a specialized statistical methodology.[58]

Quality of life also has been recognized as being an important outcome, particularly to patients with advanced disease. Quality of life is often included as a secondary outcome measure and can be combined with survival data to compare treatments in terms of quality-adjusted survival time.[59,60] In some situations, such as trials of cytostatic drugs, progression-free survival time may be considered a relevant primary outcome. In early-stage lung cancer when the treatment is potentially curative, local or distant recurrence-free survival time may be either the primary outcome measure or an important secondary outcome. For time-to-event

outcomes, a hazard ratio is the most commonly used statistic. The hazard ratio compares the relative benefits of the new treatment with the standard treatment in terms of the overall risk of the chosen end point at any point in time; values less than 1 indicate benefit with the new treatment.

Phase III trial designs are traditionally based on hypothesis testing for a difference between treatments. Typically, this approach tests the null hypothesis that there is no difference between treatments (i.e., $\theta = 1$, where θ is the unknown true hazard ratio in the population) against the alternative hypothesis that there is difference (i.e., $\theta \neq 1$ for a two-sided test of a difference in either direction, or $\theta < 1$ for a one-sided test of the superiority of the new treatment). The size of the trial is based on maximizing the chances of drawing a correct conclusion from the trial data. Trials are designed to (a) have a small chance of incorrectly rejecting the null hypothesis (i.e., a false-positive conclusion, known statistically as a type I error) by setting the decision boundary known as the significance level to 5% and (b) have a good chance (usually 90%) of rejecting the null hypothesis (at a 5% significance level) when a prespecified minimum clinically relevant treatment effect truly exists, a feature known as power (the false-negative error, known statistically as a type II error).

Noninferiority Designs

Noninferiority trials are conducted when the underlying hypothesis is that the investigational treatment may not provide additional efficacy but may benefit patients or society in terms of quality of life and cost. For example, less toxicity should improve a patient's quality of life and reduce the cost of supportive care; easier administration should be more convenient to patients, thereby improving their quality of life and reducing health service costs for administration; and a less expensive treatment would benefit society by reducing health-care costs. Demonstrating noninferiority shows that the new treatment has an acceptable level of efficacy to be adopted into clinical practice as an alternative to the current standard therapy. Use of such trial designs to study antineoplastic agents has increased in recent years; 17 noninferiority studies in patients with lung cancer were identified in a 2012 review.[61] As drugs with better outcomes are produced, it will become more difficult to develop new drugs that are superior to existing drugs, so the objective of clinical trials is likely to change.

Key examples of noninferiority trials in lung cancer include the following: (a) a randomized phase III trial comparing pemetrexed with docetaxel for patients with advanced NSCLC previously treated with chemotherapy, which resulted in Food and Drug Administration approval for pemetrexed in this setting;[62] (b) IRESSA NSCLC Trial Evaluating Response and Survival against Taxotere (INTEREST), a study in the same setting, but investigating gefitinib rather than pemetrexed;[63] and (c) a randomized phase trial comparing cisplatin and pemetrexed with cisplatin and gemcitabine as first-line treatment for advanced NSCLC.[64]

Special guidelines have been developed to address the unique challenges of designing noninferiority trials, as well as analyzing and interpreting data, and reporting the results.[65] Because the crux of this type of trial is that the new treatment is noninferior to the standard treatment, defining what that means is a crucial aspect of the design and interpretation. The trial is meant to demonstrate beyond reasonable doubt that the new treatment is not worse than the currently accepted standard of care by a small, prespecified margin, called the noninferiority margin. There are various approaches to selecting this margin, such as the conventional method and the effect-retention method.[61] The conventional method, also known as the fixed-margin method, is a subjective approach. A level of inferiority is selected that is considered to be of no clinical relevance or outweighed by other benefits of the experimental treatment. With the effect-retention

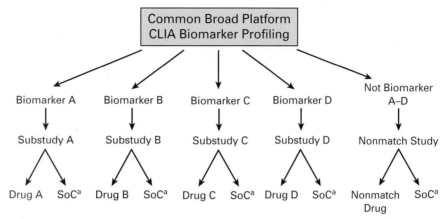

Fig. 59.4. Master Lung Protocol (Southwest Oncology Group S1400) study design schema. [a]Experimental drug or regimen could be single agent or a combination with the current standard of care (SoC). The standard of care can vary by biomarker. *CLIA*, Clinical Laboratory Improvements Amendment.

method, also known as the percent-retention or putative-placebo method, a noninferiority margin is selected that ensures a substantial fraction (typically 50%) of the benefit demonstrated for the standard treatment over placebo is still retained by the new treatment. In a review of lung cancer trials, hazard ratios for the noninferiority margin ranged from 1.18 to 1.37.[61] Ultimately, the value chosen has to be sufficiently small that the clinical community accepts the new treatment as the preferred option, given the other benefits demonstrated.

In terms of hypothesis testing, if a trial is set up to test the null hypothesis that there is no difference between treatments and the results are nonsignificant, then one can only conclude that the trial does not provide evidence of a difference between treatments. Although it is tempting to conclude that the treatments are equivalent, especially if the observed hazard ratio is close to 1, this conclusion is invalid. Therefore the hypotheses that are tested in a noninferiority trial are opposite to the hypotheses specified when testing for superiority. In a noninferiority trial, the null hypothesis is that the new treatment is inferior to the standard control treatment. The alternative research hypothesis is that the experimental treatment is not inferior to the standard control arm by the prespecified margin. The aim of a noninferiority trial is to collect data that provide sufficient evidence to reject the null hypothesis in favor of the research hypothesis; that is, if θ is the unknown true hazard ratio in the population, as specified previously, and k is the prespecified noninferiority margin, then the analysis will compare the null hypothesis that $\theta > k$ with the alternative hypothesis that $\theta < k$. These hypotheses are one-sided, which is the statistical approach usually taken; however, two-sided hypotheses can be specified in a similar way to test for equivalence rather than noninferiority. The significance level and power for the trial are selected to minimize the chance of erroneously concluding that an inferior treatment is noninferior.

The final methodologic consideration in noninferiority trials is the choice of the population included for analysis. In traditional comparative designs, the criterion standard is the intent-to-treat population, which includes all patients within their randomly assigned treatment allocation, despite what treatment they may have actually received. The intent-to-treat population is a conservative analysis strategy for assessing potential treatment benefit. Sole use of this approach in a noninferiority trial may dilute a clinically important difference between treatments, leading to an incorrect conclusion about noninferiority. Therefore the recommendation is to perform an additional analysis of the per-protocol population, which includes only the patients who have received a prespecified minimum level of treatment. Guidelines state that a robust interpretation of noninferiority can be achieved only if both analyses lead to similar conclusions and that any differences between the intent-to-treat and per-protocol analyses need careful and close examination.[66,67]

Phase II/III Designs

The phase II/III design, also known as the multiarm, multistage design, is essentially a phase III design with an early interim analysis that stops the trial for futility alone.[52,68] The primary outcome of the phase II interim analysis may be different than the phase III primary outcome. For example, a phase II/III trial may be designed to assess progression-free survival as the primary end point for the phase II component and overall survival as the primary end point for the phase III component. Patients enrolled in the phase II portion of the trial are included in the phase III trial, provided that the study does not stop for futility at the phase II analysis. The timing of the phase II interim analysis is based on phase II design properties. In contrast to standard interim monitoring plans, which are unlikely to stop early for futility under the alternative hypothesis, the phase II interim analysis typically has a 10% to 20% chance of stopping the trial for futility when the alternative hypothesis is true.

The Southwest Oncology Group (SWOG) is implementing this design in the Master Lung Protocol (SWOG S1400), which is evaluating second-line treatment of squamous cell NSCLC. In this study, multiple parallel but independent phase II/III trials will be conducted such that all clinically eligible patients are assigned to a substudy and randomly assigned to either an experimental regimen or the standard of care (Fig. 59.4). Patients are screened for a specific set of biomarkers and assigned to a biomarker-driven substudy using a targeted design if they have one of the biomarkers. If none of the target biomarkers is present, the patient is assigned to a nonmatch substudy, which is a version of an all-comers design. The design within each substudy is standardized (Fig. 59.5). The phase II interim analysis will occur once 55 progression-free survival events have occurred. If the study continues after the interim analysis, the final phase III analysis will occur after 256 deaths, that is, overall survival events in the study population. These cut points were based on a phase II design with 90% power and 10% one-sided type I error to detect a twofold increase in median progression-free survival, and a phase III design with 90% power and one-sided 2.5% type I error to detect a 50% increase in median overall survival.

Use of a phase II/III design expedites drug development by streamlining accrual and eliminating the time between phase II and phase III trials. The drawback is that continuation from phase II to phase III is based on one prespecified rule. Study sponsors

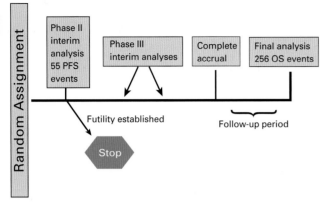

Fig. 59.5. Substudy design for the Master Lung Protocol (Southwest Oncology Group S1400). Progression-free survival (PFS) is the primary outcome for the phase II portion, and overall survival (OS) is the primary outcome for the phase III portion.

and investigators cannot review study data at phase II and then decide if they want to continue into phase III, as this would not be an independent assessment. Successful use of a phase II/III design is predicated on having adequate safety data from pilot studies, selecting the best outcome measure, and identifying potential biomarkers before the study is launched.

Biomarker-Based Trial Designs

Biomarkers can be classified as prognostic biomarkers, predictive biomarkers, or surrogate end points; some biomarkers belong in more than one category. Prognostic and predictive biomarkers provide information about individual risk classification and treatment selection, respectively, whereas biomarkers used as surrogate end points aid in evaluating the efficacy of a new treatment. It is crucial to realize that the intended usage of a biomarker determines its classification and the validation methods that are required. A prognostic biomarker predicts the natural course of the disease in a given individual, and it aids in deciding whether a patient needs an intensive, possibly toxic treatment, standard therapy, or no treatment.[69] A predictive biomarker predicts whether an individual will respond to a particular therapy, thereby facilitating individualized therapy. A surrogate end-point biomarker is used in place of a primary clinical outcome to evaluate the efficacy of a new treatment at the population level; this approach is often more cost-effective than studying a clinical outcome such as overall survival.[70]

Predictive biomarker validation is complex, and definitive validation requires the same level of evidence as the adoption of a new treatment does.[71] Thus predictive marker validation is prospective in nature, and the obvious strategy is to conduct an appropriately designed prospective randomized controlled trial. Evidence from a randomized controlled trial provides the only assurance that patient outcomes are comparable across treatment arms and are not confounded by other artifacts. However, a prospective phase III randomized controlled trial is not always possible because of ethical and logistical considerations, such as size or duration. In this case, a well-conducted, prospectively specified validation study using retrospectively collected data can provide valuable information in a timely manner to guide treatments in marker-defined patient subgroups.[72] For example, retrospective validation was used to establish that the presence of Kirsten rat sarcoma (KRAS) mutation predicted the efficacy of panitumumab and cetuximab in patients with advanced colon cancer.[73] Enrichment and all-comer designs have been used in oncology for prospective biomarker validation; variations of the all-comers design used for this purpose include hybrid designs, marker by treatment

interaction designs, sequential testing strategy designs, and adaptive analysis designs.[71,74–79]

Trial Designs for Rare Tumors

Tumors with an incidence of less than 2 per 100,000 are typically deemed rare. Lung cancer is certainly not a rare tumor but in the emerging world of stratified medicine, development of treatments will be increasingly based on small biomarker-defined subsets of patients, and the disease will be transformed into a collection of multiple rare tumors. Clinicians caring for patients with rare tumors have to make difficult treatment decisions on a daily basis, and patients with rare tumors have the same right to evidence-based decisions as patients with common tumors. The problem with the traditional approach to sample size calculations for a phase III trial in the context of rare cancers is that it demands an unfeasibly large number of patients, and a smaller trial would be underpowered and unlikely to generate the correct conclusion. Trials based on traditional designs may be possible if patients with rare tumors are recruited internationally. An example of this approach is the International Rare Cancers Initiative, which facilitates trials in a selection of rare cancers (www.irci.info).[80]

Less conventional methodologic approaches are acceptable if they improve the interpretability of trial results, and a variety of alternative approaches have been proposed.[80,81] One alternative view is to abandon the use of hypothesis testing to reach a definitive conclusion about a treatment effect and, instead, use the unbiased study data to reduce uncertainty about the size of the treatment effect. Given the premise that there is considerable uncertainty about a treatment effect, having data from a small but well-designed clinical trial reduces that uncertainty and provides information to help clinicians make necessary treatment decisions. This alternative statistical view lends itself to using a bayesian approach to analysis, but there are issues in its implementation that need to be considered.[82–85] One key issue in bayesian analysis relates to the incorporation of prior information. Strategies have been proposed to develop an evidence-based prior distribution, but in the context of rare disease, previous evidence is often of poor quality, making its use problematic.[86,87] However, the bayesian approach can still be implemented with noninformative priors. One of the great advantages of this method is that the trial results can be expressed as direct probabilities that the treatment effect is a certain size. Data reported this way can be used practically by clinicians in discussion with patients and enable evidence-based treatment decisions, whereas a nonsignificant result from hypothesis testing might simply be regarded as inconclusive or incorrectly interpreted as evidence of no treatment effect.

CONCLUSION

Clinical trial design has evolved rapidly in the last decade. The focus of oncology research has shifted from the traditional anatomic staging systems to selecting treatment based on the genetic makeup of the tumor and the patient's genotype, and predicting individual outcomes. For dose-finding trials, a preliminary assessment of efficacy along with safety has become a necessity to identify a so-called minimum effective dose to take forward into phase II trials. A better understanding of the tumor biology (e.g., identifying patient subsets and rare tumor subtypes), advancement in assay techniques, and availability of commercial kits with rapid turnaround times have enabled the use of enrichment designs in phase II and phase III trials, allowing only patients with a particular molecular profile to enroll in the trial. Tailored treatments with effective biomarker-driven hypotheses are leading to smaller clinical trials targeting larger treatment effects. Phase II/III designs using small patient subsets are becoming more popular, streamlining accrual and random assignment to maximize

59

enrollment. With integrated phase II/III designs, multiple experimental agents are assessed simultaneously against the standard of care in the phase II portion using an intermediate (or surrogate) end point. This approach eliminates the need to conduct separate, large-scale phase II trials to evaluate each experimental regimen. The promising experimental arms continue on to phase III testing, in which they are compared with the standard of care. Advances in technology such as mobile computing, electronic data capture, and integration of research records with electronic medical records have made real-time access to clinical trial and biomarker data a reality, allowing adaptive designs to take on a much greater role in clinical trials.

KEY REFERENCES

2. Elizabeth M, Hammond H, Taube SE. Issues and barriers to development of clinically useful tumor markers: a development pathway proposal. *Semin Oncol.* 2002;29(3):213–221.
3. McShane LM, Altman DG, Sauerbrei W, et al. *J Clin Oncol.* 2005;23(36):9067–9072.
10. Mandrekar SJ, Qi Y, Hillman SL, et al. Endpoints in phase II trials for advanced non-small cell lung cancer. *J Thorac Oncol.* 2010;5(1):3–9.
11. Lara PN Jr, Redman MW, Kelly K, et al. Disease control rate at 8 weeks predicts clinical benefit in advanced non-small-cell lung cancer: results from Southwest Oncology Group randomized trials. *J Clin Oncol.* 2008;26:463–467.
18. Gelmon KA, Eisenhauer EA, Harris AL, Ratain MJ, Workman P. Anticancer agents targeting signaling molecules and cancer cell environment: challenges for drug development. *J Natl Cancer Inst.* 1999;91(15):1281–1287.
23. Storer BE. Choosing a phase I design. In: Crowley J, Hoering A, eds. *Handbook of Statistics in Clinical Oncology.* Boca Raton, FL: Chapman & Hall/CRC; 2012:3–20.
41. Rogatko A, Schoeneck D, Jonas W, Tighiouart M, Khuri FR, Porter A. Translation of innovative designs into phase I trials. *J Clin Oncol.* 2007;25(31):4982–4986.
47. Bilusic M, Gulley JL. Endpoints, patient selection, and biomarkers in the design of clinical trials for cancer vaccines. *Cancer Immunol Immunother.* 2012;61(1):109–117.
50. Taylor JM, Braun TM, Li Z. Comparing an experimental agent to a standard agent: relative merits of a one-arm or randomized two-arm phase II design. *Clin Trials.* 2006;3(4):335–348.
52. Redman MW, Goldman BH, Leblanc M, Schott A, Baker LH. Modeling the relationship between progression-free survival and overall survival: the phase II/III trial. *Clin Cancer Res.* 2013;19(10):2646–2656.
53. Mandrekar SJ, An MW, Sargent DJ. A review of phase II trial designs for initial marker validation. *Contemp Clin Trials.* 2013; 36(2):597–604.
71. Mandrekar SJ, Sargent DJ. Clinical trial designs for predictive biomarker validation: theoretical considerations and practical challenges. *J Clin Oncol.* 2009;27(24):4027–4034.
75. Zhou X, Liu S, Kim ES. Bayesian adaptive design for targeted therapy development in lung cancer—a step towards personalized medicine. *Clin Trials.* 2008;5:181–193.
82. Gupta S, Faughnan ME, Tomlinson GA, Bayoumi AM. A framework for applying unfamiliar trial designs in studies of rare diseases. *J Clin Epidemiol.* 2011;64:1085–1094.
86. Billingham L, Malottki K, Steven N. Small sample sizes in clinical trials: a statistician's perspective. *Clin Invest.* 2012;2(7):655–657.

See Expertconsult.com for full list of references.

60

How to Promote and Organize Clinical Research in Lung Cancer

Fabrice Barlesi, Julien Mazieres, Yang Zhou, Roy Herbst, and Gérard Zalcman

SUMMARY OF KEY POINTS

- Despite two decades of progress, the prognosis for patients with lung cancer remains poor. Therefore forming new hypotheses and conducting clinical trials to investigate this patient population are still important.

- Accordingly, in the past 25 years, the number of clinical trials involving patients with lung cancer has increased dramatically (Fig. 60.1); however, only a minority of these trials have been conducted on an academic basis. In addition, only a few of these trials have led to a real change in practice. For example, fewer than 10 new drugs were approved for the management of cancer during 2013, with only one drug having a new indication and two drugs having an expanded indication for patients with lung cancer.[1]

- While international societies, including the International Association for the Study of Lung Cancer,[2] have encouraged patient participation in clinical trials, the number of patients actually included in such trials worldwide is very low. The actual proportion of patients with cancer who participate in oncology clinical trials is difficult to determine, usually ranging from 2% to 7% in Western countries.[1] However, if we compare the 7.5 million people who die of lung cancer worldwide per year with the reported accrual in clinical trials, the actual proportion of patients with lung cancer who are included in clinical trials worldwide is probably closer to 0.1% to 1%.

- Therefore the improvement and promotion of clinical research related to lung cancer are of crucial importance. This chapter provides some proposals that are intended to enable researchers to better organize and promote clinical trials that are designed to advance research and science toward reducing the burden of thoracic malignancies worldwide.

HOW TO ORGANIZE CLINICAL TRIALS IN LUNG CANCER

Issues

Definition of Lung Cancer Today

Does lung cancer still exist as an entity? The answer is that it probably does not, considering the progress that had been made in developing a better clinical, pathologic, and biologic definition of this disease. Consequently, including all of these patients in a single trial is irrelevant. However, most clinical studies focus on obtaining a reliable estimate of the average treatment effect in a broad population of patients. In practice, clinical trials in oncology involve a delicate balance between the need for reliable evidence for a large population and the need to integrate biomarkers and thus to focus on the population carrying these biomarkers against which the targeted therapies are supposed to be efficient. For example, many drug developments have been stopped because

of the absence of focus on predefined biomarkers. The first clinical trials analyzing the effect of epidermal growth factor receptor (EGFR)-tyrosine kinase inhibitors such as gefitinib independently of EGFR status or cetuximab with an inappropriate biomarker threshold led to disappointing results, despite the high number of patients enrolled.[3,4] Conversely, the selection of patients on the basis of the accurate biomarker (EGFR-activating mutation, anaplastic lymphoma kinase [ALK] translocation) recently led to impressive results with fewer patients.[5-7] Therefore lung cancer is now considered to comprise a mosaic of rare diseases, and clinical trials should be designed adequately.

Expectations for Quick Progress and Impact on Financial Issues

Patients are obviously waiting for rapid improvement in the treatment of the disease, and the delay between the discovery of a new biologic target, preclinical proof of principle, and the approval of a new drug (or a new strategy) is generally viewed as unacceptably long. From this perspective, at least, the expectations of drug companies are consistent with those of patients. Is this situation changing? Perhaps, indeed, the delays between the results of the first phase I study and the European Medicines Agency (EMA) and/or the US Food and Drug Administration (US FDA) approval of new biomarker-guided drugs appear shorter when compared with those for previous standard chemotherapy (Fig. 60.2). In addition, the results presented during the 2013 American Society of Clinical Oncology (ASCO) meeting by Canadian colleagues suggest that biomarker-guided treatments clearly have the greatest chance of demonstrating an activity after starting clinical development than do standard, nonbiomarker-guided, treatments.[8] Indeed, after the assessment of more than 2400 trials, the authors found that the likelihood of a new drug passing all phases of clinical testing and being approved (i.e., the cumulative clinical trial success rate) was 11%, which was less than the expected industry aggregate rate (16.5%). The success of phase III trials was found to be the biggest obstacle for drug approval, with a success rate of only 28%. Biomarker-guided targeted therapies (with a success rate of 62%) and receptor-targeted therapies (with a success rate of 31%) were found to have the highest likelihood of success in clinical trials.[8] Accordingly, Subramanian et al.[2] conducted a survey to review ongoing clinical trials involving patients with nonsmall cell lung cancer (NSCLC) as listed in the ClinicalTrials.gov registry in 2012 and found that the number of clinical trials with biomarker-based treatment selection for lung cancer had significantly increased since 2009 (from 7.9% to 25.8%; $p < 0.001$).

The costs of a clinical trial depend on many factors. An audit of industry-sponsored clinical trials in oncology recently indicated that the average cost is $165 million for basic research and discovery, $87 million for preclinical development, $130 million for a phase I trial, $190 million for a phase II trial, and $268 million for a phase III trial. It seems that the use of a validated biomarker, such as human EGFR-2 for breast cancer, reduces clinical trial risk by as much as 50%, resulting in cost savings of 27% in advanced and metastatic breast cancer.[9] This percentage

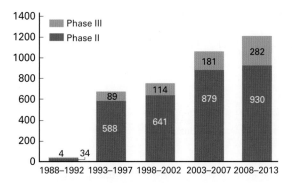

Fig. 60.1. Number of published phase II and phase III clinical trials involving lung cancer from 1988–2013.

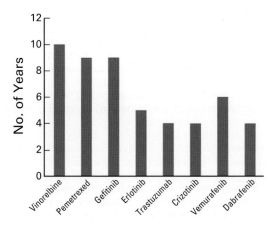

Fig. 60.2. Time (in years) between the publication of the first phase I trial and the first phase III trial for some chemotherapies and biomarker-guided treatments available for melanoma, breast cancer, and lung cancer.

is comparable with the results of a large study in which the use of biomarkers decreased the cost of drug development by 26%.[8] It is difficult to have a worldwide picture of the funding of clinical trials in oncology. However, one recent example in the United States showed how academic-sponsored clinical trials in oncology are fragile. At the time of the federal budget cuts in 2013, a survey showed that a large proportion of US oncologists consequently reduced the end points of trials (36.9%), closed or participated in fewer cooperative group trials (28.3%), postponed the launch of clinical trials (26.7%), and limited enrollment in clinical trials (23.1%).[1] Therefore adapting the design of oncology clinical trials and durably ensuring their funding are important.

Selection of Hypotheses for Clinical Trials and Impact of Biomarkers on Design

Instead of testing therapeutic strategies or new chemotherapeutic drugs, clinical researchers now face a huge amount of basic-science data and preclinical concepts. The challenge is to build the most appropriate trials to validate some of these hypotheses. A dispensable time in the building of a clinical trial is to deeply analyze the preclinical data and to anticipate all issues that may impair the development of the drugs (efficacy, toxicity, pharmacokinetics, etc.).

Advances in biotechnology and genomics gradually have uncovered the biology of lung cancer. Deeper understanding of the biology of the disease can facilitate the development of new treatments, whereas deeper understanding of the heterogeneity of the disease can facilitate the development of effective

biomarkers or diagnostic tests that can be used to select appropriate treatments for individual patients. In particular, the recent establishment of high-throughput molecular assay technologies, such as high-throughput sequencing, single-nucleotide polymorphism arrays, gene-expression microarrays, and protein arrays, has allowed for the discovery of potential new biomarkers and the development of composite genomic signatures for personalized medicine.

Consequently, different trial designs have been proposed on the basis of the incidence of a given biomarker. For example, early phase trials initially tested the efficacy of a drug in a population harboring a rare molecular abnormality such as v-raf murine sarcoma viral oncogene homolog B (BRAF) mutation or ALK translocation.[6,10] Then, randomized trials were conducted in populations with a more frequent or better characterized molecular alteration. Nevertheless, those studies can be criticized, as the prognostic value of the biomarker by itself (independent of its predictive value) is often underestimated. Therefore we again need new designs of clinical trials in oncology.

National, Multinational, and International Cooperation or Competition

Thousands of studies are carried out every year around the world, involving thousands of patients and billions of dollars of investment. In addition, conducting clinical trials, especially when the patient population is small, as is the case for the current development of the vast majority of biomarker-guided inhibitors, is necessarily competitive. First, at the time of targeted clinical trials in oncology, only centers with high-level facilities can still test and enroll patients, and, when two or more studies are in competition, substantial time and resources that otherwise could have been applied to other valuable projects inevitably will be wasted. Second, the winner is not necessarily the best treatment, as the trials are conducted sequentially. Third, there is also a competition between industrial and academic trials in that they often involve the same patients but have different trial designs. Fourth, there is competition between countries as each country has its own way of funding trials. Thus it is sometimes harder to conduct international trials because of the complexity of administrative procedures. Therefore collaborations, networks, and simplified rules are needed.

Possible Solutions
New Designs for Modern Clinical Trials

Freidlin et al.[11] recently proposed three designs for biomarker-based clinical trials (Fig. 60.3). If there are two or more existing treatment options with no definitive evidence for one being preferred, the most efficient trial design for evaluating biomarker utility is the biomarker-stratified design. Biomarker status is assigned, and two groups are established: one group is biomarker positive, and the other is biomarker negative. In each group, randomization is performed for treatment assignment. The analysis plan will be centered on determining treatment effect dependence according to the biomarker status. The biomarker-stratified design maximizes the advantage of randomization by providing unbiased estimates of benefit-to-risk ratios across different biomarker-defined subgroups and for the entire randomly assigned population. For predictive biomarkers, the biomarker-stratified design can assess whether the marker is useful for selecting the best among two or more treatments for a given patient.

In some situations, sufficiently convincing evidence based on preclinical or clinical data is available and suggests that the potential treatment benefit is limited to a certain biomarker-defined patient subgroup. In these situations, the clinical utility of the biomarker can be partially assessed in a trial with an enrichment

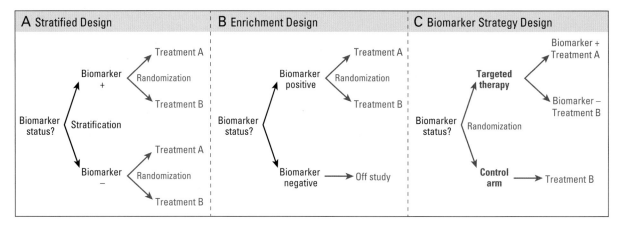

Fig. 60.3. Examples of designs for biomarker-based oncology clinical trials.

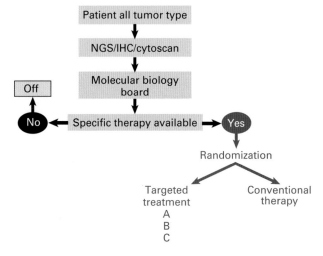

Fig. 60.4. Example of design for biomarker-based oncology clinical trials based on multigene-screening techniques. *IHC,* immunohistochemistry; *NGS,* next-generation sequencing.

design: the biomarker is evaluated in all patients, but random assignment is restricted to patients who have biomarker-positive tumors.

In the third type of trial, with a biomarker-strategy design, patients are randomly assigned to an experimental treatment arm in which the biomarker is used to determine therapy or to a control arm in which a biomarker is not used.

Because of the multiplicity of biomarkers and limited resources, some recent trials have been designed to analyze several targets and subsequently to test several dedicated drugs (Fig. 60.4). The main objectives of this type of trial are to determine the feasibility of such a wide molecular screening, the superiority of tailored treatment, and, in some cases, the effect of new drugs on selected targets. The first example of such a design is the Biomarker-integrated Approaches of Targeted Therapy for Lung Cancer Elimination (BATTLE) trial. Following an initial equal randomization period, patients with NSCLC that was refractory to chemotherapy were adaptively randomly assigned to treatment with erlotinib, vandetanib, erlotinib plus bexarotene, or sorafenib on the basis of relevant molecular biomarkers.[12] Following this trial, BATTLE-2 randomly assigned patients to erlotinib, erlotinib plus MK-2206, MK-2206 plus AZD6244, or sorafenib, stratified by Kirsten rat sarcoma (KRAS) status.[13] Other trials of the same type are currently being conducted in France and other countries. In the Molecular Screening for Cancer Treatment Optimization trial (initiated at Institut Gustave

Roussy in France), the molecular profile of patients with refractory cancer is determined using comparative genomic hybridization array and a panel of hot-spot mutations in 96 amplicons from a biopsy sample taken from a metastatic site.[14] Patients are enrolled into specific phase I trials according to the presence of a molecular abnormality. Each patient who is enrolled in the trial with a matched molecular-targeted agent is used as his or her own control for the evaluation of the efficacy of this approach. As another example, the SHIVA trial was a randomized proof-of-concept phase II trial in which therapy based on tumor molecular profiling was compared with conventional therapy in patients with refractory cancer. One hundred and ninety-five patients were randomly assigned to each arm, with a crossover at disease progression whenever possible. In the experimental arm, patients were treated with an approved molecularly targeted agent based on an actionable molecular abnormality. However, an actionable molecular abnormality might not be identified in every patient. In contrast to traditional randomized trials in oncology that are performed in a homogeneous population of patients with a specific type of tumor and in a specific setting, the goal of this trial was to look for heterogeneity in tumor types to establish the proof of concept of whether targeted agents should be developed according to their tumor molecular profile rather than according to tumor type.[15,16]

Similarly, the design just described now has been adapted to lung cancer with the SAFIR02 lung trial (Fig. 60.5). This open-label phase II randomized trial involves the use of high-throughput genome analysis as a therapeutic decision tool for patients with stage IV NSCLC that has not progressed after induction chemotherapy. The trial will compare a maintenance treatment administered according to the identified molecular anomaly of the lung tumor with a maintenance treatment administered without consideration of the tumor genome analysis; pemetrexed will be given to patients with nonsquamous cell carcinoma, and erlotinib will be given to patients with squamous cell carcinoma.

The Lung Master Protocol (Lung-MAP) trial is another study that was designed to test several targeted therapies for patients with advanced squamous cell lung cancer. The trial is a biomarker-driven phase II/III with multiple substudies that open and close independently. A common platform of next-generation DNA sequencing is used to identify a patient's actionable molecular abnormalities, and the patient is assigned to the investigational drug that targets the mutation or to a "nonmatch" substudy that consists of an immunotherapy or combination therapy.[17]

Lastly, another way to test several hypotheses in a clinical trial is to test a targeted drug in patients with several cancer types harboring the target. For example, the VE-BASKET trial tests the efficacy of vemurafenib (which is known to be efficient for the treatment of melanoma that harbors the BRAF V600E mutation)

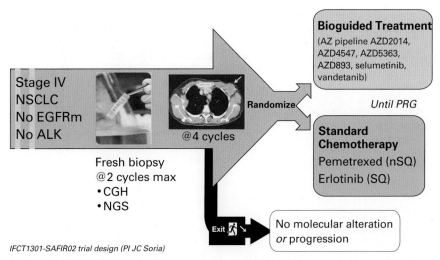

IFCT1301-SAFIR02 trial design (PI JC Soria)

Fig. 60.5. General design of the SAFIR02 lung randomized clinical trial. *ALK,* anaplastic lymphoma kinase gene; *CGH,* comparative genomic hybridization; *EGFRm,* epidermal growth factor receptor mutation; *NGS,* next-generation sequencing; *NSCLC,* nonsmall cell lung cancer; *nSQ,* nonsquamous cell carcinoma; *PRG,* progression; *SQ,* squamous cell carcinoma.

for the treatment of other solid tumors. This trial enrolls patients with histologically confirmed cancers or myelomas (excluding melanoma and papillary thyroid cancer) that harbor a BRAF V600 mutation and are refractory to standard therapy or for which standard or curative therapy does not exist.

New Designs: Mixing Avatar Models and Clinical Trials

Targeted therapies have demonstrated efficacy against specific subsets of molecularly defined cancers. Although most patients with lung cancer are stratified according to a single oncogenic driver, cancers harboring identical activating genetic mutations show large variations in their responses to the same targeted therapy.[6,18,19] The biology underlying this heterogeneity is not well understood, and the impact of coexisting genetic mutations, especially the loss of tumor suppressors, has not been fully explored. Chen et al.[20] used genetically engineered mouse models to conduct a so-called co-clinical trial that mirrors an ongoing human clinical trial in patients with KRAS-mutant lung cancers. The aim of this trial is to determine if the mitogen-activated protein kinase kinase (MEK) inhibitor selumetinib (AZD6244) increases the efficacy of docetaxel, a standard-of-care chemotherapy. The authors demonstrated that concomitant loss of either p53 (also known as TP53) or Lkb1 (also known as Stk11), two clinically relevant tumor suppressors, markedly impaired the response of KRAS-mutant cancers to docetaxel monotherapy. They observed that the addition of selumetinib provided substantial benefit for mice with lung cancer caused by KRAS and p53 mutations, but mice with KRAS and Lkb1 mutations had primary resistance to this combination therapy. These co-clinical results identified predictive genetic biomarkers that should be validated by interrogating samples from patients enrolled in the concurrent clinical trial. These studies also highlight the rationale for synchronous co-clinical trials, which is not only to anticipate the results of ongoing human clinical trials but also to generate clinically relevant hypotheses that can inform the analysis and design of human studies.

Cooperation and Networks

The issues described can be partially solved by organizing clinical research in a national and/or transnational way. Our ability to strengthen international collaborations will result in maximization of resources and the access of patients to clinical trials in oncology.

On the one hand, drug companies and clinical research organizations, which are mainly international companies, usually know how to use the various resources that are nationally or internationally available. Pending budget availability, these entities built the so-called ideal clinical and translational network needed to conduct a defined trial. The influence of clinicians, cooperative groups, and even national health authorities (except for the EMEA and FDA) on the study design is often limited.

On the other hand, academic clinical trials in oncology initially were mainly organized by local or regional centers. This organization responds first to the wishes of patients who want to be treated closer to home and second to the opportunity to easily have access to a clinical trial, as the distance from a physician's practice to the nearest clinical trial site is inversely associated with referral and recruitment.[21,22] Cooperation between centers is essential for the successful conception, funding, and performance of clinical trials in oncology. Consequently, national groups have been created to promote clinical and translational research. For example, in the United States, the National Cancer Institute (NCI) Clinical Trials Cooperative Group Program has served as the leading network for federally funded clinical research on cancer. In Asia and Europe, many countries have organized themselves according to the same model, with one or more cooperative groups involved in clinical trials focusing on lung cancer. In Europe, the European Organisation for Research and Treatment of Cancer Lung Cancer Study Group and the European Thoracic Oncology Platform are performing multinational clinical trials.

Regulatory, logistic, and financial hurdles, however, often hamper the conduct of joined trials. Working together should help researchers to overcome these barriers, with the International Association for the Study of Lung Cancer (IASLC) as a central link.

Worldwide Standardization of Oncology Clinical Trials Allowing Cross-Trial Comparisons

Besides rules regarding publication,[3,4] the issue of cross-trial comparison raises the problem of worldwide standardization of oncology clinical trials, and, more widely, clinical research in oncology. The best example in this field is the increasing number of biomarker-based prognostic and predictive studies aiming to define which subset of patients may actually benefit best from a specific drug or therapeutic strategy (Fig. 60.6). One of the major issues encountered in these studies is the reproducibility

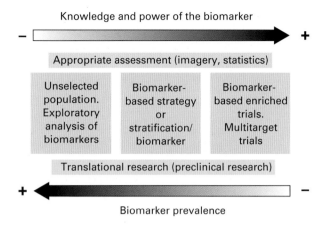

Fig. 60.6. Illustration of the different strategies to include biomarkers in the design of oncology clinical trials.

of published results, that is, the stability of the biomarkers across different series of patients, across different geographic areas, and over time. Once the question of variability of molecular assays is fixed across different laboratories, an issue that is not trivial, limiting the confusion bias is a major step of the analysis. Multivariate analyses aim to control for stratification factors of the trial and for the confounding clinical or pathologic characteristics influencing survival in the univariate analysis at a given p value (<0.1 or <0.2, depending on the study). However, the strategy of such multivariate analyses is rarely comparable within multiple trials or series, often making such comparisons hazardous.

The next step is to check that the results obtained in one specific series of patients simply could not have been obtained by chance, taking into account possible variations across different series of patients, from various geographic origins, smokers or nonsmokers, chemo-naive or not, with varying sex ratios, performance status, or ages. The first step is actually to limit the risk of false-positive results by limiting the multiplicity of analyses performed within a single series of patients. The only way is to check, before any publication, that the power calculation was prespecified, with a fixed number of analyses planned, at the initiation of the study when the trial was registered in the ClinicalTrials.gov database. Otherwise, any retrospective study with unplanned analyses, no prespecified power calculation, or no prespecified multivariate analysis strategy should be considered as only hypothesis-generating and needing external and/or prospective validation. Accordingly, multiple sequential publications over the time of prognostic studies, within the same series of patients or the same clinical trial, should be discouraged if not preplanned in the initial statistical design, or, alternatively, should be externally validated in an independent new series of patients. The use of statistically recognized techniques such as Bonferroni, Holm, or Hochberg correction,[23] which are widely used for complementary DNA microarray analyses, also should be encouraged in oncology clinical trials with biomarker-driven multiple subgroup analyses. Such methods take into account not only the multiplicity of variables but also the number of sequential analyses performed during the period of follow-up and required in subset analyses.

The reproducibility of a molecular assay analysis needs to be addressed in independent series of patients studied by distinct research groups; however, these series, to the extent possible, should be comparable with the initial series in terms of all identified clinical and pathologic variables. This external validation mainly has been used in microarray studies of NSCLC specimens, as a complete lack of concordance across studies has been reported in the numerous gene signatures published to date and claimed to be of prognostic value.[24,25] In such replication studies,

hazard ratios for death or progression based on biomarker(s) are usually inferior to those of the initial study,[26] reflecting the variability of biomarker prognostic impact, driven by the patient characteristics in each series.

Lastly, a highly significant hazard ratio for death does not mean that a prognostic signature or biomarker will be of clinical utility, as it does not imply that the accuracy of the predictive biomarker is sufficient to justify its use in clinical practice. For instance, a molecular signature with a positive predictive value of 0.80, meaning that about one-fifth of the patients with poor prognosis signature will not die, does not accurately help to predict which patients will or will not die, and therefore modify therapeutic strategy. Such clinical utility could be approached with the highest level of evidence by prospective trials with an interaction design, in which all patients are stratified according to biomarker level and then are randomly assigned to one of two treatments.[27] Standardization of biomarker studies has been theorized with international guidelines already published by the Reporting Recommendations for Tumor Marker Prognostic Studies (REMARK) group, providing an opportunity for worldwide standardization.[28]

Regulatory Issues

The primary goal of all of our research is to provide patients with new and more efficient strategies as soon as possible. Strategies that are based on drugs require approval from national or multinational agencies, such as the FDA and EMEA and their equivalents worldwide. The agencies ensure that drugs work correctly and that their health benefits outweigh their known risks. In recent studies investigating the use of biomarker-guided therapies for stage IV NSCLC, the number of patients needed to demonstrate the benefits has been relatively low (100 patients to 200 patients).[6,7] However, what is the ideal number for assessing the risks? If frequent adverse events are usually identified in phase I/Ib trials, the assessment of rare (<1%) adverse events requires more patients, leading to more time for accrual, a longer interval before results are available, and a need for more funding. What is the best way to assess the most efficient balance between benefit (rapid access of patients to a new strategy) and risk (rare but potentially severe side effects)? In the United States, ASCO has worked with partners, including the FDA and NCI, and, at its 2013 annual meeting, provided an update on its initiatives to articulate the desired end points of clinical trials that will produce results that are clinically meaningful to patients.[1] ASCO also proposed recommendations to avoid unnecessary exclusion of patients from trials, worked with the FDA to streamline data collection, and advanced the development and use of end points that will allow clinical trials to demonstrate earlier safety and efficacy.[1] In Europe and Asia, the same work probably should be done by the national agencies and the EMEA.

Financial Issues

In the United States, as a result of budget cuts affecting the National Institutes of Health (NIH), approximately 750 fewer new patients were expected to be enrolled in all clinical trials at the NIH Clinical Center hospital (Bethesda, MD, USA) in 2013,[1] illustrating how the funding of clinical trials in oncology is crucial and should be ensured. In fact, many national or international sources of funding (NCI, Translational Cancer Research, FP7, etc.) are potentially available. However, the multiplicity of the sources, the specific restrictions or exigencies related to each call for proposals, and the administrative constraints when several countries or continents are involved can make the system inefficient. Sharing experiences and training clinicians (or even cooperative group leaders) should allow researchers to overcome these difficulties, with the IASLC serving as a possible network worldwide.

TABLE 60.1 Challenges and Solutions Related to Organization of Clinical Trials in Lung Cancer

	Challenges	Possible Solutions
Lung cancer	A mosaic of molecularly defined rare diseases	New designs eventually integrating avatar models to
Quick progress	Decrease the time between biologic discoveries and available drugs	test several hypotheses simultaneously
Hypotheses	Increasing number of hypotheses to be tested on the base of the molecular alterations	
Clinical trial costs	Increasing costs	Standardization of designs and analyses of oncology
Cooperation	National and international competitions with sometimes wasted resources	clinical trials and simplification of regulatory issues

In summary, a better organization of clinical trials in thoracic oncology will help to solve numerous issues (Table 60.1).

HOW TO PROMOTE CLINICAL TRIALS

Issues

Goal and Philosophy of Different Systems

Cancer care is variably organized worldwide. In some countries, almost all patients with cancer are treated in public hospitals, whereas in others, they are treated in a private system. In addition, the costs of care are covered by national health insurance, private insurance, or both, and the payment of health-care professionals and medical structures vary widely according to these different systems. Will financial issues influence participation of patients in clinical trials? In a cohort of patients with newly diagnosed lung and colorectal cancer in the United States, the type of health insurance and whether a physician practiced at an NCI-designated cancer center or received increased income from trial enrollment were factors that were independently associated with trial enrollment.[29]

Moreover, medical structures in which financial resources are linked to the number of patients treated and the number of treatments administered may lead to reluctance to send patients to another center to participate in a clinical trial. Where applicable, a solution should be proposed to compensate these medical structures (academic network, financial compensation, etc.).

Therefore we must rethink how our systems are valorizing clinician involvement and patient participation in clinical trials to give patients the same chance to be enrolled in a clinical trial.

Increasing Difficulty of Conducting Clinical Trials

Basic regulatory requirements for conducting clinical trials are based on the Declaration of Helsinki and Good Clinical Practices. However, a major issue in achieving high-quality clinical research in thoracic oncology is to increase the level of professionalization of all health-care professionals and cancer centers.

In the end, one important remaining point is how to select centers for clinical trials.[30] Although the selection is partially based on the expected quality of the team, it is mostly based on the ability of the team to quickly include many consecutive patients, a goal that may be at odds with quality and the respect for inclusion criteria or research basic rules, especially in terms of the collection of adverse events. For example, an analysis of more than 300 randomized controlled trials indicated that the methodology for the collection of adverse events was adequately reported in only 10% of the studies.[31] In addition, clinical research organizations and sponsors also consider the aura of the principal investigator and his or her regional or national influence to meet clinical research excellence, but with no absolute guarantee.

Time and Effort

Both time and effort are required to organize centers and to enroll and treat patients in clinical trials. The income provided by industry-sponsored trials may be the compensation for these efforts, but that is not always the case for academic-sponsored trials. Nonetheless, public encouragement and efforts for funding and structuring professional clinical research also should include financial compensation for the medical time. Similarly, universities should promote such time-consuming activity; for instance, the number of annual inclusions in clinical trials could be monitored and credited to the departments and investigators responsible for such activity, either by directly refunding their structures or research staff or by taking into account such activity for continuing medical education credit or university/hospital career advancement. However, strict and clear rules with transparency should be applied to ensure that public hospital means are not used for private interest without any control but rather are used to provide broader access to innovative drugs for the largest population.

Patient Education

Several studies have evaluated the factors related to patient participation in clinical trials. While older age is associated with a lower rate of participation in clinical trials in oncology,[32] this association seems to be mostly related to the eligibility for trials. However, among eligible patients, the rate of participation among older patients is similar to that among younger patients.[33] Moreover, the impact of ethnic or racial minority status and socioeconomic characteristics on enrollment in clinical trials is debated. If the rate of participation in clinical trials in oncology is indeed lower among ethnic/racial minority populations,[32] this relationship is not significant when adjusted for socioeconomic characteristics.[34] Conversely, a low income level negatively influences the rate of participation in clinical trials in oncology.[35]

Lastly, many patients, especially in populations with a low socioeconomic status, may misunderstand trial information,[36] mainly because of less discussion of the purpose and risks associated with the trials.[37] In the same way, family members are also important, as family members in some ethnic/racial populations frequently argue against trial participation.[36]

Possible Solutions

Train Physicians Early and Continuously

The values, beliefs, and awareness of clinical trials among oncologists play an important role in the accrual of patients for clinical trials.[38] Therefore the initial training of medical students, as well as the continuous training of physicians, is important. The type of training probably should be adapted to the various specialties, as, for example, it has been suggested that medical oncologists are more likely than surgical or radiation oncologists to discuss the possibility, benefits, and risks of clinical trial enrollment with their patients.[22]

Therefore specific academic training should be offered to all clinicians (e.g., with use of e-learning) under the supervision of health agencies, universities, or collaborative groups. Several tools are already available, usually at a national level, but also

TABLE 60.2 Challenges and Solutions Related to Promotion of Clinical Trials in Lung Cancer

	Challenges	Possible Solutions
Public versus private systems	Reluctance to propose clinical trials or to send patients to dedicated centers	Better valorization of direct or indirect participation in clinical trials for clinicians
Time consumption	Proposal of and participation in clinical trials are time-consuming	Better financial and nonfinancial (career, etc.) valorization
Difficulties in conducting clinical trials	Increasing level of exigency from sponsors	Professionalization of cancer centers for clinical research. Train physicians and health-care professionals
Population and patient views of clinical trials	Low participation in clinical trials (fear, low comprehension of risks, underestimation of benefits)	Education and development of multimedia resources for trial information

through the Web. Interestingly, several drug companies joined efforts to develop a common tool including a Good Clinical Practices training of investigators. Therefore the same certificate will be valid for several trials across different drug companies.

Educate the General Population and Patients With Lung Cancer About Clinical Trials

Mancini et al.[39] reported that 43.0% of patients with breast cancer expressed mild regret and 25.8% expressed moderate to strong regret after participating in a clinical trial. A quarter of these women (25.6%) said that the doctor made the decision alone, and 13.5% said that the decision was not consistent with their own wishes. An involuntarily passive role in decision making was found to be associated with greater regret.[39] Therefore educating and informing patients are of primary importance to increase their active participation in clinical trials in oncology. Indeed, when patients feel greater self-efficacy and have more knowledge, they feel more prepared to make the decision to participate in a clinical trial. A reduced decisional conflict is also associated with the decision to enroll in a clinical trial.[40]

On a patient level, multimedia resources (audiovisual, Web, etc.) may enhance the delivery and acceptance of information regarding clinical trials.[41–44] These resources are an important source of information that also help to educate families and to enhance the communication between patients and their healthcare providers.[45]

On a larger level, business-model approaches and marketing techniques might be used.[46] Many national public or nonprofit organizations as well as drug companies have developed information tools. For example, the Center for Information and Study on Clinical Research Participation is a nonprofit organization dedicated to educating and informing the public, patients, medical and research communities, the media, and policymakers about clinical research and the role that each party plays in the process (www.ciscrp.org/patient).

Simplify Regulation

The various national cancer institutes and their equivalents worldwide, such as the NCI in the United States or the NCI in France (INCa), have used several strategies, which are used directly or indirectly, to harmonize the available resources and the opportunities offered to patients with cancer regarding clinical trials. These resources include molecular testing and labeled units for trials, to support and funding of research programs.[47–49]

Concomitantly, support should be offered to patients to travel to the specific centers where clinical trials are available. Such support is already provided in many industry-sponsored trials, but it should also be organized for academic-sponsored clinical trials.

In summary, better promotion of clinical trials will resolve many issues (Table 60.2).

CONCLUSION

Although participation in clinical trials provides patients with new therapeutic opportunities and helps physicians to implement new techniques, the number of patients with lung cancer who participate in clinical trials remains too low. The barriers are multiple, with some problems to be solved globally through a worldwide approach and others to be solved locally with the IASLC as a possible network to provide help.

KEY REFERENCES

4. Pirker R, Pereira JR, Szczesna A, et al. Cetuximab plus chemotherapy in patients with advanced non-small-cell lung cancer (FLEX): an open-label randomised phase III trial. *Lancet.* 2009;373(9674):1525–1531.
5. Rosell R, Carcereny E, Gervais R, et al. Erlotinib versus standard chemotherapy as first-line treatment for European patients with advanced EGFR mutation-positive non-small cell lung cancer (EURTAC): a multicentre, open-label, randomized phase 3 study. *Lancet Oncol.* 2012;13(3):239–246.
6. Maemondo M, Inoue A, Kobayashi K, et al. Gefitinib or chemotherapy for non-small-cell lung cancer with mutated EGFR. *N Engl J Med.* 2010;362(25):2380–2388.
7. Kwak EL, Bang YJ, Camidge DR, et al. Anaplastic lymphoma kinase inhibition in non-small-cell lung cancer. *N Engl J Med.* 2010;363(18):1693–1703.
11. Freidlin B, Sun Z, Gray R, Korn EL. Phase III clinical trials that integrate treatment and biomarker evaluation. *J Clin Oncol.* 2013;31(25):3158–3161.
13. Papadimitrakopoulou V, Lee JJ, Wistuba II, et al. The BATTLE-2 Study: a biomarker-integrated targeted therapy study in previously treated patients with advanced non-small-cell lung cancer. *J Clin Oncol.* 2016 Aug 1;pii: JCO660084. [Epub ahead of print] PubMed PMID: 27480147.
16. Le Tourneau C, Delord J, Goncalves A, et al. Molecularly targeted therapy based on tumor molecular profiling versus conventional therapy for advanced cancer (SHIVA): a multicentre, open-label, proof-of-concept, randomized, controlled phase 2 trial. *Lancet Oncol.* 2015;16(13):1324–1334.
17. Herbst RS, Gandara DR, Hirsch FR, et al. Lung Master Protocol (Lung-MAP): a biomarker-driven protocol for accelerating development of therapies for squamous cell lung cancer: SWOG 1400. *Clin Cancer Res.* 2015;21(7):1514–1524.
20. Chen Z, Cheng K, Walton Z, et al. A murine lung cancer co-clinical trial identifies genetic modifiers of therapeutic response. *Nature.* 2012;483(7391):613–617.
31. Péron J, Maillet D, Gan HK, Chen EX, You B. Adherence to CONSORT adverse event reporting guidelines in randomized clinical trials evaluating systemic cancer therapy: a systematic review. *J Clin Oncol.* 2013;31(31):3957–3963.
39. Mancini J, Genre D, Dalenc F, et al. Patients' regrets after participating in a randomized controlled trial depended on their involvement in the decision making. *J Clin Epidemiol.* 2012;65(6):635–642.
43. Dear RF, Barratt AL, Askie LM, et al. Impact of a cancer clinical trials web site on discussions about trial participation: a cluster randomized trial. *Ann Oncol.* 2012;23(7):1912–1918.

See Expertconsult.com for full list of references.

61   The Role of Advocacy Groups in Lung Cancer

Glenda Colburn, Selma Schimmel†, and Jesme Fox

SUMMARY OF KEY POINTS

- To describe the functions of advocacy.
- To describe how lung cancer advocacy groups accomplish their goals.
- To describe how they can influence lung cancer outcomes.

Advocacy is defined as the act or process of supporting a cause or proposal. Effective advocates in the health-care field influence disease awareness and education, research and drug development, public policy, and legislative and governmental issues. Cancer advocates have become an instrumental and influential force on behalf of cancer care.

Cancer advocacy is rooted in the early work of the breast cancer movement in the United States beginning in the 1970s. The political and social activism of the HIV/AIDS movement during the 1980s and 1990s further influenced US breast cancer advocacy. Foundations and charitable organizations emerged to fund efforts on behalf of breast cancer information, education, emotional support, and research. Media played an essential role, and with an engaged public, policymakers and decision makers were paying attention to the vision and demands of the breast cancer advocacy community,[1] which eventually led the way for advocacy efforts for other disease types. The common goals of cancer advocates include raising awareness and education; ensuring patient access to screening, diagnosis, and treatment; stimulating research and clinical trials; addressing the psychosocial and emotional issues associated with cancer; and empowering individuals to gain control of their disease. Advocates are directly responsible for challenging public perceptions, stigma, and disease identity; they can influence and shape research and policy agendas.

Today, in many parts of the world, cancer advocates work in conjunction with medical experts, political leaders, the pharmaceutical and biotech industries, corporations, and government and legislative representatives. Each country and region of the world presents unique issues for advocates that are based on culture, society, economics, and existing governmental and health policy infrastructures. Global patient advocacy must tailor its tactics and activities to meet and respond to these needs.

LUNG CANCER ADVOCACY GROUPS

In 2001, a global search revealed the existence of only nine not-for-profit organizations with an interest in lung cancer advocacy. Of these, only two were lung cancer specific; the others were representing generic cancer or respiratory diseases. In coming together, these organizations established the Global Lung Cancer Coalition (GLCC), an allied group of registered not-for-profit, nongovernment organizations dedicated

to improving lung cancer outcomes. By 2016, the GLCC had grown to 35 member organizations, from 25 countries, and now provides a centralized referral network to these organizations within its website. Lung Cancer Europe is a relatively new coalition, which provides a European platform for already existing lung cancer patient advocacy groups and supports the establishment of new national groups in European countries, where they do not currently exist. More information is available at http://www.lungcancereurope.eu. There are also additional lung cancer advocacy groups in the United States, and there may well be others across the world advocating in this disease.

CHALLENGES IN LUNG CANCER ADVOCACY

Despite the recent formation of several advocacy groups in lung cancer, the number of these groups is still low. Lung cancer advocacy is most developed in North America, Australia, and the European Union, in particular, the United Kingdom. We see small groups emerging elsewhere in the world, even though in Eastern Europe national lung cancer organizations are not common. As with other health-related agendas, sustaining and building advocacy groups is a challenge. Negative issues associated with lung cancer, such as those described in the following section, make it particularly difficult to advocate for change and improvement.

Lack of Advocates

Individuals who advocate for a particular disease tend to be directly affected by the disease, such as patients and caregivers. Sadly, few people with lung cancer are well enough or survive long enough to become advocates. Lung cancer is the number 1 cancer claiming more lives than any other cancer in the world and has a less than 17% 5-year survival rate. An additional issue is that compared with other common cancers, there are relatively few high-profile celebrity supporters of this disease. As such, there are relatively few lung cancer voices championing the cause.

Stigma Surrounding the Association With Tobacco

Lung cancer is often seen as self-inflicted because of its association with tobacco. An Ipsos MORI consumer poll, commissioned by the GLCC in 2011,[2] showed that, although there was national variation across the 15 countries surveyed, on average, 20% of people felt less sympathy for people with lung cancer than for people with other common cancers (Fig. 61.1). The national variation was 10% to 29%.

People with lung cancer have reported higher levels of perceived cancer-related stigma compared with people with breast or prostate cancer.[3] The belief that one has caused one's own cancer has been correlated with higher levels of guilt, shame, anxiety, and depression.[3] The stigma caused by a tobacco-related disease can create hardship for patients, many of whom suffer in silence and isolation and feel a sense of hopelessness and helplessness about their condition.[3] In fact, irrespective of whether people with lung cancer smoked or have never smoked, they feel stigmatized because of the tobacco association.[4-6]

---

†Deceased.

Lung cancer is mainly caused by smoking cigarettes and other tobacco products. Bearing this in mind, to what extent do you agree or disagree with the following statement...

I have less sympathy for people with lung cancer than people with other types of cancer

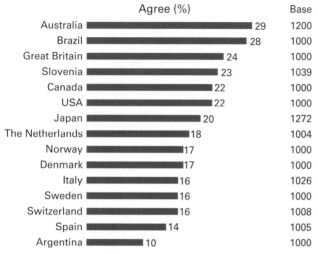

	Agree (%)	Base
Australia	29	1200
Brazil	28	1000
Great Britain	24	1000
Slovenia	23	1039
Canada	22	1000
USA	22	1000
Japan	20	1272
The Netherlands	18	1004
Norway	17	1000
Denmark	17	1000
Italy	16	1026
Sweden	16	1000
Switzerland	16	1008
Spain	14	1005
Argentina	10	1000

Fig. 61.1. Results of Global Lung Cancer Coalition/Ipsos MORI consumer poll (2011) to evaluate sympathy for people with lung cancer compared with other types of cancer.

The stigma and blame associated with lung cancer are also a contributing factor to late presentation.[7–9] Stigmatization has a negative impact on the disease and on advocacy initiatives. Central to the lung cancer advocacy community is its focus on reducing the stigma associated with this disease because it can profoundly affect not only patients in their personal identity, social life, and economic opportunities, but also their families. Many diseases are lifestyle related, yet the patients are not affected in this way. It is important that messages such as "no one deserves lung cancer" and "smoker, former smoker, or never-smoker—anyone can get lung cancer" are widely disseminated.

Low Public Profile

Because of poor outcomes overall, a lack of advocates, and a relative lack of celebrity supporters, engaging the media in lung cancer has been challenging. Journalists in many countries consider lung cancer to be depressing and so have been reluctant to report on lung cancer issues. In addition, there is a reluctance from those living with lung cancer to speak out, given the stigma and fear of self and community blame.

LUNG CANCER ADVOCACY GROUP ACTIVITY

All organizations engaging in lung cancer advocacy are different and respond to the particular culture and need of their regions or countries. However, they campaign for some or all of the following.

Integrated Tobacco Control Programs

Many lung cancer advocacy groups have an interest in disease prevention and campaign for the development and implementation of antitobacco strategies. These strategies include smoking cessation services; legislation, where necessary (e.g., to ban smoking in enclosed public places, point-of-sales advertising, cigarette vending machines, and to ensure plain packaging for cigarette packs); educational programs in schools; and public awareness campaigns, all of which underscore the importance of not smoking and the value of quitting.

Increased Funding for Lung Cancer Research

Globally, lung cancer is the most common cancer. Yet, compared with other common cancers, there has been relatively little investment in lung cancer research. The GLCC has commissioned the Institute of Cancer Policy to undertake a review of "The State of Global Lung Cancer Research."[10] As many as 32,000 published lung cancer research articles were examined, from 2085 different journals. Of these, only 5.6% of all global cancer research was in lung cancer (2013), an increase of only 1.2% since 2004. As many as 24 countries were found to be responsible for more than 95% of lung cancer research outputs. Individual country reports are available at http://www.lungcancercoalition.org. The majority of lung cancer research (53%) is focused on medicines, genetics, and biomarkers, with only 1% on supportive and palliative care issues.

In 2013, the National Cancer Research Institute reported that only 6.7% of cancer site-specific spending in the United Kingdom was on lung cancer (charities and government).[11] Although this rate represents an increase from the 3.9% spent on lung cancer in 2006, the rate is still poor despite the fact that lung cancer accounts for more than 20% of cancer deaths in the United Kingdom annually.

In 2015, Cancer Australia reported that only 5% of cancer site-specific spending in Australia was on lung cancer (charities and government).[12] Total funding to lung cancer research (including pleural mesothelioma) decreased from 2006–2008 to 2009–2011 and showed that the proportional funding to lung cancer research was very low compared with incidence, mortality, and burden of disease on the Australian population. Lung cancer accounts for 19% of cancer deaths in Australia annually.

Campaigning to increase investments in lung cancer research is a core function of lung cancer advocacy. Many lung cancer advocacy groups are also funders of research, working in conjunction with scientists and clinicians to build research capacity in the lung cancer community to ensure better future outcomes.

Increased Number of People With Lung Cancer Enrolled in Clinical Trials

Unless a person with lung cancer is being treated at a center that participates in clinical trials relevant to his or her disease, it can be very difficult to access clinical trials or even be aware of them. Many advocacy groups play a key role in this area, both in raising awareness of clinical trials in general and in directing people with lung cancer to appropriate trials and trial sites. Some advocacy groups have included links to clinical trial databases from their websites to make it easier for people with lung cancer to find appropriate trials; the lack of a national service that can provide adequate and updated information is a barrier for people who wish to participate in clinical trials. The GLCC has also collated links to websites in various countries, where details on clinical trials are available.[13]

Earlier Diagnosis

Diagnosing more people with lung cancer at an early stage, when curative treatments are an option, can save lives. In recent years, there has been increased focus on lung cancer screening. In countries where lung cancer screening is available, advocates are directing high-risk individuals to these services. Advocates are also calling for further research to evaluate the benefit of screening tools.

Raising general public awareness of the signs and symptoms associated with lung cancer is a key function of many lung cancer advocacy groups; however, there is a variety of associated signs and symptoms, so this can be a difficult task. In England, the Department of Health, in 2012, funded the national "Be Clear on Cancer—Lung Cancer" campaign.[14] This campaign, focusing on persistent cough, and results from the pilot study noted a 22% increase in the number of patients who visited their general practitioner with relevant symptoms and also noted an increase in chest computed tomography scans being performed. This campaign was repeated in 2013 and in 2014. Results of the 2012 campaign showed that an extra 700 diagnoses were made (9% higher than same period in 2011) and around 400 patients were picked up in early stage (300 of whom were offered surgery).[15] Using nationally agreed-upon guidelines, advocacy groups have produced community information such as the GLCC awareness-raising leaflets, which are translated into 13 languages and available for download.[16]

Equitable Access to Best-Practices Treatment and Care

Ensuring equitable access to the best care is of ever-increasing importance in lung cancer advocacy because of current global financial issues, pressures on health services budgets, and the rising cost of new diagnostics and therapies. It is the advocate's ultimate goal that all people with lung cancer will be treated within nationally agreed-upon treatment guidelines, that they will be offered high-quality support and information, and that they will have access to up-to-date, evidence-based diagnostics and therapies. Across regions and countries of the world, realistic expectations vary. However, using the Internet and social media, people with lung cancer are able to learn about available lung cancer treatments and technologies, but may not be able to access them, which may result in considerable distress.

The production of patient-focused information materials on all aspects of lung cancer diagnosis, treatment, and care is a core function of most advocacy groups. Such information ensures that patients and their families have a better understanding of their disease and are better equipped to make informed decisions about care. Some advocacy groups have positioned themselves as an extension to the health-care system and a supportive care service for patients and caregivers whilst away from their treating centers. Information can be delivered in many formats, such as print, the Web, DVD, and other new media formats. A challenge for all patient information providers is to ensure that these materials are current, evidence based, and easily accessible.

In recent years, financial pressures across the globe have resulted in health-care providers undertaking formal health technology assessments, particularly in the area of new developments, including targeted therapies and immunotherapies. Cancer advocacy groups play a substantial role in making sure that national health technology assessment bodies understand the importance of segmented populations, biomarkers, and issues of study crossover. In this new research area, in particular in the United States, cancer advocacy groups have taken on a key role in tissue banking and molecular testing; the National Lung Cancer Partnership has collaborated with 14 top cancer centers to form the Lung Cancer Mutation Consortium, which is the largest effort to date to promote molecular testing for people with lung cancer. Elsewhere, groups are raising awareness of new lung cancer diagnostics, evidence-based clinical pathways, and campaigning for widely available pathology services.

High-Quality Data

Underpinning all issues is the need for advocates to access high-quality, timely data on survival, quality of life, and patient experience. Such data not only provide a benchmark for the quality and outcomes of lung cancer services, but also give advocates a tool with which they can campaign for improvement and showcase best practices. A good example of this is the work of the International Cancer Benchmarking Partnership,[17] which has shown a huge variation in 1-year and 5-year survival rates in lung cancer across the study countries, prompting health-care policymakers to investigate reasons for these differences.

In November 2015, the GLCC launched a global interactive lung cancer atlas,[18] allowing clinicians and advocates to easily source and compare lung cancer data from every World Health Organization (WHO) country. Data available include mortality, incidence, survival, and other country-specific data on cancer registry, cancer planning, and implementation of the WHO Framework Convention on Tobacco Control.

An important national initiative is the United Kingdom's National Lung Cancer Audit.[19] Year after year, this audit has shown improvement in areas such as the rate of surgical resection. These audit data have been extensively used by advocacy groups in the United Kingdom, as in the Web-based Smart Map,[20] which displays the data in a patient-friendly, easily accessible format. Elsewhere, a European Respiratory Society taskforce has completed a feasibility study regarding the prospective collection of clinical data for people with lung cancer in 27 European countries. Their hope is that a Pan-European database of people with lung cancer can soon be a reality.

Help for People With Lung Cancer and Their Families

Living with the disease, the diagnosis, and treatment of cancer are traumatic events for people with cancer and their loved ones. It can be a time of a great emotional distress and can evoke a wide range of emotions. The expression of these feelings is crucial in order to cope with a diagnosis of cancer and side effects from treatment; emotional support, physical care, and practical help may be of benefit to both patients and their families.

LUNG CANCER ADVOCACY STRATEGIES

In their efforts to achieve these outcomes, advocacy groups use a variety of strategies.

Use of Mass Media, Including New Social Media

Advocacy groups are increasingly using mass media in facilitating community education and building awareness about lung cancer and its impact. Social media outlets such as Facebook allow a cost-effective broader reach into the community and for those who have been touched by lung cancer to share the messages within their networks. This form of media plays a significant role in forming and influencing people's attitudes and behavior. Common use of lung cancer-themed hashtags and approaches are becoming more visible. New technologies within social media platforms such as Thunderclaps allow advocates to amplify the message with the power of crowdsourcing and help people be heard by saying something together.

Public Awareness Campaigns

A main focus of the lung cancer advocacy community has been the November "Lung Cancer Awareness Month" initiative, initially developed in the United States by the Alliance for Lung Cancer Advocacy, Support and Education (now the Lung Cancer Alliance), and adopted by the global community in 2002. A cross-country initiative, "Shine a Light on Lung Cancer," is the largest coordinated awareness event in the world, with more than 125 vigils in the United States, 30 events in Australia, and additional vigils held in Brazil, Egypt, New Zealand, and Poland (http://www.shinealightonlungcancer.org). The purpose of each vigil is to build the lung cancer community, and each year more voices are added to this movement.

There are many methods of raising awareness of lung cancer, including public meetings and petitions, position statements, advertising, and mass publication of informational leaflets. The West Japan Oncology Group, for example, has hosted 25 public lectures in 11 cities across Japan between 2001 and 2012. These lectures on lung cancer have attracted more than 11,000 attendees, consisting of people with lung cancer (29%), their families (34%), and others. The format of the meetings has included a lecture from a key specialist on a topic (e.g., epidemiology, diagnosis, pathology, or treatment), testimony from a lung cancer survivor, and a question-and-answer period. The lectures have also gained public awareness through articles in local and national newspapers, with articles published in 89 million printed newspapers. A key product of this initiative is the creation of a guidebook for people with lung cancer.

Political Lobbying

In the United States, political lobbying by the Lung Cancer Alliance, including campaigning for legislative change and print/Web efforts to harness public opinion, has led to a $68.5 million congressional authorization for lung cancer research by the Department of Defense.[21]

Informing and Influencing Health Services Providers

Advocacy groups can play a large part in influencing health services workers to provide better care to their patients with lung cancer. Lung Foundation Australia has campaigned to support lung cancer specialist nurses in Australia, and in the United Kingdom, the Roy Castle Lung Cancer Foundation and the National Forum for Lung Cancer Nurses have developed a report on the value of lung cancer nurses.[22]

People with lung cancer who seek emotional and/or practical support from cancer organizations geared toward people with the disease may find psychologic support and programs specifically designed with the aim to help alleviate emotional distress for them and their families. Advocacy groups lead in the formation and conduct of lung cancer patient support groups, which include face-to-face and telephone formats. Other programs may include webinars, mindfulness classes, make-up sessions for women receiving treatment, relaxation technique sessions, cooking classes, and art and music therapy.

CONCLUSION

Despite recent advances, lung cancer remains a devastating disease for many people and is still characterized by much negativity and poor outcomes. Advocacy groups have much to offer in changing this picture, particularly in light of recent advances in screening for the early detection of lung cancer. There is increasing hope that more survivors will produce more advocates and a stronger global voice in this disease.

With the current research focus on biomarkers and immune therapy in lung cancer, it is clear that, over the next few years, lung cancer will be a disease of interest in the development of targeted therapy and immunotherapy treatments.

Educating patients about genomics therefore represents a new advocacy task. In addition to the direct benefits of new therapy options, this will likely mean more people with lung cancer in clinical trials, more clinicians engaged in lung cancer research, and a higher profile for the disease in general. The challenge for lung cancer advocates will be to ensure that these benefits are realized. Advocates, however, cannot make a difference in isolation. Working with scientists and health-care professionals at the local, national, and international level is much more effective and will result in a focus on local priorities. At a global level, the International Association for the Study of Lung Cancer has engaged with the advocacy movement through representation on key committees and at professional meetings. Closer collaboration can only be beneficial when working toward better future outcomes for those affected by this disease.

KEY REFERENCES

2. Global Lung Cancer Coalition. *Global Perceptions of Lung Cancer* 2016. http://www.lungcancercoalition.org/en/news/global-perceptions-lung-cancer.
4. LoConte NK, Else-Quest NM, Eickhoff J, Hyde J, Schiller JH. Assessment of guilt and shame in patients with non-small-cell lung cancer compared with patients with breast and prostate cancer. *Clin Lung Cancer*. 2008;9(3):171–178.
5. Chapple A, Ziebland S, McPherson A. Stigma, shame, and blame experienced by patients with lung cancer: qualitative study. *BMJ*. 2004;328(7454):1470.
8. Tod AM, Craven J, Allmark P. Diagnostic delay in lung cancer: a qualitative study. *J Adv Nurs*. 2008;61(3):336–343.
9. Corner J, Hopkinson J, Fitzsimmons D, Barclay S, Muers M. Is late diagnosis of lung cancer inevitable? Interview study of patients' recollections of symptoms before diagnosis. *Thorax*. 2005;60(4):314–319.
10. Aggarwal A, Lewison G, Idir S, et al. The state of lung cancer research: a global analysis. *J Thorac Oncol*. 2016;11(7):1040–1050.
15. Walters S, Benitez-Majano S, Muller P, et al. Is England closing the international gap in cancer survival? *Br J Cancer*. 2015;113:848–860.
17. Coleman MP, Forman D, Bryant H, et al. Cancer survival in Australia, Canada, Denmark, Norway, Sweden, and the UK, 1995–2007 (the International Cancer Benchmarking Partnership): an analysis of population-based cancer registry data. *Lancet*. 2011;377(9760):127–138.

See Expertconsult.com for full list of references.

62 The Role of Health Services Research in Improving the Outcomes for Patients With Lung Cancer

William J. Mackillop, Shalini K. Vinod, and Yolande Lievens

SUMMARY OF KEY POINTS

- Health services research aims to improve the outcomes to treatment for lung cancer by optimizing the accessibility, quality, and efficiency of treatment programs.
- Achieving optimal outcomes for patients with lung cancer requires that every patient should receive optimal treatment, but many patients today do not receive optimal treatment or experience optimal outcomes.
- Deviations from optimal treatment may be due to resource limitations that compromise the accessibility of treatment, to errors in clinical decision-making, or to flaws in the implementation of treatment decisions.
- Delay in the diagnosis and treatment of lung cancer is widespread. Setting standards and streamlining referral processes may reduce waiting times, but these strategies only work if there are adequate resources available to provide the necessary care.
- Lack of treatment resources may be the inevitable consequence of the low levels of funding available in low- and middle-income countries, but it also may be due to poor planning in high-income countries.
- Multidisciplinary team (MDT) management improves the quality of care for patients with lung cancer and probably improves outcomes.
- Practice guidelines improve clinical decision-making, but one size does not fit all. Patients' values and preferences must be factored into treatment decisions. Decision aids can help patients to participate in decisions about their care.
- The outcomes of surgery for lung cancer are better at high-volume centers. The same is probably true of radiotherapy. Centralizing treatment services may improve overall outcomes, if this can be achieved without compromising access to care.

Health research may be considered as a continuum of four overlapping domains: basic or biomedical research, clinical research, health services research, and population health research. Health services research is defined as a "multidisciplinary field of scientific investigation that studies how social factors, financing systems, organizational structures and processes, health technologies, and personal behaviors affect access to health care, the quality and cost of health care, and ultimately, our health and well-being."[1] Clinical research and health services research overlap to some degree, but their purposes are distinct. Clinical research is primarily intended to guide decisions of physicians about the care of individual patients, whereas health services research is intended to guide the decisions of managers and policymakers about the design and implementation of health-care programs.[2]

HOW CAN HEALTH SERVICES RESEARCH IMPROVE THE OUTCOMES FOR PATIENTS WITH LUNG CANCER?

At any point in time, the state of knowledge and the state of technology set an upper limit on what is achievable for patients with cancer. However, what is actually achieved depends not only on what would be achievable with optimal care but also on how close we come to delivering optimal care, a quantity that has been termed the attainment factor.[2] This relationship can be expressed with the following equation.

Achieved outcome = Achievable outcome × Attainment factor

Thus, outcomes can be improved by increasing the achievable outcome through innovation or by increasing the attainment factor through the optimization of health-care systems. The goal of biomedical and clinical research is to improve outcomes through innovation, whereas the goal of health services research is to improve outcomes through the optimization of health system performance. Innovation and optimization are complementary rather than competitive activities. Innovative biomedical and clinical research both have the potential to improve outcomes greatly in the long term, but health services research may offer the best opportunity of improving outcomes in the short term.[3] The optimal balance of expenditure between innovation and optimization is unknown. However, in the case of diseases such as lung cancer, for which innovative biomedical and clinical research has been slow to yield real improvements in outcome, it is important to put a high priority on health services research in order to achieve the maximum societal benefits from existing treatments.

THE THREE DIMENSIONS OF HEALTH SYSTEM PERFORMANCE

Health system performance may be characterized in three different dimensions: accessibility, quality, and efficiency.[2] Accessibility describes the extent to which patients are able to get the care they need when they need it. Quality describes the extent to which the right care is delivered in the right way. Efficiency describes the extent to which accessibility and effectiveness are optimized in relation to the resources expended. Each of these dimensions of health system performance must be optimized in order to achieve optimal outcomes. Health services research is concerned with measuring access, quality, and efficiency; understanding the factors that influence them; and discovering ways to enhance them. The three dimensions of health system performance are clearly not independent of one another. For example, interventions aimed at enhancing quality have the potential to adversely affect accessibility and/or efficiency. It is therefore unwise to focus on one dimension of health system performance without at least keeping an eye on what is happening in the other two dimensions.

Health-Care Accessibility

The term health-care accessibility originally was used narrowly to describe the ability of patients to obtain entry into the health system.[4] Today, it is used more broadly to encompass all of the factors that influence the level of use of a health service in relation to the level of need for the service in a population.[5] The concept of access has been described as representing the overall "degree of fit between the clients and the system."[6] Several factors have been shown to influence the overall degree of fit.[6] Availability describes the volume and type of services available in relation to the number of patients and their needs. Spatial accessibility describes the relationship between the location of supply of service and the location of the patients who need the service, taking into account travel times and costs.[6] Accommodation describes the extent to which the system is designed to facilitate patient access to service, for example, by operating at convenient hours or by providing lodging for those who require treatment that is only available far from their homes.[6] Affordability describes the relationship between prices and the ability of patients to pay. It also encompasses indirect costs, for example, loss of earnings during treatment that may deter use of the service.[6] Awareness describes the extent to which those who need the service are aware that it is available and that they might benefit from it.[2]

Quality in Health Care

Almost half a century ago, Donabedian[7,8] defined the quality of health care as "a property of, and a judgement upon, some definable unit of health care, and that care is divisible into at least two parts: technical and interpersonal." The quality of technical care is measured by the extent to which "the application of medical science and technology maximizes its health benefits without correspondingly increasing its risks." The quality of interpersonal care is measured by "how well the physician–patient interaction meets the socially defined norms of the relationship." Today, the Institute of Medicine describes health-care quality as "the degree to which health services for individuals and populations increase the likelihood of desired health outcomes and are consistent with current professional knowledge."[9]

Donabedian[8] also provided a framework for evaluating the quality of health care in terms of structure, process, and outcome. The term structure is defined broadly to include facilities, equipment, personnel, and organizational structures. The term process includes both the type of care that is delivered and the way in which it is delivered. The term outcome refers to the consequences of the care that has been provided. Donabedian reasoned that optimal process is necessary for optimal outcome; that adequate structure is necessary, although not sufficient, for optimal process; and that outcomes may be enhanced by identifying and correcting deficiencies in structure and/or process.

Efficiency in Health Care

The resources available for health services are always limited, even in high-income nations. What is achievable in terms of cancer control depends on the total health-care budget, on how much of that total budget is directed to cancer care, and on how efficiently the available resources are used in providing cancer care. Efficiency measures whether we are getting the best value for money from the available health-care resources. Inefficiency is said to be present when using those resources in a different way would provide greater health benefits.[10] Health economists distinguish between technical efficiency, productive efficiency, and allocative efficiency. As stated by Palmer and Torgerson,[11] "technical efficiency addresses the issue of using given resources to maximum advantage; productive efficiency of choosing different combinations of resources to achieve the maximum health benefit for a given cost; and allocative efficiency of achieving the right mixture of healthcare programs to maximize the health of society." Methods for measuring each of these quantities are well established[12] and have been used to address some important issues in the treatment of lung cancer, but the sphere of health economics is beyond the scope of this chapter and therefore we will not deal with it in detail here.

In this chapter, we will review the results of research studies that have sought to optimize the accessibility and quality of programs of care for patients with lung cancer. This work involves identifying barriers to optimal care as well as designing and evaluating interventions to overcome those barriers. However, before one can identify deviations from optimal health system performance, one must first identify appropriate indicators of performance and establish standards of performance with respect to those indicators. We will therefore begin by reviewing the prescriptive research that has been undertaken to establish standards of care for patients with lung cancer. We will distinguish between standards of care for the individual patient and standards for the operation of the health programs that are required to deliver care to a population of patients. Standards of care for the individual patient should be based, whenever possible, on the results of randomized clinical trials that directly compare the outcomes of alternative forms of treatment. Likewise, standards for the operation of health programs should be based on the results of randomized trials that directly compare the effectiveness of alternative approaches to health-care delivery or at least on the results of well-controlled observational studies. However, we will show that the empirical evidence that underpins program standards today is usually much weaker than the evidence that supports guidelines for the care of the individual patient.

STANDARDS FOR THE CARE OF INDIVIDUAL PATIENTS

For more than half a century, treatment guidelines for the management of specific clinical problems have been widely used to guide clinical decision-making.[13] In the past, guidelines were based largely on expert opinion, but it is now generally accepted that practice guidelines must be based on a thorough evaluation of all relevant evidence. This concept is the essence of evidence-based medical practice, defined by Sackett et al.[14] as "the conscientious, explicit and judicious use of current best evidence in making decisions about the care of the individual patient." Sackett et al.[15,16] also provided a useful system for the classification of the types of clinical evidence that may be available and rules for their use in creating guidelines. The Institute of Medicine (IOM) has defined practice guidelines as "systematically developed statements to assist practitioner and patient decisions about appropriate health care for specific clinical circumstances."[17]

Given the importance of practice guidelines, many individuals and agencies have sought to give direction on how to create them. The Cochrane Collaboration has been instrumental in promoting systematic reviews of the medical literature. The Collaboration provides guidance for undertaking the systematic reviews necessary to identify all of the relevant evidence, for evaluating the quality of the evidence, and for synthesizing the evidence through meta-analysis.[18,19] The IOM monograph entitled Clinical Practice Guidelines We Can Trust examines the current state of clinical practice guidelines and provides guidance on how to improve them.[20] Recognizing the societal importance of practice guidelines, government agencies have also played a role in this activity, and there also have been international efforts to optimize and harmonize the process of guidelines development.[21]

Guidelines for the Care of Individual Patients With Lung Cancer

Guidelines for the treatment of lung cancer have been developed by many different agencies and organizations around the world, including specialty societies such as the American Society of Clinical Oncology (ASCO),[22] the European Society for Medical Oncology,[23,24] the American College of Chest Physicians,[25] and the American Society for Radiation Oncology;[26] groups of healthcare institutions such as the National Comprehensive Cancer Network (NCCN) in the United States;[27,28] and government agencies such as the National Institute for Health and Care Excellence in the United Kingdom,[29] Cancer Care Ontario in Canada,[30] and the Cancer Council Australia.[31] Some of these agencies attempt to provide comprehensive guidelines that cover the entire spectrum of possible presentations of the disease,[23–25,27,29,30] whereas others have focused on providing detailed guidelines for management in specific clinical contexts.[22,26,30,31] Most guidelines are written primarily for the use of physicians, but some agencies also provide a version that targets patients directly.[28] It is recognized that practice guidelines that are created in one country may not be applicable in other societies with very different resources and/ or different populations of patients. The NCCN, an alliance of 23 major cancer centers in the United States, is now endeavoring to provide international adaptations and translations of its guidelines to make them suitable for use in countries with different levels of economic development.[32] Nonetheless, it is probably preferable for each society to develop its own guidelines. Repeating work that has already been done elsewhere may seem to be a waste of resources, but the process of guideline development is important in its own right and may have as much normative effect on practice as the guideline itself.[33]

Challenges to the Development and Application of Practice Guidelines

Variation in patient values and the biologic heterogeneity of tumors pose particular challenges for the creation and application of treatment guidelines.

Variation in Patient Values

Patients differ in their values and preferences. Treatments that offer only modest benefit but substantial toxicity may be desirable to some but not to others. Under these circumstances, there is no standard treatment, and patients and physicians are faced with the choice between what Eddy[34] described as options with preferences split. It has been shown that this is exactly the situation that prevails in decisions about the use of chemotherapy for nonsmall cell lung cancer (NSCLC). In an early study of decision-making related to the treatment of locally advanced NSCLC, Brundage et al.[35] found that patients varied widely in terms of the degree of improvement in survival that they believed would justify the added toxicity of chemotherapy.

Once it is recognized that optimal decisions depend on patient values, it becomes imperative to engage patients actively in decisions about their medical care. However, it is well known that patients with cancer, particularly lung cancer, often overestimate the potential benefits of treatment and may have little understanding of potential toxicities.[36,37] Better communication with patients about the benefits and risks of treatment is therefore necessary for patient-centered decision-making.

Since the late 1990s, there has been a sustained effort to develop and evaluate decision aids to provide patients with the information that they need in order to make informed decisions and also to provide them with ways of clarifying their values.[38] A systematic review demonstrated (1) that cancer-related decision aids usually are acceptable to patients and (2) that such aids

do help patients to make treatment choices that are based on realistic expectations of outcomes.[38] A decision aid for patients with locally advanced NSCLC, developed more than a decade ago, was favorably reviewed by patients and their physicians. The decision aid was shown to help patients understand the benefits and risks of treatment and also was shown to help them make the treatment choice that was most consistent with their values.[39–41] In a positive recent development, ASCO has created a series of decision aids for patients with lung cancer and has made them available online as a supplement to its treatment guidelines.[42]

Biologic Heterogeneity

The biologic heterogeneity of cancers and the genetic heterogeneity of the human population present ongoing challenges in the development and application of evidence-based treatment guidelines. The evidence on which the treatment of any individual patient is based is derived from reports of the outcomes observed in a reference group of similar patients who were similarly treated in the past.[43] The validity of this type of inductive reasoning depends on the degree of similarity between the present patient and the patients in the reference group. It goes without saying that this type of inference is only valid when the present patient is classified in the same way as the patients in the reference group. However, the predictive value of previous observations in the present patient also depends on the degree of similarity in the outcomes observed among the patients in the reference group. If the patients in the reference group experienced widely different outcomes, in spite of having tumors of the same origin, morphology, and extent of disease, then the benefits of treatment in the individual patient remain unpredictable.[43] As a result, there has been an unrelenting search for prognostic and predictive factors that might reduce uncertainty about the natural history of lung cancer and its response to treatment.[44] Dramatic advances in molecular genetics over the past 20 years have led to the discovery of genetic variations that are associated with tumor behavior and response to therapy. These advances have provided the basis for new targeted therapies and predictive tests that reduce the degree of uncertainty about the response to therapy in the individual patient.[45] In the context of NSCLC, for example, it has been shown that the probability of response to tyrosine kinase inhibitors is very high in patients with epidermal growth factor receptor (*EGFR*) mutations but patients without *EGFR* mutations are more likely to benefit from chemotherapy.[46] Some authors have seen these developments as heralding the start of a new era of personalized medicine. In the context of lung cancer, Gazdhar[46] describes a transition from the era when "patients with specific types and stages of cancer" were "treated according to standardized, predetermined protocols" to a new era of "individualized selection of treatment as determined by the characteristics of the patient and the tumor." In reality, these developments will not change the fundamental nature of clinical decision-making. We will still need the standardized, predetermined protocols that we call guidelines, but eligibility for treatment according to those protocols will be determined with use of new and better predictive assays.

Do Guidelines Guide Practice?

A quarter of a century ago, Lomas et al.[47] famously asked this question after the dissemination of a nationally endorsed consensus statement recommending decreases in the use of cesarean deliveries in Canada. Their answer was a qualified "no." Lomas et al.[47] found that, although one-third of the hospitals and obstetricians reported changing their practice as a consequence of the guidelines, actual practice changed very little. The authors concluded that "guidelines for practice may predispose physicians to consider changing their behavior, but unless there are other incentives or the removal of disincentives, guidelines are unlikely to affect rapid change in actual practice." It is therefore important to evaluate the extent to which guidelines for the treatment of lung cancer actually guide practice.

A number of studies have evaluated the degree of concordance between clinical practice and guidelines for the treatment of lung cancer. Some studies have assessed whether treatment recommendations were concordant with guidelines,[48,49] whereas others have assessed whether actual treatment was concordant with guidelines.[50-55]

In two recent studies, clinician recommendations for treatment were compared with the corresponding guidelines. Vinod et al.[48] evaluated the degree of concordance between treatment recommendations and Australian practice guidelines in a study involving a cohort of patients with lung cancer who were discussed in a multidisciplinary management meeting (MDM). The MDM recommendations were deemed to be concordant if the general plan of treatment that was recommended corresponded with the guidelines. The rate of concordance was 71% for overall management, 58% for surgery, 88% for radiotherapy, and 71% for chemotherapy. Couraud et al.[49] asked oncologists and pulmonologists specializing in thoracic oncology for their treatment recommendations in four hypothetical clinical scenarios and compared their recommendations with the corresponding French guidelines. Their criteria for concordance required consideration of the details of treatment, including the specific chemotherapeutic agents and the number of cycles of chemotherapy recommended. On the basis of these fairly strict criteria, the rate of concordance with the guidelines ranged from 25% to 63% in the four scenarios. Clinicians who worked in public practice were more likely to comply with the guidelines than those who worked in private practice. Overall, only 15% of clinicians applied the guidelines appropriately to all four cases, and 10% did not apply them in any of the cases.[49] Not surprisingly, these two studies illustrate that the observed degree of concordance depends on how strictly concordance is defined.

A number of population-based studies have assessed the concordance between the treatment that patients actually receive and the prevailing guidelines for the treatment of lung cancer.[50-58] In a population-based study in the United States that was initiated in 1996, Potosky et al.[50] described the treatment of NSCLC and compared the observed treatment with best practice as defined by the authors based on the evidence at the time. Overall, 52% of the patients received guideline-recommended treatment, but this rate varied significantly from 41% for patients with stage IV disease to 69% for patients with stage I and II disease ($p < 0.05$). The rate of guideline-recommended treatment was significantly lower for older patients, for patients who were single, and for the nonwhite population ($p < 0.05$).[50] A decade later, in a similar US population-based study, the actual treatment of NSCLC was compared with recommended treatment in the prevailing NCCN guidelines.[51] The rate of guideline-recommended treatment was only 42% overall, 37% for patients with stage I or II disease, 58% for those with stage III disease, and 29% for those with stage IV disease. Older patients and African-American patients were less likely to receive guideline-recommended treatment. In a population-based study from the Netherlands, de Rijke et al.[52] found that only 44% of patients with stage I–III NSCLC received guideline-recommended treatment. The rate of guideline-recommended treatment again varied according to stage and was reported to be 82% for patients with stage I or II disease, 48% for patients with stage IIIA disease, and 54% for patients with stage IIIB disease.[52] Rates of guideline-recommended treatment were significantly lower among older patients, and higher levels of comorbidity and lower Eastern Cooperative Oncology Group (ECOG) performance status were associated with a lower rate of guideline-recommended treatment for patients with stage I and II disease. Duggan et al.[53] reported very similar findings in

a population-based study in which the actual treatment of lung cancer was compared with treatment recommended in Australian guidelines. The rate of guideline-recommended treatment was 54% for patients with small cell lung cancer (SCLC) and 51% for patients with NSCLC. Increasing age and poorer ECOG performance status were associated with lower rates of guideline-recommended treatment.

Thus, population-based studies from three continents have shown that, at best, only half of all patients with lung cancer are treated according to guidelines. All of these studies showed that older patients are less likely to receive guideline-recommended treatment. Although these studies did not consistently evaluate other patient characteristics, taken together, they provide evidence that patients with poorer performance status or higher levels of comorbidity are less likely to receive guideline-recommended treatment. These general findings have been supported by the results of several similar studies in more selected populations of patients with lung cancer.[54,55] Other studies of compliance with guidelines focusing on specific clinical situations have provided similar results. Allen et al.[56] found low rates of adherence to surgical guidelines for the treatment of operable NSCLC; Salloum et al.[57] noted low rates of guideline-recommended treatment with respect to the use of chemotherapy in patients with stage II to stage IV NSCLC; and Langer et al.[58] found low rates of guideline-recommended treatment with respect to the use of concurrent chemotherapy and radiotherapy in patients with limited-stage SCLC and stage I to stage III NSCLC.

Two recent studies showed that there may be cogent reasons why patients do not receive guideline-recommended treatment. Landrum et al.[59] found that many patients who did not have surgery for the treatment of stage I or II NSCLC, as indicated in the guidelines, were either in poor health (61%) or had declined the operation (26%). Poor health was defined as encompassing advanced age, comorbidity, poor performance status, and poor lung function. In a presentation focusing on a cohort of patients with lung cancer who were discussed at an MDM, Boxer et al.[55] noted that the main reasons why patients did not receive guideline-recommended treatment were a decline in performance status (24%), large tumor volume precluding radical radiotherapy (17%), comorbidities (14%), and patient preference (13%).

Thus, discordance between practice and guidelines for cancer treatment does not always indicate inappropriate patient care. It may instead indicate that the existing guidelines do not adequately take into account variations in the health status of patients with cancer in the general population. This consideration is particularly important in the context of lung cancer, with more than 50% of patients having at least one other substantial medical problem that may affect their care.[60,61]

Does Adherence to Guidelines Improve Outcomes in the General Population?

It is important to ask whether adherence to evidence-based guidelines actually yields the improvements in outcome in the general population that would be expected on the basis of the results of the relevant clinical trials. Only a small proportion of all cases of lung cancer are included in clinical trials, and these cases are not necessarily representative of the overall population of patients with lung cancer. Furthermore, the institutions and physicians likely to engage in clinical trials are unlikely to be representative of the heath-care system as a whole.

Two studies showed that patients with lung cancer who are seen in routine practice are indeed different from those who are enrolled in clinical trials.[62,63] De Ruysscher et al.[62] found that 59% of patients with stage III NSCLC and limited-stage SCLC who were seen at their clinic would not have been eligible for entry into the clinical trials that showed a benefit from concurrent chemoradiation therapy, mainly because of their advanced age. Firat et al.[63] found that 33% of the patients who were treated with chemoradiotherapy at their center did not meet eligibility criteria for any Radiation Therapy Oncology Group (RTOG) trials being performed at the time, primarily because of weight loss or comorbidity.

Thus, there are good reasons to be concerned that the efficacy established by randomized controlled trials may not translate into an identical level of effectiveness in the general population. Some empirical studies have called into question whether adherence to guidelines is associated with better outcomes. Allen et al.[56] showed no difference in survival or mortality rates between patients who were and were not treated according to NCCN-defined surgical treatment guidelines. In a study of patients with stage I–III NSCLC, Duggan et al.[64] noted that patients who were treated in accordance with prevailing Australian guidelines experienced slightly better outcomes than those who did not receive guideline-recommended treatment, but that trend was not significant.

It has therefore been suggested that, after evidence-based guidelines have been adopted, phase IV population-based outcome studies should be done to confirm the value of the new treatment in the general population.[65] The results of a recent Canadian study were surprisingly reassuring.[66] Following the publication of the positive results of a Canadian trial of adjuvant chemotherapy for resected NSCLC, this practice was rapidly adopted in Canada.[67] Booth et al.[66] evaluated the results of a phase IV population-based study that documented the rapid adoption of adjuvant chemotherapy in Ontario and reported that such therapy was associated with an increase in survival commensurate with that expected on the basis of the results of the preceding randomized controlled trial. The fact that the results of this particular trial were reproduced in routine practice does not guarantee the generalizability of the results of other randomized controlled trials, and additional phase IV population-based outcome studies are required to evaluate the societal benefit of the adoption of other promising new treatments.[65]

To achieve optimal outcomes at the societal level, every patient must receive the correct treatment, and that treatment must be delivered correctly. Thus, in addition to practice guidelines for the selection of the appropriate treatment, additional standards are required to ensure the quality and accessibility of treatment.

QUALITY STANDARDS FOR CANCER TREATMENT PROGRAMS

General Quality Standards

In order to provide the optimal quality of treatment, the necessary structures and processes must be in place to deliver the treatment correctly. The term structure is used here to include human resources, physical resources, and organizational resources, and the term process includes all of the activities and procedures used to ensure the quality of treatment, as described earlier. Although practice guidelines target precisely defined subgroups of patients, the structures and processes required to ensure optimal quality of care are often applicable to much broader groups of patients. The same facilities usually serve the needs of diverse groups of patients, and the structures and processes that determine the quality of care are often common to many different types of cancer. Thus, the quality of the care that patients with lung cancer receive is in large measure determined by the degree of institutional adherence to general standards of practice that are applicable to the care of every patient with cancer.

The American College of Surgeons has been a leader in this field. In 1930, its Committee on the Treatment of Malignant Diseases released its first set of cancer program standards and created an accreditation program to evaluate the performance of a cancer clinic against those standards. As the management of cancer became increasingly multidisciplinary, the membership of this committee was broadened to include individuals from nonsurgical disciplines and its name was changed to the Commission on Cancer. Today, it provides a suite of program standards aimed at ensuring comprehensive, patient-centered, high-quality, multidisciplinary care for all patients with cancer.[68]

Multidisciplinary Team Management

No individual specialty has all of the knowledge and expertise necessary for optimal decision-making related to the management of a complex disease in the modern era. The primary rationale for introducing MDTs is to bring together the expertise of all of the key professional groups in making clinical decisions for individual patients.[69] Treatment decisions are made by consensus, reducing the risk that the bias of any individual physician will determine the final decision. There is usually considerable overlap in expertise among team members, providing a built-in opportunity for peer review of treatment decisions. The organized and open decision-making process provides a suitable forum for applying treatment guidelines and for identifying patients who are eligible for participation in clinical trials.[70] When several different health professionals are involved in the overall plan of care for the individual patient, the team structure fosters communication among all those involved. MDT management therefore has been recommended as a mechanism for improving the quality of care for patients with various complex diseases, including diabetes, stroke, ischemic heart disease, and cancer.[69]

On the basis of the persuasive arguments in favor of its use, the MDT approach has been widely adopted in cancer care systems throughout much of Europe, the United States, and Australia.[69] At the outset, there was very little empirical evidence that this approach actually improved the quality of patient care or the outcomes of treatment.[69] Although some observers remain skeptical about the value of MDT work,[71] accumulating evidence suggests that this approach does lead to better decision-making and that it may improve outcomes, at least for patients with certain types of cancer.[70–72] In one study from the United Kingdom, the vast majority of health professionals reported that they enjoyed working within the framework of an MDT and many reported that doing so had increased their job satisfaction.[73]

Multidisciplinary Team Management of Lung Cancer

MDT management of lung cancer is particularly important as studies have shown that practice varies widely,[74–76] that physician views are not always concordant with guidelines,[77,78] and that the different specialists involved in treatment tend to be biased in favor of their own modality of treatment.[79,80] It is also essential in the setting of lung cancer because multimodality treatment is common, pathologic subtyping is continually evolving, and patient comorbidities can have a substantial impact on the safety of therapeutic options.

The MDT should involve all of the clinicians who are involved in the diagnosis and treatment of lung cancer, including respiratory physicians, cardiothoracic surgeons, medical oncologists, radiation oncologists, palliative care physicians, and lung cancer nurses. The presence of a pathologist, radiologist, and nuclear medicine physician is also essential for accurate interpretation of the pathologic and imaging findings that underpin management recommendations. Ideally, all patients should be discussed at an MDM where all of these disciplines are represented. The presence of clinicians from different specialties should serve to reduce specialty bias in the treatment of patients and to inform colleagues of the role of different treatment modalities. The potential benefits of an MDM are increased compliance with evidence-based guidelines, improved utilization of treatment, increased referrals for psychosocial care, improved timeliness of treatment, and increased recruitment to clinical trials.

The impact of an MDM ideally would be tested in a randomized controlled trial, but this type of study is difficult to conduct for such a complex intervention. However, a number of investigators have sought to evaluate the impact of MDMs either by comparing patterns of care before and after the implementation of an MDM or by comparing cases discussed in an MDM with contemporaneous controls who were not discussed in the MDM.[81–85] Both of these approaches are susceptible to bias. The longitudinal "before-and-after" design is vulnerable to changes in case mix, staging, and management over time, whereas the use of contemporaneous controls is susceptible to bias in the selection of patients for the MDM. In analyzing the results of such observational studies, it is therefore important to control, as much as possible, other factors that may influence the choice of treatment or its outcome.

Forrest et al.[81] evaluated the impact of the introduction of a multidisciplinary lung cancer team on the treatment of patients with inoperable NSCLC.[81] The pre-MDM data were collected retrospectively for 1997, the year preceding introduction of the MDM, and the post-MDM data were collected prospectively for 2001. The authors found a significant increase in formal staging of lung cancer (81% vs. 70%; $p = 0.04$), a significant increase in the use of chemotherapy (23% vs. 7%; $p < 0.001$), a decrease in the use of palliative care alone (58% vs. 44%; $p = 0.05$), and no significant change in the use of radiotherapy. The median survival was significantly greater for patients who were discussed at the MDM (6.6 vs. 3.2 months; $p < 0.001$). The two cohorts were not balanced for stage, with the post-MDM group including fewer patients with stage IIIA disease, which one would expect to result in poorer survival.

The improvement in survival therefore was attributed to the increased use of chemotherapy. However, it seems somewhat improbable that this factor alone could have been responsible for the large difference in survival. It remains possible that differences in case mix between the groups, not fully controlled for in the analysis, may have contributed to the difference in survival.

Erridge et al.[82] compared patterns of care in Scotland before and after the implementation of a number of changes related to the treatment of lung cancer, including the introduction of MDMs at which all patients with newly diagnosed lung cancer were discussed, the introduction of management guidelines, and an increase in the number of oncologists specializing in the treatment of lung cancer. Although the overall active treatment rate was unchanged, the investigators found a significant increase in the use of curative radiotherapy (5% vs. 15%; $p < 0.001$) and chemotherapy (7% vs. 18%; $p < 0.001$) for patients with NSCLC. The median survival time improved from 4.1 to 5.2 months ($p = 0.004$). As there were multiple concurrent changes in cancer care over time, it was not possible to tease out the impact of MDMs alone.

Seeber et al.[83] compared the treatment of lung cancer before and after the implementation of an MDM videoconference that was held at a peripheral site. The investigators found that the MDM changed the treatment recommendations of the presenting team in 25% of the cases. The use of radiotherapy increased from 30% to 70% ($p = 0.001$) following the introduction of the MDM. There was no change in the use of chemotherapy, and the authors did not comment on the use of surgery.

The largest study to evaluate the impact of the introduction of an MDM at a single institution was performed by Freeman et al.,[84] who compared the care of 535 patients who were treated before the implementation of an MDM with that of 687 patients who were treated after its introduction. The investigators found increased completeness of staging (93% vs. 79%; $p < 0.0001$), greater adherence to NCCN guidelines (97% vs. 81%, $p < 0.0001$), and reduced time from diagnosis to treatment (17 vs.

29 days; $p < 0.0001$) after the introduction of the MDM. There was also greater use of neoadjuvant chemotherapy and surgical resections for patients with stage IIIA NSCLC who were treated after the introduction of the MDM.

Two studies have compared the treatment of and outcomes for patients who were discussed at an MDM with those who were not in a cohort of patients who were seen at the same center over the same time period.[85,86] Bydder et al.,[85] in a small study of patients with inoperable NSCLC, found no difference between the MDM and non-MDM subgroups in terms of treatment but reported that the MDM subgroup had a longer median survival time (280 vs. 205 days; $p = 0.05$). However, the authors noted some imbalances between the groups in terms of tumor characteristics and acknowledged that selection bias may have affected the results. In a much larger study of 988 patients who were diagnosed with lung cancer between 2005 and 2008, Boxer et al.[86] compared 504 patients who were discussed at the MDM with 484 patients who were not. The investigators found that patients in the MDM subgroup were significantly more likely to be treated with radiotherapy (66% vs. 33%, $p < 0.001$), to be treated with chemotherapy (46% vs. 29%, $p < 0.001$), and to be referred for palliative care (66% vs. 53%, $p < 0.001$). The groups did not differ with respect to the rate of surgical treatment. Multivariate analysis showed that discussion at an MDM was an independent predictor of nonsurgical treatment and palliative care referrals but was not predictive of survival. Clinician selection bias may have had some influence on these results. Patients with better performance status may have been selected for presentation at the MDM on the assumption that they would receive treatment. Unfortunately, ECOG performance status was not available for the patients in the non-MDM cohort, and the authors therefore were unable to control for this factor in the analysis. The authors tried to minimize potential bias by assigning population-derived ECOG data to compensate for this limitation, but the potential for confounding remains.

Single-arm studies also may provide some useful information about the quality of care for patients who are discussed in an MDM. Conron et al.[87] described the activity of a lung cancer multidisciplinary clinic at which 431 patients were discussed between 2002 and 2004. Management was compared with prospectively identified measures of quality of care. They found that 98% of patients with stage I to stage IIIA NSCLC have macroscopically complete surgical resection, that 100% of patients with stage IIIB NSCLC have positron emission tomography before curative chemoradiation therapy, that 84% of patients with stage IIIB NSCLC complete curative radiotherapy, that 86% of patients with stage IV NSCLC are referred for palliative chemotherapy, and that 100% and 85% of patients with limited-stage SCLC have complete staging and receive thoracic radiotherapy, respectively. In a study that was described earlier, Vinod et al.[48] found 71% concordance between MDM recommendations and guidelines, but, in a follow-up study, Boxer et al.[55] found that only 51% of patients actually received guideline-based care.

The efficacy of MDMs has been evaluated in terms of whether recommendations are translated into practice and whether deviations from these recommendations affect outcomes.[88,89] Leo et al.[88] analyzed the concordance between MDM-planned treatment and administered treatment in a study involving a cohort of French patients who were discussed in 2003 and 2004. Patients who did not receive the recommended treatment had poorer survival, although this finding did not reach significance. In the United States, Osarogiagbon et al.[89] compared the outcomes for patients with any thoracic malignancy who received treatment that was concordant or discordant with MDM recommendations. Patients who received concordant treatment had a shorter time to clinical intervention (14 vs. 25 days, $p < 0.002$) and better median survival (2.1 vs. 1.3 years, $p < 0.01$). The authors were unable to identify the reasons for discordance in their study; however,

Black race and lack of medical insurance were the two factors associated with the receipt of discordant care.

In summary, although there is no level 1 evidence to support the use of MDMs, observational studies have shown that patients who are discussed at an MDM are more likely to receive treatment (particularly radiotherapy and chemotherapy), more likely to receive potentially curative treatment, and more likely to be referred for palliative care. The increased use of all and any of these modalities, including palliative care,[90] has the potential to improve survival, although there is little direct evidence that discussion at an MDM is associated with improved survival. For these reasons, case discussion at an MDM has been adopted as an indicator of quality of lung cancer care in some jurisdictions.[91–93]

Although it is now widely accepted that multidisciplinary management is effective for improving the quality of care for patients with lung cancer, the optimal structure and operations of the MDT have yet to be defined. Taylor and Ramirez,[73] in a study commissioned by the National Cancer Action Team in the United Kingdom, recently surveyed members of multidisciplinary cancer teams, with three objectives: (1) to identify the attributes of an effective MDT, (2) to learn how best to measure MDT effectiveness, and (3) to determine what support or tools MDTs need to be most effective. More than 2000 MDT members responded to the survey, of whom 53% were physicians, 26% were nurses, and 15% were MDT coordinators. The results of the survey demonstrated a high degree of consensus about the domains that are important for effective functioning of the MDT, including the membership, leadership, and governance of the team; the physical environment of the venue, technologic resources, preparation for meetings, administration of meetings, and attendance at meetings; the decision-making process, case management, and coordination of service; data collection, analysis, and auditing of outcomes; and development and training of participants. This very useful report provides many additional details of the elements of an effective MDT from the perspective of experienced team members. It should be essential reading for any member of a cancer program who is contemplating the introduction of an MDT.[73]

If MDT care is worth doing, it is worth doing well. In England, the Improving Lung Cancer Outcomes Project brings together multidisciplinary health-care teams from different regions under the leadership of the Royal College of Physicians. A recent report from this group described a quality-improvement exercise in which each of 30 randomly selected MDTs were paired with one another in visiting the others' services for a day, attending the MDM, and reviewing audit results.[94] The most commonly identified problems concerned the way in which MDMs operated, including deficiencies in the amount of information available at the meetings, the way in which decisions were made, and methods for capturing outcomes. The teams then used standard quality-improvement methods to target specific problems that were identified in the peer-review process. Ultimately, the impact of this peer-review process will be evaluated by comparing the outcomes achieved by the 30 MDTs that participated in the intervention with outcomes achieved by MDTs that did not.[94] This exercise may prove to be a very useful approach for enhancing the effectiveness of MDT care in the future.

MDT management necessarily generates added costs, and the cost-effectiveness of this approach has not been well evaluated. One small study from the United Kingdom, which considered only the salaries of senior staff and excluded preparation time and management costs, estimated the cost of discussing each patient to be £36.6 (US$60.64),[95] whereas another study from the United Kingdom, which considered all costs, including use of audiovisual equipment, clerical time, preparation time for radiographic and pathologic examinations, and room overhead, estimated the cost per treatment plan to be £87.41 (US$144.83).[96] If multidisciplinary management really results in improvements

in treatment and outcome, then MDMs may still be very cost-effective.[96] However, the cost of MDMs is clearly not trivial and further research on MDT management should seek to find ways to enhance its efficiency as well as its effectiveness.

Modality-Specific Quality Standards for Cancer Programs

Standards that target the quality of the major modalities of cancer treatment are also necessary to ensure the optimal treatment of lung cancer. For example, both Australia and Canada have established quality standards for radiotherapy programs,[97,98] which are clearly pertinent to the optimal care of patients who have lung cancer and other malignant diseases. While these guidelines also deal with general aspects of patient care, they are most important for prescribing the structures and processes required for the safe delivery of radiotherapy, which are not stipulated in more general cancer program guidelines.[97,98]

Standards for Acceptable Patient Volumes for Cancer Programs

The results of recent studies suggest that the outcomes of cancer may be better among patients who are treated at larger institutions.[99,100] The initial observations were made in the field of cancer surgery, in which many studies have shown an inverse association between surgical mortality and the number of operations performed in a given hospital or by a given surgeon. von Meyenfeldt et al.[99] recently performed a meta-analysis to explore the relationship between volume and outcome in the surgical treatment of lung cancer. The 19 studies that were included in the analysis proved to be very heterogeneous, particularly with respect to the definition of volume categories. However, pooled estimates showed a significantly lower surgical mortality in favor of larger hospitals (odds ratio, 0.71; 95% confidence interval [CI], 0.62–0.81) but no significant difference in terms of long-term survival (odds ratio, 0.93; 95% CI, 0.84–1.03). In a subsequent study of 4460 patients who underwent surgery for the treatment of lung cancer at 436 hospitals in the United States, Kozower and Stukenborg[100] compared three alternative measures of volume for evaluating the volume-outcome relationship. The authors found no significant association between hospital procedure volume and in-hospital mortality when volume was measured as a continuous variable. A significant relationship was found when volumes were categorized into quintiles, but the magnitude of the association was small. The authors concluded that the apparent impact of hospital volume on mortality is dependent on how volume is defined, that volume is not consistently related to mortality, and that volume should not be used as a proxy measure for the quality of surgery.[100] However, Lüchtenborg et al.[101] recently found a strong and significant association between institutional volume and survival in a study from England involving 134,293 patients who had been diagnosed with NSCLC between 2004 and 2008, of whom 12,862 (9.6%) underwent surgical resection. The authors found that rates of resection are higher at high-volume hospitals, where surgery is performed more often on patients who were older and had more comorbidities. Despite these findings, survival was significantly better at hospitals at which more than 150 surgical resections were performed each year than at those at which fewer than 70 surgical resections were performed each year (hazard ratio, 0.78; 95% CI, 0.67–0.90).

There have been far fewer studies investigating the impact of case volume on the outcomes of radiotherapy, but there are good reasons to expect that a similar relationship may be found, particularly in the context of complex types of treatment. Lee et al.[102] combined the results of two RTOG trials (RTOG 91-06 and RTOG 92-04) to address this question in the context of chemoradiation therapy for inoperable lung cancer. After controlling for other prognostic factors as much as possible, the investigators found significantly better survival among patients who were treated at institutions that enrolled five or more patients each year as compared with those who were treated at lower-volume centers (31% vs. 13% at 3 years). The magnitude of this volume effect did not diminish over the study period, and the authors concluded that collective institutional experience contributed more to the difference in outcome than the learning curve effect did. The investigators did not attempt to distinguish the effect of the experience of the individual oncologist from institutional experience.

These so-called volume effects are potentially very important. If they are real, they represent an extraordinary opportunity for improving the outcomes for patients with lung cancer. Intervention studies are now urgently required to confirm that limiting treatment to high-volume facilities improves overall outcomes. Further explanatory studies are also required to try to identify the underlying differences in care that are responsible for the differences in outcomes between low- and high-volume centers. If these causative factors can be identified, then it may be possible to develop strategies to increase the quality of care at smaller centers to the level provided at the larger centers, thus avoiding the need for centralization of services, which may come at the cost of decreased accessibility.

STANDARDS FOR THE ACCESSIBILITY OF CANCER MANAGEMENT PROGRAMS

Standards for Waiting Times

Delays in the diagnosis and treatment of cancer are distressing for every patient, and there is good evidence that delays in treatment also may have an adverse impact on long-term outcomes.[103,104] Long waiting times for radiotherapy and cancer surgery have been reported in many health systems since the late 1990s,[105,106] and many jurisdictions therefore have established standards or targets for maximum acceptable waiting times. Waiting times for cancer diagnosis and treatment may be regarded as indicators of the accessibility of care or as indicators of quality.[2] Some organizations have confined themselves to setting standards for waiting times between diagnosis and treatment.[105] Others have correctly recognized that even greater delays may precede the diagnosis and therefore also have set standards for the acceptable interval between the initial presentation and consultation with the appropriate specialist.[29,107] Once waiting time targets have been established, it is important to monitor compliance with those targets and to identify factors associated with delay. Cancer care is complex, and process mapping can help to identify rate-limiting steps in patient flow.[2] Redesign of systems then may be useful for reducing treatment delays.[2] However, no amount of fine-tuning of patient flows will have any impact on waiting times for treatment if the available resources are not sufficient to meet overall demand.[2,108] A recent study in the United Kingdom showed that the introduction of waiting time targets was associated with reduced delays in consultations with lung cancer specialists, but delays in treatment persisted, primarily because of a lack of capacity to meet the demand for radiotherapy and thoracic surgery.[107]

Standards for Rates of Treatment Utilization

A long waiting list is often a symptom of inadequate resources, but the length of a waiting list provides no information about the magnitude of the shortfall between supply and demand.[2] Furthermore, the absence of a waiting list does not mean that access is optimal. Waiting lists develop only in response to inadequate availability of services. Waiting times are entirely insensitive to problems with respect to spatial accessibility, affordability, or awareness, as already noted. Problems in those dimensions of

accessibility limit demand and actually may reduce or eliminate waiting lists.[2] Thus, the absence of a waiting list does not imply that access is optimal. To ensure appropriate access to care, it is therefore also necessary to set standards for, and monitor, rates of treatment utilization.[2]

The best quantitative measure of the accessibility of any service is the rate of its appropriate utilization, that is, the proportion of patients who actually receive the treatment that they need.[2] The term need is used here as defined by Cuyler,[109] who stated that "the need for medical care exists when an individual has an illness for which there is effective and acceptable treatment." Two objective methods have been developed for estimating the appropriate rate of treatment utilization for cancer: (1) evidence-based requirements analysis and (2) criterion-based benchmarking. Much of the early work on estimating appropriate rates of cancer treatment focused on radiotherapy, probably because of well-known and widespread problems in access to radiotherapy in the 1990s. However, these methods are readily applicable to other treatment modalities.

Methods for Setting Standards for Appropriate Rates of Treatment Utilization

Evidence-Based Requirements Analysis

Evidence-based requirements analysis is an objective method that may be used to estimate the need for any medical intervention or service. In the field of oncology, it was first used by Tyldesley et al.[110] to estimate the need for radiotherapy for lung cancer. The process was as follows: first, the indications for radiotherapy were identified by means of a systematic review; next, an epidemiologic approach was used to estimate how frequently each indication for radiotherapy occurs in the population of interest; and finally, the results of the systematic review and the epidemiologic analysis were combined to estimate the appropriate rate of utilization of radiotherapy for lung cancer. The strengths of the method are that all of the involved assumptions are explicit and that models can readily be adapted to reflect the case mix in any community of interest or to explore the implications of changes in the indications for radiotherapy. The main weaknesses of the approach are that it is complex and time-consuming and that the results are only as good as the information on which it is based. This method can be expected to produce valid results only when it is applied to major cancers for which the indications for radiotherapy are well defined and there is sufficient epidemiologic information available to estimate the frequency with which each indication occurs. Other investigators have since extended the use of this method to measure the need for radiotherapy across the entire spectrum of malignant disease, and it is now being widely used to predict requirements for radiotherapy equipment.[111]

Criterion-Based Benchmarking

An alternative way of estimating the appropriate rate of utilization of any treatment is to use a series of observations to derive a so-called benchmark. In the business world, benchmarking has been defined as "measuring products against the toughest competitors or those recognized as industry leaders."[112] Similarly, the rate of treatment use in privileged communities where there are no barriers to access to treatment may serve as benchmarks for the appropriate rate of utilization. This method was first used by Barbera et al.[113] to determine the appropriate rate of utilization of radiotherapy for lung cancer. In that original study from Ontario, benchmarks for the utilization of radiotherapy were set in counties where radiotherapy centers with short waiting times were located. This inductive method, grounded in observations in the real world, provides benchmarks that are demonstrably achievable and is unlikely to overestimate the need for treatment. The estimates of the appropriate rate of use of radiotherapy derived from the benchmarking approach were almost identical to those derived from evidence-based requirements analysis.[113] This cross validation suggested that either method may reasonably be used to set utilization targets and to plan treatment capacity. The simpler benchmarking approach has been adopted by the provincial cancer agency in Ontario and is used by the Cancer Quality Council of Ontario to evaluate the performance of the provincial radiotherapy system on an ongoing basis. Shortfalls in the rates of use of radiotherapy for lung cancer in relation to benchmarks are routinely mapped at the county level and are posted on the Internet (http://www.csqi.on.ca/all_indicators/#.UnxoyeJih-w).

BARRIERS TO THE OPTIMAL CARE OF PATIENTS WITH LUNG CANCER

One of the most consistent findings in health services research is the gap between evidence and practice.[114] Even if continuous efforts are made and substantial resources are invested to improve the quality of care, it is a regretful fact that only a limited fraction of novel evidence-based health-care interventions makes it into practice, and, even then, implementation can take many years. Studies in both the United States and Europe have shown that between 30% and 50% of patients fail to receive clinical interventions that are justified according to the best scientific evidence. Conversely, 20% to 25% or more of the care that is provided is not needed and may even be harmful. While the use of inappropriate treatment may have a negative impact on patient well-being or even survival, the inappropriate consumption of resources translates into further wasting of these limited resources and placing additional burdens on overloaded health services.[114,115]

The lack of implementation of guideline-recommended treatment is in line with the observation that passive dissemination of information generally has little or no effect in terms of altering professional practices. In order to accelerate the rate at which existing and new evidence on optimal care is implemented in health-related settings around the world, it is first necessary to identify the specific barriers to change and to develop systematic and strategic approaches to address these barriers.[116,117] The process of implementing evidence-based health innovations is complex and involves the interplay of many different factors and stakeholders. Several research groups have suggested a framework to categorize these factors.

Classification of Barriers to Optimal Care

The European Assessment Subgroup on Dissemination and Impact of Technology (EUR-ASSESS) Project[117] defined three categories of barriers: (1) environmental barriers, such as political climate, lobbying by special interest groups, cultural and professional practice characteristics, and financial disincentives; (2) personal characteristic barriers, such as perception of risk, clinical uncertainty, and information overload; and (3) prevailing opinion barriers, such as standards of professional practice and opinion leaders.

Haines et al.[115] described barriers situated in different environments. Some barriers are embedded within the health-care system itself, such as lack of resources, inappropriate financial incentives, inadequate human resources (in terms of both quantity and quality), and lack of access to care. Other barriers are external to the health-care system and are found within the practice environment (e.g., time limitations, poor practice organization), the educational environment (e.g., failure of curricula to reflect research evidence, inadequate continuing medical education), the social environment (e.g., inappropriate demands and/or beliefs created by the influence of the media), or the political environment (e.g., ideologic beliefs that may be inconsistent with research evidence or dominance of short-term thinking). Lastly, the introduction and implementation of optimal care may be hampered by the interaction between practitioners (who may be insufficiently knowledgeable or influenced by the beliefs and attitudes of opinion leaders) and patients (who may demand ineffective care on the basis of their preconceptions or cultural beliefs).

Chaudoir et al.[118] categorized factors that are expected to have an impact on the implementation of innovation into five distinct levels: structural, organizational, provider, innovation, and patient. The structural level encompasses a number of factors that represent the broader sociocultural and economic context in which a specific organization is nested. The organizational level involves aspects of the organization itself in which an innovation is being implemented. These aspects include leadership effectiveness, culture or climate, and employee morale or satisfaction. The provider level relates to individual health-care providers and covers attitudes toward evidence-based practice or perceived behavioral control. The innovation level deals with aspects of the innovation itself (e.g., the relative advantage of using an innovation rather than existing practices). The patient level includes patient characteristics such as health-relevant beliefs, motivation, and personality traits.

Regardless of how barriers are defined and organized, it is clear that, in order to promote change, we must take into account the specific social, organizational, and structural setting in which health-care professionals work and address the barriers at the different levels. The most successful examples of evidence and guideline implementation have acted on predisposing factors (e.g., knowledge and attitudes in the target group), enabling factors (e.g., capacity, resources, and availability of services), and reinforcing factors (e.g., opinions and behavior of others).[119] Moreover, the roles of all key players, including policymakers, the public, patients, and service providers alike, should be addressed.[115]

Barriers to Optimal Care: Case Studies From High-Income Countries

The first important barrier relates to the knowledge and beliefs of physicians who treat lung cancer. In the mid-1990s, a Canadian study showed how the beliefs of physicians regarding the natural history of NSCLC and the response to treatment varied widely and were strongly associated with their treatment recommendations.[120] As these physicians were in charge of therapy or treatment referral, it can be postulated that such variable perceptions may have an impact on the delivered care and, potentially, on prognosis. Another study analyzed survival estimates, treatment perceptions, and referral patterns for NSCLC on the basis of a survey of pulmonologists and thoracic surgeons in the United States. The results of the survey demonstrated both overestimation and underestimation of survival as well as considerably different beliefs regarding, for example, the benefit of radiotherapy for patients with stage I to stage III disease or the benefits of chemotherapy for those with metastatic disease. The authors found that a longer time interval since training and a lower volume of patients with NSCLC were associated with beliefs discordant with evidence-based recommendations.[121] A subsequent analysis from the same group focused on physician beliefs in comparison with guidelines. Although the authors found that the vast majority of American thoracic physicians consulted and used guidelines, there were some specific therapeutic areas—for example, the use of palliative chemotherapy for patients with metastatic NSCLC—in which their personal beliefs differed considerably from the evidence.[77]

Physician beliefs and therapeutic choices are but one small part of the total picture. Examples of the complex and multifactorial interplay that can hamper optimal lung cancer treatment have been described at all stages of the disease. A study from Auckland, New Zealand, analyzed reasons for delay in the diagnosis of lung cancer.[122] Apart from two central themes (access to health services and processes of care), issues related to symptom interpretation, health beliefs, provider continuity, relationships, and perceived expertise contributed to patient and general practitioner delay. System complexity, information, and resourcing issues were identified as barriers at the primary care–secondary care interface as well as within secondary care. At the other end of the spectrum, the authors found that many individuals with advanced-stage lung cancer who perceive pain resulting from both the disease and the treatment do not want to use analgesics because of personal concerns of addiction, the cost of treatment, or lack of recommendation of analgesics from their health-care providers.[123]

Studies in the United Kingdom have shown a relationship between the accessibility of oncology services and the chance of receiving a correct diagnosis and optimal care for lung cancer. In South East England, patients with lung cancer whose first hospital attendance was at a radiotherapy center were found to be more likely to receive active treatment, radiotherapy, and chemotherapy.[124] Similarly, in Northern England, living in a deprived region (as determined with the Index of Multiple Deprivation) reduced the likelihood of obtaining a histologic diagnosis and undergoing definitive treatment for lung cancer, with the exception of chemotherapy for the treatment of small cell lung cancer.[125] These findings were further strengthened by reduced access expressed in travel time to the health service.

Socioeconomic factors are known to play an important role in the implementation of optimal care, especially if new interventions are more costly and more resource-demanding than the existing strategies, which is often the case. Whereas a lack of resources typically translates into the use of fewer, less complex, less costly, and, potentially, less qualitative treatments, the opposite scenario—i.e., more frequent use of advanced technology and costly and potentially inappropriate treatments—is found if resources are abundant.

At the individual level, physicians tend to adapt their clinical behavior to the reimbursement offered, more or less independently from the available resources.[126] If reimbursement lags behind the development of innovative treatments, which is typically the case in many European countries, the uptake of these new treatments will be hampered, even if effectiveness is proven. In contrast to data on clinical outcomes, there is often less evidence on cost-effectiveness, global budgetary impact, cultural appropriateness, and effects on health inequalities, all of which are important considerations at the macro level of health policy-making and financing.[115,127]

Barriers to Optimal Care in Low- and Middle-Income Countries

Whereas socioeconomic determinants already play a role in high-income countries, it seems evident that they have an even larger impact on health-care delivery in low- and middle-income countries. The lack of resources (e.g., to purchase medicines or to invest in radiotherapy facilities) typically represents a more important barrier in low-income countries than in most high-income settings. Besides purely financial factors, additional challenges to the use of research evidence, such as the weakness of health systems with unregulated commercial interests, the lack of professional regulation and continuing professional development, and limited access to research evidence, are found in low- and middle-income countries.[128]

Radiotherapy, one of the core modalities of lung cancer treatment, is a resource-demanding specialty and, consequently, is highly sensitive to the economic status of the country or region. An analysis of the data for 33 countries that were registered in the Directory of Radiotherapy Centers database, administered by the International Atomic Energy Agency, showed how a lower economic status, expressed as gross national income per capita, translates into a higher throughput on the machines and a relative shortage in equipment.[129] This finding is in line with the earlier observation, from the European Society for Radiotherapy and Oncology–Quantification of radiation therapy infrastructure and staffing needs (ESTRO-QUARTS) project, that guidelines for machine requirements recommend, on the average, 1 accelerator per 183,000 inhabitants in high-resource countries, compared with only 1 per 500,000 in low-resource countries.[130] Even if both examples disregard epidemiologic needs and the impact of treatment complexity, the findings suggest that, in some countries referrals for radiotherapy may be more difficult to accomplish than in other countries. Moreover, the adoption of today's standard of care in radiotherapy, requiring optimal imaging equipment and treatment machines as well as highly educated personnel, may become problematic. A patterns-of-care study in Spain showed how limitations in technology and infrastructure in the Spanish health-care system delayed the uptake of evidence-based practices related to the use of radiotherapy for lung cancer.[131] Similarly, variations in the use of specific diagnostic and treatment modalities related to radiotherapy for lung cancer in Central and Eastern European countries have been traced to shortages in equipment and the need for educational support for health-care providers in these countries.[132]

Do Variations in Patterns of Care Affect the Outcomes of Lung Cancer?

Lung cancer is the most common type of cancer worldwide. In 2012, there were an estimated 1.8 million new cases of lung cancer, representing 12.9% of all new cancers. Lung cancer is also the most important cause of cancer-related death, leading to an estimated 1.59 million deaths annually and representing 19.4% of the total cancer-related mortality.[133] The highest rates are seen in Central-Eastern and Southern Europe, Northern America, and Eastern Asia, with still very low rates in Middle Africa and Western Africa.[133] However, over the past decades, a geographic shift has occurred in terms of the absolute numbers of cases of lung cancer. Whereas in the middle of the last century lung cancer typically was a disease affecting those in industrialized countries, today 55% of the cases occur in developing regions. There is often a different pattern for men and women. In Europe, for instance, the incidence is highest among men in Central and Eastern European countries such as Hungary, Macedonia, Serbia, and Poland, and the incidence is lowest in Northern European countries, such as Finland and Sweden. The reverse holds for women, with the rates being higher in Northern Europe (e.g., Denmark and the Netherlands) and lower in Eastern Europe (e.g., Ukraine and Belarus).[134]

Because of the high fatality of lung cancer—the ratio of mortality to incidence is 0.86—with very little variability in cure rates in developed and developing countries, geographic patterns of mortality are quite similar to those of incidence.[133,134] This finding seems to suggest, at least at the macro level, that patterns of care do not have a substantial impact on the survival of patients with lung cancer. However, at the micro level (i.e., within countries or even regions), differences in care have been described, resulting in differences in outcomes.

Two studies from the Netherlands demonstrated that treatment, especially surgical intervention and the use of chemoradiation therapy for stage III NSCLC, varied by region.[76,135] Although the surgery rate tended to be higher in specialized centers or higher-volume hospitals, the variation among individual hospitals was much more distinct, suggesting that hospital characteristics per se are no guarantee of optimal treatment. Regardless of the type of hospital, however, more aggressive treatment translated into better survival.

A similar strong link between dissemination of optimal care and survival was found in a Dutch study on stereotactic ablative radiotherapy (SABR) for early-stage NSCLC in older patients. Between

1999 and 2007, before and after the introduction of SABR, an absolute increase in radiotherapy use was seen in the Amsterdam region, along with a decline in the proportion of untreated older patients and an improvement in overall survival in this population.[136] This example demonstrated how a well-structured and unobstructed introduction of a therapeutic innovation can translate into a substantial improvement in outcome. Unfortunately, as described previously, many countries in Europe currently do not have the necessary resources to support the wide dissemination of SABR, even for a proven indication such as inoperable early-stage NSCLC.[129,130] The delayed uptake of actual state-of-the-art radiotherapy techniques and the variation among countries in this regard have both been related to economic factors.[131,132]

CONCLUSION

Achieving optimal outcomes for patients with lung cancer requires that every patient receive optimal treatment. However, as we have shown, there is abundant evidence that many patients do not receive optimal treatment or experience optimal outcomes. Deviations from optimal treatment may be due to resource limitations that compromise the accessibility of treatment, to errors in clinical decision-making, or to flaws in the implementation of treatment decisions.

Problems in the accessibility of treatment may be the inevitable consequence of the low levels of health funding available in low- and middle-income countries, but they also may be due to suboptimal planning of treatment services or to the inequitable distribution of those services in high-income nations. Health services research has provided methods for needs-based system planning, which permit the design of health systems that will fully meet the needs of patients with lung cancer in high-income nations, and which also may be used to design health systems that will, as far as economically possible, meet the needs of patients in low- and middle-income countries. Health services research has demonstrated the importance of ongoing auditing of access to treatment as a way of identifying underutilization of effective treatments for lung cancer. It has also been valuable for identifying vulnerable subgroups of patients who are most likely to experience problems in obtaining access to treatment.

There is good evidence that clinical decision-making in cases of lung cancer is not always optimal. It has been shown that the treatment that patients with lung cancer receive is only concordant with evidence-based guidelines in about 50% of cases. Furthermore, some evidence indicates that such deviations may be associated with inferior outcomes. The reasons for deviation from guidelines are complex, but the personal beliefs of physicians about optimal care vary widely and discipline bias may have a substantial effect on their individual treatment recommendations. Evidence suggests that MDT management effectively overcomes discipline bias and is associated with increased compliance with evidence-based guidelines, resulting in better outcomes. Although the results of MDT management are very promising, the optimal structure and process of the team remain to be defined and the cost-effectiveness of this approach still needs to be established. Deviations from guidelines do not always mean that patients are receiving suboptimal treatment. Today's guidelines may not adequately take into consideration the overall health status or the personal values and preferences of the patient. Physicians and patients therefore may have cogent reasons for choosing to deviate from guidelines. There is a need for the development of guidelines that more fully reflect the wide variation in the health status of patients with lung cancer as well as for the wider use of decision aids that explicitly factor patient values into treatment decisions.

Factors affecting the quality of treatment delivery have been less extensively studied, but there is evidence that the outcome of surgery for lung cancer may depend on the level of experience

of the institution or the individual surgeon. This so-called volume effect still requires further study, but it does suggest that the experience and skill of the health-care team may affect the quality of care and hence the outcomes achieved. There are good reasons to extend this research beyond the field of surgery to determine whether the outcomes of other technically challenging interventions, including modern radiotherapy techniques, are also volume-dependent.

Health services research has identified many ways in which the outcomes of lung cancer can be improved by making better use of existing knowledge, technology, and resources, and we believe that research aimed at optimization of health system performance should be a high priority within any overall program of lung cancer research.

KEY REFERENCES

2. Mackillop WJ. Health services research in radiation oncology. In: Gunderson LL, Tepper JE, eds. *Clinical Radiation Oncology*. 3rd ed. Philadelphia, PA: Elsevier; 2012:203–222.
5. Aday LA, Begley C, Larson DR, Slater CH. *Evaluating the health care system: effectiveness, efficiency, and equity*. Chicago: Health Administration Press; 1998.
6. Penchansky R, Thomas JW. The concept of access: definition and relationship to consumer satisfaction. *Med Care*. 1981;19(2):127–140.
7. Donabedian A. Evaluating the quality of medical care. *Milbank Mem Fund Q*. 1966;44(3 Suppl):166–206.
14. Sackett DL, Rosenberg WM, Gray JA, Haynes RB, Richardson WS. Evidence based medicine: what it is and what it isn't. *BMJ*. 1996;312(7023):71–72.
18. Cochrane AL. *Effectiveness and efficiency: random reflections on health services*. London, UK: Nuffield Provincial Hospitals Trust; 1972.
20. Graham R, Mancher M, Wolman DM, Greenfield S, Steinberg E, eds. *Clinical practice guidelines we can trust*. Washington, DC: The National Academies Press; 2011.
21. Committee of Ministers of the Council of Europe. Developing a methodology for drawing up guidelines on best medical recommendation. http://www.leitlinien.de/mdb/edocs/pdf/literatur/coerec-2001-13.pdf.
22. American Society of Clinical Oncology. Lung cancer guidelines http://www.asco.org/guidelines/lung-cancer.
35. Brundage MD, Davidson JR, Mackillop WJ. Trading treatment toxicity for survival in locally advanced non-small cell lung cancer. *J Clin Oncol*. 1997;15(1):330–340.
36. Mackillop WJ, Stewart WE. Ginsburg AD, Stewart SS. Cancer patients' perceptions of their disease and its treatment. *Br J Cancer*. 1988;58(3):355–358.
39. Brundage MD, Feldman-Stewart D, Cosby R, et al. Phase I study of a decision aid for patients with locally advanced non–small-cell lung cancer. *J Clin Oncol*. 2001;19(5):1326–1335.
41. Brundage MD, Feldman-Stewart D, Dixon P, et al. A treatment trade-off based decision aid for patients with locally advanced non-small cell lung cancer. *Health Expect*. 2000;3(1):55–68.
42. American Society of Clinical Oncology. Decision aid. Stage IV non-small cell lung cancer (NSCLC) first-line-chemotherapy. http://www.asco.org/sites/www.asco.org/files/nsclc_first_line_decision_aid_11.12.09_0.pdf.
47. Lomas J, Anderson GM, Domnick-Pierre K, Vayda E, Enkin MW, Hannah WJ. Do practice guidelines guide practice? The effect of a consensus statement on the practice of physicians. *N Engl J Med*. 1989;321(19):1306–1311.
48. Vinod SK, Sidhom MA, Delaney GP. Do multidisciplinary meetings follow guideline-based care? *J Oncol Pract*. 2010;6(6):276–281.
50. Potosky AL, Saxman S, Wallace RB, Lynch CF. Population variations in the initial treatment of non-small-cell lung cancer. *J Clin Oncol*. 2004;22(16):3261–3268.
53. Duggan K, Vinod SK, Yeo A. Treatment patterns for lung cancer in South Western Sydney, Australia. Do patients get treated according to guidelines? *J Thorac Oncol*. 2011;6:S1447.
57. Salloum RG, Smith TJ, Jensen GA, Lafata JE. Factors associated with adherence to chemotherapy guidelines in patients with non-small cell lung cancer. *Lung Cancer*. 2012;75(2):255–260.

58. Langer CJ, Moughan J, Movsas B, et al. Patterns of care survey (PCS) in lung cancer: how well does current U.S. practice with chemotherapy in the non-metastatic setting follow the literature? *Lung Cancer.* 2005;48(1):93–102.

65. Booth CM, Mackillop WJ. Translating new medical therapies into societal benefit: the role of population-based outcome studies. *JAMA.* 2008;300(18):2177–2179.

66. Booth CM, Shepherd FA, Peng Y, et al. Adoption of adjuvant chemotherapy for non-small cell lung cancer: a population-based outcomes study. *J Clin Oncol.* 2010;28(21):3472–3478.

79. Mackillop WJ, O'Sullivan B, Ward GK. Non-small cell lung cancer: how oncologists want to be treated. *Int J Radiat Oncol Biol Phys.* 1987;13(6):929–934.

82. Erridge SC, Murray B, Price A, et al. Improved treatment and survival for lung cancer patients in South-East Scotland. *J Thoracic Oncol.* 2008;3(5):491–498.

85. Bydder S, Nowak A, Marion K, Phillips M, Atun R. The impact of case discussion at a multidisciplinary team meeting on the treatment and survival of patients with inoperable non-small cell lung cancer. *Intern Med J.* 2009;39(12):838–841.

86. Boxer MM, Vinod SK, Shafiq J, Duggan KJ. Do multidisciplinary team meetings make a difference in the management of lung cancer? *Cancer.* 2011;117(22):5112–5120.

89. Osarogiagbon RU, Phelps G, McFarlane J, Bankole O. Causes and consequences of deviation from multidisciplinary care in thoracic oncology. *J Thoracic Oncol.* 2011;6(3):510–516.

91. Hermens RP, Ouwens MM, Vonk-Okhuijsen SY, et al. Development of quality indicators for diagnosis and treatment of patients with non-small cell lung cancer: a first step toward implementing a multidisciplinary, evidence-based guideline. *Lung Cancer.* 2006;54(1):117–124.

92. Ouwens MM, Hermens RR, Termeer RA, et al. Quality of integrated care for patients with nonsmall cell lung cancer: variations and determinants of care. *Cancer.* 2007;110(8):1782–1790.

99. von Meyenfeldt EM, Gooiker GA, van Gijn W, et al. The relationship between volume or surgeon specialty and outcome in the surgical treatment of lung cancer: A systematic review and meta-analysis. *J Thorac Oncol.* 2012;7(7):1170–1178.

103. Chen Z, King W, Pearcey R, Kerba M, Mackillop WJ. The relationship between waiting time for radiotherapy and clinical outcomes: a systematic review of the literature. *Radiother Oncol.* 2008;87(1):3–16.

104. Mackillop WJ. Killing time: the consequences of delays in radiotherapy. *Radiother Oncol.* 2007;84(1):1–4.

110. Tyldesley S, Boyd C, Schulze K, Walker H, Mackillop WJ. Estimating the need for radiotherapy for lung cancer: an evidence-based, epidemiologic approach. *Int J Radiat Oncol Biol Phys.* 2001;49(4): 973–985.

113. Barbera L, Zhang-Salomons J, Huang J, Tyldesley S, Mackillop W. Defining the need for radiotherapy for lung cancer in the general population: a criterion-based, benchmarking approach. *Med Care.* 2003;41(9):1074–1085.

120. Raby B, Pater J, Mackillop WJ. Does knowledge guide practice? Another look at the management of non-small-cell lung cancer. *J Clin Oncol.* 1995;13(8):1904–1911.

125. Crawford SM, Sauerzapf V, Haynes R, Zhao H, Forman D, Jones AP. Social and geographical factors affecting access to treatment of lung cancer. *Br J Cancer.* 2009;101(6):897–901.

129. Rosenblatt E, Izewska J, Anacak Y, et al. Radiotherapy capacity in European countries: an analysis of the Directory of Radiotherapy Centres (DIRAC) database. *Lancet Oncol.* 2013;14(2):e79–e86.

130. Slotman B, Cottier B, Bentzen S, Heeren G, Lievens Y, van den Bogaert W. Overview of national guidelines for infrastructure and staffing of radiotherapy. ESTRO-QUARTS: work package 1. *Radiother Oncol.* 2005;75(3):349–354.

134. Ferlay J, Steliarova-Foucher E, Lortet-Tieulent J, et al. Cancer incidence and mortality patterns in Europe: estimates for 40 countries in 2012. *Eur J Cancer.* 2013;49(6):1374–1403.

135. Li WW, Visser O, Ubbink DT, Klomp HM, Kloek JJ, de Mol BA. The influence of provider characteristics on resection rates and survival in patients with localized non-small cell lung cancer. *Lung Cancer.* 2008;60(3):441–451.

See Expertconsult.com for full list of references.

Diagnostic Algorithms

Thomas Hensing, Isa Mambetsariev, Nicholas Campbell, and Ravi Salgia

SUMMARY OF KEY POINTS

- Mind maps are used as a tool to illustrate the principles involved in the diagnostic evaluation of a patient with known or suspected lung cancer.
- Addressed are factors important in establishing the diagnosis and defining the extent of disease; the histologic and molecular classifications of lung cancer; and the potential role for repeat biopsy in patients with acquired resistance to targeted therapies.
- Reviewed are diagnostic platforms for tumor profiling in the clinical setting and the use of these technologies in the noninvasive evaluation of surrogate tissues for both disease monitoring and early diagnosis.

The personalized treatment of lung cancer begins with an accurate diagnosis and assessment of both the extent of disease and other clinically relevant prognostic and predictive factors that are necessary to define the optimal treatment approach. Treatment decision making relies on a number of both patient- and tumor-specific factors. Lung cancer is a heterogeneous disease, and recent advances in molecular analysis and the development of targeted therapy approaches have added to the complexity of the diagnostic evaluation. In addition, revisions in the staging system, changes in the pathologic classification, and the addition of minimally invasive diagnostic modalities have increased the importance of a coordinated multidisciplinary team approach to establish both the diagnosis and the tumor stage as efficiently as possible.[1–4]

Mind mapping was developed as a technique to visually represent ideas and their nonlinear relationships.[5] Mind maps have been used as teaching tools in a number of different fields, including medical education, to present complex information and improve recall.[5,6] Originally developed by Tony Buzan, a mind map starts with a central idea or key concept, which is then linked by branches to related ideas. Mind maps include color and pictures to illustrate the intra- and inter-relationship between ideas. Unlike a linear algorithm or a concept map, a mind map begins with a central idea, and its relationships are depicted radially (i.e., radial or spider map). The information is organized hierarchically, with the most general information at the center and more detailed information depicted at the extremes of each relationship branch.

In this appendix, we use mind maps as a tool to illustrate the principles involved in the diagnostic evaluation of a patient with known or suspected lung cancer. The initial mind maps address the factors that are important in establishing the diagnosis and defining the extent of disease. Because of the growing importance of targeted therapies, we use this technique to illustrate both the histologic and molecular classifications of lung cancer. In addition, we address the potential role for repeat biopsy in patients with acquired resistance to targeted therapies. Lastly, we use mind maps to review diagnostic platforms for tumor profiling in the clinical setting and to assess the potential to use these technologies in the noninvasive evaluation of surrogate tissues for both disease monitoring and early diagnosis.

INITIAL EVALUATION

History and Physical

Fig. A.1 includes a mind map that outlines the factors that are important to address during the initial history and physical examination of a patient suspected of having lung cancer. The objectives of the initial evaluation are to estimate the probability that lung cancer is present and to assess for evidence of distant metastatic disease.[7] In addition, the initial evaluation should clarify patient-specific factors that may affect treatment decision making

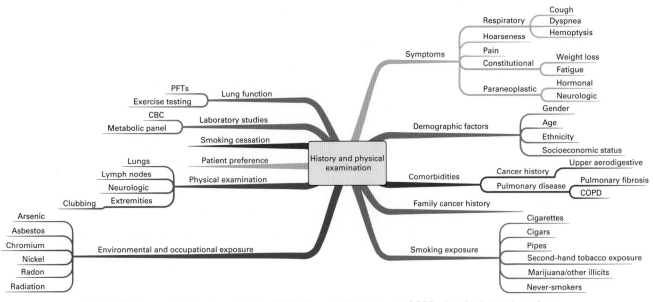

Fig. A.1. History and physical examination. *CBC,* Complete blood count; *COPD,* chronic obstructive pulmonary disease; *PFTs,* pulmonary function tests.

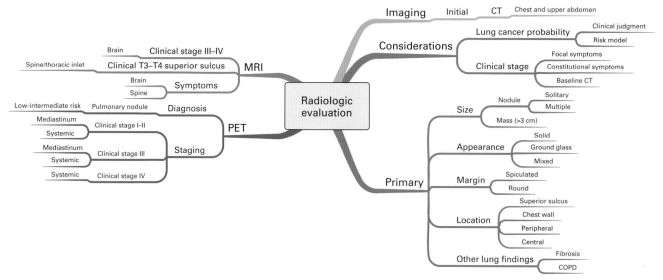

Fig. A.2. Radiographic evaluation of lung cancer. *COPD,* Chronic obstructive pulmonary disease; *CT,* computed tomography; *MRI,* magnetic resonance imaging; *PET,* positron emission tomography.

if cancer is confirmed, including comorbidities, performance status, underlying lung function, and the patient's values and goals.

The initial risk assessment for lung cancer includes an evaluation of symptoms. Most patients with lung cancer will have symptoms at presentation.[7] Symptoms may be due to the primary tumor or due to regional or distant spread of disease. Constitutional symptoms, including weight loss or fatigue, are important to consider because they may reflect an advanced stage of lung cancer. Several paraneoplastic syndromes have also been described, each with potentially unique clinical manifestations. Early recognition of a paraneoplastic process is important to minimize the risk for long-term morbidity and mortality.[7]

The most common risk factor for lung cancer remains tobacco smoking. Lung cancer is 10 to 20 times more likely to develop in individuals with a history of smoking than in persons who have never smoked.[8] The individual risk is affected by age as well as the duration and intensity of smoking.[9] Lung cancer develops in only a minority of smokers, however, so inherited factors may also play a role in lung cancer risk. Other environmental and occupational exposures are also important to consider (see Fig. A.1).[10] For example, pollution is increasingly being recognized as a risk factor for lung cancer.[11] Important personal risk factors include age, gender, ethnicity, socioeconomic status, and comorbidities, including acquired lung disease.[10] Although more men than women will die of lung cancer, the gender gap is narrowing, and lung cancer is the leading cause of cancer-related mortality among women in the United States.[12] Although the rates of lung cancer are similar for black and white women, the incidence of lung cancer is higher among black men than among white men.[12] Both the incidence of and mortality from lung cancer are higher in populations of lower socioeconomic status.[13,14]

Radiographic Evaluation

Fig. A.2 is a mind map that illustrates the radiologic evaluation. All patients should have initial computed tomography (CT) of the chest and upper abdomen that extends through the adrenal glands.[7,15] The decision to pursue additional imaging for diagnosis and staging depends on both the estimated risk of lung cancer and the initial clinical stage. When patients have focal symptoms suggestive of metastatic disease, directed imaging (e.g., magnetic resonance imaging of the spine or brain) is recommended for confirmation. The radiographic characteristics of the primary abnormality in the lung that affect the risk assessment include the size, radiographic appearance, margin, and location of this lesion,

as well as any underlying lung disease or additional lesions.[16] Positron emission tomography (PET) is used in the diagnostic evaluation to characterize pulmonary nodules considered to be at low to intermediate risk for lung cancer.[17] PET is not recommended to characterize abnormalities considered to be at high risk for lung cancer.[17] However, PET is frequently recommended for mediastinal and systemic staging in most patients, including patients with early (stage I–II), locally advanced (stage IIIA–IIIB), and metastatic (stage IV) disease. In addition to PET, magnetic resonance imaging of the brain is frequently recommended for staging of patients with clinical stage III or IV disease.[4,15]

Invasive Diagnosis

Options for tissue confirmation of the lung cancer diagnosis are outlined in Fig. A.3. Important considerations before pursuing biopsy include the probability of lung cancer and the estimated clinical stage, as well as the feasibility, risk, diagnostic yield, and the potential to obtain adequate tissue for both histologic confirmation and molecular analysis. Patient-specific factors outlined previously are also important to consider, including performance status, comorbidities, pulmonary function, and the patient's values and goals. Given the complexity of treatment decision making, multidisciplinary tumor boards are generally recommended, if available, to help coordinate the diagnostic plan.

The most important principle is to take a biopsy specimen from the most distant site of disease to confirm both diagnosis and stage.[16] If obtaining this type of specimen is not considered feasible or safe, but the patient has a high likelihood of distant metastatic disease on the basis of clinical presentation and imaging, then a biopsy specimen of the safest site is generally recommended. Solitary abnormalities at a distant metastatic site evident on PET images warrant tissue confirmation because false-positive imaging will affect both treatment planning and intent. Likewise, clinical stage III disease should be confirmed by pathologic analysis. Mediastinoscopy remains the criterion standard for pathologic confirmation of N2 and N3 disease. However, image-guided needle techniques, including endobronchial ultrasound-guided transbronchial needle aspiration and endoscopic ultrasound-guided biopsy, are increasingly being recognized as valid alternatives to mediastinoscopy for mediastinal staging.[4]

If a patient is considered to have an early stage (I–II) lung cancer, a thoracic surgery evaluation should be pursued before a needle biopsy is performed for tissue confirmation because resection could be used as the primary means of both diagnosis

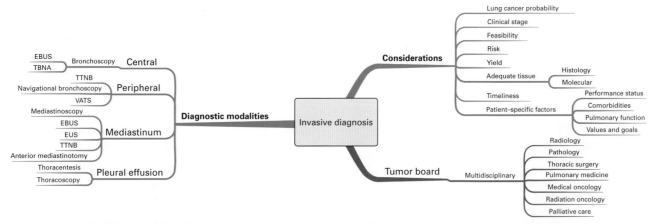

Fig. A.3. Invasive diagnosis and staging of lung cancer. *EBUS,* Endobronchial ultrasound; *EUS,* endoscopic ultrasound; *TBNA,* transbronchial needle aspiration; *TTNB,* transthoracic needle biopsy; *VATS,* video-assisted thoracoscopic surgery.

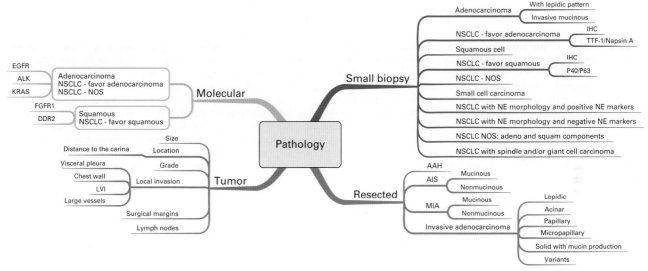

Fig. A.4. Pathology of lung cancer. *AAH,* Atypical adenomatous hyperplasia; *AIS,* adenocarcinoma in situ; *ALK,* anaplastic lymphoma kinase; *DDR2,* discoidin domain-containing receptor 2; *EGFR,* epidermal growth factor receptor; *FGFR,* fibroblast growth factor receptor; *IHC,* immunohistochemistry; *KRAS,* Kirsten rat sarcoma viral oncogene homolog; *LVI,* lymphovascular invasion; *MIA,* minimally invasive adenocarcinoma; *NE,* neuroendocrine; *NOS,* not otherwise specified; *NSCLC,* nonsmall cell lung cancer; *TTF-1,* thyroid transcription factor-1.

and treatment. If that patient is not considered a surgical candidate because of comorbidities, poor underlying lung function, or unwillingness to have an operation, then tissue confirmation should be pursued. The specific procedure will depend on tumor location as well as the other factors indicated earlier (see Fig. A.3).

PATHOLOGIC CLASSIFICATION OF LUNG CANCER

Tumor Histology

In 2011, the International Association for the Study of Lung Cancer, the American Thoracic Society, and the European Respiratory Society published a new pathologic classification system for lung cancer.[2,3] This new system is separated into two components by the method in which the tissue was obtained; standardized diagnostic criteria are provided for small biopsy specimens and cytologic specimens as well as for resected specimens. A mind map shows this new classification system (Fig. A.4). Most patients will have advanced disease at presentation, and the diagnosis will be confirmed by evaluation of a small biopsy specimen. Given the therapeutic implications, emphasis is placed on

establishing the specific histologic subtype, including adenocarcinoma, squamous cell carcinoma, and small cell carcinoma. The previous designation of large cell neuroendocrine carcinoma is now classified as nonsmall cell lung cancer (NSCLC) with neuroendocrine morphology and positive or negative neuroendocrine markers. For those tumors without classic morphologic features, the new system includes recommendations for limited special stains to determine the subtype of carcinoma beyond NSCLC, not otherwise specified. If an adenocarcinoma marker is positive (e.g., thyroid transcription factor-1), then the tumor is classified as NSCLC-favor adenocarcinoma, and if a squamous cell marker is positive (e.g., p40), then the tumor is classified as NSCLC-favor squamous cell carcinoma.

For resected specimens, the term bronchioloalveolar cell carcinoma has been discontinued, and the terms adenocarcinoma in situ and minimally invasive adenocarcinoma have been added.[3] Both of these adenocarcinomas are defined as small tumors (3 cm or less) with a lepidic growth pattern. Minimally invasive adenocarcinoma includes tumors with no more than 5 mm of invasion. Larger tumors with more than 5 mm of invasion are designated as invasive adenocarcinoma, and the subtype is determined based on the predominant growth pattern.[3] In validation studies, the proposed subtyping contained in this new system was shown to have prognostic significance.[18–20] In addition to the histologic subtype, the reporting of resected tumors should include descriptions of the size, location, grade, margins, pleural involvement, lymphovascular invasion, and lymph node involvement by station.[21]

Molecular Classification

This IASLC/ATS/ERS pathologic classification system also emphasizes the importance of molecular testing based on tumor histology.[3] An institutional multidisciplinary strategy for obtaining and processing small biopsy specimens should be established to make sure that sufficient tissue is available for both histologic classification and molecular analysis. Given the clinical validation of mutations in the epidermal growth factor receptor (EGFR) and translocations of anaplastic lymphoma kinase (ALK) as therapeutic targets, current guidelines from the American Society of Clinical Oncology and the National Comprehensive Cancer Network, as well as a joint guideline from the College of American Pathologists, International Association for the Study of Lung Cancer, and the Association for Molecular Pathology, recommend testing adenocarcinoma of the lung for these two markers at diagnosis before selecting patients for directed therapy.[22–24]

Fig. A.5 is a mind map that illustrates the molecular classification of adenocarcinoma of the lung. In addition to EGFR mutations and ALK translocations, increasing numbers of other so-called driver mutations and gene fusions have been described.[25–27] Given the limited overlap, these molecular alterations define unique subsets of lung adenocarcinoma and can potentially be used to select patients with advanced adenocarcinoma of the lung for molecularly targeted therapy as well as targeted immunotherapy indicated by increased activity of PD-1/PD-L1 pathway inhibitors.[28] Investigators from the Clinical Lung Cancer Genome Project and Network Genomic Medicine (CLCGP/NGM) characterized genome alterations in 1255 clinically annotated lung tumors.[25] Overall, more than 55% of the tumors had at least one genomic alteration

that was potentially amenable to targeted therapy. The pattern of genomic alterations differed among histologic subsets. This mind map includes an illustration of the genomic alterations that were relatively common in lung adenocarcinoma.

In addition to clinically validated genomic alterations that can be used to guide treatment selection, the recently reported KEYNOTE-024 trial validated PD-L1 protein expression by immunohistochemistry (IHC)[29,30] to guide the selection of an immune checkpoint inhibitor in the first line treatment of patients with advanced squamous and nonsquamous NSCLC. In the KEYNOTE-024 trial, 305 patients, with previously untreated advanced NSCLC with PD-L1 expression on at least 50% of tumor cells and no sensitizing mutations of EGFR or ALK translocations, were randomly assigned to receive either pembrolizumab at a fixed dose of 200 mg every 3 weeks or the investigator's choice of platinum-based chemotherapy.[28] The results of this randomized study showed a marked improvement in the median progression-free survival of 10.3 months for the pembrolizumab arm versus 6.0 months for patients treated with platinum-based chemotherapy (hazard ratio [HR] for disease progression or death, 0.50; 95% confidence interval (CI), 0.37–0.68; $p < 0.001$). The estimated rate of overall survival at 6 months also favored pembrolizumab with a rate of 80.2% versus 72.4% in the chemotherapy group (HR, 0.60; 95% C, 0.41–0.89; $p = 0.005$). This was further accentuated by a higher response rate of 44.8% in the pembrolizumab group compared to 27.8% in the chemotherapy group. Patients in the pembrolizumab arm also experienced fewer treatment-related adverse events of any grade as well as a less frequent occurrence of high-grade (grade III–V) treatment-related adverse events. The results of this study recently led to the U.S. Food and Drug Administration approval of pembrolizumab as first line therapy for patients with metastatic NSCLC whose tumors have high PD-L1 expression (Tumor Proportion Score (TPS) greater than or equal to 50%) and no EGFR or ALK genomic tumor alterations.[28]

Although no molecular targets for squamous cell carcinoma or small cell lung cancer have yet been validated, the genomic

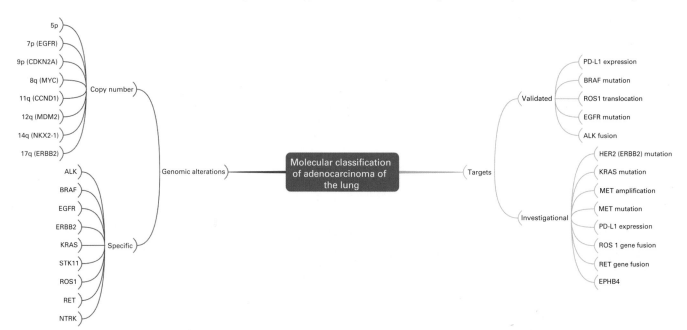

Fig. A.5. Molecular classification of adenocarcinoma of the lung. *ALK,* Anaplastic lymphoma kinase; *BRAF,* v-raf murine sarcoma viral oncogene homolog B; *CCND1,* cyclin D1; *CDKN2A,* cyclin-dependent kinase inhibitor 2A; *EGFR,* epidermal growth factor receptor; *HER2,* ERBB2 (v-erb-b2 avian erythroblastic leukemia viral oncogene homolog 2; *MDM2,* MDM2 oncogene, *E3* ubiquitin protein ligase; *MET,* MET proto-oncogene; *MYC,* v-myc avian myelocytomatosis viral oncogene homolog; *NKX2-1,* NK2 homeobox 1; *PD-L1,* programmed cell death 1 ligand 1; *RET,* ret proto-oncogene; *ROS,* c-ros oncogene 1; *STK11,* serine/threonine kinase 11.

characterization of both tumor histologies has recently been described.[31–34] This information has led to clinical trials evaluating molecular therapeutics for both tumor types. Mind maps are useful to illustrate the genomic alterations found in squamous cell carcinoma (Fig. A.6) and small cell carcinoma (Fig. A.7) of the lung, as reported in the genomic data set.[25] Both mind maps include examples of potential therapeutic targets, some of which are being evaluated in ongoing clinical trials.

In a prospective testing of the CLCGP/NGM genomics-based diagnostic algorithm,[28] genomic testing was feasible in 75% of paraffin-embedded tumor samples obtained by routine diagnostic procedures from 5145 patients with lung cancer.[28] In a multivariate analysis controlling for tumor stage and histology, the patients whose tumors had been successfully genotyped had an improvement in overall survival ($p = 0.002$) compared with patients for whom a genetic diagnosis was not feasible.[25] The improvement in survival is most likely due to improved outcomes among patients treated with molecularly selected kinase inhibitors. Although this study was not randomized, this observation supports the routine incorporation of molecular testing in the diagnosis of lung cancer for the clinical selection of patients for targeted therapy.

Repeat Biopsy for Acquired Resistance

Both intrinsic (de novo) and acquired resistance can complicate the treatment of patients with a targeted tyrosine kinase inhibitor (TKI). Acquired resistance to an EGFR inhibitor has been defined as systemic progression of disease (by Response Evaluation Criteria in Solid Tumors [RECIST] or World Health Organization [WHO] criteria) while receiving treatment with an EGFR TKI within the past 30 days in a patient whose tumor has a sensitive EGFR mutation or in a patient who had objective clinical benefit from therapy (defined as partial or complete response or more than 6 months of stable disease).[35] Potential mechanisms of resistance for both EGFR-, ROS1, and ALK-selected therapy have been described and can either be present at baseline or evolve by selective pressure during therapy.[36–39] These mechanisms of resistance for EGFR-, ROS1- and ALK-directed therapy, including include alterations in the molecular target, activation of accessory pathways, impairment in apoptotic pathways (e.g., BIM), and histologic transformation (Fig. A.8). Identification of the resistance mechanism by repeat biopsy offers the potential to identify another therapeutic target that may improve clinical outcome. In reported series, repeat biopsies to reassess the tumor histology and genomic profile have been shown to be feasible and safe.[40,41] As strategies to overcome de novo and acquired resistance become validated, repeat biopsies will likely become a standard component of the long-term management of disease in this patient population.

Molecular Diagnostic Platforms

Since the clinical validation of EGFR mutations and ALK translocations as therapeutic targets, the number of diagnostic platforms available for genomic profiling of lung cancer has increased

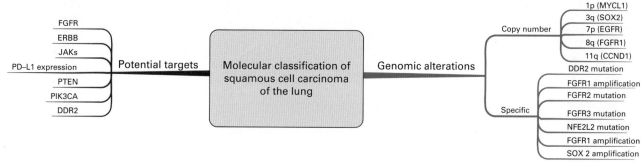

Fig. A.6. Molecular classification of squamous cell carcinoma of the lung. *CCND1,* cyclin D1; *DDR2,* discoidin domain-containing receptor 2; *EGFR,* epidermal growth factor receptor; *ERBB,* v-erb-b2 avian erythroblastic leukemia viral oncogene homolog; *FGFR,* fibroblast growth factor receptor; *JAK,* Janus kinase; *MYCL1,* L-myc-1 proto-oncogene; *NFE2L2,* nuclear factor-like 2; *PD-L1,* programmed death-ligand 1; *PIK3CA,* phosphatidylinositol-4,5-bisphosphate 3-kinase, catalytic subunit alpha; *PTEN,* phosphatase and tensin homolog; *SOX2,* SRY-box 2.

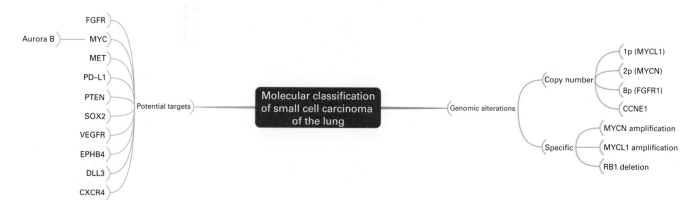

Fig. A.7. Molecular classification of small cell carcinoma of the lung. *CCNE1,* Cyclin E1; *FGFR,* fibroblast growth factor receptor; *MET,* MET proto-oncogene; *MYCL1,* L-myc-1 proto-oncogene; *MYC,* v-myc avian myelocytomatosis viral oncogene homolog; *MYCN,* v-myc avian myelocytomatosis viral oncogene neuroblastoma derived homolog; *PD-L1,* programmed cell death 1 ligand 1; *PTEN,* phosphatase and tensin homolog; *RB1,* retinoblastoma 1; *SOX2,* SRY-box 2; *VEGFR,* vascular endothelial growth factor receptor.

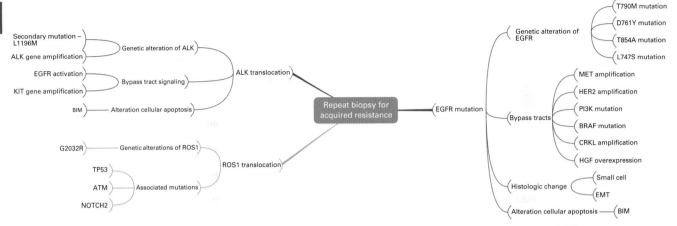

Fig. A.8. Repeat biopsy for acquired resistance. *ALK,* Anaplastic lymphoma kinase; *BIM,* BCL2-like 11; *CRKL,* v-crk avian sarcoma virus CT10 oncogene homolog-like; *BRAF,* v-raf murine sarcoma viral oncogene homolog B; *EGFR,* epidermal growth factor receptor; *EMT,* epithelial-mesenchymal transition; *HGF,* hepatocyte growth factor; *KIT,* v-kit Hardy-Zuckerman 4 feline sarcoma viral oncogene homolog; *MET,* MET proto-oncogene; *PI3K* *(PIK3CA),* phosphatidylinositol-4,5-bisphosphate 3-kinase, catalytic subunit alpha.

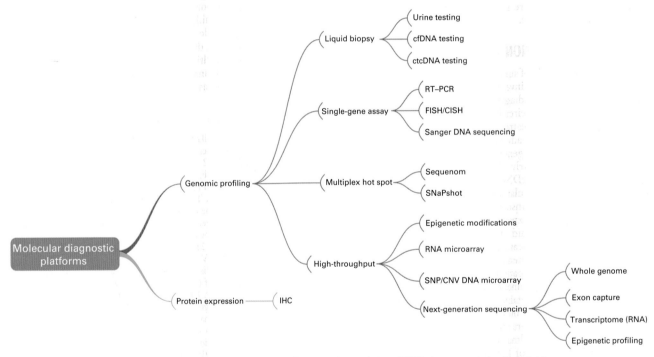

Fig. A.9. Molecular diagnostic platforms. *CNV,* Copy number variation; *CISH,* chromogenic in situ hybridization; *FISH,* fluorescence in situ hybridization; *RT-PCR,* reverse transcription polymerase chain reaction; *SNP,* single-nucleotide polymorphism.

rapidly (Fig. A.9). In the molecular testing guideline mentioned earlier, single-gene assays are recommended to select patients for EGFR or ALK TKI therapy, including testing based on polymerase chain reaction for EGFR mutation and the fluorescence in situ hybridization assay using dual-labeled break-apart probes for ALK.[23] In the case of ALK, the break-apart fluorescence in situ hybridization assay was developed and validated as a predictive biomarker in parallel with the development of crizotinib.

Multiplex genotyping platforms offer the potential to simultaneously assess many genes of interest. Both SNaPshot (Applied Biosystems, Foster City, CA, USA) and Sequenom (San Diego, CA, USA) are multiplex polymerase chain reaction–based platforms that are used to analyze tumor genomic DNA in formalin-fixed, paraffin-embedded specimens.[42] Both can analyze for selected, known hotspot mutations and oncogenes. Next-generation

sequencing (NGS) platforms are also being applied increasingly in both research and clinical settings. In addition to screening patients for therapeutically actionable targets, NGS platforms can aid in the discovery of novel drug targets. NGS platforms can be used for genome-wide characterization of tumor DNA, messenger RNA, transcription factor regions, microRNA, chromatin structure, and DNA methylation. Sequencing platforms are available for whole-genome, whole-exome, whole-transcriptome, and whole-epigenome analysis.[42] All platforms generate a large amount of sequencing data in a relatively short period of time. Analysis of these data takes longer, however, and requires a robust informatics infrastructure. The application of multiplex, high-throughput systematic genomic testing for patients with NSCLC has been shown to be feasible and to influence treatment decision making. However, the turnaround times vary, and both cost

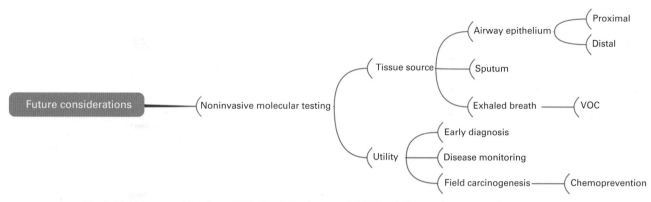

Fig. A.10. Future considerations. *CTC,* Circulating tumor cell. *VOC,* volatile organic compound.

and reimbursement remain potential limitations. Furthermore, extensive genotyping using multiplex or NGS platforms has not been shown to improve clinical outcomes in prospective trials.[42]

As our understanding of the biology of lung cancer improves, it will be feasible to determine the relevance and expression of altered proteins with immunohistochemistry. Immunohistochemistry can be used more universally than the more complex and expensive technologies.

FUTURE CONSIDERATIONS

The noninvasive analysis of surrogate tissues for molecular markers (Fig. A.10) has been investigated as a strategy for disease monitoring and for early diagnosis of lung cancer. The potential effectiveness of using circulating tumor cells to detect resistance mutations during treatment with an EGFR TKI has been described.[43-46] The recent advances in the development of high-throughput platforms for genomic analysis have also facilitated biomarker discovery for early diagnosis and molecular screening. Circulating tumor DNA(ctDNA) is a potential screening options that would allow for molecular detection of oncogene-driven targeted therapy markers in instances where invasive tissue biopsy may not be possible, cost expensive or associated with high morbidity. A non-invasive liquid biopsy would allow for physicians to periodically monitor disease progression, response to therapy, and development of treatment resistance. In a first clinic-based research study of NSCLC patients that assessed outcomes of targeted therapies using a commercially available ctDNA assay, over 80% of patients had detectable ctDNA with high concordance between paired tissue and blood for truncal oncogenic drivers, and patients with biomarkers identified in plasma had PFS in the expected range.[47] The landmark National Lung Screening Trial established the potential of low-dose CT screening to reduce mortality due to lung cancer in a high-risk population as defined by smoking history and age. However, the prevalence of lung cancer in this clinically defined population is low. The testing of surrogate tissues for molecular alterations that may be present early in the course of lung cancer has been investigated as a complement to clinical factors to improve patient selection for low-dose CT screening. This strategy has included interrogating surrogate tissues in the airway epithelium, sputum, and blood for molecular alterations as well as analyzing exhaled breath for endogenous products of cellular metabolism. Several candidate biomarkers have been discovered, although none has been validated. Prospective trials are expected to provide further information on the use of surrogate tissues for molecular analysis.

CONCLUSION

Lung cancer is a complex and heterogeneous disease. Personalized therapy requires assessment of factors specific to both the patient and tumor to help guide treatment decision making. Because

most patients will present with advanced-stage disease, tissue confirmation will usually be established with evaluation of a small biopsy specimen or cytologic examination. With the clinical validation of EGFR mutations and ALK translocations to select patients for targeted therapy, molecular characterization of tumors is becoming a standard component of the diagnostic evaluation. Furthermore, genomic changes that occur during therapy have also established the potential role for repeat biopsies to help guide the long-term care of patients. Given the complexity of the ongoing diagnostic evaluation of patients with lung cancer, integrated multidisciplinary teams have become essential to efficiently guide management decisions and the overall care of patients with this disease.

KEY REFERENCES

3. Travis WD, Brambilla E, Riely GJ. New pathologic classification of lung cancer: relevance for clinical practice and clinical trials. *J Clin Oncol.* 2013;31(8):992–1001.
5. Farrand P, Hussain F, Hennessy E. The efficacy of the "mind map" study technique. *Med Educ.* 2002;36(5):426–431.
7. Ost DE, Yeung SC, Tanoue LT, Gould MK. Clinical and organizational factors in the initial evaluation of patients with lung cancer: diagnosis and management of lung cancer, 3rd ed: American College of Chest Physicians evidence-based clinical practice guidelines. *Chest.* 2013;143(suppl 5):e121S–e241S.
9. Alberg AJ, Brock MV, Ford JG, Samet JM, Spivack SD. Epidemiology of lung cancer: diagnosis and management of lung cancer, 3rd ed: American College of Chest Physicians evidence-based clinical practice guidelines. *Chest.* 2013;143(suppl 5):e1S–e29S.
17. Gould MK, Donington J, Lynch WR, et al. Evaluation of individuals with pulmonary nodules: when is it lung cancer? Diagnosis and management of lung cancer, 3rd ed: American College of Chest Physicians evidence-based clinical practice guidelines. *Chest.* 2013;143(suppl 5):e93S–e120S.
22. Keedy VL, Temin S, Somerfield MR, et al. American Society of Clinical Oncology provisional clinical opinion: epidermal growth factor receptor (EGFR) mutation testing for patients with advanced non-small-cell lung cancer considering first-line EGFR tyrosine kinase inhibitor therapy. *J Clin Oncol.* 2011;29(15):2121–2127.
27. Govindan R, Ding L, Griffith M, et al. Genomic landscape of non-small cell lung cancer in smokers and never-smokers. *Cell.* 2012;150(6):1121–1134.
28. Reck M, Rodriguez-Abreu D, Robinson AG, et al. Pembrolizumab versus Chemotherapy for PD-L1-Positive Non-Small-Cell Lung Cancer. *N Engl J Med.* 2016.
36. Tartarone A, Lazzari C, Lerose R, et al. Mechanisms of resistance to EGFR tyrosine kinase inhibitors gefitinib/erlotinib and to ALK inhibitor crizotinib. *Lung Cancer.* 2013;81(3):328–336.
39. Awad MM, Katayama R, McTigue M, et al. Acquired resistance to crizotinib from a mutation in CD74-ROS1. *N Engl J Med.* 2013;368:2395–2401.

See Expertconsult.com for full list of references.

Index

A

AAPM. *see* American Association of Physicists in Medicine (AAPM)
Abbott Molecular, 173
Ablation
  cryoablation, 356, 357f
  irreversible electroporation, 356–357
  for localized nonsmall cell lung cancer, 355–362.e3
  mechanism of action of, 355–357
  microwave, 355–356, 356f
  radiofrequency, 355, 356f
  surveillance after, 359–360
  thermal, 358–359
  treatment considerations, 360–362
Ablation zone, technical factors influencing size of, 357–358
  heat sink, 358
  probe characteristics, 357
  tissue characteristics, 357–358
ACCP. *see* American College of Chest Physicians (ACCP)
Acetaminophen, for pain, 617
Acinar predominant invasive adenocarcinoma, 144t, 147
Acneiform (papulopustular) rash, 491, 492f, 493t, 495f
ACOSOG. *see* American College of Surgeons Oncology Group (ACOSOG)
ACR. *see* American College of Radiology (ACR)
Acromegaly, 234t
ACTB, 109t
ACTIN, 109t
ACTL6A, 109t
ACTL6B, 109t
Acute pulmonary embolism, 213, 213f
Adaptive designs, trials, 624
Adenocarcinoma, 143–150, 144t, 203f, 206f
  cells of origin and, 117
  classification in resection specimens, 144t
  colloid, 147, 148f
  conditional oncogene-driven, cells of origin in, 118
  cytologic characteristics of, 161–162, 161f
  diagnosis of, algorithm for, 159f
  diffuse pneumonic-type, 260, 263t
  driver mutations in, 27t, 467–468, 468t
  fetal, 147
  gene fusions in, 89f
  genetic abnormalities in, 480, 481t

Adenocarcinoma *(Continued)*
  genetic amplifications in, 85f
  histologic and molecular correlations in, 148
  immunohistochemistry of, 148, 149f
  impact of new classification on tumor, node, metastasis staging in, 148–149
  invasive, 144t, 146–147
    variants of, 147–148, 148f
  large cell neuroendocrine carcinoma from, markers for differentiation of, 558
  lepidic predominant invasive, 144t, 147
  micropapillary predominant, 146f, 147
  minimally invasive, 144–146, 144t, 145f
    defined, 183
  molecular classification of, 654, 654f
  molecular targets in, 431t
  multifocal pulmonary, with ground glass/lepidic features, 260, 262t
  next-generation hallmark of, 98, 100f
  papillary predominant, 144t, 147
  part-solid nonmucinous, measurement of tumor size in, 256–257
  PET imaging of, 223, 225f
  PET-CT imaging of, 231f
  primary pulmonary, with enteric differentiation, 147–148
  radiography for evaluation of, 183
  small biopsy and cytology samples for, 149–150, 149t
  solid predominant invasive, 144t, 147
Adenocarcinoma in situ (AIS), 144–145, 145f
  defined, 183
  diagnosis of, 146
Adenoma, 144t
  adrenal, 216–217, 217f
  parathyroid, 553, 553f
Adenomatous polyposis coli (APC), 164–165
Adenosquamous carcinoma, 144t, 153, 153f
Adenoviral vector (AdV) transduction, 124
Ad.HSVtk, 549
Adjuvant analgesics, for pain, 618
Adjuvant Lung Cancer Enrichment Marker Identification and Sequencing Trial (ALCHEMIST), 520
Adjuvant Lung Project Italy (ALPI), 515

Adjuvant Navelbine International Trial Association (ANITA), 515
Adrenal adenoma, 216–217, 217f
Adrenal gland imaging, 210
Adrenal metastases
  lung cancer and, 190–191
  PET imaging of, 222–223, 224f
  stereotactic ablative radiotherapy (SABR) for, 351
Adrenocorticotropic hormone syndrome, ectopic, 234t
Advertising, tobacco, 12
Advocacy, 635–638.e1
Advocacy groups, role of, 635–638.e1
Advocates, 635
Afatinib, 480
  for metastatic NSCLC, 439–440
  for nonsmall cell lung cancer, 427t, 428
  side effects of, 497
Aflibercept, 439
Age
  and patient selection for radiotherapy, 338
  and prognosis, 418
Air pollution, 6–7
Airway epithelia, neuroendocrine, 119
Airway repair, 119
Airway stenting, for central airway obstruction, 594, 594f–595f
AKT1 gene, 487
Alcohol, lung cancer and, 4
Alectinib, 441
ALK gene
  fusion of, 86–89, 87f–88f, 88t, 90t
    in lung cancer, 172, 173f
  in lung cancer, 26, 26t, 71
  rearrangement, in nonsmall cell lung cancer, 420
ALK-FISH assay, 173, 174f
Allelic-specific PCR/Scorpion ARMS, 166t
Alliance for Lung Cancer Advocacy, Support and Education, 637–638
Alpha-Tocopherol, Beta-Carotene Cancer Prevention (ATBC) Study, 77, 77t
Amatuximab (MORAb-009), 548
American Association of Physicists in Medicine (AAPM)
  IMRT Subcommittee: Guidance document on delivery, treatment planning, and clinical implementation of IMRT, 319b–320b

---

Note: Pages followed by "*b*," "*t*," and "*f*" refer to boxes, tables, and figures, respectively.

American Association of Physicists in Medicine *(Continued)*
  Task Group (TG) 6: Managing the use of fluoroscopy in medical institutions (1998), 319b–320b
  Task Group (TG) 28: Radiotherapy portal imaging quality (1987), 319b–320b
  Task Group (TG) 53: Quality assurance for clinical radiotherapy treatment planning, 319b–320b
  Task Group (TG) 58: Clinical use of electronic portal imaging, 319b–320b
  Task Group (TG) 75: Management of imaging dose during IGRT, 319b–320b
  Task Group (TG) 76: Management of respiratory motion in radiation oncology, 319b–320b
  Task Group (TG) 101: Stereotactic ablative radiation therapy (SABR), 319b–320b
  Task Group (TG) 104: Role of in-room kilovoltage x-ray imaging for patient setup and target localization (2009), 319b–320b
  Task Group (TG) 142: Quality assurance of medical accelerators, 319b–320b
  Task Group (TG) 179: Quality assurance for image-guided radiation therapy (IGRT) utilizing computed tomography (CT)-based technologies, 319b–320b
American College of Chest Physicians (ACCP), 314
  Evidence-Based Clinical Practice Guidelines: Treatment of SCLC, 319b–320b
  Evidence-Based Clinical Practice Guidelines: Treatment of stage I and II NSCLC, 319b–320b
  Evidence-Based Clinical Practice Guidelines: Treatment of stage I and III NSCLC, 319b–320b
  evidence-based practice guidelines for multiple primary lung cancers (MPLCs), 312
  guidelines on evaluation and treatment of cardiac risk factors in candidates, 266
  indications for invasive mediastinal staging and, 242
American College of Radiology (ACR)
  Appropriateness Criteria: Induction and adjuvant therapy for stage N2 non-small cell lung cancer, 319b–320b
  Appropriateness Criteria: Nonsurgical treatment for NSCLC, 319b–320b
  Appropriateness Criteria: Nonsurgical treatment for NSCLC: good performance status/definitive intent, 319b–320b
  Appropriateness Criteria: Radiation therapy for SCLC, 319b–320b

American College of Radiology *(Continued)*
  Practice Guideline: 3-D external-beam radiation planning and conformal (2011), 319b–320b
  Practice Guideline: Intensity-modulated radiation therapy (IMRT), 319b–320b
  Practice Guideline: Performance of SABR, 319b–320b
  Practice Guideline: Radiation oncology (2009), 319b–320b
  Practice Guidelines: IGRT, 319b–320b
  Technical Standard: Medical physics performance monitoring of IGRT (2009), 319b–320b
  Technical Standard: Performance of radiation oncology physics for external-beam therapy, 319b–320b
American College of Surgeons Oncology Group (ACOSOG), 314–316
American Joint Committee on Cancer (AJCC), 537, 538t
American Society for Radiation Oncology (ASTRO)
  Evidence-based Clinical Practice Guideline: Palliative thoracic radiotherapy in lung cancer, 319b–320b
  evidence-based practice guidelines for multiple primary lung cancers (MPLCs), 313
  Practice Guideline: 3-D external-beam radiation planning and conformal (2011), 319b–320b
  Practice Guideline: Intensity-modulated radiation therapy (IMRT), 319b–320b
  Practice Guideline: Performance of SABR, 319b–320b
  Practice Guidelines: IGRT, 319b–320b
American Society of Clinical Oncology (ASCO), 464
  Quality Oncology Practice Initiative (ASCO QOPI), 19
American Thoracic Society, classification of adenocarcinoma, 256–257
Amifostine, 398–399
Amitriptyline, 417
Amrubicin, 526t, 527, 532
Anaplastic lymphoma kinase (ALK), 196, 441–443, 469
  fusion, in lung cancer, 172, 173f
  in lung cancer, 164–165, 172–175
  as predictor of response to ALK inhibitors, 172–175
  rearrangements in, 479
    in NSCLC, incidence of, 173t
  testing for, 165
    assays for, 173–174
    clinical recommendation for, 175
  wild-type and various types of, 173f
Anaplastic lymphoma kinase inhibitors, 369
  side effects of, 498

Anastomosis
  bronchial, 307
  type of, 305–306
  vascular, 307
Anastrozole, 39
Anatomic pathology, classic, 143–163.e4
Ancillary testing, fixation and considerations for, 183f, 185
Anemia, 193
Anethole dithiollethione (ADT), 78t
Aneuploidy, 83–84
Angiogenesis agents, 369
Angiogenic squamous dysplasia, 150
Angiotensin-converting enzyme inhibitors, 399
Anthropometric measures, lung cancer and, 5
Antiangiogenic agents, 426–427, 494–496
Antiangiogenic therapy, 425–427
Antibodies. *see also* Monoclonal antibodies
  anti-CTLA-4, 126–127, 504–505
  antimesothelin antibody drug conjugates, 548
  anti-PD1, 499, 505–506, 506t–507t
  anti-PDL1, 505–506, 506t–507t
  anti-PD-L1, 499
Anticancer drugs, 368
Anti-CTLA-4 antibody, 504–505
Antigen-presenting cells (APC), 137–140, 138f
Anti-MAGE-A3, 520
Antimesothelin antibody drug conjugates, 548
Anti-PD1 antibodies, 499, 505–506, 506t–507t
Anti-PDL1 antibodies, 499, 505–506, 506t–507t
Anti-program death 1, 444–445
Applied Biosystems, 656–657
ARF gene, 536
Arginase, 141
Arginine-glycine-aspartic acid (RGD), 229–230
Argon plasma, 596
ARID1A, 109t
ARID1B, 109t
ARID2, 109t
Aromatase, lung cancer and, 38–39
Arylamine N-acetyltransferase (NAT2), 34
Asbestos, lung cancer and, 5
Asia, 33, 33f
Asian/Indian, 169t
Asian/Pacific Islander, 169t
Association of Molecular Pathologist (AMP), in guidelines for molecular testing, 165
ASTRO. *see* American Society for Radiation Oncology (ASTRO)
Ataxia telangiectasia mutated (ATM), 164–165
Atezolizumab, 445, 506t, 507–509
ATLAS trial, 456t, 459
Atypical adenomatous hyperplasia (AAH), 118, 145, 145f

Australia, smoking and smoking-attributable deaths in, 10
Autoantibodies, 67
Automated quantitative analysis (AQUA), of in situ protein expression, 467
Autonomic neuropathy, 194
AUY922
    phase study of, 443
    side effects of, 498–499
AVAIL trial, 460
AVAPERL trial, 452t, 454–455
AXL receptor tyrosine kinase, 164–165
AZD9291, 440

B
BAF47, 109t
BAF53A, 109t
BAF53B, 109t
BAF57, 109t
BAF60A, 109t
BAF60B, 109t
BAF60C, 109t
BAF155, 109t
BAF170, 109t
BAF180, 109t
BAF200, 109t
BAF250A, 109t
BAF250B, 109t
BAP1 gene, 536–537
Barriers to optimal care, 647–648
    case studies from high-income countries, 647–649
    classification of, 647
    in low-and-middle-income countries, 648
Basal mucous secretory cells, 117
Basaloid carcinoma, 152–153, 153f
Basic Score for bone metastases, 390
BAY94-9343, 547–548
BD (Becton, Dickinson and Company) Diagnostics, 184
Belagenpumatucel-L, 504
Benchmarking, criterion-based, 646
Best-practices treatment and care, 637
Beta-Carotene and Retinol Efficacy Trial (CARET), 77, 77t
Bevacizumab, 229–230, 438–439
    for advanced NSCLC, 44, 45t
    chemotherapy with, 369
    maintenance chemotherapy with, 455, 460
    platinum-based chemotherapy with, 425, 426t
    side effects of, 498
Bexarotene, 79
BI 1482694. *see* Olmutinib
Big Lung Trial (BLT), 515
Bimodality Lung Oncology Team (BLOT), 520–521
Biologic heterogeneity, 641
Biologic risk factors, 47
Biology
    of lung carcinogenesis, 60
    of malignant mesothelioma, 536
Biomarker-based subgroups, 622f–623f, 623–624
Biomarker-based trial designs, 626

Biomarkers
    for chemotherapy selection, 424–425
    diagnostic
        for lung cancer, 129–132, 130t–131t
        for malignant mesothelioma, 539
    for EGFR blockade, 429
    to individualize adjuvant chemotherapy, 521–523, 523f
    for lung cancer, 60f, 61–68, 62t–63t
        autoantibodies in, 67
        circulating tumor cells in, 64
        circulating tumor DNA in, 64
        currently recommended, 169–175
        cytology, 61–64
        diagnostic, 129–132, 130t–131t
        discovery techniques for, advances in, 61
        genetic changes in, 64–66
        metabolomics in, 67–68
        microRNAs as, 129–136.e2
        mitochondrial DNA in, 64
        new molecular, 175–176
        noncoding RNAs in, 64
        preclinical, 59–68.e4
        predictive, 175–176
        prognostic, 132–134, 133t, 175
        proteomics in, 66–67
        screening, 58, 58t
        specimen types of, 61
        for treatment response, 134–136, 135t
        tumor-associated antigens in, 67
        validation of, 60–61
    for malignant mesothelioma, 538–539
    molecular, 477
        measurement of, 467
        new, 175–176
    predictive
        for chemotherapy, 466–478.e3
        for lung cancer, 175–176
    prognostic, 175, 466–477
        for lung cancer, 132–134, 133t
    prognostic imaging, 539
    for radiation pneumonitis, 398
    testing
        guidelines for, 165
        sample availability and prioritization of, 168–169
Biopsy
    core-needle
        processing specimens and cell blocks, 182, 183f
        touch preparation for, 182, 182f
        TTNA and, 239
    vs. fine-needle aspiration, 179
    image-guided, 210, 212f
    repeat, 655, 656f
    tumor cellularity in, 168f
Bisphosphonates, 388
    for bone metastases, 190
    for pain, 618
Black, 169t
Bleomycin, 117
Blood disorders, paraneoplastic, 191t, 193
BMS-936558 (nivolumab), 506, 506t–507t, 509
Bone imaging, 210

Bone metastases
    Basic Score for, 390
    consensus endpoints, international, 385–386
    external-beam radiotherapy for, 383
    lung cancer and, 189–190
    palliative radiotherapy for, 385–389, 385t
    uncomplicated, external-beam radiotherapy, 386, 386f
BR.21, 437–438
Brachial plexopathy, 410t
Brachial plexus, 409–411
Brachytherapy, 385
    endobronchial, 385
    in marginally resectable stage I NSCLC, 315
BRAF gene, 46, 479
    in lung adenocarcinoma, 27t, 431, 431t
    in lung cancer, 26–27, 26t, 176
BRAF inhibitor, side effects of, 499
B-Raf kinase, 442
Brain imaging, 210
Brain metastases, 372
    alternative management approaches, 391
    lung cancer and, 190
    outcomes, 391
    palliative radiotherapy for, 390
    repeat treatment for, 391–392
    in small-cell lung carcinoma (SCLC), 379–380
Brain neurotoxicity, 412–413
BRCA1 gene, 475–476
    for advanced NSCLC, 475–476, 475f
BRD7, 109t
BRD9, 109t
Breast cancer, 406, 406f
    dosimetric factors, 406–407
Breast cancer 1 (BRCA1), 175–176
BRG1, 109t
Brief pain inventory, 617
Brigatinib, 441
BRM, 109t
Bronchial anastomosis, 307
Bronchial scraping, brushing, or washing, 160
Bronchiolo-alveolar cell carcinoma, 144
Bronchoalveolar stem cells (BASCs), 118
Bronchogenic cysts, 552, 552f
Bronchopulmonary carcinoids, 555, 556f
    adjuvant treatment of, 564
    applicability of TNM classification to, 256
    clinical characteristics of, 561
    diagnosis of, 555
    hormonal symptoms, management of, 565–566
    interferon, 566
    liver metastases-directed therapy for, 565
    metastatic, therapy for, 565
    molecularly targeted therapy for, 566
    palliative chemotherapy for, 565
    palliative radiotherapy for, 566
    prognosis of, 567–568
    from small cell lung cancer, markers for differentiation of, 558–559
    surgery of, 563–564, 566

Bronchorrhea, 186–187
Bronchoscopic balloon dilatation, 596
Bronchoscopic laser resection, for central
  airway obstruction, 593–594
Bronchoscopy
  flexible, 237
  for massive hemoptysis, 599
  navigational, 179
Bronchovascular sleeve resections,
  304–307.e1
  healing of anastomotic site after,
    304–305, 305f
  history and surgical outcomes of, 304,
    305t
  surgical techniques and controversies
    regarding, 305–306
  suturing layers, 305
  suturing method, 305
  type of anastomosis, 305–306
  type of sleeve resection, 306, 306f
Brushing or washing, bronchial, 160
Budesonide, 77, 78t
Bupropion, 20, 21t
Buzan, Tony, 651

C
Cachexia, 617
Calypso System, 326
Canada, warning about dangers of
  tobacco in, 11–12
Canadian National Consensus
  Statement, 165
Cancer
  biologic heterogeneity of, 641
  breast, 406, 406f
  lung, 30
    age-standardized death rates for
      women in Europe, 32, 32f
    biologic risk factors for, 47
    biomarkers for early detection of,
      60f, 61–68, 62t–63t
    case-control studies of, 47–48
    case-family cohort studies of, 47–48
    chemoprevention of, 69–81.e5
    chemotherapy for, 42–43
    diagnostic workup for, 233–240.e2
    diet in, 35–36
    early, 69–81.e5
    early-stage, gender as a prognostic
      factor in, 40–42, 41f
    environmental exposures in, 35
    epidemiology of, 1–8.e3, 2f, 30–33
    familial aggregation of, 47–48
    family history of, 35
    gender-related differences in, 30–45.
      e5, 31f
    genetic factors in, gender-related
      differences in, 34–35, 35f–36f
    genetic susceptibility to, 46–51.e2
    genome-wide association studies,
      50–51
    high-risk syndromes conferring
      increased risk of, 48
    human papillomavirus (HPV) in, 35
    imaging features of, 235–236
    immune dysregulation in, 137–142.
      e3
    linkage analysis of, 49–50

Cancer (Continued)
    molecular testing in, 164–177.e5
    in never-smokers, 23–29.e3, 33–34
    nonsmoking-related, 23–24
    PET imaging of, 219–232.e4,
      220f–221f
    preclinical biomarkers for, 59–68.e4
    predictive biomarkers in, 169–175
    preexisting lung disease and,
      36
    segregation analyses of, 48–49
    steroid hormones in, 36–40
    survival in, gender differences,
      41–42, 41t–42t
    susceptibility to, 33–34
    tobacco use and, 24
    twin studies of, 47
    viral factors in, 35
    tobacco-related, segregation analyses
      of, 48–49
Cancer and Leukemia Group B, VATS
  lobectomy defined by, 274
Cancer and Leukemia Group B
  (CALGB), 367, 516
  30106, phase II study, 368–369
Cancer and Leukemia Group B
  (CALGB), in radiotherapy,
  376–377
Cancer Care Ontario (CCO), 242, 244f,
  244t
Cancer Care Outcomes Research and
  Surveillance (CanCORS), 19
Cancer programs
  accessibility standards for, 646–647
  modality-specific quality standards for,
    645
  quality standards for, 643–646
  standards for acceptable patient
    volumes for, 645–646
Cancer-associated retinopathy, 194
Cancerization, 70
Cancer-related fatigue, 615–616
Carbon monoxide lung diffusion capacity
  (DLCO), 267–268
Carboplatin
  for chemotherapy-induced peripheral
    neuropathy, 414
  combination chemotherapy with
    for advanced NSCLC in elderly
      patients, 424, 424t
    with bevacizumab, 425, 426t
    for EGFR mutated NSCLC, 427,
      427t
    for locally advanced nonsmall cell
      lung cancer, 366
    for nonsmall cell lung cancer,
      420–421, 421t
  maintenance chemotherapy with
    continuation, 454–455
    historical trials, 449
    switch, 450
  for older patients, 530
  for SCLC, 525, 526t
  vs. cisplatin, for nonsmall cell lung
    cancer, 421, 421t
Carboxyaminoimidazole (CAI),
  461
Carcinoid syndrome, 192, 234t

Carcinoids, 155–157, 156f. see also
  Bronchopulmonary carcinoids
  atypical, 155, 156f
    from large cell neuroendocrine
      carcinoma, markers for
      differentiation of, 559
    markers for differentiation of, 558
  typical, 155, 156f
    from large cell neuroendocrine
      carcinoma, markers for
      differentiation of, 559
    markers for differentiation of, 558
Carcinosarcoma, 154
Cardiac risk
  preoperative estimation of, 266–267
  Revised Cardiac Risk Index (RCRI),
    266
  ThRCRI, 266
Cardiomyopathy, radiation effects on,
  405t, 407t
Cardiopulmonary exercise test (CPET),
  269–270
Cardiopulmonary resuscitation, lung
  cancer and, 618
Cardiovascular toxicity
  scoring of, 404
  types of, 404, 404f
CARET (Beta-Carotene and Retinol
  Efficacy Trial), 77, 77t
β-Carotene, 77, 77t–78t
Carotenoids, lung cancer and, 4, 4t
Case-control studies, 47–48
Case-family cohort studies, 47–48
Catenin (cadherin-associated protein),
  beta 1, 88 kDa (CTNNB1),
  164–165
CCL21, 124–125
CD4₊ helper T cells, 123
CD4⁺ T cells, TILs and, 141
CD4⁺CD25⁺ T cells, 141
CD8+ Tcells (CTLs), 123
CD28, 139
CD133-positive cells, 117–118
CDKN2A gene
  in lung cancer, 27–28
  in squamous cell NSCLC, 431t
CDKN2A/p16, 113
CDKN2/ARF, 536
Celecoxib, 78, 78t
Cell blocks, 182, 183f, 185
Cells of origin, 117
Cell-secreted inflammatory mediators, in
  TME, 122–123
Cellular immune dysregulation, 137–142.
  e3, 138f
Central airway obstruction, 590–596
  airway stenting of, 594, 594f–595f
  argon plasma, 596
  bronchoscopic balloon dilatation, 596
  bronchoscopic laser resection for,
    593–594
  chest radiographs often aid in
    diagnosis of, 592–593, 592f
  clinical findings of, 592
  covered self-expanding metal stents,
    596
  cryotherapy, 595–596
  diagnosis of, 592

Central airway obstruction (*Continued*)
emergency bronchoscopic management of, expected outcomes of, 596
endobronchial brachytherapy, 595
evaluation of patients, 593, 593t
external-beam radiotherapy, 594–595
flexible bronchoscopic examination for, 593
imaging of, 214
photodynamic therapy, 595
symptoms of lung cancer-related, 591–592
treatment modalities for, emergency management of lung cancer-related, 593
types of, presenting as emergencies, 590–591, 591f
Central nervous system disorders, 194
Ceritinib, 441
Cervical mediastinoscopy, extended, 248–249, 248f
Cetuximab, 428
drug combinations, for locally advanced nonsmall cell lung cancer, 368
maintenance therapy with, 459–460
Charlson Comorbidity Index, 265, 266t
CHART weekend less (CHARTWEL), 333
CHD13, 113
Chemoprevention, 69–81.e5
future strategies of, 80
by manipulation of lung tumor microenvironment, 126–127
primary randomized trials of, 77, 77t
secondary randomized trials of, 77–79, 78t
tertiary, 79t
trials of, 76–80, 77t–78t
Chemoradiation therapy, 364–368
chemotherapy drug combinations for, 366–367
concurrent therapy, for locally advanced nonsmall cell lung cancer, 365–366, 365t, 366f
consolidation therapy, 367
DDP-based, 366
induction therapy, for locally advanced nonsmall cell lung cancer, 367
for locally advanced nonsmall cell lung cancer, 364–368
molecularly targeted therapeutic agents, 368–369
for older individuals, 367–368, 368f
palliative, 385
platinum-based, 364
sequential and concurrent therapy, 365–366
in stage III NSCLC, 395, 396t
Chemotherapy, 435
adjuvant
benefit of, 513f
biomarkers to individualize, 521–523, 523f
cisplatin-based, 516–517, 517t
for early stage nonsmall cell lung cancer, 512–524.e4

Chemotherapy (*Continued*)
early studies of, 514
efficacy of, 517–518, 517t
large-scale studies on platinum-based, 514–517, 514t
meta-analyses, 517–518, 517t, 518f
new regimens, 519–520
for older patients, 518–519
with oral UFT, 517
platinum-based, large-scale studies on, 514–517, 514t–516t
quality of life and, 516–517
rationale for, 513
survival rates of, 515t
systematic reviews, 517–518, 517t
targeted therapy and, 519–520
agent, choice of, 436
alternating non-cross-resistant regimens, 528–529
alternative strategies of, 527–529
biomarkers for, predictive, 466–478.e3
biomarkers for selection of, 424–425
cisplatin-based, 470
combination, 420, 420t
for advanced NSCLC in elderly patients, 424, 424t
for extensive-stage SCLC, 525–527, 526t
platinum-based, 420–421, 421t
platinum-free, 422
for poor performance status patients, 531
concurrent medication, 331
CT imaging of response to, 211
dose intensification of, 527–528
drug combinations, 366–367
with EGFR TKIs in NSCLC, 169
for elderly patients, 423–424
first-line
intrapleural, 544–545
for malignant mesothelioma, 539–540
for older patients, 529–531
for small cell lung cancer, 525–529
host-related factors in, 477
induction, 367
for lung cancer, 42–43, 334
maintenance therapy
continuation, 450–455, 452t, 454f
cost-effectiveness, 463–464
history trials, 448–449
meta-analyses, 462–463, 463f
with noncytotoxic agents, 455–461
for nonsmall cell lung cancer, 422–423
patient selection for, 464
for small cell lung cancer, 529
switch, 450, 450t, 451f
for malignant mesothelioma, 539–541
with molecularly targeted agents, 437–439
neoadjuvant, 520–521, 522f
for early stage nonsmall cell lung cancer, 512–524.e4
for nonsmall cell lung cancer
duration of, 422
maintenance therapy, 422–423
neurotoxicity related to, 409–417.e2
systemic, 420, 420t

Chemotherapy (*Continued*)
platinum doublet, EGFR TKI *vs.*, in EGFR mutated NSCLC, 427, 427t
platinum-based, 422
platinum-free, 422
pooled analysis of, 518
postoperative, 371
radiotherapy and, combined, for thymic tumors, 582
retrospective analysis of, 518
role of, for locally advanced nonsmall cell lung cancer, 365
scheduling of, 436–437
second-line, 435–436, 531–533, 532t
for small cell lung cancer, neurotoxicity related to, 409–417.e2
with surgery, 518f
third and subsequent-line of, 437
for thymic tumors, 580–582
triplet, 421–422, 422t
tumor-related factors and, 466–477
Chemotherapy for Early Stages Trial (ChEST), 521, 522f
Chemotherapy-induced peripheral neuropathy, 414
chemotherapy treatments associated with, 414–415, 415t
pharmacologic therapy for, 416–417, 416t
prevention of, 415–416
Chest pain, lung cancer and, 187
Chest radiography, imaging with, for lung cancer, 202–205
blind spots on, 203, 204f–205f
computer-aided detection in, 204
dual-energy subtraction, 204–205, 207f
lung cancer missed characteristics, 204
new technology in, 204
special views, 204, 206f
technical factors in, 203
Chest radiotherapy in Extensive Stage (CREST), 379
Chest-wall reconstruction, 296
Chest-wall tumors, 295–297
computed tomography image of, 295, 296f
general principles of, 295
results and long-term survival of, 296–297
staging of, 295–296, 296f
surgical resection of, 296, 296t, 297f
China, smoking and smoking-attributable deaths in, 10
CHRNA3 gene, in lung cancer, 25
CHRNA5 gene, 25
CHRNB4 gene, 25
Chromatin remodeling, 104–116.e5
functional consequences of abnormalities in, 110
Chromatin remodeling complexes, 108–110, 108f, 109t
Chromogenic in situ hybridization, 166
Chromogranin A, for diagnosis of LCNEC, 157
Chromosomal aberrations, 559

Chronic bronchitis, lung cancer and, 6
Circulating tumor cells, 64
Circulating tumor DNA, 64
Cisplatin, 470
    adjuvant chemotherapy with
        early studies of, 514
        quality of life and, 516–517
        systematic reviews and meta-
            analyses of, 517t
    anticancer activity of, 420
    combination chemotherapy with,
        420–422, 421t
        dose-dense regimens, 528
    for locally advanced nonsmall cell lung
        cancer, 364
    maintenance chemotherapy with,
        continuation, 454–455
    neurotoxicity of, 414
    for nonsmall cell lung cancer, 420,
        420t
    for older patients, 530
    for SCLC, 525, 526t
    vs. carboplatin, for nonsmall cell lung
        cancer, 421
CK7, in lung adenocarcinoma, 148
Clara cell, 117
Class I P13Ks (phosphoinositide
    3-kinase), 479
Class III beta-tubulin (TUBB3), 175–176
Clinical trials. see Research
Club cell, 117
c-MET gene, 482
cMET inhibitors, 490
CO1686. see Rociletinib
Coamplification at lower denaturation
    temperature-PCR, 165–166
Cobalt Therapy Systems, 324
Cobas, 166t
Cochrane collaboration, 640
Cochrane systematic review, 513
Coffee, lung cancer and, 3
Cognitive disturbance, 410t
College of American Pathologists (CAP),
    185
    in guidelines for molecular testing, 165
Colloid adenocarcinoma, 147, 148f
Common Terminology Criteria for
    Adverse Events (CTCAE), 393,
    395t, 404, 405t, 409, 410t
Comorbidity
    Charlson Comorbidity Index, 265,
        266t
    and patient selection for radiotherapy,
        338
    patient-related factors, 418
    preoperative evaluation of, 265–266
Comparative genomic hybridization, 166
Completely portal robotic operations
    (CPRs), 283, 284t
Computed tomography (CT)
    after thermal ablation, 359–360, 360f
    for biopsy, 210
    blind spots on, 206, 208f
    characteristics of lung cancers missed
        on, 206
    chest-wall tumors image in, 295, 296f
    cone-beam, 326
    FDG-PET-CT, 227–231, 227f

Computed tomography (Continued)
    imaging with, 205–206
        of response to therapy, 211–213
    low-dose (LDCT), 52, 54t, 72
        improvements in, 76
        recommended algorithm, for
            management of findings, 73f
        screening for lung cancer, 76
    lung cancer detection, 59
    lung cancer staging, 206–210
        adrenal gland imaging, 210
        bone imaging, 210
        brain imaging, 210
        liver imaging, 210
        lymph node (N) descriptors,
            209–210
        mediastinum, direct invasion of, 208
        metastasis (M) descriptors, 210,
            211f–212f
        pleura, direct invasion of, 207
        postobstructive collapse or
            pneumonitis, 209
        satellite nodules, 208–209
        tumor (T) descriptors, 207, 209f
    for massive hemoptysis, 599
    morphologic features on, 235t
    for neuroendocrine tumors, 561
    neurologic effects of, 410
    new technology in, 206
        computer-aided detection, 206,
            208f
        maximum intensity projection, 206
    PET-CT, 227, 227f, 230f, 231,
        359–360, 361f–362f
    radiotherapy and, 320, 341
Computer Motion's system, 283
Concentration impairment, 410t
Concurrent chemoradiation therapy,
    365, 365t, 366f
    induction chemotherapy to, 367
    with third-generation anticancer
        agents, 366t
Conditional oncogene-driven
    adenocarcinoma, 118
Continuous hyperfractionated
    accelerated radiotherapy (CHART),
    333
Core-needle biopsy, 210
    processing specimens and cell blocks,
        182, 183f
    touch preparation for, 182, 182f
    TTNA and, 239
    vs. fine-needle aspiration, 179
Coronary artery disease, 403
Corticosteroids, for pain, 618
Cost-effectiveness, 463–464
Cough, 616
    lung cancer and, 186–187
    suppression, 616
Covered self-expanding metal stents, 596
CPET. see Cardiopulmonary exercise test
    (CPET)
Cranial irradiation, prophylactic
    in extensive disease, 380–381
    neurotoxicity of, 379–380
    for small-cell lung cancer, 379–380
Cranial radiation, prophylactic,
    neurotoxicity of, 413

CREB-binding protein (CREBBP),
    164–165
CREST. see Chest radiotherapy in
    Extensive Stage (CREST)
Criterion-based benchmarking, for lung
    cancer, 646
Crizotinib, 172, 441, 443, 469
    side effects of, 498
c-Ros oncogene 1, 483–484
CRS-207, 548
Cryoablation, mechanism of action of,
    356, 357f
Cryotherapy, 595–596
Cullin 3 (CUL3), 164–165
Current smoker, definition of, 23
Cushing syndrome, 192
CyberKnife, 324, 326
Cycleave PCR, 166t
Cyclin-dependent kinase, 488–489
Cyclin-dependent kinase inhibitor
    (CDKN2A), in lung cancer,
    164–165
Cyclooxygenase (COX) inhibition, in
    lung cancer, 124
Cyclooxygenase (COX-2) inhibitors, 80
Cyclophosphamide
    for extensive-stage SCLC, 525, 526t,
        527
    for poor performance status patients,
        531
CYP3A, 477
Cystic masses, benign, 552
Cysts
    bronchogenic, 552, 552f
    esophageal, 552
    pericardial, 552
Cytochrome P450, 477, 500
Cytokeratin markers, 558
Cytokines, immunosuppressive, 546
Cytokines and angiogenic factors (CAFs),
    78–79
Cytology
    liquid-based, 160–161, 184
    of lung cancer, 61–64
        molecular analysis, 161
        special staining and
            immunocytochemistry, 161
    neuroendocrine tumors, 556–557
    samples, 101–102
Cytoreductive surgery, 542–544
Cytotoxic T cells, 123
Cytotoxic T-lymphocyte-associated
    antigen 4 (CTLA-4), 126–127, 139,
    139f, 444–445, 504, 546
Cytotoxins, hypoxic, 335

D

da Vinci Surgical System (Intuitive
    Surgical Inc.), 283–284
Dabrafenib, 442
    side effects of, 499
Dacomitinib, 440
DC-based vaccines, for lung cancer, 126
DDR2 gene, 484
    in lung cancer, 26–27, 26t
Deep venous thrombosis, 193
Delayed radiation myelopathy, 411
Denaturing HPLC, 166t

Dendritic cell-based immunotherapy, 546–547, 547f
Dendritic cells, 124–125, 139–140
Denosumab, 388
  for bone metastases, 190
Dermatologic disorders, paraneoplastic, 191–192, 191t
Dermatomyositis, 191
Dexamethasone, for fatigue, 616
Diagnosis
  earlier, 636–637
  endoscopic techniques for, 237–239
  future considerations, 657
  invasive, 652–653, 653f
Diagnostic algorithms, 651
Diagnostic platforms, 655–657, 656f
Diagnostic workup, 233–240.e2
  changes in, 76
Diaphragmatic paralysis, lung cancer and, 189
Diarrhea
  consequences and management of, 497
  EGFR TKI-induced, 496
  incidence and effect of, 496–497
  mechanism of, 496
Diet, lung cancer and, 36
Dietary factors, lung cancer and, 3–4
Diff Quik stain, 184
Diffuse idiopathic pulmonary neuroendocrine cell hyperplasia (DIPNECH), 155
Digital clubbing, 191
Discoidin domain receptors (DDRs), 484
Disseminated intravascular coagulopathy, 193
DLCO. see Carbon monoxide lung diffusion capacity (DLCO)
DNA
  circulating tumor, 64
  mitochondrial, 64
  radiation damage, 330
DNA hypermethylation, in lung cancer, 111–114, 112f
DNA hypomethylation, in lung cancer, 111–115
DNA methylation, 104–116.e5, 110–111
  in lung cancer in never-smokers, 27–28
DNA template, or single DNA molecules, massively parallel, 166
Docetaxel
  adjuvant chemotherapy with, 519
  combination chemotherapy with
    for EGFR mutated NSCLC, 427, 427t
    for malignant mesothelioma, 541t
    for nonsmall cell lung cancer, 420–421, 421t
  for locally advanced nonsmall cell lung cancer, 367
  maintenance chemotherapy with
    continuation, 454
    switch, 450
  neurotoxicity of, 414
  for nonsmall cell lung cancer, 420, 420t
  phase II studies of, 435
  thymidylate synthase and, 476

Doxorubicin
  dose-dense regimens of, 528
  for extensive-stage SCLC, 525, 526t
Drinking water contamination, 7
Drug development. see also specific drugs
  phase I trial, 621
  phase II trial, 622–624, 622f
  phase II/III designs, 625–626
Drug toxicity, chemotherapy and, 211
Dry skin (xerosis), 491t, 494t
Duloxetine, 416, 416t
Durvalumab, 445
Dutch Lung Cancer Study Group, 379
Dysphagia, lung cancer and, 189
Dyspnea, 187, 616

E
E1A-binding protein p300 (EP300), 164–165
E4599 trial, 460
E5508 trial, 460
Early phase trials, 621–622, 621f
East Asians, 25–27
Eastern Cooperative Oncology Group (ECOG), 514–515
Echinoderm microtubule-associated protein-like 4 and anaplastic lymphoma kinase (EMLA-ALK), as molecularly targeted therapeutic agents, 368–369
ECOG score, in patient selection for radiotherapy, 337
Effusions, pleural, in malignant mesothelioma, 537, 537f
EGFR gene, 25, 26t, 46
  in adenocarcinoma, 431, 431t
  amplification of, 84
  in lung cancer, 64, 70–71
  mutations
    assay for, 165–166
    clinical-pathologic characteristics in, 169t
    detection, commonly used methods for, 166t
    for EGFR TKI therapy, 169–172, 170t
    in lung adenocarcinomas, 169t
    in lung cancer, 164–165
    for NSCLCs, 169
    testing, 165
  in nonsmall cell lung cancer, 420
EGFR TKIs. see Tyrosine kinase inhibitors (TKIs), EGFR
Elderly patients
  chemoradiation therapy for, 367–368, 368f
  chemotherapy for, 424, 424t
  first-line chemotherapy for, 529–531
  nonsmall cell lung cancer in, management of, 423–424
Elective nodal irradiation (ENI), 377
Electronic portal imaging, 326
Electroporation, irreversible, 356–357, 358f
ELUXA trial program, 440–441
Emerging technologies, 101
Emphysema, lung cancer and, 6
Encephalomyelitis, 194, 234t

Endobronchial brachytherapy, 385, 595
Endobronchial needle aspiration, 237
Endobronchial ultrasound (EBUS), 236, 250–252, 251f
  combined with EUS, 238–239
  mediastinal evaluation, 538
Endobronchial ultrasound-guided fine-needle aspiration (EBUS-FNA), 237
Endobronchial ultrasound-guided transbronchial needle aspiration (EBUS-TBNA), 237, 241, 251, 251f
Endocrine phenomena, paraneoplastic, 191t, 192–193
Endoscopic ultrasound (EUS), 236, 250–252
  combined with EBUS, 238–239
  mediastinal evaluation, 538
Endoscopic ultrasound-guided fine-needle aspiration (EUS-FNA), 250
Endoscopic ultrasound-guided needle aspiration (EUS-NA), 241
Endothelial hyperplasia lesions, 118
Endovascular embolization, 600–601, 601f–602f
  complications of, 602t
Endovascular stenting, for SVCS, 188–189
EndoWrist instruments, 283–284
End-point considerations, clinical trials, 622–623
End-to-end anastomosis, 305–306
Environmental exposures, lung cancer and, 35
Environmental tobacco smoke, 11
Environmental toxins, lung cancer in never-smokers and, 24
Enzastaurin, 78, 78t
EORTC trial, 456t
EPH receptor A3 (EPHA3), 164–165
EPH receptor A5 (EPHA5), 164–165
EPH7 gene, 164–165
Epidemiology, of lung cancer, 30–33
  in Asia, 33, 33f
  in Europe, 32–33, 32f
  in United States, 30–32, 31f
Epidermal growth factor receptor (EGFR), 34–35, 196, 335–336, 434, 468–469
  blockade of
    biomarkers for, 429
    in NSCLC, 427–430
  as molecularly targeted therapeutic agents, 368–369
  monoclonal antibody against, 428–429
  mutations, 468–469
    consequences of, 469
    in NSCLC, 469t
  nonsmall cell lung cancer and, 358–359, 427
  overexpression of, 341, 468
  somatic mutations in, 479
  upregulation of, 368
  wild-type, 468

Epidermal growth factor receptor (EGFR) inhibitors, 46
  dermatologic side effects of, 491–496, 491t, 492f
  dose-modification strategy for, 492–494, 496f
  gastrointestinal side effects of, 496–497
  maintenance therapy with, 455–460, 456t
  for NSCLC, 43, 44t
  pulmonary side effects of, 497–498
  second-and third-generation, 439–441
Epidermal growth factor vaccine, 504
Epidural tumors, resection of, 301, 301f
Epigenetics
  genetic interactions, 105, 106f
  of lung cancer, 104–116.e5, 107f, 115t, 197
  mechanisms of, 105f
Epigenome, 97–98
Epirubicin, for malignant mesothelioma, 541t
Epithelial cell adhesion molecule-based technology, 174
Epithelial-to-mesenchymal transition (EMT), 121–122
Epithelium, normal-appearing, 122
ERACLE trial, 455
ERBB2 gene, 164–165
  amplification of, 84–85
ERCC1 gene, 425
  in advanced NSCLC, 472, 473f–474f
  thymidylate synthase and, 476
Erlotinib, 368, 427
  epidermal growth factor receptor tyrosine kinase inhibitor, 455
  gastrointestinal side effects of, 496–497
  IFCT-GFPC 0502 trial of, 454
  as maintenance therapy, 459
  second-line treatment with, 437–438
  for squamous cell carcinoma, 439–440
  vs. platinum doublet chemotherapy, for nonsmall cell lung cancer, 427, 427t
ERS/ESTS. see European Respiratory Society/European Society of Thoracic Surgeons (ERS/ESTS)
Esophageal cysts, 552
Esophagitis, radiation-induced, 399, 402f
Esophagus toxicity, 399–403
  acute, of thoracic radiotherapy, 393–408.e4
  clinical factors in, 401–402
  dosimetric factors, 400–401
  grading, 399–400, 401f
  late
    scoring, 399t
    of thoracic radiotherapy, 393–408.e4
Estrogen, nongenomic signaling, and interactions with growth factor receptor signaling pathways, 39–40, 39f
Estrogen receptors, lung cancer and, 36–38, 37f
ESTRO-QUARTS project, 648
Ethnic differences, in targeted therapy side effects, 500

Ethnicity, and prognosis, 419
Etoposide
  combination chemoradiation therapy with, for locally advanced nonsmall cell lung cancer, 367
  combination chemotherapy with dose-dense regimens, 528
    for extensive-stage SCLC, 525, 526t
    for poor performance status patients, 531
EUR-ASSESS Project, 647
Europe, 32–33, 32f
European Association of Nuclear Medicine, 225
European Organisation for Research and Treatment of Cancer (EORTC), 370, 375, 515
  cardiac toxicity, scoring system, 404, 405t
  late esophagus toxicity scoring, 399–400, 399t
European Organization for research and Treatment of Cancer Quality of Life Questionnaire (EORTC-LC-13), 615
European Randomized Trial of Tarceva versus Chemotherapy (EURTAC), 165–166
European Respiratory Society (ERS), 637
  classification of adenocarcinoma, 256–257
European Respiratory Society/European Society of Thoracic Surgeons (ERS/ESTS), guidelines on evaluation and treatment of cardiac risk factors in candidates, 266
European Society for Medical Oncology (ESMO), 464
  Clinical Practice Guidelines: early-stage and locally advanced NSCLC, 319b–320b
  Clinical Practice Guidelines: SCLC, 319b–320b
  evidence-based practice guidelines for multiple primary lung cancers (MPLCs), 312
  in guidelines for biomarker testing, 165
European Society of Thoracic Surgeons (ESTS), indications for invasive mediastinal staging and, 242
European Union, 32–33, 32f
EUROSCAN study, 79
Ever-smokers, 23, 28t
Evidence-based requirements analysis, 646
Evidence-based tobacco dependence treatment, delivery of, in cancer settings, 19
ExacTrac, 326
Excision repair cross-complementation group 1 (ERCC1), 195, 466–467, 470–475
  mRNA expression, 44, 44f
Excision repair cross-complementing rodent repair deficiency, complementation group 1 (ERCC1), 175–176

Exercise testing, 268–270
Extended lymph node dissection, 245t
Extended mediastinoscopy, 249
Extensive disease, prophylactic cranial irradiation in, 380–381
External-beam radiotherapy, 383
  for bone metastases, uncomplicated, 386, 386f
  for central airway obstruction, 594–595
  complicated, 386–387
  hemibody, 387–388
  indications for, 386–387
  minimally invasive techniques and, 388
  with other modalities, 388–389
  regimens, 383
  repeat radiation, 384–385, 388–389
  side effects of, 383–384, 388
  systemic therapy and, 388
Extracellular ice crystals, 356
Extrapleural pneumonectomy, 542–545, 543f, 543t, 545f
Extrathymic second malignancy, 570

F
^{18}F fluoromisonidazole (FMISO), 231
^{18}F FPPRGD2, 229–230
F-2-deoxy-D-glucose uptake, in patient selection for radiotherapy, 340–341
^{18}F-AH111585. see ^{18}-F-fluciclatide
Familial aggregation, 47–48
Family history, 35
Fatigue, 615–616
  and patient selection for radiotherapy, 339
FDG-PET, 219–220
  for LD-SCLC, 377–378
FDG-PET-CT, 227–231, 227f
Female Lung Cancer Consortium in Asia (FLCCA), 34
Fenretinide, 77–78, 78t
Fetal adenocarcinoma, 147
^{18}-F-fluciclatide, 229–230, 231f
^{18}F-galacto-RGD, 229–230
FGFR gene, 487
FGFR1 gene, 164–165, 483
  amplification of, 85–86
FGFR2 gene, 483
  in lung cancer, 26–27, 26t
FGFR3 gene, 483
Fibroblast growth factor receptor (FGFR), 483
Fibroblast growth factor receptor 1 (FGFR1), 196
Fibroblast growth factor receptor 2 (FGFR2), 164–165
Fibroblast growth factor receptor 4 (FGFR4), 164–165
Fibrosis, pulmonary, 395t
"Field cancerization," 122
Fine-needle aspiration
  algorithm for optimizing samples, 180, 181f
  endobronchial ultrasound (EBUS), 237
  endoscopic ultrasound (EUS), 250
  samples, 160
  slide preparation for, 180–182, 182f
  steps for processing, 181b
  vs. core-needle biopsy, 179

Finite-element methods, 323
Firefly Fluorescence Imaging (Intuitive
 Surgical Inc.), 283–284
First-generation sequencing, 95–96
FLEX trial, 459–460
Flexible bronchoscopy, 237
 for central airway obstruction
  examination, 593
Fluorescence in situ hybridization
 (FISH), 166, 167f
 ALK-FISH assay, 173, 174f
3'-deoxy-3'-fluorothymidine (FLT)
 PET, 228, 230f
5-Fluorouracil, 476
Fluticasone, 78t
Folic acid, 78t
Foretinib, 490
Forkhead box P1 (FOXP1), 164–165
Formalin-fixed paraffin-embedded
 (FFPE) tissue, 165
Formalin-fixed samples, 101
Former smoker, definition of, 23
FoxP3, 141
Fractionation
 accelerated
  clinical applications of, 333
  schedules, in lung cancer, 333
 conventional, 332
Fracture, pathologic, 386
Fragilis, 338
Fragment length, and RFLP analysis,
 166t
Frailty, and patient selection for
 radiotherapy, 338
Frameshift mutations, 95
Framework Convention on Tobacco
 Control (FCTC), 9
France, 32–33, 32f
Freeze-thaw cycle, 356
Fruits, lung cancer and, 3
Fulvestrant, 38
Functional Assessment of Cancer
 Therapy-Lung (FACT-L), 615
Future directions
 in chemoprevention, 80
 for lung cancer diagnosis, 657
 for maintenance chemotherapy
  for nonsmall cell lung cancer,
  464–465
 for microRNAs, 136
 for next-generation sequencing, 103
 for radiotherapy, 335
 for tobacco use treatment, 20–22

G
Gabapentin, 416–417, 416t
Ganetespib, 443–444
Gefitinib, 368, 459
 gastrointestinal side effects of, 496
 second-line treatment with, 437, 437t
 vs. platinum doublet chemotherapy,
  for nonsmall cell lung cancer, 427,
  427t
Gemcitabine
 for advanced NSCLC in elderly
  patients, 424, 424t
 combination chemotherapy with
  with bevacizumab, 425, 426t

Gemcitabine (Continued)
 for EGFR mutated NSCLC,
  427–428, 427t
 in elderly patients, 424, 424t
 for nonsmall cell lung cancer,
  420–422, 421t, 424, 424t
 maintenance chemotherapy with
  continuation, 450–454
  historical trials, 449
  switch, 450
 for malignant mesothelioma, 540, 546
 for nonsmall cell lung cancer, 135,
  420, 420t
 phase II studies of, 435
Gender differences
 in advanced NSCLC, 43, 44t
 in early-stage lung cancer, 40–42
 in lung cancer, 30–45.e5, 31f
Gene amplification, as mechanism of
 oncogenesis, 84–86, 85f. see also
 specific genes
 EGFR, 84
 ERBB2, 84–85
 FGFR1, 86
 MET, 85
 PIK3CA, 85–86
Gene copy number, 166
Gene expression arrays, 196–197
Gene expression profiling, 65, 476–477
Gene expression signatures, 336
Gene hypermethylation, 65–66
Gene mutations. see also specific genes
 epidermal growth factor receptor
  (EGFR), 468–469, 469t
 frameshift, 95
 indels, 95
 in lung cancer, 65, 165–166
 missense, 95
 nonsense, 95
 and patient selection for radiotherapy,
  341
 silent, 95
 in smokers vs. never-smokers, 98, 99f
 splicing, 95
Gene silencing, 71
Gene structure, changes in, 166
Gene therapy, for malignant
 mesothelioma, 549
General thoracic operation, definition
 of, 283
Genetic abnormalities, in lung cancer,
 164–165
Genetic alterations. see also Gene
 mutations
 epigenetic interactions and, 105, 106f
 in lung cancer, 105
 in squamous cell lung cancer, 98, 101f
 at SWI/SNF chromatin remodeling
  factors, 108f, 109–110, 109t
Genetic changes, in lung cancer, 64–66
Genetics
 epigenetic interactions, 105, 106f
 of lung cancer, 25
 in never-smokers, 25
 susceptibility to lung cancer, 46–51.e2
Genome organizers, 105f
Genome-wide association studies, 50–51
Genome-wide molecular changes, 27

Genomic technologies, 95–96
Genomics, for lung cancer, 65
Genotyping, MALDI-TOF MS-base,
 166t
Germ cell tumors, 550–551, 551f
 nonseminomatous, 551
Germany, 32–33, 32f
Giant cell carcinoma, 154
Gilbert syndrome, 477
Global Adult Tobacco Survey, 10–11
Global Analysis of Pemetrexed in SCLC,
 527
Global Health Professions Student
 Survey, 10–11
Global Lung Cancer Coalition (GLCC),
 635, 636f
Global School Personnel Survey, 10–11
Global Tobacco Surveillance System,
 10–11
Global Youth Tobacco Survey, 10–11
Glutathione S-transferase (GSTM1), 34
GNAS complex locus (GNAS), 164–165
Goiter, substernal, 552–553, 553f
Golden Grading System, 390
Gottron papules, 191
Graded Prognostic Assessment (GPA),
 390
 disease-specific, 390
Granulocytosis, 234t
Granulomas, 184
Ground-glass nodules, 235
Growth factor receptor signaling
 pathways, 39–40, 39f
Guidelines, 641–642. see also specific
 guidelines
 for biomarker testing, 165
 for care of individual lung cancer
  patients, 641
 general population outcomes and,
  642–643
 for molecular testing, 165
 for tobacco use treatment, 20

H
Hadron Therapy Systems, 324
Hair abnormalities, 491t, 492, 493f
Hampton Hump sign, 213
Hand-foot skin reaction, 494–495, 496f
Health care
 accessibility of, 640
 development and application of
  practice guidelines, 641
 efficiency in, 640
 quality in, 640
 standards for care of individual,
  640–643
Health services providers, 638
Health services research, 639–650.e3
Health system performance, three
 dimensions of, 639–640
Heart, radiation injury, 403–407
 management of, 407
 pathophysiology of, 403–404, 403f
 prevention of, 407
Heart disease, radiation-associated, 404,
 405t
Heart imaging, 403–404, 404f
Heart toxicity, grading of, 404–407

Heat shock protein 90, 488
Heat-shock protein 90 inhibitors, 443–444
 side effects of, 498–499
Heat-shock proteins chaperone antigenic peptides, 361
Heat sink, 358
Hedgehog signaling, 119
HeliScope, 101
Helper T cells, 123
Hematologic disorders, 570
 paraneoplastic, 191t, 193
Hemibody external-beam radiation, 387–388
Hemoptysis, 233–234
 local tumor growth and, 187
 massive, 596–602
Hepatocyte growth factor, 490
Hepatocyte growth factor receptor, 442–443
Hepatocyte growth factor receptor-MET, 482–483
HER1 gene, 468
HER2 gene, 431t
Heterozygosity, loss of, 559
High-quality oncology care, 19
High-resolution melting analysis, 166t
Hispanic, 169t
Histology
 importance in treatment of NSCLC, 423
 in nonsmall cell lung cancer, 419
 small specimens, 178–185.e2
 of thymic tumors, 573–576
 tumor, 653–654
Histone deacetylase inhibitors, 115
Histone modifications, 105–108
Histone-modifying enzymes, 106, 107t
HLA-A gene, 431t
Hoarseness, in lung cancer, 187–188
Hodgkin disease, 406, 407t
Hodgkin lymphoma, 551–552
Hormonal symptoms, of bronchopulmonary carcinoid, 565–566
Hormone replacement therapy (HRT), lung cancer and, 38
Hormones, lung cancer and, 4–5
Horner syndrome, 189, 233–234
HOX family, 113
HPV-16, lung cancer and
HPV-18, lung cancer and
HSVtk gene, 549
Human epidermal growth factor receptor type 2 (HER2), 480–481
Human epidermal growth factor receptor type 3 (HER3), 481–482
Human leukocyte antigen (HLA), 139
Human papillomavirus (HPV), lung cancer and, 35
 in never-smokers, 24
Humoral hypercalcemia of malignancy (HHM), 192–193
Humoral immune dysregulation, 137–142.e3, 138f
Hungary, 32–33, 32f
Hypercalcemia, 192–193, 234, 234t
Hypercoagulation states, 193

Hyperfractionated accelerated radiotherapy (HART), 333, 364
Hyperfractionation, clinical applications of, 332
Hypersensitivity reaction, 491t
Hypertrophic pulmonary osteoarthropathy, 191
Hypofractionated radiation schedules, 333
Hypofractionation, 364
Hyponatremia, 192, 234t
Hypoxia, tumor, 335
Hypoxic cell radiosensitizers, 335
Hypoxic cytotoxins, 335

IFCT-GFPC 0502 trial, 452t, 454, 456t
Ifosfamide, 421–422, 422t
Illumina, 96
Iloprost, 78, 78t
Imaging. *see also specific modalities*
 adrenal gland, 210
 bone, 210
 brain, 210
 of central airway obstruction, 214
 conventional, 199–218.e3
 electronic portal, 326
 heart, 403–404, 404f
 liver, 210
 massive pleural effusions, 606
 of neuroendocrine tumors, 561–563
 prognostic biomarkers, 539
 of pulmonary embolism, 213
 radiotherapy planning and, technical advances in, 328
 of superior vena cava syndrome, 214, 214f
Imaging systems, 320
Immobilization devices, for radiotherapy, 321
Immune checkpoint inhibition, 546
Immune checkpoint inhibitors, 444, 504–509
 PD-1/PD-L-1, 369
Immune dysfunction, cigarette smoking and, 142
Immune dysregulation
 cellular, 137–142.e3
 cigarette smoking and, 140, 142
 humoral, 137–142.e3
 in lung cancer, 137–142.e3, 138f
Immune effector cells, 122–123
Immune-modulating agents, 533
Immunization, intratumoral, for lung cancer, 126
Immunohistochemistry (IHC)
 of ALK rearrangement, 172–175
 optimization of specimens for, 182–183
 in protein expression, 165
 sample processing and analysis in, 168
 tissue requirements for, 167–168
Immunologic dysfunction, in patients with lung cancer, 501–502, 502f
Immunostimulatory monoclonal antibodies, 126–127
Immunosuppressive cytokines, 546
Immunosurveillance, 501

Immunotherapy
 dendritic cell-based, 546–547, 547f
 for lung cancer, 501–511.e3, 176
  use of, supporting evidence for, 502
 mesothelin-targeted, 547–548
 for nonsmall cell lung cancer, 432, 461–462, 502
 PD1 ligand (PDL1), 501
 program death-1 (PD1), 501
Implanted markers, with radiofrequency guidance, 326
In vitro studies of stem cells, 117–120.e2
In vivo studies of stem cells, 117–120.e2
Indels, 95
India, smoking and smoking-attributable deaths in, 10
Indoor air pollution, 6–7
 lung cancer in never-smokers and, 24
Induction therapy, measurement of tumor size after, 257
Industrial robots, 283
Infections. *see also specific infections*
 lung cancer and, 5
 testing for, 184
Inferior mediastinoscopy, 250
Inflammatory cytokines, 617
Inflammatory mediators, 122–123
INFORM trial, 456t
Inhibin beta A (INHBA), 164–165
INI1, 109t
Insulin-like growth factor, 490
αvβ3 integrin, 229–230
Intensity-modulated radiation therapy (IMRT), 324–326, 325f
Intensive care unit, lung cancer and, 618
Interferon, 566
Interleukin-2 (IL-2), 125
Interleukin-6 (IL-6), 125
Interleukin-10 (IL-10), 140
International Adjuvant Lung Cancer Trial (IALT), 515
International Agency for Research on Cancer Lung Cancer Consortium (IARC), 319b–320b
International Association for the Study of Lung Cancer (IASLC), 19
 classification of adenocarcinoma proposed by, 256–257
 database for eight edition, 253, 254t
 guidelines for molecular testing, 165, 185
 lymph node stations, 241–242
 map of regional lymph nodes, 238f, 242f
 regional lymph node map, 255, 257f
 Staging and Prognostic Factors Committee, 255
International Atomic Energy Agency, 318
International Cancer Benchmarking Partnership, 637
International Commission on Radiation Units and Measurements (ICRU), 321–322
International Mesothelioma Interest Group staging system, 537, 538t
International Tailored Chemotherapy Adjuvant Trial, 523, 523f

Interstitial lung disease, 497–498
  incidence of, 497
  management of, 497–498
Intrafraction imaging approaches, 326
Intrapleural therapy, 544–545
Intrapulmonary metastases, of lung
  cancer, 260, 262t
Intratumoral immunization, for lung
  cancer, 126
Intuitive Surgical Inc., 283
Invasion
  locoregional, 219
  visceral pleural, 255f, 262
Invasive adenocarcinoma, 144t, 146–147
  variants of, 147–148, 148f
Invasive mucinous adenocarcinoma, 147,
  148f
Invasive staging
  indications for, mediastinal, 242–244
  required lymph node stations for,
    245
  techniques for, 245–252
Ionizing radiation, 5. *see also* Radiation
Ipilimumab, 444, 490, 504–505, 533–534
  for nonsmall cell lung cancer, 432
Iressa NSCLC Trial Evaluating
    Response and Survival *versus*
    Taxotere (INTEREST), 437
Irinotecan, 477
  combination chemotherapy with,
    525–527, 526t
  for nonsmall cell lung cancer, 420,
    420t
Irinotecan, radiotherapy with, 367
Irreversible electroporation, mechanism
  of action of, 356–357, 358f
Isothiocyanates, lung cancer and, 4, 4f
Isotretinoin, 78t–79t
Italian Association of Medical Oncology/
    Italian Society of Pathology and
    Cytopathology, 165
Italy, 32–33, 32f

J

Jackman criteria, 429
Janus Kinase 2 (JAK2), 164–165
Japan, smoking and smoking-attributable
  deaths in, 10
Japan Clinical Oncology Group (JCOG),
  375
JCOG. *see* Japan Clinical Oncology
  Group (JCOG)
JMEN trial, 448, 450, 451f
  evaluation of pemetrexed, 450
Joule-Thompson effect, 356

K

Karnofsky, David A., 330–331
Karnofsky score, and patient selection for
  radiotherapy, 337
KEAP1 gene, 431t
Kelch-like ECH-associated protein 1
    (KEAP1), 164–165
Ketamine, 417
Keyhole limpet hemocyanin, 547
Ki-67, 196
Kinase insert domain receptor (KDR),
  164–165

KRAS gene, 46, 196, 469
  in adjacent histologically normal-
    appearing lung, 122
  in lung adenocarcinoma, 431t
  in lung cancer, 25, 26t, 70–71,
    164–165
  mutations in, 25, 442
  in nonsmall cell lung cancer, 420

L

Lambert-Eaton Myasthenic syndrome
    (LEMS), 194
Lambert-Eaton syndrome, 234t
Laparoscopy, 537
Lapatinib, 480
Large cell carcinoma, 144t, 154–155,
  155f
Large cell neuroendocrine carcinoma
    (LCNEC), 156f, 157, 556t
  from adenocarcinoma, markers for
    differentiation of, 558
  adjuvant treatment of, 564–565
  atypical and typical carcinoids from,
    markers for differentiation of, 559
  chromosomal aberrations in, 559
  classification of, 555, 556t
  clinical characteristics, 561
  combined, 567, 567f
  cytology, 556–557
  diagnosis of, 555–559
  differential diagnosis of, 557–559
  heterozygosity, loss of, 559
  histology of, 556, 557f
  imaging of, 561
  metastatic, therapy for, 566–567
  microarray comparison, 560
  molecular biology of, 559
  molecularly targeted therapies for, 567
  mutation analysis of, 560, 560t
  pathways, 560–561
  prognosis, 567–568
  from small cell lung cancer, markers
    for differentiation of, 559
  from squamous cell carcinoma,
    markers for differentiation of, 558
  staging of, 561
  surgery of, 562t, 564
Laser capture microdissection (LCM),
  168
L-BLP25, 503
LCSG. *see* Lung Cancer Study Group
    (LCSG) trial
Leiomyoma, 553, 553f
Lemur tyrosine kinase 2 (LMTK2),
  164–165
Lepidic predominant adenocarcinoma
    (term), 144
Lepidic predominant invasive
    adenocarcinoma, 144t, 147
Leptomeningeal carcinomatosis, in
    NSCLC, 190
let-7, 129, 130t, 134
let-7a, 130t
Leukocyte receptor tyrosine kinase
    (LTK), 164–165
Leukocytosis, 193
Lhermitte sign, 411
Limbic encephalitis, 194

Linear accelerator, 323–324, 323f
Linear-quadratic model, 330–331, 334
Linkage analysis, 49–50
Lipids, lung cancer and, 4
Liquid biopsies, 102–103, 102f
Liquid-based cytology, 160–161
Liquid-based preparations, 184
Liver imaging, 210
Liver metastases
  lung cancer and, 190–191
  stereotactic ablative radiotherapy
    (SABR) for, 351
  therapy directed against, 565
Lobar collapse, postobstructive, 209
Lobbying, political, 638
Lobectomy
  radical, 289, 291f
  for small lung cancers, 293, 293f
  VATS, 274
Lobe-specific systematic lymph node
    dissection, 244, 245t
Local tumor growth, symptoms and signs
    of, 186–187
Locoregional invasion, PET imaging of,
    219
Lopez model, 9–10, 10f
Loss of heterozygosity, 64–65, 70
Low public profile, 636
Low-density lipoprotein receptor-related
    protein 1B (LRP1B), 164–165
Low-dose radiation computed
    tomography (LDCT), 52, 54t, 72
  improvements in, 76
  recommended algorithm for
    management of findings, 73f
  screening for lung cancer, 76
    eligibility for, 72–74, 74t
    meeting or exceeding NLST
      favorable outcomes, 75
Low-technology tests, 268–269
Lung
  function, and patient selection for
    radiotherapy, 330–331
  normal, 117
  rodent fetal, 117
Lung adenocarcinoma. *see*
    Adenocarcinoma
Lung Adjuvant Cisplatin Evaluation
    (LACE), 517
Lung cancer, 30, 434–435. *see also specific
    types*
  adrenal gland metastases and, 190–191
  advanced, prognostic/predictive role of
    gender in, 42–45
  agents and clinical development, 505f,
    504–509
  age-standardized death rates for
    women in Europe, 32, 32f
  amplification as mechanism of
    oncogenesis in, 84–86, 85f–86f
    EGFR, 84
    ERBB2, 84–85
    FGFR1, 86
    MET, 85
    PIK3CA, 85–86
  barriers to optimal care for, 647–648
    case studies from high-income
      countries, 647–649

Lung cancer (*Continued*)
classification of, 647
in low-and-middle-income
countries, 648
best-practices treatment and care for,
637
biologic heterogeneity, 641
biologic risk factors for, 47
biomarker-based subgroups,
622f–623f, 623–624
biomarker-based trial designs, 626
biomarkers for
diagnostic, 129–132, 130t–131t
early detection of, 60f, 61–68
microRNAs as, 129–136.e2
preclinical, 59–68.e4
prognostic, 132–134, 133t
for treatment response, 134–136,
135t
brain metastases and, 190
cardiopulmonary resuscitation and,
618
case-control studies of, 47–48
case-family cohort studies of, 47–48
CD133-positive stem-like population
in, isolation of, 117–118
characteristics missed on radiography,
204
checkpoint inhibitors, 504–506
chemoprevention of, 69–81.e5,
126–127
trials, 76–80
chemotherapy for, 42–43
chest pain and, 187
chest-confined, 233–240.e2
classic anatomic pathology and,
143–163.e4
classification of, 653–657
diffuse pneumonic-type lung
adenocarcinoma, 260, 263t
metachronous primary lung cancers,
260, 262t
multifocal pulmonary
adenocarcinomas, with ground
glass/lepidic features, 260, 262t
with multiple lesions, 260, 263t
separate tumor nodules of
same histopathologic type
(intrapulmonary metastases),
260, 262t
synchronous primary lung cancers,
260, 262t
tumor, node, and metastasis (TNM),
eight edition of, 253–264.e1
clinical and molecular prognostication
of, 194–197, 195t
clinical features of, 233–234
clinical presentation and prognostic
factors in, 186–198.e6, 187t
clinical research in, 628–634.e2, 629f
clinical trial methodology, 620–627.e2
clinical trial organization
clinical trials and impact of
biomarkers on design, selection
of hypotheses for, 629
cooperation and networks, 631
definition of, 628
financial issues, 632–633

Lung cancer (*Continued*)
issues in, 628–629
mixing avatar models and clinical
trials, 631
modern clinical trials, designs for,
629–631, 630f–631f
national, multinational, and
international cooperation/
competition, 629
quick progress and impact on
financial issues, expectations
for, 628–629, 629f
regulatory issues, 632
solutions for, 629–633
worldwide standardization, of
oncology clinical trials allowing
cross-trial comparisons,
631–632, 632f, 633t
clinical trial promotion
conducting clinical trials, increasing
difficulty of, 633
educate general population and
patients with, 634
goal and philosophy of different
systems, 633
issues in, 633
patient education, 633
simplify regulation, 634, 634t
solutions, 633–634
time and effort, 633
train physician early and
continuously, 633–634
combination strategy, 509–510, 510f
conventional imaging of, 199–218.e3
with chest radiographs, 202–205
with CT, 205–206
of emergent conditions in, 213–214
with MRI, 214–215
copy number abnormalities in, 82–94.
e4
cough and, 186–187
criterion-based benchmarking, 646
current classification of, 144t
cytologic analysis of, 160–162
bronchial scraping, brushing, or
washing, 160
fine-needle aspiration samples, 160
liquid-based cytology, 160–161
molecular analysis of cytology
specimens, 161
pleural fluid or washing materials,
160
special staining and
immunocytochemistry of
cytology specimens, 161
sputum smears, 160
cytologic characteristics of each
histologic type of, 161–162
adenocarcinoma, 161–162, 161f
small cell lung cancer, 161f, 162
squamous cell carcinoma, 161f,
162
data from patients with radiotherapy-
associated cardiac toxicity,
405–406
descriptive epidemiology of, 1, 2f, 3t
development and application of
practice guidelines, 641

Lung cancer (*Continued*)
diagnosis of
future considerations in, 657f
invasive, 652–653, 653f
use of immunohistochemistry for,
158–160, 159f
diagnostic approach for, 236–239
diagnostic workup for, 233–240.e2
changes in, 76
diaphragmatic paralysis and, 189
diet in, 35–36
distant metastasis of, 221–223, 222f
DNA hypermethylation in, 111–114,
112f
DNA hypomethylation in, 111–115
driver mutations in, 26t
dysphagia and, 189
dyspnea and, 187
earlier diagnosis of, 636–637
early, management of, 69–81.e5
early detection of, 59–61
early phase trials, 621–622, 621f
early stage
gender as a prognostic factor in,
40–42, 41f
and pulmonary metastases,
328
enrolled in clinical trial, increased
number of people with, 636
environmental exposures in, 35–36
epidemiology of, 1–8.e3, 2f, 30–33
in Asia, 33, 33f
in Europe, 32–33, 32f
in United States, 30–32, 31f
epigenetic events in, 104–116.e5
epigenetic therapy for, 115–116,
115t
evidence-based requirements analysis,
646
extended resections for, 295–303.e2
extended resections for,
bronchovascular sleeve resections,
304–307.e1
familial aggregation of, 47–48
family history of, 35
first-line PD1 inhibition, 508–509
funding for, 636
gender-related differences in, 30–45.
e5, 31f
gene fusions in, 82–94.e4
general quality standards for, 643
genetic abnormalities in, 164–165
genetic alterations in, 105
genetic factors in, gender-related
differences in, 34–35, 35f–36f
genetic susceptibility to, 46–51.e2
genome-wide association studies,
50–51
guidelines for care of individual
patients with, 641
health services research, 639–650.e3
help for people with, 637
hemoptysis and, 187
high-risk syndromes conferring an
increased risk of, 48
histone modifications in, 105–108
history in, 234–235, 651–652, 651f
human papillomavirus (HPV) in, 35

Lung cancer (*Continued*)

imaging of
CT, 235, 235t
features of, 235–236
PET, 219–232.e4, 220f–221f
immune dysfunction in, 137–142.e3
immunologic dysfunction in, 501–502, 502f
immunotherapy for, 501–511.e3
use of, supporting evidence for, 502
incidence of, 199
initial evaluation of, 651–653
initial phase I study, 506–507
and intensive care unit, 618
intrathoracic spread of, symptoms and signs of, 187–189
linkage analysis of, 49–50
liver metastases and, 190–191
locally advanced, 328
local-regional spread of, symptoms and signs of, 187–189
locoregional invasion by, 219
Lopez model on, 9–10, 10f
marginally resectable
patients with, 314, 315t
surgical management of, 314–317.e1
melanoma-associated antigen-A3 vaccine, 502–503
metastatic spread of. *see also* Metastases
symptoms and signs of, 189–191
and microenvironment, 121–128.e4
miRNAs in, 129–136
molecular classification of, 654–655, 654f–655f
molecular testing in, 164–177.e5
morphologic features of, 235t
mortality, 143
tobacco control impact on, 10f, 12–16, 13f–17f
mucinous glycoprotein-1 vaccines, 503–504
multidisciplinary team management, 643–645
multiple primary, staging system for, 309, 310t
mutational events in, 95–103.e2, 100f
in never-smokers, 23–29.e3, 33–34
clinical-pathologic features of, 24–25
DNA methylation, 27–28
East Asian individuals, molecular characteristics of, 25–27
epidemiology of, 23–24
genetics of, 25
genome-wide molecular changes in, 27
known or suspected etiologic factors of, 24
preneoplastic changes in, 27
new specific rules for, 256–260
new targets for therapy in, 479–489. e6, 489
nonreceptor targets of, 485–489
cyclin-dependent kinase, 488–489
heat shock protein 90, 488
mammalian target of rapamycin, 487–488
mitogen activated protein kinase-MEK, 486

Lung cancer (*Continued*)

phosphoinositide 3-kinase, 486–487
protein kinase B-AKT, 487
RAS, 485
v-Raf murine sarcoma viral oncogene homolog B-BRAF, 485–486
nonsmall cell. *see* Nonsmall cell lung cancer (NSCLC)
nonsmoking-related, 23–24
oligometastases from, 350–351
outcomes of
benefits of cessation on, 18–19
guidelines for improvement, in general population, 642–643
health services research and, 639
smoking cessation and, 11
variations in patterns of care, 648–649
palliative care in, role of, 608–619.e8
palliative radiotherapy for, 382–392.e3
Pancoast syndrome and, 189
paraneoplastic syndromes of, 191–194, 191t, 234
pathologic classification of, 653–657, 653f
pathology samples for molecular testing of, 160
pericardial effusion and, 188, 188f
pharmacogenomics in, 466–478.e3
phase I trial, 621
phase II trials, 622–624, 622f
phase II/III and phase III trials, 624–626
phase II/III designs, 625–626, 625f–626f
physical examination in, 651–652, 651f
pleural effusion and, 188, 188f
predictive biomarkers in, 169–175
preexisting lung disease and, 36
prevalence of, persistent smoking among patients with, 18–19
prevention
primary, 76
secondary, 76–77
tertiary, 79t
primary, 199
prognosis for, 223–226
programs
accessibility standards for, 646–647
modality-specific quality standards for, 645
quality standards for, 643–646
standards for acceptable patient volumes for, 645–646
public profile, 636
radiobiology of, 330–336.e2
radiographic evaluation of, 652, 652f
radiologic presentation of, 199
radiotherapy for
dose calculation for, 322–323
future directions in, 328
quality assurance for, 327–328, 327f
technical requirements for, 318–329. e2
resection of, robotic surgery techniques and results for, 283–288.e1

Lung cancer (*Continued*)

resection of, video-assisted techniques results of, 274–282.e2
risk factors for, 1–7
alcohol as, 4
anthropometric measures as, 5
dietary, 3–4
drinking water contamination as, 7
hormones as, 4–5
indoor air pollution as, 6–7
infections as, 5
ionizing radiation as, 5
medical conditions and treatment as, 6
occupational exposures as, 5–6, 6t
outdoor air pollution as, 7, 7t
smokeless tobacco products as, 3
tobacco smoking as, 1–3
screening for, 52–58.e3, 53t, 72–75
biomarkers in, 58, 58t
overdiagnosis in, 56
participant selection in, 53–54
pulmonary nodules in, 54–56
randomized trials, summary of, 54
smoking cessation and, 56–58
second-line randomized studies establishing PD1/PDL1 inhibition as standard care, 507–508
segregation analyses of, 48–49
size, 219
small, 291–292, 292f
small cell. *see* Small cell lung cancer (SCLC)
spinal cord metastases or spinal compression and, 190
stage I
sublobar, limited resection for, 291–293
surgical resection of, 289–294.e2
stage II
sublobar, limited resection for, 291–293
surgical resection of, 289–294.e2
staging of, 653f
with CT, 206–210, 209f
endoscopic techniques for, 237–239
with MRI, 215–217, 215f–216f
with PET, 219–223, 220f–222f
TNM, 238f
stem cells and, 117–120.e2
steroid hormones in, 36–40
aromatase in, 38–39
estrogen receptors in, 36–38, 37f
progesterone receptors in, 40
stridor and, 187
structural changes leading to oncogenesis in, 86–93
ALK fusion in, 86–89, 87f–88f, 88t, 90t
other fusions in, 93
RET fusion in, 91–93, 92t–93t
ROS1 fusion in, 87f, 89–91, 90t, 92t
superior vena cava syndrome and, 188–189, 189f
surgery
evolution of, 289–290, 290f

Lung cancer (*Continued*)
surgery of
preoperative functional evaluation of candidates, 265–273.e3
survival in, gender differences, 41–42, 41t–42t
susceptibility to, 33–34
and balancing antagonistic pathways, 71–72
SWI/SNF chromatin remodeling factors in, 108f, 109–110, 109t
symptoms, managing of, 615–618
synchronous and metachronous, management of, 308–313.e2
targeted therapies for, 43–45, 44f, 44t
therapeutic targets of, 480–489, 481t
therapy for, implications for, 40
thoracic symptoms of, 382–385
tobacco use and, 24
treatment of
by manipulation of lung tumor microenvironment, 126–127
prognostic/predictive role of gender in, 42–43
resources for, 319b–320b
response to, 134–136
utilization standard rates for, 646
trial designs for rare tumors, 626
tumor histology of, 653–654
tumor-related factors in, 466–477
twin studies of, 47
vaccines for, 502–504
variation in patients values, 641
viral factors in, 35
waiting time, standards for, 646
wheezing and, 187
in women
incidence of, 32
mortality rate of, 30
Lung cancer advocacy, 635–638.e1
challenges in, 635–636
groups, 635
lack of, 635
strategies, 637–638
Lung Cancer Alliance, 75, 638
Lung Cancer Awareness Month, 637–638
Lung cancer emergencies, 590–607.e4
Lung Cancer Mutation Consortium (LCMC), 176, 431, 431t
Lung Cancer Screening Framework, 75
Lung cancer specialist, helping patients to stop tobacco use, 18–19
Lung Cancer Study Group (LCSG) trial, 314–315
Lung Cancer Symptom Scale (LCSS), 615
Lung carcinogenesis, 121–122
biology of, 60
Lung disease
interstitial, 497–498
preexisting, 36
Lung resection
for epidural tumors, 301, 301f
extended, 304–307.e1, 295–303.e2
results of, 290–291
for stage I lung cancer, 289–294.e2
for stage II lung cancer, 289–294.e2

Lung resection (*Continued*)
sublobar, limited
oncologic considerations for, 292–293
for stage I and II lung cancer, 291–292
surgical margin, 291–292, 292f
technical and pathologic consideration for, 291–292
Lung toxicity, 393–394
Lung tumor microenvironment, 121
adjacent histologically normal-appearing epithelium, 122
cellular components of, 122–127
developing, 122–123
field component of, 122
manipulation of, 126–127
soluble components of, 122–123, 125–127
structural components of, 123
Lung tumors, 143, 357–358
complications from cryotherapy of, 359
neuroendocrine, 155–158, 156f
tumor (T) descriptors, 207, 209f
LUX-Lung 3 trials, 165–166
Lymph nodes
definitions of mediastinal, 245t
descriptors for staging, 209–210, 219–221, 262–263
CT, 209–210, 210f
innovations in, 254–255, 255f–257f, 258t
MRI, 216, 216f
dissection of
extended, 244, 245t
lobe-specific systematic, 244, 245t
mediastinal, 244, 245t
mediastinal
assessment of, 244, 245t
choice of staging technique in, 245
staging, 244
staging, definitions of, 244
metastases, stereotactic ablative radiotherapy (SABR) for, 351–352
regional, PET imaging of, 219–221
stations, 241–242, 243t
Lymphadenectomy
mediastinoscopic, 246
TEMLA in, 246
VAMLA in, 246
Lymphoepithelioma-like carcinoma (LELC), 158
Lymphoma
Hodgkin, 551–552
non-Hodgkin, 552
systemic symptoms of, 551–552, 551f
Lymphoproliferative disorders, 184

M

MAGE-A3, 502–503
Magnetic resonance imaging (MRI)
for lung cancer, 214–215
of response to therapy, 217
use in staging, 215–217
neurologic effects of, 410
for radiotherapy, 321

Major histocompatibility complex (MHC), 137, 138f–139f
Malignancy
extrathymic second, 570
lung cancer
chemoprevention of, 69–81.e5
diagnostic workup for, 233–240.e2
early, 69–81.e5
imaging of, 235–236
Malignant mesothelioma, 536–549.e4
biology of, 536
biomarkers of, 538–539
chemotherapy for, 539–541
first-line, 539–540
repeat induction therapy, 541t
timing on, 540
cytoreductive surgery for, 542–544
diagnosis of, 537
gene therapy for, 549
intrapleural therapy for, 544–545
laparoscopy in, 537
mediastinal evaluation in, 538
mesothelin-targeted therapy for, 547–548
palliative surgery for, 541–542
second-line, 540–541
repeat induction therapy, 541t
staging of, 537–538, 538t
surgery for, 541–545
thoracoscopy in, 537
viral therapy against, 548–549
Malnutrition, lung cancer and, 339
Mammalian target of rapamycin (mTOR), 479–480, 487–488
Marlex mesh with methylmethacrylate (MMM) sandwich technique, 296
Mass media, 637
MassARRAY, 166t
Masses
benign cystic, 552
mediastinal, 550, 551t
Massive hemoptysis, 596–602
approach to diagnosis, 599, 599f
bronchoscopy, 599–600
clinical assessment, initial resuscitation, and stabilization, 598
computed tomography, 599
definition of, 597
endovascular embolization, 600–601, 601f–602f
etiology of, 597
outcomes, 602
surgery, 602
treatment of, 599–600
vascular source of bleeding in, 597–598, 598t
Massive pleural effusions, 602–607
chest imaging of, 606
clinical presentation of, 603
definitive management of, 606–607
etiology and pathogenesis of, 602–603
histologic analysis of, 606
initial management of, 603
initial presentation of, 603, 604f–605f
initial therapeutic intervention for, 603–606, 604f

Massive pleural effusions (*Continued*)
  medical thoracoscopy and video-assisted thoracoscopic surgery, 606
  pleural fluid analysis for, 606
  pleural physiology, 602
  pleurodesis and indwelling pleural catheter, 606–607
  serial thoracentesis, 606
  subsequent management, 606
Matuzumab, 428–429
MDX-1106/ONO-4538 (nivolumab), 506, 506t–507t, 509
MDX-1108, OPDIVO (nivolumab), 507–508
Meat, lung cancer and, 3
Mediastinal lymph node dissection, 245t, 249
  choice of staging technique, 245
  definitions of, 245t, 249
Mediastinal lymph node staging, definitions of, 244
Mediastinal tumors, 550–554.e1
  differential diagnosis of, 550, 551t
  surgical approach, 553–554
  systemic symptom of, 550, 551t
Mediastinoscopy, 245–246
  complications of, 246
  extended cervical, 248–249, 248f
  inferior, 250
  limitations of, 246
  results of, 246
  retrosternal or prevascular, 249
  technical variants for mediastinoscopic lymphadenectomy, 246
  technique for, 245–246, 245f–247f
  variants of extended, 249
Mediastinotomy, parasternal, 246–248, 248f
Mediastinum
  direct invasion of, 208
  evaluation in, 538
  invasive staging of, 241–252.e2
    indications for, 242–244, 243t
    recommendations for, 242, 244f
    restaging, 252
  lymph node anatomy of, 241
  lymph node staging of, 244
  preoperative assessment of, 241
  restaging of, 252
  staging of, invasive, 241–252.e2, 244t
Medical conditions, lung cancer and, 6
Medical Research Council (MRC), 521, 522f, 528
Medical thoracoscopy and video-assisted thoracoscopic surgery, 606
Medical treatment, lung cancer and, 6
Medication, concurrent, 338
Medroxyprogesterone, for lung cancer, 40
MEK, 486
MEK inhibitors, side effects of, 499
MEK1, 479
Melanoma-associated antigen-A3 vaccine, 502–503
Men, lung cancer in
  survival in, 41–42, 41t–42t
  in United States, 30, 31f

MER, 484–485
Mesothelin vaccine, 548
Mesothelin-directed CAR therapy, 548
Mesothelin-targeted therapy, 547–548
Mesothelioma
  immunomodulation of, 546, 547f
  immunotherapy of, 545–549
  malignant, 536–549.e4
  pleural, 536
    extrapleural pneumonectomy for, 542–543, 543f, 543t
    pleurectomy/decortication for, 543–544
MET, 442–443
MET gene, 164–165, 469–470
  amplification of, 85, 431t
MET inhibitor, 498
Metabolic phenomena, paraneoplastic, 191t, 192–193
Metabolomics, 67–68
Metachronous lung cancers, management of, 308–313.e2
Metachronous primary lung cancers, 260, 262t, 310–311
  evaluation of, 310
  incidence of, 310, 311t
  pneumonectomy and, 311
  surgical resection and outcome of, 310, 311t
Metals, lung cancer and, 5–6
Metastases
  adrenal
    lung cancer and, 190–191
    PET imaging of, 222–223, 224f
    stereotactic ablative radiotherapy (SABR) for, 351
  bone
    Basic Score for, 390
    consensus endpoints, international, 385–386
    external-beam radiotherapy for, 383
    lung cancer and, 189–190
    palliative radiotherapy for, 385–389, 385t
    uncomplicated, external-beam radiotherapy, 386, 386f
  brain, 372
    alternative management approaches, 391
    lung cancer and, 190
    outcomes, 391
    palliative radiotherapy for, 390
    repeat treatment for, 391–392
    in small-cell lung carcinoma (SCLC), 379–380
  descriptors for staging, 210, 211f–212f, 263–264
    CT, 210, 211f–212f
    innovations in, 255–256, 259f
    MRI, 216–217, 217f–218f
  distant, PET imaging of, 221–223, 223f
  liver
    lung cancer and, 190–191
    stereotactic ablative radiotherapy (SABR) for, 351
    therapy directed against, 565
  in mediastinal lymph nodes, 241

Metastatic bronchopulmonary carcinoid, therapy for, 565
Metastatic disease, 210, 211f–212f
  vs. multiple primary lung cancers, 308–312, 309t
Metastatic large cell neuroendocrine carcinoma, therapy for, 566–567
METex14, 443
Methotrexate, 531
MGMT, 113
Microarray comparison, 560
Microenvironment, and lung cancer, 121–128.e4
Micrometastatic dissemination, of cancer cells, 512
Micronutrients, 72
  lung cancer and, 4
Micropapillary predominant adenocarcinoma, 146f, 147
MicroRNAs (miRNAs), 129, 136, 197
  future perspectives for, 136
  hypermethylation of, 113
  in lung cancer, 64, 71, 129–136
    as diagnostic biomarkers, 129–132, 130t–131t
    as prognostic biomarkers, 132–134, 133t
    treatment response biomarkers, 134–136, 135t
  miR-4423, 125–126
Microsatellite instability, 64–65, 82–83
Microtubule-associated protein 4 (MAP4/3K3), 164–165
Microwave ablation, mechanism of action of, 355–356, 356f
Mind maps, 651
Minimally invasive adenocarcinoma (MIA), 144–146, 144t, 145f
  definition of, 183
  diagnosis of, 146
Minimally invasive techniques, 388
Mini-Mental Status Exam (MMSE), 412
Missense mutations, 95
MISSION trial, 439
Mitochondrial DNA, 64
Mitogen activated protein kinase (MAPK), 442, 486
Mitomycin, 365
Mitomycin C, 335
MLL2 gene, 431t
MMM. *see* Marlex mesh with methylmethacrylate (MMM) sandwich technique
Modern dose-escalation studies, 337–338
Molecular biology, of neuroendocrine tumors, 559–561
Molecular biomarkers, 477
  measurement of, 467
Molecular changes, genome-wide, 27
Molecular classification
  of adenocarcinoma, 654, 654f
  of small cell carcinoma, 654–655, 655f
  of squamous cell carcinoma, 654–655, 655f
Molecular diagnostic platforms, 655–657, 656f

Molecular markers
  new, 175–176
  and prognosis, 420
Molecular testing
  assay platforms in, 165–166
  guidelines for, 165, 185
  optimization of specimens for, 183
  pathology samples for, 160
  preanalytic factors in, 167–168
  sample processing and analysis in, 168
  tissue requirements for, 167–168
Molecularly targeted therapy
  agents for, 368–369
  bronchopulmonary carcinoid, 566
  for large cell neuroendocrine
    carcinoma, 567
MONET 1, 461
Monoclonal antibodies
  dermatologic side effects of, 491–496
  against EGFR, 428–429
  immunostimulatory, 126
Monte Carlo methods, 323
MORAb-009, 548
Morphine, for dyspnea, 616
Mucinous glycoprotein-1 vaccines,
  503–504
Mucositis, 491t
Multidisciplinary team management, 643
  care of, 645
  efficacy of, 644–645
  impact of, 644
  of lung cancer, 643–645
Multifocal pulmonary adenocarcinomas,
  with ground glass/lepidic features,
  260, 262t
Multiple lesions, lung cancers
  classification with, 260, 263t
Multiple nodules, management of,
  308–313.e2
Multiple organ metastases, stereotactic
  ablative radiotherapy (SABR) for,
  353
Multiple primary lung cancers (MPLCs)
  concept of, 308
  differentiating, from metastatic
    disease, 308–312, 309t
  evidence-based practice guidelines,
    312–313
  in lung cancer staging system, 309,
    310t
  metachronous primary lung cancers,
    310–311
    evaluation of, 310
    incidence of, 310, 311t
    pneumonectomy and, 311
    surgical resection and outcome of,
      310, 311t
  patient evaluation of, 309–310
    surgical resection and outcome,
      309–310, 310t–311t
  stereotactic body radiotherapy,
    311–312, 312t
  synchronous primary lung cancer, 309
Multiple VEGF receptor inhibitors, 461
Multiplex genotyping platforms, 656–657
Multivariate analysis, 516
Musculoskeletal disorders,
  paraneoplastic, 191–192, 191t

Mutations. *see* Gene mutations
MutS homolog 2 (MSH2), 175–176
Myasthenia gravis, 569–570
Myelitis, radiation, 411
Myeloid-derived suppressor cells
  (MDSCs), 141
Myeloid/lymphoid or mixed-lineage
  leukemia (MLL) genes, 164–165
Myelopathy, radiation, 411
Myelosuppression, chemotherapy and,
  334
Myocardium, injury for, 403

N
Nab-paclitaxel, 414–415, 423
N-Acetylcysteine, 78t–79t, 79
National Cancer Database, 376
National Cancer Institute (NCI),
  Common Terminology Criteria for
  Adverse Events (CTCAE), 409, 410t
National Cancer Institute of Canada,
  519–520
National Cancer Institute of Canada-
  Cancer Treatment Group (NCIC-
  CTG), 528
National Cancer Institute-American
  Association for Cancer Research
  (NCI-AACR), 19
National Cancer Institute's Surveillance,
  Epidemiology, and End Results
  (SEER) Program, 379
National Comprehensive Cancer
  Network (NCCN), 73f, 74t
  Clinical Practice Guidelines in
    Oncology: Nonsmall cell lung
    cancer (NSCLC), 319b–320b
  Clinical Practice Guidelines in
    Oncology: Small cell lung cancer
    (SCLC), 319b–320b
National Consensus of the Spanish
  Society of Medical Oncology, in
  guidelines for biomarker testing, 165
National Lung Cancer Audit, 637
National Lung Screening Trial (NLST),
  52, 72, 75t, 657
Navigational bronchoscopy, 179
NCAM/CD56, for SCLC, 157–158
Necitumumab, 460
Needle aspiration
  combined EBUS and EUS needle
    aspiration, 238–239
  endobronchial (EBNA), 237
  endobronchial ultrasound (EBUS), 237
  endoscopic ultrasound (EUS), 237–238
  fine-needle
    algorithm for optimizing samples,
      180, 181f
    slide preparation for, 180–182, 182f
    steps for processing, 181b
    vs. core-needle biopsy, 179
  transbronchial, 237
  transthoracic (TTNA), 237
NELSON (Dutch-Belgian Randomized
  Lung Cancer Screening Trial),
  74–75, 75t
Neoadjuvant Taxol Carboplatin Hope
  (NATCH), 521
Neoplastic lesions, in SCLC, 119

Neuralgia, 410t
Neuroblastoma RAS viral (v-ras)
  oncogenes homolog (NRAS), in
  lung cancer, 164–165
Neurocognitive complications, 414–417
Neuroendocrine carcinoma, large cell,
  156f, 157
Neuroendocrine hedgehog signaling, and
  SCLC, 119
Neuroendocrine thymic tumor, 576
  recommended management of, 588
Neuroendocrine tumors, 155–158, 156f
  adjuvant treatment of, 564–566
  chromosomal aberrations in, 559
  classification of, 555, 556t
  clinical characteristics, 561
  cytology, 556–557
  diagnosis of, 555–559
  differential diagnosis of, 557–559
  heterozygosity, loss of, 559
  histology of, 555–556
  imaging of, 561–563
    computed tomography, 561
    findings, 563t
    positron emission tomography, 561
    somatostatin receptor scintigraphy,
      563, 563t
  of lung, 555–568.e6
  microarray comparison, 560
  molecular biology, 559–561
  mutation analysis, 560, 560t
  pathways, 560–561
  staging of, 561
  surgery of, 563–564
  therapy for, 563–567
Neurofibroma, 552
Neurofibromatosis 1 (NF1), 164–165
Neurofibromatosis type 2, 536
Neurogenic tumor, 552, 552f
Neurologic syndromes, paraneoplastic,
  191t, 193–194
Neuromyotonia, 570
Neuropathic pain, 386–387
Neuropathy
  chemotherapy-induced, 414
  sensory, 234t
Neurotoxicity
  of prophylactic cranial irradiation,
    379–380
  related to radiotherapy and
    chemotherapy, 409–417.e2
Neurotrophic tyrosine kinase, receptor,
  type 3 (NTRK3), 164–165
Never-smokers
  definition of, 23
  lung cancer in, 23–29.e3, 28t
  lung cancer in, susceptibility to, 33–34
  mutations in, 98, 99f
New Zealand, smoking and smoking-
  attributable deaths in, 10
Next-generation sequencing (NGS),
  95–96, 97f
  applications of, 96–98
  future directions for, 103
  in lung adenocarcinoma, 98
  in lung cancer, 98–99
  massively parallel, 166, 166t
  platform used for, 96

NF2 gene, 536
NFE2L2 gene, 431t
Nicotine inhalation system, 21t
Nicotine lozenge, 21t
Nicotine nasal spray, 21t
Nicotine patch, 21t
Nicotine polacrilex gum, 21t
Nintedanib, 426, 439
Nivolumab (BMS-936558, MDX-
    1106/ONO-4538, MDX-1108,
    OPDIVO), 499, 506–509, 506t–507t
    for nonsmall cell lung cancer, 127, 432
Nodules. *see also* Pulmonary nodules
    ground-glass, 235
    multiple, management of, 308–313.e2
    satellite, 208–209
Noncytotoxic agents, maintenance
    therapy with, 455–461
Non-Hodgkin lymphoma, 552
Noninferiority trials, 624–625
Nonsense mutations, 95
Nonsmall cell lung cancer (NSCLC),
    37, 117–119, 199, 201f, 203f–204f,
    207f–208f, 210f, 434–435, 501
    advanced
        algorithm therapy in, 438f
        bevacizumab treatment of, 44, 45t
        in elderly patients, 423–424, 424t
        triplets for, 421–422, 422t
    ALK-rearranged, 430–431
    antiangiogenic for, 519
    biomarkers for, treatment response,
        134–135
    brain metastases in, 372
    cardiac toxicity related to, 407t
    chemoradiation therapy for
        radiation pneumonitis, 395, 396t,
            398f
        toxicity results in, 401t
    chemotherapy for
        duration of, 422
        maintenance therapy, 422–423
        neurotoxicity related to, 409–417.e2
        platinum-based, 134–135, 422
        platinum-free, 422
        prognostic/predictive role of gender
            in, 42–45
        systemic, 420
        triplet, 421–422, 422t
    Collaborative Group, 365
    combination chemotherapy against,
        ERCC1 and RRM1 for, 472
    CTLA-4 in, 139
    docetaxel for, 436
    early-stage
        adjacent histologically normal-
            appearing lung and, 122
        adjuvant chemotherapy for,
            512–524.e4
        neoadjuvant chemotherapy for,
            512–524.e4
        surgery for, 512
    EGFR mutation in, 469, 469t
    epidermal growth factor receptor
        (EGFR) and, 358–359
    fractionation schedule for, 331
    gemcitabine for, 135
    hyperfractionation for, role of, 332

Nonsmall cell lung cancer (*Continued*)
    imaging of, with PET, 219, 220f–224f,
        225
    immunotherapy for, 432, 461–462, 502
    interleukin-10 in, 140
    key signal transduction pathways in,
        479–480, 480f
    localized
        ablation options for, 355–362.e3
        treatment considerations of,
            360–361
    locally advanced
        chemoradiation therapy for,
            364–368
        radiotherapy for, 363–373.e3
        vaccination treatment, 501
    maintenance chemotherapy for,
        448–465.e4
        history trials, 448–449
        modern trials, 450–462
        with noncytotoxic agents for,
            455–461
        questions and future studies,
            464–465
        switch, 450, 450t, 451f
    management of elderly patients with,
        423–424, 424t
    MDSC in, 141–142
    metastatic, afatinib for, 439–440
    molecular characterization of, 431
    next-generation sequencing in, 98
    palliative radiotherapy for, 392
    patient selection for radiotherapy in,
        338
    PCI for, 372t
    pemetrexed for, 135
    platinum-based chemotherapy for,
        134–135
        phase II and III clinical trials,
            446t
    prognostic factors in, 418–420
    prophylactic cranial irradiation for,
        372
    radical resection for, 513t
    radiochemotherapy for
        late esophagus toxicity in, 400t
        toxicity results in, 401t
    radiotherapy for
        biologically effective dose, 331–332
        neurotoxicity related to, 409–417.e2
    randomized phase III trial for, 435
    role of surgery in, 369, 370t
    Southwest Oncology Group (SWOG)
        on, 368
    squamous cell, 431t
    stage I, 342–354.e4
        clinical assessment of, 343
        diagnosis of, before SABR, 343
        marginally resectable, 314
        salvage therapies, 349
        staging of, before SABR, 343
        standard treatment for, 314
        technical overview for radiation
            oncologist in, 344–345
        in thermal ablation, 358
        treatment planning of, 344, 345t
    stage III, concurrent chemoradiation
        therapy, 395

Nonsmall cell lung cancer (*Continued*)
    staging of, with PET, 219–220,
        220f–223f
    standard of care for, 358
    stereotactic ablative radiotherapy
        (SABR) for stage I, 342
        alternatives to, 349
        background and definitions of,
            342–343
        for central lesions, 347, 347f
        clinical results of, 345–347,
            345t–346t
        diagnosis and staging before, 343
        follow-up after, 347–349, 347f–350f
        implementation of, 343
    sublobar resection in treatment of,
        314–315
    of superior sulcus, 298, 299t
    surgically resected, 139–140
    systemic chemotherapy for, 420
    systemic therapy for, 418–433.e6
    TGF-β in, 140
    treatment delivery for, 324–326
        conformal radiotherapy, 324–326,
            325f
        hadron therapy, 326
        image-guided radiotherapy, 326
        2-D planning simulation, 324
    treatment of
        advanced, 420–423
        algorithm for, 418, 419f
        biomarkers for response to, 134–135
        importance of histology in, 423
    tumor stroma inflammatory cells in,
        140–141
    VATS lobectomies as treatment for, 274
Non-TNM staging systems, 572, 574b
North Central Cancer Treatment
    Group, 529
NOTCH 1/2 gene, 164–165
NOTCH gene, 164–165
Notch signaling, in maintenance of stem
    cell populations, 118–119
NOTCH1 gene, 431t
NSCLC. *see* Nonsmall cell lung cancer
    (NSCLC)
NSCLC Meta-analysis Collaborative
    Group, 518f, 521
Nuclear factor, erythroid 2-like 2
    (NFE2L2), 164–165
Nucleotide excision repair (NER),
    incision stage of, 470, 471f
Nucleotide excision repair system, 195
NUT carcinoma, 158
Nutrition, and patient selection for
    radiotherapy, 339

O
Occupational exposures, 5–6, 6t, 24
Occupational toxins, and lung cancer in
    never-smokers, 24
Older patients. *see* Elderly patients
Oligometastases
    from lung cancer, 350–351
    stereotactic ablative radiotherapy
        (SABR) for
        in adrenal gland, 351
        clinical results of, 351–353

Oligometastases (*Continued*)
  immune effects of, 351
  in liver, 351
  in lymph nodes, 351–352
  in multiple organs, 353
  in vertebrae, 352–353, 352f
Olmutinib, 440
Onartuzumab, 443
Oncimmune LLC, 67
"Oncogene addiction," 468
Oncogene-driven adenocarcinoma, conditional, 118
Oncogenes, 196
Oncogenesis
  amplification as mechanism of, 84–86, 85f–86f
    EGFR, 84
    ERBB2, 84–85
    FGFR1, 86
    MET, 85
    PIK3CA, 85–86
  structural changes leading to, 86–93
    ALK fusion in, 86–89, 87f–88f, 88t, 90t
    RET fusion in, 91–93, 92t–93t
    ROS1 fusion in, 87f, 89–91, 90t, 92t
Oncology, palliative care and, philosophical differences between, 608–609
Oncology care, high-quality, 19
Oncolytic viral therapy, 548–549
OPCML, 113
Opsoclonus-Myoclonus, 194
Osimertinib, 440
Osteoarthropathy, hypertrophic pulmonary, 191
Outdoor air pollution, 7, 7t
Overdiagnosis, and screening for lung cancer, 56

P
p16 gene, 70
p16/cyclin D1/ Rb pathway, 560–561
P21 protein (Cdc42/Rac)-activated kinase 3 (PAK3), 164–165
p53 gene, 27, 46, 560
Pacific Biosciences, 101
Paclitaxel
  combination chemotherapy with
    for advanced NSCLC in elderly patients, 424, 424t
    with bevacizumab, 425, 426t
    for locally advanced nonsmall cell lung cancer, 366
    for nonsmall cell lung cancer, 420–421, 421t
  maintenance chemotherapy with
    continuation, 455
    historical trials, 449
  for nonsmall cell lung cancer, 420, 420t
  phase II studies of, 435
  for SCLC, 525, 526t
Paclitaxel sensory neuropathy, 414
Pain
  chest, 187
  neuropathic, 386–387
  in palliative care, 617–618

Palliative care
  assessing symptoms and quality of life in lung cancer, 614–615, 615b
  barriers to integrating, into cancer care, 613–614
  cachexia and anorexia, 617
  communication, 610–612
  cough, 616
  definition of, 608
  dyspnea, 616
  early integration of, into oncology, benefits of, 612–613
  end-of-life care, 614
  fatigue, 615–616
  health care economics, 612–613
  lung cancer
    and cardiopulmonary resuscitation, 618
    and intensive care unit, 618
  in lung cancer, role of, 608–619.e8
  lung cancer symptoms, managing of, 615–618
  pain, 617–618
  patient-related outcomes and, 612
  philosophical differences between oncology and, 608–609
  quality of life and, 612
  rehabilitation, 612
  structure of, 609, 609b
  studies documenting benefits to integrating, into cancer care, 613
  survival, 613
  symptoms of, 609–610, 611b
Palliative care interdisciplinary teams, 609, 610b
Palliative chemoradiation therapy, 385
Palliative chemotherapy, bronchopulmonary carcinoid, 565
Palliative pleurectomy, 542
Palliative radiotherapy
  for bone metastases, 385–389
  for bronchopulmonary carcinoid, 566
  for lung cancer, 382–392.e3
  for thoracic symptoms, 382–385
Palliative surgery, for malignant mesothelioma, 541–542
Pancoast, Henry, 298
Pancoast syndrome, lung cancer and, 189
Pancoast tumors, 298–302
  anatomic definition of, 298
  historical background of, 298, 298t
  multimodality treatment of, 298–300, 299t
  pretreatment evaluation of, 298, 299f
  technical approaches to resection, 300–302
    anterior approaches, 301–302, 302f
    posterior (Paulson) approach, 300–301, 301f
    vertebral body and epidural tumors, 301, 301f
Papanicolaou stain, 184
Papillary predominant adenocarcinoma, 144t, 147
Papillomas, 144t
Papulopustular (acneiform) eruption, 491, 492f, 493t

Parallel progression model, of lung cancer, 121–122
PARAMOUNT trial, 452t, 454, 454f, 465
Paraneoplastic neurologic syndromes (PNSs), 193–194
Paraneoplastic syndromes, 191–194, 191t, 234, 234t
  blood disorders, 193
    anemia, 193
    deep venous thrombosis and thromboembolism, 193
    disseminated intravascular coagulopathy, 193
    hypercoagulation states, 193
    leukocytosis, 193
    thrombocytosis, 193
    thrombotic microangiopathy, 193
  dermatologic or musculoskeletal disorders, 191–192
    dermatomyositis, 191
    hypertrophic pulmonary osteoarthropathy and digital clubbing, 191
    polymyositis, 191–192
    rare skin disorders, 191
  endocrine and metabolic phenomena, 192–193
    carcinoid syndrome, 192
    Cushing syndrome, 192
    hypercalcemia, 192–193
    syndrome of inappropriate antidiuretic hormone secretion, 192
  neurologic, 193–194
    central nervous system, 194
    neuromuscular group of peripheral nervous system, 194
    peripheral nervous system, 194
Parasternal mediastinotomy, 246–248, 248f
Parathyroid adenoma, 553, 553f
Paresthesia, 410t
Paronychia, 491–492, 491t, 492f, 494t, 495f
Participant selection, in screening for lung cancer, 53–54
Pathologic fracture, 386
Pathology, of lung cancer, 653f
Patient-related factors, 337–339
Patients values, variations in, 641
Pattern recognition receptor agonists (PRRago), 126
Pattern recognition receptors (PRRs), 126
Paulson approach, 300–301, 301f
Pazopanib, 369
PBRM1, 109t
PD1 monoclonal antibody, side effects of, 499–500
PD1/PDL1 inhibition, second-line randomized studies for, as standard care, 507–508
PDL1 expression, and association with response, 509
PD-L1 monoclonal antibody, side effects of, 499–500

Pembrolizumab (MK-3475, Keytruda), 445, 499–500, 506–509, 506t–507t
  for NSCLC, 127
Pemetrexed
  anticancer effects of, 425
  combination chemotherapy with
    for locally advanced nonsmall cell lung cancer, 367
    for SCLC, 525, 526t
  maintenance chemotherapy with
    continuation, 454, 454f
    switch, 450
  for malignant mesothelioma, 541t
  for nonsmall cell lung cancer, 450
  for NSCLC, 135
  phase II studies of, 436
  response to, 135
  thymidylate synthase and, 476
  in advanced NSCLC, 476
Pentoxifylline, 399
Performance status
  and patient selection for radiotherapy, 337
  poor
    first-line chemotherapy with, 531
    management of patients with, 424
  prognosis and, 418
Perfusion defects, 403
Pericardial cysts, 552
Pericardial effusion, lung cancer and, 188, 188f
Pericardioscopy, subxiphoid, 250
Pericarditis, radiation-associated, 404, 405t
Peripheral motor neuropathy, 410t
Peripheral nervous system disorders, paraneoplastic, 194
  neuromuscular group, 194
Peripheral neuropathy, chemotherapy-induced, 414
Peripheral sensory neuropathy, 410t
PET. see Positron emission tomography
Pharmacogenomics, 466–478.e3
Pharmacotherapy, for smoking cessation, 11, 20, 21t
Phase I trial design, 621
Phase II trials, 622–624, 622f
Phase III trials, 624–626
Phase II/III designs, 625–626, 625f–626f
Phase II/III trials, 624–626
Phosphatase and tensin homolog (PTEN), 164–165
Phosphatidylinositol 3-kinase subunits (PIK3C), 176
Phosphatidylinositol-4, 5-bisphosphate 3-kinase, catalytic subunit alpha (PI3KCA), 164–165
Phosphoinositide 3-kinase (P13K), 479, 486–487
Phosphoinositide-dependent kinase 1 (PDDK1), 479–480
Photodynamic therapy, 595
  intracavitary, 544
Photon transport correction methods, 322
Physical activity, and patient selection for radiotherapy, 339
Physical examination, 651–652

Physician's Health Study, 77
PIK3CA gene
  amplification of, 85–86
  in squamous cell NSCLC, 431t
Pimonidazole, 335
Platelet-derived growth factor receptor
  alpha polypeptide (PDGFRA), 164–165
  beta polypeptide (PDGFR1), 164–165
Platinum compounds, 420–421
Platinum-based chemotherapy
  adjuvant, large-scale studies on, 514–517, 514t–516t
  combination chemotherapy with, with bevacizumab, 425, 426t
  intrapleural, 544
  neoadjuvant, 520
  for NSCLC, 134–135
    phase II and III clinical trials, 446t
  response to, 134–135
  for SCLC, 134
  with targeted agents, 425
  vs. platinum-free chemotherapy, for nonsmall cell lung cancer, 422
Platinum-doublet chemotherapy, 435
Pleomorphic cell carcinoma, 154
Pleura, direct invasion of, 207
Pleural drainage, 541–542
Pleural effusions
  lung cancer and, 188, 188f
  in malignant mesothelioma, 537, 537f
Pleural fluid accumulation, 188
Pleural fluid analysis, 606
Pleural fluid or washing materials, 160
Pleural manometry, 603–605
Pleural mesothelioma, 536
  extrapleural pneumonectomy for, 542–543, 543t
  malignant, biology of, 536
  pleurectomy/decortication for, 543–544, 543f, 544t
Pleurectomy, palliative, 542
Pleurectomy/decortication, 543–544, 543f, 544t
Pleurodesis and indwelling pleural catheter, 606–607
PNA-LNA PCR clamp, 166t
Pneumonectomy
  in EORTC trial, 370
  extrapleural, 542–545, 543f, 543t, 545f
  metachronous tumors following, 311
Pneumonitis, 209
  grading criteria, 395t
  radiation, 395–399
Pneumothorax, as complications of thermal ablation, 359
PointBreak trial, 452t, 454–455
Poland, 32–33, 32f
Political lobbying, 638
Pollution. see Air pollution
Polycyclic aromatic hydrocarbons, 6, 199
Polymerase chain reaction (PCR), 522
Polymyositis, 191–192
Positron emission tomography (PET)
  boost trial, 365f
  FDG-PET-CT, 227–231, 227f
  18F-fluciclatide PET-CT, 229–230, 231f

Positron emission tomography
  (Continued)
  FLT PET, 228
  lung cancer imaging, 219–232.e4, 220f–223f
  lung cancer staging, 219–223, 220f–223f
  metrics, radiotherapy and, 341
  for neuroendocrine tumors, 561
  novel tracers for, 228–231
  for radiotherapy, 320–321
  standardized protocol for, 225
  therapeutic response, 226–227
Positron emission tomography-computed tomography (PET-CT), 227, 227f, 230f, 231, 359–360, 361f–362f
Postdiscontinuation therapy, 454
Postobstructive collapse, 209
Postoperative anticoagulant therapy, in pulmonary artery angioplasty, 307
Postoperative Radiation Therapy (PORT) meta-analysis, 513
ppoDLCO. see Predicted postoperative carbon monoxide lung diffusion capacity (ppoDLCO)
ppoFEV1. see Predicted postoperative forced expiratory volume in 1 second (ppoFEV1)
Practice Guideline: Intensity-modulated radiation therapy (IMRT) (ACR and ASTRO), 319b–320b
Precachexia, 617
Predicted postoperative carbon monoxide lung diffusion capacity (ppoDLCO), 267–268
Predicted postoperative forced expiratory volume in 1 second (ppoFEV1), 267
Preneoplastic changes, of lung cancer in never-smokers, 27
Prevascular mediastinoscopy, retrosternal or, 249
Prevention, chemoprevention, 69–81.e5
Primary carcinoma, of pulmonary origin, 199
Primary pulmonary adenocarcinoma, with enteric differentiation, 147–148
Progesterone receptors, lung cancer and, 40
Prognostic factors, in nonsmall cell lung cancer, 418–420
Program death 1 ligand, 444–445
Programmed cell death 1 (PD-1), 138f–139f, 139
Promotion
  bans on tobacco promotion, 12
  of clinical trials, 633–634
PRONOUNCE study, 452t, 455
Prophylactic cranial irradiation, 372
Prophylactic cranial radiation, 372
Prostate, Lung, Colorectal, and Ovarian (PLCO) screening trial, 53, 74
Protein expression, 165
Protein kinase B (AKT), 479–480, 487
Protein kinases, 196
Protein markers, 66
Protein tyrosine phosphatase, receptor type, D (PTPRD), 164–165

Proteomic analysis, for lung cancer, 197
Proteomics, 66–67
Proton-pump inhibitors, for cough, 616
Proto-oncogene tyrosine-protein kinase (MER), 484–485
Pruritus, 491t, 494t
PTEN gene
  loss of, 118
  in lung cancer, 26–27, 26t
  in squamous cell NSCLC, 431t
Public awareness campaigns, 637–638
Pulmonary artery angioplasty
  history and surgical outcomes of, 304, 305t
  postoperative anticoagulant therapy in, 307
  surgical techniques and controversies regarding, 306–307
Pulmonary artery resections, reconstructions and, 306–307
Pulmonary blastoma, 154
Pulmonary embolism, imaging of, 213
Pulmonary fibrosis, 395t
Pulmonary function, in patient selection for radiotherapy, 338
Pulmonary function tests, 394–395
Pulmonary metastases, early stage lung cancer and, 328
Pulmonary neuroendocrine, 555
Pulmonary nodules
  characterization of, 214–215
  identification of, 214
  and screening for lung cancer, 54–56
    baseline probabilistic risk prediction of, 55–56
    longitudinal surveillance in, 55f, 56, 57f
  solitary, characterization of, 199–202, 200f
Pulmonary rehabilitation, preoperative, 271
Pulmonary system, acute and late toxicities of thoracic radiotherapy, 393–408.e4
Pulmonary toxicity, 393–395
Pure ground-glass lesions, 200
Pyrosequencing, 166t

Q

Quality assurance
  for clinical radiotherapy treatment planning (AAPM)(TG 53), 319b–320b
  high-quality data, 637
  for image-guided radiation therapy (IGRT) utilizing computed tomography (CT)-based technologies (AAPM)(TG 179), 319b–320b
  for lung cancer radiotherapy, 327–328, 327f
  of medical accelerators (AAPM)(TG 142), 319b–320b
  modality-specific quality standards, 645
  of stereotactic ablative radiotherapy (SABR), 343

Quality of life, 387
  and adjuvant cisplatin-based chemotherapy, 516–517
Quality standards, for cancer treatment programs, 643–646
Quantitative Analysis of Normal Tissue Effects in the Clinic, 340

R

Racotumomab, 461, 504
RADES I, 390
RADES II, 390
RADIANT trial, 520
Radiation
  cell survival, 330
  damage, biologic effects of, 330
  linear-quadratic model of, 330–331
  low-dose, 52, 54t, 72, 73f, 74t
  prophylactic cranial, 413
  repeat, 332–334, 384–385, 388–389
  response
    biomarkers predictive of, 335–336
    modification of, 334–335
  treatment planning, with FDG-PET-CT, 227–231, 227f
  volumes of, 377–378
Radiation esophagitis, 400
  acute, management of, 403
  clinical factors in, 401–402
  combined dosimetric and clinical factors of, 402
  dosimetric factors in, 400–401, 402f
  management of, 402–403
  pathophysiology of, 399
  prevention of, 402–403
Radiation injury, to heart, 403–407
Radiation myelitis, 411
Radiation myelopathy, 411
Radiation pneumonitis, 395–399
  clinical factors of, 396–397
  combined dosimetric and clinical factors, 397–398, 397f–398f
  in concurrent chemoradiation therapy in stage III NSCLC, 395, 396t, 398f
  dosimetric factors, 396
  grading criteria, 395t
  predict incidence of, 397f
  prevention and management of, 398–399
  stages of, 393
  treatment of, 399
  vs. cardiac injury, 407
Radiation Therapy Oncology Group (RTOG)
  brachial plexus contouring atlas, 410
  Graded Prognostic Assessment (GPA), 390
  late esophagus toxicity, scoring system, 399–400
  phase III trial, 363
  pneumonitis grading criteria, 395t
  Recursive Partitioning index (RPA), 390
  studies in patient selection for radiotherapy, 337–338
Radiation-associated heart disease, 404, 405t

Radiobiology
  four Rs of, 331
  of lung cancer, 330–336.e2
  of stereotactic ablative radiotherapy, 334
Radiochemotherapy
  concurrent
    late esophagus toxicity in, 400, 400t
    toxicity results in, 401t
  for nonsmall cell lung cancer
    late esophagus toxicity in, 400, 400t
    toxicity results in, 400, 401t
Radiofrequency ablation, for localized nonsmall cell lung cancer, 355, 356f
Radiographic evaluation, of lung cancer, 652, 652f
Radiosensitizer, hypoxic cell, 335
Radiosurgery, stereotactic, 388
Radiotherapy
  adjuvant, role of, 513–514
  age and frailty in, 338
  altered fractionation schedules and, 364
  alternative fractionation schedules and dose escalation of, 332–334
  anaplastic lymphoma kinase inhibitors in, 369
  antiangiogenesis agents in, 369
  biomarkers predictive of, response to, 335–336
  for bone metastases, 385–389
  brain metastases and prophylactic cranial radiation in, 372
  Cancer and Leukemia Group B (CALGB) studies in, 376–377
  cardiovascular toxicity, 404
  chemotherapy regimen combined with, 378–379
  clinical trials utilizing molecular compounds with combined chemoradiotherapy for, 367t
  combined modality, 363–373.e3, 407
  computed tomography in, 341
  considerations for, 371–372, 371t
  continuous hyperfractionated accelerated radiotherapy (CHART), 333
  conventionally fractionated, 330–332
  CT imaging of response to, 211–213, 213f
  dose of, 376–377
    biologically effective, 331–332
    escalation, 332–334
    limits, 333
    for locally advanced nonsmall cell lung cancer, 363–364
  epidermal growth factor receptor in, 368–369
  equipment for
    computed tomography, 320
    imaging and stimulation systems, 320
    immobilization, 321
    magnetic resonance imaging, 321
    positron emission tomography, 320–321
    target and normal tissue delineation, 321–322
    treatment planning systems, 321
    2-D simulation, 320

Radiotherapy (*Continued*)
extensive disease for, 379
external-beam, 361–362
for bone metastases, 385–389, 385t
hemibody, 387–388
minimally invasive techniques and, 388
with other modalities, 388–389
side effects of, 388
systemic therapy and, 388
for thoracic symptoms, 383
F-2-deoxy-D-glucose uptake in, 340–341
fractionation, 376–377
accelerated, schedules, 333
conventional, 332
hyperfractionation, 332
for locally advanced nonsmall cell lung cancer, 363–364
schedules, alternative, 332–334
future directions of, 335
hyperfractionated, 332
hyperfractionated accelerated radiotherapy (HART), 333
hypofractionation, 364
image-guided, 326
imaging technical advances in, 328
immune check point inhibitors (PD-1/PD-L-1) in, 369
individualizing treatment, 328
induction and consolidation therapy, 367
locoregional treatment with, 369–372
lung cancer
dose calculation for, 322–323
equipment of, 320–324
future directions in, 328
quality assurance, 327–328, 327f
technical requirements for, 318–329.e2
mean lung dose (MLD), 331
molecular factors in, 338–339
molecularly targeted therapeutic agents in, 368–369
motion management, 326–327, 327f
mutation status in, 341
NCI-C trial in, 375–376
neurocognitive complications of, 414–417
neurotoxicity from, 409–414
for nonsmall cell lung cancer
cardiac toxicity related to, 407t
neurotoxicity related to, 409–417.e2
outcome measurements of, 373, 373t
palliative
with brain metastases, 390
for bronchopulmonary carcinoid, 566
indications for, 383
for lung cancer, 382–392.e3
regimens, 383, 384t
side effects of, 383–384
for thoracic symptoms, 382–385
whole-brain radiotherapy, 390–391
pathophysiology of, 393, 394f
patient selection for, 337–341.e3
patient-related factors in, 337–339
performance status in, 337

Radiotherapy (*Continued*)
perfusion defects in, 403
planning, 383–385
technical advances in, 328
positron emission tomography metrics in, 341
postoperative, 386, 387f
prophylactic cranial irradiation in, 379–380
radiated volume, 340
radiation treatment volumes of, 377–378
repeat, 384–385, 388–389
for small cell lung cancer
management, 374–381.e3
neurotoxicity related to, 409–417.e2
stereotactic ablative, 334
suggested dose/volume limits for the heart, 407t
thoracic, 379
toxicities of, 393–408.e4
for thymic tumors, 579–580
timing question in, 375–376
toxicity of, 340
treatment delivery systems, 323–324
tumor-related factors for, 339–341
whole-brain, 390–391
toxicity of, 391
Radiotherapy-induced brachial plexopathy (RIBP), 409–410
Radon, exposure to, lung cancer and, 35
Ramucirumab, 439
side effects of, 498
Random sampling, 244
Randomized and single-arm designs, 623
RAP80, and *BRCA1*, for advanced NSCLC, 475–476, 475f
Rapid on-site evaluation (ROSE), 179–180, 180f
RARB, 113
RAR-β gene, 71
Rare tumors, trial designs for, 626
RAS, 485
RAS gene, 164–165
RAS/RAF/MAPK pathway, 479
RASSF1A, 113
RB1 gene, 431t
RCRI. *see* Revised Cardiac Risk Index (RCRI)
Real time/TaqMan PCR, 166t
Reassortment, 331
Recall radiation pneumonitis, 398
Receptor tyrosine kinase (ROS1), 164–165
Receptor tyrosine kinases (RTKs), 479–485
c-Ros oncogene 1, 483–484
discoidin domain receptors, 484
fibroblast growth factor receptor, 483
hepatocyte growth factor receptor-MET, 482–483
human epidermal growth factor receptor type 2, 480–481
human epidermal growth factor receptor type 3, 481–482
proto-oncogene tyrosine-protein kinase (MER), 484–485
rearranged during transfection-RET, 484

Receptor tyrosine kinases (*Continued*)
tropomysin receptor kinase, 485
tyrosine-protein kinase receptor UFO (AXL), 484–485
Recurrent thymic tumors, 587–588
diagnosis of, 587–588
treatment of, 588
Recursive Partitioning index (RPA), 390
Refametinib, 499
Regulator of G-protein signaling 17 (*RGS17*) gene, 25
Regulatory RNAs, 104, 105f
Reoxygenation, 331
Repair, 331
Repeat radiation, 332–334, 384–385, 388–389
Replacement smokers, 12
Repopulation, 331
Research. *see also specific trials*
adaptive designs, 624
biomarker-based subgroups, 622f–623f, 623–624
biomarker-based trial designs, 626
clinical trial methodology, 620–627.e2
early phase trials, 621–622, 621f
end-point considerations, 622–623
epigenetic therapy trials, 115, 115t
funding for, 636
high-quality data in, 637
lung cancer clinical trial organization
clinical trials and impact of biomarkers on design, selection of hypotheses for, 629
cooperation and networks, 631
definition of, 628
financial issues, 632–633
issues in, 628–629
mixing avatar models and clinical trials, 631
modern clinical trials, designs for, 629–631, 630f–631f
national, multinational, and international cooperation/competition, 629
quick progress and impact on financial issues, expectations for, 628–629, 629f
regulatory issues, 632
solutions for, 629–633
worldwide standardization, of oncology clinical trials allowing cross-trial comparisons, 631–632, 632f, 633t
lung cancer clinical trial promotion
conducting clinical trials, increasing difficulty of, 633
educate general population and patients with, 634
goal and philosophy of different systems, 633
issues in, 633
patient education, 633
simplify regulation, 634, 634t
solutions, 633–634
time and effort, 633
train physician early and continuously, 633–634
lung cancer screening trials, 75t

Research (*Continued*)
noninferiority trials, 624–625
phase I trial, 621
phase II trials, 622–624, 622f
phase III trials, 624–626
phase II/III designs, 625–626, 625f–626f
phase II/III trials, 624–626
randomized trial designs, 623
single-arm designs, 623
traditional designs, 624
trial designs for rare tumors, 626
in vitro study of stem cells, 117–120.e2
in vivo study of stem cells, 117–120.e2
Resection. *see also* Surgical resection
of epidural tumors, 301, 301f
minimally invasive, for thymoma, 578–579
pulmonary artery, and reconstructions, 306–307
of vertebral body, 301, 301f
Resistance, acquired, 655
RET, 484
RET gene, 164–165
fusion of, 91–93, 92t–93t
in lung cancer, 71
translocation, 431t
Retinoblastoma (RB1), 164–165
9-cis-Retinoic acid, 77–78, 78t
13-cis-Retinoic acid, 78, 78t
Retinopathy, 234t
Retinyl palmitate, 79, 79t
"Reverse telescope," 305–306
Revised Cardiac Risk Index (RCRI), 266
RGS17 gene, 25
Ribonucleotide reductase M1 (RRM1), 175–176, 195, 424–425, 466–467, 470–475
RNA binding motif protein 10 (RBM10), 164–165
RNAs
microRNAs
in lung cancer, 129–136
miR-4423, 125–126
noncoding, 64
regulatory, 104, 105f
small nucleolar, 64
Robotic lobectomy
general concepts of, 286
mediastinal lymph node dissection, 286
left side, 286
right side, 286
operating room configuration, 284–285, 284f
patient positioning, 285, 285f
port placement/docking, 285, 285f
sequence of port placement, 285–286, 285f–286f
technical aspects of, 284–286
Robotic surgery
completely portal robotic operations (CPRs), 283
definitions of, 283, 284t
general concepts, 286
history of, 283–284
mediastinal lymph node dissection, 286

Robotic surgery (*Continued*)
operating room configuration for, 284–285, 284f
console, 284
robot/bed, 284, 285f
surgical team, 284–285
outcomes of, 287t, 288
long-term results, 288
short-term results, 288
patient positioning for, 285, 285f
port placement/docking of, 285, 285f
sequence of port placement of, 285–286, 285f–286f
technical aspects, 284–286
techniques and results for resection of lung cancer, 283–288.e1
Robotic system, definition of, 283
Robotic thoracic operation, definition of, 283
Robotic-assisted operation, 283, 284t
Roche 454, 96
Roche Molecular Diagnostics, 165–166
Rociletinib, 440
ROS1, 442
ROS1 gene, 470
fusion of, 87f, 89–91, 90t, 91f, 92t
in lung adenocarcinoma, 26
in lung cancer, 71
translocation, 431t
Rovalpituzumab, 534
Royal Marsden Hospital, 530
RPA. *see* Recursive Partitioning index (RPA)
RRM1 gene, in advanced NSCLC, 472, 473f–474f

S
Salivary gland tumors, 144t
Salivary gland-type tumors, 158
Sampling, navigational bronchoscopy for, 179
Sampling/samples. *see also* Specimens
of biomarkers for testing, 168–169
fine-needle aspiration, 160
pathology samples for molecular testing, 160
random, 244, 245t
systematic, 244, 245t
Sanger sequencing method, 165, 166t
Sarcomatoid carcinoma, 144t, 153f, 154
Satellite cell proliferation, 617
Satellite nodules, 208–209
SATURN trial, 448, 456t, 458, 458f
SCLC. *see* Small cell lung cancer (SCLC)
Scleroderma, risk for, in radiotherapy, 338
Screening, 52–58.e3, 53t, 72–75, 75t
biomarkers in, 58, 58t
overdiagnosis in, 56
participant selection in, 53–54
pulmonary nodules in, 54–56
baseline probabilistic risk prediction of, 55–56
longitudinal surveillance in, 55f, 56, 57f
randomized trials, summary of, 54
smoking cessation and, 56–58
trials, 54

Second-line therapy, for systemic options, 434–447.e5
anaplastic lymphoma kinase as, 441–443
B-Raf kinase, 442
KRAS, 442
MET, 442–443
ROS1, 442
chemotherapy, 435–436
choice of agent for, 436
cytotoxic T-lymphocyte associated antigen 4 as, 444–445
anti-program death 1 and program death 1 ligand, 444–445
heat-shock protein 90 inhibitors as, 443–444
history of, 435
immune checkpoint inhibitors as, 444
novel targets of, 439–441
second-and third-generation epidermal growth factor receptor inhibitors, 439–441
phase I and phase II trials of, 435
scheduling of chemotherapy for, 436–437
third and subsequent-line of chemotherapy, 437
treatment with molecularly targeted agents, 437–439
epidermal growth factor receptor tyrosine kinase inhibitors as, for wild-type EGFR tumors, 438, 438f
erlotinib as, 437–438
gefitinib as, 437
vascular endothelial growth factor inhibitors as, 438–439
Segmentectomy, 316
for small lung cancers, 293, 293f
video-assisted thoracoscopic surgery (VATS), 293
Segregation analyses, of lung cancer, 48–49
Selumetinib, 442, 499
Semi-Markov model, 463–464
Seminoma, 550–551
Sensory neuropathy, 194
chemotherapy-induced, 414
subacute, 234t
Sequencing
first-generation, 95–96
next-generation, 95–96, 97f
in suboptimal samples, 101–103
targeted, 97
third-generation, 101
whole-exome, 97
whole-genome, 96
Sequencing platforms, 656–657
Sequenom, 656–657
Sequential chemoradiation therapy, 365, 365t, 366f
Serial thoracentesis, 606
Serine/threonine kinase 11 (STK11), 164–165
"Shine a Light on Lung Cancer," 637–638
Shuttle Walk Test, 268–269

Signal transduction pathways, 479–480, 480f
Silent mutations, 95
Silica, lung cancer and, 6
Silver in situ hybridization, 166
Single-molecule real-time technology, 101
Single-nucleotide polymorphisms (SNPs), 477
6-Minute Walking Test, 268
Skin disorders, rare, 191
Sleeve resection, 307
    bronchovascular, 304–307.e1
    double, first reconstructed in, 307
    type of, 306, 306f
Slide preparation, for fine-needle aspirate, 180–182
Slit homolog 2 (SLIT2), 164–165
Small cell lung cancer (SCLC), 555–568. e6, 119, 156f, 157–158, 199
    applicability of TNM classification to, 256
    biomarkers for, treatment response, 134
    brain metastases, 379
    bronchopulmonary carcinoid from, differentiation of, 558–559
    chemotherapy for
        maintenance therapy, treatment duration and, 529
        neurotoxicity related to, 409–417.e2
    classification of, 555, 556t
    cytologic characteristics of, 161f, 162
    diagnosis of, 555–559
    differential diagnosis of, 557–559
    elderly patients with, 380
    elective nodal irradiation (ENI) in, 377
    extensive-stage
        combination chemotherapy for, 525–527
        first-line chemotherapy for, 525–529, 526t
        new drugs for, 533–534
        second-line chemotherapy for, 531–533, 532t
        survival trends, 530f
        thoracic radiotherapy for, 379
        treatment of, 525–535.e5
    gene mutation in, 164–165
    high-risk syndromes conferring increased risk of, 48
    histology of, 555–556
    large cell neuroendocrine carcinoma from, markers for differentiation of, 559
    limited disease (LD), 374
        ^{18}F-2-deoxy-D-glucose (FDG)-PET for, 377–378
    management of, 374
    molecular classification of, 654–655, 655f
    mutation analysis, 560
    neuroendocrine hedgehog signaling in, 119
    next-generation sequencing in, 98–99
    nonmetastatic disease, treatment for, 374
    origin of, 119

Small cell lung cancer (Continued)
    palliative radiotherapy for, 392
    PCI, as standard of care in, 381
    platinum-based chemotherapy response, 134
    prophylactic cranial irradiation for, 379–380
    radiotherapy for, 374–381.e3
        neurotoxicity related to, 409–417.e2
    selected targets and agents for, 534t
    thoracic radiotherapy for, 379
    TNM classifications, 374
    tumor heterogeneity and, 119
Small samples, 180
Small specimens
    algorithm for processing, 180, 181f, 181b
    management of, 178–185.e2, 179f
    optimization for, 180–183, 182f
    triage for ancillary studies, 180–184, 181f
SMARCA2, 109t
SMARCA4, 109t
SMARCB1, 109t
SMARCC1, 109t
SMARCC2, 109t
SMARCD1, 109t
SMARCD2, 109t
SMARCD3, 109t
SMARCE1, 109t
SMARCF1, 109t
Smart Map, 637
Smear preparation, 180–182, 182f
Smokeless tobacco products, 3
Smokers, 98, 99f
Smoking. *see* Tobacco smoking
Smoking and Health (US Surgeon General), 18
Smoking cessation
    pharmacotherapy for, 20, 21t
    preoperative, 270–271
    and screening for lung cancer, 56–58
SN-38, 477
SN-38 glucuronide (SN-38G), 477
Snail, 125–126
SNaPshot (Applied Biosystems), 656–657
SNaPshot PCR, 166t
SNF5, 109t
Social Media, 637
Society of Thoracic Surgeons (STS), 274
SOLiD platform, 96
Solid predominant invasive adenocarcinoma, 144t, 147
Solitary pulmonary nodule characterization, 199–202, 200f
    adipose content, 201
    borders, 201
    calcification, 201
    cavitation, 201–202, 203f
    density, 200
    enhancement, 201
    ground-glass opacity, 200–201, 201f–202f
    location, 202
    multiplicity, 202
    shape, 201, 203f
    size, 200

Solute carrier family 38, member 3 (SLC38A3), 164–165
Somatostatin receptor scintigraphy, 563
Sorafenib, dermatologic side effects of, 494–495, 496f
Southwest Oncology Group (SWOG), 525–527
    S9900 study, 520–521
    SWOG 0819 trial, 459–460
SOX family, *of genes*, 46
Spain, 32–33, 32f
Spanish Lung Cancer Group, 527–528
Spanish Society of Pathology, in guidelines for biomarker testing, 165
SP-C/CCA double-positive cells, 118
Specimens. *see also* Sampling
    core-needle biopsy
        processing, 182
        touch preparation for, 182, 182f
    small
        algorithm for processing, 180, 181f, 181b
        management of, 178–185.e2, 179f
        optimization for, 180–183, 182f
        triage for ancillary studies, 180–184, 181f
    types, 61
Spinal compression, lung cancer and, 190
Spinal cord, neurotoxicity of, 411–412
Spinal cord compression, 389
    repeat radiotherapy for, 389
Spinal cord metastases, lung cancer and, 190
Spindle cell carcinoma, 153f, 154
Splicing, 95
Spread through alveolar spaces (STAS) invasion, 147
Sputum smears, 160
Squamous cell adenocarcinoma, gene amplifications in, 86f
Squamous cell carcinoma, 119, 144t, 150–153
    ASF-type, 150, 152f
    cytologic characteristics of, 161f, 162
    early invasive, 150
    genetic abnormalities in, 480, 481t
    genetic alterations in, 98, 101f
    hilar-type, 150
    immunohistochemistry of, 151–152
    keratinizing, 150–152, 152f
    large cell neuroendocrine carcinoma, markers for differentiation of, 558
    molecular classification of, 654–655, 655f
    molecular targets in, 431t
    in never-smokers, 24
    nonkeratinizing, 150–152, 152f
    peripheral-type, 150
    preinvasive lesions of, 150, 151f
SQUIRE trial, 460
SRY (sex determining region Y)-box 2 (SOX2), 164–165
SS1P, 547–548
Staging
    of chest-wall tumors, 295–296
    choice of, technique, 245
    endoscopic techniques for, 237–239

Staging (*Continued*)
  invasive
    indications for, mediastinal, 242–244
    required lymph node stations for, 245
    techniques for, 245–252
  with PET, 219–223, 220f
  restaging, 252
  technique
    lymph node stations and choice of, 241–242
    surgical, 245–252
  tumor, node, metastasis (TNM)
    lymph node descriptors, 219–221
    metastases (M) descriptor, 221
    T descriptor, 219
Stair-Climbing Test, 269
Standard mediastinoscopy, 241
Standardization, of clinical trials, 631–632, 632f
Standards of care, modality-specific quality standards, 645
Stem cells, 117–120.e2
  maintenance of, 118–119
  naphthalene-resistant, 117
  in vitro and in vivo studies of, 117–120.e2
Stereotactic ablative radiotherapy (SABR), 334
  for bone metastases, 190
  dose fractionation and prescription for, 344
  effects of, 334
  linear-quadratic model, 334
  mechanisms of cell killing, 334
  motion management strategy for, 344
  multifraction, 335
  for oligometastases
    in adrenal gland, 351
    clinical results of, 351–353
    immune effects of, 351
    in liver, 351
    in lymph nodes, 351–352
    in multiple organs, 353
    in vertebrae, 352–353, 352f
  patient immobilization for, 345
  protocol development of, 343
  quality assurance of, 343
  radiobiology of, 334
  results of, reproducibility of, 349
  set-up for, 345
  single-fraction, 335
  spinal cord tolerance, 412
  for stage I nonsmall cell lung cancer, 342–343
    alternatives to, 349
    background and definitions of, 342–343
    for central lesions, 347, 347f
    clinical results of, 345–347, 345t–346t
    diagnosis and staging before, 343
    follow-up after, 347–349, 347f–350f
    implementation of, 343
    target volume concept, 344
    target volume definition in, 344
    toxicity in, 346–347, 346f
    universal survival curve, 334

Stereotactic body radiotherapy (SBRT), 311–312, 312t, 342, 343f
Stereotactic radiosurgery, 388
Steroid hormones, in lung cancer, 36–40
  aromatase in, 38–39
  estrogen receptors in, 36–38, 37f
  progesterone receptors in, 40
Steroids, 399
Stigma, tobacco, 635–636
Stimulation systems, 320
STK11 gene, 26–27, 26t, 46
Stridor, lung cancer and, 187
Stroma, 123
Subacute cerebellar degeneration, 194
Sublobar resection, 289, 290f
  impact of, on lung function and morbidity, 315–316
  indication for, 293
  limited, 291–293, 292f
  optimization of oncologic outcomes with, 316
  role of, in treatment of nonsmall cell lung cancer, 314–315
  for stage I and II lung cancer, 291–293
  vs. other local therapies, 316
Submucosal suture, for cartilaginous portion of bronchus, 305
Suboptimal samples, sequencing in, 101–103
Substernal goiter, 552–553, 553f
Subxiphoid pericardioscopy, 250
Sulindac, 78, 78t
Sunitinib, 439
Superior sulcus, nonsmall cell lung cancer of, 298, 299t
Superior vena cava syndrome (SVCS), 234
  imaging of, 214, 214f
  lung cancer and, 188–189, 189f
Superposition/convolution methods, 322
SurePath (BD Diagnostics), 184
Surgery
  advantages and disadvantages of, 371
  considerations for, 371–372, 371t
  cytoreductive, 542–544
  locoregional treatment with, 369–372
  for lung cancer, evolution of, 289–290, 290f
  for malignant mesothelioma, 541–545
  for massive hemoptysis, 602
  for neuroendocrine tumors, 563–564
  palliative, for malignant mesothelioma, 541–542
  preoperative functional evaluation of candidates, 265–273.e3
    algorithms, 270, 271f–272f
    carbon monoxide lung diffusion capacity, 267–268
    cardiac risk estimation, 266–267
    comorbidity estimation, 265–266, 266t
    exercise testing, 268–270
    pulmonary rehabilitation, 271
    smoking cessation, 270–271
    video-assisted thoracoscopic surgery, 268
  randomized trials of, 369–370
  for thymoma, 577–579

Surgical resection
  results of, 290–291
  for stage I lung cancer, 289–294.e2
  for stage II lung cancer, 289–294.e2
  sublobar, 289, 290f
    for stage I and II lung cancer, 291–292
  for thymoma, 577, 577f
Surgical robots, 283
Surgical staging techniques, 245–252
Surveillance, Epidemiology and End Results (SEER), 35
Surveillance, Epidemiology and End Results (SEER)-Medicare, 342
Surveillance, for thermal ablation, 359–360
Sweden, smoking and smoking-attributable deaths in, 10
SWI/SNF chromatin remodeling complex, in lung cancer, 108f, 109–110, 109t
SWI/SNF-related, matrix-associated, actin-dependent regulator of chromatin, subfamily a, member 4 (SMARCA4), 164–165
Switch maintenance chemotherapy, 450, 450t, 451f, 456t
  concept of, 448
  evidence of efficacy of, 465
Synaptophysin, for diagnosis of LCNEC, 157
Synchronous lung cancers, 309
  management of, 308–313.e2
Synchronous primary lung cancers, 260, 262t
Syndrome of inappropriate antidiuretic hormone secretion, 192
Systemic lupus erythematosus, risk for, in radiotherapy, 338
Systemic therapy
  external-beam radiotherapy and, 388
  front-line options, in nonsmall cell lung cancer, 418–433.e6

T cells
  cytotoxic, 123
  helper, 123
  in mesothelioma, 546
  regulation of, 137, 138f, 139
  regulatory, in developing lung tumor microenvironment, 123–124
T790M mutation, 469
Tamoxifen, lung cancer and, 38
Tangential resection, 306–307, 306f
Targeted gene sequencing, 97
Targeted therapies. *see also specific agents*
  adjuvant chemotherapy and, 519–520
  for lung cancer, 43–45, 44f, 44t
  side effects of, ethnic differences in, 500
  toxicities of, management of, 490–500
Taxes, tobacco, raising, 12
Tea, lung cancer and, 3
Tecemotide (L-BLP25), 503
Telescope anastomosis, 305–306
Teratoma, benign, 550
TERT gene, 25

TFINE study, 454
TG4010 vaccine, 503–504
TGF-β tyrosine kinase inhibitors, 399
Thalidomide, chemoradiation therapy with, 369
The Cancer Genome Atlas (TCGA), 96, 431, 431t
Therapeutic response, imaging of, with PET, 226–227
Thermal ablation
   in combination with adjunctive therapies, 361–362
   complications of, 359
   computed tomography after, 359–360, 360f
   ideal candidate for, 360–361
   immunologic effects of, 361
   indications for, 358–359
   outcomes of, 359–360, 360t
   positron emission tomography-computed tomography after, 359–360, 361f–362f
   surveillance, 359–360
   survival and recurrence of, 359
ThinPrep (Hologic Inc.), 184
Third-generation sequencing, 101
Thoracic radiotherapy, 374
   early initiation of, 376
   for extensive disease, 379
   external-beam radiotherapy, 383
   palliative, 383, 384f
      indications for, 383
      regimens, 383, 384t
      side effects of, 383–384
   pulmonary toxicity of, 393–395
   toxicities of, 393–408.e4
Thoracic Revised Cardiac Risk Index (ThRCRI), 266
Thoracic symptoms, 382–385
Thoracoscopic surgery, video-assisted (VATS), 249–250
   comparison with open lobectomy, 275–281
   definition of, 274–275
   lobectomy, 274
      defined by The Cancer and Leukemia Group B, 274
      discussion, 281
      robotic vs., 281
      as treatment for nonsmall cell lung cancer, 274
   for lung cancer, 268
   outcomes of, 275–281
      long-term, 276–280, 279t, 280f
      short-term, 275–276, 276t, 277f–279f, 278t
   patient selection for, 274–275, 275t
   specific issues, 280–281
      ability to tolerate adjuvant chemotherapy, 281
      learning curve, 281
      node dissection/staging N1 and N2, 280
Thoracoscopy, 249–250
   in malignant mesothelioma, 537
ThRCRI. see Thoracic Revised Cardiac Risk Index (ThRCRI)

3-D conformal radiotherapy, 324–326, 325f
Thrombocytosis, 193, 234t
Thromboembolism, 193, 234t
Thrombotic microangiopathy, 193
Through-and-through suture, for cartilaginous portion of bronchus, 305
Thymic carcinoma, 575–576, 576t, 583–584
   clinical presentation and diagnosis of, 583–585, 583f
   histologic classification of, 585
   histology of, 583–584
   neuroendocrine thymic tumor, 584
   prognostic factors, recurrence, and follow-up, 586t, 587
   recommended management of, 588
   staging system, 575t, 584–585
   survival and prognostic factors, 584, 585t
   treatment of, 580f, 584–587, 586f, 586t
Thymic tumors, 569–589.e4
   global efforts, 588–589
   histology of, 573–576
   management of, 588
   outcome measures, 576, 576t
   polychemotherapy regimens for, 581t
   prognostic factors, 576–577, 577t
   recommended management of, 588
   recurrence of, 588
Thymidylate synthase, 476, 523
Thymoma, 569–573
   associated systemic diseases, 571f, 571t
   chemotherapy, 580–582
      exclusive, 582, 582t
      postoperative, 582
      primary, 581–582, 581t
      radiotherapy and, combined, 582
   demographics and clinical presentation, 569–570, 570f
   diagnostic imaging techniques, 570–571
   extent of resection, 577
   histologic diagnosis, 571–572
   histology of, 573–575
   imaging during follow-up, 571
   mediastinal biopsy techniques, 572
   minimally invasive resection for, 578–579
   non-TNM staging systems, 572, 574b
   radiotherapy, 579–580
      definitive, 580
      postoperative, 579–580, 580f
      preoperative, 579
   recommended management of, 588
   recurrent thymic tumors, 587–588
   stage IVA, 575f, 579, 579f
   staging systems, 572–573
   surgery, 577–579
   surgical approach, 577, 577f
   surgical biopsies, 572
   surgical management of stage III, 578, 578f
   targeted therapy, 582–583
   TNM-based staging systems, 572–573, 575t
   treatment of, 577–583, 580f

Thymoma (Continued)
   type A, 573, 575f
   type B, 573
   type B2, 573
   type B3, 573, 575f
Thyroid transcription factor-1 (TTF-1), in adenocarcinomas, 148, 149f
Time management, standards for waiting times, 646
Tirapazamine, 335
Tivantinib, 443, 500
TNM classification. see Tumor, node, and metastasis (TNM) classification
Tobacco, 635–636
Tobacco advertising, 12
Tobacco consumption, lung cancers and, 339
Tobacco control and primary prevention, 9–17.e1
   21st century tobacco-control measures, 10–16
      combination of, 12
      enforce bans on tobacco advertising, promotion, and sponsorship, 12
      monitor tobacco use and prevention, 10–11
      offer help to quit tobacco use, 11
      protect people from tobacco smoke, 11
      raising taxes on tobacco, 12
      warning about dangers of tobacco, 11–12
   Framework Convention on Tobacco Control (FCTC) in, 9
   Global Tobacco Surveillance System for, 10–11
   impact on lung cancer mortality, 10f, 12–16, 13f–17f
   measures to assist with implementation of, 10t
   MPOWER strategy for, 12–13
   tobacco epidemic, historical context, 9–10, 10f
Tobacco control programs, 636
Tobacco dependence, treatment of
   evidence-based, delivery of, 19
   in lung cancer care, 19–20
Tobacco products, smokeless, 3
Tobacco smoke
   lung carcinogen interactions, 3
   second-hand, 3, 11
Tobacco smoking
   cessation of, benefits of, on lung cancer outcomes, 18–19
   confounding effects of, 3
   effects of, according to histology, gender, and race, 2–3
   epidemic of, 9–10, 10f
   and immune dysregulation, 142
   and lung cancer, 1–3
   in patient selection for radiotherapy, 339
   persistent
      factors associated with, 19
      prevalence of, 18–19
      risk of, 18–19
   protecting people from, 11

Tobacco use
  assessment of, 19
    in lung cancer care, 18–22.e2
  helping to quit, 11
  and prevention, policies in, monitoring
    of, 10–11
  treatment of
    future directions for, 20–22
    guidelines for, 20
    integrating evidence-based,
      19
    in lung cancer care, 18–22.e2
Tobacco-related cancers, segregation
  analyses of, 48–49
Toll-like receptors (TLRs), 126
Tomatoes, lung cancer and, 36
TomoTherapy, 324
Topical BAK-PLO, 416t, 417
Topotecan, combination chemotherapy
  with, 525, 526t, 532–533
Touch preparation, for core-needle
  biopsy, 182, 182f
Toxicity
  cardiovascular, 404
  esophagus, 399–403
  long-term, of prophylactic cranial
    irradiation, 380–381
  lung, 393–394
  neurological, of prophylactic cranial
    irradiation, 379–380
  neurotoxicity, related to radiotherapy
    and chemotherapy, 409–417.e2
  radiated volume and, 340
  in stereotactic ablative radiotherapy
    (SABR), 346–347, 346f
  of thoracic radiotherapy, 393–408.e4
  of whole-brain radiotherapy, 391
Toxins, environmental and occupational,
  24
TP53 (p53) gene, 27, 46, 431t
TP63 gene, 25
Traditional designs, phase III trial,
  624
Trametinib, 499
Transbronchial needle aspiration
  (TBNA), 237
  EBUS-TBNA, 241, 251, 251f
Transcervical extended mediastinal
  lymphadenectomy (TEMLA), 242,
  246
Transcriptome, 97
Transfection, rearranged during, RET,
  484
Transforming growth factor-β (TGF-β),
  140, 393
  in developing lung TME, 125
Transthoracic needle aspiration
  (TTNA), 237
Treatment response, biomarkers for,
  134–136, 135t
Tremelimumab, 444, 546
Trial designs, for rare tumors,
  626
Tripe palm, 191
Tropomycin receptor kinase, 485
Trousseau syndrome, 193
Tuberin (TSC2), 479–480
Tuberin-hamartin (TSC1), 479–480

β-Tubulin, 425, 476
Tumor, node, and metastasis (TNM)
  classification
  of lung cancer, 253–264.e1
    for bronchopulmonary carcinoids, 256
    categories, subcategories and
      descriptors of, 259t–260t
    implications for clinical practice,
      260–264
    International Association for the
      Study of Lung Cancer database
      for, 253, 254t
    for small cell lung cancer, 256
    stage grouping, 256, 259t–260t, 261f
    T, N, and M descriptors,
      innovations in, 253–256
  of malignant tumors, 253
  of small-cell lung carcinomas (SCLCs),
    374
  for thymoma, 572–573, 575t
Tumor-associated antigens, 67
Tumor bulk, 371–372
Tumor cell proliferation, 196
Tumor-derived soluble factors, 140
Tumor heterogeneity, and SCLC, 119
Tumor histology, 653–654
Tumor hypoxia, 335
Tumor-infiltrating lymphocytes (TILs),
  123, 139–141
Tumor microenvironment (TME), in
  lung, 121, 127
  components of
    cellular, 122–127
    field, 122
    soluble, 122–123, 125–127
    structural, 123
  developing, 122–123
  manipulation of, 126–127
Tumor necrosis factor-related apoptosis-
  inducing ligand (TRAIL), 135–136
Tumor protein 53 (P53), 164–165
Tumor protein p63 (TP63), 164–165
Tumor-related brachial plexopathy
  (TRBP), 409–410
Tumors
  chest-wall, 295–303.e2, 295–297
  classification of, that do not fit in
    descriptors, 256, 261t
  descriptors for staging, 207, 219
    CT and, 207, 209f
    innovations in, 253–254, 254f–255f
    MRI and, 215–216, 215f–216f
  neurogenic, 552, 552f
  rare, trial designs for, 626
  thymic, 569–589.e4
Tumor stage, and prognosis, 419
Tumor suppressor genes, 196
Twin studies, 47
2-D treatment planning simulation, for
  nonsmall cell lung cancer, 324
Tyrosine kinase inhibitors (TKIs),
  164–165, 426
  EGFR, 427–428, 427t
    dermatologic side effects of, 491–494
    dose-modification strategy for,
      492–494, 496f
    gastrointestinal side effects of,
      496–497

Tyrosine kinase inhibitors *(Continued)*
    in nonsmall cell lung cancer,
      427–428, 427t
    pulmonary side effects of, 497–498
    resistance to, 429–430
    second-line treatment with, for wild-
      type EGFR tumors, 438, 438f
Tyrosine-protein kinase receptor UFO
  (AXL), 484–485

U
U2 small nuclear RNA auxiliary factor 1
  (U2AF1), 164–165
UFT, 517
UGT1A1*28 (uridine diphosphate
  glucuronosyltransferase 1A1), 477
Ultrasound
  endobronchial (EBUS), 237, 250–252,
    251f, 538
  endobronchial ultrasound-guided
    transbronchial needle aspiration
    (EBUS-TBNA), 241, 251, 251f
  endoscopic, 250–252
  endoscopic ultrasound (EUS), 237,
    538
  mediastinal evaluation, 538
United Kingdom
  age-standardized death rates for
    women in, 32–33, 32f
  smoking and smoking-attributable
    deaths in, 10
  smoking cessation in, 13, 15f
  warning about dangers of tobacco in,
    11–12
United States
  lung cancer in
    epidemiology of, 30–32, 31f
  warning about dangers of tobacco in,
    11–12
Universal survival curve, 334
Uridine diphosphate
  glucuronosyltransferase 1A1
  (UGT1A1*28), 477
US Intergroup 91-0001 trial, 79
US Public Health Service Treating
  Tobacco Use and Dependence
  Clinical Practice Guideline, 20
US Surgeon General, 18

V
Vaccination
  for nonsmall cell lung cancer, 502–505
  with WT1, 547
Vaccines, mesothelin, 548
Valve disease, radiation-associated, 404,
  405t
Vandetanib, 439
  for lung cancer, 44
Varenicline, 20, 21t
Vascular anastomosis, 307
Vascular endothelial growth factor
  receptor (VEGFR), 426
Vascular endothelial growth factor
  (VEGF) inhibitors
  adjuvant chemotherapy with, 519
  second-line treatment with, 438–439
Vascular endothelial growth factor
  (VEGF) targeted agents, 460–461

Vascular endothelium, 334
VATS. *see* Video-assisted thoracoscopic surgery (VATS)
Vegetables, lung cancer and, 3
Vemurafenib, side effects of, 499
Venlafaxine, 416–417, 416t
Ventana Medical Systems, 173
V-erb-b2 avian erythroblastic leukemia viral oncogene homolog (ERBB) 4, 164–165
VeriStrat assay, 429
Vertebrae metastases, stereotactic ablative radiotherapy (SABR) for, 352f
Vertebral body, resection of, 301, 301f
Video-assisted mediastinal lymphadenectomy (VAMLA), 242, 246
Video-assisted thoracoscopic surgery (VATS), 249–250, 268, 316
  comparison with open lobectomy, 275–281
  definition of, 274–275
  lobectomy, 274
    defined by The Cancer and Leukemia Group B, 274
    discussion, 281
    robotic *vs*., 281
    as treatment for nonsmall cell lung cancer, 274
  outcomes of, 275–281
    long-term, 276–280, 279t, 280f
    short-term, 275–276, 276t, 277f–279f, 278t
  patient selection for, 274–275, 275t
  specific issues, 280–281
    ability to tolerate adjuvant chemotherapy, 281
    learning curve, 281
    node dissection/staging N1 and N2, 280
Videomediastinoscopy, 241
Vinblastine, 365
Vinca alkaloids vindesine, phase II studies of, 435
Vincristine
  dose-dense regimens of, 528
  for extensive-stage SCLC, 525, 526t
  for poor performance status patients, 531

Vindesine
  combination chemotherapy with, for nonsmall cell lung cancer, 420, 421t
  radiotherapy with, 365
Vinorelbine
  for advanced NSCLC in elderly patients, 423
  in chemotherapy-induced peripheral neuropathy, 414
  combination chemotherapy with
    in elderly patients, 424, 424t
    for nonsmall cell lung cancer, 420–421, 421t
    for malignant mesothelioma, 541t
    for nonsmall cell lung cancer, 420, 420t
  phase II studies of, 435
  radiotherapy with, 364
Visceral pleural invasion, 255f, 262
  definition of, 254
VITAL study (phase III), 439
Vitamin B_{12}, 77–78, 78t
Vitamin E, 399
Vitamins, 72
Vocal cord paralysis, 187–188
Volatile organic compounds, 67–68
Volumetric modulated radiation therapy (VMAT), 322, 324–326, 325f
v-raf murine sarcoma viral oncogene homolog B (BRAF), 164–165, 485–486
Vysis ALK Break Apart FISH probe kit, 431
Vysis LSI ALK Break Apart FISH Probe Kit (Abbott Molecular), 173

W

Washing, bronchial, 160
Weight loss, lung cancer and, 339
West Japan Thoracic Oncology Group Trial 0203, 458
Westermark sign, 213
Wheezing, lung cancer and, 187
Whites, 169t
Whole-brain radiotherapy, 390–391
  dose fractionation, 390–391
  neurotoxic effects, 412
  planning, 390–391
  toxicity of, 391

Whole-exome gene sequencing, 97
Whole-genome sequencing, 96
WJTOG 0203 trial, 456t
Wnt signaling, in maintenance of stem cell populations, 118–119
Women
  lung cancer in
    age-standardized death rates, 32, 32f
    survival in, 41–42, 41t–42t
    in United States, 30, 31f
  never-smokers, 23–24
Women's Health Study, 77
World Health Organization (WHO)
  Framework Convention on Tobacco Control (FCTC) of, 9
  Global Adult Tobacco Survey by, 10–11
  Global Health Professions Student Survey by, 10–11
  Global School Personnel Survey by, 10–11
  Global Tobacco Surveillance System by, 10–11
  Global Youth Tobacco Survey, 10–11
  histologic types of thymic tumors, 575, 576t
  MPOWER strategy by, 12–13
  nonmucinous adenocarcinoma classification, 256–257
WT1 protein, 547

X

Xerosis (dry skin), 491t, 494t

Z

ZEAL study (third), of vandetanib, 439
Zinc finger, MYND-type containing 10 (ZMYND10/BLU), 164–165
ZODIAC study (second), of vandetanib, 439
Zoledronic acid, for bone metastases, 190
Zubrod, C. Gordon, 330–331
Zubrod score, and patient selection for radiotherapy, 337